NEW YORK REVIEW BOOKS
CLASSICS

THE ANATOMY
OF MELANCHOLY

ROBERT BURTON (1577–1640) was born in Leicestershire and educated at Oxford, where he became librarian of Christ's Church College, a position he held for life. He was also the vicar of St. Thomas, Oxford, and the rector of Seabrave, Leicestershire. The first edition of *The Anatomy of Melancholy* appeared in 1621 and was an immediate popular success. Burton continued to revise and add to his great book, which went through a further five editions, until his death.

WILLIAM H. GASS was born in Fargo, North Dakota, in 1924. He is the author of five works of fiction, among them *Omensetter's Luck* and *The Tunnel*, and six volumes of criticism. He lives in St. Louis, where he is the director of the International Writer's Center.

D0813241

THE ANATOMY
OF MELANCHOLY

ROBERT BURTON

Edited and with an Introduction by
HOLBROOK JACKSON

And with a new Introduction by
WILLIAM H. GASS

NEW YORK REVIEW BOOKS

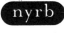

New York

THIS IS A NEW YORK REVIEW BOOK
PUBLISHED BY THE NEW YORK REVIEW OF BOOKS
435 Hudson Street, New York, NY 10014
www.nyrb.com

Library of Congress Cataloging-in-Publication Data
Burton, Robert, 1577–1650
    The anatomy of melancholy / Robert Burton ; introduction by William H.
Gass.
       p. cm.
    Includes bibliographical references and index.
    ISBN 0-940322-66-8 (pbk. : alk. paper)
    1. Melancholy. I. Title
PR2223 .A1 2001
616.89—dc21

                                            00–069101

ISBN 978-0-940322-66-0

Book design by Lizzie Scott
Printed in the United States of America on acid-free paper.
10 9 8

CONTENTS

Contents

INTRODUCTION

DURING the early seventeenth century men everywhere in Europe were beginning to realize that the institutions that had seemed to offer them hope and keep them from care were actually making them fearful of their fate, and encouraging them to trade their lives for lies. The world was now wider than anyone had previously imagined—ships had sailed it round; the heavens were on quite another course than had been sworn to; social organizations were being drastically revised and power was slipping from popes to princes, from the universal Church to the secular State; former methods of deciding things were now utterly up in the air; rude and vigorous vernaculars were driving back Latin everywhere (Dante, Descartes, Hobbes would ennoble several vulgar tongues by their employment); people were lifting their heads from canonical books to look boldly around, and what they saw first were errors, plentiful as leaves. Delight and despair took turns managing their moods.

The past is never lightly thrown off, though it often seems doffed like a hat with a flourish or carelessly tossed like a cape into a corner; it is only a cap that's been removed, only an old coat there in its puddle. Young men were watching the new day dawn with old minds, and traditional intentions. Robert Burton (1577–1640) boldly chastises the clergy for their ceremonious pomp, hypocritical zeal, and scandalous lapses, but it is the pomp, the zeal, the lapses he is after, and he is careful to keep his new faith clear of the old church's ritual forms and corporate grip. Sir Thomas Browne was rewarded for his royalist loyalties with a knighthood, and his most popular book, about vulgar errors, the *Pseudodoxia Epidemica*, omitted a number of crucial ones, while he keeps helpfully at hand the "unspeakable mysteries" of the Scriptures; Descartes aimed to set his religion back on sound foundations, even if he did make its bones dance, and rightly feared Bruno's burning at the stake; Burton's skepticism, like Montaigne's, and Descartes' later, is persistent but programmatic, an epistemological strategy not a deep state of mind; Thomas Hobbes, playing both sides of the English Civil War to perfection, would place Cromwell's face on the giant whose image would serve to front his *Leviathan* (a body politic literally made of a crowd of bodies squeezed into the outline of a sovereign), while on that Protestant head he impressed a Catholic crown; Bacon, More, and Montaigne all sought ways to release Science to follow every scent Nature might emit so long as it never treed Divinity.

Of all the habits that were hard to break, being bookish was perhaps the most difficult. Now, in addition to the scriptures, there would be all the classical authors you had the opportunity to cite—the honor of the first quote in Burton's address to the reader goes to Seneca—thereby showing generosity in the "loan" of the resources of your library and by your readiness to "spread the word," just as you also took good care to gather books and manuscripts, diligently copying passages from the volumes which had to pass through, rather than remain in, your hands. Guided by a genius, the pages of a commonplace book could be transformed into an original and continuously argued text as Ben Jonson did with *Discoveries* —a form which Burton's *Anatomy* sometimes resembles though it never mimics.

These new authorities, who often elbow Matthew, Mark, Luke, and John to one side, supply evidence of two kinds: first, of the breadth of the author's learning, and second, of the rightness of his opinions, because the facts that matter are still those mostly found in books, not those picked like posies out of a meadow or distilled in an alembic; moreover, the words themselves are magical; you cannot have too many of them; they are like spices brought back from countries so far away they're even out of sight of seas; words that roll, Poloniously, into the reader's ken in lists that subside only to resume in no time at all with words even more exotic, redolent, or chewy; for instance the names and kinds of terrestrial devils that lurk about to pester us: lares, lemurs, genii, satyrs, fauns, fairies, wood-nymphs, trolls, and foliots, those visitors to forlorn houses, about whom you may not be familiar, who make "strange noises in the night, howl sometimes pitifully, and then laugh again, cause great flame and sudden lights, fling stones, rattle chains," and if you wake to find your beard shaved and your chin smooth, they will be the impish cause.

To ridicule superstition or succumb to it, embrace the new learning or belabor it, celebrate change or condemn it, relate every tale or tell none; or, more characteristically, to quote, testify, enlarge upon every subject with such serious thoroughness there could be no response but laughter: in Robert Burton these impulses blow like winds; no one was ever more an arena for the contest between what was pagan and what was pious, what seemed demonstrable to science and mathematics or what seemed sensible upon textual scrutiny and harmonious with settled doctrine, than this nonconformist clergyman, this quiet monkish man who would pursue secular studies behind the walls of a famous college, a skeptic whose credulity was a welcome you could count on, a pessimist and melancholic whose great celebrational comedy will last as many years as its thousand pages.

Robert Burton may have momentarily put aside his pen on December 5, 1620, to declare his work done; however, since sales were solid and five fresh editions needed, he let his baby grow from gigantic to gargantuan. We have ourselves continued to manufacture material for his *Melancholy*, and were Burton as immortal as his book he could keep the

Anatomy routinely up to date with the distraughts, foul humors, and tragedies that trouble us today and will beset us tomorrow. What the present reader may find strange is Burton's eager allowance of hearsay and observation, myth and science, superstition and common sense, to help him in his hunt for causes, and provide more than cosmetic in the makeup of his explanations: not merely citing heredity, disease, dotage, and personal loss as sources of melancholy, while displaying a skepticism as ardent as his faith; but blaming God, evil angels as well as devils, a bad balance among the four humors, the discoveries of chiromancy and physiognomy, indurate dishes and sharp sauces, unsuitable parents, odors of the earth, even the stars themselves.

What may strike one as quaint and unfashionable at one time may be the latest wisdom to another. When I was first engaged to Robert Burton's book (my copy's flyleaf says Dec. 1944), the mother's womb was sturdier and more insulated than it is believed to be now, so, when I read that if the mother "be over-dull, heavy, angry, peevish, discontented, and melancholy, not only at the time of conception, but even all the while she carries the child in her womb . . . her son will be so likewise affected," I thought the risks overstated; for wasn't the moat of amniotic fluid about the baby nearly unswimmable?—what else was it there for?—but I would not think so now—now everything, including noise, gets through, and, unless it is the music of Mozart, wreaks havoc.

Unlike Erasmus' famous work, this is no praise of folly; it is, however, a parade of them: every day in Burton's year is St. Patrick's, bands brag in the streets, beer is the only proffered drink, and the beer is green. Moreover the parade has a settled order of march; the word "anatomy" signifying its dissected analytical layout, its deployment of commentary descending through partitions, sections, members, into subsections, and adding to those body parts appendices, poetic addresses, a daunting synopsis, and a preface nearly the length of an ordinary book. The analytical outline should not daunt. Burton pays as much attention to his own schematisms as he pays to the syntax of his sentences. Imposing indeed are his interconnections, but it is rather as if a net had been flung down on top of fish who continue to roil and flop freely about beneath it.

Nor is there much that's melancholy, in our present sense of the word, about the *Anatomy*; and the principle reason for this is that the illnesses Burton discusses and the causes and cures he proposes have not, in the main, been drawn from bedsides, battlefields, or courts, but from books and reports, descriptions and disquisitions; for it is easy, even agreeable, while enjoying the safety of the page, to face without qualms a situation and its solution as they are set down in some chronicle or almanac, harsh or bizarre as they may combine to be, when in life what it is being reported may encourage harrowing practices and produce deplorable pains, such as drilling a hole in a patient's skull to release noxious vapors that have gathered there, or latterly, prevailing on leeches to bleed a body already badly in need of its blood.

What is not secondhand are Burton's pages on the melancholies of the scholar, the vices of princes, and the deficiencies of the Catholic Church. He has both read and lived these —through an impending Civil War, contending clergies, the machinations of a parliament seeking new powers, and royals protecting traditional privileges. Yet when one's nose is in a book it is as alive and alert as if it smelled smoke in the house or anticipated the serving of soup—more so, because it is bent over concepts; it is breathing Forms; it is becoming acquainted with minds. For Burton, learning is the disease that will cure his other ailments the way consolidating your debts will bring due only one—still crushing—lump sum payment.

But Thomas Hobbes, who had Burton and Browne and Montaigne in view, was of a different, and, as usual, impressively put opinion:

From whence it happens, that they which trust to books,
do as they that cast up many little summes into a greater,
without considering whether those little summes were
rightly cast up or not; and at last finding the errour visible, and not mistrusting their first grounds, know not
which way to cleere themselves; but spend time in fluttering over their bookes; as birds that entring by the
chimney, and finding themselves inclosed in a chamber, flutter at the false light of a glasse window, for
want of wit to consider which way they came in."
[*Leviathan*, Pt. 1, Ch. 4]

If he could have had his way, Burton would have preferred
to be a poet and playwright, and he does write a comedy in
Latin verse his students perform in the Hall of Oxford's
Christ Church in 1617. We have several samples of his occa-
sionally charming doggerel in front of us, one with the well-
known refrain, "None so sweet"—so sad, so sour, so harsh,
so damned—"as melancholy." He would also have preferred
to write in Latin, but publishers were increasingly reluctant
to constrict their sales to the rich and learned; what, after
all, was the vernacular to Dante, Descartes, and Hobbes but
a paddle to place across the rumps of the schoolmen and
punish their inhibiting pedantries? The languages of Italian,
French, and English were those of increasingly secular states
and their mercantile interests. Robert Burton would also seek
a popular public, but under a protective nom de plume, in the
shelter of a life whose movements rose and fell as calmly as a
cork amidst the tumults of the times.

If Burton had wanted us to know who the author of the
Anatomy was, he should not have chosen a pseudonym behind which to hide (as he, himself, says); yet if he had not
wanted us to know who he was (as he claims) he should
not have chosen a name like "Democritus" behind which to
pretend to conceal himself, for that name plainly points to-

ward a position on the nature of things that is material, quantitative, and scientific; moreover one that soon would have, in the strengthening temper of the time, two great spokesmen—Thomas Hobbes and René Descartes—to represent the rational spirits of Galileo and Copernicus in whom the Renaissance was realized. But it is the life and character of Democritus (taken from authorities as unreliable as ancient) that our coy author wishes to suggest bear a semblance to his own, and that his epithet, "the laughing philosopher," is one Burton also deserves: the sage's quiet, solitary regularities, his ardent devotion to his studies, the elevation that philosophy confers upon his occupations, such as Burton's ministry allowed, and with an interest in mathematics they could share, the enjoyment of rueful laughter, as well as a fondness for the rhetoric of skepticism—the same with men like Montaigne, Lipsius, and Muret, who left their busy lives to dwell in sheltered cells where their amusement at human behavior would disturb not even the sobriety of birds.

As Democritus Junior, Burton is free to parade folly after folly past Democritus Senior's amused yet scornful eye. The operative phrase is "what would he have said" were he to have thought X, felt Y, seen Z; although the indictment that follows the question has been drawn up by Burton alone. Concerning wars, for instance (the dots signify omitted quotations):

> What would he have said to see, hear, and read so many bloody battles, so many thousands slain at once, such streams of blood able to turn mills, through the mad guilt of one person, or to make sport for princes, without any just cause ... whilst statesmen themselves in the meantime are secure at home, pampered with all delights and pleasures, take their ease, and follow their lusts, not considering what intolerable misery poor soldiers endure, their often wounds, hunger, thirst, etc.,

the lamentable cares, torments, calamities and oppressions, that accompany such proceedings . . .

The book was so popular it went into six editions during Burton's lifetime, and its gratified author was eager to doff his anonymity after the first. It should have been popular. Although it gave expression to the pains of the people (always a kind of comfort), his *Anatomy* recounted so many sorts of follies that most of them had to have been performed or believed by others rather than ourselves; we could then happily send a hearty guffaw around the common table like a pitcher of ale, and drink to the dunces who had so deluded themselves as to think thus, do such. When the mind enters a madhouse, Burton shows, however sane it was when it went in, and however hard it struggles to remain sane while there, it can only make the ambient madness more monstrous, more absurd, more bizarrely laughable by its efforts to be rational.

For a contemporary Robert Burton whom we might imagine sitting down now with unwearying zeal and sorrow to record our melancholy lot, there'd be no lack of data either, and the sections he'd have planned for his book would fill up faster than a thimble. What about bad diets as a cause of nervous illness? Both Burtons would have room for that. Or foul air? They could jointly bewail it. Or immoderate exercise? Or a love of gambling? Nothing unfamiliar there, nor with the desperations of imprisonment or the glooms that follow prolonged study, or the despairs impoverishment brings on. What of the consequences, both devious and direct, of festering discontents, of local resentments and historic hatreds, concerning which we have always had an apparently inexhaustible supply? Or the dangerous delusions brought on by self-love and vain-glory in an era of shameless self-promotion like our own? Surely our obsession with sex and what Burton calls its artificial allurements would shock our scholar, while the space in the plan of his book set aside for the miasmas of religion would find sects jostling one another for booths from which to sell their latest absurdities and repeatedly boast of their unique merits and cry aloud their bewares.

Burton himself will pretend to be a plain speaker, and plainly enough he does speak, if one considers the time, and the artificiality of his predecessors; but when he says that his book is "writ with as small deliberation as I do ordinarily speak, without all affectation of big words, fustian phrases, jingling terms, tropes, strong lines, that like Acestes' arrows caught fire as they flew, strains of wit, brave heats, elogies, hyperbolical exornations, elegancies, etc., which many so much affect," what are we now to think? "Strong lines" refers to a preference orators had, in that time, for balance, gnomic terseness, and an elevation of thought and diction which could seem, when it failed, to yield the artificial, riddling, and bombastic; nevertheless, Burton's looseness can only be called "exuberance" now, "celebration," and indicative of a nominalism that feels that if every person huddling under an umbrella is not named they shall have no protection.

One can only listen. Robert the Ranter rails. It is delicious.

To see [we are still in this rhetorical mode of address, so it is Democritus Senior who is the imagined observer] a man turn himself into all shapes like a chameleon, or as Proteus . . . to act twenty parts and persons at once for his advantage, to temporize and vary like Mercury the planet, good with good, bad with bad; having a several face, garb, and character for every one he meets; of all religions, humours, inclinations; to fawn like a spaniel . . . rage like a lion, bark like a cur, fight like a dragon, sting like a serpent, as meek as a lamb, and yet again grin like a tiger, weep like a crocodile, insult over some, and yet other domineer over him, here command, there crouch, tyrannize in one place, be

baffled in another, a wise man at home, a fool abroad to
make others merry.

The sentence indeed does unravel, but into a flouncy
tuffet, not into a maze or a strew. Meaning, motion, and emo-
tion are superbly fused. It achieves the tone of a tirade that, in
the midst of its fury, smiles at itself—recognizes itself as a
recital of fearful changeabilities and confident clichés. I am
also tempted to admire (for it may be merely a textual error,
of which in the *Anatomy* there are so many) the odd and
awkward phrase "and yet other domineer over him" as a
creative misprint for "let." In its anger, its energy, its rhythm,
its terminological greed, its sermoniacal excoriations, this
prose is a seedbed for the high semi-sacred styles of Browne's
Urn Burial and Taylor's *Holy Dying*.

Be prepared to proceed slowly and you will soon go swiftly
enough. Read a member a day; it will chase gloom away. The
late section on religious melancholy has been particularly admired. I also have a special fondness for Burton's pages on
museums and libraries. But above all, it is the width of the
world that can be seen from one college window that amazes
me; what a love of all life can be felt by one who has lived it
sitting in a chair; and Robert Burton's unashamed display of
his lust for the word—his desire to name each thing, and find
a song in which each thing can be sung—is a passion that we
might emulate to our assuredly better health.

—WILLIAM H. GASS

INTRODUCTION
TO THE 1932 EDITION

IT IS IRONICAL that a treatise of melancholy should have become one of the great entertainments among English writings; but the irony is accidental, for if the author of *The Anatomy of Melancholy* was not precisely of the breed of Mark Tapley he was no hypochondriac, and had no intention of compiling a doleful work. Robert Burton was a good-humoured pessimist, and unless he himself had told us we should not have guessed that he was addicted to a melancholy, lamentable enough for him, but most fortunate for us because it was the first cause of a delightful book. For proof of his fundamental amiability we must recall Bishop Kennett's story which tells how Burton, when the melancholy weighed upon him, would leave his study in Christ Church, Oxford, stroll down to Folly Bridge and recreate himself by listening to the vigorous back-chat of the bargees. He confesses, however, that he wrote the *Anatomy* to relieve his own melancholy. We do not know whether the disease yielded to the treatment, but we do know that, for over three centuries, his work has been a prophylactic against the megrims, and his kindly if irascible soul still goes marching on in successive editions of his masterpiece, blazing new trails of pleasure among the generations succeeding that which was enriched by his presence.

There are few details of his life, and few are necessary, for if ever the author were embodied in a book or if ever book were the presentment of an author, that author was Robert Burton and that book *The Anatomy of Melancholy*. The biographical facts are that he was born at Lindley Hall in Leicestershire on

8th February, 1577, the fourth of a family of nine; that he went
to the Free School at Sutton Coldfield and later to Nuneaton
Grammar School; that he entered Brasenose College in 1593,
was elected a student of Christ Church in 1599, took his B.D.
in 1614, became Vicar of St. Thomas, Oxford, two years later,
and was presented with the living of Seagrave in Leicestershire, by his patron George, Lord Berkeley, in 1630. He was a
ready versifier in both Latin and English, contributed to several academic anthologies, and in his thirty-first year wrote
Philosophaster, a satirical comedy in Latin verse. This, his
first sustained work, was rewritten in 1615 and performed by
the students in the Hall of Christ Church in 1617.[1] *The
Anatomy of Melancholy* was published in 1621, and went
through five editions during the author's life. The last edition
which he saw through the press was that of 1638, for in the
following year he died at the age of sixty-three and was buried
in the Cathedral of the University where his brother William,
author of the *Description of Leicestershire* (1622), erected a
monument to his memory in the form of a portrait bust,
tinted to the life, after the manner of those times.

His life was uneventful. "I have lived," he says, "a silent,
sedentary, solitary, private life, *mihi & musis* in the University as long almost as *Xenocrates* in *Athens, ad senectam
fere*, to learn wisdom as he did, penned up most part in my
study." This we may accept literally, although he was a parson, and for some years a pluralist parson, with the duties of
his incumbencies, which he probably reduced by delegation
or neglect. Yet it would be unsafe to conclude that even so
large and complicated a work as the *Anatomy* was necessarily a whole-time job. Diligence and an enjoyment of drudgery
can accomplish miracles in the spare time of a busy life.

---

1. *Philosophaster* remained in MS. until 1862, when it was edited by William Edward
Buckley and published by the Roxburghe Club. The first translation was made by
Paul Jordan-Smith and published by Stanford University, California, in 1931.

Burton may have been reclusive, but he was no hermit. Apart from his position as a clerk in Holy Orders, there is evidence of other activities: he was librarian of his college, and for a year at least, a Clerk of Oxford Market. Primarily, however, he was a scholar and a bookman agreeably cloistered in his own rooms, with plenty of books,[2] or in the admirable library of "the most flourishing College in Europe," or the Bodleian, endeavouring by his researches into the causes and cure of melancholy to be more than "a drone" or "an unprofitable and unworthy member of so learned and noble a society," and to avoid writing "that which should be in any way dishonourable to such a royal and ample foundation."

Such a man might have lapsed into pedantry; but although he uses a pedantic method his outlook is far from it, and he himself has few of the vices of the schoolman. Nor is his solemn vocation reflected in his style. The *Anatomy*, indeed, is often unparsonic; even his admonitions are tolerant and urbane, whilst his conversation was said to be lively, although, as Thomas Hearne is careful to record, "very innocent." But of such details we know little, for it is a curious fact that, although a familiar figure in the university life of his day and a popular author, he shared with Shakespeare an almost complete immunity from contemporary gossip. Beyond the documentary evidence of his offices and the few autobiographical details dotted about his book, no contemporary references of any importance have come to light, and Burton had been dead over fifty years before Anthony à Wood's character of him appeared in the *Athenæ Oxonienses*. Wood never met him, but talked with those who had. But even then the Oxford historian is not essential, for as likely a character could be drawn from the hints and admissions in Burton's own book.

"He was," says Anthony Wood, "an exact Mathematician,

2. He owned about 2,000 volumes, which he bequeathed to the library of his College and the Bodleian.

a curious calculator of Nativities, a general read Scholar, a thro'-pac'd Philologist, and one that understood the surveying of Lands well. As he was by many accounted a severe student, a devourer of Authors, a melancholy and humorous Person; so by others, who knew him well, a Person of great honesty, plain dealing and Charity. I have heard some of the Ancients of Christ Church often say that his Company was very merry, facete and juvenile, and no man did surpass him for his ready and dextrous interlarding his common discourses among them with Verses from the Poets or Sentences from classical Authors, which being then the fashion in the University, made his Company more acceptable."

We know how he looked from his portraits, of which there are three: a painting in oils at Brasenose, the engraved miniature by Le Blon in the emblematic frontispiece of the *Anatomy*, and the painted bust in the Cathedral at Oxford. From these sources we may compose a portrait of our English Democritus among his books in the agreeable setting of a famous and already venerable college: a thick-set, plumpish man, with dark brown beard of formal cut; there is a satiric glint in the large eyes, and intelligence and memory are revealed in the monumental forehead; his nose is enterprising and he has the snap mouth of the well-opinioned, corrected by an indulgent nether lip. It is the face of a character such as England often produced in those days and sometimes even now: a competent, thoughtful, self-sufficient face, with a hint of shyness which might indicate a preference for a sheltered life rather than a life of adventure, unless it were adventures among books. And from this composite presentment we may safely infer a genial yet reclusive, diffident yet self-opinionated man, who might be friendly but not demonstrative, tolerant yet irascible, and who would suffer fools sadly rather than gladly.

Yet when we have said all and listened attentively to Anthony Wood we have not probed very far into the soul of

Robert Burton. We have not yet divined that entity which is he and none other. The Anatomist is, indeed, somewhat of a paradox. Like most interesting men, he is not quite consistent. He preaches the happy mean and does not practise it. His book is always excessive. He overloads every statement. It is the most sententious book ever written, yet it reads trippingly as a novel. It is packed with common sense and uncommon nonsense. He is never tired of apologizing for his long-windedness, and immediately starts expatiating again. He fears that he will go too far in his exposition of love-melancholy, and does. He was never married, but marriage has no mysteries for him. He laughs at humanity and weeps over the sorrows and stupidities of men. He is scientifical and superstitious at one and the same time. He is as frank as a pornographer and as mincing as a prude. He mixes facetiæ with theology. He is not a deliberate humorist, yet he is often funnier than the professional wag. He is most frivolous when he is most earnest, and when he is frank and colloquial he is most profound. Like Whitman, he is large and multitudinous. He spills himself and the whole of ancient learning into his book and adroitly turns the medley into an ordered theme which, because of its great size, may weary his reader but never bore him.

Robert Burton was a bookman first and last. He lived among books and upon them, and devoted the greater part of his life to the writing of an epitome or quintessence of the books of all times. His treatise is the legitimate offspring of a bookish mind, and although it is largely a distillation of authors it is an original work. The *Anatomy* looks like a crude assembly of quotations and it is indeed a vast mobilization of the notions and expressions of others, yet it is not they but the rifler who is revealed on every page, it is he, not they, who peeps from behind every quotation. The reason is clear. He is an artist in literary mosaic, using the shreds and patches he has torn from the work of others to make a picture emphatically his own. Books are his raw material. Other artists fashion images out of clay, contrive fabrics and forms of stone, symphonies of words, sounds, or pigments. Burton makes a cosmos out of quotations. He raids the writings of the past, which he often finds neglected or in ruins, and re-assembles them in a structure of his own, much as the ruins of Rome were pillaged by the builders of the Renaissance and worked into the temples and palaces of a new civilization.

His apologies for this fascinating literary structure seem superfluous, but they are due neither to mock modesty nor to a sense of inferiority. Burton never lacked proper conceit. He was convinced of his ability to accomplish his task and he believed in his own sagacity. Authors rarely compile works running into half a million words without being encouraged by the conviction that they are doing something worth doing. His apologetics were, of course, a convention; no seventeenth century work was complete without a prefatory vindication. He not only excuses himself for his subject and his manner of presenting it, he apologizes even for his title. He wrote about melancholy not solely, it would seem, to re-lieve himself of that distemper, as he asserts in one place, but because he thought it "a subject most necessary and com-modious, less common and controversial than Divinity, which I do acknowledge to be the queen of professions." His title to-day seems explicit enough. It is unnecessary for him to cite precedents, for anatomies were almost as common then as anthologies are now. But if it is a little odd, he will let it stand, since "it is a kind of policy in these days to prefix a phantastical title to a book which is to be sold—for as larks come down to a day—net, many vain readers will tarry and stand gazing, like silly passengers, at an antic picture in a painter's shop, that will not look at a judicious piece." For the same reason he commits his treatise, in the main, to the Eng-lish language. "It was not mine intent," he says, "to prosti-tute my muse in English," but if he had composed his work in Latin he could not have got it printed: "Any scurrile pamphlet is welcome to our mercenary stationers in English," he complains, "but in Latin they will not deal." But we do not join him in reviling those mercenary publishers, for if they had not thought of their profits they would have robbed us of ours, and Burton, like so many flourishing wits, would lie smothered in oblivion.

His style is peculiar only as it is linked with a method which demands lavish quotation and citation. He is a master of both these arts. The quantity, audacity, and aptness of his quotations have always astounded and refreshed his readers; and he is easily the greatest collector and coordinator of apophthegms in an age which had many notable specialists in that craft. Stripped, however, of these characteristic and entertaining encumbrances, Burton's prose is direct and normal. It has a brisk, staccato style, which guarantees the fluency of his long and leisurely book. He is often charged with eccentricity; but if we allow for the inevitable quaintness created by time such a charge cannot be upheld. Burton is a self-conscious quoter and a deviser of processions of glittering words and epithets, but he is no mere phrase-maker. He does not invent a phrase for its own sake, and then stand back to admire it as one feels Browne doing and Donne doing. His style is too colloquial for that. It is like good talk. You can hear the cadence of a disputatious yet friendly voice tirelessly advising and expounding, but always redeemed from monotony by an apt twist or a whimsical turn, and when these fail, he brings up his reserves of curious tales which he marshals with ingenuity and gusto.

The *Anatomy* is great in size and scope. It ranges over all times and places, diving into the past, dipping into the future, and even glancing ironically at the present. Although his theme is melancholy, he contrives by a method of intermission and digression to glance at almost every human interest or endeavour. The work is thus a commentary upon the life and habits of the human race. It is a bridge between medieval and modern thought: the swan song of authoritarian scholasticism (all that Glanvill condemned in his *Scepsis Scientifica*), and an anticipation of the method of deduction from observed facts. He adopts the traditional form of the conspectus of his time. The work is arranged in three "partitions" and numerous "sections," "members," and "subsections," the titles and sub-titles being set out synoptically at the beginning of each part. In addition to the parts and chapters proper there are several admitted "digressions," often the size of a treatise, and "a satirical Preface conducing to the ... Discourse" which fills seventy-eight pages, folio, in the definitive edition.

Sir William Osler described the *Anatomy* as "the greatest medical treatise written by a layman." But apart from the main theme there are sections which, although organically related to it, are complete essays in themselves. Some of these do pioneer work. The long and fascinating chapter called "A Digression of Air" is the first essay in climatology, and the section on "Religious Melancholy" is the first study of that subject. His psychological study of sex anticipates Havelock Ellis, and his repudiation of romantic love, Bernard Shaw; his chapters on "Jealousy" contain all the ingredients of the post-war problem-novel; whilst buried in the famous preface is a Utopia which suggests Wells. Burton is revealed as a sound political economist, a little-Englander, a protectionist, an opponent of monopolies, an enemy of war, an advocate of better highways, the extension of inland waterways, the reclamation of marshlands, the building of garden villages, and the granting of old age pensions.

The Anatomy of Melancholy is one of those books which possess something like human character and behaviour, the kind of book which seems to have grown. Few books are more definitely or more curiously imbued with their authorship. The *Anatomy* is Burton, and Burton the *Anatomy*. To read it is to read him: to read him is to talk with him, to know him as we know the great persons of fiction, or those few writers who have so projected themselves into their works as to have achieved for their own personalities what the great novelists and dramatists have achieved for the characters of their stories and plays. Burton, like Montaigne, Pepys, and Lamb, has made a fiction of himself, stranger and more interesting than fact.

It was born in 1621, when Burton was forty-five: a small quarto, of nearly nine hundred pages, exceedingly plump for its size. During the following seventeen years it continued to grow and improve through four editions, 1624, 1628, 1632, and 1638, each in small folio, but, after the author's death in 1639–40, decline began. Inferior printing and paper set in with the edition of 1651, the first reprint after Burton's death and the last to contain his corrections. In 1660 another edition appears, still more degenerate in character, and the seventeenth-century editions end with the lanky folio of 1676, from which all charm and character have gone. There were no further editions for a hundred and twenty-four years. No book of the century exhibits more clearly the personal influence of author upon printer. The hand of Burton is revealed in all the editions up to 1638. There are innumerable changes, often small and even whimsical, sometimes considerable, which bear evidence of a taste and fancy other than what at that time spontaneously issued even from the Oxford printing office. The author, true bookman as he was, must have had many an exciting wrangle with his publishers, Henry Cripps and Leonard Lichfield, "Printer to the famous University," coming out, as I gather, victoriously, for he has contrived also to leave his own mark upon the typography of the book into which he had put so much of himself.

The appreciation of Burton is a test of bookishness, and although he has never lacked readers, even during the dark age, 1677–1799, when no edition of the *Anatomy* appeared, there have not been lacking those who have belittled and misrepresented him. I am not concerned at the moment with his defence, even if it were necessary, which it is not, for there is no reason why any one should read him unless he wishes to do so. Burton is for the Burtonian. But it is necessary to refer to the misrepresenters, both ancient and modern, because many of them have sinned ignorantly. Critics and commentators have not always taken the trouble to read, still less understand the book, hence much popular nonsense, of which Hallam's description of the *Anatomy* as "a sweeping of the miscellaneous literature from the Bodleian Library," and Lowell's

> A mire ankle-deep of deliberate confusion,
> Made up of old jumbles of classic allusion,

are typical specimens.

Burton has been oftener damned with faint praise than scoffed at by the ignorantly learned. I know of only one downright depreciator, the Manx poet, T. E. Brown. In a vigorous and humourless essay, contributed to the *New Review* in 1895, this minor poet and major schoolmaster can find no good word for our good Burton. His learning is but a "parade," the "product of omnivorous folio-bolting and quarto-gulping, urged on and sustained by inordinate vanity"; his method naught but a "pseudo-method," a mere "affectation of method and order." Brown concedes, however, that Burton has "slanging power . . . a wondrous hurly-burly of invective"; and his conclusion reveals a sneaking, if slightly priggish regard. Like Charles Lamb, he is opposed to reprints of the *Anatomy*. "I do not know a more heartless sight than the reprint of the *Anatomy of Melancholy*," says Lamb. "What need was there of unearthing the bones of that fantastic old great man, to expose them in a winding-sheet of the newest fashion to modern censure? What hapless stationer could dream of Burton ever becoming popular?" Brown is not so generous or so romantic. An old Burton has a charm, he admits, but only "in an old library; old dust embalms it, old memories haunt it. It is worth seeking there": and he thinks it ought to be read there *in situ*. "Neglect, decay," he admonishes, "must be the fate of all such ponderous eccentricities. And to smarten them up, and turn them out spick-and-span, radiant and raw, into the forum of literature, is a doubtful sort of proceeding. They belong to the cave, and scholars are their natural friends and custodians. Leave them to the scholars." Brown was wrong, but there is evidence that he had at least read his Burton.

His appreciators extend from his own day to ours. He received honourable mention from Anthony Wood, and he gets a good word even from malicious Thomas Hearne, who incidentally gives a hint of the fallen prestige of the *Anatomy* during the first half of the eighteenth century. "No book sold better formerly," he writes in his diary (1734), "than Burton's *Anatomy of Melancholy*, in which there is a great variety of learning, so that it hath been a common-place for filchers. It hath a great many impressions, and the bookseller got an estate by it; but now 'tis disregarded, and a good fair copy (although of the seventh impression) may be purchased for one shilling, well bound. . . ." Twenty years later, Dr. Thomas Herring, Archbishop of Canterbury, told a friend to "look into" the *Anatomy*, as Burton was "one of the pleasantest, the most learned and the most full of sterling sense. . . . The wits of Queen Anne's reign, and the beginning of George the first's were not a little beholden to him."

The legend of Burton as a crib for the lazy and a mine for the creative is well established. The *Anatomy* is a lucky-bag, whether you are a plagiarist, legitimately predatory, or an adventurous reader, like Dr. Johnson, whom it "took out of bed two hours sooner than he wanted to rise." Many authors of genius have rifled Burton to the advantage of our literature. John Ferriar, in his *Illustrations of Sterne*, reproves Laurence

Sterne for incorporating into *Tristram Shandy* so much of the *Anatomy*, "once the favourite of the learned and the witty, and a source of surreptitious learning to many others." Wharton's discovery that Milton was not above taking hints from Burton, when composing *Il Penseroso*, is the occasion for a neat appreciation of the *Anatomy*: "The writer's variety of learning, his quotations from scarce and curious books, his pedantry sparkling with rude wit and shapeless elegance, miscellaneous matter, intermixture of agreeable tales and illustrations, and perhaps, above all, the singularities of his feelings cloathed in an uncommon quaintness of style, have contributed to render it, even to modern readers, a valuable repository of amusement and information."

These references indicate continuous interest over a period which knew not Burton in person or in a new edition. With the turn of the century the *Anatomy* comes once more into favour. Byron tells Moore that it is the most useful book "to a man who wishes to acquire a reputation of being well read, with the least trouble." But Lamb was probably its rediscoverer. It was well within his zone of research and appreciation. He composes an amusing pastiche of its style, and it is doubtless through him that Keats and his friends hear of it. Charles Brown gives the poet a copy of the 1813 edition in 1819. Keats reads the volume through "carefully, with pen in hand, scoring the margins constantly," annotating, and indexing special passages on the last fly-leaf. In the very year of the gift he writes "Lamia," which is based upon a well-known passage in the *Anatomy*. From then until now interest in the book grows. Dibdin possesses "the cubical quarto of 1621, the tapering folio of 1678 [*sic*], and all the intermediate editions," and "these copies were all bound in picked russia by Faulkner; for then, Charles Lewis 'was not.'" "What an extraordinary book it is," he exclaims, "and what an extraordinary portion of it is the chapter on 'Love Melancholy'! I was grateful for the octavo reprint of it, which has gone through two editions: but Burton has not yet been clothed in the editorial garb which ought to encircle his shoulders." A hundred years have passed away, and although over forty editions of the *Anatomy* have appeared, Dibdin's wish has not yet been carried out. But Burton is not without honour even in our hurried days, for he has perhaps more readers now than ever he had, and in the last decade Mr. Francis Meynell has admitted him into the distinguished company of the Nonesuch Press. An American edition with "an all-English text" has been published under the editorship of Mr. Floyd Dell and Mr. Paul Jordan-Smith, and now the *Anatomy* achieves apotheosis as a popular classic in the honoured ranks of Everyman's Library.

—HOLBROOK JACKSON

NOTE ON THE TEXT

THE FACT that no manuscript exists of *The Anatomy of Melancholy* has placed Burton, like Shakespeare, at the mercy of editors and printers. Burton himself was confessedly careless in the revision of the printed sheets, and preferred in each successive edition to add new matter rather than correct the old. The work thus swelled; and even the first posthumous edition, the sixth, includes a number of additions and corrections which Burton intended to have incorporated himself, had he lived. The present text follows the sixth edition, collated with the fifth, which is superior in point of typography. Many egregious misprints, some of which were perpetuated even into the nineteenth century, have been cleared away; but it has been taken into account that numerous errors, especially of quotation, were Burton's own, and these it would be presumptuous and anachronistic to remove. Considerable use has been made of the edition of the nineteenth century, which commands the most attention: that of the Rev. A. R. Shilleto in 1893. Several emendations to this edition have been made by Professor Edward Bensly in the Ninth and Tenth Series of *Notes and Queries*, and to his understanding of Burton the present editor wishes to make acknowledgment. As in later reprints of The *Anatomy* since the edition of 1800, the choice of type, punctuation, and spelling in this edition has been in the interest of clarity and agreeableness to a present-day reader. Where it does not interfere with Burton's own paraphrase, translations have been added to the quotations from Latin and Greek, and a glossary of archaic words follows the third partition. Burton's annotations, printed originally in the margin, have for clearance of the text been printed at the end of each partition, together with a few notes by the present editor [in square brackets].

THE ANATOMY
OF MELANCHOLY

DEMOCRITUS JUNIOR AD LIBRUM SUUM

VADE liber, qualis, non ausim dicere, felix,
  Te nisi felicem fecerit Alma dies.
Vade tamen quocunque lubet, quascunque per oras,
  Et Genium Domini fac imitere tui.
I blandas inter Charites, mystamque saluta
  Musarum quemvis, si tibi lector erit.
Rura colas, urbem, subeasve palatia regum,
  Submisse, placide, te sine dente geras.
Nobilis, aut si quis te forte inspexerit heros,
  Da te morigerum, perlegat usque lubet.
Est quod Nobilitas, est quod desideret heros,
  Gratior hæc forsan charta placere potest.
Si quis morosus Cato, tetricusque Senator,
  Hunc etiam librum forte videre velit,
Sive magistratus, tum te reverenter habeto;
  Sed nullus; muscas non capiunt aquilæ.
Non vacat his tempus fugitivum impendere nugis,
  Nec tales cupio; par mihi lector erit.
Si matrona gravis casu diverterit istuc,
  Illustris domina, aut te Comitissa legat:
Est quod displiceat, placeat, quod forsitan illis,
  Ingerere his noli te modo, pande tamen.
At si virgo tuas dignabitur inclyta chartas
  Tangere, sive schedis hæreat illa tuis:
Da modo te facilem, et quædam folia esse memento
  Conveniant oculis quæ magis apta suis.
Si generosa ancilla tuos aut alma puella
  Visura est ludos, annue, pande lubens.
Dic utinam nunc ipse meus (nam diligit istas)
  In præsens esset conspiciendus herus.[1]
Ignotus notusve mihi de gente togata
  Sive aget in ludis, pulpita sive colet,
Sive in Lycæo, et nugas evolverit istas,
  Si quasdam mendas viderit inspiciens,
Da veniam Authori, dices; nam plurima vellet
  Expungi, quæ jam displicuisse sciat.
Sive Melancholicus quisquam, seu blandus Amator,
  Aulicus aut Civis, seu bene comptus Eques
Huc appellat, age et tuto te crede legenti,
  Multa istic forsan non male nata leget.
Quod fugiat, caveat, quodque amplexabitur, ista
  Pagina fortassis promere multa potest.

3

At si quis Medicus coram te sistet, amice
    Fac circumspecte, et te sine labe geras:
Inveniet namque ipse meis quoque plurima scriptis,
    Non leve subsidium quæ sibi forsan erunt.
Si quis Causidicus chartas impingat in istas,
    Nil mihi vobiscum, pessima turba vale;
Sit nisi vir bonus, et juris sine fraude peritus,
    Tum legat, et forsan doctior inde siet.
Si quis cordatus, facilis, lectorque benignus
    Huc oculos vertat, quæ velit ipse legat;
Candidus ignoscet, metuas nil, pande libenter,
    Offensus mendis non erit ille tuis,
Laudabit nonnulla.   Venit si Rhetor ineptus,
    Limata et tersa, et qui bene cocta petit,
Claude citus librum; nulla hic nisi ferrea verba,
    Offendent stomachum quæ minus apta suum.
At si quis non eximius de plebe poeta,
    Annue; namque istic plurima ficta leget.
Nos sumus e numero, nullus mihi spirat Apollo,
    Grandiloquus Vates quilibet esse nequit.
Si criticus Lector, tumidus Censorque molestus,
    Zoilus et Momus, si rabiosa cohors:
Ringe, freme, et noli tum pandere, turba malignis
    Si occurrat sannis invidiosa suis:
Fac fugias; si nulla tibi sit copia eundi
    Contemnes, tacite scommata quæque feres.
Frendeat, allatret, vacuas gannitibus auras
    Impleat, haud cures; his placuisse nefas.
Verum age si forsan divertat purior hospes,
    Cuique sales, ludi, displiceantque joci,
Objiciatque tibi sordes, lascivaque: dices,
    Lasciva est Domino et Musa jocosa tuo,
Nec lasciva tamen, si pensitet omne; sed esto;
    Sit lasciva licet pagina, vita proba est.
Barbarus, indoctusque rudis spectator in istam
    Si messem intrudat, fuste fugabis eum,
Fungum pelle procul (jubeo), nam quid mihi fungo?
    Conveniunt stomacho non minus ista suo.
Sed nec pelle tamen; læto omnes accipe vultu,
    Quos, quas, vel quales, inde vel unde viros.
Gratus erit quicunque venit, gratissimus hospes
    Quisquis erit, facilis difficilisque mihi.
Nam si culparit, quædam culpasse juvabit,
    Culpando faciet me meliora sequi.
Sed si laudarit, neque laudibus efferar ullis,
    Sit satis hisce malis opposuisse bonum.
Hæc sunt quæ nostro placuit mandare libello,
    Et quæ dimittens dicere jussit Herus.

DEMOCRITUS JUNIOR TO HIS BOOK

Go forth, my book, into the open day;
    Happy, if made so by its garish eye.
O'er earth's wide surface take thy vagrant way,
    To imitate thy master's genius try.
The Graces three, the Muses nine salute,
    Should those who love them try to con thy lore.
The country, city seek, grand thrones to boot,
    With gentle courtesy humbly bow before.
Should nobles gallant, soldiers frank and brave
    Seek thy acquaintance, hail their first advance:
From twitch of care thy pleasant vein may save,
    May laughter cause or wisdom give perchance.
Some surly Cato, senator austere,
    Haply may wish to peep into thy book:
Seem very nothing—tremble and revere:
    No forceful eagles, butterflies e'er look.
They love not thee: of them then little seek,
    And wish for readers triflers like thyself.
Of ludeful matron watchful catch the beck,
    Or gorgeous countess full of pride and pelf.
They may say "Pish!" and frown, and yet read on:
    Cry odd, and silly, coarse, and yet amusing.
Should dainty damsels seek thy page to con,
    Spread thy best stores: to them be ne'er refusing:
Say, "Fair one, master loves thee dear as life;
    Would he were here to gaze on thy sweet look."
Should known or unknown student, free'd from strife
    Of logic and the schools, explore my book:
Cry, "Mercy, critic, and thy book withhold:
    Be some few errors pardon'd though observ'd:
An humble author to implore makes bold,
    Thy kind indulgence, even undeserv'd."
Should melancholy wight or pensive lover,
    Courtier, snug cit, or carpet knight so trim
Our blossoms cull, he 'll find himself in clover,
    Gain sense from precept, laughter from our whim.
Should learned leech with solemn air unfold
    Thy leaves, beware, be civil, and be wise:
Thy volume many precepts sage may hold,
    His well-fraught head may find no trifling prize.
Should crafty lawyer trespass on our ground,
    Caitiffs avaunt! disturbing tribe away!

5

Unless (white crow) an honest one be found;
  He 'll better, wiser go for what we say.
Should some ripe scholar, gentle and benign,
  With candour, care, and judgment thee peruse:
Thy faults to kind oblivion he 'll consign;
  Nor to thy merit will his praise refuse.
Thou may'st be searched for polish'd words and verse
  By flippant spouter, emptiest of praters:
Tell him to seek them in some mawkish verse:
  My periods are all rough as nutmeg graters.
The dogg'rel poet, wishing thee to read,
  Reject not; let him glean thy jests and stories.
His brother I, of lowly sembling breed:
  Apollo grants to few Parnassian glories.
Menac'd by critic with sour furrowed brow,
  Momus or Zoilus or Scotch reviewer:
Ruffle your heckle, grin and growl and vow:
  Ill-natured foes you thus will find the fewer.
When foul-mouth'd senseless railers cry thee down,
  Reply not: fly, and show the rogues thy stern:
They are not worthy even of a frown:
  Good taste or breeding they can never learn;
Or let them clamour, turn a callous ear,
  As though in dread of some harsh donkey's bray.
If chid by censor, friendly though severe,
  To such explain and turn thee not away.
Thy vein, says he perchance, is all too free;
  Thy smutty language suits not learned pen:
Reply, "Good Sir, throughout, the context see;
  Thought chastens thought; so prithee judge again.
Besides, although my master's pen may wander
  Through devious paths, by which it ought not stray,
His life is pure, beyond the breath of slander:
  So pardon grant; 'tis merely but his way."
Some rugged ruffian makes a hideous rout—
  Brandish thy cudgel, threaten him to baste;
The filthy fungus far from thee cast out;
  Such noxious banquets never suit my taste.
Yet, calm and cautious, moderate thy ire,
  Be ever courteous should the case allow—
Sweet malt is ever made by gentle fire:
  Warm to thy friends, give all a civil bow.
Even censure sometimes teaches to improve,
  Slight frosts have often cured too rank a crop;
So, candid blame my spleen shall never move,
  For skilful gard'ners wayward branches lop.
Go then, my book, and bear my words in mind;
Guides safe at once, and pleasant them you 'll find.]

THE ARGUMENT OF THE FRONTISPIECE

Ten distinct squares here seen apart,
Are joined in one by cutter's art.

I

Old Democritus under a tree,
Sits on a stone with book on knee;
About him hang there many features,
Of cats, dogs, and such-like creatures,
Of which he makes anatomy,
The seat of black choler to see.
Over his head appears the sky,
And Saturn, Lord of melancholy.

II

To the left a landscape of Jealousy,
Presents itself unto thine eye.
A kingfisher, a swan, an hern,
Two fighting-cocks you may discern,
Two roaring bulls each other hie,
To assault concerning venery.
Symbols are these; I say no more,
Conceive the rest by that 's afore.

III

The next of Solitariness,
A portraiture doth well express,
By sleeping dog, cat: buck and doe,
Hares, conies in the desert go:
Bats, owls the shady bowers over,
In melancholy darkness hover.
Mark well: if 't be not as 't should be,
Blame the bad cutter, and not me.

IV

I' th' under column there doth stand
Inamorato with folded hand;
Down hangs his head, terse and polite,
Some ditty sure he doth indite.

7

His lute and books about him lie,
As symptoms of his vanity.
If this do not enough disclose,
To paint him, take thyself by th' nose.

V

Hypocondriacus leans on his arm,
Wind in his side doth him much harm,
And troubles him full sore, God knows,
Much pain he hath and many woes.
About him pots and glasses lie,
Newly brought from 's apothecary.
This Saturn's aspects signify,
You see them portray'd in the sky.

VI

Beneath them kneeling on his knee,
A Superstitious man you see:
He fasts, prays, on his idol fixt,
Tormented hope and fear betwixt:
For hell perhaps he takes more pain,
Than thou dost heaven itself to gain.
Alas poor soul, I pity thee,
What stars incline thee so to be?

VII

But see the Madman rage downright
With furious looks, a ghastly sight.
Naked in chains bound doth he lie,
And roars amain, he knows not why.
Observe him; for as in a glass,
Thine angry portraiture it was.
His picture keep still in thy presence;
'Twixt him and thee there 's no difference.

VIII, IX

Borage and Hellebore fill two scenes,
Sovereign plants to purge the veins
Of melancholy, and cheer the heart,
Of those black fumes which make it smart;
To clear the brain of misty fogs,
Which dull our senses, and soul clogs.
The best medicine that e'er God made
For this malady, if well assay'd.

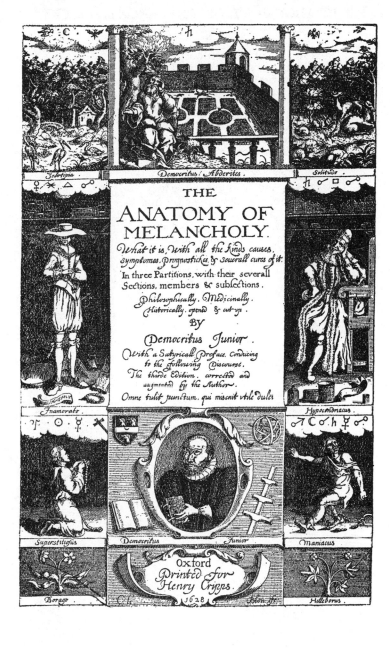

THE
ANATOMY OF
MELANCHOLY.
What it is, With all the kinds, causes,
symptomes, prognostickes, & severall cures of it.
In three Partitions, with their severall
Sections, members & subsections.
Philosophically, Medicinally,
Historically, opened & cut vp.
By
Democritus Junior.
With a Satyricall Preface, conducing
to the following Discourse.
The thirde Edition, corrected and
augmented by the Author.
Omne tulit punctum, qui miscuit vtile dulci.

Oxford
Printed for
Henry Cripps.
1628

Iealousia.

Democritus Abderites.

Solitudo.

Inamorato.

Hypocondriacus.

Superstitiosus.

Democritus   Junior.

Maniacus.

Borage.

Hellleborus.

x

Now last of all to fill a place,
Presented is the Author's face;
And in that habit which he wears,
His image to the world appears.
His mind no art can well express,
That by his writings you may guess.
It was not pride, nor yet vainglory
(Though others do it commonly),
Made him do this: if you must know,
The printer would needs have it so.
Then do not frown or scoff at it,
Deride not, or detract a whit,
For surely as thou dost by him,
He will do the same again.
Then look upon 't, behold and see,
As thou lik'st it, so it likes thee.
And I for it will stand in view,
Thine to command, reader, adieu.

THE AUTHOR'S ABSTRACT OF MELANCHOLY,

Διαλογικῶs

WHEN I go musing all alone,
Thinking of divers things fore-known
When I build castles in the air,
Void of sorrow and void of fear,
Pleasing myself with phantasms sweet,
Methinks the time runs very fleet.
    All my joys to this are folly,
    Naught so sweet as melancholy.
When I lie waking all alone,
Recounting what I have ill done,
My thoughts on me then tyrannize,
Fear and sorrow me surprise,
Whether I tarry still or go,
Methinks the time moves very slow.
    All my griefs to this are jolly,
    Naught so sad as melancholy.
When to myself I act and smile,
With pleasing thoughts the time beguile,
By a brook side or wood so green,
Unheard, unsought for, or unseen,
A thousand pleasures do me bless,
And crown my soul with happiness.
    All my joys besides are folly,
    None so sweet as melancholy.
When I lie, sit, or walk alone,
I sigh, I grieve, making great moan,
In a dark grove, or irksome den,
With discontents and Furies then,
A thousand miseries at once
Mine heavy heart and soul ensconce,
    All my griefs to this are jolly,
    None so sour as melancholy.
Methinks I hear, methinks I see,
Sweet music, wondrous melody,
Towns, palaces, and cities fine;
Here now, then there; the world is mine,
Rare beauties, gallant ladies shine,
Whate'er is lovely or divine.
    All other joys to this are folly,
    None so sweet as melancholy.

Methinks I hear, methinks I see,
Ghosts, goblins, fiends; my phantasy
Presents a thousand ugly shapes,
Headless bears, black men, and apes,
Doleful outcries, and fearful sights,
My sad and dismal soul affrights.
    All my griefs to this are jolly,
      None so damn'd as melancholy.
Methinks I court, methinks I kiss,
Methinks I now embrace my miss.
O blessed days, O sweet content,
In Paradise my time is spent.
Such thoughts may still my fancy move,
So may I ever be in love.
    All my joys to this are folly,
      Naught so sweet as melancholy.
When I recount love's many frights,
My sighs and tears, my waking nights,
My jealous fits; O mine hard fate
I now repent, but 'tis too late.
No torment is so bad as love,
So bitter to my soul can prove.
    All my griefs to this are jolly,
      Naught so harsh as melancholy.
Friends and companions get you gone,
'Tis my desire to be alone;
Ne'er well but when my thoughts and I
Do domineer in privacy.
No gem, no treasure like to this,
'Tis my delight, my crown, my bliss.
    All my joys to this are folly,
      Naught so sweet as melancholy.
'Tis my sole plague to be alone,
I am a beast, a monster grown,
I will no light nor company,
I find it now my misery.
The scene is turn'd, my joys are gone,
Fear, discontent, and sorrows come.
    All my griefs to this are folly,
      Naught so fierce as melancholy.
I 'll not change life with any king,
I ravisht am: can the world bring
More joy, than still to laugh and smile,
In pleasant toys time to beguile?
Do not, O do not trouble me,
So sweet content I feel and see.
    All my joys to this are folly,
      None so divine as melancholy.

I 'll change my state with any wretch,
Thou canst from gaol or dunghill fetch;
My pain 's past cure, another hell,
I may not in this torment dwell!
Now desperate I hate my life,
Lend me a halter or a knife;
    All my griefs to this are jolly,
    Naught so damn'd as melancholy.

DEMOCRITUS JUNIOR TO THE READER

GENTLE READER, I presume thou wilt be very inquisitive to know what antic or personate actor this is, that so insolently intrudes upon this common theatre to the world's view, arrogating another man's name; whence he is, why he doth it, and what he hath to say. Although, as he said,[1] *Primum si noluero, non respondebo, quis coacturus est?* I am a free man born, and may choose whether I will tell; who can compel me? if I be urged, I will as readily reply as that Egyptian in Plutarch,[2] when a curious fellow would needs know what he had in his basket, *Quum vides velatam, quid inquiris in rem absconditam?* It was therefore covered, because he should not know what was in it. Seek not after that which is hid; if the contents please thee, " and be for thy use, suppose the Man in the Moon, or whom thou wilt, to be the author ";[3] I would not willingly be known. Yet in some sort to give thee satisfaction, which is more than I need, I will show a reason, both of this usurped name, title, and subject. And first of the name of Democritus ; lest any man by reason of it should be deceived, expecting a pasquil, a satire, some ridiculous treatise (as I myself should have done), some prodigious tenent, or paradox of the earth's motion, of infinite worlds, *in infinito vacuo, ex fortuita atomorum collisione*, in an infinite waste, so caused by an accidental collision of motes in the sun, all which Democritus held, Epicurus and their master Leucippus of old maintained, and are lately revived by Copernicus, Brunus, and some others. Besides, it hath been always an ordinary custom, as Gellius observes,[4] " for later writers and impostors to broach many absurd and insolent fictions under the name of so noble a philosopher as Democritus, to get themselves credit, and by that means the more to be respected," as artificers usually do, *Novo qui marmori ascribunt Praxitelen suo* [who sign the name of Praxiteles on a new statue of their own]. 'Tis not so with me.

> *Non hic Centauros, non Gorgonas, Harpyasque*
> *Invenies, hominem pagina nostra sapit.*[5]
>
> No Centaurs here, or Gorgons look to find,
> My subject is of man and humankind.

Thou thyself art the subject of my discourse.

Quicquid agunt homines, votum, timor, ira, voluptas,
Gaudia, discursus, nostri farrago libelli.[1]

Whate'er men do, vows, fears, in ire, in sport,
Joys, wand'rings, are the sum of my report.

My intent is no otherwise to use his name, than Mercurius
Gallobelgicus, Mercurius Britannicus, use the name of Mercury,
Democritus Christianus,[2] etc.; although there be some other
circumstances for which I have masked myself under this vizard,
and some peculiar respects which I cannot so well express, until
I have set down a brief character of this our Democritus, what
he was, with an epitome of his life.

Democritus, as he is described by Hippocrates[3] and Laertius,[4]
was a little wearish old man, very melancholy by nature, averse
from company in his latter days, and much given to solitariness,[5]
a famous philosopher in his age, *coævus* with Socrates,[6] wholly
addicted to his studies at the last, and to a private life:
writ many excellent works, a great divine, according to the
divinity of those times, an expert physician, a politician, an
excellent mathematician, as *Diacosmus*[7] and the rest of his works
do witness. He was much delighted with the studies of husbandry, saith Columella,[8] and often I find him cited by Constantinus[9] and others treating of that subject. He knew the
natures, differences of all beasts, plants, fishes, birds; and, as
some say, could understand the tunes and voices of them.[10]
In a word, he was *omnifariam doctus*, a general scholar, a great
student; and to the intent he might better contemplate, I find
it related by some,[11] that he put out his eyes, and was in his old
age voluntarily blind, yet saw more than all Greece besides, and
writ of every subject,[12] *Nihil in toto opificio naturæ, de quo non
scripsit* [there was nothing in the whole range of nature about
which he did not write]. A man of an excellent wit, profound
conceit; and to attain knowledge the better in his younger
years he travelled to Egypt and Athens,[13] to confer with learned
men, "admired of some, despised of others."[14] After a
wandering life, he settled at Abdera, a town in Thrace, and
was sent for thither to be their law-maker, recorder, or town
clerk as some will; or as others, he was there bred and born.
Howsoever it was, there he lived at last in a garden in the
suburbs, wholly betaking himself to his studies and a private
life, "saving that sometimes he would walk down to the haven,[15]
and laugh heartily at such variety of ridiculous objects, which
there he saw."[16] Such a one was Democritus.

But in the meantime, how doth this concern me, or upon what reference do I usurp his habit? I confess, indeed, that to compare myself unto him for aught I have yet said, were both impudency and arrogancy. I do not presume to make any parallel, *antistat mihi millibus trecentis* [he is immeasurably ahead of me], *parvus sum, nullus sum, altum nec spiro, nec spero* [1] [I am insignificant, a nobody, with little ambition and small prospects]. Yet thus much I will say of myself, and that I hope without all suspicion of pride, or self-conceit, I have lived a silent, sedentary, solitary, private life, *mihi et musis* [for myself and my studies] in the university, as long almost as Xenocrates in Athens, *ad senectam fere* [practically to old age] to learn wisdom as he did, penned up most part in my study. For I have been brought up a student in the most flourishing college of Europe, *augustissimo collegio,* [2] and can brag with Jovius, [3] almost, *in ea luce domicilii Vaticani, totius orbis celeberrimi, per 37 annos multa opportunaque didici* [for 37 years I have made good use of my opportunities for study in the world-renowned library of the Vatican]; for thirty years I have continued (having the use of as good libraries as ever he had [4]) a scholar, and would be therefore loath, either by living as a drone to be an unprofitable or unworthy member of so learned and noble a society, or to write that which should be anyway dishonourable to such a royal and ample foundation. Something I have done, though by my profession a divine, yet *turbine raptus ingenii,* as he [5] said, out of a running wit, an unconstant, unsettled mind, I had a great desire (not able to attain to a superficial skill in any) to have some smattering in all, to be *aliquis in omnibus, nullus in singulis* [a somebody in general knowledge, a nobody in any one subject], which Plato commends, [6] out of him Lipsius approves and furthers, [7] " as fit to be imprinted in all curious wits, not to be a slave of one science, or dwell altogether in one subject, as most do, but to rove abroad, *centum puer artium* [one who can turn his hand to anything], to have an oar in every man's boat, to taste of every dish, and sip of every cup," [8] which, saith Montaigne, [9] was well performed by Aristotle and his learned countryman Adrian Turnebus. This roving humour (though not with like success) I have ever had, and like a ranging spaniel, that barks at every bird he sees, leaving his game, I have followed all, saving that which I should, and may justly complain, and truly, *qui ubique est, nusquam est* [he who is everywhere is nowhere], which Gesner did in modesty, [10] that I have read

many books, but to little purpose, for want of good method ;
I have confusedly tumbled over divers authors in our libraries,
with small profit for want of art, order, memory, judgment.
I never travelled but in map or card, in which my unconfined
thoughts have freely expatiated, as having ever been especially
delighted with the study of cosmography. Saturn was lord of
my geniture, culminating, etc., and Mars principal significator
of manners, in partile conjunction with mine ascendant ; both
fortunate in their houses, etc.[1] I am not poor, I am not rich ;
nihil est, nihil deest, I have little, I want nothing : all my
treasure is in Minerva's tower. Greater preferment as I could
never get, so am I not in debt for it, I have a competency (*laus
Deo*) from my noble and munificent patrons, though I live still
a collegiate student, as Democritus in his garden, and lead a
monastic life, *ipse mihi theatrum* [sufficient entertainment to
myself], sequestered from those tumults and troubles of the
world, *et tanquam in specula positus* (as he said[2]), in some
high place above you all, like *Stoicus sapiens, omnia sæcula,
præterita præsentiaque videns, uno velut intuitu* [the Stoic philosopher, surveying with one sweep all ages down to the present],
I hear and see what is done abroad, how others run, ride,
turmoil, and macerate themselves in court and country,[3] far
from those wrangling lawsuits, *aulæ vanitatem, fori ambitionem,
ridere mecum soleo* [I laugh to myself at the vanities of the
court, the intrigues of public life], I laugh at all ; "only secure
lest my suit go amiss, my ships perish," corn and cattle miscarry,
trade decay, "I have no wife nor children good or bad to provide
for."[4]   A mere spectator of other men's fortunes and adventures,
and how they act their parts, which methinks are diversely
presented unto me, as from a common theatre or scene. I hear
new news every day, and those ordinary rumours of war, plagues,
fires, inundations, thefts, murders, massacres, meteors, comets,
spectrums, prodigies, apparitions, of towns taken, cities besieged
in France, Germany, Turkey, Persia, Poland, etc., daily musters
and preparations, and such-like, which these tempestuous times
afford, battles fought, so many men slain, monomachies, shipwrecks, piracies, and sea-fights, peace, leagues, stratagems, and
fresh alarums. A vast confusion of vows, wishes, actions, edicts,
petitions, lawsuits, pleas, laws, proclamations, complaints,
grievances are daily brought to our ears. New books every day,
pamphlets, currantoes, stories, whole catalogues of volumes of
all sorts, new paradoxes, opinions, schisms, heresies, controversies in philosophy, religion, etc. Now come tidings of weddings,

maskings, mummeries, entertainments, jubilees, embassies, tilts
and tournaments, trophies, triumphs, revels, sports, plays : then
again, as in a new shifted scene, treasons, cheating tricks,
robberies, enormous villainies in all kinds, funerals, burials,
deaths of princes, new discoveries, expeditions: now comical,
then tragical matters. To-day we hear of new lords and officers
created, to-morrow of some great men deposed, and then again
of fresh honours conferred ; one is let loose, another imprisoned ;
one purchaseth, another breaketh ; he thrives, his neighbour
turns bankrupt ; now plenty, then again dearth and famine ;
one runs, another rides, wrangles, laughs, weeps, etc. Thus
I daily hear, and such-like, both private and public news; amidst
the gallantry and misery of the world—jollity, pride, perplexities
and cares, simplicity and villainy; subtlety, knavery, candour
and integrity, mutually mixed and offering themselves—I rub
on *privus privatus* [in complete privacy] ; as I have still lived,
so I now continue, *statu quo prius*, left to a solitary life and
mine own domestic discontents : saving that sometimes, *ne
quid mentiar* [not to conceal anything], as Diogenes went into
the city and Democritus to the haven to see fashions, I did for
my recreation now and then walk abroad, look into the world,
and could not choose but make some little observation, *non
tam sagax observator, ac simplex recitator* [less by way of shrewd
remark than of simple statement of fact], not as they did,
to scoff or laugh at all, but with a mixed passion.

> *Bilom sæpe, jocum vestri movere tumultus.*[1]
>
> [Your fond heats have been,
> How oft ! the objects of my mirth and spleen.]

I did sometime laugh and scoff with Lucian, and satirically
tax with Menippus, lament with Heraclitus, sometimes again
I was *petulanti splene cachinno*[2] [with mocking temper moved
to laughter loud], and then again, *urere bilis jecur*[3] [my liver
was aflame with gall], I was much moved to see that abuse
which I could not mend. In which passion howsoever I may
sympathize with him or them, 'tis for no such respect I shroud
myself under his name ; but either in an unknown habit to
assume a little more liberty and freedom of speech, or if you
will needs know, for that reason and only respect which Hippocrates relates at large in his Epistle to Damagetus, wherein he
doth express, how coming to visit him one day, he found
Democritus in his garden at Abdera, in the suburbs, under a
shady bower,[4] with a book on his knees, busy at his study,[5]

sometimes writing, sometimes walking. The subject of his book was melancholy and madness ; about him lay the carcasses of many several beasts, newly by him cut up and anatomized; not that he did contemn God's creatures, as he told Hippocrates, but to find out the seat of this *atra bilis*, or melancholy, whence it proceeds, and how it was engendered in men's bodies, to the intent he might better cure it in himself, and by his writings and observations teach others how to prevent and avoid it.[1] Which good intent of his, Hippocrates highly commended : Democritus Junior is therefore bold to imitate, and because he left it unperfect, and it is now lost, *quasi succenturiator Democriti* [as a substitute for Democritus], to revive again, prosecute, and finish in this treatise.

You have had a reason of the name. If the title and inscription offend your gravity, were it a sufficient justification to accuse others, I could produce many sober treatises, even sermons themselves, which in their fronts carry more phantastical names. Howsoever, it is a kind of policy in these days, to prefix a phantastical title to a book which is to be sold ; for, as larks come down to a day-net, many vain readers will tarry and stand gazing like silly passengers at an antic picture in a painter's shop, that will not look at a judicious piece. And, indeed, as Scaliger observes,[2] " nothing more invites a reader than an argument unlooked for, unthought of, and sells better than a scurrile pamphlet," *tum maxime cum novitas excitat palatum* [most of all when it has the spice of novelty]. "Many men," saith Gellius,[3] " are very conceited in their inscriptions," " and able " (as Pliny quotes out of Seneca[4]) "to make him loiter by the way that went in haste to fetch a midwife for his daughter, now ready to lie down." For my part, I have honourable precedents for this which I have done:[5] I will cite one for all, Anthony Zara, *Pap. Episc.*, his Anatomy of Wit, in four sections, members, subsections, etc., to be read in our libraries.

If any man except against the matter or manner of treating of this my subject, and will demand a reason of it, I can allege more than one. I write of melancholy, by being busy to avoid melancholy. There is no greater cause of melancholy than idleness, " no better cure than business," as Rhasis holds :[6] and howbeit *stultus labor est ineptiarum*, to be busy in toys is to small purpose, yet hear that divine Seneca, better *aliud agere quam nihil*, better do to no end than nothing. I writ therefore, and busied myself in this playing labour, *otiosaque diligentia ut vitarem torporem feriandi* [to escape the ennui of idleness by a leisurely kind of employment], with Vectius in Macrobius, *atque otium in utile verterem negotium* [and so turn leisure to good account].

Simul et jucunda et idonea dicere vitæ,
Lectorem delectando simul atque monendo.[1]

[At once to profit and delight mankind,
And with the pleasing have th' instructive joined.]

To this end I write, like them, saith Lucian, that " recite to trees, and declaim to pillars for want of auditors": as Paulus Ægineta ingenuously confesseth, "not that anything was unknown or omitted, but to exercise myself," [2] which course if some took, I think it would be good for their bodies, and much better for their souls; or peradventure as others do, for fame, to show myself (*Scire tuum nihil est, nisi te scire hoc sciat alter* [your own knowledge is nothing unless another also knows that you know]). I might be of Thucydides' opinion, "To know a thing and not to express it, is all one as if he knew it not." [3]   When I first took this task in hand, *et quod ait ille,*[4] *impellente genio negotium suscepi* [and, as he saith, I undertook the work from some inner impulse], this I aimed at, *vel ut lenirem animum scribendo,*[5] [or] to ease my mind by writing; for I had *gravidum cor, fœdum caput,* a kind of imposthume in my head, which I was very desirous to be unladen of, and could imagine no fitter evacuation than this.   Besides, I might not well refrain, for *ubi dolor, ibi digitus,* one must needs scratch where it itches. I was not a little offended with this malady, shall I say my mistress Melancholy, my Egeria, or my *malus genius* [evil genius]? and for that cause, as he that is stung with a scorpion, I would expel *clavum clavo* [a nail with a nail], comfort one sorrow with another, idleness with idleness,[6] *ut ex vipera theriacum* [as an antidote out of a serpent's venom], make an antidote out of that which was the prime cause of my disease.   Or as he did, of whom Felix Plater speaks,[7] that thought he had some of Aristophanes' frogs in his belly, still crying *Brecececex, coax, coax, oop, oop,* and for that cause studied physic seven years, and travelled over most part of Europe to ease himself; to do myself good I turned over such physicians as our libraries would afford, or my private friends impart,[8] and have taken this pains.   And why not?   Cardan professeth he wrote his book *de Consolatione* after his son's death, to comfort himself; so did Tully write of the same subject with like intent after his daughter's departure, if it be his at least, or some impostor's put out in his name, which Lipsius probably suspects. Concerning myself, I can peradventure affirm with Marius in Sallust, "That which others hear or read of, I felt and practised myself; they get their knowledge by books, I mine by melancholizing." [1] *Experto crede Roberto.* Something I can speak out of experience, *ærumnabilis experientia me docuit* [sorrowful experience has taught me]; and with her in the poet, *Haud ignara mali miseris succurrere disco,*[2] I would help others out of a fellow-feeling; and, as that virtuous lady did of old, "being a leper herself, bestow all her portion to build an hospital for lepers," [3] I will spend my time and knowledge, which are my greatest fortunes, for the common good of all.

Yea, but you will infer that this is *actum agere,*[4] an unnecessary work, *cramben bis coctam apponere,*[5] the same again and again in other words. To what purpose? "Nothing is omitted that may well be said," [6] so thought Lucian in the like theme. How many excellent physicians have written just volumes and elaborate tracts of this subject! No news here; that which I have is stolen from others, *Dicitque mihi mea pagina, fur es* [7] [my page cries out to me, You are a thief]. If that severe doom of Synesius be true, "It is a greater offence to steal dead men's labours than their clothes," [8] what shall become of most writers? I hold up my hand at the bar among others, and am guilty of felony in this kind, *habes confitentem reum* [the defendant pleads guilty], I am content to be pressed with the rest. 'Tis most true, *tenet insanabile multos scribendi cacoethes,*[9] and "there is no end of writing of books," [10] as the wise man found of old, in this scribbling age [11] especially, wherein "the number of books is without number" (as a worthy man saith [12]), "presses be oppressed," and out of an itching humour that every man hath to show himself, desirous of fame and honour [13] (*scribimus indocti doctique* [we all write, learned and ignorant alike]), he will write no matter what, and scrape together it boots not whence. "Bewitched with this desire of fame,[14] *etiam mediis in morbis* [even in the midst of illness]," to the disparagement of their health, and scarce able to hold a pen, they must say something, "and get themselves a name," saith Scaliger, "though it be to the downfall and ruin of many others." [15] To be counted writers, *scriptores ut salutentur* [to be addressed as authors], to be thought and held polymaths and polyhistors, *apud imperitum vulgus* [among the ignorant crowd], *ob ventosæ nomen artis* [to get a name for a worthless talent], to get a paper-kingdom:

nulla spe quæstus sed ampla famæ [with no hope of gain but great hope of fame], in this precipitate, ambitious age, *nunc ut est sæculum, inter immaturam eruditionem, ambitiosum et præceps* ('tis Scaliger's censure[1]); and they that are scarce auditors, *vix auditores*, must be masters and teachers, before they be capable and fit hearers.   They will rush into all learning, *togatam, armatam* [civil or military], divine, human authors, rake over all indexes and pamphlets for notes, as our merchants do strange havens for traffic, write great tomes, *cum non sint re vera doctiores, sed loquaciores*, whenas they are not thereby better scholars, but greater praters.   They commonly pretend public good, but as Gesner observes,[2] 'tis pride and vanity that eggs them on; no news or aught worthy of note, but the same in other terms. *Ne feriarentur fortasse typographi, vel ideo scribendum est aliquid ut se vixisse testentur* [they have to write to keep the printers occupied, or even to show that they are alive].   As apothecaries we make new mixtures every day, pour out of one vessel into another; and as those old Romans robbed all the cities of the world to set out their bad-sited Rome, we skim off the cream of other men's wits, pick the choice flowers of their tilled gardens to set out our own sterile plots. *Castrant alios ut libros suos per se graciles alieno adipe suffarciant* (so Jovius inveighs[3]): they lard their lean books with the fat of others' works. *Ineruditi fures* [unlettered thieves], etc.   A fault that every writer finds, as I do now, and yet faulty themselves, *trium literarum homines*,[4] all thieves; they pilfer out of old writers to stuff up their new comments, scrape Ennius' dung-hills, and out of Democritus' pit,[5] as I have done.   By which means it comes to pass, "that not only libraries and shops are full of our putid papers, but every close-stool and jakes,"[6] *Scribunt carmina quæ legunt cacantes*; they serve to put under pies, to lap spice in,[7] and keep roast-meat from burning.   "With us in France," saith Scaliger,[8] "every man hath liberty to write, but few ability.   Heretofore learning was graced by judicious scholars, but now noble sciences are vilified by base and illiterate scribblers,"[9] that either write from vainglory, need, to get money, or as parasites to flatter and collogue with some great men, they put out *burras, quisquiliasque ineptiasque*[10] [trifles, trash, nonsense].   "Amongst so many thousand authors you shall scarce find one, by reading of whom you shall be any whit better, but rather much worse,"[11] *quibus inficitur potius, quam perficitur*, by which he is rather infected than anyway perfected.

> *Qui talia legit,*
> *Quid didicit tandem, quid scit nisi somnia, nugas ?* [1]
>
> [Who reads such stuff, what does he learn to know
> Save idle dreams and vain frivolities?]

So that oftentimes it falls out (which Callimachus taxed of old) a great book is a great mischief. Cardan finds fault with Frenchmen and Germans,[2] for their scribbling to no purpose; *Non, inquit, ab edendo deterreo, modo novum aliquid inveniant,* he doth not bar them to write, so that it be some new invention of their own; but we weave the same web still, twist the same rope again and again; or if it be a new invention, 'tis but some bauble or toy which idle fellows write, for as idle fellows to read, and who so cannot invent? "He must have a barren wit, that in this scribbling age can forge nothing."[3] "Princes show their armies, rich men vaunt their buildings, soldiers their manhood, and scholars vent their toys ";[4] they must read, they must hear whether they will or no.

> *Et quodcunque semel chartis illeverit, omnes*
> *Gestiet a furno redeuntes scire lacuque,*
> *Et pueros et anus.*[5]
>
> What once is said and writ, all men must know,
> Old wives and children as they come and go.

"What a company of poets hath this year brought out!" as Pliny complains to Sossius Senecio; "this April every day some or other have recited."[6] What a catalogue of new books all this year, all this age (I say), have our Frankfort marts, our domestic marts brought out! Twice a year, *proferunt se nova ingenia et ostentant,*[7] we stretch our wits out, and set them to sale, *magno conatu nihil agimus* [we do nothing with a great expenditure of energy]. So that, which Gesner much desires,[8] if a speedy reformation be not had, by some prince's edicts and grave supervisors, to restrain this liberty, it will run on *in infinitum. Quis tam avidus librorum helluo ?* [Where can we find such a glutton of books?], who can read them? As already, we shall have a vast chaos and confusion of books, we are oppressed with them,[9] our eyes ache with reading, our fingers with turning.[10] For my part I am one of the number, *nos numerus sumus*: I do not deny it, I have only this of Macrobius to say for myself, *Omne meum, nihil meum,* 'tis all mine, and none mine. As a good housewife out of divers fleeces weaves one piece of cloth, a bee gathers wax and honey out of many flowers, and makes a new bundle of all, *Floriferis ut apes in saltibus omnia libant* [as bees in flowery glades sip from each cup], I have laboriously collected this cento out of divers writers,[1] and that *sine injuria*, I have wronged no authors, but given every man his own; which Hierome so much commends in Nepotian,[2] he stole not whole verses, pages, tracts, as some do nowadays, concealing their authors' names, but still said this was Cyprian's, that Lactantius', that Hilarius', so said Minucius Felix, so Victorinus, thus far Arnobius: I cite and quote mine authors (which, howsoever some illiterate scribblers account pedantical, as a cloak of ignorance, and opposite to their affected fine style, I must and will use), *sumpsi, non surripui* [I have taken, not filched]; and what Varro, *lib. 3 de re rust.*, speaks of bees, *minime maleficæ nullius opus vellicantes faciunt deterius* [they do little harm, and damage no one in extracting honey], I can say of myself, Whom have I injured?   The matter is theirs most part, and yet mine, *apparet unde sumptum sit* [it is plain whence it was taken] (which Seneca approves), *aliud tamen quam unde sumptum sit apparet*, [yet it becomes something different in its new setting]; which nature doth with the aliment of our bodies incorporate, digest, assimilate, I do *concoquere quod hausi* [assimilate what I have swallowed], dispose of what I take.   I make them pay tribute to set out this my *Macaronicon*, the method only is mine own; I must usurp that of Wecker *e Ter., nihil dictum quod non dictum prius, methodus sola artificem ostendit*,[3] we can say nothing but what hath been said, the composition and method is ours only, and shows a scholar. Oribasius, Aetius, Avicenna, have all out of Galen, but to their own method, *diverso stilo, non diversa fide*.   Our poets steal from Homer; he spews, saith Ælian, they lick it up.   Divines use Austin's words *verbatim* still, and our story-dressers do as much; he that comes last is commonly best,

> *donec quid grandius ætas*
> *Postera sorsque ferat melior.*
>
> [Till a later age,
> More favoured, shall produce a nobler page.]

Though there were many giants of old in physic and philosophy, yet I say with Didacus Stella,[4] "A dwarf standing on the shoulders of a giant may see farther than a giant himself"; I may likely add, alter, and see farther than my predecessors; and it is no greater prejudice for me to indite after others, than for Ælianus Montaltus, that famous physician, to write *de morbis capitis* [about diseases of the head] after Jason Pratensis,

Heurnius, Hildesheim, etc., many horses to run in a race, one logician, one rhetorician, after another. Oppose then what thou wilt,

Allatres licet usque nos et usque,
Et gannitibus improbis lacessas,

[Though you bark at me as much as you please, and growl threateningly,]

I solve it thus. And for those other faults of barbarism, Doric dialect, extemporanean style, tautologies, apish imitation, a rhapsody of rags gathered together from several dung-hills,[1] excrements of authors, toys and fopperies confusedly tumbled out, without art, invention, judgment, wit, learning, harsh, raw, rude, phantastical, absurd, insolent, indiscreet, ill-composed, indigested, vain, scurrile, idle, dull, and dry; I confess all ('tis partly affected), thou canst not think worse of me than I do of myself. 'Tis not worth the reading, I yield it, I desire thee not to lose time in perusing so vain a subject, I should be peradventure loath myself to read him or thee so writing; 'tis not *operæ pretium* [worth while]. All I say is this, that I have precedents for it,[2] which Isocrates calls *perfugium iis qui peccant* [a refuge for sinners], others as absurd, vain, idle, illiterate, etc. *Nonnulli alii idem fecerunt,* others have done as much, it may be more, and perhaps thou thyself, *Novimus et qui te, etc.* [we know someone who has seen you also]. We have all our faults; *scimus, et hanc veniam, etc.* [we know and beg pardon], 'thou censurest me, so have I done others, and may do thee,[3] *Cædimus, inque vicem, etc.* [we smite, and in turn, etc.], 'tis *lex talionis, quid pro quo.* Go now, censure, criticize, scoff, and rail.

Nasutus sis usque licet, sis denique nasus :
Non potes in nugas dicere plura meas,
Ipse ego quam dixi, etc.[4]

Wert thou all scoffs and flouts, a very Momus,
Than we ourselves, thou canst not say worse of us.

Thus, as when women scold, have I cried whore first, and in some men's censures I am afraid I have overshot myself; *Laudare se vani, vituperare stulti* [self-praise is boastful, self-depreciation foolish], as I do not arrogate, I will not derogate. *Primus vestrum non sum, nec imus,* I am none of the best, I am none of the meanest of you. As I am an inch, or so many feet, so many parasangs, after him or him, I may be peradventure an ace before thee. Be it therefore as it is, well or ill, I have assayed, put myself upon the stage; I must abide the censure, I may not escape it. It is most true, *stilus virum arguit*, our style bewrays us, and as hunters find their game by the trace, so is a man's genius descried by his works;[1] *multo melius ex sermone quam lineamentis de moribus hominum judicamus* [we can judge a man's character much better from his conversation than his physiognomy]; 'twas old Cato's rule. I have laid myself open (I know it) in this treatise, turned mine inside outward: I shall be censured, I doubt not; for, to say truth with Erasmus, *nihil morosius hominum judiciis*, there 's naught so peevish as men's judgments; yet this is some comfort, *ut palata, sic judicia*, our censures are as various as our palates.

> *Tres mihi convivæ prope dissentire videntur,*
> *Poscentes vario multum diversa palato, etc.*[2]

> [Three guests I have, dissenting at my feast,
> Requiring each to gratify his taste
> With different food.]

Our writings are as so many dishes, our readers guests, our books like beauty, that which one admires another rejects; so are we approved as men's fancies are inclined. *Pro captu lectoris habent sua fata libelli* [the fate of books depends on the fancy of the reader]. That which is most pleasing to one is *amaracum sui*, most harsh to another. *Quot homines, tot sententiæ*, so many men, so many minds: that which thou condemnest he commends Quod petis, id sane est invisum acidumque duobus[3] [what attracts you, others find sour and repulsive]. He respects matter, thou art wholly for words; he loves a loose and free style, thou art all for neat composition, strong lines, hyperboles, allegories; he desires a fine frontispiece, enticing pictures, such as Hieron. Natali the Jesuit hath cut to the Dominicals,[4] to draw on the reader's attention, which thou rejectest; that which one admires, another explodes as most absurd and ridiculous. If it be not point-blank to his humour, his method, his conceit, *si quid forsan omissum, quod is animo conceperit, si quæ dictio*,[5] etc., if aught be omitted, or added, which he likes, or dislikes, thou art *mancipium paucæ lectionis*, an idiot, an ass, *nullus es*, or *plagiarius*, a trifler, a trivant, thou art an idle fellow; or else it is a thing of mere industry, a collection without wit or invention, a very toy. *Facilia sic putant omnes quæ jam facta, nec de salebris cogitant, ubi via strata*[6] [when a thing has once been done, people think it easy; when the road is made, they forget how rough the way used to be]; so men

are valued, their labours vilified by fellows of no worth themselves, as things of naught, who could not have done as much.
Unusquisque abundat sensu suo, every man abounds in his own
sense; and whilst each particular party is so affected, how
should one please all?

> *Quid dem? quid non dem? Renuis tu quod jubet ille.*[1]
>
> [What courses must I choose?
> What not? What he would order you refuse.]

How shall I hope to express myself to each man's humour and
conceit, or to give satisfaction to all?[2] Some understand too
little, some too much, *qui similiter in legendos libros, atque in
salutandos homines irruunt, non cogitantes quales, sed quibus vestibus
induti sint* [they pay their respects to books on the same
principle as to people, judging not by the character but by
the outer garb], as Austin observes,[3] not regarding what, but
who write, *orexin habet auctoris celebritas*[4] [the author's name
creates a demand], not valuing the metal, but the stamp that is
upon it, *cantharum aspiciunt, non quid in eo* [they look only
at the jar, not at its contents]. If he be not rich, in great
place, polite and brave, a great doctor, or full-fraught with
grand titles, though never so well qualified, he is a dunce; but,
as Baronius hath it of Cardinal Caraffa's works,[5] he is a mere
hog that rejects any man for his poverty. Some are too partial,
as friends to overween, others come with a prejudice to carp,
vilify, detract, and scoff (*qui de me forsan, quicquid est, omni
contemptu contemptius judicant* [who perhaps regard anything
I produce as utterly beneath contempt]); some as bees for honey,
some as spiders to gather poison. What shall I do in this
case? As a Dutch host, if you come to an inn in Germany
and dislike your fare, diet, lodging, etc., replies in a surly tone,
Aliud tibi quæras diversorium,[6] If you like not this, get you
to another inn: I resolve, if you like not my writing, go read
something else. I do not much esteem thy censure, take thy
course, 'tis not as thou wilt, not as I will, but when we have both
done, that of Plinius Secundus to Trajan[7] will prove true,
"Every man's witty labour takes not, except the matter,
subject, occasion, and some commending favourite happen to
it." If I be taxed, exploded by thee and some such, I shall
haply be approved and commended by others, and so have
been (*Expertus loquor*), and may truly say with Jovius in like
case[8] (*absit verbo jactantia* [without boasting]), *heroum quorundam, pontificum, et virorum nobilium familiaritatem et amicitiam*

*gratasque gratias, et multorum bene laudatorum laudes sum inde
promeritus* [1] [I have on this account been honoured with the
intimate friendship of prominent military men, clergymen, and
nobles, and have earned their favour along with the praises of
many persons of repute]; as I have been honoured by some
worthy men, so have I been vilified by others, and shall be.
At the first publishing of this book, which Probus of Persius'
Satires, [2] *editum librum continuo mirari homines, atque avide
deripere cœperunt* [when the book first appeared, people opened
their eyes, and began eagerly to pick holes in it], I may in
some sort apply to this my work; the first, second, and third
edition were suddenly gone, eagerly read, and, as I have said,
not so much approved by some as scornfully rejected by others.
But it was Democritus his fortune, *Idem admirationi et irrisioni
habitus* [3] [he was the object both of admiration and scorn].
'Twas Seneca's fate, that superintendent of wit, learning, judgment, *ad stuporem doctus* [4] [amazingly learned], the best of
Greek and Latin writers in Plutarch's opinion; "that renowned
corrector of vice," as Fabius terms him, [5] "and painful omniscious philosopher, that writ so excellently and admirably well,"
could not please all parties, or escape censure. How is he
vilified by Caligula, [6] A. Gellius, Fabius, and Lipsius himself, his
chief propugner! *In eo pleraque perniciosa,* saith the same
Fabius, many childish tracts and sentences he hath, *sermo
illaboratus,* too negligent often and remiss, as A. Gellius observes,
*oratio vulgaris et protrita, dicaces et ineptæ sententiæ, eruditio
plebeia* [a homely and commonplace style, far-fetched and
foolish ideas, mediocre learning], an homely shallow writer as
he is. *In partibus spinas et fastidia habet* [he is very involved
and stilted in parts], saith Lipsius; [7] and, as in all his other
works, so especially in his epistles, *aliæ in argutiis et ineptiis
occupantur, intricatus alicubi, et parum compositus, sine copia
rerum hoc fecit* [some are full of idle subtleties; sometimes he is
involved and ill arranged, and this without any great wealth
of matter], he jumbles up many things together immethodically,
after the Stoics' fashion, *parum ordinavit, multa accumulavit,*
etc. If Seneca be thus lashed, and many famous men that
I could name, what shall I expect? How shall I, that am *vix
umbra tanti philosophi* [scarce the shadow of so great a philo-
sopher], hope to please? "No man so absolute," Erasmus
holds, [8] "to satisfy all, except antiquity, prescription, etc., set
a bar." But as I have proved in Seneca, this will not always
take place, how shall I evade? 'Tis the common doom of all

writers, I must (I say) abide it; I seek not applause; *Non ego
ventosæ venor suffragia plebis* [1] [I court not the favour of the
fickle crowd]; again, *non sum adeo informis* [I am not so ugly],
I would not be vilified.[2]

> *Laudatus abunde,*
> *Non fastiditus si tibi, lector, ero.*[3]

[Sufficient praise for me if thou disdainest me not, O worthy reader.]

I fear good men's censures, and to their favourable acceptance
I submit my labours,

> *et linguas mancipiorum*
> *Contemno.*[4]

[I scorn the talk of slaves.]

As the barking of a dog, I securely contemn those malicious and
scurrile obloquies, flouts, calumnies of railers and detractors;
I scorn the rest. What therefore I have said, *pro tenuitate
mea* [to the best of my poor ability], I have said.

One or two things yet I was desirous to have amended if I
could, concerning the manner of handling this my subject, for
which I must apologize, *deprecari*, and upon better advice give
the friendly reader notice. It was not mine intent to prostitute
my muse in English, or to divulge *secreta Minervæ*, but to have
exposed this more contract in Latin, if I could have got it
printed. Any scurrile pamphlet is welcome to our mercenary
stationers in English; they print all,

> *cuduntque libellos*
> *In quorum foliis vix simia nuda cacaret;*

but in Latin they will not deal; which is one of the reasons
Nicholas Car, in his oration of the paucity of English writers,
gives, that so many flourishing wits are smothered in oblivion,
lie dead and buried in this our nation.[5] Another main fault is,
that I have not revised the copy, and amended the style, which
now flows remissly, as it was first conceived; but my leisure
would not permit; *Feci nec quod potui, nec quod volui*, I confess
it is neither as I would, nor as it should be.

> *Cum relego scripsisse pudet, quia plurima cerno*
> *Me quoque quæ fuerant judice digna lini.*[6]

> When I peruse this tract which I have writ,
> I am abash'd, and much I hold unfit.

Et quod gravissimum [and what is most serious], in the matter
itself, many things I disallow at this present, which when I writ,

Non eadem est ætas, non mens [1] [I was younger and more foolish]; I would willingly retract much, etc., but 'tis too late, I can only crave pardon now for what is amiss.

I might indeed (had I wisely done), observed that precept of the poet, *Nonumque prematur in annum* [keep back your work for nine years before printing], and have taken more care: or, as Alexander the physician would have done by lapis lazuli, fifty times washed before it be used, I should have revised, corrected, and amended this tract; but I had not (as I said) that happy leisure, no amanuenses or assistants.   Pancrates in Lucian,[2] wanting a servant as he went from Memphis to Coptus in Egypt, took a door-bar, and after some superstitious words pronounced (Eucrates the relater was then present) made it stand up like a serving-man, fetch him water, turn the spit, serve in supper, and what work he would besides; and when he had done that service he desired, turned his man to a stick again.   I have no such skill to make new men at my pleasure, or means to hire them; no whistle to call like the master of a ship, and bid them run, etc.   I have no such authority, no such benefactors, as that noble Ambrosius was to Origen,[3] allowing him six or seven amanuenses to write out his dictates; I must for that cause do my business myself, and was therefore enforced, as a bear doth her whelps, to bring forth this confused lump; I had not time to lick it into form, as she doth her young ones, but even so to publish it as it was first written, *quicquid in buccam venit* [whatever came uppermost], in an extemporean style, as I do commonly all other exercises,[4] *effudi quicquid dictavit genius meus* [I poured out whatever came into my mind], out of a confused company of notes, and writ with as small deliberation as I do ordinarily speak, without all affectation of big words, fustian phrases, jingling terms, tropes, strong lines, that like Acestes' arrows caught fire as they flew,[5] strains of wit, brave heats, elogies, hyperbolical exornations, elegancies, etc., which many so much affect.   I am *aquæ potor* [6] [a water-drinker], drink no wine at all, which so much improves our modern wits, a loose, plain, rude writer, *ficum voco ficum et ligonem ligonem* [I call a fig a fig and a spade a spade], and as free, as loose, *idem calamo quod in mente* [what my mind thinks my pen writes], I call a spade a spade,[7] *animis hæc scribo, non auribus* [I write for the mind, not the ear], I respect matter, not words; remembering that of Cardan, *verba propter res, non res propter verba* [words should minister to matter, not vice versa], and seeking with Seneca, *quid scribam, non quemadmodum*, rather what than how to write: for as Philo thinks, "He that is conversant about matter neglects words, and those that excel in this art of speaking have no profound learning." [1]

> *Verba nitent phaleris, at nullas verba medullas*
> *Intus habent.* [2]

[Their words well tricked, but void of pith within.]

Besides, it was the observation of that wise Seneca, "When you see a fellow careful about his words, and neat in his speech, know this for a certainty, that man's mind is busied about toys, there's no solidity in him." [3] *Non est ornamentum virile concinnitas* [prettiness is not a masculine adornment]: as he said of a nightingale, *Vox es, praeterea nihil* [you are a voice and nothing more], etc. I am therefore in this point a professed disciple of Apollonius, a scholar of Socrates, [4] I neglect phrases, and labour wholly to inform my reader's understanding, not to please his ear; 'tis not my study or intent to compose neatly, which an orator requires, but to express myself readily and plainly as it happens. So that as a river runs sometimes precipitate and swift, then dull and slow; now direct, then *per ambages* [winding]; now deep, then shallow; now muddy, then clear; now broad, then narrow; doth my style flow: now serious, then light; now comical, then satirical; now more elaborate, then remiss, as the present subject required, or as at that time I was affected. And if thou vouchsafe to read this treatise, it shall seem no otherwise to thee than the way to an ordinary traveller, sometimes fair, sometimes foul; here champaign, there enclosed; barren in one place, better soil in another: by woods, groves, hills, dales, plains, etc. I shall lead thee *per ardua montium, et lubrica vallium, et roscida cespitum, et glebosa camporum* [5] [over steep mountains, slippery glades, wet grass, and sticky fields], through variety of objects, that which thou shalt like and surely dislike.

For the matter itself or method, if it be faulty, consider I pray you that of Columella, *Nihil perfectum, aut a singulari consummatum industria* [nothing can be perfected or completed by the efforts of a single individual], no man can observe all, much is defective no doubt, may justly be taxed, altered, and avoided in Galen, Aristotle, those great masters. *Boni venatoris* (one holds [6]) *plures feras capere, non omnes*, he is a good huntsman can catch some, not all: I have done my endeavour. Besides, I dwell not in this study, *Non hic sulcos ducimus, non hoc pulvere desudamus* [I am not driving a furrow here, this is not my field of labour], I am but a smatterer, I confess, a stranger, here and there I pull a flower;[1] I do easily grant, if a rigid censurer should criticize on this which I have writ, he should not find three sole faults, as Scaliger in Terence, but three hundred. So many as he hath done in Cardan's Subtleties, as many notable errors as Gul. Laurembergius, a late professor of Rostock, discovers in that Anatomy of Laurentius,[2] or Barocius the Venetian in Sacroboscus. And although this be a sixth edition, in which I should have been more accurate, corrected all those former escapes, yet it was *magni laboris opus*, so difficult and tedious, that, as carpenters do find out of experience, 'tis much better build a new sometimes, than repair an old house; I could as soon write as much more as alter that which is written. If aught therefore be amiss (as I grant there is), I require a friendly admonition, no bitter invective, *Sint Musis socii Charites, Furia omnis abesto*[3] [let the Graces come with the Muses, but let the Furies keep away], otherwise, as in ordinary controversies, *funem contentionis nectamus, sed cui bono?* We may contend, and likely misuse each other, but to what purpose? We are both scholars, say,

Arcades ambo,
Et cantare pares, et respondere parati.[4]

[Both young Arcadians, both alike inspir'd
To sing and answer as the song requir'd.]

If we do wrangle, what shall we get by it? Trouble and wrong ourselves, make sport to others. If I be convict of an error, I will yield, I will amend. *Si quid bonis moribus, si quid veritati dissentaneum, in sacris vel humanis literis a me dictum sit, id nec dictum esto* [if I have said anything contrary to good morals or to truth as expressed either in sacred or profane letters, let it be regarded as unsaid]. In the meantime I require a favourable censure of all faults omitted, harsh compositions, pleonasms of words, tautological repetitions (though Seneca bear me out, *nunquam nimis dicitur, quod nunquam satis dicitur* [that is never said too often, which cannot be said often enough]), perturbations of tenses, numbers, printers' faults, etc. My translations are sometimes rather paraphrases than interpretations, *non ad verbum* [not literal], but, as an author, I use more liberty, and that's only taken which was to my purpose. Quotations are often inserted in the text, which makes the style more harsh, or in the margin as it happened. Greek authors, Plato, Plutarch.

Athenæus, etc., I have cited out of their interpreters, because the original was not so ready. I have mingled *sacra profanis* [sacred with profane], but I hope not profaned, and in repetition of authors' names, ranked them *per accidens* [as they occurred], not according to chronology; sometimes neoterics before ancients, as my memory suggested. Some things are here altered, expunged in this sixth edition, others amended, much added, because many good authors in all kinds are come to my hands since,[1] and 'tis no prejudice, no such indecorum or oversight.

Nunquam ita quicquam bene subducta ratione ad vitam fuit,
Quin res, ætas, usus, semper aliquid apportent novi,
Aliquid moneant, ut illa quæ scire te credas, nescias,
Et quæ tibi putaris prima, in exercendo ut repudias.[2]

Ne'er was aught yet at first contriv'd so fit,
But use, age, or something would alter it;
Advise thee better, and, upon peruse,
Make thee not say, and what thou tak'st refuse.

But I am now resolved never to put this treatise out again; *Ne quid nimis* [not too much of anything], I will not hereafter add, alter, or retract; I have done. The last and greatest exception is, that I, being a divine, have meddled with physic.

Tantumne est ab re tua otii tibi,
Aliena ut cures, eaque nihil quæ ad te attinent?[3]

which Menedemus objected to Chremes; have I so much leisure, or little business of mine own, as to look after other men's matters which concern me not? What have I to do with physic? *Quod medicorum est promittant medici* [let doctors look after their own job]. The Lacedæmonians were once in counsel about state matters,[4] a debauched fellow spake excellent well, and to the purpose, his speech was generally approved: a grave senator steps up, and by all means would have it repealed, though good, because *dehonestabatur pessimo auctore*, it had no better an author; let some good man relate the same, and then it should pass. This counsel was embraced, *factum est*, and it was registered forthwith, *Et sic bona sententia mansit, malus auctor mutatus est* [and so the good plan was retained, the bad counsellor was dismissed]. Thou sayest as much of me, *stomachosus* [peevish] as thou art, and grantest peradventure this which I have written in physic, not to be amiss, had another done it, a professed physician, or so; but why should I meddle with this tract? Hear me speak. There be many other subjects,

I do easily grant, both in humanity and divinity, fit to be treated of, of which had I written *ad ostentationem* only, to show myself, I should have rather chosen, and in which I have been more conversant, I could have more willingly luxuriated, and better satisfied myself and others; but that at this time I was fatally driven upon this rock of melancholy, and carried away by this by-stream, which, as a rillet, is deducted from the main channel of my studies, in which I have pleased and busied myself at idle hours, as a subject most necessary and commodious. Not that I prefer it before divinity, which I do acknowledge to be the queen of professions, and to which all the rest are as handmaids, but that in divinity I saw no such great need. For had I written positively, there be so many books in that kind, so many commentators, treatises, pamphlets, expositions, sermons, that whole teams of oxen cannot draw them; and had I been as forward and ambitious as some others, I might have haply printed a sermon at Paul's Cross, a sermon in St. Mary's Oxon, a sermon in Christ Church, or a sermon before the right honourable, right reverend, a sermon before the right worshipful, a sermon in Latin, in English, a sermon with a name, a sermon without, a sermon, a sermon, etc. But I have been ever as desirous to suppress my labours in this kind, as others have been to press and publish theirs. To have written in controversy had been to cut off an hydra's head, *lis litem generat*,[1] one [dispute] begets another, so many duplications, triplications, and swarms of questions *in sacro bello hoc quod stili mucrone agitur* [in this sacred war which is waged with the pen], that having once begun, I should never make an end. One had much better, as Alexander the Sixth, Pope, long since observed, provoke a great prince than a begging friar,[2] a Jesuit, or a seminary priest, I will add, for *inexpugnabile genus hoc hominum*, they are an irrefragable society, they must and will have the last word; and that with such eagerness, impudence, abominable lying, falsifying, and bitterness in their questions they proceed, that as he said, *Furorne cæcus, an rapit vis acrior, an culpa? responsum dute.*[3] Blind fury, or error, or rashness, or what it is that eggs them, I know not; I am sure many times, which Austin perceived long since,[4] *tempestate contentionis, serenitas caritatis obnubilatur*, with this tempest of contention the serenity of charity is overclouded, and there be too many spirits conjured up already in this kind in all sciences, and more than we can tell how to lay, which do so furiously rage, and keep such a racket, that as Fabius said,[5] "It had been much better for some of them to have been born dumb, and altogether illiterate, than so far to dote to their own destruction."

> *At melius fuerat non scribere, namque tacere*
> *Tutum semper erit.*

[Better it had been not to write at all:
From saying naught no mischief can befall.]

'Tis a general fault, as Severinus the Dane complains in physic, "Unhappy men as we are, we spend our days in unprofitable questions and disputations," intricate subtleties, *de lana caprina* [about a goat's fleece], about moonshine in the water, "leaving in the meantime those chiefest treasures of nature untouched, wherein the best medicines for all manner of diseases are to be found, and do not only neglect them ourselves, but hinder, condemn, forbid, and scoff at others, that are willing to inquire after them."[1]   These motives at this present have induced me to make choice of this medicinal subject.

If any physician in the meantime shall infer, *Ne sutor ultra crepidam,*[2] and find himself grieved that I have intruded into his profession, I will tell him in brief, I do not otherwise by them than they do by us, if it be for their advantage.   I know many of their sect which have taken orders in hope of a benefice, 'tis a common transition, and why may not a melancholy divine, that can get nothing but by simony, profess physic?   Drusianus, an Italian (Crusianus, but corruptly, Trithemius calls him), "because he was not fortunate in his practice, forsook his profession, and writ afterwards in divinity."[3]   Marsilius Ficinus was *semel et simul,* a priest and a physician at once, and T. Linacre in his old age took orders.[4]   The Jesuits profess both at this time, divers of them *permissu superiorum* [by the permission of the superiors], chirurgeons, panders, bawds, and midwives, etc.   Many poor country vicars, for want of other means, are driven to their shifts, to turn mountebanks, quacksalvers, empirics, and if our greedy patrons hold us to such hard conditions as commonly they do, they will make most of us work at some trade, as Paul did, at last turn taskers, maltsters, costermongers, graziers, sell ale as some have done, or worse. Howsoever, in undertaking this task, I hope I shall commit no great error or indecorum; if all be considered aright, I can vindicate myself with Georgius Braunus and Hieronymus Hemingius, those two learned divines; who (to borrow a line or two of mine elder brother[5]), drawn by a "natural love, the one of pictures and maps, prospectives and chorographical delights, writ that ample Theatre of Cities; the other to the study of genealogies, penned *Theatrum Genealogicum*." Or else I can excuse my studies with Lessius the Jesuit in like case.[1] It is a disease of the soul on which I am to treat, and as much appertaining to a divine as to a physician, and who knows not what an agreement there is betwixt these two professions? A good divine either is or ought to be a good physician, a spiritual physician at least, as our Saviour calls Himself, and was indeed (Matt. iv, 23; Luke v, 18; Luke vii, 21). They differ but in object, the one of the body, the other of the soul, and use divers medicines to cure: one amends *animam per corpus* [the soul through the body], the other *corpus per animam* [the body through the soul] as our Regius Professor of Physic well informed us in a learned lecture of his not long since.[2] One helps the vices and passions of the soul, anger, lust, desperation, pride, presumption, etc., by applying that spiritual physic; as the other uses proper remedies in bodily diseases. Now this being a common infirmity of body and soul, and such a one that hath as much need of a spiritual as a corporal cure, I could not find a fitter task to busy myself about, a more apposite theme, so necessary, so commodious, and generally concerning all sorts of men, that should so equally participate of both, and require a whole physician. A divine in this compound mixed malady can do little alone, a physician in some kinds of melancholy much less, both make an absolute cure.

> *Alterius sic altera poscit opem.*[3]
>
> [When in friendship joined,
> A mutual succour in each other find.]

And 'tis proper to them both, and I hope not unbeseeming me, who am by my profession a divine, and by mine inclination a physician. I had Jupiter in my sixth house; I say with Beroaldus, *non sum medicus, nec medicinæ prorsus expers* [I am not a doctor, yet have some knowledge of medicine], in the theoric of physic I have taken some pains, not with an intent to practise, but to satisfy myself, which was a cause likewise of the first undertaking of this subject.

If these reasons do not satisfy thee, good reader, as Alexander Munificus, that bountiful prelate, sometime Bishop of Lincoln, when he had built six castles, *ad invidiam operis eluendam*, saith Mr. Camden,[4] to take away the envy of his work (which very words Nubrigensis hath of Roger the rich Bishop of Salisbury, who in King Stephen's time built Sherborne Castle, and that of Devizes), to divert the scandal or imputation which might be thence inferred, built so many religious houses; if this my discourse be over-medicinal, or savour too much of humanity, I promise thee that I will hereafter make thee amends in some treatise of divinity. But this I hope shall suffice, when you have more fully considered of the matter of this my subject, *rem substratam*, melancholy, madness, and of the reasons following, which were my chief motives: the generality of the disease, the necessity of the cure, and the commodity or common good that will arise to all men by the knowledge of it, as shall at large appear in the ensuing preface. And I doubt not but that in the end you will say with me, that to anatomize this humour aright, through all the members of this our *microcosmos*, is as great a task as to reconcile those chronological errors in the Assyrian monarchy, find out the quadrature of a circle, the creeks and sounds of the north-east or north-west passages, and all out as good a discovery as that hungry Spaniard's[1] of *Terra Australis Incognita*, as great a trouble as to perfect the motion of Mars and Mercury, which so crucifies our astronomers, or to rectify the Gregorian calendar. I am so affected for my part, and hope as Theophrastus did by his Characters, "that our posterity, O friend Polycles, shall be the better for this which we have written, by correcting and rectifying what is amiss in themselves by our examples, and applying our precepts and cautions to their own use."[2] And as that great captain Zisca would have a drum made of his skin when he was dead, because he thought the very noise of it would put his enemies to flight, I doubt not but that these following lines, when they shall be recited, or hereafter read, will drive away melancholy (though I be gone) as much as Zisca's drum could terrify his foes. Yet one caution let me give by the way to my present or future reader, who is actually melancholy, that he read not the symptoms or prognostics in this following tract,[3] lest by applying that which he reads to himself, aggravating, appropriating things generally spoken to his own person (as melancholy men for the most part do), he trouble or hurt himself, and get in conclusion more harm than good. I advise them therefore warily to peruse that tract; *Lapides loquitur* (so said Agrippa, *de occ. Phil.*[4]), *et caveant lectores ne cerebrum iis excutiat* [he discourses stones, and the readers must beware lest he break their heads]. The rest I doubt not they may securely read, and to their benefit. But I am over-tedious, I proceed.

Of the necessity and generality of this which I have said, if any man doubt, I shall desire him to make a brief survey of the world, as Cyprian adviseth Donat; "supposing himself to be transported to the top of some high mountain, and thence to behold the tumults and chances of this wavering world, he cannot choose but either laugh at, or pity it." [1] St. Hierome, out of a strong imagination, being in the wilderness, conceived with himself that he then saw them dancing in Rome; and if thou shalt either conceive, or climb to see, thou shalt soon perceive that all the world is mad, that it is melancholy, dotes; that it is (which Epichthonius Cosmopolites expressed not many years since in a map) made like a fool's head (with that motto, *Caput helleboro dignum* [a head requiring hellebore]); a crazed head, *cavea stultorum*, a fools' paradise, or as Apollonius, a common prison of gulls, cheaters, flatterers, etc., and needs to be reformed. Strabo, in the ninth book of his Geography, compares Greece to the picture of a man, which comparison of his Nic. Gerbelius, in his exposition of Sophianus' map, approves; the breast lies open from those Acroceraunian hills in Epirus to the Sunian promontory in Attica; Pagæ and Megara are the two shoulders; that Isthmus of Corinth the neck; and Peloponnesus the head. If this allusion hold, 'tis sure a mad head; Morea may be Moria [Folly]; and to speak what I think, the inhabitants of modern Greece swerve as much from reason and true religion at this day, as that Morea doth from the picture of a man. Examine the rest in like sort, and you shall find that kingdoms and provinces are melancholy, cities and families, all creatures, vegetal, sensible, and rational, that all sorts, sects, ages, conditions, are out of tune, as in Cebes' Table, *omnes errorem bibunt*, before they come into the world, they are intoxicated by error's cup, from the highest to the lowest have need of physic, and those particular actions in Seneca,[2] where father and son prove one another mad, may be general; Porcius Latro shall plead against us all. For indeed who is not a fool, melancholy, mad? *Qui nil molitur inepte*,[3] who is not brain-sick? Folly, melancholy, madness, are but one disease, delirium is a common name to all. Alexander Gordonius, Jason Pratensis, Savonarola, Guianerius, Montaltus, confound them as differing *secundum magis et minus*; so doth David (Ps. lxxv, 4), "I said unto the fools, deal not so madly," and 'twas an old Stoical paradox, *omnes stultos insanire*,[4] all fools are mad, though some madder than others. And who is not a fool, who is free from melancholy? Who is not touched more or less in habit or disposition? If in disposition, "ill dispositions beget habits, if they persevere," saith Plutarch,[1] habits either are or turn to diseases. 'Tis the same which Tully maintains in the second of his Tusculans, *omnium insipientum animi in morbo sunt, et perturbatorum*, fools are sick, and all that are troubled in mind: for what is sickness, but as Gregory Tholosanus defines it, "a dissolution or perturbation of the bodily league, which health combines":[2] and who is not sick, or ill disposed? In whom doth not passion, anger, envy, discontent, fear, and sorrow reign? Who labours not of this disease? Give me but a little leave, and you shall see by what testimonies, confessions, arguments I will evince it, that most men are mad, that they had as much need to go a pilgrimage to the Anticyræ (as in Strabo's time they did[3]) as in our days they run to Compostella, our Lady of Sichem, or Loretto to seek for help; that it is like to be as prosperous a voyage as that of Guiana, and that there is much more need of hellebore than of tobacco.

That men are so misaffected, melancholy, mad, giddy-headed, hear the testimony of Solomon (Eccles. ii, 12): "And I turned to behold wisdom, madness and folly," etc.; and v. 23: "All his days are sorrow, his travail grief, and his heart taketh no rest in the night." So that, take melancholy in what sense you will, properly or improperly, in disposition or habit, for pleasure or for pain, dotage, discontent, fear, sorrow, madness, for part or all, truly or metaphorically, 'tis all one. Laughter itself is madness according to Solomon, and as St. Paul hath it, "Worldly sorrow brings death." "The hearts of the sons of men are evil, and madness is in their hearts while they live" (Eccles. ix, 3). Wise men themselves are no better (Eccles. i, 18): "In the multitude of wisdom is much grief, and he that increaseth wisdom increaseth sorrow." He hated life itself, nothing pleased him, he hated his labour (chap. ii, 17); all, as he concludes, is "sorrow, grief, vanity, vexation of spirit."[4] And though he were the wisest man in the world, *sanctuarium sapientiæ* [a shrine of wisdom], and had wisdom in abundance, he will not vindicate himself, or justify his own actions. "Surely I am more foolish than any man, and have not the understanding of a man in me" (Prov. xxx, 2). Be they Solomon's words, or the words of Agur, the son of Jakeh, they are canonical. David, a man after God's own heart, confesseth as much of himself (Ps. lxxiii, 21, 22): "So foolish was I and ignorant, I was even as a beast before thee"; and condemns all for fools (Ps. liii; xxxii, 9; xlix, 20). He compares them to "beasts, horses, and mules, in which there is no understanding." The Apostle Paul

accuseth himself in like sort (2 Cor. xi, 21): "I would you would
suffer a little my foolishness, I speak foolishly." "The whole
head is sick," saith Esay,[1] "and the heart is heavy" (chap. i, 5);
and makes lighter of them than of oxen and asses, "the ox
knows his owner," etc. Read Deut. xxxii, 6; Jer. iv; Amos iii,
1; Ephes. v, 6. "Be not mad, be not deceived; foolish Galatians,
who hath bewitched you?" How often are they branded with
this epithet of madness and folly! No word so frequent amongst
the Fathers of the Church and divines; you may see what an
opinion they had of the world, and how they valued men's
actions.

I know that we think far otherwise, and hold them most
part wise men that are in authority, princes, magistrates, rich
men, they are wise men born, all politicians and statesmen
must needs be so, for who dare speak against them?[2] And on
the other, so corrupt is our judgment, we esteem wise and
honest men fools. Which Democritus well signified in an epistle
of his to Hippocrates: the Abderites "account virtue madness,"[3]
and so do most men living. Shall I tell you the reason of it?
Fortune and Virtue, Wisdom and Folly, their seconds, upon a
time contended in the Olympics; every man thought that
Fortune and Folly would have the worst, and pitied their cases;
but it fell out otherwise.[4] Fortune was blind and cared not
where she stroke, nor whom, without laws, *andabatorum instar*
[like blind gladiators], etc. Folly, rash and inconsiderate,
esteemed as little what she said or did. Virtue and Wisdom
gave place, were hissed out and exploded by the common
people, Folly and Fortune admired, and so are all their followers
ever since:[5] knaves and fools commonly fare and deserve best in
worldlings' eyes and opinions. Many good men have no better
fate in their ages: Achish (1 Sam. xxi, 14) held David for a
madman. Elisha[6] and the rest were no otherwise esteemed.
David was derided of the common people (Ps. lxxi, 6): "I am become a monster to many." And generally we are accounted
fools for Christ (1 Cor. iv, 10). "We fools thought his life madness, and his end without honour" (Wisd. v, 4). Christ and
His Apostles were censured in like sort (John x; Mark iii; Acts
xxvi). And so were all Christians in Pliny's time, *fuerunt et alii
similis dementiæ*[7] [there were others similarly crazed], etc.,
and called not long after, *vesaniæ sectatores, eversores hominum,
polluti novatores, fanatici, canes, malefici, venefici, Galilæi
homunciones*[8] [devotees of madness, destroyers of society,
blasphemous innovators, fanatics, dogs, criminals, poisoners,

Galilean manikins], etc. 'Tis an ordinary thing with us to account honest, devout, orthodox, divine, religious, plain-dealing men idiots, asses, that cannot or will not lie and dissemble, shift, flatter, *accommodare se ad eum locum ubi nati sunt* [adapt themselves to the station in which they were born], make good bargains, supplant, thrive, *patronis inservire, solennes ascendendi modos apprehendere, leges, mores, consuetudines recte observare, candide laudare, fortiter defendere, sententias amplecti, dubitare de nullis, credere omnia, accipere omnia, nihil reprehendere, cæteraque quæ promotionem ferunt et securitatem, quæ sine ambage felicem reddunt hominem, et vere sapientem apud nos* [fawn upon their patrons, learn the usual methods of getting on, be scrupulous in the observance of laws, manners, customs, praise in glowing terms, defend with vigour, adopt others' opinions, doubt nothing, believe everything, endure everything, resent nothing, and do all the other things which lead to promotion and safe position, which make a man fortunate beyond all question, and truly wise, according to our notions]; that cannot temporize as other men do, hand and take bribes, etc.,[1] but fear God, and make a conscience of their doings. But the Holy Ghost, that knows better how to judge, He calls them fools. "The fool hath said in his heart" (Ps. liii, 1). "And their ways utter their folly" (Ps. xlix, 13). "For what can be more mad, than for a little worldly pleasure to procure unto themselves eternal punishment?"[2] as Gregory and others inculcate unto us.

Yea, even all those great philosophers the world hath ever had in admiration, whose works we do so much esteem, that gave precepts of wisdom to others, inventors of arts and sciences, Socrates the wisest man of his time by the Oracle of Apollo, whom his two scholars, Plato[3] and Xenophon,[4] so much extol and magnify with those honourable titles, "best and wisest of all mortal men, the happiest, and most just"; and as Alcibiades incomparably commends him;[5] Achilles was a worthy man, but Brasidas and others were as worthy as himself; Antenor and Nestor were as good as Pericles, and so of the rest; but none present, before or after Socrates, *nemo veterum neque eorum qui nunc sunt* [none of the ancients nor of those of our own day], were ever such, will match, or come near him. Those seven wise men of Greece, those British Druids, Indian Brachmanni, Ethiopian Gymnosophists, Magi of the Persians, Apollonius (of whom Philostratus, *non doctus, sed natus sapiens*, wise from his cradle), Epicurus, so much admired by his scholar Lucretius:

Qui genus humanum ingenio superavit, et omnes
Perstrinxit stellas exortus ut ætherius sol.

Whose wit excell'd the wits of men as far,
As the sun rising doth obscure a star.

Or that so much renowned Empedocles:

Ut vix humana videatur stirpe creatus.[1]

[So that he scarce seems sprung from human stock.]

All those of whom we read such hyperbolical elogiums,[2] as
of Aristotle, that he was wisdom itself in the abstract, a miracle
of nature,[3] breathing libraries, as Eunapius of Longinus, lights
of nature, giants for wit, quintessence of wit, divine spirits,
eagles in the clouds, fallen from heaven, gods, spirits, lamps of
the world, dictators, *Nulla ferant talem secla futura virum* [No
future age shall such a man produce], monarchs, miracles,
superintendents of wit and learning, *Oceanus, Phœnix, Atlas,*
monstrum, portentum hominis, orbis universi musæum, ultimus
humanæ naturæ conatus, naturæ maritus [Oceanus, Phœnix,
Atlas, a prodigy, a marvel of a man, a museum of the whole
world, the supreme product of humanity, the spouse of Nature],

merito cui doctior orbis
Submissis defert fascibus imperium.

[To whom the learned world,
As to its rightful monarch, homage pays.]

As Ælian writ of Protagoras and Gorgias, we may say of them
all, *tantum a sapientibus abfuerunt, quantum a viris pueri* [they
could no more be called wise than boys men], they were children
in respect, infants, not eagles, but kites; novices, illiterate,
eunuchi sapientiæ.   And although they were the wisest, and
most admired in their age, as he censured Alexander, I do them,
there were 10,000 in his army as worthy captains (had they
been in place of command), as valiant as himself; there were
myriads of men wiser in those days, and yet all short of what
they ought to be.   Lactantius, in his book of Wisdom,[4] proves
them to be dizzards, fools, asses, madmen, so full of absurd and
ridiculous tenents and brain-sick positions, that to his thinking
never any old woman or sick person doted worse.   Democritus
took all from Leucippus, and left, saith he, "the inheritance of
his folly to Epicurus,"[5] *insanienti dum sapientiæ,* etc.[6]   The
like he holds of Plato, Aristippus, and the rest, making
no difference "betwixt them and beasts, saving that they
could speak."[7]   Theodoret, in his tract *de cur. Græc. affect.,*[8]

manifestly evinces as much of Socrates, whom though that oracle
of Apollo confirmed to be the wisest man then living, and
saved him from the plague, whom 2000 years have admired, of
whom some will as soon speak evil as of Christ, yet *re vera* [in
reality], he was an illiterate idiot, as Aristophanes calls him,[1]
irrisor et ambitiosus [a scoffer and fond of praise], as his
master Aristotle terms him, *scurra Atticus* [an Attic buffoon],
as Zeno, an enemy to all arts and sciences,[2] as Athenæus, to
philosophers and travellers, an opinative ass, a caviller, a kind
of pedant; for his manners, as Theod. Cyrensis describes him,
a sodomite,[3] an atheist (so convict by Anytus), *iracundus et
ebrius, dicax* [hot-tempered, a heavy drinker, quarrelsome],
etc., a pot-companion, by Plato's own confession, a sturdy
drinker; and that of all others he was most sottish, a very
madman in his actions and opinions. Pythagoras was part
philosopher, part magician, or part witch. If you desire to
hear more of Apollonius, a great wise man, sometime paralleled
by Julian the Apostate to Christ, I refer you to that learned
tract of Eusebius against Hierocles, and for them all to Lucian's
Piscator, Icaromenippus, Necyomantia: their actions, opinions
in general were so prodigious, absurd, ridiculous, which they
broached and maintained, their books and elaborate treatises
were full of dotage, which Tully *ad Atticum* long since observed,
delirant plerumque scriptores in libris suis [writers mostly rave
in their books], their lives being opposite to their words, they
commended poverty to others, and were most covetous themselves, extolled love and peace, and yet persecuted one another
with virulent hate and malice. They could give precepts for
verse and prose, but not a man of them (as Seneca tells them
home[4]) could moderate his affections. Their music did show
us *flebiles modos* [sad airs], etc., how to rise and fall, but they
could not so contain themselves as in adversity not to make
a lamentable tone. They will measure ground by geometry,
set down limits, divide and subdivide, but cannot yet prescribe
quantum homini satis [how much is enough for a man], or keep
within compass of reason and discretion. They can square
circles, but understand not the state of their own souls, describe
right lines and crooked, etc., but know not what is right in
this life, *quid in vita rectum sit ignorant*; so that as he said,
Nescio an Anticyram ratio illis destinet omnem, I think all the
Anticyræ will not restore them to their wits. If these men
now,[5] that held Zenodotus' heart, Crates' liver,[6] Epictetus' lanthorn, were so sottish, and had no more brains than so many

beetles, what shall we think of the commonalty? what of the rest?

Yea, but will you infer, that is true of heathens, if they be conferred with Christians (1 Cor. iii, 19): "The wisdom of this world is foolishness with God," "earthly and devilish," as James calls it (iii, 15). "They were vain in their imaginations, and their foolish heart was full of darkness" (Rom. i, 21). "When they professed themselves wise, became fools" (v. 22). Their witty works are admired here on earth, whilst their souls are tormented in hell-fire. In some sense, *Christiani Crassiani*, Christians are Crassians, and if compared to that wisdom, no better than fools. *Quis est sapiens? Solus Deus*, Pythagoras replies.[1] "God is only wise" (Rom. xvi), Paul determines, "only good," as Austin well contends, "and no man living can be justified in His sight." "God looked down from heaven upon the children of men, to see if any did understand" (Ps. liii, 2, 3), but all are corrupt, err. "None doth good, no, not one" (Rom. iii, 12). Job aggravates this (iv, 18): "Behold, he found no steadfastness in his servants, and laid folly upon his angels"; (v. 19,) "How much more on them that dwell in houses of clay!" In this sense we are all fools, and the Scripture alone is *arx Minervæ*[2] [the citadel of Minerva], we and our writings are shallow and unperfect. But I do not so mean; even in our ordinary dealings we are no better than fools. "All our actions," as Pliny told Trajan,[3] "upbraid us of folly," our whole course of life is but matter of laughter: we are not soberly wise; and the world itself, which ought at least to be wise by reason of his antiquity, as Hugo de Prato Florido will have it,[4] *semper stultizat*, "is every day more foolish than other; the more it is whipped, the worse it is, and as a child will still be crowned with roses and flowers." We are apish in it, *asini bipedes* [two-legged asses], and every place is full *inversorum Apuleiorum*, of metamorphosed and two-legged asses,[5] *inversorum Silenorum* [of metamorphosed Silenuses], childish, *pueri instar bimuli, tremula patris dormientis in ulna* [like a two-year-old child, sleeping on its father's arm]. Jovianus Pontanus, *Antonio Dial.*, brings in some laughing at an old man, that by reason of his age was a little fond, but as he admonisheth there, *Ne mireris, mi hospes, de hoc sene*, marvel not at him only, for *tota hæc civitas delirat*, all our town dotes in like sort, we are a company of fools.[6] Ask not with him in the poet, *Larvæ hunc intemperiæ insaniæque agitant senem?*[7] What madness ghosts this old man? but, What madness ghosts us all? For we are *ad unum omnes,* all mad, *semel insanivimus omnes,* not once, but always so, *et semel, et simul, et semper,* ever and altogether as bad as he; and not *senex bis puer, delira anus* [an old man is in his second boyhood, an old woman dotes], but say it of us all, *semper pueri,* young and old, all dote, as Lactantius proves out of Seneca; and no difference betwixt us and children, saving that *majora ludimus, et grandioribus pupis,* they play with babies of clouts and such toys, we sport with greater baubles. We cannot accuse or condemn one another, being faulty ourselves, *deliramenta loqueris,* you talk idly, or as Mitio upbraided Demea, *insanis, aufer te* [1] [you are mad, away with you], for we are as mad our own selves, and it is hard to say which is the worst. Nay, 'tis universally so; *Vitam regit fortuna, non sapientia* [2] [life is governed by chance, not wisdom].

When Socrates had taken great pains to find out a wise man,[3] and to that purpose had consulted with philosophers, poets, artificers, he concludes all men were fools; and though it procured him both anger and much envy, yet in all companies he would openly profess it. When Supputius in Pontanus [4] had travelled all over Europe to confer with a wise man, he returned at last without his errand, and could find none. Cardan concurs with him: "Few there are (for aught I can perceive) well in their wits." [5] So doth Tully: "I see everything to be done foolishly and unadvisedly." [6]

> *Ille sinistrorsum, hic dextrorsum, unus utrique*
> *Error, sed variis illudit partibus omnes.*

> One reels to this, another to that wall ;
> 'Tis the same error that deludes them all.

They dote all, but not alike, Μανία γὰρ οὐ πᾶσιν ὁμοία, not in the same kind. "One is covetous, a second lascivious, a third ambitious, a fourth envious, etc.," [7] as Damasippus the Stoic hath well illustrated in the poet:

> *Desipiunt omnes æque ac tu.* [8]

> [And they who call you fool, with equal claim
> May plead an ample title to the name.]

'Tis an inbred malady in every one of us, there is *seminarium stultitiæ,* a seminary of folly, "which, if it be stirred up, or get ahead, will run *in infinitum,* and infinitely varies, as we ourselves are severally addicted," saith Balthasar Castilio: [9] and cannot so easily be rooted out, it takes such fast hold, as Tully holds, *altæ radices stultitiæ* [deep are the roots of folly], so we are bred, and so we continue.[1] Some say there be two main defects of wit, error and ignorance, to which all others are reduced; by ignorance we know not things necessary, by error we know them falsely. Ignorance is a privation, error a positive act. From ignorance comes vice, from error heresy, etc. But make how many kinds you will, divide and subdivide, few men are free, or that do not impinge on some one kind or other. *Sic plerumque agitat stultos inscitia* [2] [so are the foolish commonly a prey to ignorance], as he that examines his own and other men's actions shall find.

Charon in Lucian,[3] as he wittily feigns, was conducted by Mercury to such a place, where he might see all the world at once; after he had sufficiently viewed, and looked about, Mercury would needs know of him what he had observed. He told him that he saw a vast multitude and a promiscuous, their habitations like molehills, the men as emmets, "he could discern cities like so many hives of bees, wherein every bee had a sting, and they did naught else but sting one another, some domineering like hornets bigger than the rest, some like filching wasps, others as drones." Over their heads were hovering a confused company of perturbations, hope, fear, anger, avarice, ignorance, etc., and a multitude of diseases hanging, which they still pulled on their pates. Some were brawling, some fighting, riding, running, *sollicite ambientes, callide litigantes* [earnestly suing or cunningly disputing], for toys and trifles, and such momentany things; their towns and provinces mere factions, rich against poor, poor against rich, nobles against artificers, they against nobles, and so the rest. In conclusion, he condemned them all for madmen, fools, idiots, asses, *O stulti, quænam hæc est amentia?* O fools, O madmen! he exclaims, *insana studia, insani labores*, etc., mad endeavours, mad actions, mad, mad, mad, *O seclum insipiens et infacetum*,[4] a giddy-headed age. Heraclitus the philosopher, out of a serious meditation of men's lives, fell a-weeping, and with continual tears bewailed their misery, madness, and folly. Democritus, on the other side, burst out a-laughing, their whole life seemed to him so ridiculous, and he was so far carried with this ironical passion, that the citizens of Abdera took him to be mad, and sent therefore ambassadors to Hippocrates the physician, that he would exercise his skill upon him. But the story is set down at large by Hippocrates, in his Epistle to Damagetus, which, because it is not impertinent to this discourse, I will insert verbatim almost as it is delivered by Hippocrates himself, with all the circumstances belonging unto it.

When Hippocrates was now come to Abdera, the people of the city came flocking about him, some weeping, some entreating of him that he would do his best. After some little repast, he went to see Democritus, the people following him, whom he found (as before) in his garden in the suburbs all alone, "sitting upon a stone under a plane tree, without hose or shoes, with a book on his knees, cutting up several beasts, and busy at his study." [1] The multitude stood gazing round about to see the congress. Hippocrates, after a little pause, saluted him by his name, whom he resaluted, ashamed almost that he could not call him likewise by his, or that he had forgot it. Hippocrates demanded of him what he was doing: he told him that he was "busy in cutting up several beasts, to find out the cause of madness and melancholy." [2] Hippocrates commended his work, admiring his happiness and leisure. "And why," quoth Democritus, "have not you that leisure?" "Because," replied Hippocrates, "domestical affairs hinder, necessary to be done for ourselves, neighbours, friends; expenses, diseases, frailties and mortalities which happen; wife, children, servants, and such businesses which deprive us of our time." At this speech Democritus profusely laughed (his friends and the people standing by, weeping in the meantime, and lamenting his madness). Hippocrates asked the reason why he laughed. He told him, "At the vanities and the fopperies of the time, to see men so empty of all virtuous actions, to hunt so far after gold, having no end of ambition; to take such infinite pains for a little glory, and to be favoured of men; to make such deep mines into the earth for gold, and many times to find nothing, with loss of their lives and fortunes. Some to love dogs, others horses, some to desire to be obeyed in many provinces, and yet themselves will know no obedience.[3] Some to love their wives dearly at first, and after a while to forsake and hate them; [4] begetting children, with much care and cost for their education, yet when they grow to man's estate, to despise, neglect, and leave them naked to the world's mercy.[5] Do not these behaviours express their intolerable folly? [6] When men live in peace, they covet war, detesting quietness, deposing kings, and advancing others in their stead,[7] murdering some men to beget children of their wives. How many strange humours are in men! When they are poor and needy, they seek riches, and when they have them, they do not enjoy them, but hide them underground, or else wastefully spend them. O wise Hippocrates, I laugh at such things being done, but much more when no good comes of them, and when they are done to so ill purpose. There is no truth or justice found amongst them, for they daily plead one against another, the son against the father and the mother, brother against brother, kindred and friends of the same quality;[1] and all this for riches, whereof after death they cannot be possessors. And yet, notwithstanding, they will defame and kill one another, commit all unlawful actions, contemning God and men, friends and country. They make great account of many senseless things, esteeming them as a great part of their treasure, statues, pictures, and such-like movables, dear-bought, and so cunningly wrought, as nothing but speech wanteth in them,[2] and yet they hate living persons speaking to them.[3] Others affect difficult things; if they dwell on firm land they will remove to an island, and thence to land again, being no way constant to their desires. They commend courage and strength in wars, and let themselves be conquered by lust and avarice; they are, in brief, as disordered in their minds as Thersites was in his body. And now, methinks, O most worthy Hippocrates, you should not reprehend my laughing, perceiving so many fooleries in men; for no man will mock his own folly, but that which he seeth in a second, and so they justly mock one another.[4] The drunkard calls him a glutton whom he knows to be sober. Many men love the sea, others husbandry; briefly, they cannot agree in their own trades and professions, much less in their lives and actions."

When Hippocrates heard these words so readily uttered, without premeditation, to declare the world's vanity, full of ridiculous contrariety, he made answer, "That necessity compelled men to many such actions, and divers wills ensuing from divine permission, that we might not be idle, being nothing is so odious to them as sloth and negligence. Besides, men cannot foresee future events, in this uncertainty of human affairs; they would not so marry, if they could foretell the causes of their dislike and separation; or parents, if they knew the hour of their children's death, so tenderly provide for them; or an husbandman sow, if he thought there would be no increase; or a merchant adventure to sea, if he foresaw shipwreck; or be a magistrate, if presently to be deposed. Alas, worthy Democritus, every man hopes the best, and to that end he doth it, and therefore no such cause, or ridiculous occasion, of laughter."

Democritus, hearing this poor excuse, laughed again aloud,

perceiving he wholly mistook him, and did not well understand what he had said concerning perturbations and tranquillity of the mind. "Insomuch that, if men would govern their actions by discretion and providence, they would not declare themselves fools as now they do, and he should have no cause of laughter; but" (quoth he) "they swell in this life as if they were immortal, and demi-gods, for want of understanding. It were enough to make them wise, if they would but consider the mutability of this world, and how it wheels about, nothing being firm and sure. He that is now above, to-morrow is beneath; he that sate on this side to-day, to-morrow is hurled on the other; and not considering these matters, they fall into many inconveniences and troubles, coveting things of no profit and thirsting after them, tumbling headlong into many calamities. So that if men would attempt no more than what they can bear, they should lead contented lives and, learning to know themselves, would limit their ambition;[1] they would perceive then that nature hath enough without seeking such superfluities and unprofitable things, which bring nothing with them but grief and molestation. As a fat body is more subject to diseases, so are rich men to absurdities and fooleries, to many casualties and cross inconveniences. There are many that take no heed what happeneth to others by bad conversation, and therefore overthrow themselves in the same manner through their own fault, not foreseeing dangers manifest. These are things (O more than mad," quoth he) "that give me matter of laughter, by suffering the pains of your impieties, as your avarice, envy, malice, enormous villainies, mutinies, unsatiable desires, conspiracies, and other incurable vices; besides your dissimulation and hypocrisy,[2] bearing deadly hatred one to the other, and yet shadowing it with a good face, flying out into all filthy lusts, and transgressions of all laws, both of nature and civility. Many things which they have left off, after a while they fall to again, husbandry, navigation; and leave again, fickle and unconstant as they are. When they are young, they would be old; and old, young. Princes commend a private life,[3] private men itch after honour; a magistrate commends a quiet life, a quiet man would be in his office, and obeyed as he is: and what is the cause of all this, but that they know not themselves? Some delight to destroy, one to build, another to spoil one country to enrich another and himself.[4] In all these things they are like children,[5] in whom is no judgment or counsel, and resemble beasts, saving that beasts are better than

they, as being contented with nature. When shall you see a
lion hide gold in the ground, or a bull contend for better
pasture? [1] When a boar is thirsty, he drinks what will serve
him, and no more; and when his belly is full, ceaseth to eat:
but men are immoderate in both; as in lust, they covet carnal
copulation at set times, men always, ruinating thereby the
health of their bodies. And doth it not deserve laughter to see
an amorous fool torment himself for a wench; weep, howl for a
misshapen slut, a dowdy sometimes, that might have his choice
of the finest beauties? Is there any remedy for this in physic?
I do anatomize and cut up these poor beasts,[2] to see these
distempers, vanities, and follies, yet such proof were better made
on man's body, if my kind nature would endure it: who from
the hour of his birth is most miserable, weak, and sickly;[3] when
he sucks he is guided by others, when he is grown great prac-
tiseth unhappiness and is sturdy, and when old, a child again,
and repenteth him of his life past."[4] And here being interrupted
by one that brought books, he fell to it again, that all were
mad, careless, stupid. "To prove my former speeches, look into
courts, or private houses. Judges give judgment according to
their own advantage, doing manifest wrong to poor innocents
to please others.[5] Notaries alter sentences, and for money
lose their deeds. Some make false moneys; others counterfeit
false weights. Some abuse their parents, yea, corrupt their own
sisters; others make long libels and pasquils, defaming men of
good life, and extol such as are lewd and vicious. Some rob
one, some another; magistrates make laws against thieves, and
are the veriest thieves themselves.[6] Some kill themselves,
others despair, not obtaining their desires. Some dance, sing,
laugh, feast and banquet, whilst others sigh, languish, mourn
and lament, having neither meat, drink, nor clothes. Some
prank up their bodies, and have their minds full of execrable
vices.[7] Some trot about to bear false witness, and say anything for money;[8] and though judges know of it, yet for a
bribe they wink at it, and suffer false contracts to prevail
against equity. Women are all day a-dressing, to pleasure
other men abroad, and go like sluts at home, not caring to
please their own husbands whom they should. Seeing men
are so fickle, so sottish, so intemperate, why should not I laugh
at those to whom folly seems wisdom, will not be cured, and
perceive it not?"[9]

It grew late: Hippocrates left him; and no sooner was he
come away, but all the citizens came about flocking, to know

how he liked him. He told them in brief, that notwithstanding those small neglects of his attire, body, diet, the world had not a wiser, a more learned, a more honest man, and they were much deceived to say that he was mad.[1]

Thus Democritus esteemed of the world in his time, and this was the cause of his laughter: and good cause he had.

> *Olim jure quidem, nunc plus, Democrite, ride;*
> *Quin rides ? vita hæc nunc mage ridicula est.*[2]

> Democritus did well to laugh of old,
> Good cause he had, but now much more ;
> This life of ours is more ridiculous
> Than that of his, or long before.

Never so much cause of laughter as now, never so many fools and madmen. 'Tis not one Democritus will serve turn to laugh in these days; we have now need of a "Democritus to laugh at Democritus";[3] one jester to flout at another, one fool to fleer at another: a great stentorian Democritus, as big as that Rhodian Colossus. For now, as Sarisburiensis said in his time,[4] *totus mundus histrionem agit,* the whole world plays the fool; we have a new theatre, a new scene, a new Comedy of Errors, a new company of personate actors; *Volupiæ sacra* [the rites of the goddess of pleasure] (as Calcagninus willingly feigns in his Apologues) are celebrated all the world over, where all the actors were madmen and fools, and every hour changed habits, or took that which came next.[5] He that was a mariner to-day, is an apothecary to-morrow; a smith one while, a philosopher another, *in his Volupiæ ludis* [in these fêtes of the goddess of pleasure]; a king now with his crown, robes, sceptre, attendants, by and by drove a loaded ass before him like a carter, etc. If Democritus were alive now, he should see strange alterations, a new company of counterfeit vizards, whifflers, Cuman asses, maskers, mummers, painted puppets, outsides, fantastic shadows, gulls, monsters, giddy-heads, butterflies. And so many of them are indeed (if all be true that I have read [6]). For when Jupiter and Juno's wedding was solemnized of old, the gods were all invited to the feast, and many noble men besides. Amongst the rest came Chrysalus, a Persian prince, bravely attended, rich in golden attires, in gay robes, with a majestical presence, but otherwise an ass. The gods, seeing him come in such pomp and state, rose up to give him place, *ex habitu hominem metientes* [measuring the man by his garb]; but Jupiter, perceiving what he was, a light, fantastic, idle fellow, turned him and his proud followers into butterflies:[1] and so they continue still (for aught I know to the contrary) roving about in pied coats, and are called chrysalides by the wiser sort of men: that is, golden outsides, drones, flies, and things of no worth. Multitudes of such, etc.

Ubique invenies
Stultos avaros, sycophantas prodigos.
[You will find everywhere miserly fools and spendthrift sycophants.]

Many additions, much increase of madness, folly, vanity, should Democritus observe, were he now to travel, or could get leave of Pluto to come see fashions, as Charon did in Lucian, to visit our cities of Moronia Pia and Moronia Felix:[2] sure I think he would break the rim of his belly with laughing. *Si foret in terris rideret Democritus* [were Democritus alive, how would he laugh!], *seu,*[3] etc.

A satirical Roman in his time thought all vice, folly, and madness were all at full sea, *Omne in præcipiti vitium stetit*[4] [every vice was in headlong career].

Josephus the historian taxeth his countrymen Jews for bragging of their vices, publishing their follies, and that they did contend amongst themselves who should be most notorious in villainies;[5] but we flow higher in madness, far beyond them,

Mox daturi progeniem vitiosiorem,[6]

[And yet with crimes to us unknown,
Our sons shall mark the coming age their own,]

and the latter end (you know whose oracle it is) is like to be worst. 'Tis not to be denied, the world alters every day; *Ruunt urbes, regna transferuntur* [cities fall, kingdoms are transferred], etc., *variantur habitus, leges innovantur* [fashions change, laws are altered], as Petrarch observes,[7] we change language, habits, laws, customs, manners, but not vices, not diseases, not the symptoms of folly and madness, they are still the same. And as a river, we see, keeps the like name and place, but not water, and yet ever runs, *Labitur et labetur in omne volubilis ævum;*[8] our times and persons alter, vices are the same, and ever will be; look how nightingales sang of old, cocks crowed, kine lowed, sheep bleated, sparrows chirped, dogs barked, so they do still; we keep our madness still, play the fools still, *nec dum finitus Orestes* [and the play is not yet finished]; we are of the same humours and inclinations as our predecessors were; you shall find us all alike, much at one, we and our sons, *Et nati natorum, et qui nascuntur ab illis,* and so shall our posterity continue to the last. But to speak of times present.

If Democritus were alive now, and should but see the superstition of our age, our religious madness,[1] as Meteran calls it, *religiosam insaniam*,[2] so many professed Christians, yet so few imitators of Christ; so much talk of religion, so much science, so little conscience; so much knowledge, so many preachers, so little practice; such variety of sects, such have and hold of all sides, *obvia signis Signa* [3] [standards ranged against standards], etc., such absurd and ridiculous traditions and ceremonies; if he should meet a Capuchin,[4] a Franciscan, a pharisaical Jesuit, a man-serpent, a shave-crowned monk in his robes, a begging friar, or see their three-crowned Sovereign Lord the Pope, poor Peter's successor, *servus servorum Dei* [the servant of the servants of God], to depose kings with his foot, to tread on emperors' necks, make them stand barefoot and bare-legged at his gates, hold his bridle and stirrup, etc. (O that Peter and Paul were alive to see this!); if he should observe a prince creep so devoutly to kiss his toe,[5] and those red-cap cardinals, poor parish priests of old, now princes' companions; what would he say? *Cœlum ipsum petitur stultitia* [folly seeks entrance to heaven itself]. Had he met some of our devout pilgrims going barefoot to Jerusalem, our Lady of Loretto, Rome, St. Iago, St. Thomas' Shrine, to creep to those counterfeit and maggot-eaten relics; had he been present at a Mass, and seen such kissing of paxes, crucifixes, cringes, duckings, their several attires and ceremonies, pictures of saints, indulgences, pardons, vigils, fasting, feasts, crossing, knocking, kneeling at Ave-Maries, bells, with many such,[6] *jucunda rudi spectacula plebi* [fine spectacles to please the mob], praying in gibberish, and mumbling of beads. Had he heard an old woman say her prayers in Latin, their sprinkling of holy water, and going a procession:

Incedunt monachorum agmina mille;
Quid memorem vexilla, cruces, idolaque culta, etc.; [7]

[Monks in thousands marching along, with banners, crosses, images, and so forth;]

their breviaries, bulls, hallowed beans, exorcisms, pictures, curious crosses, fables and bables; had he read the Golden Legend, the Turks' Alcoran, or Jews' Talmud, the Rabbins' Comments, what would he have thought? How dost thou think he might have been affected? Had he more particularly

examined a Jesuit's life amongst the rest, he should have seen
an hypocrite profess poverty, and yet possess more goods
and lands than many princes, to have infinite treasures and
revenues;[1] teach others to fast, and play the gluttons themselves; like watermen, that row one way and look another. Vow
virginity, talk of holiness, and yet indeed a notorious bawd,
and famous fornicator, *lascivum pecus* [a wanton creature],
a very goat.[2] Monks by profession,[3] such as give over the
world, and the vanities of it, and yet a Machiavellian rout
interested in all matters of state:[4] holy men, peace-makers, and
yet composed of envy, lust, ambition, hatred, and malice; firebrands, *adulta patriæ pestis* [a full-grown scourge of their
country], traitors, assassinates, *hac itur ad astra* [in this way
heaven is won], and this is to supererogate, and merit heaven
for themselves and others. Had he seen, on the adverse side,
some of our nice and curious schismatics in another extreme
abhor all ceremonies, and rather lose their lives and livings
than do or admit anything papists have formerly used, though
in things indifferent (they alone are the true Church, *sal terræ,
cum sint omnium insulsissimi* [the salt of the earth, though
they are of all people the most insipid]); formalists, out of
fear and base flattery, like so many weather-cocks turn round,
a rout of temporizers, ready to embrace and maintain all that
is or shall be proposed in hope of preferment; another Epicurean
company, lying at lurch as so many vultures, watching for a
prey of Church goods, and ready to rise by the downfall of any:
as Lucian said in like case, what dost thou think Democritus
would have done, had he been spectator of these things?[5]
Or had he but observed the common people follow like so
many sheep one of their fellows drawn by the horns over a
gap, some for zeal, some for fear, *quo se cunque rapit tempestas*
[wherever they are whirled along], to credit all, examine
nothing, and yet ready to die before they will abjure any of
those ceremonies to which they have been accustomed; others
out of hypocrisy frequent sermons, knock their breasts, turn
up their eyes, pretend zeal, desire reformation, and yet professed usurers, gripers, monsters of men, harpies, devils in their
lives, to express nothing less.
What would he have said to see, hear, and read so many
bloody battles, so many thousands slain at once, such streams
of blood able to turn mills, *unius ob noxam furiasque* [through
the mad guilt of one person], or to make sport for princes, without any just cause, "for vain titles" (saith Austin), "precedency,

some wench, or such-like toy, or out of desire of domineering, vainglory, malice, revenge, folly, madness," [1] (goodly causes all, *ob quas universus orbis bellis et cædibus misceatur* [for plunging the whole world into an orgy of war and slaughter]), whilst statesmen themselves in the meantime are secure at home, pampered with all delights and pleasures, take their ease, and follow their lusts, not considering what intolerable misery poor soldiers endure, their often wounds, hunger, thirst, etc., the lamentable cares, torments, calamities, and oppressions that accompany such proceedings, they feel not, take no notice of it. "So wars are begun, by the persuasion of a few deboshed, hair-brain, poor, dissolute, hungry captains, parasitical fawners, unquiet Hotspurs, restless innovators, green heads, to satisfy one man's private spleen, lust, ambition, avarice, etc."; *tales rapiunt scelerata in prælia causæ* [such causes bring on war with all its crimes]. *Flos hominum* [the flower of mankind], proper men, well proportioned, carefully brought up, able both in body and mind, sound, led like so many beasts to the slaughter in the flower of their years, pride, and full strength, without all remorse and pity, sacrificed to Pluto, killed up as so many sheep, for devils' food, 40,000 at once.[2] At once, said I, that were tolerable, but these wars last always, and for ages; nothing so familiar as this hacking and hewing, massacres, murders, desolations; *ignoto cœlum clangore remugit* [the skies re-echo the unwonted noise], they care not what mischief they procure, so that they may enrich themselves for the present; they will so long blow the coals of contention, till all the world be consumed with fire. The siege of Troy lasted ten years, eight months; there died 870,000 Grecians, 670,000 Trojans at the taking of the city, and after were slain 276,000 men, women, and children of all sorts.[3] Cæsar killed a million, Mahomet the second Turk 300,000 persons;[4] Sicinius Dentatus fought in an hundred battles, eight times in single combat he overcame, had forty wounds before, was rewarded with 140 crowns, triumphed nine times for his good service. M. Sergius had 32 wounds; Scæva, the centurion, I know not how many; every nation had their Hectors, Scipios, Cæsars, and Alexanders. Our Edward the Fourth was in 26 battles afoot:[5] and as they do all, he glories in it, 'tis related to his honour. At the siege of Hierusalem, 1,100,000 died with sword and famine. At the battle of Cannæ, 70,000 men were slain, as Polybius records,[6] and as many at Battle Abbey with us; and 'tis no news to fight from sun to sun, as they did, as Constantine and Licinius, etc. At the siege of Ostend (the devil's academy), a poor town in respect, a small fort, but a great grave, 120,000 men lost their lives, besides whole towns, dorps, and hospitals, full of maimed soldiers; there were engines, fireworks, and whatsoever the devil could invent to do mischief with 2,500,000 iron bullets shot of 40 pound weight, three or four millions of gold consumed. "Who" (saith mine author) "can be sufficiently amazed at their flinty hearts, obstinacy, fury, blindness, who, without any likelihood of good success, hazard poor soldiers, and lead them without pity to the slaughter, which may justly be called the rage of furious beasts, that run without reason upon their own deaths?"[1] *quis malus genius, quæ furia, quæ pestis,* etc.,[2] what plague, what fury brought so devilish, so brutish a thing as war first into men's minds? Who made so soft and peaceable a creature, born to love, mercy, meekness, so to rave, rage like beasts, and run on to their own destruction? How may Nature expostulate with mankind, *Ego te divinum animal finxi*, etc., I made thee an harmless, quiet, a divine creature! how may God expostulate, and all good men! yet, *horum facta* (as one condoles[3]) *tantum admirantur, et heroum numero habent* [these alone are admired for their deeds and counted as heroes]: these are the brave spirits, the gallants of the world, these admired alone, triumph alone, have statues, crowns, pyramids, obelisks to their eternal fame, that immortal genius attends on them, *hac itur ad astra*. When Rhodes was besieged, *fossæ urbis cadaveribus repletæ sunt,*[4] the ditches were full of dead carcasses: and as when the said Solyman, Great Turk, beleaguered Vienna, they lay level with the top of the walls. This they make a sport of, and will do it to their friends and confederates, against oaths, vows, promises, by treachery or otherwise; *dolus an virtus? quis in hoste requirat?*[5] [guile or valour? against an enemy, 'tis all one], leagues and laws of arms (*silent leges inter arma*[6] [amid the clash of arms the law is mute]), for their advantage, *omnia jura, divina, humana, proculcata plerumque sunt*, God's and men's laws are trampled underfoot, the sword alone determines all; to satisfy their lust and spleen, they care not what they attempt, say, or do, *Rara fides probitasque viris qui castra sequuntur*[7] ['tis rare to find faith or honour among those who go to war]. Nothing so common as to have "father fight against the son, brother against brother, kinsman against kinsman, kingdom against kingdom, province against province, Christians against Christians":[8] *a quibus nec unquam cogitatione fuerunt læsi*, of whom they never had offence in thought, word, or deed. Infinite treasures consumed, towns burned, flourishing cities sacked and ruinated, *quodque animus meminisse horret* [and what the mind shudders to remember], goodly countries depopulated and left desolate, old inhabitants expelled, trade and traffic decayed, maids deflowered, *Virgines nondum thalamis jugatæ, Et comis nondum positis ephebi* [maidens not yet married and youths not yet come to man's estate]; chaste matrons cry out with Andromache, *Concubitum mox cogar pati ejus, qui interemit Hectorem*,[1] they shall be compelled peradventure to lie with them that erst killed their husbands: to see rich, poor, sick, sound, lords, servants, *eodem omnes incommodo macti*, consumed all or maimed, etc., *et quicquid gaudens scelere animus audet, et perversa mens* [and whatever a criminal mind and perverted disposition can prompt], saith Cyprian, and whatsoever torment, misery, mischief, hell itself, the devil, fury and rage can invent to their own ruin and destruction;[2] so abominable a thing is war, as Gerbelius concludes, *adeo fœda et abominanda res est bellum, ex quo hominum cædes, vastationes*,[3] etc., the scourge of God, cause, effect, fruit, and punishment of sin, and not *tonsura humani generis* [the mere pruning of the human race], as Tertullian calls it, but *ruina* [its destruction]. Had Democritus been present at the late civil wars in France, those abominable wars— *bellaque matribus detestata* [wars, of mothers loathed]—"where, in less than ten years, ten thousand men were consumed," saith Collignius, twenty thousand churches overthrown;[4] nay, the whole kingdom subverted (as Richard Dinoth adds[5]): so many myriads of the commons were butchered up, with sword, famine, war, *tanto odio utrinque ut barbari ad abhorrendam lanienam obstupescerent*, with such feral hatred, the world was amazed at it: or at our late Pharsalian fields, in the time of Henry the Sixth, between the Houses of Lancaster and York, an hundred thousand men slain, one writes;[6] another, ten thousand families were rooted out,[7] "that no man can but marvel," saith Comineus, "at that barbarous immanity, feral madness, committed betwixt men of the same nation, language, and religion." *Quis furor, O cives?*[8] "Why do the Gentiles so furiously rage?" saith the Prophet David (Ps. ii, 1). But we may ask, why do the Christians so furiously rage? *Arma volunt, quare poscunt, rapiuntque juventus?*[9] [Why do the youth call for war and rush to arms?] Unfit for Gentiles, much less for us so to tyrannize, as the Spaniards in the West Indies, that killed up in forty-two years (if we may believe Bartholomæus à Casa,[10] their own bishop) twelve millions of men, with stupend and exquisite torments; neither should I lie (said he) if I said fifty millions. I omit those French massacres, Sicilian Evensongs, the Duke of Alva's tyrannies,[1] our gunpowder machinations, and that fourth fury, as one calls it,[2] the Spanish Inquisition, which quite obscures those ten persecutions; *sævit toto Mars impius orbe*[3] [the ruthless rage of war spreads o'er the world]. Is not this *mundus furiosus*, a mad world, as he terms it,[4] *insanum bellum?* are not these madmen, as Scaliger concludes, *qui in prælio acerba morte, insaniæ suæ memoriam pro perpetuo teste relinquunt posteritati,*[5] which leave so frequent battles as perpetual memorials of their madness to all succeeding ages? Would this, think you, have enforced our Democritus to laughter, or rather made him turn his tune, alter his tone, and weep with Heraclitus,[6] or rather howl, roar, and tear his hair in commiseration, stand amazed;[7] or as the poets feign, that Niobe was for grief quite stupefied, and turned to a stone? I have not yet said the worst, that which is more absurd and mad, in their tumults, seditions, civil and unjust wars,[8] *quod stulte suscipitur, impie geritur, misere finitur*[9] [begun in folly, continued in crime, and ended in misery]. Such wars I mean; for all are not to be condemned, as those phantastical anabaptists vainly conceive. Our Christian tactics are all out as necessary as the Roman *acies*, or Grecian phalanx; to be a soldier is a most noble and honourable profession (as the world is), not to be spared, they are our best walls and bulwarks, and I do therefore acknowledge that of Tully to be most true,[10] "All our civil affairs, all our studies, all our pleading, industry, and commondation, lies under the protection of warlike virtues, and whensoever there is any suspicion of tumult, all our arts cease." Wars are most behoveful, and *bellatores agricolis civitati sunt utiliores* [fighting men are more useful to the State than husbandmen] as Tyrius defends:[11] and valour is much to be commended in a wise man; but they mistake most part, *auferre, trucidare, rapere, falsis nominibus virtutem vocant*, etc. ('twas Galgacus' observation in Tacitus), they term theft, murder, and rapine, virtue, by a wrong name; rapes, slaughters, massacres, etc., *jocus et ludus*, are pretty pastimes, as Ludovicus Vives notes. "They commonly call the most hair-brain bloodsuckers, strongest thieves, the most desperate villains, treacherous rogues, inhuman murderers, rash, cruel and dissolute caitiffs, courageous and generous spirits, heroical and worthy captains, brave men-at-arms,[12] valiant and renowned soldiers, possessed with a brute

persuasion of false honour," [1] as Pontus Heuter in his Burgundian
History complains. By means of which it comes to pass that
daily so many voluntaries offer themselves, leaving their sweet
wives, children, friends, for sixpence (if they can get it) a day,
prostitute their lives and limbs, desire to enter upon breaches,
lie sentinel, perdu, give the first onset, stand in the fore-front
of the battle, marching bravely on, with a cheerful noise of
drums and trumpets, such vigour and alacrity, so many banners
streaming in the air, glittering armours, motions of plumes,
woods of pikes and swords, variety of colours, cost and magnificence, as if they went in triumph, now victors to the Capitol,
and with such pomp as when Darius' army marched to meet
Alexander at Issus. Void of all fear, they run into imminent
dangers, cannon's mouth, etc., *ut vulneribus· suis ferrum hostium
hebetent* [to blunt the enemy's sword on their own flesh], saith
Barletius,[2] to get a name of valour, honour and applause, which
lasts not neither, for it is but a mere flash this fame, and like
a rose, *intra diem unum extinguitur*, 'tis gone in an instant. Of
fifteen thousand proletaries slain in a battle, scarce fifteen are
recorded in history, or one alone, the general perhaps, and after
a while his and their names are likewise blotted out, the whole
battle itself is forgotten. Those Grecian orators, *summa vi
ingenii et eloquentiæ* [with great genius and eloquence], set out
the renowned overthrows at Thermopylæ, Salamis, Marathon,
Mycale, Mantinea, Chæronæa, Platæa. The Romans record their
battle at Cannæ, and Pharsalian Fields, but they do but record,
and we scarce hear of them. And yet this supposed honour,
popular applause, desire of immortality by this means, pride
and vainglory spurs them on many times rashly and unadvisedly,
to make away themselves and multitudes of others. Alexander
was sorry because there were no more worlds for him to conquer; he is admired by some for it, *animosa vox videtur, et regia,*
'twas spoken like a prince; but as wise Seneca censures him,[3]
'twas *vox inquissima et stultissima,* 'twas spoken like a bedlam
fool; and that sentence which the same Seneca appropriates to
his father Philip and him, I apply to them all, *non minores
fuere pestes mortalium quam inundatio, quam conflagratio, quibus,*[4]
etc., they did as much mischief to mortal men as fire and water,
those merciless elements, when they rage. Which is yet more
to be lamented, they persuade them this hellish course of life
is holy, they promise heaven to such as venture their lives *bello
sacro* [in a sacred war], and that by these bloody wars, as
Persians,[5] Greeks, and Romans of old, as modern Turks do now

their commons, to encourage them to fight, *ut cadant infeliciter* [1]
[to die miserably (? *feliciter*, "happily")], "if they die in
the field, they go directly to heaven, and shall be canonized
for saints" (O diabolical invention!), put in the chronicles,
in perpetuam rei memoriam, to their eternal memory: whenas
in truth, as some hold, it were much better (since wars are the
scourge of God for sin, by which he punisheth mortal men's
peevishness and folly) such brutish stories were suppressed,
because *ad morum institutionem nihil habent*, they conduce not
at all to manners, or good life.[2]   But they will have it thus
nevertheless, and so they "put a note of divinity upon the most
cruel and pernicious plague of humankind,"[3] adore such men
with grand titles, degrees, statues, images, honour, applaud,
and highly reward them for their good service, no greater glory
than to die in the field.[4]   So Africanus is extolled by Ennius;
Mars, and Hercules,[5] and I know not how many besides of old,
were deified, went this way to heaven, that were indeed bloody
butchers, wicked destroyers, and troublers of the world, prodigious monsters, hell-hounds, feral plagues, devourers, common
executioners of humankind, as Lactantius truly proves, and
Cyprian to Donatus, such as were desperate in wars, and precipitately made away themselves (like those Celts in Damascene, with ridiculous valour, *ut dedecorosum putarent muro
ruenti se subducere*, [so that they thought it] a disgrace to
run away for a rotten wall, now ready to fall on their heads),
such as will not rush on a sword's point, or seek to shun a
cannon's shot, are base cowards, and no valiant men.   By
which means, *madet orbis mutuo sanguino*, the earth wallows
in her own blood, *sævit amor ferri et scelerati insania belli* [6]
[a mad lust for war with all its horrors is rampant], and for
that which, if it be done in private, a man shall be rigorously
executed, "and which is no less than murder itself; if the
same fact be done in public in wars, it is called manhood, and
the party is honoured for it." [7]   *Prosperum et felix scelus
virtus vocatur* [8] [vice, when successful, is called virtue].   We
measure all as Turks do, by the event, and most part, as
Cyprian notes, in all ages, countries, places, *sævitiæ magnitudo
impunitatem sceleris acquirit*, the foulness of the fact vindicates
the offender.   One is crowned for that for which another is tormented: *Ille crucem sceleris pretium tulit, hic diadema;* [9] made
a knight, a lord, an earl, a great duke (as Agrippa notes [10]) for
which another should have hung in gibbets, as a terror to
the rest:

et tamen alter,
Si fecisset idem, caderet sub judice morum.[1]

[Had another done the same, he would have been brought up
before the censor.]

A poor sheep-stealer is hanged for stealing of victuals, compelled
peradventure by necessity of that intolerable cold, hunger, and
thirst, to save himself from starving: but a great man in office
may securely rob whole provinces,[2] undo thousands, pill and
poll, oppress *ad libitum*, flay, grind, tyrannize, enrich himself by
spoils of the commons, be uncontrollable in his actions, and
after all, be recompensed with turgent titles, honoured for his
good service, and no man dare find fault, or mutter at it.[3]

How would our Democritus have been affected to see a wicked
caitiff, or "fool, a very idiot, a funge, a golden ass, a monster of
men, to have many good men, wise men, learned men to attend
upon him with all submission, as an appendix to his riches,[4]
for that respect alone, because he hath more wealth and money,
and to honour him with divine titles and bombast epithets,"
to smother him with fumes and eulogies, whom they know to be a
dizzard, a fool, a covetous wretch, a beast, etc., "because he is
rich"![5]   To see *sub exuviis leonis onagrum* [an ass in a lion's skin],
a filthy loathsome carcass, a Gorgon's head puffed up by parasites, assume this unto himself, glorious titles, in worth an
infant, a Cuman ass, a painted sepulchre, an Egyptian temple!
To see a withered face, a diseased, deformed, cankered complexion, a rotten carcass, a viperous mind and Epicurean soul
set out with orient pearls, jewels, diadems, perfumes, curious
elaborate works, as proud of his clothes as a child of his new
coats; and a goodly person, of an angelic divine countenance,
a saint, an humble mind, a meek spirit, clothed in rags, beg, and
now ready to be starved!   To see a silly contemptible sloven
in apparel, ragged in his coat, polite in speech, of a divine
spirit, wise; another neat in clothes, spruce, full of courtesy,
empty of grace, wit, talk nonsense!

To see so many lawyers, advocates, so many tribunals, so
little justice; so many magistrates, so little care of common
good; so many laws, yet never more disorders; *tribunal litium
segetem* [the court a crop of lawsuits], the tribunal a labyrinth, so many thousand suits in one court sometimes, so
violently followed!   To see *injustissimum sæpe juri præsiden-
tem, impium religioni, imperitissimum eruditioni, otiosissimum
labori, monstrosum humanitati* [the greatest wrongdoer often
administering justice, the most impious in charge of religion,

the most ignorant presiding over learning, the most idle over employment, and the most heartless over the distribution of charity]! To see a lamb executed, a wolf pronounce sentence,[1] *latro* [a robber] arraigned, and *fur* [a thief] sit on the bench, the judge severely punish others, and do worse himself, *eundem furtum facere et punire*,[2] *rapinam plectere, quum sit ipse raptor* [3] [the same man commit the theft and punish it, punish robbery and be himself a robber]! Laws altered, misconstrued, interpreted pro and con, as the judge is made by friends, bribed, or otherwise affected as a nose of wax, good to-day, none to-morrow;[4] or firm in his opinion, cast in his! Sentence prolonged, changed, *ad arbitrium judicis* [at the pleasure of the judge], still the same case, "one thrust out of his inheritance, another falsely put in by favour, false deeds or wills." [5] *Incisæ leges negliguntur*, laws are made and not kept; or if put in execution, they be some silly ones that are punished.[6] As put case it be fornication, the father will disinherit or abdicate his child, quite cashier him (Out, villain, begone, come no more in my sight); a poor man is miserably tormented with loss of his estate perhaps, goods, fortunes, good name, for ever disgraced, forsaken, and must do penance to the utmost; a mortal sin, and yet, make the worst of it, *Numquid aliud fecit*, saith Tranio in the poet,[7] *nisi quod faciunt summis nati generibus ?* he hath done no more than what gentlemen usually do. *Neque novum, neque mirum, neque secus quam alii solent* [8] ['tis neither new nor strange nor different from what others do]. For in a great person, right worshipful sir, a right honourable grandee, 'tis not a venial sin, no, not a peccadillo, 'tis no offence at all, a common and ordinary thing, no man takes notice of it; he justifies it in public, and peradventure brags of it,

> *Nam quod turpe bonis, Titio, Seioque, decebat Crispinum.*[9]
>
> [For what would be base in good men, Titius, and Seius, became Crispinus.]

Many poor men, younger brothers, etc., by reason of bad policy and idle education (for they are likely brought up in no calling), are compelled to beg or steal, and then hanged for theft;[10] than which what can be more ignominious? *non minus enim turpe principi multa supplicia, quam medico multa funera* [a prince is no less discredited by frequent sentences on his subjects than a doctor by frequent deaths among his patients], 'tis the governor's fault; *libentius verberant quam docent*, as

schoolmasters do, rather correct their pupils than teach them when
they do amiss. "They had more need provide there should be
no more thieves and beggars, as they ought with good policy,
and take away the occasions, than let them run on as they do
to their own destruction":[1] root out likewise those causes of
wrangling, a multitude of lawyers, and compose controversies,
lites lustrales et seculares [age-long lawsuits], by some more
compendious means. Whereas now for every toy and trifle
they go to law, *mugit litibus insanum forum, et sævit invicem
discordantium rabies*[2] [the courts are a bedlam, and the fury
of litigants knows no bounds], they are ready to pull out one
another's throats; and for commodity "to squeeze blood," saith
Hierome, "out of their brother's heart,"[3] defame, lie, disgrace,
backbite, rail, bear false witness, swear, forswear, fight and
wrangle, spend their goods, lives, fortunes, friends, undo one
another, to enrich an harpy advocate, that preys upon them
both, and cries *Eia Socrates! eia Xanthippe!*[4] or some corrupt
judge, that like the kite in Æsop, while the mouse and frog
fought, carried both away.[5] Generally they prey one upon
another as so many rávenous birds, brute beasts, devouring
fishes, no medium, *omnes hic aut captantur aut captant; aut
cadavera quæ lacerantur, aut corvi qui lacerant,*[6] either deceive
or be deceived; tear others or be torn in pieces themselves;
like so many buckets in a well, as one riseth another falleth,
one's empty, another's full; his ruin is a ladder to the third;
such are our ordinary proceedings. What's the market? A
place, according to Anacharsis, wherein they cozen one another,[7]
a trap; nay, what's the world itself? A vast chaos, a confusion
of manners, as fickle as the air, *domicilium insanorum* [a mad-
house], a turbulent troop full of impurities, a mart of walking
spirits, goblins, the theatre of hypocrisy, a shop of knavery,
flattery, a nursery of villainy, the scene of babbling, the school
of giddiness, the academy of vice;[8] a warfare, *ubi velis nolis
pugnandum, aut vincas aut succumbas* [where you have to fight
whether you will or no, and either conquer or go under], in
which kill or be killed; wherein every man is for himself, his
private ends, and stands upon his own guard. No charity,
love, friendship, fear of God, alliance, affinity, consanguinity,
Christianity, can contain them, but if they be anyways
offended, or that string of commodity be touched, they fall
foul.[9] Old friends become bitter enemies on a sudden for toys
and small offences, and they that erst were willing to do all
mutual offices of love and kindness, now revile and persecute

one another to death, with more than Vatinian hatred, and
will not be reconciled. So long as they are behoveful, they
love, or may bestead each other, but when there is no more
good to be expected, as they do by an old dog, hang him up
or cashier him: which Cato [1] counts a great indecorum, to use
men like old shoes or broken glasses, which are flung to the
dunghill; he could not find in his heart to sell an old ox, much
less to turn away an old servant: but they, instead of recompense,
revile him, and when they have made him an instrument of
their villainy, as Bajazet the Second, Emperor of the Turks, did
by Acomethes Bassa,[2] make him away, or instead of reward,
hate him to death, as Silius was served by Tiberius.[3]
In a word, every man for his own ends. Our *summum
bonum* is commodity, and the goddess we adore *Dea
Moneta*, Queen Money, to whom we daily offer sacrifice, which
steers our hearts, hands, affections, all:[4] that most powerful
goddess, by whom we are reared, depressed, elevated, esteemed
the sole commandress of our actions,[5] for which we pray, run,
ride, go, come, labour, and contend as fishes do for a crumb
that falleth into the water. It is not worth, virtue (that's
bonum theatrale [a theatrical good]), wisdom, valour, learning,
honesty, religion, or any sufficiency for which we are respected,
but money, greatness, office, honour, authority;[6] honesty is
accounted folly; knavery, policy; men admired out of opinion,[7]
not as they are, but as they seem to be: such shifting, lying,
cogging, plotting, counterplotting, temporizing, flattering,
cozening, dissembling, "that of necessity one must highly
offend God if he be conformable to the world," *Cretizare cum
Crete* [to do at Crete as the Cretans do], "or else live in contempt, disgrace, and misery." [8] One takes upon him temperance, holiness, another austerity, a third an affected kind of
simplicity, whenas indeed he, and he, and he, and the rest are
hypocrites, ambidexters,[9] outsides, so many turning pictures,
a lion on the one side, a lamb on the other.[10] How would
Democritus have been affected to see these things!

To see a man turn himself into all shapes like a chameleon, or
as Proteus, *omnia transformans sese in miracula rerum* [who
transformed himself into every possible shape], to act twenty
parts and persons at once for his advantage, to temporize and
vary like Mercury the planet, good with good, bad with bad;
having a several face, garb, and character for every one
he meets; of all religions, humours, inclinations; to fawn like
a spaniel, *mentitis et mimicis obsequiis* [with feigned and

hypocritical observance], rage like a lion, bark like a cur, fight like a dragon, sting like a serpent, as meek as a lamb, and yet again grin like a tiger, weep like a crocodile, insult over some, and yet others domineer over him, here command, there crouch, tyrannize in one place, be baffled in another, a wise man at home, a fool abroad to make others merry.

To see so much difference betwixt words and deeds, so many parasangs betwixt tongue and heart, men like stage-players act variety of parts, give good precepts to others, [to] soar aloft, whilst they themselves grovel on the ground.[1]

To see a man protest friendship, kiss his hand, *quem mallet truncatum videre*[2] [whom he would like to see decapitated], smile with an intent to do mischief, or cozen him whom he salutes,[3] magnify his friend unworthy with hyperbolical elogiums; his enemy, albeit a good man, to vilify and disgrace him, yea, all his actions, with the utmost livor and malice can invent.[4]

To see a servant able to buy out his master, him that carries the mace more worth than the magistrate,[5] which Plato, *lib.* 11 *de leg.*, absolutely forbids, Epictetus abhors. An horse that tills the land fed with chaff, an idle jade have provender in abundance;[6] him that makes shoes go barefoot himself, him that sells meat almost pined; a toiling drudge starve, a drone flourish.

To see men buy smoke for wares, castles built with fools' heads, men like apes follow the fashions in tires, gestures, actions: if the king laugh, all laugh:

> *Rides? majore cachinno*
> *Concutitur, flet si lacrimas conspexit amici.*[7]

[Should you smile, a heartier laughter shakes his sides; he sees you weep, and tears drop from his eyes.]

Alexander stooped, so did his courtiers;[8] Alphonsus turned his head, and so did his parasites. Sabina Poppæa, Nero's wife, wore amber-coloured hair, so did all the Roman ladies in an instant, her fashion was theirs.[9]

To see men wholly led by affection, admired and censured out of opinion without judgment: an inconsiderate multitude, like so many dogs in a village, if one bark, all bark without a cause: as fortune's fan turns, if a man be in favour, or commended by some great one, all the world applauds him; if in disgrace, in an instant all hate him,[10] and as at the sun when he is eclipsed, that erst took no notice, now gaze and stare upon him.

To see a man wear his brains in his belly,[1] his guts in his head, an hundred oaks on his back, to devour an hundred oxen at a meal, nay more, to devour houses and towns, or as those Anthropophagi, to eat one another.[2]

To see a man roll himself up like a snowball, from base beggary to right worshipful and right honourable titles, unjustly to screw himself into honours and offices; another to starve his genius, damn his soul to gather wealth, which he shall not enjoy, which his prodigal son melts and consumes in an instant.[3]

To see the κακοζηλίαν [unhappy rivalry] of our times, a man bend all his forces, means, time, fortunes, to be a favourite's favourite's favourite, etc., a parasite's parasite's parasite, that may scorn the servile world as having enough already.

To see an hirsute beggar's brat, that lately fed on scraps, crept and whined, crying to all, and for an old jerkin ran of errands, now ruffle in silk and satin, bravely mounted, jovial and polite, now scorn his old friends and familiars, neglect his kindred, insult over his betters, domineer over all.

To see a scholar crouch and creep to an illiterate peasant for a meal's meat; a scrivener better paid for an obligation, a falconer receive greater wages than a student: a lawyer get more in a day than a philosopher in a year, better reward for an hour than a scholar for a twelvemonth's study; him that can paint Thais, play on a fiddle, curl hair,[4] etc., sooner get preferment than a philologer or a poet.

To see a fond mother, like Æsop's ape, hug her child to death; a wittol wink at his wife's honesty, and too perspicuous in all other affairs;[5] one stumble at a straw, and leap over a block; rob Peter, and pay Paul; scrape unjust sums with one hand, purchase great manors by corruption, fraud and cozenage, and liberally to distribute to the poor with the other, give a remnant to pious uses, etc.; penny wise, pound foolish; blind men judge of colours; wise men silent, fools talk; find fault with others, and do worse themselves;[6] denounce that in public which he doth in secret;[7] and which Aurelius Victor gives out of Augustus, severely censure that in a third, of which he is most guilty himself.

To see a poor fellow, or an hired servant, venture his life for his new master that will scarce give him his wages at year's end; a country colone toil and moil, till and drudge for a prodigal idle drone, that devours all the gain, or lasciviously consumes with phantastical expenses; a nobleman in a bravado to encounter death, and for a small flash of honour to cast away

himself; a worldling tremble at an executor, and yet not fear
hell-fire; to wish and hope for immortality, desire to be happy,
and yet by all means avoid death, a necessary passage to bring
him to it.

To see a foolhardy fellow, like those old Danes *qui decollari
malunt quam verberari*, [who would] die rather than be punished,
in a sottish humour embrace death with alacrity, yet scorn to
lament his own sins and miseries, or his dearest friends'
departures.[1]

To see wise men degraded, fools preferred; one govern towns
and cities, and yet a silly woman overrules him at home; command a province, and yet his own servants or children prescribe
laws to him,[2] as Themistocles' son did in Greece; "What I will"
(said he) "my mother wills, and what my mother wills, my father
doth."[3] To see horses ride in a coach, men draw it; dogs devour
their masters; towers build masons; children rule; old men go
to school; women wear the breeches; sheep demolish towns,
devour men,[4] etc.; and in a word, the world turned upside
downward! *O viveret Democritus!* [would Democritus were
alive again!]

To insist in every particular were one of Hercules' labours,
there's so many ridiculous instances as motes in the sun.[5]
Quantum est in rebus inane! [How much vanity there is in
things!] And who can speak of all? *Crimine ab uno disce
omnes* [from one charge learn all], take this for a taste.

But these are obvious to sense, trivial and well known, easy
to be discerned. How would Democritus have been moved,
had he seen the secrets of their hearts![6] If every man had a
window in his breast, which Momus would have had in Vulcan's
man, or, that which Tully so much wished, it were written in
every man's forehead, *quid quisque de republica sentiret*, what
he thought; or that it could be effected in an instant, which
Mercury did by Charon in Lucian, by touching of his eyes, to
make him discern *semel et simul rumores et susurros* [forthwith
rumours and whispers],

> *Spes hominum cæcas, morbos, votumque labores,*
> *Et passim toto volitantes æthere curas:*

> Blind hopes and wishes, their thoughts and affairs,
> Whispers and rumours, and those flying cares;

that he could *cubiculorum obductas foras recludere et secreta
cordium penetrare* [unlock the doors of bedchambers and read
inmost thoughts], which Cyprian desired,[7] open doors and locks,

shoot bolts, as Lucian's Gallus did with a feather of his tail: or
Gyges' invisible ring, or some rare perspective glass, or otacousticon, which would so multiply *species* [appearances] that a man
might hear and see all at once (as Martianus Capella's Jupiter
did in a spear which he held in his hand, which did present
unto him all that was daily done upon the face of the earth),[1]
observe cuckolds' horns, forgeries of alchemists, the philosopher's
stone, new projectors, etc., and all those works of darkness,
foolish vows, hopes, fears, and wishes, what a deal of laughter
would it have afforded! He should have seen windmills in one
man's head, an hornet's nest in another. Or had he been
present with Icaromenippus in Lucian at Jupiter's whispering
place, and heard one pray for rain, another for fair weather;
one for his wife's, another for his father's death, etc., "to ask
that at God's hand which they are abashed any man should
hear," [2] how would he have been confounded! Would he,
think you, or any man else, say that these men were well in
their wits? *Hæc sani esse hominis quis sanus juret Orestes?*
Can all the hellebore in the Anticyræ cure these men? No,
sure, "an acre of hellebore will not do it." [3]

That which is more to be lamented, they are mad like Seneca's
blind woman, and will not acknowledge, or seek for any cure of
it,[4] for *pauci vident morbum suum, omnes amant* [few see their
own diseases, and all are attached to them]. If our leg or arm
offend us, we covet by all means possible to redress it; and if we
labour of a bodily disease, we send for a physician; [5] but for
the diseases of the mind, we take no notice of them.[6] Lust
harrows us on the one side; envy, anger, ambition on the other.
We are torn in pieces by our passions, as so many wild horses,
one in disposition, another in habit; one is melancholy, another
mad; and which of us all seeks for help, doth acknowledge his
error, or knows he is sick? [7] As that stupid fellow put out
the candle because the biting fleas should not find him, he
shrouds himself in an unknown habit, borrowed titles, because
nobody should discern him. Every man thinks with himself,
Egomet videor mihi sanus [I regard myself as sane], I am well,
I am wise, and laughs at others. And 'tis a general fault
amongst them all, that which our forefathers have approved,
diet, apparel, opinions, humours, customs, manners, we deride
and reject in our time as absurd. Old men account juniors
all fools,[8] when they are mere dizzards; and as to sailors
terræque urbesque recedunt, they move, the land stands still;
the world hath much more wit, they dote themselves. Turks

deride us, we them; Italians Frenchmen, accounting them
light-headed fellows; the French scoff again at Italians, and at
their several customs; Greeks have condemned all the world
but themselves of barbarism, the world as much vilifies them
now; we account Germans heavy, dull fellows, explode many
of their fashions; they as contemptibly think of us; Spaniards
laugh at all, and all again at them. So are we fools and
ridiculous, absurd in our actions, carriages, diet, apparel,
customs, and consultations; we scoff and point one at another,[1]
whenas in conclusion all are fools, "and they the veriest
asses that hide their ears most."[2]   A private man, if he be
resolved with himself, or set on an opinion, accounts all idiots
and asses that are not affected as he is, *nil rectum, nisi quod
placuit sibi, ducit*,[3] that are not so minded (*quodque volunt
homines se bene velle putant*[4] [men ever count their own desires
as right]), all fools that think not as he doth; he will not say
with Atticus, *Suam cuique sponsam, mihi meam*, let every man
enjoy his own spouse; but his alone is fair, *suus amor*, etc., and
scorns all in respect of himself, will imitate none, hear none
but himself,[5] as Pliny said, a law and example to himself.[6]
And that which Hippocrates, in his Epistle to Dionysius, reprehended of old, is verified in our times, *Quisque in alio superfluum
esse censet, ipse quod non habet nec curat*, that which he hath
not himself or doth not esteem, he accounts superfluity, an
idle quality, a mere foppery in another: like Æsop's fox, when
he had lost his tail, would have all his fellow foxes cut off theirs.
The Chinese say that we Europeans have one eye, they themselves two, all the world else is blind (though Scaliger accounts
them brutes too, *merum pecus* [mere cattle]);[7] so thou and thy
sectaries are only wise, others indifferent, the rest beside themselves, mere idiots and asses.   Thus, not acknowledging our
own errors and imperfections, we securely deride others, as if
we alone were free, and spectators of the rest, accounting it an
excellent thing, as indeed it is, *aliena optimum frui insania*,
to make ourselves merry with other men's obliquities, whenas
he himself is more faulty than the rest, *mutato nomine, de te
fabula narratur* [change but the name, the tale applies to you],
he may take himself by the nose for a fool; and which one calls
maximum stultitiæ specimen [a gross exhibition of folly], to be
ridiculous to others, and not to perceive or take notice of it, as
Marsyas was when he contended with Apollo, *non intelligens se
deridiculo haberi* [not perceiving that he was being made a
laughing-stock], saith Apuleius;[8] 'tis his own cause, he is a

convict madman, as Austin well infers, "In the eyes of wise
men and angels he seems like one that to our thinking walks
with his heels upward." [1] So thou laughest at me, and I at
thee, both at a third; and he returns that of the poet upon us
again, *Hei mihi, insanire me aiunt, quum ipsi ultro insaniant.*[2]
We accuse others of madness, of folly, and are the veriest
dizzards ourselves. For it is a great sign and property of a fool
(which Eccles. x, 3, points at) out of pride and self-conceit to
insult, vilify, condemn, censure, and call other men fools (*Non
videmus manticæ quod a tergo est* [we do not see what we have
on our backs]), to tax that in others of which we are most
faulty; teach that which we follow not ourselves: for an inconstant man to write of constancy, a profane liver prescribe
rules of sanctity and piety, a dizzard himself make a treatise of
wisdom, or with Sallust to rail downright at spoilers of countries,
and yet in office to be a most grievous poller himself.[3] This
argues weakness, and is an evident sign of such parties' indiscretion. *Peccat uter nostrum cruce dignius?*[4] [Which of us
deserves more to be crucified?] "Who is the fool now?" Or
else peradventure in some places we are all mad for company, and so 'tis not seen; *Societas erroris et dementiæ pariter
absurditatem et admirationem tollit* [folly and madness, when
widely diffused, cease to be either ridiculous or strange]. 'Tis
with us, as it was of old (in Tully's censure at least[5]) with C.
Fimbria in Rome, a bold, hair-brain, mad fellow, and so
esteemed of all, such only excepted that were as mad as
himself: now in such a case there is no notice taken of it.[6]

> *Nimirum insanus paucis videatur; eo quod*
> *Maxima pars hominum morbo jactatur eodem.*

> When all are mad, where all are like opprest,
> Who can discern one madman from the rest?

But put case they do perceive it, and someone be manifestly
convicted of madness, he now takes notice of his folly, be it in
action, gesture, speech,[7] a vain humour he hath in building,
bragging, jangling, spending, gaming, courting, scribbling,
prating, for which he is ridiculous to others, on which he dotes,
he doth acknowledge as much:[8] yet with all the rhetoric thou
hast, thou canst not so recall him, but to the contrary notwithstanding, he will persevere in his dotage. 'Tis *amabilis insania,
et mentis gratissimus error* [a lovable madness, a most pleasing
aberration], so pleasing, so delicious, that he cannot leave it:[9]
He knows his error, but will not seek to decline it; tell him

what the event will be, beggary, sorrow, sickness, disgrace,
shame, loss, madness, yet "an angry man will prefer vengeance,
a lascivious his whore, a thief his booty, a glutton his belly,
before his welfare." [1] Tell an epicure, a covetous man, an
ambitious man of his irregular course, wean him from it a little,
Pol me occidistis amici, he cries anon, you have undone him, and
as "a dog to his vomit," [2] he returns to it again; no persuasion
will take place, no counsel, say what thou canst,

> *Clames licet et mare cœlo*
> *Confundas,*
>
> [Though you shout enough to make the welkin ring,]

surdo narras [your words fall on deaf ears]; demonstrate as
Ulysses did to Elpenor and Gryllus, and the rest of his companions, "those swinish men," [3] he is irrefragable in his humour,
he will be a hog still; bray him in a mortar, he will be the same.
If he be in an heresy, or some perverse opinion, settled as some
of our ignorant papists are, convince his understanding, show
him the several follies and absurd fopperies of that sect, force
him to say, *veris vincor* [I bow to facts], make it as clear as the
sun, he will err still, peevish and obstinate as he is; [4] and as he
said, *si in hoc erro, libenter erro, nec hunc errorem auferri mihi
volo* [5] [if I am wrong in this, I am glad to be wrong, I do not
wish to be weaned from this error]; I will do as I have done,
as my predecessors have done, and as my friends now do: [6] I
will dote for company. Say now, are these men mad or no? [7]
Heus age, responde [8] [answer, I say], are they ridiculous? *cedo
quemvis arbitrum* [take any judge you please], are they *sanæ
mentis,* sober, wise, and discreet? have they common sense? *uter
est insanior horum?* [9] [which of these two is the madder?] I
am of Democritus' opinion for my part, I hold them worthy to be
laughed at; a company of brain-sick dizzards, as mad as Orestes
and Athamas, [10] that they may go "ride the ass," and all sail along
to the Anticyræ in the "ship of fools" for company together.
I need not much labour to prove this which I say otherwise than
thus, make any solemn protestation, or swear, I think you will
believe me without an oath; say at a word, are they fools? I
refer it to you, though you be likewise fools and madmen yourselves, and I as mad to ask the question; for what said our
comical Mercury?

> *Justum ab injustis petere insipientia est.* [11]
>
> ['Tis folly to expect justice from the unjust.]

I 'll stand to your censure yet, what think you?

But forasmuch as I undertook at first, that kingdoms, provinces, families, were melancholy as well as private men, I will examine them in particular, and that which I have hitherto dilated at random, in more general terms, I will particularly insist in, prove with more special and evident arguments, testimonies, illustrations, and that in brief. *Nunc accipe quare desipiant omnes æque ac tu* [1] [now hear why all are as mad as you]. My first argument is borrowed from Solomon, an arrow drawn out of his sententious quiver (Prov. iii, 7), "Be not wise in thine own eyes." And xxvi, 12, "Seest thou a man wise in his own conceit? more hope is of a fool than of him." Isaiah pronounceth a woe against such men (chap. v, 21), "that are wise in their own eyes, and prudent in their own sight." For hence we may gather that it is a great offence, and men are much deceived that think too well of themselves, an especial argument to convince them of folly. "Many men" (saith Seneca) "had been without question wise, had they not had an opinion that they had attained to perfection of knowledge already, even before they had gone half-way," [2] too forward, too ripe, *præproperi*, too quick and ready, *cito prudentes, cito pii, cito mariti, cito patres, cito sacerdotes, cito omnis officii capaces et curiosi* [3] [in a trice they are wise, they are pious, they are husbands, fathers, priests, qualified and ambitious for every station], they had too good a conceit of themselves, and that marred all; of their worth, valour, skill, art, learning, judgment, eloquence, their good parts; all their geese are swans, and that manifestly proves them to be no better than fools. In former times they had but seven wise men, now you can scarce find so many fools. Thales sent the golden tripos, which the fishermen found and the oracle commanded to be "given to the wisest," [4] to Bias, Bias to Solon, etc. If such a thing were now found, we should all fight for it, as the three goddesses did for the golden apple, we are so wise: we have women politicians, children metaphysicians; every silly fellow can square a circle, make perpetual motions, find the philosopher's stone, interpret *Apocalypsis*, make new theorics, a new system of the world, new logic, new philosophy, etc. *Nostra utique regio*, saith Petronius, "our country is so full of deified spirits, divine souls, that you may sooner find a god than a man amongst us," [5] we think so well of ourselves; and that is an ample testimony of much folly.

My second argument is grounded upon the like place of Scripture, which though before mentioned in effect, yet for some reasons is to be repeated (and by Plato's good leave, I

may do it, δὶς τὸ καλὸν ῥηθὲν οὐδὲν βλάπτει[1] [there is no harm
in saying a good thing twice]). "Fools" (saith David) "by reason
of their transgressions," etc. (Ps. cvii, 17). Hence Musculus
infers all transgressors must needs be fools. So we read (Rom. ii),
"Tribulation and anguish on the soul of every man that doeth
evil"; but all do evil. And Isaiah lxv, 14, "My servants shall
sing for joy, and ye[2] shall cry for sorrow of heart, and vexation
of mind." 'Tis ratified by the common consent of all philosophers.
"Dishonesty" (saith Cardan) "is nothing else but folly and madness." *Probus quis nobiscum vivit?*[3] Show me an honest man.
Nemo malus qui non stultus [there is no criminal who is not also
a fool], 'tis Fabius' aphorism to the same end. If none honest,
none wise, then all fools. And well may they be so accounted:
for who will account him otherwise, *qui iter adornat in occidentem,
quum properaret in orientem,* that goes backward all his life,
westward, when he is bound to the east? or hold him a wise
man (saith Musculus[4]) "that prefers momentany pleasures to
eternity, that spends his master's goods in his absence, forthwith to be condemned for it?" *Nequitquam sapit qui sibi non
sapit* [in vain is he wise who is not wise for himself]. Who will
say that a sick man is wise, that eats and drinks to overthrow
the temperature of his body? Can you account him wise or
discreet that would willingly have his health, and yet will do
nothing that should procure or continue it?   Theodoret, out of
Plotinus the Platonist, "holds it a ridiculous thing for a man
to live after his own laws, to do that which is offensive to God,
and yet to hope that He should save him: and when he voluntarily neglects his own safety, and contemns the means, to think
to be delivered by another."[5] Who will say these men are wise?
   A third argument may be derived from the precedent. All men
are carried away with passion, discontent, lust, pleasures, etc.,[6]
they generally hate those virtues they should love, and love
such vices they should hate. Therefore more than melancholy,
quite mad, brute beasts, and void of reason, so Chrysostom
contends; or rather dead and buried alive, as Philo Judæus
concludes it for a certainty,[7] of all such that are carried away
with passions, or labour of any disease of the mind. "Where is
fear and sorrow," there, Lactantius stiffly maintains, "wisdom
cannot dwell."[8]

*Qui cupiet, metuet quoque porro,
Qui metuens vivit, liber mihi non erit unquam.*

[Who hath desires must ever fearful be;
Who lives in fear cannot be counted free.]

Seneca and the rest of the Stoics are of opinion that, where is any the least perturbation, wisdom may not be found. "What more ridiculous," as Lactantius urges, "than to hear how Xerxes whipped the Hellespont, threatened the mountain Athos, and the like?" [1] To speak *ad rem*, who is free from passion? [2] *Mortalis nemo est quem non attingat dolor, morbusve* as Tully [3] determines out of an old poem, no mortal men can avoid sorrow and sickness, and sorrow is an inseparable companion from melancholy. Chrysostom pleads farther yet, that they are more than mad, very beasts, stupefied and void of common sense: "For how" (saith he) "shall I know thee to be a man, when thou kickest like an ass, neighest like a horse after women, ravest in lust like a bull, ravenest like a bear, stingest like a scorpion, rapest like a wolf, as subtle as a fox, as impudent as a dog? Shall I say thou art a man, that hast all the symptoms of a beast? How shall I know thee to be a man? By thy shape? That affrights me more, when I see a beast in likeness of a man." [4]

Seneca [5] calls that of Epicurus *magnificam vocem*, an heroical speech, "A fool still begins to live," and accounts it a filthy lightness in men, every day to lay new foundations of their life, but who doth otherwise? One travels, another builds; one for this, another for that business, and old folks are as far out as the rest; *O dementem senectutem!* [alas for the madness of old age!], Tully exclaims. Therefore young, old, middle age, all are stupid, and dote.

Æneas Sylvius, [6] amongst many other, sets down three special ways to find a fool by. He is a fool that seeks that he cannot find: he is a fool that seeks that which being found will do him more harm than good: he is a fool that, having variety of ways to bring him to his journey's end, takes that which is worst. If so, methinks most men are fools; examine their courses, and you shall soon perceive what dizzards and madmen the major part are.

Beroaldus will have drunkards, afternoon-men, and such as more than ordinarily delight in drink, to be mad. The first pot quencheth thirst, so Panyasis the poet determines in Athenæus; *secunda Gratiis, Horis et Dionyso*, the second makes merry; the third for pleasure; *quarta ad insaniam*, the fourth makes them mad. If this position be true, what a catalogue of madmen shall we have! what shall they be that drink four times four? *Nonne supra omnem furorem, supra omnem insaniam reddunt insanissimos?* [Does not drink render them insane beyond all fury and madness?] I am of his opinion, they are more than mad, much worse than mad.

The Abderites condemned Democritus for a madman, because
he was sometimes sad, and sometimes again profusely merry.[1]
Hac patria (saith Hippocrates) *ob risum furere et insanire dicunt,*
his countrymen hold him mad because he laughs; and therefore "he desires him to advise all his friends at Rhodes, that
they do not laugh too much, or be over-sad." [2]   Had those
Abderites been conversant with us, and but seen what fleering
and grinning there is in this age, they would certainly have
concluded, we had been all out of our wits.[3]

Aristotle in his Ethics holds *felix idemque sapiens,* to be wise
and happy are reciprocal terms, *bonus idemque sapiens honestus*
[the honourable man is both good and wise].   'Tis Tully's
paradox, "wise men are free, but fools are slaves," [4] liberty is
a power to live according to his own laws, as we will ourselves.
Who hath this liberty? who is free?

> *Sapiens sibique imperiosus,*
> *Quem neque pauperies, neque mors, neque vincula terrent,*
> *Responsare cupidinibus, contemnere honores*
> *Fortis, et in seipso totus teres atque rotundus.*[5]

> He is wise that can command his own will,
> Valiant and constant to himself still,
> Whom poverty nor death, nor bands can fright,
> Checks his desires, scorns honours,.just and right.

But where shall such a man be found?   If nowhere, then
e diametro, we are all slaves, senseless, or worse.   *Nemo malus
felix* [no wicked man is happy].   But no man is happy in
this life, none good, therefore no man wise.   *Rari quippe
boni*[6] [good men are few and far between].   For one virtue
you shall find ten vices in the same party; *pauci Promethei, multi
Epimethei* [there are few Prometheuses, many Epimetheuses].
We may peradventure usurp the name, or attribute it to others
for favour, as Carolus Sapiens, Philippus Bonus, Lodovicus
Pius,[7] etc., and describe the properties of a wise man, as Tully
doth an orator, Xenophon Cyrus, Castilio a courtier, Galen
temperament, an aristocracy is described by politicians.   But
where shall such a man be found?

> *Vir bonus et sapiens, qualem vix repperit unum*
> *Millibus e multis hominum consultus Apollo.*

> A wise, a good man in a million,
> Apollo consulted could scarce find one.

A man is a miracle of himself, but Trismegistus adds, *Maximum
miraculum homo sapiens,* a wise man is a wonder: *multi thyrsigeri,*

pauci Bacchi [many carry the thyrsus, but there are few Bacchuses].

Alexander when he was presented with that rich and costly casket of King Darius, and every man advised him what to put in it, he reserved it to keep Homer's works, as the most precious jewel of human wit, and yet Scaliger [1] upbraids Homer's Muse, *nutricem insanæ sapientiæ*, a nursery of madness, impudent as a court lady, that blushes at nothing.[2] Jacobus Mycillus, Gilbertus Cognatus, Erasmus, and almost all posterity admire Lucian's luxuriant wit, yet Scaliger rejects him in his censure, and calls him the Cerberus of the Muses. Socrates, whom all the world so much magnified, is by Lactantius and Theodoret condemned for a fool. Plutarch extols Seneca's wit beyond all the Greeks, *nulli secundus*, yet Seneca saith of himself, "When I would solace myself with a fool, I reflect upon myself, and there I have him." [3] Cardan, in his sixteenth book of Subtleties, reckons up twelve supereminent, acute philosophers, for worth, subtlety, and wisdom: Archimedes, Galen, Vitruvius, Archytas Tarentinus, Euclid, Geber, that first inventor of algebra, Alkindus the mathematician, both Arabians, with others. But his *triumviri terrarum* [great triumvirate] far beyond the rest, are Ptolemæus, Plotinus, Hippocrates. Scaliger, *Exercitat.* 224, scoffs at this censure of his, calls some of them carpenters and mechanicians, he makes Galen *fimbriam Hippocratis*, a skirt of Hippocrates; and the said Cardan [4] himself elsewhere condemns both Galen and Hippocrates for tediousness, obscurity, confusion. Paracelsus will have them both mere idiots, infants in physic and philosophy. Scaliger and Cardan admire Suisset the calculator, *qui pene modum excessit humani ingenii* [whose talents were almost superhuman], and yet Lod. Vives [5] calls them *nugas Suisseticas*: and Cardan, opposite to himself in another place, contemns those ancients in respect of times present, *majoresque nostros ad præsentes collatos juste pueros appellari* [6] [and says our forbears compared with the present generation might fairly be called boys]. In conclusion, the said Cardan [7] and Saint Bernard will admit none into this catalogue of wise men, but only prophets and apostles;[8] how they esteem themselves, you have heard before. We are worldly-wise, admire ourselves, and seek for applause: but hear Saint Bernard, *Quanto magis foras es sapiens, tanto magis intus stultus efficeris, etc., in omnibus es prudens, circa teipsum insipiens:* [9] the more wise thou art to others, the more fool to thyself. I may not deny but that there is some folly approved, a divine fury, a

I—D 886

holy madness, even a spiritual drunkenness in the saints of God themselves; *sanctam insaniam* Bernard calls it (though not as blaspheming Vorstius,[1] would infer it as a passion incident to God Himself, but) familiar to good men, as that of Paul (2 Cor.), "he was a fool," etc., and (Rom. ix) he wisheth himself "to be anathematized for them." Such is that drunkenness which Ficinus speaks of, when the soul is elevated and ravished with a divine taste of that heavenly nectar, which poets deciphered by the sacrifice of Dionysus; and in this sense, with the poet, *insanire lubet*, as Austin exhorts us, *ad ebrietatem se quisque paret*,[2] let's all be mad and drunk.[3] But we commonly mistake, and go beyond our commission, we reel to the opposite part, we are not capable [4] of it, and as he said [5] of the Greeks, *Vos Græci semper pueri* [you Greeks are all boys], *vos Britanni, Galli, Germani, Itali* [you British, French, Germans, Italians], etc., you are a company of fools.

Proceed now *a partibus ad totum*, or from the whole to parts, and you shall find no other issue; the parts shall be sufficiently dilated in this following Preface. The whole must needs follow by a sorites or induction. Every multitude is mad,[6] *bellua multorum capitum* [a many-headed beast], precipitate and rash without judgment, *stultum animal*, a roaring rout. Roger Bacon proves it out of Aristotle,[7] *Vulgus dividi in oppositum contra sapientes, quod vulgo videtur verum, falsum est:* that which the commonalty accounts true, is most part false, they are still opposite to wise men, but all the world is of this humour (*vulgus*), and thou thyself art *de vulgo*, one of the commonalty, and he, and he, and so are all the rest; and therefore, as Phocion concludes, to be approved in naught you say or do, mere idiots and asses. Begin then where you will, go backward or forward, choose out of the whole pack, wink and choose, you shall find them all alike, "never a barrel better herring." [8]

Copernicus, Atlas his successor, is of opinion the earth is a planet, moves and shines to others, as the moon doth to us. Digges, Gilbert, Keplerus, Origanus, and others, defend this hypothesis of his in sober sadness, and that the moon is inhabited: if it be so that the earth is a moon, then are we also giddy, vertiginous and lunatic within this sublunary maze.

I could produce such arguments till dark night: if you should hear the rest,

Ante diem clauso component vesper Olympo:

[The day would sooner than the tale be done:]

but, according to my promise, I will descend to particulars. This melancholy extends itself not to men only, but even to vegetals and sensibles. I speak not of those creatures which are saturnine, melancholy by nature, as lead and such-like minerals, or those plants, rue, cypress, etc., and hellebore itself, of which Agrippa treats,[1] fishes, birds, and beasts, hares, conies, dormice, etc., owls, bats, nightbirds, but that artificial, which is perceived in them all. Remove a plant, it will pine away, which is especially perceived in date trees, as you may read at large in Constantine's Husbandry, that antipathy betwixt the vine and the cabbage, wine and oil. Put a bird in a cage, he will die for sullenness, or a beast in a pen, or take his young ones or companions from him, and see what effect it will cause. But who perceives not these common passions of sensible creatures, fear, sorrow, etc.? Of all other, dogs are most subject to this malady, insomuch some hold they dream as men do, and through violence of melancholy run mad; I could relate many stories of dogs that have died for grief, and pined away for loss of their masters, but they are common in every author.[2]

Kingdoms, provinces, and politic bodies are likewise sensible and subject to this disease, as Boterus in his Politics hath proved at large.[3] "As in human bodies" (saith he) "there be divers alterations proceeding from humours, so there be many diseases in a commonwealth, which do as diversely happen from several distempers," as you may easily perceive by their particular symptoms. For where you shall see the people civil, obedient to God and princes, judicious, peaceable and quiet, rich, fortunate, and flourish,[4] to live in peace, in unity and concord, a country well tilled, many fair-built and populous cities, *ubi incolæ nitent*, [where,] as old Cato said,[5] the people are neat, polite and terse, *ubi bene beateque vivunt* [where they live well and happily], which our politicians make the chief end of a commonwealth; and which Aristotle, *Polit. lib. 3, cap. 4*, calls *commune bonum*[6] [the common weal], Polybius, *lib. 6, optabilem et selectum statum* [an enviable and ideal condition], that country is free from melancholy; as it was in Italy in the time of Augustus, now in China, now in many other flourishing kingdoms of Europe. But whereas you shall see many discontents, common grievances, complaints, poverty, barbarism, beggary, plagues, wars, rebellions, seditions, mutinies, contentions, idleness, riot, epicurism, the land lie untilled, waste, full of bogs, fens, deserts, etc., cities decayed, base and poor towns, villages depopulated, the people squalid, ugly, uncivil; that kingdom, that country, must needs be discontent, melancholy, hath a sick body, and had need to be reformed.

Now that cannot well be effected, till the causes of these maladies be first removed, which commonly proceed from their own default, or some accidental inconvenience: as to be sited in a bad clime, too far north, sterile, in a barren place, as the desert of Libya, deserts of Arabia, places void of waters, as those of Lop and Belgian in Asia, or in a bad air, as at Alexandretta, Bantam, Pisa, Durazzo, St. John de Ulloa, etc., or in danger of the sea's continual inundations, as in many places of the Low Countries and elsewhere, or near some bad neighbours, as Hungarians to Turks, Podolians to Tartars, or almost any bordering countries, they live in fear-still, and by reason of hostile incursions are oftentimes left desolate.   So are cities by reason of wars,[1] fires, plagues, inundations, wild beasts,[2] decay of trades, barred havens, the sea's violence, as Antwerp may witness of late, Syracuse of old, Brundusium in Italy, Rye and Dover with us, and many that at this day suspect the sea's fury and rage, and labour against it as the Venetians to their inestimable charge.   But the most frequent maladies are such as proceed from themselves, as first when religion and God's service is neglected, innovated or altered, where they do not fear God, obey their prince, where atheism, Epicurism, sacrilege, simony, etc., and all such impieties are freely committed, that country cannot prosper.   When Abraham came to Gerar, and saw a bad land, he said, sure the fear of God was not in that place.   Cyprian Echovius,[3] a Spanish chorographer, above all other cities of Spain, commends Barcino,[4] "in which there was no beggar, no man poor, etc., but all rich, and in good estate," and he gives the reason, "because they were more religious than their neighbours."   Why was Israel so often spoiled by their enemies, led into captivity, etc., but for their idolatry, neglect of God's word, for sacrilege, even for one Achan's fault?   And what shall we expect that have such multitudes of Achans, church robbers, simoniacal patrons, etc.? how can they hope to flourish, that neglect divine duties, that live most part like epicures?

Other common grievances are generally noxious to a body politic; alteration of laws and customs, breaking privileges, general oppressions, seditions, etc., observed by Aristotle,[5] Bodine, Boterus, Junius, Arnisæus, etc. I will only point at some of the chiefest.   *Impotentia gubernandi, ataxia,* confusion, ill government, which proceeds from unskilful, slothful, griping, covetous, unjust, rash, or tyrannizing magistrates, when they are fools, idiots, children, proud, wilful, partial, indiscreet, oppressors, giddy heads, tyrants, not able or unfit to manage such offices:[1] many noble cities and flourishing kingdoms by that means are desolate, the whole body groans under such heads,[2] and all the members must needs be disaffected, as at this day those goodly provinces in Asia Minor, etc., groan under the burden of a Turkish government; and those vast kingdoms of Muscovia, Russia, under a tyrannizing duke.[3] Who ever heard of more civil and rich populous countries than those of Greece, Asia Minor, "abounding with all wealth, multitudes of inhabitants, force, power, splendour, and magnificence?"[4] and that miracle of countries, the Holy Land, that in so small a compass of ground[5] could maintain so many towns, cities, produce so many fighting men? Egypt, another paradise, now barbarous and desert, and almost waste, by the despotical government of an imperious Turk, *intolerabili servitutis jugo premitur* [is subjected to an intolerable servitude] (one saith[6]); not only fire and water, goods or lands, *sed ipse spiritus ab insolentissimi victoris pendet nutu*, [but] such is their slavery, their lives and souls depend upon his insolent will and command: a tyrant that spoils all wheresoever he comes, insomuch that an historian complains, "If an old inhabitant should now see them, he would not know them, if a traveller, or stranger, it would grieve his heart to behold them."[7] Whereas Aristotle notes, *Novæ exactiones, nova onera imposita*,[8] new burdens and exactions daily come upon them, like those of which Zosimus, *lib. 2*, so grievous, *ut viri uxores, patres filios prostituerent ut exactoribus e quæstu*, etc., they must needs be discontent, *hinc civitatum gemitus et ploratus*, as Tully holds,[9] hence come those complaints and tears of cities, "poor, miserable, rebellious, and desperate subjects," as Hippolytus adds;[10] and as a judicious countryman of ours observed not long since, in a survey of that great Duchy of Tuscany,[11] the people lived much grieved and discontent, as appeared by their manifold and manifest complainings in that kind: "That the state was like a sick body which had lately taken physic, whose humours are not yet well settled, and weakened so much by purging, that nothing was left but melancholy."

Whereas the princes and potentates are immoderate in lust, hypocrites, epicures, of no religion, but in show: *Quid hypocrisi fragilius?* what so brittle and unsure? what sooner subverts their estates than wandering and raging lusts on their subjects' wives, daughters? to say no worse. That they should *facem præferre*, lead the way to all virtuous actions, are the ringleaders oftentimes of all mischief and dissolute courses, and by that means their countries are plagued, "and they themselves often ruined, banished, or murdered by conspiracy of their subjects,"[1] as Sardanapalus was, Dionysius Junior, Heliogabalus, Periander, Pisistratus, Tarquinius, Timocrates, Childericus, Appius Claudius, Andronicus, Galeacius Sforsia,[2] Alexander Medices, etc.

Whereas the princes or great men are malicious, envious, factious, ambitious, emulators, they tear a commonwealth asunder, as so many Guelfs and Ghibellines disturb the quietness of it, and with mutual murders let it bleed to death;[3] our histories are too full of such barbarous inhumanities, and the miseries that issue from them.

Whereas they be like so many horse-leeches, hungry, griping, corrupt, covetous,[4] *avaritiæ mancipia* [slaves of avarice], ravenous as wolves (for as Tully writes, *Qui præest prodest, et qui pecudibus præest, debet eorum utilitati inservire* [to rule is to serve; he who rules sheep must devote himself to their interests]), or such as prefer their private before the public good (for as he said [5] long since, *Res privatæ publicis semper officere* [private interest always interferes with public service]); or whereas they be illiterate, ignorant, empirics in policy, *ubi deest facultas, virtus* (Aristot. *Pol.* 5, *cap.* 8), *et scientia* [6] [deficient in talents, character, and knowledge], wise only by inheritance, and in authority by birthright, favour, or for their wealth and titles; there must needs be a fault, a great defect:[7] because, as an old philosopher affirms,[8] such men are not always fit: "Of an infinite number, few alone are senators, and of those few, fewer good, and of that small number of honest, good, and noble men, few that are learned, wise, discreet and sufficient, able to discharge such places"; it must needs turn to the confusion of a state.

For as the princes are, so are the people;[9] *Qualis rex, talis grex*: and which Antigonus right well said of old, *qui Macedoniæ regem erudit, omnes etiam subditos erudit*,[10] he that teacheth the King of Macedon, teacheth all his subjects, is a true saying still:

> For princes are the glass, the school, the book,
> Where subjects' eyes do learn, do read, do look.

> *Velocius et citius nos*
> *Corrumpunt vitiorum exempla domestica, magnis*
> *Cum subeant animos auctoribus.*

> [Domestic examples of vice corrupt us more swiftly
> and sooner, when in stirring our passions they
> are backed by the example of the great.]

Their examples are soonest followed, vices entertained; if they be profane, irreligious, lascivious, riotous, epicures, factious, covetous, ambitious, illiterate, so will the commons most part be idle, unthrifts, prone to lust, drunkards, and therefore poor and needy (ἡ πενία στάσιν ἐμποιεῖ καὶ κακουργίαν, for poverty begets sedition and villainy), upon all occasions ready to mutiny and rebel, discontent still, complaining, murmuring, grudging, apt to all outrages, thefts, treasons, murders, innovations, in debt, shifters, cozeners, outlaws, *profligatæ famæ ac vitæ* [of bad repute and dissolute life]. It was an old politician's aphorism, "They that are poor and bad envy rich, hate good men, abhor the present government, wish for a new, and would have all turned topsy-turvy." [1] When Catiline rebelled in Rome, he got a company of such debauched rogues together, they were his familiars and coadjutors, and such have been your rebels most part in all ages, Jack Cade, Tom Straw, Kett and his companions.

Where they be generally riotous and contentious, where there be many discords, many laws, many lawsuits, many lawyers, and many physicians, it is a manifest sign of a distempered, melancholy state, as Plato long since maintained: [2] for where such kind of men swarm, they will make more work for themselves, and that body politic diseased, which was otherwise sound. A general mischief in these our times, an insensible plague, and never so many of them: "which are now multiplied" (saith Mat. Geraldus, a lawyer himself) "as so many locusts, not the parents, but the plagues of the country, and for the most part a supercilious, bad, covetous, litigious generation of men, [3] *crumenimulga natio*, etc., a purse-milking nation, a clamorous company, gowned vultures, [4] *qui ex injuria vivunt et sanguine civium* [5] [who live by robbing and killing their fellow-citizens], thieves and seminaries of discord; worse than any pollers by the highway side, *auri accipitres, auri exterebronides, pecuniarum hamiolæ, quadruplatores, curiæ harpagones, fori tintinnabula, monstra hominum, mangones*, etc., that take upon them to make peace, but are indeed the very disturbers of our peace, a company of irreligious harpies, scraping, griping catchpoles (I mean our common hungry pettifoggers, *rabulas forenses*, love and honour in the meantime all good laws, and worthy lawyers, that are so many oracles and pilots of a well-governed commonwealth [6]), without art, without judgment, that do more harm, as Livy said, [7] *quam bella externa, fames, morbive*, than sickness, wars, hunger, diseases; "and cause a most incredible destruction of a commonwealth," saith Sesellius, [8] a famous civilian sometime in Paris.   As ivy doth by an oak, embrace it so long, until it hath got the heart out of it, so do they by such places they inhabit; no counsel at all, no justice, no speech to be had, *nisi eum premulseris* [unless you grease his palm], he must be fee'd still, or else he is as mute as a fish, better open an oyster without a knife.   *Experto crede* (saith Sarisburiensis [1]), *in manus eorum millies incidi, et Charon immitis qui nulli pepercit unquam, his longe clementior est:* "I speak out of experience, I have been a thousand times amongst them, and Charon himself is more gentle than they; he is contented with his single pay, but they multiply still, they are never satisfied"; [2] besides, they have *damnificas linguas,* as he terms it, *nisi funibus argenteis vincias* [ruinous tongues, unless you bind them with silver chains], they must be fee'd to say nothing, and get more to hold their peace than we can to say our best. [3]   They will speak their clients fair, and invite them to their tables, but, as he follows it, "of all injustice there is none so pernicious as that of theirs, which, when they deceive most, will seem to be honest men." [4] They take upon them to be peacemakers, *et fovere causas humilium* [to espouse the cause of the lowly], to help them to their right, *patrocinantur afflictis* [they champion the oppressed], but all is for their own good, *ut loculos pleniorum exhauriant* [5] [to drain the purses of the wealthy], they plead for poor men gratis, but they are but as a stale to catch others.   If there be no jar, they can make a jar, [6] out of the law itself find still some quirk or other, to set them at odds, and continue causes so long, *lustra aliquot* [for decades], I know not how many years before the cause is heard, and when 'tis judged and determined, by reason of some tricks and errors it is as fresh to begin, after twice seven years sometimes, as it was at first; and so they prolong time, delay suits, till they have enriched themselves and beggared their clients.   And, as Cato inveighed against Isocrates' scholars, [7] we may justly tax our wrangling lawyers, they do *consenescere in litibus* [grow old over a lawsuit], are so litigious and busy here on earth, that I think they will plead their clients' causes hereafter, some of them in hell.   Simlerus complains amongst the Switzers of the advocates in his time, that when they should make an end, they began controversies, and "protract their causes many years, persuading them their title is good, till their patrimonies be consumed, and that they have spent more in seeking than the thing is worth, or they shall get by the recovery." [8]   So that he that goes to law, as the proverb is, holds a wolf by the ears,[1] or as a sheep in a storm runs for shelter to a briar, if he prosecute his cause he is consumed, if he surcease his suit he loseth all;[2] what difference? They had wont heretofore, saith Austin, to end matters *per communes arbitros* [by arbitration]; and so in Switzerland (we are informed by Simlerus), "they had some common arbitrators or daysmen in every town, that made a friendly composition betwixt man and man, and he much wonders at their honest simplicity, that could keep peace so well, and end such great causes by that means."[3] At Fez in Africa, they have neither lawyers nor advocates; but if there be any controversies amongst them, both parties, plaintiff and defendant, come to their Alfakins or chief judge, "and at once, without any further appeals or pitiful delays, the cause is heard and ended."[4] Our forefathers, as a worthy chorographer of ours observes,[5] had wont *pauculis cruculis aureis*, with a few golden crosses, and lines in verse, [to] make all conveyances, assurances. And such was the candour and integrity of succeeding ages, that a deed (as I have oft seen) to convey a whole manor was *implicite* contained in some twenty lines or thereabouts; like that schede or *scytala Laconica*,[6] so much renowned of old in all contracts, which Tully so earnestly commends to Atticus,[7] Plutarch in his *Lysander*, Aristotle, *Polit.*, Thucydides, *lib.* 1, Diodorus[8] and Suidas approve and magnify for that laconic brevity in this kind; and well they might, for, according to Tertullian,[9] *certa sunt paucis*, there is much more certainty in fewer words. And so was it of old throughout: but now many skins of parchment will scarce serve turn; he that buys and sells a house must have a house full of writings, there be so many circumstances, so many words, such tautological repetitions of all particulars (to avoid cavillation, they say); but we find, by our woeful experience, that to subtle wits it is a cause of much more contention and variance, and scarce any conveyance so accurately penned by one, which another will not find a crack in, or cavil at; if any one word be misplaced, any little error, all is disannulled. That which is law to-day is none to-morrow; that which is sound in one man's opinion is most faulty to another; that, in conclusion, here is nothing amongst us but contention and confusion, we bandy one against another. And that which long since Plutarch complained of them in Asia,[10] may be verified in our times. "These men here assembled, come not to sacrifice to their gods, to offer Jupiter their first-fruits, or merriments to Bacchus; but a yearly disease exasperating Asia hath brought them hither, to make an end of their controversies and lawsuits." 'Tis *multitudo perdentium et pereuntium*, a destructive rout that seek one another's ruin. Such most part are our ordinary suitors, termers, clients; new stirs every day, mistakes, errors, cavils, and at this present, as I have heard, in some one court I know not how many thousand causes: no person free, no title almost good, with such bitterness in following, so many slights, procrastinations, delays, forgery, such cost (for infinite sums are inconsiderately spent), violence and malice, I know not by whose fault, lawyers, clients, laws, both or all: but as Paul reprehended the Corinthians long since,[1] I may more positively infer now: "There is a fault amongst you, and I speak it to your shame; Is there not a wise man amongst you, to judge between his brethren?[2] but that a brother goes to law with a brother." And Christ's counsel concerning lawsuits was never so fit to be inculcated as in this age: "Agree with thine adversary quickly,"[3] etc. (Matt. v, 25).

I could repeat many such particular grievances, which must disturb a body politic. To shut up all in brief, where good government is, prudent and wise princes, there all things thrive and prosper, peace and happiness is in that land: where it is otherwise, all things are ugly to behold, incult, barbarous, uncivil, a paradise is turned to a wilderness. This island amongst the rest, our next neighbours the French and Germans, may be a sufficient witness, that in a short time, by that prudent policy of the Romans, was brought from barbarism; see but what Cæsar reports of us, and Tacitus of those old Germans; they were once as uncivil as they in Virginia, yet by planting of colonies and good laws, they became, from barbarous outlaws, to be full of rich and populous cities, as now they are, and most flourishing kingdoms.[4]   Even so might Virginia, and those wild Irish, have been civilized long since, if that order had been heretofore taken, which now begins, of planting colonies, etc. I have read a discourse,[5] printed *anno* 1612, "discovering the true causes why Ireland was never entirely subdued, or brought under obedience to the Crown of England, until the beginning of his Majesty's happy reign." Yet if his reasons were thoroughly scanned by a judicious politician, I am afraid he would not altogether be approved, but that it would turn to the dishonour of our nation, to suffer it to lie so long waste. Yea, and if some travellers should see (to come nearer home) those rich United Provinces of Holland, Zealand, etc., over against us; those neat cities and populous towns, full of most industrious artificers, so much land recovered from the sea,[1] and so painfully preserved by those artificial inventions, so wonderfully approved, as that of Bemster in Holland, *ut nihil huic par aut simile invenias in toto orbe*, saith Bertius the geographer, all the world cannot match it, so many navigable channels from place to place, made by men's hands, etc.,[2] and on the other side so many thousand acres of our fens lie drowned, our cities thin, and those vile, poor, and ugly to behold in respect of theirs, our trades decayed, our still running rivers stopped, and that beneficial use of transportation wholly neglected, so many havens void of ships and towns, so many parks and forests for pleasure, barren heaths, so many villages depopulated, etc., I think sure he would find some fault.

I may not deny but that this nation of ours doth *bene audire apud exteros* [is highly reputed abroad], is a most noble, a most flourishing kingdom, by common consent of all geographers,[3] historians, politicians, 'tis *unica velut arx* [a peerless stronghold], and which Quintius in Livy said of the inhabitants of Peloponnesus may be well applied to us, we are *testudines testa sua inclusi*, like so many tortoises in our shells, safely defended by an angry sea, as a wall on all sides. Our island hath many such honourable elogiums; and as a learned countryman of ours right well hath it, "Ever since the Normans' first coming into England, this country, both for military matters and all other of civility, hath been paralleled with the most flourishing kingdoms of Europe and our Christian world," [4] a blessed, a rich country, and one of the Fortunate Isles: and for some things preferred before other countries,[5] for expert seamen, our laborious discoveries, art of navigation, true merchants, they carry the bell away from all other nations, even the Portugals and Hollanders themselves; "without all fear," saith Boterus, "furrowing the ocean winter and summer, and two of their captains, with no less valour than fortune, have sailed round about the world." [6] We have besides many particular blessings,[7] which our neighbours want, the Gospel truly preached, church discipline established, long peace and quietness, free from exactions, foreign fears, invasions, domestical seditions, well manured, fortified by art and nature, and now most happy in that fortunate union of England and Scotland,[8] which our forefathers have laboured to effect, and desired to see. But in which we excel all others, a wise, learned, religious king, another Numa, a second Augustus, a true Josiah; most worthy senators, a learned clergy, an obedient commonalty, etc. Yet amongst many roses some thistles grow, some bad weeds and enormities, which much disturb the peace of this body politic, eclipse the honour and glory of it, fit to be rooted out, and with all speed to be reformed.

The first is idleness, by reason of which we have many swarms of rogues and beggars, thieves, drunkards, and discontented persons (whom Lycurgus in Plutarch calls *morbos reipublicæ*, the boils of the commonwealth), many poor people in all our towns, *civitates ignobiles*, as Polydore [1] calls them, base-built cities, inglorious, poor, small, rare in sight, ruinous, and thin of inhabitants. Our land is fertile, we may not deny, full of all good things, and why doth it not then abound with cities, as well as Italy, France, Germany, the Low Countries? Because their policy hath been otherwise, and we are not so thrifty, circumspect, industrious. Idleness is the *malus genius* [evil genius] of our nation. For as Boterus [2] justly argues, fertility of a country is not enough, except art and industry be joined unto it. According to Aristotle, riches are either natural or artificial; natural are good land, fair mines, etc., artificial are manufactures, coins, etc. Many kingdoms are fertile, but thin of inhabitants, as that Duchy of Piedmont in Italy, which Leander Albertus so much magnifies for corn, wine, fruits, etc., yet nothing near so populous as those which are more barren. "England," saith he, "London only excepted, hath never a populous city, and yet a fruitful country." [3] I find 46 cities and walled towns in Alsatia, a small province in Germany, 50 castles, an infinite number of villages, no ground idle, no, not rocky places or tops of hills are untilled, as Munster informeth us. [4] In Greichgea, a small territory on the Necker, 24 Italian miles over, I read of 20 walled towns, innumerable villages, each one containing 150 houses most part, besides castles and noblemen's palaces. [5] I observe in Turinge [6] in Dutchland (twelve miles over by their scale) 12 counties, and in them 144 cities, 2000 villages 144 towns, 250 castles. [7] In Bavaria 34 cities, 46 towns, etc. [8] *Portugallia interamnis*, [9] a small plot of ground, hath 1460 parishes, [10] 130 monasteries, 200 bridges. Malta, a barren island, yields 20,000 inhabitants. But of all the rest, I admire Lues Guicciardine's relations of the Low Countries. Holland hath 26 cities, 400 great villages; Zealand, 10 cities, 102 parishes; Brabant, 26 cities, 102 parishes; Flanders, 28 cities, 90 towns, 1154 villages, besides abbeys, castles, etc. The Low Countries generally have three cities at least for one of ours, and those far more populous and rich: and what is the cause, but their industry and excellency in all manner of trades; their commerce, which is maintained by a multitude of tradesmen, so many excellent channels made by art, and opportune havens, to which they build their cities? all which we have in like measure, or at least may have. But their chiefest loadstone, which draws all manner of commerce and merchandise, which maintains their present estate, is not fertility of soil, but industry that enricheth them, the gold mines of Peru or Nova Hispania may not compare with them. They have neither gold nor silver of their own, wine nor oil, or scarce any corn growing in those United Provinces, little or no wood, tin, lead, iron, silk, wool, any stuff almost, or metal; and yet Hungary, Transylvania, that brag of their mines, fertile England, cannot compare with them. I dare boldly say, that neither France, Tarentum, Apulia, Lombardy, or any part of Italy, Valence in Spain, or that pleasant Andalusia, with their excellent fruits, wine and oil, two harvests, no, not any part of Europe, is so flourishing, so rich, so populous, so full of good ships, of well-built cities, so abounding with all things necessary for the use of man. 'Tis our Indies, an epitome of China, and all by reason of their industry, good policy, and commerce. Industry is a loadstone to draw all good things; that alone makes countries flourish, cities populous, and will enforce by reason of much manure, which necessarily follows, a barren soil to be fertile and good,[1] as sheep, saith Dion, mend a bad pasture.[2]

Tell me, politicians, why is that fruitful Palestina, noble Greece, Egypt, Asia Minor, so much decayed, and (mere carcasses now) fallen from that they were? The ground is the same, but the government is altered, the people are grown slothful, idle, their good husbandry, policy, and industry is decayed. *Non fatigata aut effeta humus,* as Columella well informs Sylvinus, *sed nostra fit inertia,* etc.[3] [the soil is not worked out or exhausted, but is barren only through our sloth]. May a man believe that which Aristotle in his Politics, Pausanias, Stephanus, Sophianus, Gerbelius relate of old Greece? I find heretofore seventy cities in Epirus overthrown by Paulus Æmilius, a goodly province in times past, now left desolate of good towns and almost inhabitants.[4] Sixty-two cities in Macedonia in Strabo's time. I find thirty in Laconia, but now scarce so many villages, saith Gerbelius. If any man from Mount Taygetus should view the country round about, and see *tot delicias, tot urbes per Peloponnesum dispersas,* so many delicate and brave-built cities, with such cost and exquisite cunning, so neatly set out in Peloponnesus, he should perceive them now ruinous and overthrown, burnt, waste, desolate, and laid level with the ground.[1] *Incredibile dictu* ['tis not to be believed], etc. And as he laments, *Quis talia fando Temperet a lacrimis? Quis tam durus aut ferreus* [Who, telling such a tale, can refrain from tears? Who is so stony-hearted, etc.], (so he prosecutes it). Who is he that can sufficiently condole and commiserate these ruins? Where are those 4000 cities of Egypt, those 100 cities in Crete? Are they now come to two? What saith Pliny and Ælian of old Italy? There were in former ages 1166 cities: Blondus and Machiaval both grant them now nothing near so populous and full of good towns as in the time of Augustus (for now Leander Albertus can find but 300 at most), and if we may give credit to Livy, not then so strong and puissant as of old: "They mustered seventy legions in former times, which now the known world will scarce yield." [2] Alexander built seventy cities in a short space for his part, our Sultans and Turks demolish twice as many, and leave all desolate. Many will not believe but that our island of Great Britain is now more populous than ever it was; yet let them read Bede, Leland, and others, they shall find it most flourished in the Saxon Heptarchy, and in the Conqueror's time was far better inhabited than at this present. See that Domesday Book, and show me those thousands of parishes which are now decayed, cities ruined, villages depopulated, etc. The lesser the territory is, commonly the richer it is. *Parvus sed bene cultus ager* [a small farm, but well tilled]. As those Athenian, Lacedæmonian, Arcadian, Elean, Sicyonian, Messenian, etc., commonwealths of Greece make ample proof, as those imperial cities and free states of Germany may witness, those cantons of Switzers, Rheti, Grisons, Walloons, territories of Tuscany, Luke and Senes [3] of old, Piedmont, Mantua, Venice in Italy, Ragusa, etc.

That prince, therefore, as Boterus adviseth,[4] that will have a rich country and fair cities, let him get good trades, privileges, painful inhabitants, artificers, and suffer no rude matter unwrought, as tin, iron, wool, lead, etc., to be transported out of his country—a thing in part seriously attempted amongst us, but not effected.[5] And because industry of men, and multitude of trade, so much avails to the ornament and enriching of a kingdom, those ancient Massilians would admit no man into their city that had not some trade.[6] Selim, the first Turkish emperor,[7] procured a thousand good artificers to be brought from Tauris to Constantinople. The Polanders indented with Henry, Duke of Anjou, their new-chosen king, to bring with him an hundred families of artificers into Poland. James the First in Scotland (as Buchanan writes[1]) sent for the best artificers he could get in Europe, and gave them great rewards to teach his subjects their several trades. Edward the Third, our most renowned king, to his eternal memory brought clothing first into this island, transporting some families of artificers from Gaunt hither. How many goodly cities could I reckon up, that thrive wholly by trade, where thousands of inhabitants live singular well by their fingers' ends! As Florence in Italy by making cloth of gold; great Milan by silk and all curious works; Arras in Artois by those fair hangings; many cities in Spain, many in France, Germany, have none other maintenance, especially those within the land. Mecca, in Arabia Petræa, stands in a most unfruitful country, that wants water, amongst the rocks (as Vertomannus describes it), and yet it is a most elegant and pleasant city, by reason of the traffic of the east and west.[2] Ormus in Persia is a most famous mart-town, hath naught else but the opportunity of the haven to make it flourish. Corinth, a noble city (*lumen Græciæ*, Tully calls it, the eye of Greece), by reason of Cenchreæ and Lechæum, those excellent ports, drew all that traffic of the Ionian and Ægean Seas to it; and yet the country about it was *curva et superciliosa*, as Strabo terms it,[3] rugged and harsh. We may say the same of Athens, Actium, Thebes, Sparta, and most of those towns in Greece. Nuremberg in Germany is sited in a most barren soil, yet a noble imperial city, by the sole industry of artificers and cunning trades; they draw the riches of most countries to them, so expert in manufactures, that, as Sallust long since gave out of the like, *sedem animæ in extremis digitis habent*, their soul, or *intellectus agens*, was placed in their fingers' ends; and so we may say of Basil, Spires, Cambrai, Frankfort, etc. It is almost incredible to speak what some write of Mexico and the cities adjoining to it, no place in the world at their first discovery more populous; [what] Mat. Riccius, the Jesuit,[4] and some others, relate of the industry of the Chinese, most populous countries, not a beggar or an idle person to be seen, and how by that means they prosper and flourish. We have the same means, able bodies, pliant wits, matter of all sorts, wool, flax, iron, tin, lead, wood, etc., many excellent subjects to work upon, only industry is wanting. We send our best commodities beyond the seas, which they make good use of to their necessities, set themselves a-work about, and severally improve, sending the same to us back at dear rates, or else make toys and baubles of the tails of them, which they sell to us again, at as great a reckoning as the whole. In most of our cities, some few excepted, like Spanish loiterers,[1] we live wholly by tippling-inns and ale-houses; malting are their best ploughs, their greatest traffic to sell ale. Meteran and some others object to us that we are no whit so industrious as the Hollanders: "Manual trades" (saith he) "which are more curious or troublesome, are wholly exercised by strangers: they dwell in a sea full of fish, but they are so idle, they will not catch so much as shall serve their own turns, but buy it of their neighbours."[2] Tush! *Mare liberum*[3] [the sea is free], they fish under our noses, and sell it to us when they have done, at their own prices.

Pudet hæc opprobria nobis
Et dici potuisse, et non potuisse refelli.

I am ashamed to hear this objected by strangers, and know not how to answer it.

Amongst our towns, there is only London that bears the face of a city,[4] *Epitome Britanniæ*,[5] a famous emporium, second to none beyond seas, a noble mart: but *sola crescit decrescentibus aliis* [it grows only at the expense of the rest]; and yet, in my slender judgment, defective in many things. The rest (some few excepted [6]) are in mean estate, ruinous most part, poor, and full of beggars, by reason of their decayed trades, neglected or bad policy, idleness of their inhabitants, riot, which had rather beg or loiter, and be ready to starve, than work.

I cannot deny but that something may be said in defence of our cities, that they are not so fair built (for the sole magnificence of this kingdom (concerning buildings) hath been of old in those Norman castles and religious houses), so rich, thick-sited, populous, as in some other countries;[7] besides the reasons Cardan gives, *Subtil. lib.* 9, we want wine and oil, their two harvests, we dwell in a colder air, and for that cause must a little more liberally feed of flesh,[8] as all northern countries do: our provisions will not therefore extend to the maintenance of so many; yet notwithstanding we have matter of all sorts, an open sea for traffic, as well as the rest, goodly havens. And how can we excuse our negligence, our riot, drunkenness, etc., and such enormities that follow it? We have excellent laws enacted, you will say, severe statutes, houses of correction, etc., to small purpose it seems; it is not houses will serve, but cities of correction; our trades generally ought to be reformed, wants supplied.[1] In other countries they have the same grievances, I confess, but that doth not excuse us, wants,[2] defects, enormities, idle drones, tumults, discords, contention, lawsuits, many laws made against them to repress those innumerable brawls and lawsuits, excess in apparel, diet, decay of tillage, depopulations, especially against rogues, beggars,[3] Egyptian vagabonds (so termed at least), which have swarmed all over Germany, France, Italy, Poland,[4] as you may read in Munster,[5] Cranzius, and Aventinus; as those Tartars and Arabians at this day do in the eastern countries: yet such has been the iniquity of all ages, as it seems to small purpose. *Nemo in nostra civitate mendicus esto* [let there be no beggars in our state], saith Plato: he will have them purged from a commonwealth,[6] "as a bad humour from the body," [7] that are like so many ulcers and boils, and must be cured before the melancholy body can be eased.

What Carolus Magnus, the Chinese, the Spaniards, the Duke of Saxony, and many other states, have decreed in this case, read Arnisæus, *cap.* 19; Boterus, *lib.* 8, *cap.* 2; Osorius, *De rebus gest. Eman. lib.* 11. When a country is overstocked with people, as a pasture is oft overlaid with cattle, they had wont in former times to disburden themselves by sending out colonies, or by wars, as those old Romans; or by employing them at home about some public buildings, as bridges, roadways, for which those Romans were famous in this island; as Augustus Cæsar did in Rome, the Spaniards in their Indian mines, as at Potosi in Peru, where some thirty thousand men are still at work, six thousand furnaces ever boiling, etc., aqueducts, bridges, havens, those stupend works of Trajan,[8] Claudius at Ostia,[9] Dioclesiani Thermæ,[10] Fucinus Lacus,[11] that Piræus in Athens, made by Themistocles, ampitheatrums of curious marble, as at Verona, Civitas Philippi and Heraclea in Thrace, those Appian and Flaminian Ways, prodigious works all may witness; and rather than they should be idle,[12] as those Egyptian Pharaohs, Mœris, and Sesostris did,[13] to task their subjects to build unnecessary pyramids, obelisks, labyrinths, channels, lakes, gigantic works all, to divert them from rebellion, riot, drunkenness, *quo scilicet alantur et ne vagando laborare desuescant* [14] [that they might support themselves and not become vagrants and idlers].

Another eyesore is that want of conduct and navigable rivers, a great blemish, as Boterus,[15] Hippolytus à Collibus,[16] and other politicians hold, if it be neglected in a commonwealth. Admirable cost and charge is bestowed in the Low Countries on this behalf, in the duchy of Milan, territory of Padua, in France,[1] Italy, China, and so likewise about corrivations of water to moisten and refresh barren grounds, to drain fens, bogs, and moors. Masinissa made many inward parts of Barbary and Numidia in Africa, before his time incult and horrid, fruitful and bartable by this means. Great industry is generally used all over the eastern countries in this kind, especially in Egypt, about Babylon and Damascus, as Vertomannus and Gotardus Arthus [2] relate; about Barcelona, Segovia, Murcia, and many other places of Spain, Milan in Italy; by reason of which their soil is much improved, and infinite commodities arise to the inhabitants.

The Turks of late attempted to cut that isthmus betwixt Africa and Asia, which Sesostris and Darius,[3] and some Pharaohs of Egypt, had formerly undertaken, but with ill success, as Diodorus Siculus records,[4] and Pliny, for that the Red Sea, being three cubits higher than Egypt,[5] would have drowned all the country, *cœpto destiterant*, they left off; yet as the same Diodorus writes,[6] Ptolemy renewed the work many years after, and absolved in it a more opportune place.

That Isthmus of Corinth was likewise undertaken to be made navigable by Demetrius, by Julius Cæsar, Nero, Domitian, Herodes Atticus, to make a speedy passage, and less dangerous, from the Ionian and Ægean Seas; [7] but because it could not be so well effected, the Peloponnesians built a wall like our Picts' Wall about Schœnus, where Neptune's temple stood, and in the shortest cut over the Isthmus, of which Diodorus, *lib*. II, Herodotus, *lib*. 8, *Uran*. Our latter writers call it Hexamilium, which Amurath the Turk demolished, the Venetians, *anno* 1453, repaired in fifteen days with thirty thousand men. Some, saith Acosta, would have a passage cut from Panama to Nombre de Dios in America. Thuanus and Serres, the French historians, speak of a famous aqueduct in France, intended in Henry the Fourth's time, from the Loire to the Seine, and from Rhodanus to Loire. The like to which was formerly assayed by Domitian the emperor, from Arar to Moselle, which Cornelius Tacitus speaks of in the thirteenth of his Annals, after by Charles the Great and others.[8] Much cost hath in former times been bestowed in either new making or mending channels of rivers, and their passages (as Aurelianus did by Tiber to make it navigable to Rome, to convey corn from

Egypt to the city, *vadum alvei tumentis effodit*, saith Vopiscus, *et Tiberis ripas extruxit* [he deepened the bed of the river, and banked up the sides], he cut fords, made banks, etc.), decayed havens, which Claudius the emperor, with infinite pains and charges, attempted at Ostia, as I have said, the Venetians at this day to preserve their city. Many excellent means to enrich their territories have been fostered, invented in most provinces of Europe, as planting some Indian plants amongst us, silkworms; the very mulberry leaves in the plains of Granada yield thirty thousand crowns per annum to the King of Spain's coffers, besides those many trades and artificers that are busied about them in the kingdom of Granada, Murcia, and all over Spain.[1] In France a great benefit is raised by salt, etc. Whether these things might not be as happily attempted with us, and with like success, it may be controverted, silkworms (I mean), vines, fir-trees, etc. Cardan exhorts Edward the Sixth to plant olives, and is fully persuaded they would prosper in this island. With us, navigable rivers are most part neglected; our streams are not great, I confess, by reason of the narrowness of the island, yet they run smoothly and even, not headlong, swift, or amongst rocks and shelves, as foaming Rhodanus and Loire in France, Tigris in Mesopotamia, violent Durius [2] in Spain, with cataracts and whirlpools, as the Rhine and Danubius, about Schaffhausen, Laufenburg, Linz, and Krems, to endanger navigators; or broad, shallow, as Neckar in the Palatinate, Tibris in Italy; but calm and fair as Arar in France, Hebrus in Macedonia, Eurotas in Laconia, they gently glide along, and might as well be repaired, many of them (I mean Wye, Trent, Ouse, Thamesis at Oxford, the defect of which we feel in the meantime) as the river of Lea from Ware to London. B[ishop] Atwater of old, or, as some will, Henry I, made a channel from Trent to Lincoln, navigable, which now, saith Mr. Camden, is decayed,[3] and much mention is made of anchors, and such-like monuments found about old Verulamium; [4] good ships have formerly come to Exeter, and many such places, whose channels, havens, ports, are now barred and rejected. We contemn this benefit of carriage by waters, and are therefore compelled in the inner parts of this island, because portage is so dear, to eat up our commodities ourselves, and live like so many boars in a sty, for want of vent and utterance.

We have many excellent havens, royal havens, Falmouth, Portsmouth, Milford, etc., equivalent, if not to be preferred, to that Indian Havana, old Brundusium in Italy, Aulis in Greece,

Ambracia in Acarnania, Suda in Crete, which have few ships in them, little or no traffic or trade, which have scarce a village on them, able to bear great cities, *sed viderint politici* [but this is a matter for our statesmen]. I could here justly tax many other neglects, abuses, errors, defects among us and in other countries, depopulations, riot, drunkenness, etc., and many such, *quæ nunc in aurem susurrare non libet* [which I would not now so much as whisper]. But I must take heed, *ne quid gravius dicam*, that I do not overshoot myself. *Sus Minervam* [the sow would teach Minerva], I am forth of my element, as you peradventure suppose; and sometimes *veritas odium parit* [truth makes enemies], as he said, "verjuice and oatmeal is good for a parrot." For as Lucian said of an historian, I say of a politician: he that will freely speak and write must be for ever no subject, under no prince or law, but lay out the matter truly as it is, not caring what any can, will, like or dislike.

We have good laws, I deny not, to rectify such enormities, and so in all other countries, but it seems not always to good purpose. We had need of some general visitor in our age, that should reform what is amiss; a just army of Rosy-cross men,[1] for they will amend all matters (they say), religion, policy, manners, with arts, sciences, etc.; another Attila, Tamerlane, Hercules, to strive with Achelous, *Augeæ stabulum purgare* [to cleanse the Augean stables], to subdue tyrants, as he did Diomedes and Busiris:[2] to expel thieves, as he did Cacus and Lacinius: to vindicate poor captives, as he did Hesione: to pass the torrid zone, the deserts of Libya, and purge the world of monsters and Centaurs: or another Theban Crates to reform our manners, to compose quarrels and controversies, as in his time he did, and was therefore adored for a god in Athens. "As Hercules purged the world of monsters, and subdued them, so did he fight against envy, lust, anger, avarice, etc., and all those feral vices and monsters of the mind."[3] It were to be wished we had some such visitor, or, if wishing would serve, one had such a ring or rings as Timolaus desired in Lucian,[4] by virtue of which he should be as strong as ten thousand men, or an army of giants, go invisible, open gates and castle doors, have what treasure he would, transport himself in an instant to what place he desired, alter affections, cure all manner of diseases, that he might range over the world, and reform all distressed states and persons, as he would himself. He might reduce those wandering Tartars in order, that infest China on the one side, Muscovy, Poland, on the other; and tame the vagabond Arabians that rob and spoil those eastern countries, that they should never use more caravans, or janizaries to conduct them. He might root out barbarism out of America, and fully discover *Terra Australis Incognita*,[1] find out the north-east and north-west passages, drain those mighty Mæotian fens, cut down those vast Hercynian woods, irrigate those barren Arabian deserts, etc., cure us of our epidemical diseases, *scorbutum, plica, morbus Neapolitanus*, etc., end all our idle controversies, cut off our tumultuous desires, inordinate lusts, root out atheism, impiety, heresy, schism, and superstition, which now so crucify the world, catechize gross ignorance, purge Italy of luxury and riot, Spain of superstition and jealousy, Germany of drunkenness, all our northern countries of gluttony and intemperance, castigate our hard-hearted parents, masters, tutors; lash disobedient children, negligent servants; correct these spendthrifts and prodigal sons, enforce idle persons to work, drive drunkards off the ale-house, repress thieves, visit corrupt and tyrannizing magistrates, etc. But as L. Licinius taxed Timolaus, you may us. These are vain, absurd, and ridiculous wishes not to be hoped: all must be as it is, Boccalinus may cite commonwealths to come before Apollo, and seek to reform the world itself by commissioners,[2] but there is no remedy, it may not be redressed, *desinent homines tum demum stultescere quando esse desinent* [men will cease to be fools only when they cease to be men], so long as they can wag their beards, they will play the knaves and fools.

Because, therefore, it is a thing so difficult, impossible, and far beyond Hercules' labours to be performed; let them be rude, stupid, ignorant, incult, *lapis super lapidem sedeat* [let stone sit on stone], and as the apologist will, *Resp. tussi et graveolentia laboret, mundus vitio*[3] [let the State cough and choke, the world be corrupt], let them be barbarous as they are, let them tyrannize, epicurize, oppress, luxuriate, consume themselves with factions, superstitions, lawsuits, wars, and contentions, live in riot, poverty, want, misery;[4] rebel, wallow as so many swine in their own dung, with Ulysses' companions, *stultos jubeo esse libenter* [I give them full permission to be fools]. I will yet, to satisfy and please myself, make an Utopia of mine own, a New Atlantis, a poetical commonwealth of mine own, in which I will freely domineer, build cities, make laws, statutes, as I list myself. And why may I not? *Pictoribus atque poetis*, etc.[5]—you know what liberty poets ever had, and besides, my predecessor Democritus was a politician, a recorder of Abdera,

a law-maker, as some say; and why may not I presume so much
as he did? Howsoever I will adventure. For the site, if you
will needs urge me to it, I am not fully resolved, it may be in
Terra Australis Incognita, there is room enough (for of my knowledge neither that hungry Spaniard,[1] nor Mercurius Britannicus,
have yet discovered half of it), or else one of these floating
islands in Mare del Zur,[2] which, like the Cyanean Isles in the
Euxine Sea, alter their place, and are accessible only at set
times, and to some few persons; or one of the Fortunate Isles,
for who knows yet where, or which they are? There is room
enough in the inner parts of America and northern coasts of
Asia.   But I will choose a site, whose latitude shall be forty-five
degrees (I respect not minutes) in the midst of the temperate
zone, or perhaps under the Equator, that paradise of the world,
ubi semper virens laurus [where the laurel is ever green], etc.,
where is a perpetual spring: [3] the longitude for some reasons
I will conceal.   Yet "be it known to all men by these presents,"
that if any honest gentleman will send in so much money as
Cardan allows an astrologer for casting a nativity, he shall be
a sharer, I will acquaint him with my project; or if any worthy
man will stand for any temporal or spiritual office or dignity
(for, as he said of his archbishopric of Utopia, 'tis *sanctus
ambitus* [a sacred ambition], and not amiss to be sought
after), it shall be freely given without all intercessions, bribes,
letters, etc., his own worth shall be the best spokesman; and
because we shall admit of no deputies or advowsons, if he be
sufficiently qualified, and as able as willing to execute the place
himself, he shall have present possession.   It shall be divided
into twelve or thirteen provinces, and those by hills, rivers,
roadways, or some more eminent limits exactly bounded.
Each province shall have a metropolis, which shall be so
placed as a centre almost in a circumference, and the rest
at equal distances, some twelve Italian miles asunder, or there-
about, and in them shall be sold all things necessary for the
use of man, *statis horis et diebus* [at stated hours and on stated
days]; no market towns, markets or fairs, for they do but
beggar cities (no village shall stand above six, seven, or eight
miles from a city); except those emporiums which are by the
seaside, general staples, marts, as Antwerp, Venice, Bergen of
old, London, etc.   Cities most part shall be situated upon
navigable rivers or lakes, creeks, havens; and for their form,
regular, round, square, or long square,[4] with fair, broad, and
straight streets,[5] houses uniform, built of brick and stone, like

Bruges, Brussels, Rhegium Lepidi, Berne in Switzerland, Milan, Mantua, Crema, Cambalu in Tartary, described by M. Polus, or that Venetian Palma. I will admit very few or no suburbs, and those of baser building, walls only to keep out man and horse, except it be in some frontier towns, or by the seaside, and those to be fortified after the latest manner of fortification,[1] and situated upon convenient havens, or opportune places. In every so built city, I will have convenient churches, and separate places to bury the dead in, not in churchyards; a *citadella* (in some, not all) to command it, prisons for offenders, opportune market-places of all sorts, for corn, meat, cattle, fuel, fish, commodious courts of justice, public halls for all societies, bourses, meeting-places, armouries,[2] in which shall be kept engines for quenching of fire, artillery gardens, public walks, theatres, and spacious fields allotted for all gymnics, sports, and honest recreations, hospitals of all kinds, for children, orphans, old folks, sick men, madmen, soldiers, pest-houses, etc., not built *precario* [as a favour], or by gouty benefactors, who, when by fraud and rapine they have extorted all their lives, oppressed whole provinces, societies, etc., give something to pious uses, build a satisfactory almshouse, school, or bridge, etc., at their last end, or before perhaps, which is no otherwise than to steal a goose and stick down a feather, rob a thousand to relieve ten; and those hospitals so built and maintained, not by collections, benevolences, donaries, for a set number (as in ours), just so many and no more at such a rate, but for all those who stand in need, be they more or less, and that *ex publico ærario* [at the public expense], and so still maintained; *non nobis solum nati sumus* [we are not born for ourselves alone], etc. I will have conduits of sweet and good water aptly disposed in each town, common granaries,[3] as at Dresden in Misnia, Stettin in Pomerland, Nuremberg, etc.; colleges of mathematicians, musicians, and actors, as of old at Lebedus in Ionia, alchemists,[4] physicians, artists, and philosophers, that all arts and sciences may sooner be perfected and better learned; and public historiographers, as amongst those ancient Persians, *qui in commentarios referebant quæ memorantu digna gerebantur*,[5] informed and appointed by the State to register all famous acts, and not by each insufficient scribbler, partial or parasitical pedant, as in our times. I will provide public schools of all kinds, singing, dancing, fencing, etc., especially of grammar and languages, not to be taught by those tedious precepts ordinarily used, but by use, example, conversation,[6] as travellers learn abroad, and nurses teach their children: as I will have all such places, so will I ordain public governors, fit officers to each place, treasurers, ædiles, quæstors, overseers of pupils, widows' goods, and all public houses, etc.,[1] and those once a year to make strict accounts of all receipts, expenses, to avoid confusion, *et sic fiet ut non absumant* (as Pliny to Trajan), *quod pudeat dicere* [and in this way there will be no squandering, if you will pardon my mentioning such a thing]. They shall be subordinate to those higher officers and governors of each city, which shall not be poor tradesmen and mean artificers, but noblemen and gentlemen, which shall be tied to residence in those towns they dwell next, at such set times and seasons: for I see no reason (which Hippolytus complains of[2]) "that it should be more dishonourable for noblemen to govern the city than the country, or unseemly to dwell there now than of old. I will have no bogs, fens, marshes, vast woods, deserts, heaths, commons, but all enclosed[3] (yet not depopulated, and therefore take heed you mistake me not); for that which is common, and every man's, is no man's; the richest countries are still enclosed, as Essex, Kent, with us, etc., Spain, Italy; and where enclosures are least in quantity, they are best husbanded, as about Florence in Italy, Damascus in Syria, etc., which are liker gardens than fields.[4] I will not have a barren acre in all my territories, not so much as the tops of mountains: where nature fails, it shall be supplied by art: lakes and rivers shall not be left desolate.[5] All common highways, bridges, banks, corrivations of waters, aqueducts, channels, public works, building, etc., out of a common stock,[6] curiously maintained and kept in repair; no depopulations, engrossings, alterations of wood, arable, but by the consent of some supervisors that shall be appointed for that purpose, to see what reformation ought to be had in all places, what is amiss, how to help it, *Et quid quæque ferat regio, et quid quæque recuset* [what each region will or will not produce], what ground is aptest for wood, what for corn, what for cattle, gardens, orchards, fishponds, etc., with a charitable division in every village (not one domineering house greedily to swallow up all, which is too common with us), what for lords, what for tenants;[7] and because they shall be better encouraged to improve such lands they hold, manure, plant trees, drain, fence, etc., they shall have long leases, a known rent, and known fine, to free them from those intolerable exactions of tyrannizing landlords. These supervisors shall likewise appoint what quantity of land in each manor is fit for the lord's demesnes, what for holding of tenants, how it ought to be husbanded—*Ut Magnetes equis, Minyæ gens cognita remis* [1] [as the Magnesians are famed for their horses, the Argonauts for oarsmanship]—how to be manured, tilled, rectified,

Hic segetes veniunt, illic felicius uvæ,
Arborei fœtus alibi, atque injussa virescunt
Gramina, [2]
[Here corn, and here the vine is better grown;
Here fruits abound and grasses spring unsown,]

and what proportion is fit for all callings, because private professors are many times idiots, ill husbands, oppressors, covetous, and know not how to improve their own, or else wholly respect their own, and not public good.

Utopian parity is a kind of government to be wished for rather than effected, *Respub. Christianopolitana,* [3] Campanella's City of the Sun, and that New Atlantis, [4] witty fictions, but mere chimeras, and Plato's community in many things is impious, absurd, and ridiculous, it takes away all splendour and magnificence. I will have several orders, degrees of nobility, and those hereditary, not rejecting younger brothers in the meantime, for they shall be sufficiently provided for by pensions, or so qualified, brought up in some honest calling, they shall be able to live of themselves. I will have such a proportion of ground belonging to every barony; he that buys the land shall buy the barony, he that by riot consumes his patrimony and ancient demesnes shall forfeit his honours. [5] As some dignities shall be hereditary, so some again by election, or by gift (besides free offices, pensions, annuities), like our bishoprics, prebends, the bassas' palaces in Turkey, the procurators' houses and offices in Venice, [6] which, like the golden apple, shall be given to the worthiest and best deserving both in war and peace, as a reward of their worth and good service, as so many goals for all to aim at (*honos alit artes* [honour is an encouragement to art]), and encouragement to others. For I hate these severe, unnatural, harsh, German, French, and Venetian decrees, which exclude plebeians from honours; be they never so wise, rich, virtuous, valiant, and well qualified, they must not be patricians, but keep their own rank; this is *naturæ bellum inferre* [to make war on nature], odious to God and men, I abhor it. My form of government shall be monarchical;

Nunquam libertas gratior extat,
Quam sub rege pio, etc. [7]
[Liberty is ne'er more sweet than when vouchsafed by a
virtuous prince.]

Few laws, but those severely kept, plainly put down, and in the mother tongue, that every man may understand. Every city shall have a peculiar trade or privilege, by which it shall be chiefly maintained: and parents shall teach their children, one of three at least, bring up and instruct them in the mysteries of their own trade.[1] In each town these several tradesmen shall be so aptly disposed, as they shall free the rest from danger or offence: fire-trades, as smiths, forge-men, brewers, bakers, metal-men, etc., shall dwell apart by themselves: dyers, tanners, fellmongers, and such as use water, in convenient places by themselves: noisome or fulsome for bad smells, as butchers' slaughterhouses, chandlers, curriers, in remote places and some back lanes. Fraternities and companies I approve of, as merchants' bourses, colleges of druggers, physicians, musicians, etc., but all trades to be rated in the sale of wares, as our clerks of the market do bakers and brewers; corn itself, what scarcity soever shall come, not to exceed such a price. Of such wares as are transported or brought in, if they be necessary, commodious, and such as nearly concern man's life, as corn, wood, coal, etc.,[2] and such provision we cannot want, I will have little or no custom paid, no taxes; but for such things as are for pleasure, delight, or ornament, as wine, spice, tobacco, silk, velvet, cloth of gold, lace, jewels, etc., a greater impost. I will have certain ships sent out for new discoveries every year, and some discreet men appointed to travel into all neighbour kingdoms by land,[3] which shall observe what artificial inventions and good laws are in other countries, customs, alterations, or aught else, concerning war or peace, which may tend to the common good. Ecclesiastical discipline, *penes episcopos* [in the hands of the bishops], subordinate as the other. No impropriations, no lay patrons of church livings, or one private man, but common societies, corporations, etc., and those rectors of benefices to be chosen out of the universities, examined and approved, as the *literati* in China. No parish to contain above a thousand auditors. If it were possible, I would have such priests as should imitate Christ, charitable lawyers should love their neighbours as themselves, temperate and modest physicians, politicians contemn the world, philosophers should know themselves, noblemen live honestly, tradesmen leave lying and cozening, magistrates corruption, etc.; but this is impossible, I must get such as I may. I will therefore have of lawyers, judges, advocates, physicians, chirurgeons, etc., a set number,[4] and every man, if it be possible.

to plead his own cause, to tell that tale to the judge which he
doth to his advocate,[1] as at Fez in Africa, Bantam, Aleppo,
Ragusa, *suam quisque causam dicere tenetur* [every one is expected to plead his own cause].   Those advocates, chirurgeons,
and physicians [2] which are allowed, to be maintained out of the
common treasure,[3] no fees to be given or taken upon pain of
losing their places; or if they do, very small fees, and when the
cause is fully ended.[4] He that sues any man shall put in a
pledge, which, if it be proved he hath wrongfully sued his adversary, rashly or maliciously, he shall forfeit and lose.[5]   Or else,
before any suit begin, the plaintiff shall have his complaint
approved by a set delegacy to that purpose; if it be of moment,
he shall be suffered as before to proceed, if otherwise, they shall
determine it.   All causes shall be pleaded *suppresso nomine*,
the parties' names concealed, if some circumstances do not
otherwise require.   Judges and other officers shall be aptly
disposed in each province, villages, cities, as common arbitrators
to hear causes and end all controversies, and those not single,
but three at least on the bench at once, to determine or give
sentence, and those again to sit by turns or lots, and not to
continue still in the same office.   No controversy to depend
above a year, but without all delays and further appeals to be
speedily dispatched, and finally concluded in that time allotted.
These and all other inferior magistrates to be chosen as the
literati in China,[6] or by those exact suffrages of the Venetians,[7]
and such again not to be eligible, or capable of magistracies,
honours, offices, except they be sufficiently qualified for learning,[8]
manners, and that by the strict approbation of deputed
examinators: first scholars to take place, then soldiers;[9] for I
am of Vegetius his opinion, a scholar deserves better than a
soldier, because *unius ætatis sunt quæ fortiter fiunt, quæ vero
pro utilitate reipub. scribuntur, æterna:* a soldier's work lasts
for an age, a scholar's for ever.   If they misbehave themselves,
they shall be deposed,[10] and accordingly punished, and whether
their offices be annual or otherwise,[11] once a year they shall be
called in question, and give an account; for men are partial
and passionate, merciless, covetous, corrupt, subject to love,
hate, fear, favour, etc., *omne sub regno graviore regnum* [every
throne is subject to a greater throne]: like Solon's Areopagites,
or those Roman censors, some shall visit others, and be visited
invicem [in turn] themselves,[12] they shall oversee that no
prowling officer, under colour of authority, shall insult over
his inferiors,[13] as so many wild beasts, oppress, domineer, flay,

grind, or trample on, be partial or corrupt, but that there be
æquabile jus, justice equally done, live as friends and brethren
together; and which Sesellius would have and so much desires
in his kingdom of France,[1] "a diapason and sweet harmony of
kings, princes, nobles, and plebeians so mutually tied and
involved in love, as well as laws and authority, as that they
never disagree, insult or encroach one upon another." If any
man deserve well in his office he shall be rewarded,

> *Quis enim virtutem amplectitur ipsam,*
> *Præmia si tollas?*

[For take away the prize, and who chooses virtue for its
own sake?]

He that invents anything for public good in any art or science,
writes a treatise, or performs any noble exploit at home or
abroad,[2] shall be accordingly enriched,[3] honoured, and preferred.[4]
I say with Hannibal in Ennius, *Hostem qui feriet erit mihi Cartha-
ginensis* [whoever strikes down an enemy shall be in my eyes
a Carthaginian], let him be of what condition he will, in all
offices, actions, he that deserves best shall have best.

Tilianus in Philonius, out of a charitable mind no doubt,
wished all his books were gold and silver, jewels and precious
stones, to redeem captives, set free prisoners, and relieve all
poor distressed souls that wanted means;[5] religiously done, I
deny not, but to what purpose? Suppose this were so well done,
within a little after, though a man had Crœsus' wealth to bestow,
there would be as many more. Wherefore I will suffer no
beggars, rogues, vagabonds, or idle persons at all,[6] that cannot
give an account of their lives how they maintain themselves.[7]
If they be impotent, lame, blind, and single, they shall be
sufficiently maintained in several hospitals, built for that purpose; if married and infirm, past work, or by inevitable loss or
some such-like misfortune cast behind, by distribution of corn,
house-rent free, annual pensions or money,[8] they shall be
relieved, and highly rewarded for their good service they have
formerly done; if able, they shall be enforced to work. "For
I see no reason" (as he said [9]) "why an epicure or idle drone, a
rich glutton, a usurer, should live at ease, and do nothing, live
in honour, in all manner of pleasures, and oppress others, whenas in the meantime a poor labourer, a smith, a carpenter, an
husbandman that hath spent his time in continual labour, as
an ass to carry burdens, to do the commonwealth good, and
without whom we cannot live, shall be left in his old age to beg

or starve, and lead a miserable life worse than a jument."[1]   As
all conditions shall be tied to their task, so none shall be overtired, but have their set times of recreations and holidays,
indulgere genio [to follow their own bent], feasts and merry
meetings, even to the meanest artificer, or basest servant, once
a week to sing or dance (though not all at once), or do whatsoever he shall please;[2] like that *Sacarum festum*[3] amongst the
Persians, those Saturnals in Rome, as well as his master.   If
any be drunk, he shall drink no more wine or strong drink in a
twelvemonth after.[4]   A bankrupt shall be *catomidiatus in
Amphitheatro*,[5] publicly shamed, and he that cannot pay his
debts, if by riot or negligence he have been impoverished, shall
be for a twelvemonth imprisoned; if in that space his creditors
be not satisfied, he shall be hanged.[6]   He that commits sacrilege
shall lose his hands;[7] he that bears false witness, or is of
perjury convict, shall have his tongue cut out, except he
redeem it with his head.   Murder, adultery,[8] shall be punished
by death, but not theft, except it be some more grievous
offence, or notorious offenders:[9] otherwise they shall be condemned to the galleys, mines, be his slaves whom they have
offended, during their lives.   I hate all hereditary slaves, and
that *duram Persarum legem* [hard law of the Persians], as
Brisonius calls it;[10] or as Ammianus, *impendio formidatas et
abominandas leges, per quas ob noxam unius omnis propinquitas
perit*,[11] hard law that wife and children, friends and allies,
should suffer for the father's offence.

No man shall marry until he be 25,[12] no woman till she be 20,
nisi aliter dispensatum fuerit[13] [without a dispensation].   If
one die, the other party shall not marry till six months after;[14]
and because many families are compelled to live niggardly,
exhaust and undone by great dowers, none shall be given at
all,[15] or very little, and that by supervisors rated, they that are
foul shall have a greater portion; if fair, none at all, or very
little: howsoever, not to exceed such a rate as those supervisors
shall think fit.[16]   And when once they come to those years,
poverty shall hinder no man from marriage, or any other
respect, but all shall be rather enforced than hindered,[17] except
they be dismembered, or grievously deformed,[18] infirm, or
visited with some enormous hereditary disease in body or mind;
in such cases upon a great pain or mulct, man or woman shall
not marry,[19] other order shall be taken for them to their content.[20]
If people overabound, they shall be eased by colonies.[21]

No man shall wear weapons in any city.[22]   The same attire shall be kept, and that proper to several callings, by which they shall be distinguished. *Luxus funerum* [display at funerals] shall be taken away, that intempestive expense moderated,[1] and many others. Brokers, takers of pawns, biting usurers, I will not admit; yet because *hic cum hominibus non cum diis agitur*, we converse here with men, not with gods, and for the hardness of men's hearts, I will tolerate some kind of usury.[2] If we were honest, I confess, *si probi essemus*, we should have no use of it, but being as it is, we must necessarily admit it. Howsoever most divines contradict it (*Dicimus inficias, sed vox ea sola reperta est* [we say "no" with our lips, but do not mean it]), it must be winked at by politicians. And yet some great doctors approve of it, Calvin, Bucer, Zanchius, P. Martyr, because by so many grand lawyers, decrees of emperors, princes' statutes, customs of commonwealths, churches' approbations, it is permitted, etc., I will therefore allow it. But to no private persons, nor to every man that will, to orphans only, maids, widows, or such as by reason of their age, sex, education, ignorance of trading, know not otherwise how to employ it; and those so approved, not to let it out apart, but to bring their money to a common bank which shall be allowed in every city,[3] as in Genoa, Geneva, Nuremberg, Venice, at 5, 6, 7, not above 8 per centum,[4] as the supervisors, or *ærarii præfecti*, shall think fit. And as it shall not be lawful for each man to be an usurer that will, so shall it not be lawful for all to take up money at use, not to prodigals and spendthrifts, but to merchants, young tradesmen, such as stand in need, or know honestly how to employ it, whose necessity, cause, and condition the said supervisors shall approve of.[5]

I will have no private monopolies, to enrich one man and beggar a multitude, multiplicity of offices, of supplying by deputies;[6] weights and measures the same throughout, and those rectified by the *Primum mobile* and sun's motion, threescore miles to a degree according to observation, 1000 geometrical paces to a mile, five foot to a pace, twelve inches to a foot, etc., and from measures known it is an easy matter to rectify weights, etc., to cast up all, and resolve bodies by algebra, stereometry. I hate wars if they be not *ad populi salutem*, upon urgent occasion. *Odimus accipitrem, quia semper vivit in armis* [we hate the hawk, because it is for ever at war]. Offensive wars, except the cause be very just, I will not allow of.[7] For I do highly magnify that saying of Hannibal to Scipio, in Livy: "It had been a blessed thing for you and us,

if God had given that mind to our predecessors, that you had
been content with Italy, we with Africa. For neither Sicily
nor Sardinia are worth such cost and pains, so many fleets and
armies, or so many famous captains' lives." [1] *Omnia prius
tentanda*, fair means shall first be tried. *Peragit tranquilla
potestas, Quod violenta nequit* [2] [peaceful pressure accomplishes
more than violence]. I will have them proceed with all moderation: but hear you, Fabius my general, not Minucius, *nam qui
consilio nititur plus hostibus nocet, quam qui sine animi ratione,
viribus* [3] [for strategy can inflict greater blows on the enemy
than uncalculating force]. And in such wars to abstain as much
as is possible from depopulations, burning of towns, massacring
of infants, etc. [4] For defensive wars, I will have forces still
ready at a small warning, by land and sea, a prepared navy,
soldiers *in procinctu, et quam Bonfinius apud Hungaros suos
vult, virgam ferream* [5] [ready for action, and, as Bonfinius desired
for his Hungarians, an iron rod], and money, which is *nervus
belli* [the sinews of war], still in a readiness, and a sufficient
revenue, a third part as in old Rome and Egypt, [6] reserved for
the commonwealth; to avoid those heavy taxes and impositions,
as well to defray this charge of wars, as also all other public
defalcations, expenses, fees, pensions, reparations, chaste sports,
feasts, donaries, rewards, and entertainments. All things in
this nature especially I will have maturely done, and with
great deliberation: [7] *ne quid temere, ne quid remisse ac timide
fiat* [8] [without rashness, yet with courage and determination];
Sed quo feror hospes? [but I am drifting too far]. To prosecute
the rest would require a volume. *Manum de tabella* [I must call
a halt], I have been over-tedious in this subject; I could have
here willingly ranged, but these straits wherein I am included
will not permit.

From commonwealths and cities I will descend to families,
which have as many corsives and molestations, as frequent
discontents as the rest. Great affinity there is betwixt a
political and economical body; they differ only in magnitude
and proportion of business (so Scaliger writes [9]); as they have
both likely the same period, as Bodine [10] and Peucer [11] hold, out
of Plato, six or seven hundred years, so many times they have
the same means of their vexation and overthrows; as namely,
riot, a common ruin of both, riot in building, riot in profuse
spending, riot in apparel, etc., be it in what kind soever, it
produceth the same effects. A chorographer of ours, [12] speaking
obiter of ancient families, why they are so frequent in the north,

continue so long, are so soon extinguished in the south, and so few, gives no other reason but this, *luxus omnia dissipavit*, riot hath consumed all. Fine clothes and curious buildings came into this island, as he notes in his annals, not so many years since; *non sine dispendio hospitalitatis*, to the decay of hospitality. Howbeit, many times that word is mistaken, and under the name of bounty and hospitality is shrouded riot and prodigality; and that which is commendable in itself well used, hath been mistaken heretofore, is become by his abuse the bane and utter ruin of many a noble family. For some men live like the rich glutton, consuming themselves and their substance by continual feasting and invitations, with Axylus in Homer, [1] keep open house for all comers, giving entertainment to such as visit them, keeping a table beyond their means,[2] and a company of idle servants (though not so frequent as of old), are blown up on a sudden, and, as Actæon was by his hounds, devoured by their kinsmen, friends, and multitude of followers. It is a wonder that Paulus Jovius relates of our northern countries, what an infinite deal of meat we consume on our tables; [3] that I may truly say, 'tis not bounty, not hospitality, as it is often abused, but riot in excess, gluttony and prodigality; a mere vice; it brings in debt, want, and beggary, hereditary diseases, consumes their fortunes, and overthrows the good temperature of their bodies. To this I might here well add their inordinate expense in building, those phantastical houses, turrets, walks, parks, etc., gaming, excess of pleasure, and that prodigious riot in apparel, by which means they are compelled to break up house, and creep into holes. Sesellius, in his Commonwealth of France, gives three reasons why the French nobility were so frequently bankrupts: "First, because they had so many lawsuits and contentions one upon another, which were tedious and costly; by which means it came to pass that commonly lawyers bought them out of their possessions. A second cause was their riot; they lived beyond their means, and were therefore swallowed up by merchants." [4] (La Nove, a French writer, yields five reasons of his countrymen's poverty, to the same effect almost, and thinks verily, if the gentry of France were divided into ten parts, eight of them would be found much impaired, by sales, mortgages, and debts, or wholly sunk in their estates.) "The last was immoderate excess in apparel, which consumed their revenues." How this concerns and agrees with our present state, look you. But of this elsewhere. As it is in a man's body, if either head, heart, stomach, liver, spleen, or any one part be misaffected, all the rest suffer with it: so is it with this economical body. If the head be naught, a spendthrift, a drunkard, a whoremaster, a gamester, how shall the family live at ease? *Ipsa si cupiat salus servare, prorsus non potest hanc familiam,*[1] as Demea said in the comedy, Safety herself cannot save it. A good, honest, painful man many times hath a shrew to his wife, a sickly, dishonest, sloth- ful, foolish, careless woman to his mate, a proud, peevish flirt, a liquorish, prodigal quean, and by that means all goes to ruin: or if they differ in nature, he is thrifty, she spends all, he wise, she sottish and soft; what agreement can there be? what friend- ship? Like that of the thrush and swallow in Æsop, instead of mutual love, kind compellations, whore and thief is heard, they fling stools at one another's heads. *Quæ intemperies vexat hanc familiam?*[2] [What madness has come over this family?] All enforced marriages commonly produce such effects, or if on their behalfs it be well, as to live and agree lovingly together, they may have disobedient and unruly children, that take ill courses to disquiet them, "their son is a thief, a spendthrift, their daughter a whore";[3] a stepmother[4] or a daughter-in- law distempers all; or else for want of means,[5] many tortures arise, debts, dues, fees, dowries, jointures, legacies to be paid, annuities issuing out, by means of which they have not where- withal to maintain themselves in that pomp as their predecessors have done, bring up or bestow their children to their callings, to their birth and quality, and will not descend to their present fortunes.[6] Oftentimes, too, to aggravate the rest, con- cur many other inconveniences, unthankful friends, decayed friends, bad neighbours, negligent servants, *servi furaces, versi- pelles, callidi, occlusa sibi mille clavibus reserant, furtimque raptant, consumunt, liguriunt*[7] [thievish slaves, sly cunning varlets, they break through a thousand bolts, they steal, they eat up, they take the tit-bits]; casualties, taxes, mulcts, chargeable offices, vain expenses, entertainments, loss of stock, enmities, emulations, frequent invitations, losses, suretyship, sickness, death of friends, and that which is the gulf of all, improvidence, ill husbandry, disorder and confusion, by which means they are drenched on a sudden in their estates, and at unawares preci- pitated insensibly into an inextricable labyrinth of debts, cares, woes, want, grief, discontent, and melancholy itself.

I have done with families, and will now briefly run over some few sorts and conditions of men. The most secure, happy, jovial, and merry in the world's esteem are princes and great

men, free from melancholy: but for their cares, miseries, suspicions, jealousies, discontents, folly and madness, I refer you
to Xenophon's *Tyrannus*, where King Hiero discourseth at
large with Simonides the poet of this subject.   Of all others
they are most troubled with perpetual fears, anxieties, insomuch
that, as he said in Valerius,[1] "If thou knewest with what cares
and miseries this robe were stuffed, thou wouldst not stoop to
take it up."   Or put case they be secure and free from fears and
discontents, yet they are void of reason too oft, and precipitate
in their actions;[2] read all our histories, *quos de stultis prodidere
stulti* [which fools have written about fools], Iliads, Æneids,
Annals, and what is the subject?

> *Stultorum regum, et populorum continet æstus.*
>
> [The giddy tumults and the foolish rage
> Of kings and people.]

How mad they are, how furious, and upon small occasions,
rash and inconsiderate in their proceedings, how they dote,
every page almost will witness:

> *Delirant reges, plectuntur Achivi.*
>
> [When doting monarchs urge
> Unsound resolves, their subjects feel the scourge.]

Next in place, next in miseries and discontents, in all manner
of hair-brain actions, are great men; *procul a Jove, procul a
fulmine* [the farther from Jove, the farther from the lightning],
the nearer the worse.   If they live in court, they are up and
down, ebb and flow with their prince's favours, *Ingenium vultu
statque caditque suo* [their talent rises or falls with his smile or
frown], now aloft, to-morrow down, as Polybius describes them,[3]
"like so many casting-counters, now of gold, to-morrow of
silver, that vary in worth as the computant will; now they
stand for units, to-morrow for thousands; now before all,
and anon behind."   Beside, they torment one another with
mutual factions, emulations: one is ambitious, another enamoured, a third in debt, a prodigal, overruns his fortunes, a
fourth solicitous with cares, gets nothing, etc.   But for these
men's discontents, anxieties, I refer you to Lucian's tract, *De
mercede conductis*, Æneas Sylvius (*libidinis et stultitiæ servos*[4]
[slaves of lust and folly] he calls them), Agrippa, and many
others.

Of philosophers and scholars *priscæ sapientiæ dictatores* [the
dictators of ancient learning], I have already spoken in general

terms, those superintendents of wit and learning, men above men, those refined men, minions of the Muses,

> *mentemque habere queis bonam*
> *Et esse corculis* [1] *datum est.* [2]

[Who have been vouchsafed good brains and quick minds.]

These acute and subtle sophisters, so much honoured, have as much need of hellebore as others. [3] *O medici, mediam pertundite venam* [4] [physicians, open the middle vein]. Read Lucian's *Piscator*, and tell how he esteemed them; Agrippa's Tract of the Vanity of Sciences; nay, read their own works, their absurd tenents, prodigious paradoxes, *et risum teneatis amici?* [and can you contain your laughter, friends?] You shall find that of Aristotle true, *nullum magnum ingenium sine mixtura dementiæ* [no great wit without some admixture of madness], they have a worm as well as others; you shall find a phantastical strain, a fustian, a bombast, a vainglorious humour, an affected style, etc., like a prominent thread in an uneven woven cloth, run parallel throughout their works. And they that teach wisdom, patience, meekness, are the veriest dizzards, hair-brains, and most discontent. "In the multitude of wisdom is grief, and he that increaseth wisdom, increaseth sorrow." [5] I need not quote mine author. They that laugh and contemn others, condemn the world of folly, deserve to be mocked, are as giddy-headed, and lie as open as any other. Democritus, that common flouter of folly, [6] was ridiculous himself; barking Menippus, scoffing Lucian, satirical Lucilius, Petronius, Varro, Persius, etc., may be censured with the rest; *Loripedem rectus derideat, Æthiopem albus* [let the straight man deride the crookshank, the white man the blackamoor]. Bale, Erasmus, Hospinian, Vives, Kemnisius, explode as a vast ocean of *obs* and *sols*, [7] school divinity. A labyrinth of intricable questions, [8] unprofitable contentions, *incredibilem delirationem* [an incredible doting], one calls it. If school divinity be so censured, *subtilis Scotus, lima veritatis, Occam irrefragabilis, cujus ingenium vetera omnia ingenia subvertit* [9] [the subtle Scotus, who was the file of truth, the infallible Occam who confuted all the ancients], etc., Baconthorpe, Doctor Resolutus, and *Corculum Theologiæ* [the keenest of theological brains], Thomas himself, Doctor Seraphicus, *cui dictavit angelus* [10] [whose writings an angel dictated], etc., what shall become of humanity? *Ars stulta* [foolish Art], what can she plead? what can her followers say for

themselves? Much learning *cere-diminuit-brum*,[1] hath cracked
their sconce, and taken such root that *tribus Anticyris caput
insanabile*, hellebore itself can do no good, nor that renowned
lanthorn of Epictetus,[2] by which if any man studied, he should
be as wise as he was. But all will not serve; rhetoricians *in
ostentationem loquacitatis multa agitant*, out of their volubility
of tongue will talk much to no purpose; orators can persuade
other men what they will, *quo volunt, unde volunt* [to go where
they will, whence they will], move, pacify, etc., but cannot
settle their own brains. What saith Tully? *Malo indisertam
prudentiam quam loquacem stultitiam* [I prefer sense without
eloquence to folly with it]; and, as Seneca seconds him,[3] a wise
man's oration should not be polite or solicitous. Fabius esteems
no better of most of them,[4] either in speech, action, gesture,
than as men beside themselves, *insanos declamatores* [crazy
rhetoricians]; so doth Gregory, *Non mihi sapit qui sermone,
sed qui factis sapit* [I judge wisdom not from speech but from
action]. Make the best of him, a good orator is a turncoat,
an evil man, *bonus orator pessimus vir*, his tongue is set to
sale, he is a mere voice, as he said of a nightingale,[5] *dat sine
mente sonum* [all sound and no sense], an hyperbolical liar, a
flatterer, a parasite, and as Ammianus Marcellinus will, a
corrupting cozener, one that doth more mischief by his fair
speeches than he that bribes by money;[6] for a man may with
more facility avoid him that circumvents by money, than he
that deceives with glozing terms; which made Socrates so much
abhor and explode them.[7] Fracastorius, a famous poet, freely
grants all poets to be mad;[8] so doth Scaliger;[9] and who doth
not? *Aut insanit homo, aut versus facit* [he's mad or making
verses], Hor. *Sat. 7, lib. 2. Insanire lubet, i.e. versus componere*
['tis one's humour to be mad, i.e. to write verse], Virg. *Ecl. 3*,
so Servius interprets it, all poets are mad, a company of bitter
satirists, detractors, or else parasitical applauders: and what is
poetry itself but, as Austin holds, *vinum erroris ab ebriis
doctoribus propinatum* [the wine of error presented by drunken
teachers]? You may give that censure of them in general,
which Sir Thomas More once did of Germanus Brixius' poems
in particular:

*Vehunter
In rate stultitiæ, sylvam habitant furiæ.*

[They sail in the bark of folly, they inhabit the grove
of madness.]

Budæus, in an epistle of his to Lupsetus, will have civil law

to be the tower of wisdom; another honours physic, the quintessence of nature: a third tumbles them both down, and sets
up the flag of his own peculiar science. Your supercilious critics,
grammatical triflers, note-makers, curious antiquaries, find out
all the ruins of wit, *ineptiarum delicias* [exquisite follies],
amongst the rubbish of old writers; *Pro stultis habent nisi aliquid
sufficiant invenire, quod in aliorum scriptis vertant vitio,*[1] all
fools with them that cannot find fault; they correct others,
and are hot in a cold cause, puzzle themselves to find out how
many streets in Rome, houses, gates, towers, Homer's country,
Æneas' mother, Niobe's daughters, *an Sappho publica fuerit?
ovum prius exstiterit an gallina?*[2] *etc., et alia quæ dediscenda essent
scire, si scires* [whether Sappho was a courtesan; whether the
the egg came first or the hen; and similar nonsense which, even
if one had learnt it, ought to be forgotten], as Seneca holds;[3]
what clothes the senators did wear in Rome, what shoes, how
they sat, where they went to the close-stool, how many dishes
in a mess, what sauce, which for the present for an historian
to relate, according to Lodovic. Vives,[4] is very ridiculous, is
to them most precious elaborate stuff, they admired for it, and
as proud, as triumphant in the meantime for this discovery,
as if they had won a city, or conquered a province; as rich as
if they had found a mine of gold ore. *Quosvis auctores absurdis
commentis suis percacant et stercorant*, one saith, they bewray
and daub a company of books and good authors with their
absurd comments, *correctorum sterquilinia* Scaliger calls them,[5]
and show their wit in censuring others, a company of foolish
note-makers, humble-bees, dors, or beetles, *inter stercora ut pluri
mum versantur*, they rake over all those rubbish and dunghills,
and prefer a manuscript many times before the Gospel itself,
Thesaurum criticum[6] before any treasure, and with their *delea-
turs, alii legunt sic, meus codex sic habet* [omit, some read, my MS.
reads], with their *postremæ editiones* [last editions], annotations,
castigations, etc., make books dear, themselves ridiculous, and
do nobody good, yet if any man dare oppose or contradict, they
are mad, up in arms on a sudden, how many sheets are written
in defence, how bitter invectives, what apologies! *Epiphyllides
hæ sunt et meræ nugæ*[7] [these are poor grapes, mere trifles].
But I dare say no more of, for, with, or against them, because
I am liable to their lash as well as others. Of these and the
rest of our artists and philosophers, I will generally conclude
they are a kind of madmen, as Seneca esteems of them,[8] to
make doubts and scruples, how to read them truly, to mend

old authors, but will not mend their own lives, or teach us *ingenia sanare, memoriam officiorum ingerere, ac fidem in rebus humanis retinere*, to keep our wits in order, or rectify our manners. *Numquid tibi demens videtur, si istis operam impenderit?* Is not he mad that draws lines with Archimedes, whilst his house is ransacked and his city besieged, when the whole world is in combustion, or we whilst our souls are in danger (*mors sequitur, vita fugit* [death follows, life flies]), to spend our time in toys, idle questions, and things of no worth?

That lovers are mad, I think no man will deny.[1] *Amare simul et sapere* [to love and to be wise], *ipsi Jovi non datur*, Jupiter himself cannot intend both at once.

> *Non bene conveniunt, nec in una sede morantur*
> *Majestas et amor.*[2]
>
> [Majesty and love pull different ways;
> Where one is throned, the other never stays.]

Tully, when he was invited to a second marriage, replied, he could not *simul amare et sapere*, be wise and love both together. *Est Orcus ille, vis est immedicabilis, est rabies insana*,[3] love is madness, a hell, an incurable disease; *impotentem et insanam libidinem* Seneca calls it,[4] an impotent and raging lust. I shall dilate this subject apart; in the meantime let lovers sigh out the rest.

Nevisanus the lawyer holds it for an axiom, "most women are fools," [5] *consilium feminis invalidum* [6] [women's judgment is weak]; Seneca, men, be they young or old; who doubts it? Youth is mad, as Elius in Tully, *stulti adolescentuli*, old age little better, *deliri senes*, etc. Theophrastus, in the 107th year of his age, said he then began to be wise, *tum sapere cœpit*, and therefore lamented his departure.[7] If wisdom came so late, where shall we find a wise man? Our old ones dote at threescore and ten. I would cite more proofs, and a better author; but for the present, let one fool point at another. Nevisanus hath as hard an opinion of rich men,[8] "Wealth and wisdom cannot dwell together," [9] *stultitiam patiuntur opes* [wealth and folly can go together], and they do commonly *infatuare cor hominis*,[10] besot men;[11] and as we see it, "fools have fortune": *Sapientia non invenitur in terra suaviter viventium* [12] [wisdom is not found in the land of those who live at ease]. For beside a natural contempt of learning which accompanies such kind of men, innate idleness (for they will take no pains), and which Aristotle observes,[1] *ubi mens plurima, ibi minima fortuna* [where there is most wit there is least wealth], *ubi plurima fortuna, ibi mens perexigua*, great wealth and little wit go commonly together: they have as much brains some of them in their heads as in their heels; besides this inbred neglect of liberal sciences and all arts, which should *excolere mentem*, polish the mind, they have most part some gullish humour or other, by which they are led; one is an epicure, an atheist, a second a gamester, a third a whoremaster (fit subjects all for a satirist to work upon);

> *Hic nuptarum insanit amoribus, hic puerorum;*[2]
>
> [One burns to madness for the wedded dame;
> Unnatural lusts another's heart inflame;]

one is mad of hawking, hunting, cocking; another of carousing, horse-riding, spending; a fourth of building, fighting, etc.[3] *Insanit veteres statuas Damasippus emendo* [Damasippus hath a craze for buying old statues], Damasippus hath an humour of his own, to be talked of: Heliodorus the Carthaginian another.[4] In a word, as Scaliger concludes of them all, they are *statuæ erectæ stultitiæ*, the very statues or pillars of folly. Choose out of all stories him that hath been most admired, you shall still find *multa ad laudem, multa ad vituperationem magnifica* [there is much to praise, but also much to blame], as Berosus of Semiramis;[5] *omnes mortales militia, triumphis, divitiis, etc., tum et luxu, cæde, cæterisque vitiis antecessit* [she surpassed all men in military achievements and wealth, but also in profligacy, cruelty, and other vices]; as she had some good, so had she many bad parts.

Alexander, a worthy man, but furious in his anger, overtaken in drink; Cæsar and Scipio, valiant and wise, but vainglorious, ambitious; Vespasian, a worthy prince, but covetous; Hannibal, as he had mighty virtues, so had he many vices:[6] *unam virtutem mille vitia comitantur* [one virtue accompanied by a thousand vices], as Machiavel of Cosmus Medices,[7] he had two distinct persons in him. I will determine of them all, they are like these double or turning pictures; stand before which, you see a fair maid on the one side, an ape on the other, an owl; look upon them at the first sight, all is well; but further examine, you shall find them wise on the one side and fools on the other; in some few things praiseworthy, in the rest incomparably faulty. I will say nothing of their diseases, emulations, discontents, wants, and such miseries: let Poverty plead the rest in Aristophanes' *Plutus*.

Covetous men, amongst others, are most mad, they have all

the symptoms of melancholy, fear, sadness, suspicion, etc.,[1] as
shall be proved in his proper place.

Danda est hellebori multo pars maxima avaris.

[Misers make whole Anticyra their own;
Its hellebore reserv'd for them alone.]

And yet methinks prodigals are much madder than they, be
of what condition they will, that bear a public or private purse;
as a Dutch writer censured Richard, the rich Duke of Cornwall,
suing to be emperor, for his profuse spending,[2] *qui effudit
pecuniam ante pedes principium Electorum sicut aquam,* that
scattered money like water; I do censure them. *Stulta Anglia*
(saith he), *quæ tot denariis sponte est privata, stulti principes
Alemanniæ, qui nobile jus suum pro pecunia vendiderunt* [foolish
Britain, to lose so much money without need; foolish princes
of Germany, to sell their proud privileges for pelf]. Spendthrifts, bribers, and bribe-takers are fools, and so are all they
that cannot keep, disburse, or spend their moneys well.[3]

I might say the like of angry, peevish, envious, ambitious;
Anticyras melior sorbere meracas[4] [you were better to swallow
the Anticyræ undiluted]; epicures, atheists, schismatics, heretics;
hi omnes habent imaginationem læsam [they have all a diseased
imagination] (saith Nymannus), "and their madness shall be
evident" (2 Tim. iii, 9). Fabatus, an Italian, holds seafaring
men all mad; "the ship is mad, for it never stands still; the
mariners are mad, to expose themselves to such imminent
dangers: the waters are raging mad, in perpetual motion; the
winds are as mad as the rest, they know not whence they
come, whither they would go: and those men are maddest of all
that go to sea; for one fool at home, they find forty abroad."[5]
He was a madman that said it, and thou peradventure as mad
to read it. Felix Platerus[6] is of opinion all alchemists are
mad, out of their wits; Athenæus[7] saith as much of fiddlers, *et
musarum luscinias* [and those nightingales of the Muses],
musicians, *omnes tibicines insaniunt* [all flute-players are mad],
ubi semel efflant, avolat illico mens,[8] in comes music at one ear,
out goes wit at another. Proud and vainglorious persons are
certainly mad; and so are lascivious;[9] I can feel their pulses
beat hither; horn-mad some of them, to let others lie with
their wives, and wink at it.

To insist in all particulars[10] were an Herculean task, to reckon
up[11] *insanas substructiones, insanos labores, insanum luxum,*[12]
mad labours, mad books, endeavours, carriages, gross ignorance,

ridiculous actions, absurd gestures; *insanam gulam, insana jurgia* [mad gluttony, mad disputes], *insaniam villarum*, as Tully terms them, madness of villages, stupend structures; as those Egyptian pyramids, labyrinths, and sphinxes, which a company of crowned asses, *ad ostentationem opum* [to show off their wealth], vainly built, when neither the architect nor king that made them, or to what use and purpose, are yet known: to insist in their hypocrisy, inconstancy, blindness, rashness, *dementem temeritatem*, fraud, cozenage, malice, anger, impudence, ingratitude, ambition, gross superstition, *tempora infecta et adulatione sordida*,[1] as in Tiberius' times, such base flattery, stupend, parasitical fawning and colloguing, etc., brawls, conflicts, desires, contentions, it would ask an expert Vesalius to anatomize every member. Shall I say Jupiter himself, Apollo, Mars, etc., doted? and monster-conquering Hércules, that subdued the world and helped others, could not relieve himself in this, but mad he was at last. And where shall a man walk, converse with whom, in what province, city, and not meet with Signior Deliro,[2] or Hercules Furens, Mænades, and Corybantes? Their speeches say no less. *E fungis nati homines* [3] [they were men born from mushrooms], or else they fetched their pedigree from those that were struck by Samson with the jawbone of an ass; or from Deucalion and Pyrrha's stones, for *durum genus sumus, marmorei sumus*,[4] we are stony-hearted, and savour too much of the stock: as if they had all heard that enchanted horn of Astolpho, that English duke in Ariosto, which never sounded but all his auditors were mad, and for fear ready to make away with themselves; or landed in the mad haven in the Euxine Sea of *Daphne insana*, which had a secret quality to dementate; [5] they are a company of giddy-heads, afternoon-men, it is midsummer moon still, and the dog-days last all the year long, they are all mad. Whom shall I then except? Ulricus Huttenus' *Nemo*; [6] *nam, Nemo omnibus horis sapit, Nemo nascitur sine vitiis, Crimine Nemo caret, Nemo sorte sua vivit contentus, Nemo in amore sapit, Nemo bonus, Nemo sapiens, Nemo est ex omni parti beatus* [Nobody; for Nobody is sensible at all times; Nobody is born without fault; Nobody is free from blame; Nobody lives content with his own lot; Nobody is sane in love; Nobody is good, Nobody wise; Nobody is completely happy], etc., and therefore Nicholas Nemo, or Monsieur Nobody, shall go free. *Quid valeat Nemo, Nemo referre potest* [Nobody can say what Nobody is capable of]. But whom shall I except in the second place? such as are silent; *vir sapit qui pauca loquitur* [he is a wise man who says little]; no better way to avoid folly and madness than by taciturnity.[1] Whom in a third? all senators, magistrates; for all fortunate men are wise, and conquerors valiant, and so are all great men, *non est bonum ludere cum diis* [it is not good to play tricks with the gods], they are wise by authority, good by their office and place, *his licet impune pessimos esse* [they are privileged to be as bad as they like] (some say), we must not speak of them, neither is it fit; *per me sint omnia protinus alba* [everything shall be stainless for all that I shall say], I will not think amiss of them. Whom next? Stoics? *Sapiens Stoicus* [the Stoic is wise], and he alone is subject to no perturbations, as Plutarch scoffs at him, "he is not vexed with torments, or burnt with fire, foiled by his adversary, sold of his enemy: though he be wrinkled, sand-blind, toothless, and deformed, yet he is most beautiful, and like a god, a king in conceit, though not worth a groat."[2] "He never dotes, never mad, never sad, drunk, because virtue cannot be taken away," as Zeno holds, "by reason of strong apprehension,"[3] but he was mad to say so. *Anticyræ cœlo huic est opus aut dolabra*[4] [he needs either the climate of Anticyra or a pickaxe], he had need to be bored, and so had all his fellows, as wise as they would seem to be. Chrysippus himself liberally grants them to be fools as well as others, at certain times, upon some occasions, *amitti virtutem ait per ebrietatem, aut atribilarium morbum*, it [virtue] may be lost by drunkenness or melancholy; he may be sometimes crazed as well as the rest: *ad summum sapiens nisi quum pituita molesta*[5] [unfailingly wise save when troubled with the phlegm]. I should here except some Cynics, Menippus, Diogenes, that Theban Crates; or to descend to these times, that omniscious, only wise fraternity of the Rosy Cross,[6] those great theologues, politicians, philosophers, physicians, philologers, artists, etc., of whom St. Bridget, Abbas Joacchimus, Leicenbergius, and such divine spirits have prophesied, and made promise to the world, if at least there be any such (Hen. Neuhusius makes a doubt of it,[7] Valentinus Andreas,[8] and others), or an Elias Artifex their Theophrastian master; whom though Libavius and many deride and carp at, yet some will have to be "the renewer of all arts and sciences,"[9] reformer of the world, and now living, for so Johannes Montanus Strigoniensis, that great patron of Paracelsus, contends, and certainly avers "a most divine man,"[10] and the quintessence of wisdom wheresoever he is; for he, his fraternity, friends, etc., are all "betrothed to wisdom,"[11] if we may believe their disciples and followers. I must needs except Lipsius and the Pope, and expunge their name out of the catalogue of fools. For besides that parasitical testimony of Dousa,

> *A sole exoriente Mæotidas usque paludes,*
> *Nemo est qui Justo se æquiparare queat,*

[From the rising sun to the Mæotid Sea, not one can put himself on a level with Justus [1]],

Lipsius saith of himself, that he was *humani generis quidam pædagogus voce et stylo,*[2] a grand signior, a master, a tutor of us all, and for thirteen years he brags how he sowed wisdom in the Low Countries, as Ammonius the philosopher sometime did in Alexandria, *cum humanitate literas et sapientiam cum prudentia* [3] [polite learning and practical philosophy]: *antistes sapientiæ* [a master of wisdom], he shall be *sapientum octavus* [the eighth wise man]. The Pope is more than a man, as his parasites [4] often make him, a demi-god, and besides His Holiness cannot err, *in Cathedra* belike: and yet some of them have been magicians, heretics, atheists, children, and as Platina saith of John XXII, *Etsi vir literatus, multa stoliditatem et lævitatem præ se ferentia egit, stolidi et socordis vir ingenii,* a scholar sufficient, yet many things he did foolishly, lightly. I can say no more then in particular, but in general terms to the rest, they are all mad, their wits are evaporated, and, as Ariosto feigns (*lib. 34*), kept in jars above the moon.

> Some lose their wits with love, some with ambition,
> Some following lords and men of high condition.[5]
> Some in fair jewels rich and costly set,
> Others in poetry their wits forget.
> Another thinks to be an alchemist,
> Till all be spent, and that his number's mist.

Convict fools they are, madmen upon record; and I am afraid past cure many of them, *crepunt inguina,*[6] the symptoms are manifest, they are all of Gotham parish:

> *Quum furor haud dubius, quum sit manifesta phrenesis.*[7]

[Since their madness is incontestable, their delirium plain.]

What remains then but to send for *lorarios,* those officers to carry them all together for company to Bedlam, and set Rabelais to be their physician.[8]

If any man shall ask in the meantime, who I am that so boldly censure others, *Tu nullane habes vitia?* have I no faults? Yes, more than thou hast, whatsoever thou art.[9] *Nos numerus sumus* [I am of the number], I confess it again, I am as foolish, as mad as any one.

> *Insanus vobis videor, non deprecor ipse,*
> *Quo minus insanus,*[1]
>
> [You think me mad, I make no objection.]

I do not deny it, *demens de populo dematur* [let the madman be removed from society]. My comfort is, I have more fellows, and those of excellent note. And though I be not so right or so discreet as I should be, yet not so mad, so bad neither, as thou perhaps takest me to be.

To conclude, this being granted, that all the world is melancholy, or mad, dotes, and every member of it, I have ended my task, and sufficiently illustrated that which I took upon me to demonstrate at first. At this present I have no more to say. *His sanam mentem Democritus* [Democritus wishes them sanity], I can but wish myself and them a good physician, and all of us a better mind.

And although, for the above-named reasons, I had a just cause to undertake this subject, to point at these particular species of dotage, that so men might acknowledge their imperfections, and seek to reform what is amiss; yet I have a more serious intent at this time; and to omit all impertinent digressions, to say no more of such as are improperly melancholy, or metaphorically mad, lightly mad, or in disposition, as stupid, angry, drunken, silly, sottish, sullen, proud, vainglorious, ridiculous, beastly, peevish, obstinate, impudent, extravagant, dry, doting, dull, desperate, harebrain, etc., mad, frantic, foolish, heteroclites, which no new hospital [2] can hold, no physic help: my purpose and endeavour is, in the following discourse to anatomize this humour of melancholy, through all his parts and species, as it is an habit, or an ordinary disease, and that philosophically, medicinally, to show the causes, symptoms, and several cures of it, that it may be the better avoided; moved thereunto for the generality of it, and to do good, it being a disease "so frequent," as Mercurialis observes, "in these our days";[3] "so often happening," saith Laurentius, "in our miserable times,"[4] as few there are that feel not the smart of it. Of the same mind is Ælian Montaltus, Melancthon,[5] and others; Julius Cæsar Claudinus calls it "the fountain of all other diseases, and so common in this crazed age of ours, that scarce one in a thousand is free from it";[6] and that splenetic, hypochondriacal wind especially, which proceeds from the spleen and short ribs. Being then a disease so grievous, so common, I know not wherein to do a more general service, and spend my time better, than to prescribe means how to prevent and cure so universal a malady, an epidemical disease, that so often, so much, crucifies the body and mind.

If I have overshot myself in this which hath been hitherto said, or that it is, which I am sure some will object, too phantastical, "too light and comical for a divine, too satirical for one of my profession," I will presume to answer, with Erasmus [1] in like case, 'Tis not I, but Democritus, *Democritus dixit*: you must consider what it is to speak in one's own or another's person, an assumed habit and name—a difference betwixt him that affects or acts a prince's, a philosopher's, a magistrate's, a fool's part, and him that is so indeed—and what liberty those old satirists have had; it is a cento collected from others; not I, but they that say it.

> *Dixero si quid forte jocosius, hoc mihi juris*
> *Cum veniâ dabis.* [2]

[Yet some indulgence I may justly claim,
If too familiar with another's fame.]

Take heed you mistake me not. If I do a little forget myself, I hope you will pardon it. And to say truth, why should any man be offended, or take exceptions at it?

> *Licuit, semperque licebit,*
> *Parcere personis, dicere de vitiis.*

It lawful was of old, and still will be,
To speak of vice, but let the name go free.

I hate their vices, not their persons. If any be displeased, or take aught unto himself, let him not expostulate or cavil with him that said it (so did Erasmus excuse himself to Dorpius,[3] *si parva licet componere magnis* [to compare small things with great]), and so do I; "but let him be angry with himself, that so betrayed and opened his own faults in applying it to himself: if he be guilty and deserve it, let him amend, whoever he is, and not be angry." [4] "He that hateth correction is a fool" (Prov. xii, 1). If he be not guilty, it concerns him not; it is not my freeness of speech, but a guilty conscience, a galled back of his own that makes him winch.

> *Suspicione si quis errabit sua,*
> *Et rapiet ad se, quod erit commune omnium,*
> *Stulte nudabit animi conscientiam.*

[If any, thinking that himself is meant,
Shall take offence at what is aimed at large.
The more fool he, for all the world will see
His guilty conscience.]

I deny not this which I have said savours a little of Democritus;
quamvis ridentem dicere verum quid vetat?[1] one may speak in
jest, and yet speak truth.   It is somewhat tart, I grant it; *acriora
orexim excitant embammata*, as he said, sharp sauces increase
appetite, *nec cibus ipse juvat morsu fraudatus aceti*[2] [food is
not enjoyable without a dash of vinegar].   Object then, and
cavil what thou wilt, I ward all with Democritus' buckler, his
medicine shall salve it;[3] strike where thou wilt, and when:
Democritus dixit, Democritus will answer it.   It was written by
an idle fellow, at idle times, about our Saturnalian or Dionysian
feasts, when, as he said, *nullum libertati periculum est* [there is
no danger to liberty], servants in old Ròme had liberty to say
and do what them list.   When our countrymen sacrificed to
their goddess Vacuna,[4] and sat tippling by their Vacunal fires.
I writ this, and published this.   Οὔτις ἔλεγεν [no one has said
it], it is *neminis nihil* [nothing by nobody].   The time, place,
persons, and all circumstances apologize for me, and why may
I not then be idle with others, speak my mind freely?   If you
deny me this liberty, upon these presumptions I will take it:
I say again, I will take it.

> *Si quis est qui dictum in se inclementius*
> *Existimavit esse, sic existimet.*[5]

[If any one thinks he has been insulted, let him think so.]

If any man take exceptions, let him turn the buckle of his
girdle,[6] I care not.   I owe thee nothing (reader), I look for no
favour at thy hands, I am independent, I fear not.

No, I recant, I will not, I care, I fear, I confess my fault,
acknowledge a great offence,

> *Motos præstat componere fluctus.*

[Let's first assuage the troubled waves.]

I have overshot myself, I have spoken foolishly, rashly, unadvisedly, absurdly, I have anatomized mine own folly.   And
now methinks upon a sudden I am awaked as it were out of a
dream; I have had a raving fit, a phantastical fit, ranged up and
down, in and out, I have insulted over most kind of men,
abused some, offended others, wronged myself; and now being
recovered, and perceiving mine error, cry with Orlando,[7] *Solvite
me*, pardon, *O boni* [good friends], that which is past, and I
will make you amends in that which is to come; I promise
you a more sober discourse in my following treatise.

If through weakness, folly, passion, discontent,[8] ignorance,

I have said amiss, let it be forgotten and forgiven. I acknowledge that of Tacitus to be true,[1] *Asperæ facetiæ, ubi nimis ex
vero traxere, acrem sui memoriam relinquunt,* a bitter jest leaves
a sting behind it: and as an honourable man observes, "They
fear a satirist's wit, he their memories."[2]   I may justly suspect
the worst; and though I hope I have wronged no man, yet in
Medea's words I will crave pardon.

> *Illud jam voce extrema peto,*
> *Ne si qua noster dubius effudit dolor,*
> *Maneant in animo verba, sed melior tibi*
> *Memoria nostri subeat, hæc iræ data*
> *Obliterentur.*

> And in my last words this I do desire,
> That what in passion I have said, or ire,
> May be forgotten, and a better mind
> Be had of us, hereafter as you find.

I earnestly request every private man, as Scaliger did Cardan,
not to take offence.   I will conclude in his lines, *Si me cognitum
haberes, non solum donares nobis has facetias nostras, sed etiam
indignum duceres, tam humanum animum, lene ingenium, vel
minimam suspicionem deprecari oportere.*   If thou knewest my
modesty and simplicity,[3] thou wouldst easily pardon and forgive
what is here amiss, or by thee misconceived.   If hereafter,
anatomizing this surly humour, my hand slip, as an unskilful
prentice I lance too deep, and cut through skin and all at
unawares, make it smart, or cut awry, pardon a rude hand, an
unskilful knife,[4] 'tis a most difficult thing to keep an even tone, a
perpetual tenor, and not sometimes to lash out; *difficile est
satiram non scribere* [it is hard not to write a satire], there be
so many objects to divert, inward perturbations to molest, and
the very best may sometimes err; *aliquando bonus dormitat
Homerus* [sometimes that excellent Homer takes a nap], it is
impossible not in so much to overshoot; *opere in longo fas
est obrepere somnum* [over such a long work a little sleep is
permissible].   But what needs all this?   I hope there will
no such cause of offence be given; if there be, *Nemo aliquid
recognoscat, nos mentimur omnia*[5] [let no one take these things
to himself, they are all but fiction].   I'll deny all (my last
refuge), recant all, renounce all I have said, if any man except,
and with as much facility excuse as he can accuse; but I presume
of thy good favour, and gracious acceptance (gentle reader).
Out of an assured hope and confidence thereof, I will begin.

LECTORI MALE FERIATO

Tu 'vero cave, sis, edico quisquis·es, ne temere sugilles auctorem
hujusce operis, aut cavillator irridcas.   Immo ne vel ex aliorum
censura tacite obloquaris (vis dicam verbo) ne quid nasutulus
inepte improbes, aut falso fingas.   Nam si talis revera sit,
qualem præ se fert Junior Democritus, seniori Democrito saltem
affinis, aut ejus genium vel tantillum sapiat, actum de te,
censorem æque ac delatorem aget e contra (*petulanti splene cum
sit*), sufflabit te in jocos, comminuet in sales, addo etiam, et Deo
Risui te sacrificabit.[1]

Iterum moneo, ne quid cavillere, ne dum Democritum Juniorem
conviciis infames, aut ignominiose vituperes, de te non male
sentientem, tu idem audias ab amico cordato, quod olim vulgus
Abderitanum ab Hippocrate,[2] concivem bene meritum et popu-
larem suum Democritum pro insano habens.   *Ne tu Democrite
sapis, stulti autem et insani Abderitæ.*

Abderitanæ pectora plebis habes.[3]

Hæc te paucis admonitum volo (male feriate Lector) abi.

[TO THE READER WHO EMPLOYS HIS LEISURE ILL

Whoever you may be, I caution you against rashly defaming
the author of this work, or cavilling in jest against him.   Nay,
do not silently reproach him in consequence of others' censure,
nor employ your wit in foolish disapproval or false accusation.
For, should Democritus Junior prove to be what he professes,
even a kinsman of his elder namesake, or be ever so little of the
same kidney, it is all up with you: he will become both accuser
and judge of you in his petulant spleen, will dissipate you in
jests, pulverize you with witticisms, and sacrifice you, I can
promise you, to the God of Mirth.

Again I warn you against cavilling, lest, while you calumniate
or disgracefully disparage Democritus Junior, who has no ani-
mosity against you, you should hear from some judicious friend

the very words the people of Abdera heard of old from Hippocrates, when they held their well-deserving and popular fellow-
citizen to be a madman: "Truly, it is you, Democritus, that are
wise, while the people of Abdera are fools and madmen." You
have no more sense than the people of Abdera. Having given
you this warning in a few words, O reader who employ your
leisure ill, farewell.]

HERACLITE, fleas, misero sic convenit ævo,
  Nil nisi turpe vides, nil nisi triste vides.
Ride etiam, quantumque lubet, Democrite, ride
  Non nisi vana vides, non nisi stulta vides.
Is fletu, hic risu modo gaudeat, unus utrique
  Sit licet usque labor, sit licet usque dolor.
Nunc opus est (nam totus eheu jam desipit orbis)
  Mille Heraclitis, milleque Democritis.
Nunc opus est (tanta est insania) transeat omnis
  Mundus in Anticyras, gramen in helleborum.

[WEEP, Heraclitus; here is food for tears
In this sad world of ours, where naught appears
  Save what is vile and full of bitterness.
Yet thou, Democritus, with equal right
At this same world mayest laugh with all thy might
  To see such dotage and such craziness.
With tears and laughter, each as seemed him best,
These two one aim pursued, one grief expressed.
They for their day sufficed; but since, mankind
Is grown to be more vicious and more blind,
And now had need that there should come to life
A thousand such; now madness is so rife
That to Anticyra all the world should pass,
And hellebore should sprout instead of grass.]

THE SYNOPSIS OF THE FIRST PARTITION

In diseases, consider,
Sect. 1,
Memb. 1,

Their causes. *Subs.* 1.
- Impulsive; Sin, concupiscence, etc.
- Instrumental; Intemperance, all second causes, etc.

Or

Definition, Member, Division. *Subs.* 2.

Of the body 300, which are
- Epidemical, as plague, plica, etc.
  - or
- Particular, as gout, dropsy, etc.

Or

Of the head or mind. *Subs.* 3.

In disposition; as all perturbations, evil affection, etc.

Or

Habits as *Subs.* 4.
- Dotage.
- Frenzy.
- Madness.
- Ecstasy.
- Lycanthropia.
- Chorus Sancti Viti.
- Hydrophobia.
- Possession or obsession of devils.
- Melancholy.   See Y.

Y
Melancholy; in which consider

Its Equivocations, in Disposition, Improper, etc.   *Subsect.* 5.

Memb. 2. To its explication, a digression of anatomy in which observe parts of *Subs.* 1.

Body hath parts *Subs.* 1.
- contained as
  - Humours, 4. Blood, phlegm, etc.
  - Spirits; vital, natural, animal.
- or
- containing
  - Similar; spermatical, or flesh, bones, nerves, etc. *Subs.* 3.
  - Dissimilar; brain, heart, liver, etc. *Subs.* 4.

Soul and its faculties, as
- Vegetal.   *Subs.* 5.
- Sensible.   *Subs.* 6, 7, 8.
- Rational.   *Subsect.* 9, 10, 11.

Memb. 3.

Its definition, name, difference, *Subs.* 1.

The part and parties affected, affection, etc.   *Subs.* 2.

The matter of melancholy, natural, unnatural, etc.   *Subs.* 4.

Species, or kinds, which are

Proper to parts, as
- Of the head alone, Hypochondriacal, or windy melancholy. Of the whole body.
  - with their several causes, symptoms, prognostics, cures.

Or

Indefinite; as love-melancholy, the subject of the third Partition.

Its causes in general.   *Sect.* 2, A.

Its symptoms or signs.   *Sect.* 3, B.

Its prognostics or indications.   *Sect.* 4, C.

Its cures; the subject of the second Partition.

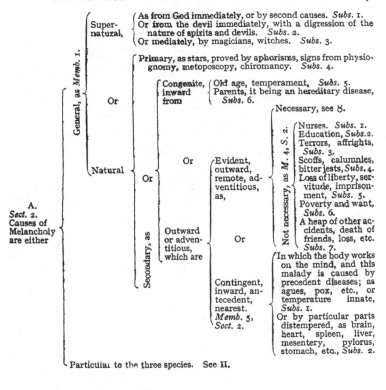

A. Sect. 2. Causes of Melancholy are either

General, as Memb. 1.

- Supernatural,
  - As from God immediately, or by second causes. *Subs.* 1.
  - Or from the devil immediately, with a digression of the nature of spirits and devils. *Subs.* 2.
  - Or mediately, by magicians, witches. *Subs.* 3.
- Or Natural
  - Primary, as stars, proved by aphorisms, signs from physiognomy, metoposcopy, chiromancy. *Subs.* 4.
  - Or Secondary, as
    - Or Congenite, inward from
      - Old age, temperament, *Subs.* 5.
      - Parents, it being an hereditary disease, *Subs.* 6.
    - Or Outward or adventitious, which are
      - Or Evident, outward, remote, adventitious, as,
        - Necessary, see 8.
        - Not necessary, as *M.* 4, *S.* 2.
          - Nurses. *Subs.* 1.
          - Education, *Subs.* 2.
          - Terrors, affrights, *Subs.* 3.
          - Scoffs, calumnies, bitter jests, *Subs.* 4.
          - Loss of liberty, servitude, imprisonment, *Subs.* 5.
          - Poverty and want, *Subs.* 6.
          - A heap of other accidents, death of friends, loss, etc. *Subs.* 7.
      - Or Contingent, inward, antecedent, nearest. *Memb.* 5, *Sect.* 2.
        - In which the body works on the mind, and this malady is caused by precedent diseases; as agues, pox, etc., or temperature innate, *Subs.* 1.
        - Or by particular parts distempered, as brain, heart, spleen, liver, mesentery, pylorus, stomach, etc., *Subs.* 2.

Particular to the three species. See II.

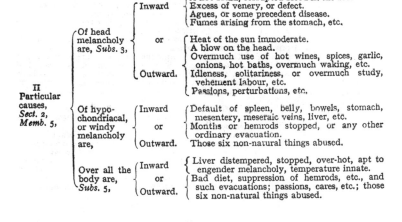

II Particular causes, *Sect.* 2, *Memb.* 5,

- Of head melancholy are, *Subs.* 3,
  - Inward
    - Innate humour, or from distemperature adust.
    - A hot brain, corrupted blood in the brain.
    - Excess of venery, or defect.
    - Agues, or some precedent disease.
    - Fumes arising from the stomach, etc.
  - or Outward.
    - Heat of the sun immoderate.
    - A blow on the head.
    - Overmuch use of hot wines, spices, garlic, onions, hot baths, overmuch waking, etc.
    - Idleness, solitariness, or overmuch study, vehement labour, etc.
    - Passions, perturbations, etc.
- Of hypochondriacal, or windy melancholy are,
  - Inward
    - Default of spleen, belly, bowels, stomach, mesentery, meseraic veins, liver, etc.
    - Months or hemrods stopped, or any other ordinary evacuation.
  - or Outward.
    - Those six non-natural things abused.
- Over all the body are, *Subs.* 5,
  - Inward
    - Liver distempered, stopped, over-hot, apt to engender melancholy, temperature innate.
  - or Outward.
    - Bad diet, suppression of hemrods, etc., and such evacuations; passions, cares, etc.; those six non-natural things abused.

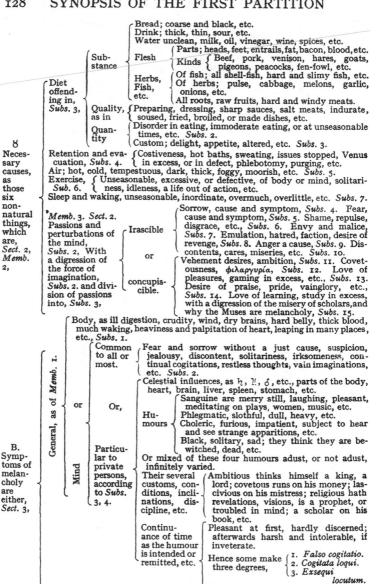

8 Necessary causes, as those six non-natural things, which are, *Sect. 2, Memb.* 2,

Diet offending in, *Subs.* 3,

Substance

Bread; coarse and black, etc.
Drink; thick, thin, sour, etc.
Water unclean, milk, oil, vinegar, wine, spices, etc.

Flesh
Parts; heads, feet, entrails, fat, bacon, blood, etc.
Kinds { Beef, pork, venison, hares, goats, pigeons, peacocks, fen-fowl, etc.

Herbs, Fish, etc.
Of fish; all shell-fish, hard and slimy fish, etc.
Of herbs; pulse, cabbage, melons, garlic, onions, etc.
All roots, raw fruits, hard and windy meats.

Quality, as in
Preparing, dressing, sharp sauces, salt meats, indurate, soused, fried, broiled, or made dishes, etc.

Quantity
Disorder in eating, immoderate eating, or at unseasonable times, etc. *Subs.* 2.
Custom; delight, appetite, altered, etc. *Subs.* 3.

Retention and evacuation, *Subs.* 4.
Costiveness, hot baths, sweating, issues stopped, Venus in excess, or in defect, phlebotomy, purging, etc.

Air; hot, cold, tempestuous, dark, thick, foggy, moorish, etc. *Subs.* 5.

Exercise, *Sub.* 6.
Unseasonable, excessive, or defective, of body or mind, solitariness, idleness, a life out of action, etc.

Sleep and waking, unseasonable, inordinate, overmuch, overlittle, etc. *Subs.* 7.

Memb. 3. *Sect.* 2. Passions and perturbations of the mind, *Subs.* 2, With a digression of the force of imagination, *Subs.* 2. and division of passions into, *Subs.* 3,

Irascible or concupiscible.

Sorrow, cause and symptom, *Subs.* 4. Fear, cause and symptom, *Subs.* 5. Shame, repulse, disgrace, etc., *Subs.* 6. Envy and malice, *Subs.* 7. Emulation, hatred, faction, desire of revenge, *Subs.* 8. Anger a cause, *Subs.* 9. Discontents, cares, miseries, etc. *Subs.* 10.

Vehement desires, ambition, *Subs.* 11. Covetousness, φιλαργυρία, *Subs.* 12. Love of pleasures, gaming in excess, etc., *Subs.* 13. Desire of praise, pride, vainglory, etc., *Subs.* 14. Love of learning, study in excess, with a digression of the misery of scholars, and why the Muses are melancholy, *Subs.* 15.

B. Symptoms of melancholy are either, *Sect.* 3,

General, as of *Memb.* 1.

Body, as ill digestion, crudity, wind, dry brains, hard belly, thick blood, much waking, heaviness and palpitation of heart, leaping in many places, etc., *Subs.* 1.

Mind
Common to all or most.
Fear and sorrow without a just cause, suspicion, jealousy, discontent, solitariness, irksomeness, continual cogitations, restless thoughts, vain imaginations, etc. *Subs.* 2.

Or,
Celestial influences, as ♄, ♃, ♂, etc., parts of the body, heart, brain, liver, spleen, stomach, etc.

Humours
Sanguine are merry still, laughing, pleasant, meditating on plays, women, music, etc.
Phlegmatic, slothful, dull, heavy, etc.
Choleric, furious, impatient, subject to hear and see strange apparitions, etc.
Black, solitary, sad; they think they are bewitched, dead, etc.
Or mixed of these four humours adust, or not adust, infinitely varied.

Particular to private persons, according to *Subs.* 3, 4.

Their several customs, conditions, inclinations, discipline, etc.
Ambitious thinks himself a king, a lord; covetous runs on his money; lascivious on his mistress; religious hath revelations, visions, is a prophet, or troubled in mind; a scholar on his book, etc.

Continuance of time as the humour is intended or remitted, etc.
Pleasant at first, hardly discerned; afterwards harsh and intolerable, if inveterate.

Hence some make three degrees,
1. *Falso cogitatio.*
2. *Cogitata loqui.*
3. *Exsequi locutum.*

By fits, or continuate, as the object varies, pleasing, or displeasing.

Simple, or as it is mixed with other diseases, apoplexies, gout, *caninus appetitus,* etc., so the symptoms are various.

Particular symptoms to the three distinct species. *Sect.* 3, *Memb.* 2.

Head melancholy. *Subs.* 1.

In body — Headache, binding and heaviness, vertigo, lightness, singing of the ears, much waking, fixed eyes, high colour, red eyes, hard belly, dry body; no great sign of melancholy in the other parts.

Or

In mind. — Continual fear, sorrow, suspicion, discontent, superfluous cares, solicitude, anxiety, perpetual cogitation of such toys they are possessed with, thoughts like dreams, etc.

Hypochondriacal, or windy melancholy. *Subs.* 2.

In body — Wind, rumbling in the guts, belly-ache, heat in the bowels, convulsions, crudities, short wind, sour and sharp belchings, cold sweat, pain in the left side, suffocation, palpitation, heaviness of the heart, singing in the ears, much spittle, and moist, etc

Or

In mind. — Fearful, sad, suspicious, discontent, anxiety, etc. Lascivious by reason of much wind, troublesome dreams, affected by fits, etc.

Over all the body. *Subs.* 3.

In body — Black, most part lean, broad veins, gross, thick blood, their hemrods commonly stopped, etc.

Or

In mind. — Fearful, sad, solitary, hate light, averse from company, fearful dreams, etc.

Symptoms of nuns', maids', and widows' melancholy, in body and mind, etc.

A reason of these symptoms. *Memb.* 3.

Why they are so fearful, sad, suspicious without a cause, why solitary, why melancholy men are witty, why they suppose they hear and see strange voices, visions, apparitions.

Why they prophesy, and speak strange languages; whence comes their crudity, rumbling, convulsions, cold sweat, heaviness of heart, palpitation, cardiaca, fearful dreams, much waking, prodigious fantasies.

C Prognostics of melancholy. *Sect.* 4.

Tending to good, as
- Morphew, scabs, itch, breaking out, etc.
- Black jaundice.
- If the hemrods voluntarily open.
- If varices appear.

Tending to evil, as
- Leanness, dryness, hollow-eyed, etc.
- Inveterate melancholy is incurable.
- If cold, it degenerates often into epilepsy, apoplexy, dotage, or into blindness.
- If hot, into madness, despair, and violent death.

Corollaries and questions
- The grievousness of this above all other diseases. The diseases of the mind are more grievous than those of the body.
- Whether it be lawful, in this case of melancholy, for a man to offer violence to himself. *Neg.*
- How a melancholy or mad man, offering violence to himself, is to be censured.

THE FIRST PARTITION

THE FIRST SECTION, MEMBER, SUBSECTION

Man's Excellency, Fall, Miseries, Infirmities; The causes of them

MAN, the most excellent and noble creature of the world, "the principal and mighty work of God, wonder of Nature," as Zoroaster calls him; *audacis naturæ miraculum* [Nature's boldest and most marvellous stroke], "the marvel of marvels," [1] as Plato; "the abridgment and epitome of the world," [2] as Pliny; *Microcosmus*, a little world, a model of the world, sovereign lord of the earth, viceroy of the world, sole commander and governor of all the creatures in it; [3] to whose empire they are subject in particular, and yield obedience; far surpassing all the rest, not in body only, but in soul; *Imaginis imago*, [4] created [5] to God's own image, [6] to that immortal and incorporeal substance, with all the faculties and powers belonging unto it; was at first pure, divine, perfect, happy, "created after God in true holiness and righteousness"; [7] *Deo congruens* [fitted for divinity], free from all manner of infirmities, and put in Paradise, to know God, to praise and glorify Him, to do His will, *Ut dis consimiles parturiat deos* [that being like the gods he may beget gods] (as an old poet saith) to propagate the Church.

But this most noble creature, *Heu tristis et lachrymosa commutatio* (one exclaims [8]), O pitiful change! is fallen from that he was, and forfeited his estate, become *miserabilis homuncio*, a castaway, a caitiff, one of the most miserable creatures of the world, if he be considered in his own nature, an unregenerate man, and so much obscured by his fall that (some few relics excepted) he is inferior to a beast; "Man in honour that understandeth not, is like unto beasts that perish," [9] so David esteems him: a monster by stupend metamorphoses, a fox, a dog, a hog, what not? [10] *Quantum mutatus ab illo!* How much altered from that he was! before blessed and happy, now miserable and accursed; "He must eat his meat in sorrow," [11] subject to death and all manner of

130

infirmities, all kind of calamities. "Great travail is created
for all men, and an heavy yoke on the sons of Adam, from the
day that they go out of their mother's womb, unto that day they
return to the mother of all things. Namely, their thoughts and
fear of their hearts, and their imagination of things they wait
for, and the day of death; from him that sitteth in the glorious
throne, to him that sitteth beneath in the earth and ashes;
from him that is clothed in blue silk and weareth a crown,
to him that is clothed in simple linen. Wrath, envy, trouble,
and unquietness, and fear of death, and rigour, and strife,
and such things come to both man and beast, but seven-
fold to the ungodly." [1] All this befalls him in this life, and
peradventure eternal misery in the life to come.

The impulsive cause of these miseries in man, this privation or
destruction of God's image; the cause of death and diseases, of
all temporal and eternal punishments, was the sin of our first
parent Adam, in eating of the forbidden fruit, by the devil's
instigation and allurement.[2] His disobedience, pride, ambition, intemperance, incredulity, curiosity; from whence proceeded original sin and that general corruption of mankind, as
from a fountain flowed all bad inclinations and actual transgressions, which cause our several calamities inflicted upon us
for our sins. And this, belike, is that which our fabulous poets
have shadowed unto us in the tale of Pandora's box, which, being
opened through her curiosity, filled the world full of all manner
of diseases.[3] It is not curiosity alone, but those other crying
sins of ours, which pull these several plagues and miseries upon
our heads. For *ubi peccatum, ibi procella* [where the sin is, there is
the storm], as Chrysostom well observes.[4] "Fools, by reason of
their transgression, and because of their iniquities, are afflicted." [5]
"Fear cometh like sudden desolation, and destruction like a
whirlwind, affliction and anguish," [6] because they did not
fear God. "Are you shaken with wars?" as Cyprian well urgeth
to Demetrius, "are you molested with dearth and famine? is
your health crushed with raging diseases? is mankind generally
tormented with epidemical maladies? 'tis all for your sins " [7]
(Hag. i, 9, 10; Amos i; Jer. vii). God is angry, punisheth and
threateneth, because of their obstinacy and stubbornness, they
will not turn unto Him. "If the earth be barren then for want
of rain, if, dry and squalid, it yield no fruit, if your fountains
be dried up, your wine, corn, and oil blasted, if the air be
corrupted, and men troubled with diseases, 'tis by reason of
their sins": [8] which like the blood of Abel cry loud to heaven

for vengeance. Lam. v, 15: "That we have sinned, therefore
our hearts are heavy." Is. lix, 11, 12: "We roar like bears,
and mourn like doves, and want health, etc., for our sins and
trespasses." But this we cannot endure to hear or to take
notice of (Jer. ii, 30): "We are smitten in vain and receive no
correction"; and (chap. v, 3): "Thou has stricken them, but they
have not sorrowed; they have refused to receive correction;
they have not returned." "Pestilence he hath sent, but they
have not turned to him" (Amos iv). Herod could not abide
John Baptist,[1] nor Domitian endure Apollonius to tell the
causes of the plague at Ephesus, his injustice, incest, adultery,
and the like.[2]

To punish therefore this blindness and obstinacy of ours as
a concomitant cause and principal agent, is God's just judgment in bringing these calamities upon us, to chastise us, I say,
for our sins, and to satisfy God's wrath. For the law requires
obedience or punishment, as you may read at large (Deut. xxviii,
15): "If they will not obey the Lord, and keep his commandments and ordinances, then all these curses shall come upon
them. Cursed in the town and in the field, etc.[3] Cursed in
the fruit of the body, etc.[4] The Lord shall send thee
trouble and shame, because of thy wickedness."[5] And a
little after, "The Lord shall smite thee with the botch of
Egypt, and with emrods, and scab, and itch, and thou canst
not be healed.[6] With madness, blindness, and astonishing of
heart."[7] This Paul seconds (Rom. ii, 9): "Tribulation and
anguish on the soul of every man that doth evil." Or else these
chastisements are inflicted upon us for our humiliation, to
exercise and try our patience here in this life, to bring us home,
to make us to know God ourselves, to inform and teach us
wisdom. "Therefore is my people gone into captivity, because
they had no knowledge; therefore is the wrath of the Lord
kindled against his people, and he hath stretched out his hand
upon them."[8] He is desirous of our salvation, *nostræ salutis
avidus*, saith Lemnius,[9] and for that cause pulls us by the ear
many times, to put us in mind of our duties: "That they which
erred might have understanding" (as Isaiah speaks, xxix, 24),
"and so to be reformed."[10] "I am afflicted, and at the point of
death," so David confesseth of himself (Ps. lxxxviii, 15, 9); "mine
eyes are sorrowful through mine affliction"; and that made
him turn unto God. Great Alexander in the midst of all his
prosperity, by a company of parasites deified, and now made
a god, when he saw one of his wounds bleed, remembered that

he was but a man, and remitted of his pride. *In morbo recolligit se animus*, as Pliny well perceived;[1] "In sickness the mind reflects upon itself, with judgment surveys itself, and abhors its former courses"; insomuch that he concludes to his friend Marius, "that it were the period of all philosophy, if we could so continue sound, or perform but a part of that which we promised to do, being sick."[2] "Whoso is wise, then, will consider these things," as David did (Ps. cvii, verse last); and whatsoever fortune befall him, make use of it. If he be in sorrow, need, sickness, or any other adversity, seriously to recount with himself, why this or that malady, misery, this or that incurable disease is inflicted upon him; it may be for his good, *sic expedit*,[3] as Peter said of his daughter's ague. Bodily sickness is for his soul's health, *periisset nisi periisset*, had he not been visited, he had utterly perished; for "the Lord correcteth him whom he loveth, even as a father doth his child in whom he delighteth."[4] If he be safe and sound on the other side, and free from all manner of infirmity; *et cui*

> *Gratia, forma, valetudo contingat abunde*
> *Et mundus victus, non deficiente crumena;*[5]

And that he have grace, beauty, favour, health,
A cleanly diet, and abound in wealth;

yet in the midst of his prosperity, let him remember that caveat of Moses, "Beware that he do not forget the Lord his God";[6] that he be not puffed up, but acknowledge them to be his good gifts and benefits, and "the more he hath, to be more thankful"[7] (as Agapetianus adviseth), and use them aright.

Now the instrumental causes of these our infirmities are as diverse as the infirmities themselves; stars, heavens, elements, etc., and all those creatures which God hath made, are armed against sinners. They were indeed once good in themselves, and that they are now many of them pernicious unto us, is not in their nature, but our corruption, which hath caused it. For, from the fall of our first parent Adam, they have been changed, the earth accursed, the influence of stars altered, the four elements, beasts, birds, plants, are now ready to offend us. "The principal things for the use of man, are water, fire, iron, salt, meal, wheat, honey, milk, oil, wine, clothing, good to the godly, to the sinners turned to evil" (Ecclus. xxxix, 26). "Fire, and hail, and famine, and dearth, all these are created for vengeance" (Ecclus. xxxix, 29).

The heavens threaten us with their comets, stars, planets, with their great conjunctions, eclipses, oppositions, quartiles, and such unfriendly aspects; the air with his meteors, thunder and lightning, intemperate heat and cold, mighty winds, tempests, unseasonable weather; from which proceed dearth, famine, plague, and all sorts of epidemical diseases, consuming infinite myriads of men. At Cairo in Egypt, every third year (as it is related by Boterus,[1] and others), 300,000 die of the plague; and 200,000 in Constantinople, every fifth or seventh at the utmost. How doth the earth terrify and oppress us with terrible earthquakes, which are most frequent in China, Japan, and those eastern climes,[2] swallowing up sometimes six cities at once! How doth the water rage with his inundations, irruptions, flinging down towns, cities, villages, bridges, etc., besides shipwrecks! whole islands are sometimes suddenly overwhelmed with all their inhabitants in Zealand,[3] Holland, and many parts of the continent drowned, as the Lake Erne in Ireland.[4] *Nihilque præter arcium cadavera patenti cernimus freto*[5] [we see nothing save the wreckage of cities upon the spreading waters]. In the fens of Friesland, 1230, by reason of tempests, the sea drowned *multa hominum millia, et jumenta sine numero*[6] [many thousands of human beings and cattle without number], all the country almost, men and cattle in it. How doth the fire rage, that merciless element, consuming in an instant whole cities! What town of any antiquity or note hath not been once, again and again, by the fury of this merciless element, defaced, ruinated, and left desolate? In a word,

> *Ignis pepercit, unda mergit, aeris*
> *Vis pestilentis æquori ereptum necat,*
> *Bello superstes, tabidus morbo perit.*[7]

Whom fire spares, sea doth drown; whom sea,
Pestilent air doth send to clay;
Whom war 'scapes, sickness takes away.

To descend to more particulars, how many creatures are at deadly feud with men! lions, wolves, bears, etc., some with hoofs, horns, tusks, teeth, nails. How many noxious serpents and venomous creatures, ready to offend us with stings, breath, sight, or quite kill us! How many pernicious fishes, plants, gums, fruits, seeds, flowers, etc., could I reckon up on a sudden, which by their very smell, many of them, touch, taste, cause some grievous malady, if not death itself! Some make mention of a thousand several poisons: but these are but trifles in respect. The greatest enemy to man is man, who by the devil's instiga-

tion is still ready to do mischief, his own executioner, a wolf,
a devil to himself and others.[1]   We are all brethren in Christ,
or at least should be, members of one body, servants of one
Lord, and yet no fiend can so torment, insult over, tyrannize,
vex, as one man doth another.   Let me not fall therefore (saith
David, when wars, plague, famine were offered) into the hands
of men, merciless and wicked men:

> *Vix sunt homines hoc nomine digni,*
> *Quamque lupi sævæ plus feritatis habent.*[2]

[Though men in shape, they scarce deserve the name;
Their savagery doth put the wolves to shame.]

We can most part foresee these epidemical diseases, and likely
avoid them.   Dearths, tempests, plagues, our astrologers foretell
us;   earthquakes, inundations, ruins of houses, consuming
fires, come by little and little, or make some noise beforehand;
but the knaveries, impostures, injuries, and villainies of men no
art can avoid.   We can keep our professed enemies from our
cities by gates, walls, and towers, defend ourselves from thieves
and robbers by watchfulness and weapons; but this malice of
men, and their pernicious endeavours, no caution can divert,
no vigilancy foresee, we have so many secret plots and devices
to mischief one another.

Sometimes by the devil's help, as magicians, witches; sometimes by impostures, mixtures,[3] poisons, stratagems, single
combats, wars, we hack and hew, as if we were *ad internecionem
nati*, like Cadmus' soldiers born to consume one another.   'Tis
an ordinary thing to read of an hundred and two hundred
thousand men slain in a battle; besides all manner of tortures,
brazen bulls, racks, wheels, strappadoes, guns, engines, etc.   *Ad
unum corpus humanum supplicia plura quam membra:* we
have invented more torturing instruments than there be several
members in a man's body, as Cyprian well observes.[4]   To come
nearer yet, our own parents by their offences, indiscretion, and
intemperance, are our mortal enemies.   "The fathers have eaten
sour grapes, and the children's teeth are set on edge." [5]   They
cause our grief many times, and put upon us hereditary diseases,
inevitable infirmities: they torment us, and we are ready to
injure our posterity:

> *mox daturi progeniem vitiosiorem,*[6]

[And yet with crimes to us unknown,
Our sons shall mark the coming age their own.]

and the latter end of the world, as Paul foretold,[7] is still like to

be the worst. We are thus bad by nature, bad by kind, but
far worse by art, every man the greatest enemy unto himself.
We study many times to undo ourselves, abusing those good
gifts which God hath bestowed upon us, health, wealth, strength,
wit, learning, art, memory to our own destruction: *Perditio tua
ex te* [1] [thy destruction is from thyself]. As Judas Maccabæus
killed Apollonius with his own weapons,[2] we arm ourselves to
our own overthrows; and use reason, art, judgment, all that
should help us, as so many instruments to undo us. Hector
gave Ajax a sword, which, so long as he fought against enemies,
served for his help and defence; but after he began to hurt
harmless creatures with it, turned to his own hurtless bowels.
Those excellent means God hath bestowed on us, well employed,
cannot but much avail us; but if otherwise perverted, they ruin
and confound us: and so by reason of our indiscretion and
weakness they commonly do, we have too many instances.
This St. Austin acknowledgeth of himself in his humble Confessions: "Promptness of wit, memory, eloquence, they were
God's good gifts, but he did not use them to His glory." If you
will particularly know how, and by what means, consult
physicians, and they will tell you that it is in offending in
some of those six non-natural things, of which I shall dilate
more at large;[3] they are the causes of our infirmities, our surfeiting and drunkenness, our immoderate, insatiable lust and
prodigious riot. *Plures crapula quam gladius* is a true saying,
the board consumes more than the sword. Our intemperance
it is that pulls so many several incurable diseases upon our
heads, that hastens old age,[4] perverts our temperature, and
brings upon us sudden death. And last of all, that which
crucifies us most, is our own folly, madness (*quos Jupiter perdit,
dementat;* by subtraction of His assisting grace God permits it),
weakness, want of government, our facility and proneness in
yielding to several lusts, in giving way to every passion and
perturbation of the mind: by which means we metamorphose
ourselves and degenerate into beasts. All which that prince of
poets [5] observed of Agamemnon, that when he was well pleased,
and could moderate his passion, he was *os oculosque Jovi par*:
like Jupiter in feature, Mars in valour, Pallas in wisdom, another
god; but when he became angry, he was a lion, a tiger, a dog,
etc., there appeared no sign or likeness of Jupiter in him; so
we, as long as we are ruled by reason, correct our inordinate
appetite, and conform ourselves to God's word, are as so many
saints: but if we give reins to lust, anger, ambition, pride, and

follow our own ways, we degenerate into beasts, transform ourselves, overthrow our constitutions, provoke God to anger,[1]
and heap upon us this of melancholy, and all kinds of incurable
diseases, as a just and deserved punishment of our sins.

SUBSECT. II.—*The Definition, Number, Division of Diseases*

What a disease is, almost every physician defines.   Fernelius
calleth it an "affection of the body contrary to nature";[2]
Fuchsius and Crato, "an hindrance, hurt, or alteration of any
action of the body, or part of it";[3]   Tholosanus, "a dissolution
of that league which is between body and soul, and a perturbation of it, as health [is] the perfection and makes to the preservation of it";[4]   Labeo, in A. Gellius, "an ill habit of the body,
opposite to nature, hindering the use of it";[5] others otherwise,
all to this effect.

How many diseases there are, is a question not yet determined; Pliny reckons up 300 from the crown of the head to the
sole of the foot:[6] elsewhere he saith, *morborum infinita multitudo,*
their number is infinite.   Howsoever it was in those times, it
boots not; in our days I am sure the number is much augmented:

> *Macies et nova febrium*
> *Terris incubuit cohors.*[7]

[New wasting maladies have swarmed upon mankind.]

For besides many epidemical diseases unheard of, and altogether
unknown to Galen and Hippocrates, as *scorbutum*, smallpox,
plica, sweating sickness, *morbus Gallicus*, etc., we have many
proper and peculiar almost to every part.

No man amongst us so sound, of so good a constitution,
that hath not some impediment of body or mind.   *Quisque
suos patimur manes*, we have all our infirmities, first or
last, more or less.   There will be peradventure in an age,
or one of a thousand, like Zenophilus the musician in Pliny,[8]
that may haply live 105 years without any manner of
impediment; a Pollio Romulus, that can preserve himself
"with wine and oil";[9] a man as fortunate as Q. Metellus,
of whom Valerius so much brags; a man as healthy as
Otto Herwardus, a senator of Augsburg in Germany, whom
Leovitius the astrologer brings in for an example and instance
of certainty in his art;[10] who, because he had the significators
in his geniture fortunate, and free from the hostile aspects of
Saturn and Mars, being a very old man, "could not remember

that ever he was sick." [1]   Paracelsus [2] may brag that he could
make a man live 400 years or more, if he might bring him up
from his infancy, and diet him as he list; and some physicians
hold, that there is no certain period of man's life; but it may
still by temperance and physic be prolonged.   We find in the
meantime, by common experience, that no man can escape,
but that of Hesiod is true: [3]

Πλείη μὲν γὰρ γαῖα κακῶν, πλείη δὲ θάλασσα,
Νοῦσοι δ' ἀνθρώποισιν ἐφ' ἡμέρῃ ἠδ' ἐπὶ νυκτὶ
Αὐτόματοι φοιτῶσι.

Th' earth 's full of maladies, and full the sea,
Which set upon us both by night and day.

If you require a more exact division of these ordinary diseases
which are incident to men, I refer you to physicians; [4] they
will tell you of acute and chronic, first and secondary, *lethales*,
salutares, errant, fixed, simple, compound, connexed, or conse-
quent, belonging to parts or the whole, in habit, or in disposition, etc.   My division at this time (as most befitting my
purpose) shall be into those of the body and mind.   For them
of the body, a brief catalogue of which Fuschius hath made
(*Institut. lib.* 3, *sect.* 1, *cap.* 11), I refer you to the voluminous
tomes of Galen, Aretæus, Rhasis, Avicenna, Alexander, Paulus,
Aetius, Gordonerius; and those exact neoterics, Savanarola,
Capivaccius, Donatus Altomarus, Hercules de Saxonia, Mercurialis, Victorius Faventinus, Wecker, Piso, etc., that have
methodically and elaborately written of them all.   Those of the
mind and head I will briefly handle, and apart.

Subsect. III.—*Division of the Diseases of the Head*

These diseases of the mind, forasmuch as they have their
chief seat and organs in the head, are commonly repeated
amongst the diseases of the head, which are divers, and vary
much according to their site.   For in the head, as there be
several parts, so there be divers grievances, which according
to that division of Heurnius [5] (which he takes out of Arculanus),
are inward or outward (to omit all others which pertain to eyes
and ears, nostrils, gums, teeth, mouth, palate, tongue, wesel,
chops, face, etc.) belonging properly to the brain, as baldness,
falling of hair, furfur, lice, etc.   Inward belonging to the skins
next to the brain, called *dura* and *pia mater*, as all headaches,
etc.,[6] or to the ventricles, cauls, kells, tunicles, creeks, and parts

of it, and their passions, as *caro*,[1] vertigo, incubus, apoplexy, falling sickness. The diseases of the nerves, cramps, stupor, convulsion, tremor, palsy; or belonging to the excrements of the brain, catarrhs, sneezing, rheums, distillations: or else those that pertain to the substance of the brain itself, in which are conceived frenzy, lethargy, melancholy, madness, weak memory, *sopor* or coma, *vigilia* [sleeplessness], and *vigil coma*.[2] Out of these again I will single such as properly belong to the phantasy, or imagination, or reason itself, which Laurentius[3] calls the diseases of the mind; and Hildesheim, *morbos imaginationis, aut rationis læsæ* [diseases of the imagination, or of injured reason], which are three or four in number, frenzy, madness, melancholy, dotage, and their kinds: as hydrophobia, lycanthropia, *chorus Sancti Viti, morbi dæmoniaci* [St. Vitus's dance, possession of devils], which I will briefly touch and point at, insisting especially in this of melancholy, as more eminent than the rest, and that through all his kinds, causes, symptoms, prognostics, cures: as Lonicerus hath done *de apoplexia*, and many other of such particular diseases. Not that I find fault with those which have written of this subject before, as Jason Pratensis, Laurentius, Montaltus, T. Bright, etc., they have done very well in their several kinds and methods; yet that which one omits, another may haply see; that which one contracts, another may enlarge. To conclude with Scribanius,[4] "that which they had neglected, or perfunctorily handled, we may more thoroughly examine; that which is obscurely delivered in them, may be perspicuously dilated and amplified by us," and so made more familiar and easy for every man's capacity, and the common good, which is the chief end of my discourse.

SUBSECT. IV.—*Dotage, Madness, Frenzy, Hydrophobia, Lycanthropia, Chorus Sancti Viti, Ecstasis*

Dotage, fatuity, or folly, is a common name to all the following species, as some will have it. Laurentius[5] and Altomarus[6] comprehended madness, melancholy, and the rest under this name, and call it the *summum genus* of them all. If it be distinguished from them, it is natural or ingenite, which comes by some defect of the organs, and overmuch brain, as we see in our common fools; and is for the most part intended or remitted in particular men, and thereupon some are wiser than others: or else it is acquisite, an appendix

or symptom of some other disease, which comes or goes; or if it
continue, a sign of melancholy itself.

Phrenitis, which the Greeks derive from the word φρήν,
is a disease of the mind, with a continual madness or dotage,
which hath an acute fever annexed, or else an inflammation of the brain, or the membranes or kells of it, with an
acute fever, which causeth madness and dotage.   It differs
from melancholy and madness, because their dotage is without
an ague: this continual, with waking, or memory decayed, etc.
Melancholy is most part silent, this clamorous; and many such-
like differences are assigned by physicians.

Madness, frenzy, and melancholy are confounded by
Celsus, and many writers; others leave out frenzy, and
make madness and melancholy but one disease, which
Jason Pratensis [1] especially labours, and that they differ only
secundum majus or *minus,* in quantity alone, the one being a
degree to the other, and both proceeding from one cause.   They
differ *intenso et remisso gradu,* saith Gordonius,[2] as the humour is
intended or remitted.   Of the same mind is Aretæus,[3] Alexander
Trallianus, Guianerius, Savonarola, Heurnius;   and   Galen
himself writes promiscuously of them both by reason of their
affinity: but most of our neoterics do handle them apart, whom
I will follow in this treatise.   Madness is therefore defined to
be a vehement dotage, or raving without a fever, far more violent
than melancholy, full of anger and clamour, horrible looks,
actions, gestures, troubling the patients with far greater vehemency both of body and mind, without all fear and sorrow, with
such impetuous force and boldness that sometimes three or
four men cannot hold them.   Differing only in this from frenzy,
that it is without a fever, and their memory is most part better.
It hath the same causes as the other, as choler adust, and blood
incensed, brains inflamed, etc.   Fracastorius adds a due
time and full age to this definition, to distinguish it from
children, and will have it confirmed impotency, to separate it
from such as accidentally come and go again, as by taking henbane, nightshade, wine, etc.[4]   Of this fury there be divers
kinds: ecstasy, which is familiar with some persons, [5] as Cardan
saith of himself, he could be in one when he list; in which the
Indian priests deliver their oracles, and the witches in Lapland,
as Olaus Magnus writeth (*lib.* 3, *cap.* 18), *ecstasi omnia prædicere,*
answer all questions in an ecstasy you will ask; as what your
friends do, where they are, how they fare, etc.   The other species
of this fury are enthusiasms, revelations, and visions, so often

mentioned by Gregory and Beda in their works; obsession or possession of devils, sibylline prophets, and poetical furies; such as come by eating noxious herbs, tarantulas stinging, etc., which some reduce to this. The most known are these: lycanthropia, hydrophobia, *chorus Sancti Viti*.

Lycanthropia, which Avicenna calls *cucubuth*, others *lupinam insaniam*, or wolf-madness, when men run howling about graves and fields in the night, and will not be persuaded but that they are wolves, or some such beasts. Aetius [1] and Paulus [2] call it a kind of melancholy; but I should rather refer it to madness as most do. Some make a doubt of it whether there be any such disease. Donat. ab Altomari saith that he saw two of them in his time.[3] Wierus tells a story of such a one at Padua 1541,[4] that would not believe to the contrary but that he was a wolf. He hath another instance of a Spaniard, who thought himself a bear. Forestus confirms as much by many examples; [5] one amongst the rest of which he was an eye-witness at Alcmaar in Holland, a poor husbandman that still hunted about graves, and kept in churchyards, of a pale, black, ugly, and fearful look. Such belike, or little better, were King Prœtus' daughters, that thought themselves kine.[6] And Nebuchadnezzar in Daniel, as some interpreters hold, was only troubled with this kind of madness. This disease perhaps gave occasion to that bold assertion of Pliny, "some men were turned into wolves in his time, and from wolves to men again"; [7] and to that fable of Pausanias, of a man that was ten years a wolf and afterwards turned to his former shape; to Ovid's tale of Lycaon,[8] etc. He that is desirous to hear of this disease, or more examples, let him read Austin in his 18th book *de Civitate Dei, cap.* 5; Mizaldus, *cent.* 5, 77; Sckenkius, *lib.* 1; Hildesheim, *Spicil.* 2, *de mania*; Forrestus, *lib.* 10, *de morbis cerebri*; Olaus Magnus; Vincentius Bellovacensis, *Spec. nat. lib.* 31, *cap.* 122; Pierius, Bodine, Zuinger, Zeilger, Peucer, Wierus, Sprenger, etc. This malady, said Avicenna, troubleth men most in February, and is nowadays frequent in Bohemia and Hungary, according to Hcurnius.[9] Scheretzius will have it common in Livonia. They lie hid most part all day, and go abroad in the night, howling at graves and deserts; "they have usually hollow eyes, scabbed legs and thighs, very dry and pale," [10] saith Altomarus; [11] he gives a reason there of all the symptoms, and sets down a brief cure of them.

Hydrophobia is a kind of madness, well known in every village, which comes by the biting of a mad dog, or scratching,

saith Aurelianus;[1] touching or smelling alone sometimes, as
Sckenkius proves,[2] and is incident to many other creatures as
well as men: so called because the parties affected cannot endure
the sight of water, or any liquor, supposing still they see a mad
dog in it. And which is more wonderful, though they be very
dry (as in this malady they are), they will rather die than
drink. Cælius Aurelianus,[3] an ancient writer, makes a doubt
whether this hydrophobia be a passion of the body or the mind.
The part affected is the brain: the cause, poison that comes from
the mad dog, which is so hot and dry that it consumes all the
moisture in the body. Hildesheim[4] relates of some that died
so mad; and being cut up, had no water, scarce blood, or any
moisture left in them. To such as are so affected, the fear of
water begins at fourteen days after they are bitten, to some
again not till forty or sixty days after: commonly, saith Heurnius, they begin to rave, fly water and glasses, to look red and
swell in the face, about twenty days after (if some remedy be
not taken in the meantime) to lie awake, to be pensive, sad, to
see strange visions, to bark and howl, to fall into a swoon, and
oftentimes fits of the falling sickness. Some say, little things
like whelps will be seen in their urines.[5] If any of these signs
appear, they are past recovery. Many times these symptoms will
not appear till six or seven months after, saith Codronchus;[6] and
sometimes not till seven or eight years, as Guianerius; twelve
as Albertus; six or eight months after, as Galen holds. Baldus
the great lawyer died of it: an Augustine friar and a woman in
Delft, that were Forestus' patients,[7] were miserably consumed
with it. The common cure in the country (for such at least as
dwell near the seaside) is to duck them over head and ears
in sea-water; some use charms: every goodwife can prescribe
medicines. But the best cure to be had in such cases is from the
most approved physicians; they that will read of them may
consult with Dioscorides, *lib.* 6, *cap.* 37, Heurnius, Hildesheim,
Capivaccius, Forestus, Sckenkius, and before all others
Codronchus, an Italian, who hath lately written two exquisite
books on the subject.

Chorus Sancti Viti, or St. Vitus' dance; the lascivious dance,
Paracelsus calls it,[8] because they that are taken from it can do
nothing but dance till they be dead or cured. It is so called,
for that the parties so troubled were wont to go to St. Vitus for
help, and after they had danced there awhile, they were certainly freed.[9] 'Tis strange to hear how long they will dance,
and in what manner, over stools, forms, tables; even great-

bellied women sometimes (and yet never hurt their children) will dance so long that they can stir neither hand nor foot, but seem to be quite dead. One in red clothes they cannot abide. Music above all things they love, and therefore magistrates in Germany will hire musicians to play to them, and some lusty sturdy companions to dance with them. This disease hath been very common in Germany, as appears by those relations of Sckenkius,[1] and Paracelsus in his book of Madness, who brags how many several persons he hath cured of it. Felix Platerus, *de mentis alienat. cap.* 3, reports of a woman in Basil whom he saw, that danced a whole month together. The Arabians call it a kind of palsy. Bodine, in his 5th book *de Repub. cap.* 1, speaks of this infirmity; Monavius in his last epistle to Scoltzius, and in another to Dudithus, where you may read more of it.

The last kind of madness or melancholy, is that demoniacal (if I may so call it) obsession or possession of devils, which Platerus and others would have to be preternatural: stupend things are said of them, their actions, gestures, contortions, fasting, prophesying, speaking languages they were never taught, etc. Many strange stories are related of them, which because some will not allow (for Deacon and Darrel have written large volumes on this subject pro and con) I voluntarily omit.

Fuchsius, *Institut. lib.* 3, *sec.* 1, *cap.* 11, Felix Plater,[2] Laurentius,[3] add to these another fury that proceeds from love, and another from study, another divine or religious fury; but these more properly belong to melancholy; of all which I will speak apart,[4] intending to write a whole book of them.

SUBSECT. V.—*Melancholy in Disposition, improperly so called. Equivocations*

Melancholy, the subject of our present discourse, is either in disposition or habit. In disposition, is that transitory melancholy which goes and comes upon every small occasion of sorrow, need, sickness, trouble, fear, grief, passion, or perturbation of the mind, any manner of care, discontent, or thought, which causeth anguish, dullness, heaviness, and vexation of spirit, any ways opposite to pleasure, mirth, joy, delight, causing frowardness in us, or a dislike. In which equivocal and improper sense, we call him melancholy that is dull, sad, sour, lumpish, ill-disposed, solitary, anyway moved or displeased. And from these melancholy dispositions, no man living is free, no Stoic, none so wise, none so happy, none so patient,

so generous, so godly, so divine, that can vindicate himself; [1]
so well composed, but more or less, some time or other, he feels
the smart of it.   Melancholy in this sense is the character of
mortality.   "Man that is born of a woman, is of short continuance, and full of trouble." [2]   Zeno, Cato, Socrates himself,
whom Ælian so highly commends for a moderate temper, that
"nothing could disturb him, but going out, and coming in, still
Socrates képt the same serenity of countenance, what misery
soever befell him," [3] (if we may believe Plato his disciple) was
much tormented with it.   Q. Metellus, in whom Valerius gives
instance of all happiness, "the most fortunate man then living,
born in that most flourishing city of Rome, of noble parentage,
a proper man of person, well qualified, healthful, rich, honourable, a senator, a consul, happy in his wife, happy in his children,"
etc., [4] yet this man was not void of melancholy, he had his
share of sorrow.   Polycrates Samius, [5] that flung his ring into
the sea, because he would participate of discontent with others,
and had it miraculously restored to him again shortly after, by
a fish taken as he angled, was not free from melancholy dispositions.   No man can cure himself; the very gods had bitter
pangs, and frequent passions, as their own poets put upon them. [6]
In general, "as the heaven, so is our life, sometimes fair,
sometimes overcast, tempestuous and serene; as in a
rose, flowers and prickles; in the year itself, a temperate
summer sometimes, a hard winter, a drouth, and then again
pleasant showers: so is our life intermixed with joys, hopes,
fears, sorrows, calumnies." [7]   *Invicem cedunt dolor et voluptas*,
there is a succession of pleasure and pain.

Medio de fonte leporum,
Surgit amari aliquid quod in ipsis floribus angat. [8]

[From out the very fountain of delight,
Rises some gall, our merriment to blight.]

"Even in the midst of laughing there is sorrow" (as Solomon
holds [9]): even in the midst of all our feasting and jollity, as
Austin infers in his Com. on the Forty-first Psalm, [10] there is
grief and discontent.   *Inter delicias semper aliquid sævi nos*
strangulat [in the midst of our enjoyment something harsh
chokes us]; for a pint of honey thou shalt here likely find a
gallon of gall, for a dram of pleasure a pound of pain, for an
inch of mirth an ell of moan; as ivy doth an oak, these miseries
encompass our life, and 'tis most absurd and ridiculous for
any mortal man to look for a perpetual tenor of happiness in

his life. Nothing so prosperous and pleasant, but it hath some
bitterness in it, some complaining, some grudging;[1] it is all
γλυκύπικρον [bitter-sweet], a mixed passion, and like a chequer-
table, black and white men; families, cities, have their falls and
wanes, now trines, sextiles, then quartiles and oppositions. We
are not here as those angels, celestial powers and bodies, sun
and moon, to finish our course without all offence, with such
constancy, to continue for so many ages: but subject to
infirmities, miseries, interrupt, tossed and tumbled up and
down, carried about with every small blast, often molested and
disquieted upon each slender occasion, uncertain, brittle, and so
is all that we trust unto.[2] "And he that knows not this is not
armed to endure it, is not fit to live in this world" (as one condoles
our time), "he knows not the condition of it, where with a
reciprocal tie pleasure and pain are still united, and succeed
one another in a ring."[3] *Exi e mundo*, get thee gone hence,
if thou canst not brook it; there is no way to avoid it, but to
arm thyself with patience, with magnanimity,[4] to oppose thyself
unto it, to suffer affliction as a good soldier of Christ, as Paul
adviseth,[5] constantly to bear it.   But forasmuch as so few can
embrace this good counsel of his, or use it aright, but rather as
so many brute beasts give a way to their passion, voluntarily
subject and precipitate themselves into a labyrinth of cares,
woes, miseries, and suffer their souls to be overcome by them,
cannot arm themselves with that patience as they ought to do,
it falleth out oftentimes that these dispositions become habits, and
"many affects contemned" (as Seneca notes [6]) "make a disease."
Even as "one distillation, not yet grown to custom, makes
a cough, but continual and inveterate causeth a consumption of
the lungs"; so do these our melancholy provocations: and
according as the humour itself is intended or remitted in men,
as their temperature of body, or rational soul, is better able to
make resistance; so are they more or less affected. For that
which is but a flea-biting to one, causeth insufferable torment
to another; and which one by his singular moderation and well-
composed carriage can happily overcome, a second is no whit
able to sustain, but upon every small occasion of misconceived
abuse, injury, grief, disgrace, loss, cross, rumour, etc. (if solitary
or idle), yields so far to passion, that his complexion is altered,
his digestion hindered, his sleep gone, his spirits obscured, and
his heart heavy, his hypochondries misaffected; wind, crudity
on a sudden overtake him, and he himself overcome with
melancholy. As it is with a man imprisoned for debt, if once

in the jail, every creditor will bring his action against him, and there likely hold him; if any discontent seize upon a patient, in an instant all other perturbations (for *qua data porta ruunt* [they rush out wherever there is an opening]) will set upon him, and then like a lame dog or broken-winged goose he droops and pines away, and is brought at last to that ill habit or malady of melancholy itself. So that as the philosophers make eight degrees of heat and cold,[1] we may make eighty-eight of melancholy, as the parts affected are diversely seized with it, or have been plunged more or less into this infernal gulf, or waded deeper into it. But all these melancholy fits, howsoever pleasing at first, or displeasing, violent and tyrannizing over those whom they seize on for the time; yet these fits I say, or men affected, are but improperly so called, because they continue not, but come and go, as by some objects they are moved.[2] This melancholy of which we are to treat, is a habit, *morbus sonticus* or *chronicus*, a chronic or continuate disease, a settled humour, as Aurelianus [3] and others [4] call it, not errant, but fixed; and as it was long increasing, so now being (pleasant, or painful) grown to an habit, it will hardly be removed.

SECT. I. MEMB. II.

Subsect. I.—*Digression of Anatomy*

Before I proceed to define the disease of melancholy, what it is, or to discourse further of it, I hold it not impertinent to make a brief digression of the anatomy of the body and faculties of the soul, for the better understanding of that which is to follow; because many hard words will often occur, as myrach, hypocondries, hemrods, etc., imagination, reason, humours, spirits, vital, natural, animal, nerves, veins, arteries, chylus, pituita; which by the vulgar will not so easily be perceived, what they are, how cited, and to what end they serve. And besides, it may peradventure give occasion to some men to examine more accurately, search farther into this most excellent subject, and thereupon with that royal prophet to praise God ("for a man is fearfully and wonderfully made, and curiously wrought"[5]), that have time and leisure enough, and are sufficiently informed in all other worldly businesses as to make a good bargain, buy and sell, to keep and make choice of a fair hawk, hound, horse, etc. But for such matters as concern the knowledge of themselves, they are wholly ignorant and careless; they know not what this body and soul are, how combined, of what parts and faculties they consist, or how a man differs from a dog. And what can be more ignominious and filthy (as Melancthon well inveighs[1]) "than for a man not to know the structure and composition of his own body, especially since the knowledge of it tends so much to the preservation of his health and information of his manners?" To stir them up therefore to this study, to peruse those elaborate works of Galen,[2] Bauhinus, Plater, Vesalius, Fallopius, Laurentius, Remelinus, etc., which have written copiously in Latin; or that which some of our industrious countrymen have done in our mother tongue, not long since, as that translation of Columbus,[3] and *Microcosmographia*,[4] in thirteen books, I have made this brief digression. Also because Wecker,[5] Melancthon,[6] Fernelius,[7] Fuchsius,[8] and those tedious tracts *de Anima* (which have more compendiously handled and written of this matter) are not at all times ready to be had, to give them some small taste, or notice of the rest, let this epitome suffice.

SUBSECT. II.—*Division of the Body, Humours, Spirits*

Of the parts of the body there may be many divisions: the most approved is that of Laurentius,[9] out of Hippocrates: which is, into parts contained, or containing. Contained, are either humours or spirits.

A humour is a liquid or fluent part of the body, comprehended in it, for the preservation of it; and is either innate or born with us, or adventitious and acquisite. The radical or innate is daily supplied by nourishment, which some call cambium, and make those secondary humours of ros and gluten to maintain it: or acquisite, to maintain these four first primary humours, coming and proceeding from the first concoction in the liver, by which means chylus is excluded. Some divide them into profitable and excrementitious. But Crato,[10] out of Hippocrates, will have all four to be juice, and not excrements, without which no living creature can be sustained: which four, though they be comprehended in the mass of blood, yet they have their several affections, by which they are distinguished from one another, and from those adventitious, peccant, or diseased humours, as Melancthon calls them.[11]

Blood is a hot, sweet, temperate, red humour, prepared in the meseraic veins, and made of the most temperate parts of the chylus in the liver, whose office is to nourish the whole body, to give it strength and colour, being dispersed by the veins through every part of it. And from it spirits are first begotten in the heart, which afterwards by the arteries are communicated to the other parts.

Pituita, or phlegm, is a cold and moist humour, begotten of the colder part of the chylus (or white juice coming out of the meat digested in the stomach), in the liver; his office is to nourish and moisten the members of the body which, as the tongue, are moved, that they be not over-dry.

Choler is hot and dry, bitter, begotten of the hotter parts of the chylus, and gathered to the gall: it helps the natural heat and senses, and serves to the expelling of excrements.

Melancholy, cold and dry, thick, black, and sour, begotten of the more feculent part of nourishment, and purged from the spleen, is a bridle to the other two hot humours, blood and choler, preserving them in the blood, and nourishing the bones. These four humours have some analogy with the four elements, and to the four ages in man.

To these humours you may add serum, which is the matter of urine, and those excrementitious humours of the third concoction, sweat and tears.

Spirit is a most subtle vapour, which is expressed from the blood, and the instrument of the soul, to perform all his actions; a common tie or medium between the body and the soul, as some will have it; or as Paracelsus, a fourth soul of itself.[1] Melancthon holds the fountain of these spirits to be the heart, begotten there; and afterward conveyed to the brain, they take another nature to them. Of these spirits there be three kinds, according to the three principal parts, brain, heart, liver; natural, vital, animal. The natural are begotten in the liver, and thence dispersed through the veins, to perform those natural actions. The vital spirits are made in the heart of the natural, which by the arteries are transported to all the other parts: if the spirits cease, then life ceaseth, as in a syncope or swooning. The animal spirits, formed of the vital, brought up to the brain, and diffused by the nerves to the subordinate members, give sense and motion to them all.

SUBSECT. III.—*Similar Parts*

Containing parts, by reason of their more solid substance, are either homogeneal or heterogeneal, similar or dissimilar;

so Aristotle divides them, *lib.* 1, *cap.* 1, *de hist. animal.*;
Laurentius, *cap.* 20, *lib.* 1. Similar, or homogeneal, are such
as, if they be divided, are still severed into parts of the same
nature, as water into water. Of these some be spermatical,
some fleshy or carnal. Spermatical are such as are immediately
begotten of the seed, which are bones, gristles, ligaments,
membranes, nerves, arteries, veins, skins, fibres or strings, fat.[1]

The bones are dry and hard, begotten of the thickest
of the seed, to strengthen and sustain other parts: some say
there be 304, some 307, or 313 in man's body. They have
no nerves in them, and are therefore without sense.

A gristle is a substance softer than bone, and harder than the
rest, flexible, and serves to maintain the parts of motion.

Ligaments are they that tie the bones together, and other
parts to the bones, with their subserving tendons. Membranes'
office is to cover the rest.

Nerves, or sinews, are membranes without, and full of marrow
within; they proceed from the brain, and carry the animal
spirits for sense and motion. Of these some be harder, some
softer; the softer serve the senses, and there be seven pair of
them. The first be the optic nerves, by which we see; the
second move the eyes; the third pair serve for the tongue to
taste; the fourth pair for the taste in the palate; the fifth belong
to the ears; the sixth pair is most ample, and runs almost over
all the bowels; the seventh pair moves the tongue. The harder
sinews serve for the motion of the inner parts, proceeding from
the marrow in the back, of whom there be thirty combinations,
seven of the neck, twelve of the breast, etc.

Arteries are long and hollow, with a double skin to
convey the vital spirits; to discern which the better, they say
that Vesalius the anatomist was wont to cut up men alive.
They arise in the left side of the heart, and are principally two,
from which the rest are derived, aorta and venosa:[2] aorta is
the root of all the other, which serve the whole body; the other
goes to the lungs, to fetch air to refrigerate the heart.

Veins are hollow and round, like pipes, arising from the
liver, carrying blood and natural spirits; they feed all the
parts. Of these there be two chief, *vena porta* and *vena cava*,
from which the rest are corrivated. That *vena porta* is a vein
coming from the concave of the liver, and receiving those
meseraical veins, by whom he takes the chylus from the stomach
and guts, and conveys it to the liver. The other derives blood
from the liver to nourish all the other dispersed members. The

branches of that *vena porta* are the meseraical and hæmorrhoids. The branches of the *cava* are inward or outward. Inward, seminal or emulgent. Outward, in the head, arms, feet, etc., and have several names.

Fibræ are strings, white and solid, dispersed through the whole member, and right, oblique, transverse, all which have their several uses. Fat is a similar part, moist, without blood, composed of the most thick and unctuous matter of the blood. The skin covers the rest, and hath *cuticulam*, or a little skin, under it.[1] Flesh is soft and ruddy, composed of the congealing of blood, etc.

SUBSECT. IV.—*Dissimilar Parts*

Dissimilar parts are those which we call organical or instrumental, and they be inward or outward. The chiefest outward parts are situate forward or backward: forward, the crown and foretop of the head, skull, face, forehead, temples, chin, eyes, ears, nose, etc., neck, breast, chest, upper and lower part of the belly, hypochondries, navel, groin, flank, etc.; backward, the hinder part of the head, back, shoulders, sides, loins, hipbones, *os sacrum*, buttocks, etc. Or joints, arms, hands, feet, legs, thighs, knees, etc. Or common to both, which, because they are obvious and well known, I have carelessly repeated, *eaque præcipua et grandiora tantum; quod reliquum ex libris de anima qui volet, accipiat* [and then only the larger and more important; the rest can be found in books on anatomy].

Inward organical parts, which cannot be seen, are divers in number, and have several names, functions, and divisions; but that of Laurentius is most notable, into noble or ignoble parts.[2] Of the noble there be three principal parts, to which all the rest belong, and whom they serve—brain, heart, liver; according to whose site, three regions, or a threefold division, is made of the whole body. As first of the head, in which the animal organs are contained, and brain itself, which by his nerves gives sense and motion to the rest, and is, as it were, a privy counsellor and chancellor to the heart. The second region is the chest, or middle belly, in which the heart as king keeps his court, and by his arteries communicates life to the whole body. The third region is the lower belly, in which the liver resides as a legate *a latere*, with the rest of those natural organs, serving for concoction, nourishment, expelling of excrements. This lower region is distinguished from the upper by the midriff, or

diaphragma, and is subdivided again by some[1] into three concavities or regions, upper, middle, and lower.   The upper of
the hypochondries, in whose right side is the liver, the left the
spleen; from which is denominated hypochondriacal melancholy.
The second of the navel and flanks, divided from the first by
the rim.   The last of the watercourse, which is again subdivided
into three other parts.   The Arabians make two parts of this
region, epigastrium and hypogastrium, upper or lower.   Epigastrium they call *myrach*, from whence comes *myrachialis melancholia*, sometimes mentioned of them.   Of these several regions
I will treat in brief apart; and first of the third region, in which
the natural organs are contained.

But you that are readers, in the meantime "suppose you were
now brought into some sacred temple, or majestical palace" (as
Melancthon saith), "to behold not the matter only, but the
singular art, workmanship, and counsel of this our great Creator.
And 'tis a pleasant and profitable speculation, if it be considered
aright." [2]   The parts of this region, which present themselves
to your consideration and view, are such as serve to nutrition
or generation.   Those of nutrition serve to the first or second
concoction; as the œsophagus or gullet, which brings meat and
drink into the stomach.   The ventricle or stomach, which is
seated in the midst of that part of the belly beneath the midriff,
the kitchen, as it were, of the first concoction, and which turns
our meat into chylus.   It hath two mouths, one above, another
beneath   The upper is sometimes taken for the stomach itself;
the lower and nether door (as Wooker calls it) is named pylorus.
This stomach is sustained by a large kell or caul, called omen-
tum; which some will have the same with peritoneum, or rim of
the belly.   From the stomach to the very fundament are produced the guts, or intestina, which serve a little to alter and
distribute the chylus and convey away the excrements.   They
are divided into small and great, by reason of their site and
substance, slender or thicker: the slender is duodenum, or whole
gut, which is next to the stomach, some twelve inches long,
saith Fuchsius.[3]   Jejunum, or empty gut, continuate to the
other, which hath many meseraic veins annexed to it, which
take part of the chylus to the liver from it.   Ilion, the third,
which consists of many crinkles, which serves with the rest to
receive, keep, and distribute the chylus from the stomach..
The thick guts are three, the blind gut, colon, and right gut.
The blind is a thick and short gut, having one mouth, in which
the ilion and colon meet: it receives the excrements, and conveys

them to the colon. This colon hath many windings, that the
excrements pass not away too fast: the right gut is straight,
and conveys the excrements to the fundament, whose lower part
is bound up with certain muscles called sphincters, that the
excrements may be the better contained, until such time as a
man be willing to go to the stool. In the midst of these guts is
situated the mesenterium or midriff, composed of many veins,
arteries, and much fat, serving chiefly to sustain the guts. All
these parts serve the first concoction. To the second, which
is busied either in refining the good nourishment or expelling
the bad, is chiefly belonging the liver, like in colour to con-
gealed blood, the shop of blood, situate in the right hypochondry,
in figure like to a half-moon—*generosum membrum*, Melancthon
styles it, a generous part; it serves to turn the chylus to blood,
for the nourishment of the body. The excrements of it are
either choleric or watery, which the other subordinate parts
convey. The gall, placed in the concave of the liver, extracts
choler to it: the spleen, melancholy; which is situate on the left
side, over against the liver, a spongy matter, that draws this
black choler to it by a secret virtue, and feeds upon it, conveying
the rest to the bottom of the stomach, to stir up appetite, or
else to the guts as an excrement. That watery matter the two
kidneys expurgate by those emulgent veins and ureters. The
emulgent draw this superfluous moisture from the blood; the
two ureters convey it to the bladder, which, by reason of his
site in the lower belly, is apt to receive it, having two parts,
neck and bottom: the bottom holds the water, the neck is
constringed with a muscle, which, as a porter, keeps the water
from running out against our will.

Members of generation are common to both sexes, or peculiar
to one; which, because they are impertinent to my purpose,
I do voluntarily omit.

Next in order is the middle region, or chest, which comprehends the vital faculties and parts; which (as I have said) is
separated from the lower belly by the diaphragma or midriff,
which is a skin consisting of many nerves, membranes; and
amongst other uses it hath, is the instrument of laughing.
There is also a certain thin membrane, full of sinews, which
covereth the whole chest within, and is called pleura, the seat
of the disease called pleurisy, when it is inflamed; some add a
third skin, which is termed mediastinus, which divides the chest
into two parts, right and left. Of this region the principal part
is the heart, which is the seat and fountain of life, of heat, of

spirits, of pulse and respiration, the sun of our body, the king and sole commander of it, the seat and organ of all passions and affections. *Primum vivens, ultimum moriens*, it lives first and dies last in all creatures. Of a pyramidical form, and not much unlike to a pineapple; a part worthy of admiration, that can yield such variety of affections, by whose motion it is dilated or contracted, to stir and command the humours in the body:[1] as in sorrow, melancholy; in anger, choler; in joy, to send the blood outwardly; in sorrow, to call it in; moving the humours as horses do a chariot. This heart, though it be one sole member, yet it may be divided into two creeks right and left. The right is like the moon increasing, bigger than the other part, and receives blood from *vena cava*, distributing some of it to the lungs to nourish them; the rest to the left side, to engender spirits. The left creek hath the form of a cone, and is the seat of life, which, as a torch doth oil, draws blood unto it, begetting of it spirits and fire; and as fire in a torch, so are spirits in the blood; and by that great artery called aorta it sends vital spirits over the body, and takes air from the lungs by that artery which is called venosa; so that both creeks have their vessels, the right two veins, the left two arteries, besides those two common anfractuous ears, which serve them both; the one to hold blood, the other air, for several uses. The lungs is a thin, spongy part, like an ox-hoof (saith Fernelius [2]), the town-clerk or crier (one terms it), the instrument of voice, as an orator to a king;[3] annexed to the heart, to express his thoughts by voice. That it is the instrument of voice is manifest, in that no creature can speak, or utter any voice, which wanteth these lights. It is, besides, the instrument of respiration, or breathing; and its office is to cool the heart, by sending air unto it, by the venosal artery, which vein comes to the lungs by that *aspera arteria*, which consists of many gristles, membranes, nerves, taking in air at the nose and mouth, and by it likewise exhales the fumes of the heart.

In the upper region serving the animal faculties, the chief organ is the brain, which is a soft, marrowish, and white substance, engendered of the purest part of seed and spirits, included by many skins, and seated within the skull or brain-pan; and it is the most noble organ under heaven, the dwelling-house and seat of the soul, the habitation of wisdom, memory, judgment, reason, and in which man is most like unto God; and therefore nature hath covered it with a skull of hard bone, and two skins or membranes, whereof the one is called *dura mater*, or meninx, the other *pia mater*. The *dura mater* is next to the skull, above the other, which includes and protects the brain. When this is taken away, the *pia mater* is to be seen, a thin membrane, the next and immediate cover of the brain, and not covering only, but entering into it. The brain itself is divided into two parts, the fore and hinder part; the fore part is much bigger than the other, which is called the little brain in respect of it. This fore part hath many concavities distinguished by certain ventricles, which are the receptacles of the spirits, brought hither by the arteries from the heart, and are there refined to a more heavenly nature, to perform the actions of the soul. Of these ventricles there be three—right, left, and middle. The right and left answer to their site, and beget animal spirits; if they be anyway hurt, sense and motion ceaseth. These ventricles, moreover, are held to be the seat of the common sense. The middle ventricle is a common concourse and cavity of them both, and hath two passages—the one to receive pituita, and the other extends itself to the fourth creek; in this they place imagination and cogitation, and so the three ventricles of the fore part of the brain are used. The fourth creek behind the head is common to the cerebel, or little brain, and marrow of the backbone, the last and most solid of all the rest, which receives the animal spirits from the other ventricles, and conveys them to the marrow in the back, and is the place where they say the memory is seated.

SUBSECT. V.—*Of the Soul and her Faculties*

According to Aristotle,[1] the soul is defined to be ἐντελέχεια, *perfectio et actus primus corporis organici, vitam habentis in potentia*, the perfection or first act of an organical body, having power of life, which most philosophers approve.[2] But many doubts arise about the essence, subject, seat, distinction, and subordinate faculties of it. For the essence and particular knowledge, of all other things it is most hard (be it of man or beast) to discern, as Aristotle himself,[3] Tully,[4] Picus Mirandula,[5] Tolet,[6] and other neoteric philosophers confess. "We can understand all things by her, but what she is we cannot apprehend." [7] Some therefore make one soul, divided into three principal faculties; others, three distinct souls: which question of late hath been much controverted by Piccolomineus and Zabarel. Paracelsus will have four souls, adding to the three grand faculties a spiritual soul:[8] which opinion of his Campanella, in his book *de sensu rerum*,[1] much labours to demonstrate and prove, because carcasses bleed at the sight of the murderer; with many such arguments; and some again, one soul of all creatures whatsoever, differing only in organs;[2] and that beasts have reason as well as men, though, for some defect of organs, not in such measure. Others make a doubt whether it be all in all, and all in every part; which is amply discussed in Zabarel amongst the rest. The common division of the soul is into three principal faculties — vegetal, sensitive, and rational,[3] which make three distinct kinds of living creatures: vegetal plants, sensible beasts, rational men. How these three principal faculties are distinguished and connected, *humano ingenio inaccessum videtur*, is beyond human capacity, as Taurellus,[4] Philip, Flavius, and others suppose. The inferior may be alone, but the superior cannot subsist without the other; so sensible includes vegetal, rational both; which are contained in it (saith Aristotle) *ut trigonus in tetragono*, as a triangle in a quadrangle.

Vegetal, the first of the three distinct faculties, is defined to be a "substantial act of an organical body, by which it is nourished, augmented, and begets another like unto itself." In which definition, three several operations are specified— *altrix, auctrix, procreatrix*; the first is nutrition, whose object is nourishment, meat, drink, and the like;[5] his organ the liver in sensible creatures; in plants, the root or sap. His office is to turn the nutriment into the substance of the body nourished, which he performs by natural heat. This nutritive operation hath four other subordinate functions or powers belonging to it: attraction, retention, digestion, expulsion.

Attraction is a ministering faculty, which, as a loadstone doth iron, draws meat into the stomach, or as a lamp doth oil;[6] and this attractive power is very necessary in plants, which suck up moisture by the root, as another mouth, into the sap, as a like stomach.

Retention keeps it, being attracted unto the stomach until such time it be concocted; for if it should pass away straight, the body could not be nourished.

Digestion is performed by natural heat; for as the flame of a torch consumes oil, wax, tallow, so doth it alter and digest the nutritive matter. Indigestion is opposite unto it, for want of natural heat. Of this digestion there be three differences: maturation, elixation, assation.

Maturation is especially observed in the fruits of trees; which are then said to be ripe when the seeds are fit to be sown again. Crudity is opposed to it, which gluttons, epicures, and idle persons are most subject unto, that use no exercise to stir natural heat, or else choke it, as too much wood puts out a fire.

Elixation is the seething of meat in the stomach, by the said natural heat, as meat is boiled in a pot; to which corruption or putrefaction is opposite.

Assation is a concoction of the inward moisture by heat; his opposite is semiustulation.

Besides these three several operations of digestion there is a four-fold order of concoction: mastication, or chewing in the mouth; chylification of this so chewed meat in the stomach; the third is in the liver, to turn this chylus into blood, called sanguification; the last is assimilation, which is in every part.

Expulsion is a power of nutrition by which it expels all superfluous excrements, and relics of meat and drink, by the guts, bladder, pores; as by purging, vomiting, spitting, sweating, urine, hairs, nails, etc.

As this nutritive faculty serves to nourish the body, so doth the augmenting faculty (the second operation or power of the vegetal faculty) to the increasing of it in quantity, according to all dimensions, long, broad, thick, and to make it grow till it come to his due proportion and perfect shape; which hath his period of augmentation, as of consumption; and that most certain, as the poet observes:

Stat sua cuique dies, breve et irreparabile tempus
Omnibus est vitæ.

A term of life is set to every man,
Which is but short, and pass it no one can.

The last of these vegetal faculties is generation, which begets another by means of seed like unto itself, to the perpetual preservation of the species. To this faculty they ascribe three subordinate operations: the first to turn nourishment into seed, etc.

Necessary concomitants or affections of this vegetal faculty are life, and his privation, death. To the preservation of life the natural heat is most requisite, though siccity and humidity, and those first qualities, be not excluded. This heat is likewise in plants, as appears by their increasing, fructifying, etc., though not so easily perceived. In all bodies it must have radical moisture to preserve it, that it be not consumed;[1] to which preservation our clime, country, temperature, and the good or bad use of those six non-natural things avail much. For as this natural heat and moisture decays, so doth our life itself; and if not prevented before by some violent accident, or interrupted through our own default, is in the end dried up by old age, and extinguished by death for want of matter, as a lamp for defect of oil to maintain it.

SUBSECT. VI.—*Of the Sensible Soul*

Next in order is the sensible faculty, which is as far beyond the other in dignity as a beast is preferred to a plant, having those vegetal powers included in it. 'Tis defined "an act of an organical body, by which it lives, hath sense, appetite, judgment, breath, and motion." His object in general is a sensible or passible quality, because the sense is affected with it. The general organ is the brain, from which principally the sensible operations are derived. This sensible soul is divided into two parts, apprehending or moving. By the apprehensive power we perceive the species of sensible things, present or absent, and retain them as wax doth the print of a seal. By the moving the body is outwardly carried from one place to another, or inwardly moved by spirits and pulse. The apprehensive faculty is subdivided into two parts, inward or outward. Outward, as the five senses, of touching, hearing, seeing, smelling, tasting, to which you may add Scaliger's sixth sense of titillation, if you please; or that of speech, which is the sixth external sense, according to Lullius. Inward are three—common sense, phantasy, memory. Those five outward senses have their object in outward things only, and such as are present, as the eye sees no colour except it be at hand, the ear [no] sound. Three of these senses are of commodity, hearing, sight, and smell; two of necessity, touch and taste, without which we cannot live. Besides the sensitive power is active or passive; active in sight, the eye sees the colour; passive when it is hurt by his object, as the eye by the sunbeams; according to that axiom, *Visibile forte destruit sensum* [excessive brightness in an object destroys the sight]; or if the object be not pleasing, as a bad sound to the ear, a stinking smell to the nose, etc.

Of these five senses, sight is held to be most precious, and the best, and that by reason of his object; it sees the whole body at once; by it we learn, and discern all things, a sense most excellent for use. To the sight three things are required, the object, the organ, and the medium. The object in general is visible, or that which is to be seen, as colours, and all shining bodies. The medium is the illumination of the air which comes from light,[1] commonly called *diaphanum*; for in dark we cannot see. The organ is the eye, and chiefly the apple of it, which by those optic nerves, concurring both in one, conveys the sight to the common sense. Betwixt the organ and object a true distance is required, that it be not too near, or too far off. Many excellent questions appertain to this sense, discussed by philosophers: as whether this sight be caused *intra mittendo, vel extra mittendo*, etc., by receiving in the visible species, or sending of them out, which Plato,[2] Plutarch,[3] Macrobius,[4] Lactantius,[5] and others dispute. And besides it is the subject of the perspectives, of which Alhazen the Arabian, Vitellio, Roger Bacon, Baptista Porta, Guidus Ubaldus, Aquilonius, etc., have written whole volumes.

Hearing, a most excellent outward sense, "by which we learn and get knowledge." His object is sound, or that which is heard; the medium, air; organ, the ear. To the sound, which is a collision of the air, three things are required: a body to strike, as the hand of a musician; the body strucken, which must be solid and able to resist, as a bell, lute-string, not wool, or sponge; the medium, the air, which is inward or outward; the outward, being struck or collided by a solid body, still strikes the next air, until it come to that inward natural air, which as an exquisite organ is contained in a little skin formed like a drum-head, and struck upon by certain small instruments like drum-sticks, conveys the sound by a pair of nerves, appropriated to that use, to the common sense, as to a judge of sounds. There is a great variety and much delight in them; for the knowledge of which consult with Boethius and other musicians.

Smelling is an "outward sense, which apprehends by the nostrils drawing in air"; and of all the rest it is the weakest sense in men. The organ in the nose, or two small hollow pieces of flesh a little above it: the medium, the air to men, as water to fish: the object, smell, arising from a mixed body resolved, which, whether it be a quality, fume, vapour, or exhalation, I will not now dispute, or of their differences, and how they are caused. This sense is an organ of health, as sight and hearing, saith A. Gellius,[6] are of discipline; and that by avoiding bad smells, as by choosing good, which do as much alter and affect the body many times as diet itself.

Taste, a necessary sense, "which perceives all savours by the tongue and palate, and that by means of a thin spittle, or watery juice." His organ is the tongue with his tasting nerves;

the medium, a watery juice; the object, taste or savour, which is a quality in the juice, arising from the mixture of things tasted. Some make eight species or kinds of savour, bitter, sweet, sharp, salt, etc., all which sick men (as in an ague) cannot discern, by reason of their organs misaffected.

Touch, the last of the senses, and most ignoble, yet of as great necessity as the other, and of as much pleasure. This sense is exquisite in men, and by his nerves dispersed all over the body, perceives any tactile quality. His organ the nerves; his object those first qualities, hot, dry, moist, cold; and those that follow them, hard, soft, thick, thin, etc. Many delightsome questions are moved by philosophers about these five senses, their organs, objects, mediums, which for brevity I omit.

SUBSECT. VII.—*Of the Inward Senses*

Inner senses are three in number, so called because they be within the brain-pan, as common sense, phantasy, memory. Their objects are not only things present, but they perceive the sensible species of things to come, past, absent, such as were before in the sense. This common sense is the judge or moderator of the rest, by whom we discern all differences of objects; for by mine eye I do not know that I see, or by mine ear that I hear, but by my common sense, who judgeth of sounds and colours: they are but the organs to bring the species to be censured; so that all their objects are his, and all their offices are his. The fore-part of the brain is his organ or seat.

Phantasy, or imagination, which some call estimative, or cogitative (confirmed, saith Fernelius,[1] by frequent meditation), is an inner sense which doth more fully examine the species perceived by common sense, of things present or absent, and keeps them longer, recalling them to mind again, or making new of his own. In time of sleep this faculty is free, and many times conceive strange, stupend, absurd shapes, as in sick men we commonly observe. His organ is the middle cell of the brain; his objects all the species communicated to him by the common sense, by comparison of which he feigns infinite other unto himself. In melancholy men this faculty is most powerful and strong, and often hurts, producing many monstrous and prodigious things, especially if it be stirred up by some terrible object, presented to it from common sense or memory. In poets and painters imagination forcibly works, as appears by their several fictions, antics, images: as Ovid's house of Sleep,

Psyche's palace in Apuleius, etc. In men it is subject and
governed by reason, or at least should be; but in brutes it hath
no superior, and is *ratio brutorum*, all the reason they have.

Memory lays up all the species which the senses have brought
in, and records them as a good register, that they may be forth-
coming when they are called for by phantasy and reason. His
object is the same with phantasy, his seat and organ the back
part of the brain.

The affections of these senses are sleep and waking, common
to all sensible creatures. "Sleep is a rest or binding of the outward senses, and of the common sense, for the preservation of
body and soul" (as Scaliger defines it [1]); for when the common
sense resteth, the outward senses rest also. The phantasy
alone is free, and his commander, reason: as appears by those
imaginary dreams, which are of divers kinds, natural, divine,
demoniacal, etc., which vary according to humours, diet,
actions, objects, etc., of which Artemidorus, Cardanus, and
Sambucus, with their several interpretators, have written great
volumes. This ligation of senses proceeds from an inhibition
of spirits, the way being stopped by which they should come;
this stopping is caused of vapours arising out of the stomach,
filling the nerves, by which the spirits should be conveyed.
When these vapours are spent, the passage is open, and the
spirits perform their accustomed duties: so that "waking is the
action and motion of the senses, which the spirits dispersed over
all parts cause."

SUBSECT. VIII.—*Of the Moving Faculty*

This moving faculty is the other power of the sensitive soul,
which causeth all those inward and outward animal motions in
the body. It is divided into two faculties, the power of appetite,
and of moving from place to place. This of appetite is threefold, so some will have it; natural, as it signifies any such inclination, as of a stone to fall downward, and such actions as retention,
expulsion, which depend not on sense, but are vegetal, as the
appetite of meat and drink, hunger and thirst. Sensitive is
common to men and brutes. Voluntary, the third, or intel-
lective, which commands the other two in men, and is a curb
unto them, or at least should be, but for the most part is
captivated and overruled by them; and men are led like beasts
by sense, giving reins to their concupiscence and several lusts.
For by this appetite the soul is led or inclined to follow that

good which the senses shall approve, or avoid that which they
hold evil: his object being good or evil, the one he embraceth,
the other he rejecteth; according to that aphorism, *omnia
appetunt bonum*, all things seek their own good, or at least
seeming good.   This power is inseparable from sense, for where
sense is, there is likewise pleasure and pain.   His organ is the
same with the common sense, and is divided into two powers
or inclinations, concupiscible or irascible: or (as one translates
it [1]) "coveting, anger invading, or impugning." Concupiscible
covets always pleasant and delightsome things, and abhors
that which is distasteful, harsh, and unpleasant.   Irascible,
quasi aversans per iram et odium,[2] as avoiding it with anger and
indignation.   All affections and perturbations arise out of
these two fountains, which, although the Stoics make light of,
we hold natural, and not to be resisted.   The good affections
are caused by some object of the same nature; and if present,
they procure joy, which dilates the heart and preserves the
body: if absent, they cause hope, love, desire, and concupiscence.
The bad are simple or mixed: simple for some bad object present,
as sorrow, which contracts the heart, macerates the soul, subverts the good estate of the body, hindering all the operations
of it, causing melancholy, and many times death itself; or future,
as fear.   Out of these two arise those mixed affections and
passions of anger, which is a desire of revenge; hatred, which is
inveterate anger; zeal, which is offended with him who hurts
that he loves; and ἐπιχαιρεκακία, a compound affection of joy
and hate, when we rejoice at other men's mischief, and are
grieved at their prosperity; pride, self-love, emulation, envy,
shame, etc., of which elsewhere.

Moving from place to place is a faculty necessarily following
the other.   For in vain were it otherwise to desire and to abhor,
if we had not likewise power to prosecute or eschew, by moving
the body from place to place: by this faculty therefore we locally
move the body, or any part of it, and go from one place to
another.   To the better performance of which, three things are
requisite: that which moves; by what it moves; that which is
moved.   That which moves is either the efficient cause, or end.
The end is the object which is desired or eschewed; as in a dog
to catch a hare, etc.   The efficient cause in man is reason,
or his subordinate phantasy, which apprehends good or bad
objects: in brutes imagination alone, which moves the appetite,
the appetite this faculty, which by an admirable league of
nature, and by mediation of the spirit, commands the organ

by which it moves: and that consists of nerves, muscles, cords, dispersed through the whole body, contracted and relaxed as the spirits will, which move the muscles, or nerves in the midst of them,[1] and draw the cord, and so *per consequens* the joint, to the place intended. That which is moved is the body or some member apt to move. The motion of the body is diverse, as going, running, leaping, dancing, sitting, and such-like, referred to the predicament of *situs* [position]. Worms creep, birds fly, fishes swim; and so of parts, the chief of which is respiration or breathing, and is thus performed. The outward air is drawn in by the vocal artery, and sent by mediation of the midriff to the lungs, which, dilating themselves as a pair of bellows, reciprocally fetch it in and send it out to the heart to cool it; and from thence now being hot, convey it again, still taking in fresh. Such a like motion is that of the pulse, of which, because many have written whole books, I will say nothing.

Subsect. IX.—*Of the Rational Soul*

In the precedent subsections I have anatomized those inferior faculties of the soul; the rational remaineth, "a pleasant, but a doubtful subject" (as one terms it [2]), and with the like brevity to be discussed. Many erroneous opinions are about the essence and original of it; whether it be fire, as Zeno held; harmony, as Aristoxenus; number, as Xenocrates; whether it be organical or inorganical; seated in the brain, heart, or blood; mortal or immortal; how it comes into the body. Some hold that it is *ex traduce*, as Phil. 1 *de Anima*, Tertullian, Lactantius, *de opific. Dei, cap.* 19; Hugo, *lib. de Spiritu et Anima*; Vincentius Bellovac. *Spec. natural. lib.* 23, *cap.* 2 *et* 11; Hippocrates, Avicenna, and many late writers;[3] that one man begets another, body and soul; or as a candle from a candle, to be produced from the seed: otherwise, say they, a men begets but half a man, and is worse than a beast that begets both matter and form; and besides, the three faculties of the soul must be together infused, which is most absurd, as they hold, because in beasts they are begot, the two inferior I mean, and may not be well separated in men. Galen supposeth the soul *crasin esse*, to be the temperature itself;[4] Trismegistus, Musæus, Orpheus, Homer, Pindarus, Pherecydes Syrius, Epictetus, with the Chaldees and Egyptians, affirmed the soul to be immortal, as did those British Druids of old.[5] The Pythagoreans defend metempsychosis and *palingenesia*, that souls go from one body to another,[6] *epota*

prius Lethes unda [after a draught of the waters of Lethe],
as men into wolves, bears, dogs, hogs, as they were inclined in
their lives, or participated in conditions:

> *Inque ferinas*
> *Possumus ire domus, pecudumque in corpora condi.*[1]

> [In beasts and cattle we may find abode,
> And in their shapes become incorporate.]

Lucian's cock[2] was first Euphorbus, a captain:

> *Ille ego (nam memini) Trojani tempore belli,*
> *Panthoides Euphorbus eram,*[3]

> [At Troy, I well recall, in former life,
> Euphorbus, son of Panthous, was I,]

a horse, a man, a sponge. Julian the Apostate thought Alexander's soul was descended into his body:[4] Plato *in Timæo*, and
in his *Phædo* (for aught I can perceive), differs not much from
this opinion, that it was from God at first, and knew all, but
being enclosed in the body, it forgets, and learns anew, which he
calls *reminiscentia*, or recalling, and that it was put into the body
for a punishment; and thence it goes into a beast's, or man's,
as appears by his pleasant fiction *de sortitione animarum* [of the
allotment of souls], *lib.* 10 *de Rep.*, and after ten thousand years
is to return into the former body again.[5]

> *Post varios annos, per mille figuras,*
> *Rursus ad humanæ fertur primordia vitæ.*[6]

> [After many years, and many transformations, he again
> commences life as a human being.]

Others deny the immortality of it, which Pomponatius of Padua
decided out of Aristotle not long since, Plinius Avunculus,[7] *cap.*
7, *lib.* 2, *et lib.* 7, *cap.* 55; Seneca, *lib.* 7, *Epist. ad Lucilium,*
epist. 55; Dicæarchus *in Tull. Tusc.*; Epicurus, Aratus, Hippocrates, Galen; Lucretius, *lib.* 1:

> *Præterea gigni pariter cum corpore, et una*
> *Crescere sentimus, pariterque senescere mentem;*

> [The mind, we see, is with the body born,
> Grows with its growth, and with its years is worn;]

Averroes, and I know not how many neoterics. "This question
of the immortality of the soul is diversely and wonderfully
impugned and disputed, especially among the Italians of late,"[8]
saith Jab. Colerus, *lib. de immort. animæ, cap.* 1. The Popes
themselves have doubted of it: Leo Decimus, that Epicurean
Pope, as some record of him,[9] caused this question to be

discussed pro and con before him, and concluded at last, as a
profane and atheistical moderator, with that verse of Cornelius
Gallus, *Et redit in nihilum, quod fuit ante nihil:* it began of
nothing and in nothing it ends. Zeno and his Stoics, as Austin
quotes him,[1] supposed the soul so long to continue, till the body
was fully putrefied, and resolved into *materia prima*: but after
that, *in fumos evanescere,* to be extinguished and vanished;
and in the meantime, whilst the body was consuming, it wandered
all abroad, *et e longinquo multa annunciare* [announced many
things from afar], and (as that Clazomenian Hermotimus
averred) saw pretty visions, and suffered I know not what.

> *Errant exsangues sine corpore et ossibus umbræ.*[2]

> [As bloodless shades, devoid of bone and flesh,
> They flit about.]

Others grant the immortality thereof, but they make many
fabulous fictions in the meantime of it, after the departure from
the body: like Plato's Elysian Fields, and that Turkey paradise.
The souls of good men they deified; the bad (saith Austin)
became devils,[3] as they supposed; with many such absurd
tenents, which he hath confuted. Hierome, Austin, and other
Fathers of the Church, hold that the soul is immortal, created
of nothing, and so infused into the child or embryo in his mother's
womb, six months after the conception;[4] not as those of brutes,
which are *ex traduce,* and dying with them vanish into nothing.
To whose divine treatises, and to the Scriptures themselves, I
rejourn all such atheistical spirits, as Tully did Atticus, doubting
of this point, to Plato's *Phædo.* Or if they desire philosophical
proofs and demonstrations, I refer them to Niphus', Nic.
Faventinus' tracts of this subject, to Fran. and John Picus
in digress. sup. 3 de Anima, Tholosanus, Eugubinus, to Soto,
Canus, Thomas, Pererius, Dandinus, Colerus, to that elaborate
tract in Zanchius, to Tolet's sixty reasons, and Lessius' twenty-
two arguments, to prove the immortality of the soul. Campanella, *lib. de sensu rerum,* is large in the same discourse,
Albertinus the Schoolman, Jacob. Nactantus, *tom. 2 op.,*
handleth it in four questions, Antony Brunus, Aonius Palearius,
Marinus Marcennus, with many others. This reasonable soul,
which Austin calls a spiritual substance moving itself, is defined
by philosophers to be "the first substantial act of a natural,
human, organical body, by which a man lives, perceives, and
understands, freely doing all things, and with election." Out of
which definition we may gather that this rational soul includes

the powers, and performs the duties, of the two other which are contained in it, and all three faculties make one soul, which is inorganical of itself, although it be in all parts, and incorporeal, using their organs, and working by them. It is divided into two chief parts, differing in office only, not in essence: the understanding, which is the rational power apprehending; the will, which is the rational power moving: to which two all the other rational powers are subject and reduced.

SUBSECT. X.—*Of the Understanding*

"Understanding is a power of the soul, by which we perceive, know, remember, and judge, as well singulars as universals, having certain innate notices or beginnings of arts, a reflecting action, by which it judgeth of his own doings and examines them." [1] Out of this definition (besides his chief office, which is to apprehend, judge all that he performs, without the help of any instruments or organs) three differences appear betwixt a man and a beast. As first, the sense only comprehends singularities, the understanding universalities. Secondly, the sense hath no innate notions. Thirdly, brutes cannot reflect upon themselves. Bees indeed make neat and curious works, and many other creatures besides; but when they have done, they cannot judge of them. His object is God, *Ens*, all nature, and whatsoever is to be understood: which successively it apprehends. The object first moving the understanding is some sensible thing; after, by discoursing, the mind finds out the corporeal substance, and from thence the spiritual. His actions (some say) are apprehension, composition, division, discoursing, reasoning, memory, which some include in invention, and judgment. The common divisions are, of the understanding: agent and patient; speculative and practic; in habit or in act; simple or compound. The agent is that which is called the wit of man, acumen or subtlety, sharpness of invention, when he doth invent of himself without a teacher, or learns anew, which abstracts those intelligible species from the phantasy, and transfers them to the passive understanding, "because there is nothing in the understanding which was not first in the sense." [2] That which the imagination hath taken from the sense, this agent judgeth of, whether it be true or false; and being so judged he commits it to the passible to be kept. The agent is a doctor or teacher, the passive a scholar; and his office is to keep and further judge of such things as are committed to his charge; as a bare and razed table[1] at first, capable of all forms and notions.   Now these notions are twofold, actions or habits: actions, by which we take notions of and perceive things; habits, which are durable lights and notions, which we may use when we will.   Some reckon up eight kinds of them: sense, experience, intelligence, faith, suspicion, error, opinion, science; to which are added art, prudency, wisdom: as also synteresis,[2] *dictamen rationis* [the dictate of reason], conscience; so that in all there be fourteen species of the understanding, of which some are innate, as the three last mentioned; the other are gotten by doctrine, learning, and use.   Plato will have all to be innate: Aristotle reckons up but five intellectual habits: two speculative, as that intelligence of the principles and science of conclusion; two practic, as prudency, whose end is to practise, art to fabricate; wisdom to comprehend the use and experiments of all notions and habits whatsoever.   Which division of Aristotle (if it be considered aright) is all one with the precedent; for three being innate, and five acquisite, the rest are improper, imperfect, and in a more strict examination excluded.   Of all these I should more amply dilate, but my subject will not permit. Three of them I will only point at, as more necessary to my following discourse.

Synteresis, or the purer part of the conscience, is an innate habit, and doth signify "a conservation of the knowledge of the law of God and Nature, to know good or evil."   And (as our divines hold) it is rather in the understanding than in the will. This makes the major proposition in a practic syllogism. The *dictamen rationis* is that which doth admonish us to do good or evil, and is the minor in the syllogism.   The conscience is that which approves good or evil, justifying or condemning our actions, and is the conclusion of the syllogism: as in that familiar example of Regulus the Roman, taken prisoner by the Carthaginians, and suffered to go to Rome, on that condition he should return again, or pay so much for his ransom.   The synteresis proposeth the question; his word, oath, promise, is to be religiously kept, although to his enemy, and that by the law of nature.   "Do not that to another which thou wouldest not have done to thyself."[3]   *Dictamen* applies it to him, and dictates this or the like: "Regulus, thou wouldst not another man should falsify his oath, or break promise with thee"; conscience concludes, "Therefore, Regulus, thou dost well to perform thy promise, and oughtest to keep thine oath."   More of this in Religious Melancholy.

SUBSECT. XI.—*Of the Will*

Will is the other power of the rational soul, "which covets or
avoids such things as have been before judged and apprehended
by the understanding."[1] If good, it approves; if evil, it abhors
it: so that his object is either good or evil. Aristotle calls this
our rational appetite; for as, in the sensitive, we are moved to
good or bad by our appetite, ruled and directed by sense; so
in this we are carried by reason. Besides, the sensitive appetite
hath a particular object, good or bad; this an universal, immaterial: that respects only things delectable and pleasant;
this honest. Again, they differ in liberty. The sensual appetite
seeing an object, if it be a convenient good, cannot but desire
it; if evil, avoid it; but this is free in his essence, "much now
depraved, obscured, and fallen from his first perfection; yet in
some of his operations still free,"[2] as to go, walk, move at his
pleasure, and to choose whether it will do or not do, steal or not
steal. Otherwise, in vain were laws, deliberations, exhortations,
counsels, precepts, rewards, promises, threats and punishments:
and God should be the author of sin. But in spiritual things
we will no good,[3] prone to evil (except we be regenerate, and
led by the spirit), we are egged on by our natural concupiscence,
and there is ἀταξία, a confusion in our powers, "our whole will
is averse from God and His law,"[4] not in natural things only,
as to eat and drink, lust, to which we are led headlong by our
temperature and inordinate appetite,

> *Nec nos obniti contra, nec tendere tantum*
> *Sufficimus,*[5]
>
> [To make a stand and manfully resist
> Our force avails not,]

we cannot resist, our concupiscence is originally bad, our heart
evil, the seat of our affections captivates and enforceth our will;
so that in voluntary things we are averse from God and goodness,
bad by nature, by ignorance worse,[6] by art, discipline, custom,
we get many bad habits, suffering them to domineer and
tyrannize over us; and the devil is still ready at hand with his
evil suggestions, to tempt our depraved will to some ill-disposed
action, to precipitate us to destruction, except our will be swayed
and counterpoised again with some divine precepts and good
motions of the spirit, which many times restrain, hinder, and
check us, when we are in the full career of our dissolute courses.
So David corrected himself, when he had Saul at a vantage.

Revenge and malice were as two violent oppugners on the one side; but honesty, religion, fear of God, withheld him on the other.

The actions of the will are *velle* and *nolle*, to will and nill: which two words comprehend all, and they are good or bad, accordingly as they are directed, and some of them freely performed by himself; although the Stoics absolutely deny it, and will have all things inevitably done by destiny, imposing a fatal necessity upon us, which we may not resist; yet we say that our will is free in respect of us, and things contingent, howsoever (in respect of God's determinate counsel) they are inevitable and necessary. Some other actions of the will are performed by the inferior powers which obey him, as the sensitive and moving appetite; as to open our eyes, to go hither and thither, not to touch a book, to speak fair or foul: but this appetite is many times rebellious in us, and will not be contained within the lists of sobriety and temperance. It was (as I said) once well agreeing with reason, and there was an excellent consent and harmony betwixt them, but that is now dissolved, they often jar, reason is overborne by passion: *Fertur equis auriga, nec audit currus habenas* [the driver is whirled along, the steeds obey not the rein], as so many wild horses run away with a chariot, and will not be curbed. We know many times what is good, but will not do it, as she said:

> *Trahit invitam nova vis, aliudque cupido,*
> *Mens aliud suadet.*[1]

Lust counsels one thing, reason another, there is a new reluctancy in men.

> *Odi, nec possum cupiens non esse quod odi.*[2]
>> [I loathe it, yet cannot abate
>> To be the very thing I hate.]

We cannot resist, but as Phædra confessed to her nurse, *quæ loqueris, vera sunt, sed furor suggerit sequi pejora* [3] [thou speakest truth, yet my passion drives me to follow the worse course]: she said well and true, she did acknowledge it, but headstrong passion and fury made her to do that which was opposite. So David knew the filthiness of his fact, what a loathsome, foul, crying sin adultery was, yet notwithstanding he would commit murder, and take away another man's wife, enforced against reason, religion, to follow his appetite.

Those natural and vegetal powers are not commanded by will at all; for "who can add one cubit to his stature?" These other may, but are not: and thence come all those headstrong passions,

violent perturbations of the mind; and many times vicious
habits, customs, feral diseases; because we give so much way
to our appetite, and follow our inclination, like so many beasts.
The principal habits are two in number, virtue and vice, whose
peculiar definitions, descriptions, differences, and kinds are
handled at large in the ethics, and are, indeed, the subject of
moral philosophy.

MEMB. III

SUBSECT. I.—*Definition of Melancholy, Name, Difference*

HAVING thus briefly anatomized the body and soul of man,
as a preparative to the rest, I may now freely proceed to treat
of my intended subject, to most men's capacity; and after many
ambages, perspicuously define what this melancholy is, show
his name and differences. The name is imposed from the
matter, and disease denominated from the material cause:
as Bruel observes, Μελαυχολία, *quasi* Μέλαινα χολή, from black
choler. And whether it be a cause or an effect, a disease or
symptom, let Donatus Altomarus and Salvianus decide; I will
not contend about it. It hath several descriptions, notations,
and definitions. Fracastorius, in his second book of Intellect,
calls those melancholy "whom abundance of that same depraved
humour of black choler hath so misaffected, that they become
mad thence, and dote in most things, or in all, belonging to
election, will, or other manifest operations of the understanding." [1] Melanelius out of Galen, Ruffus, Aetius, describe it to
be "a bad and peevish disease, which makes men degenerate
into beasts"; [2] Galen, "a privation or infection of the middle
cell of the head," etc., defining it from the part affected, which
Hercules de Saxonia approves,[3] *lib.* 1, *cap.* 16, calling it "a
depravation of the principal function"; Fuchsius, *lib.* 1, *cap.* 23;
Arnoldus, *Breviar. lib.* 1, *cap.* 18; Guianerius, and others:
"by reason of black choler," Paulus adds. Halyabbas simply
calls it a "commotion of the mind"; Aretæus, "a perpetual
anguish of the soul, fastened on one thing, without an ague"; [4]
which definition of his Mercurialis, *de affect. cap. lib.* 1, *cap.* 10,
taxeth: but Ælianus Montaltus defends, *lib. de morb. cap.* 1,
de melan., for sufficient and good. The common sort define it
to be "a kind of dotage without a fever, having for his ordinary

companions fear and sadness, without any apparent occasion.
So doth Laurentius, *cap.* 4; Piso, *lib.* 1, *cap.* 43; Donatus Altomarus, *cap.* 7 *Art. medic.*; Jacchinus, *in com. in lib.* 9 *Rhasis
ad Almansor. cap.* 15; Valesius, *Exerc.* 17; Fuchsius, *Institut.* 13,
sec. 1, *cap.* 11, etc., which common definition, howsoever approved
by most, Hercules de Saxonia will not allow of,[1] nor David
Crusius, *Theat. morb. Herm. lib.* 2, *cap.* 6; he holds it unsufficient,
"as rather showing what it is not, than what it is," [2] as omitting
the specifical difference, the phantasy and brain: but I descend
to particulars. The *summum genus* is dotage, or "anguish of
the mind," saith Aretæus; "of a principal part," Hercules
de Saxonia adds, to distinguish it from cramp and palsy, and
such diseases as belong to the outward sense and motions;
"depraved," to distinguish it from folly and madness [3] (which
Montaltus makes *angor animi*, to separate), in which those
functions are not depraved, but rather abolished; "without an
ague" is added by all, to sever it from frenzy, and that melancholy which is in a pestilent fever. "Fear and sorrow" make
it differ from madness; "without a cause" is lastly inserted, to
specify it from all other ordinary passions of "fear and sorrow."
We properly call that dotage, as Laurentius interprets it, "when
some one principal faculty of the mind, as imagination or
reason, is corrupted, as all melancholy persons have." [4]   It is
without a fever, because the humour is most part cold and dry,
contrary to putrefaction.   Fear and sorrow are the true characters and inseparable companions of most melancholy, not all,
as Hercules de Saxonia, *tract. posthumo de Melancholia, cap.* 2,
well excepts; for to some it is most pleasant, as to such as
laugh most part; some are bold again, and free from all manner
of fear and grief, as hereafter shall be declared.

SUBSECT. II.—*Of the Part affected.   Affection.   Parties affected*

Some difference I find amongst writers, about the principal
part affected in this disease, whether it be the brain, or heart,
or some other member.   Most are of opinion that it is the
brain: for being a kind of dotage, it cannot otherwise be but
that the brain must be affected, as a similar part, be it by
consent or essence,[5] not in his ventricles, or any obstructions
in them, for then it would be an apoplexy, or epilepsy, as
Laurentius well observes,[6] but in a cold, dry distemperature of
it in his substance, which is corrupt and become too cold, or
too dry, or else too hot, as in madmen and such as are inclined

to it: and this Hippocrates confirms,[1] Galen, [the] Arabians, and most of our new writers. Marcus de Oddis (in a consultation of his, quoted by Hildesheim[2]) and five others there cited are of the contrary part; because fear and sorrow, which are passions, be seated in the heart. But this objection is sufficiently answered by Montaltus,[3] who doth not deny that the heart is affected (as Melanelius proves out of Galen[4]) by reason of his vicinity, and so is the midriff and many other parts. They do *compati* [sympathize], and have a fellow-feeling by the law of nature: but forasmuch as this malady is caused by precedent imagination, with the appetite, to whom spirits obey, and are subject to those principal parts, the brain must needs primarily be misaffected, as the seat of reason; and then the heart, as the seat of affection. Capivaccius[5] and Mercurialis have copiously discussed this question, and both conclude the subject is the inner brain, and from thence it is communicated to the heart and other inferior parts, which sympathize and are much troubled, especially when it comes by consent, and is caused by reason of the stomach, or myrach, as the Arabians term it, whole body, liver, or spleen, which are seldom free,[6] pylorus, meseraic veins, etc. For our body is like a clock; if one wheel be amiss, all the rest are disordered, the whole fabric suffers: with such admirable art and harmony is a man composed, such excellent proportion, as Lodovicus Vives in his Fable of Man hath elegantly declared.

As many doubts almost arise about the affection,[7] whether it be imagination or reason alone, or both. Hercules de Saxonia proves it out of Galen, Aetius, and Altomarus, that the sole fault is in imagination.[8] Bruel is of the same mind. Montaltus in his second chapter of Melancholy confutes this tenent of theirs, and illustrates the contrary by many examples: as of him that thought himself a shell-fish, of a nun, and of a desperate monk that would not be persuaded but that he was damned; reason was in fault as well as imagination, which did not correct this error: they make away themselves oftentimes, and suppose many absurd and ridiculous things. Why doth not reason detect the fallacy, settle and persuade, if she be free? Avicenna therefore holds both corrupt,[9] to whom most Arabians sub-scribe. The same is maintained by Aretæus,[10] Gordonius,[11] Guianerius, etc. To end the controversy, no man doubts of imagination, but that it is hurt and misaffected here; for the other I determine with Albertinus Bottonus,[12] a doctor of Padua, that it is "first in imagination, and afterwards in reason,

if the disease be inveterate, or as it is more or less of continuance";
but by accident, as Herc. de Saxonia adds: "Faith, opinion,
discourse, ratiocination, are all accidentally depraved by the
default of imagination." [1]

To the part affected, I may here add the parties, which shall
be more opportunely spoken of elsewhere, now only signified.
Such as have the Moon, Saturn, Mercury misaffected in their
genitures; such as live in over-cold or over-hot climes; such as
are born of melancholy parents; as offend in those six non-
natural things, are black, or of a high sanguine complexion,
that have little heads,[2] that have a hot heart, moist brain, hot
liver and cold stomach, have been long sick; such as are
solitary by nature, great students, given to much contemplation, lead a life out of action, are most subject to melancholy.
Of sexes both, but men more often; yet women misaffected are
far more violent, and grievously troubled.[3]   Of seasons of the
year, the autumn is most melancholy.   Of peculiar times: old
age, from which natural melancholy is almost an inseparable
accident; but this artificial malady is more frequent in such as
are of a middle age.[4]   Some assign forty years, Gariopontus
thirty.   Jobertus excepts neither young nor old from this
adventitious.   Daniel Sennertus involves all of all sorts, out of
common experience, *in omnibus omnino corporibus cujuscunque
constitutionis dominatur* [5] [it attacks all persons of whatever
constitution].   Aetius and Aretæus [6] ascribe into the number
"not only discontented, passionate, and miserable persons,
swarthy, black; but such as are most merry and pleasant,
scoffers, and high coloured." [7]   "Generally," saith Rhasis, "the
finest wits and most generous spirits are before other obnoxious
to it"; [8] I cannot except any complexion, any condition, sex,
or age, but fools [9] and Stoics, which, according to Synesius,[10]
are never troubled with any manner of passion, but as Anacreon's
cicada, *sine sanguine et dolore; similes fere diis sunt* [without
blood or feeling; they are almost like the gods].   Erasmus
vindicates fools from this melancholy catalogue, because they
have most part moist brains and light hearts; "they are free
from ambition, envy, shame, and fear; they are neither troubled
in conscience, nor macerated with cares, to which our whole life
is most subject." [11]

SUBSECT. III.—*Of the Matter of Melancholy*

Of the matter of melancholy, there is much question betwixt
Avicenna and Galen, as you may read in Cardan's Contradictions,[1]
Valesius' Controversies,[2] Montanus, Prosper Calenus, Capivaccius, Bright,[3] Ficinus,[4] that have written either whole tracts,
or copiously of it in their several treatises of this subject.
"What this humour is, or whence it proceeds, how it is engendered in the body, neither Galen nor any old writer hath
sufficiently discussed,"[5] as Jacchinus thinks: the neoterics
cannot agree. Montanus, in his Consultations, holds melancholy to be material or immaterial: and so doth Arculanus.
The material is one of the four humours before mentioned, and
natural; the immaterial or adventitious, acquisite, redundant,
unnatural, artificial; which Hercules de Saxonia will have reside
in the spirits alone, and to proceed from a "hot, cold, dry, moist
distemperature, which, without matter, alters the brain and
functions of it."[6] Paracelsus wholly rejects and derides this
division of four humours and complexions, but our Galenists
generally approve of it, subscribing to this opinion of Montanus.

This material melancholy is either simple or mixed; offending
in quantity or quality, varying according to his place, where it
settleth, as brain, spleen, meseraic veins, heart, womb, and
stomach; or differing according to the mixture of those natural
humours amongst themselves, or four unnatural adust humours,
as they are diversely tempered and mingled. If natural melancholy abound in the body, which is cold and dry, "so that it
be more than the body is well able to bear, it must needs be
distempered," saith Faventius, "and diseased";[7] and so the
other, if it be depraved, whether it arise from that other melancholy of choler adust, or from blood, produceth the like effects,
and is, as Montaltus contends, if it come by adustion of humours,
most part hot and dry. Some difference I find, whether this
melancholy matter may be engendered of all four humours,
about the colour and temper of it. Galen holds it may be
engendered of three alone, excluding phlegm, or pituita, whose
true assertion Valesius and Menardus[8] stiffly maintain, and so
doth Fuchsius,[9] Montaltus, Montanus.[10] How (say they) can
white become black? But Hercules de Saxonia, *lib. post. de
mela. cap.* 8, and Cardan[11] are of the opposite part (it may be
engendered of phlegm, *etsi raro contingat*, though it seldom
come to pass); so is Guianerius,[12] and Laurentius, *cap.* 1, with
Melancthon in his book *de Anima*, and chap. of Humours; he calls

it *asininam*, dull, swinish melancholy, and saith that he was an eye-witness of it: so is Wecker.[1] From melancholy adust ariseth one kind; from choler another, which is most brutish; another from phlegm, which is dull; and the last from blood, which is best. Of these some are cold and dry, others hot and dry, varying according to their mixtures, as they are intended and remitted.[2] And indeed, as Rodericus à Fons., *cons. 12, lib.* 1, determines, ichors and those serous matters being thickened become phlegm, and phlegm degenerates into choler, choler adust becomes *æruginosa melancholia* [rusty melancholy], as vinegar out of purest wine putrefied or by exhalation of purer spirits is so made, and becomes sour and sharp; and from the sharpness of this humour proceeds much waking, troublesome thoughts and dreams, etc., so that I conclude as before. If the humour be cold, it is, saith Faventinus, "a cause of dotage, and produceth milder symptoms: if hot, they are rash, raving mad, or inclining to it."[3] If the brain be hot, the animal spirits are hot; much madness follows, with violent actions: if cold, fatuity and sottishness (Capivaccius).[4] "The colour of this mixture varies likewise according to the mixture, be it hot or cold; 'tis sometimes black, sometimes not"[5] (Altomarus). The same Melanelius proves out of Galen; and Hippocrates in his book of Melancholy (if at least it be his), giving instance in a burning coal, "which when it is hot, shines; when it is cold, looks black; and so doth the humour."[6] This diversity of melancholy matter produceth diversity of effects. If it be within the body, and not putrefied, it causeth black jaundice;[7] if putrefied, a quartan ague; if it break out to the skin, leprosy; if to parts, several maladies, as scurvy, etc. If it trouble the mind, as it is diversely mixed, it produceth several kinds of madness and dotage: of which in their place.

SUBSECT. IV.—*Of the Species or Kinds of Melancholy*

When the matter is diverse and confused, how should it otherwise be but that the species should be diverse and confused? Many new and old writers have spoken confusedly of it, confounding melancholy and madness, as Heurnius,[8] Guianerius, Gordonius, Sallustius Salvianus, Jason Pratensis, Savonarola, that will have madness no other than melancholy in extent, differing (as I have said) in degrees. Some make two distinct species, as Ruffus Ephesius, an old writer, Constantinus Africanus, Aretæus, Aurelianus,[9] Paulus Ægineta: others acknowledge a

multitude of kinds, and leave them indefinite, as Aetius in his
Tetrabiblos,[1] Avicenna,[2] *lib.* 3, *fen.* 1, *tract* 4, *cap.* 18; Arculanus,
cap. 16, *in* 9 *Rhasis*; Montanus, *Med.part.* 1. "If natural melancholy
be adust, it maketh one kind; if blood, another; if choler, a third,
differing from the first; and so many several opinions there are
about the kinds, as there be men themselves."[3] Hercules de
Saxonia sets down two kinds, "material and immaterial; one from
spirits alone, the other from humours and spirits."[4] Savonarola,
rub. 11, *tract.* 6, *cap.* 1, *de ægritud. capitis*, will have the kinds
to be infinite; one from the myrach, called *myrachialis* of the
Arabians; another *stomachalis*, from the stomach; another from
the liver, heart, womb, hemrods: "one beginning, another consummate."[5] Melancthon seconds him:[6] "As the humour is
diversely adust and mixed, so are the species diverse"; but what
these men speak of species I think ought to be understood of
symptoms, and so doth Arculanus interpret himself:[7] infinite
species, *id est*, symptoms; and in that sense, as Jo. Gorrhæus
acknowledgeth in his Medicinal Definitions, the species are
infinite, but they may be reduced to three kinds by reason of
their seat; head, body, and hypochondries. This threefold
division is approved by Hippocrates in his book of Melancholy
(if it be his, which some suspect), by Galen, *lib.* 3 *de loc. affectis*,
cap. 6; by Alexander, *lib.* 1, *cap.* 16; Rhasis, *lib.* 1 *Continent.*,
Tract. 9, *lib.* 1, *cap.* 16; Avicenna, and most of our new writers.
Th. Erastus makes two kinds; one perpetual, which is head-
melancholy; the other interrupt, which comes and goes by fits,
which he subdivides into the other two kinds, so that all comes
to the same pass. Some again make four or five kinds, with
Rodericus à Castro, *de morbis mulier. lib.* 2, *cap.* 3, and Lod.
Mercatus, who in his second book *de mulier. affect. cap.* 4, will
have that melancholy of nuns, widows, and more ancient maids
to be a peculiar species of melancholy differing from the rest:
some will reduce enthusiasts, ecstatical and demoniacal persons
to this rank, adding love-melancholy to the first,[8] and lycanthropia. The most received division is into three kinds. The
first proceeds from the sole fault of the brain, and is called
head-melancholy; the second sympathetically proceeds from
the whole body, when the whole temperature is melancholy:
the third ariseth from the bowels, liver, spleen, or membrane
called mesenterium, named hypochondriacal or windy melancholy, which Laurentius[9] subdivides into three parts, from those
three members, hepatic, splenetic, meseraic. Love-melancholy,
which Avicenna calls *ilishi*, and lycanthropia, which he calls

cucubuth, are commonly included in head-melancholy; but of this last, which Gerardus de Solo calls amorous, and most knight-melancholy, with that of religious melancholy, *virginum et viduarum* [of maids and widows], maintained by Rod. à Castro and Mercatus, and the other kinds of love-melancholy, I will speak of apart by themselves in my third partition. The three precedent species are the subject of my present discourse, which I will anatomize and treat of through all their causes, symptoms, cures, together and apart; that every man that is in any measure affected with this malady may know how to examine it in himself, and apply remedies unto it.

It is a hard matter, I confess, to distinguish these three species one from the other, to express their several causes, symptoms, cures, being that they are so often confounded amongst themselves, having such affinity that they can scarce be discerned by the most accurate physicians, and so often intermixed with other diseases that the best experienced have been plunged. Montanus, *consil.* 26, names a patient that had this disease of melancholy and *caninus appetitus* both together; and, *consil.* 23, with vertigo; Julius Cæsar Claudinus with stone, gout, jaundice;[1] Trincavellius with an ague, jaundice, *caninus appetitus*, etc. Paulus Regoline,[2] a great doctor in his time, consulted in this case, was so confounded with a confusion of symptoms, that he knew not to what kind of melancholy to refer it. Trincavellius,[3] Fallopius, and Francanzanus, famous doctors in Italy, all three conferred with about one party at the same time, gave three different opinions. And in another place, Trincavellius being demanded what he thought of a melancholy young man to whom he was sent for, ingenuously confessed that he was indeed melancholy, but he knew not to what kind to reduce it. In his seventeenth consultation there is the like disagreement about a melancholy monk. Those symptoms, which others ascribe to misaffected parts and humours, Herc. de Saxonia[4] attributes wholly to distempered spirits, and those immaterial, as I have said. Sometimes they cannot well discern this disease from others. In Reinerus Solenander's Counsels, *sect.* 3, *consil.* 5, he and Dr. Brande both agreed that the patient's disease was hypochondriacal melancholy. Dr. Matholdus said it was asthma, and nothing else. Solenander and Guarionius,[5] lately sent for to the melancholy Duke of Cleve, with others, could not define what species it was, or agree amongst themselves. The species are so confounded, as in Cæsar Claudinus his forty-fourth consultation for a Polonian

count; in his judgment "he laboured of head melancholy, and
that which proceeds from the whole temperature, both at once."[1]
I could give instance of some that have had all three kinds
semel et simul [all together], and some successively. So that
I conclude of our melancholy species, as many politicians do of
their pure forms of commonwealths,[2] monarchies, aristocracies,
democracies, are most famous in contemplation, but in practice
they are temperate and usually mixed (so Polybius informeth
us[3]), as the Lacedæmonian, the Roman of old, German now,
and many others. What physicians say of distinct species in
their books it much matters not, since that in their patients'
bodies they are commonly mixed. In such obscurity, therefore, variety and confused mixture of symptoms, causes, how
difficult a thing is it to treat of several kinds apart; to make
any certainty or distinction among so many casualties, dis-
tractions, when seldom two men shall be like affected *per
omnia* [in all respects] ! 'Tis hard, I confess, yet nevertheless
I will adventure through the midst of these perplexities, and,
led by the clue or thread of the best writers, extricate myself
out of a labyrinth of doubts and errors, and so proceed to
the causes.

SECT. II. MEMB. I.

SUBSECT. I.—*Causes of Melancholy. God a Cause*

"IT is in vain to speak of cures, or think of remedies, until
such time as we have considered of the causes," so Galen prescribes Glauco:[4] and the common experience of others confirms
that those cures must be imperfect, lame, and to no purpose,
wherein the causes have not first been searched, as Prosper
Calenius well observes in his tract *de atra bile* to Cardinal
Cœsius.[5] Insomuch that Fernelius puts "a kind of necessity
in the knowledge of the causes, and without which it is impossible to cure or prevent any manner of disease."[6] Empirics
may ease, and sometimes help, but not throughly root out;
sublata causa tollitur effectus, as the saying is, if the cause be
removed, the effect is likewise vanquished. It is a most difficult thing (I confess) to be able to discern these causes whence
they are, and in such variety to say what the beginning was.[7]
He is happy that can perform it aright.[8] I will adventure to
guess as near as I can, and rip them all up, from the first to the

last, general and particular, to every species, that so they may
the better be described.

General causes are either supernatural or natural. Supernatural are from God and His angels, or by God's permission
from the devil and his ministers. That God Himself is a
cause for the punishment of sin, and satisfaction of His justice,
many examples and testimonies of holy Scriptures make evident
unto us. Ps. cvii, 17: "Foolish men are plagued for their offence,
and by reason of their wickedness." Gehazi was strucken with
leprosy (2 Reg. v, 27); Jehoram with dysentery and flux, and
great diseases of the bowels (2 Chron. xxi, 15); David plagued
for numbering his people (1 Chron. xxi); Sodom and Gomorrah
swallowed up. And this disease is peculiarly specified (Ps.
cvii, 12), "He brought down their heart through heaviness";
(Deut. xxviii, 28), "He struck them with madness, blindness,
and astonishment of heart"; "An evil spirit was sent by the
Lord upon Saul, to vex him";[1] Nebuchadnezzar did eat grass
like an ox, and his "heart was made like the beasts of the
field."[2]   Heathen stories are full of such punishments. Lycurgus, because he cut down the vines in the country, was by
Bacchus driven into madness: so was Pentheus and his mother
Agave for neglecting their sacrifice. Censor Fulvius ran mad
for untiling Juno's temple, to cover a new one of his own, which
he had dedicated to Fortune,[3] "and was confounded to death
with grief and sorrow of heart."[4]   When Xerxes would have
spoiled Apollo's temple at Delphi of those infinite riches it
possessed, a terrible thunder came from heaven and struck
four thousand men dead, the rest ran mad.[5]   A little after, the
like happened to Brennus, lightning, thunder, earthquakes, upon
such a sacrilegious occasion.[6]   If we may believe our pontifical
writers, they will relate unto us many strange and prodigious
punishments in this kind, inflicted by their saints. How Clodoveus, sometime King of France, the son of Dagobert, lost his
wits for uncovering the body of St. Denis;[7] and how a sacrilegious Frenchman, that would have stolen a silver image of
St. John, at Birgburge, became frantic on a sudden, raging,
and tyrannizing over his own flesh;[8] of a Lord of Radnor,
that coming from hunting late at night, put his dogs into St.
Avan's Church (Llan Avan they called it), and rising betimes
next morning, as hunters use to do, found all his dogs
mad, himself being suddenly strucken blind;[9] of Tiridates, an
Armenian king, for violating some holy nuns, that was punished
in like sort, with loss of his wits. But poets and papists may

go together for fabulous tales; let them free their own credits:
howsoever they feign of their Nemesis, and of their saints, or
by the devil's means may be deluded, we find it true that
ultor a tergo Deus,[1] "He is God the avenger," as David styles
Him;[2] and that it is our crying sins that pull this and many
other maladies on our own heads; that He can by His angels,
which are His ministers, strike and heal (saith Dionysius) whom
He will;[3] that He can plague us by His creatures, sun, moon,
and stars, whom He useth as His instruments, as a husbandman
(saith Zanchius) doth a hatchet: hail, snow, winds, etc.—*Et
conjurati veniunt in classica venti*[4] [the winds in a band answer
His summons]—as in Joshua's time, as in Pharaoh's reign in
Egypt, they are but as so many executioners of His justice.
He can make the proudest spirits stoop, and cry out with
Julian the Apostate, *Vicisti, Galilæe*;[5] or with Apollo's priest in
Chrysostom,[6] *O cœlum! O terra!* [O heaven! O earth!] *unde
hostis hic?* what an enemy is this? and pray with David,
acknowledging his power, "I am weakened and sore broken,
I roar for the grief of mine heart, mine heart panteth,"
etc. (Ps. xxxviii, 8); "O Lord, rebuke me not in thine
anger, neither chastise me in thy wrath" (Ps. xxxviii, 1);
"Make me to hear joy and gladness, that the bones which
thou hast broken may rejoice" (Ps. li, 8); "Restore to me
the joy of thy salvation, and stablish me with thy free spirit"
(Ps. li, 12). For these causes belike Hippocrates[7] would have
a physician take special notice whether the disease come not
from a divine supernatural cause, or whether it follow the
course of nature. But this is further discussed by Fran. Valesius,
de sacr. philos. cap. 8, Fernelius,[8] and J. Cæsar Claudinus,[9]
to whom I refer you, how this place of Hippocrates is to be
understood. Paracelsus is of opinion that such spiritual diseases
(for so he calls them) are spiritually to be cured, and not otherwise. Ordinary means in such cases will not avail: *Non est
reluctandum cum Deo* [we must not struggle with God]. When
that monster-taming Hercules overcame all in the Olympics,
Jupiter at last in an unknown shape wrestled with him; the
victory was uncertain, till at length Jupiter descried himself,
and Hercules yielded. No striving with supreme powers. *Nil
uvat immensos Cratero promittere montes* [it avails not to promise
Craterus gold mines for a cure], physicians and physic can
do no good, "we must submit ourselves unto the mighty hand
of God, acknowledge our offences, call to Him for mercy."[10]
If He strike us, *una eademque manus vulnus opemque feret* [the

same hand will inflict the wound and provide the remedy], as
it is with them that are wounded with the spear of Achilles,
He alone must help; otherwise our diseases are incurable, and
we not to be relieved.

SUBSECT. II.—*A Digression of the Nature of Spirits, Bad
Angels, or Devils, and how they cause Melancholy*

How far the power of spirits and devils doth extend, and
whether they can cause this, or any other disease, is a serious
question, and worthy to be considered: for the better understanding of which, I will make a brief digression of the nature
of spirits. And although the question be very obscure, according to Postellus, "full of controversy and ambiguity," [1] beyond
the reach of human capacity, *fateor excedere vires intentionis
meæ*, saith Austin,[2] I confess I am not able to understand it,
finitum de infinito non potest statuere [the finite cannot decide
about the infinite], we can sooner determine with Tully (*De
nat. deorum*), *quid non sint, quam quid sint* [what they are not
than what they are], our subtle schoolmen, Cardans, Scaligers,
profound Thomists, *Fracastoriana et Ferneliana acies*, are weak,
dry, obscure, defective in these mysteries, and all our quickest
wits, as an owl's eyes at the sun's light, wax dull, and are
not sufficient to apprehend them; yet, as in the rest, I will
adventure to say something to this point. In former times, as
we read (Acts xxiii), the Sadducees denied that there were any
such spirits, devils, or angels. So did Galen the physician, the
Peripatetics, even Aristotle himself, as Pomponatius stoutly
maintains, and Scaliger in some sort grants, though Dandinus
the Jesuit, *Com. in lib. 2 de anima*, stiffly denies it; *substantiæ
separatæ* [abstract substances] and intelligences are the same
which Christians call angels, and Platonists devils, for they
name all the spirits *dæmones*, be they good or bad angels, as
Julius Pollux, *Onomasticon, lib. 1, cap. 1*, observes. Epicures
and atheists are of the same mind in general, because they
never saw them. Plato, Plotinus, Porphyrius, Iamblichus,
Proclus, insisting in the steps of Trismegistus, Pythagoras, and
Socrates, make no doubt of it: nor Stoics, but that there are
such spirits, though much erring from the truth. Concerning
the first beginning of them, the Talmudists say that Adam had
a wife called Lilis, before he married Eve, and of her he begat
nothing but devils.[3] The Turks' Alcoran is altogether as absurd
and ridiculous in this point:[4] but the Scripture informs us

Christians, how Lucifer, the chief of them, with his associates, fell from heaven for his pride and ambition;[1] created of God, placed in heaven, and sometime an angel of light, now cast down into the lower aerial sublunary parts, or into hell, "and delivered into chains of darkness to be kept unto damnation" (2 Pet. ii, 4). There is a foolish opinion which some hold, that they are the souls of men departed; good and more noble were deified, the baser grovelled on the ground, or in the lower parts, and were devils; the which, with Tertullian, Porphyrius the philosopher, M. Tyrius, *ser.* 27, maintains. "These spirits," he saith, "which we call angels and devils, are naught but souls of men departed, which either through love and pity of their friends yet living, help and assist them, or else persecute their enemies, whom they hated,"[2] as Dido threatened to persecute Æneas:

> *Omnibus umbra locis adero : dabis, improbe, pœnas.*
>
> [My angry ghost, arising from the deep,
> Shall haunt thee waking, and disturb thy sleep.]

They are (as others suppose) appointed by those higher powers to keep men from their nativity, and to protect or punish them as they see cause: and are called *boni* and *mali genii* by the Romans; heroes, lares if good, lemures or larvæ if bad, by the Stoics; governors of countries, men, cities, saith Apuleius: *Deos appellant qui ex hominum numero juste ac prudenter vitæ curriculo gubernato, pro numine, postea ab hominibus præditi fanis et ceremoniis vulgo admittuntur, ut in Ægypto Osiris*[3] [they call gods those who, having as men lived justly and wisely on earth, are after their death deified, and honoured with temples and rites, like Osiris in Egypt], etc. *Præstites* [protectors], Capella calls them, "which protected particular men as well as princes." Socrates had his *dæmonium saturninum et igneum* [saturnine and fiery familiar spirit], which of all spirits is best *ad sublimes cogitationes animum erigentem* [for stirring the mind to sublime reflections], as the Platonists supposed; Plotinus his; and we Christians our assisting angel, as Andreas Victorellus, a copious writer of this subject, Lodovicus de La-Cerda, the Jesuit, in his voluminous tract *de Angelo Custode*, Zanchius, and some divines think. But this absurd tenent of Tyrius, Proclus confutes at large in his book *de anima et dæmone*.

Psellus,[4] a Christian, and sometime tutor (saith Cuspinian) to Michael Parapinatius, Emperor of Greece, a great observer of the nature of devils, holds they are corporeal, and have

"aerial bodies, that they are mortal, live and die,"[1] (which
Martianus Capella likewise maintains, but our Christian philosophers explode), "that they are nourished and have excrements,
that they feel pain if they be hurt" (which Cardan confirms, and
Scaliger justly laughs him to scorn for; *Si pascantur aere, cur
non pugnant ob puriorem aera?* [If they feed on air, why do
they not fight for purer air?], etc.) "or stroken":[2] and if their
bodies be cut, with admirable celerity they come together
again. Austin, *in Gen. lib.* 3, *lib. arbit.*, approves as much,
mutato casu corpora in deteriorem qualitatem aeris spissioris
[conversely, their bodies can be changed to an air of inferior
and coarser quality]; so doth Hierome, *Comment. in Epist. ad
Ephes. cap.* 3, Origen, Tertullian, Lactantius, and many ancient
Fathers of the Church: that in their fall their bodies were changed
into a more aerial and gross substance. Bodine, *lib.* 4 *Theatri
Naturæ*, and David Crusius, *Hermeticæ Philosophiæ lib.* 1, *cap.* 4,
by several arguments proves angels and spirits to be corporeal:
*Quicquid continetur in loco corporeum est: At spiritus continetur
in loco, ergo* [whatever occupies space is corporeal; spirit occupies
space, therefore, etc.]. *Si spiritus sunt quanti, erunt corporei:
At sunt quanti, ergo. Sunt finiti, ergo quanti* [If spirits are
quantities, they must be corporeal; but they are quantities,
therefore . . . They are finite, therefore quantitative], etc.
Bodine goes farther yet, and will have these *animæ separatæ*
[abstract souls], genii, spirits, angels, devils, and so likewise
souls of men departed, if corporeal (which he most eagerly
contends), to be of some shape, and that absolutely round, like
sun and moon, because that is the most perfect form, *quæ nihil
habet asperitatis, nihil angulis incisum, nihil anfractibus invo-
lutum, nihil eminens, sed inter corpora perfecta est perfectissimum*[3]
[which has no rough edges, no corners, no twists, no projections,
but is the most perfect of shapes]; therefore all spirits are
corporeal, he concludes, and in their proper shapes round.
That they can assume other aerial bodies, all manner of shapes
at their pleasures, appear in what likeness they will themselves,
that they are most swift in motion, can pass many miles in an
instant, and so likewise transform bodies of others into what
shape they please, and with admirable celerity remove them
from place to place[4] (as the angel did Habakkuk to Daniel,[5]
and as Philip the Deacon was carried away by the Spirit, when
he had baptized the eunuch; so did Pythagoras and Apollonius
remove themselves and others, with many such feats); that
they can represent castles in the air, palaces, armies, spectrums,

prodigies, and such strange objects to mortal men's eyes, cause
smells, savours, etc.,[1] deceive all the senses; most writers of
this subject credibly believe; and that they can foretell future
events, and do many strange miracles.　Juno's image spake
to Camillus, and Fortune's statue to the Roman matrons, with
many such.　Zanchius, Bodine, Spondanus, and others, are of
opinion that they cause a true metamorphosis, as Nebuchadnezzar was really translated into a beast, Lot's wife into a
pillar of salt, Ulysses' companions into hogs and dogs by
Circe's charms; turn themselves and others, as they do witches,
into cats, dogs, hares, crows, etc.　Strozzius Cicogna hath
many examples, *lib. 3 Omnif. mag. cap.* 4 *et* 5, which he
there confutes, as Austin likewise doth, *de Civ. Dei, lib.* 18.
That they can be seen when, and in what shape, and to whom
they will, saith Psellus, *tametsi nil tale viderim, nec optem videre*,
though he himself never saw them nor desired it; and use sometimes carnal copulation (as elsewhere I shall prove more at
large [2]) with women and men.　Many will not believe they can
be seen, and if any man shall say, swear, and stiffly maintain,
though he be discreet and wise, judicious and learned, that he
hath seen them, they account him a timorous fool, a melancholy
dizzard, a weak fellow, a dreamer, a sick or a mad man, they
contemn him, laugh him to scorn, and yet Marcus of his credit
told Psellus that he had often seen them.　And Leo Suavius,
a Frenchman, *cap.* 8, *in Commentar. lib.* 1 *Paracelsi de vita longa*,
out of some Platonists, will have the air to be as full of them as
snow falling in the skies, and that they may be seen, and withal
sets down the means how men may see them: *Si irreverberatis
oculis sole splendente versus cœlum continuaverint obtutus* [by
looking steadfastly at the sky, in bright sunshine, without
blinking], etc., and saith moreover he tried it, *præmissorum
feci experimentum*, and it was true that the Platonists said.
Paracelsus confesseth that he saw them divers times, and
conferred with them, and so doth Alexander ab Alexandro,
"that he so found it by experience, whenas before he doubted
of it."[3]　Many deny it, saith Lavater, *de spectris, part.* 1, *cap.* 2,
and *part.* 2, *cap.* 11, "because they never saw them themselves";
but as he reports at large all over his book, especially *cap.* 19, *part.*
1, they are often seen and heard, and familiarly converse with
men, as Lod. Vives assureth us, innumerable records, histories,
and testimonies evince in all ages, times, places, and all travellers besides;[4] in the West Indies and our northern climes,
nihil familiarius quam in agris et urbibus spiritus videre, audire

qui vetent, jubeant [nothing is more common than to see spirits
both in town and country, and to hear them ordering or forbidding something], etc. Hieronymus, *vita Pauli,* Basil, *ser.* 40,
Nicephorus, Eusebius, Socrates, Sozomenus,[1] Jacobus Boissardus
in his tract *de spirituum apparitionibus,* Petrus Loyerus, *lib. de
spectris,* Wierus, *lib.* 1, have infinite variety of such examples of
apparitions of spirits, for him to read that further doubts, to
his ample satisfaction. One alone I will briefly insert. A
nobleman in Germany was sent ambassador to the King of
Sweden (for his name, the time, and such circumstances, I refer
you to Boissardus, mine author[2]). After he had done his
business, he sailed to Livonia, on set purpose to see those
familiar spirits, which are there said to be conversant with
men and do their drudgery works. Amongst other matters,
one of them told him where his wife was, in what room, in what
clothes, what doing, and brought him a ring from her, which at
his return, *non sine omnium admiratione* [to the general surprise],
he found to be true; and so believed that ever after, which before
he doubted of. Cardan, *lib.* 19 *de subtil.,* relates of his father,
Facius Cardan, that after the accustomed solemnities, *ann.* 1491,
13 August, he conjured up seven devils in Greek apparel, about
forty years of age, some ruddy of complexion, and some pale,
as he thought; he asked them many questions, and they made
ready answer, that they were aerial devils, that they lived and
died as men did, save that they were far longer lived (seven or
eight hundred years[3]); they did as much excel men in dignity
as we do juments, and were as far excelled again of those that
were above them; our governors and keepers they are, moreover,[4] which Plato in *Critias* delivered of old,[5] and subordinate
to one another, *ut enim homo homini, sic dæmon dæmoni dominatur* [for as man rules man, so devil rules devil], they rule
themselves as well as us, and the spirits of the meaner sort had
commonly such offices, as we make horsekeepers, neatherds,
and the basest of us overseers of our cattle; and that we can
no more apprehend their natures and functions than a horse
a man's. They knew all things, but might not reveal them to
men; and ruled and domineered over us, as we do over our
horses; the best kings amongst us, and the most generous
spirits, were not comparable to the basest of them. Sometimes
they did instruct men, and communicate their skill, reward
and cherish, and sometimes again terrify and punish, to keep
them in awe, as they thought fit, *nihil magis cupientes* (saith
Lysius, *Phys. Stoicorum*) *quam adorationem hominum* [longing

for nothing more than the worship of mankind]. The same
author, Cardan, in his *Hyperchen*, out of the doctrine of Stoics,
will have some of these genii (for so he calls them) to be desirous
of men's company, very affable and familiar with them, as
dogs are; others, again, to abhor as serpents, and care not for
them.[1]   The same, belike, Trithemius calls *igneos et sublunares,
qui nunquam demergunt ad inferiora, aut vix ullum habent in
terris commercium* [fiery and sublunar, who never descend to
the lower sphere, and have little to do with the earth]. "Generally they far excel men in worth, as a man the meanest worm;
though some of them are inferior to those of their own rank in
worth as the black guard in a prince's court, and to men again
as some degenerate, base, rational creatures are excelled of
brute beasts." [2]

That they are mortal, besides these testimonies of Cardan,
Martianus, etc., many other divines and philosophers hold, *post
prolixum tempus moriuntur omnes* [they all die after a great
lapse of time]; the Platonists[3] and some Rabbins, Porphyrius,
and Plutarch, as appears by that relation of Thamus: "The
great God Pan is dead";[4] Apollo Pythius ceased; and so the rest.
St. Hierome, in the life of Paul the Eremite, tells a story how
one of them appeared to St. Anthony in the wilderness, and
told him as much.   Paracelsus, of our late writers, stiffly maintains that they are mortal, live and die as other creatures do.[5]
Zozimus, *lib.* 2, farther adds, that religion and policy dies and
alters with them.   The Gentiles' gods, he saith, were expelled
by Constantine,[6] and together with them *imperii Romani
majestas et fortuna interiit, et profligata est*, the fortune and
majesty of the Roman Empire decayed and vanished; as that
heathen in Minucius formerly bragged, when the Jews were
overcome by the Romans, the Jews' God was likewise captivated
by that of Rome;[7] and Rabshakeh to the Israelites, no God
should deliver them out of the hands of the Assyrians.   But
these paradoxes of their power, corporeity, mortality, taking
of shapes, transposing bodies, and carnal copulations, are
sufficiently confuted by Zanch. *cap.* 10, *lib.* 4; Pererius, in his
Comment, and Tostatus' questions on the 6th of Gen.; Th. Aquin.,
St. Austin, Wierus, Th. Erastus, Delrio, *tom.* 2, *lib.* 2, *quæst.* 29;
Sebastian Michaelis, *cap.* 2 *de spiritibus*, Dr. Rainolds, *Lect.* 47.
They may deceive the eyes of men, yet not take true bodies, or
make a real metamorphosis; but as Cicogna proves at large,
they are *illusoriæ et præstigiatrices transformationes* [8] (*Omnif.
mag. lib.* 4, *cap.* 4), mere illusions and cozenings, like that tale

of *Pasetis obolus* in Suidas, or that of Autolycus, Mercury's son that dwelt in Parnassus, who got so much treasure by cozenage and stealth. His father Mercury, because he could leave him no wealth, taught him many fine tricks to get means, for he could drive away men's cattle, and if any pursued him, turn them into what shapes he would,[1] and so did mightily enrich himself, *hoc astu maximam prædam est adsecutus*. This, no doubt, is as true as the rest; yet thus much in general Thomas, Durand, and others grant, that they have understanding far beyond men, can probably conjecture and foretell many things;[2] they can cause and cure most diseases, deceive our senses; they have excellent skill in all arts and sciences; and that the most illiterate devil is *quovis homine scientior* (more knowing than any man), as Cicogna maintains out of others.[3] They know the virtues of herbs, plants, stones, minerals, etc., of all creatures, birds, beasts, the four elements, stars, planets; can aptly apply and make use of them as they see good; perceiving the causes of all meteors, and the like. *Dant se coloribus* (as Austin hath it[4]), *accommodant se figuris, adhærent sonis, subjiciunt se odoribus, infundunt se saporibus* [they insert themselves into colours, shapes, sounds, smells, and tastes], *omnes sensus etiam ipsam intelligentiam dæmones fallunt*, they deceive all our senses, even our understanding itself at once. They can produce miraculous alterations in the air, and most wonderful effects, conquer armies, give victories, help, further, hurt, cross, and alter human attempts and projects (*Dei permissu*) as they see good themselves.[5] When Charles the Great intended to make a channel betwixt the Rhine and Danubius, look what his workmen did in the day, these spirits flung down in the night,[6] *ut conatu rex desisteret, pervicere* [they succeeded in making the king desist from his attempt]. Such feats can they do. But that which Bodine, *lib.* 4 *Theat. nat.*, thinks (following Tyrius belike, and the Platonists), they can tell the secrets of a man's heart, *aut cogitationes hominum*, is most false; his reasons are weak, and sufficiently confuted by Zanch., *lib.* 4, *cap.* 9; Hierome, *lib.* 2 *Com. in Mat. ad cap.* 15, Athanasius, *Quæst.* 27 *ad Antiochum Principem*, and others.

As for those orders of good and bad devils, [that] which the Platonists hold is altogether erroneous, and those ethnics' *boni* and *mali genii* [good and bad genii] are to be exploded: these heathen writers agree not in this point among themselves, as Dandinus notes, *An sint mali non conveniunt*[7] [they are not agreed as to whether there are any bad]; some will have all spirits good

or bad to us by a mistake; as if an ox or horse could discourse,
he would say the butcher was his enemy because he killed him,
the grazier his friend because he fed him; an hunter preserves
and yet kills his game, and is hated nevertheless of his game;
nec piscatorem piscis amare potest [the fish cannot love the
fisherman], etc. But Iamblichus, Psellus, Plutarch, and most
Platonists acknowledge bad, *et ab eorum maleficiis cavendum*
[and we should beware of their wickedness], for they are enemies
of mankind, and this Plato learned in Egypt, that they quar-
relled with Jupiter, and were driven by him down to hell.[1]
That which Apuleius,[2] Xenophon, and Plato contend of
Socrates' *dæmonium*, is most absurd: that which Plotinus of
his, that he had likewise *deum pro dæmonio* [a god for his
familiar spirit]; and that which Porphyry concludes of them
all in general, if they be neglected in their sacrifice they are
angry; nay more, as Cardan in his *Hyperchen* will, they feed
on men's souls: *Elementa sunt plantis elementum, animalibus
plantæ, hominibus animalia, erunt et homines aliis, non autem
diis, nimis enim remota est eorum natura a nostra, quapropter
dæmonibus* [minerals are food for plants, plants for animals,
animals for men; men will also be food for other creatures, but
not for gods, for their nature is far removed from ours; it must
therefore be for devils]; and so, belike, that we have so many
battles fought in all ages, countries, is to make them a feast, and
their sole delight: but to return to that I said before, if displeased
they fret and chafe (for they feed, belike, on the souls of beasts, as
we do on their bodies), and send many plagues amongst us; but if
pleased, then they do much good; is as vain as the rest, and confuted by Austin, *lib.* 9, *cap.* 8, *de Civ. Dei.*, Euseb., *lib.* 4 *Præpar.
Evang. cap.* 6, and others. Yet thus much I find, that our
schoolmen and other divines make nine kinds of bad spirits,[3]
as Dionysius hath done of angels. In the first rank are those
false gods of the Gentiles, which were adored heretofore in
several idols, and gave oracles at Delphi, and elsewhere;
whose prince is Beelzebub. The second rank is of liars and
equivocators, as Apollo Pythius and the like. The third are
those vessels of anger, inventors of all mischief; as that Theuth
in Plato; Esay calls them vessels of fury;[4] their prince is
Belial. The fourth are malicious revenging devils; and their
prince is Asmodæus. The fifth kind are cozeners, such as
belong to magicians and witches; their prince is Satan. The
sixth are those aerial devils that corrupt the air and cause
plagues, thunders, fires, etc.; spoken of in the Apocalypse,[5]

and Paul to the Ephesians names them the princes of the air;
Meresin [1] is their prince.   The seventh is a destroyer, captain
of the Furies, causing wars, tumults, combustions, uproars,
mentioned in the Apocalypse, and called Abaddon.   The eighth
is that accusing or calumniating devil, whom the Greeks call
Διάβολος, that drives men to despair.   The ninth are those
tempters in several kinds, and their prince is Mammon.   Psellus
makes six kinds, yet none above the moon; Wierus, in his
Pseudomonarchia Dæmonis, out of an old book, makes many
more divisions and subordinations, with their several names,
numbers, offices, etc., but Gazæus, cited by Lipsius,[2] will have
all places full of angels, spirits, and devils, above and beneath
the moon,[3] ætherial and aerial, which Austin cites out of
Varro, *lib. 7 de Civ. Dei, cap.* 6, "the celestial devils above, and
aerial beneath," or, as some will, gods above, *semidei* or half-
gods beneath, lares, heroes, genii, which climb higher, if they
lived well, as the Stoics held, but grovel on the ground as they
were baser in their lives, nearer to the earth: and are manes,
lemures, lamiæ, etc.   They will have no place void, but all full
of spirits, devils, or some other inhabitants;[4] *plenum cœlum,
aer, aqua, terra, et omnia sub terra* [full is the sky, the air, the
sea, the earth, and all beneath the earth], saith Gazæus;
though Anthony Rusca, in his book *de Inferno, lib.* 5, *cap.* 7,
would confine them to the middle region, yet they will have
them everywhere, "not so much as an hairbreadth empty in
heaven, earth, or waters, above or under the earth."[5]   The air
is not so full of flies in summer as it is at all times of invisible
devils: this Paracelsus [6] stiffly maintains, and that they have
every one their several chaos; others will have infinite worlds,
and each world his peculiar spirits, gods, angels, and devils
to govern and punish it.

> *Singula nonnulli credunt quoque sidera posse
> Dici orbes, terramque appellant sidus opacum,
> Cui minimus divum præsit.*[7]

> [Some, too, believe that each star may also be called a
>   world, and regard this earth as a dark star over
>   which the least of the gods presides.]

Gregorius Tholosanus makes seven kinds of ætherial spirits or
angels,[8] according to the number of the seven planets, Saturnine, Jovial, Martial, of which Cardan discourseth, *lib.* 20 *de
subtil.*; he calls them *substantias primas* [primary substances];
Olympicos dæmones Trithemius, qui præsunt zodiaco [Trithemius

calls them Olympian spirits which rule the zodiac], etc.,
and will have them to be good angels above, devils beneath
the moon; their several names and offices he there sets down,
and, which Dionysius of angels, will have several spirits for
several countries, men, offices, etc., which live about them,
and as so many assisting powers cause their operations; will
have, in a word, innumerable, as many of them as there be stars
in the skies.   Marsilius Ficinus seems to second this opinion,[1]
out of Plato, or from himself, I know not (still ruling their
inferiors, as they do those under them again, all subordinate,
and the nearest to the earth rule us, whom we subdivide into
good and bad angels, call gods or devils, as they help or hurt
us, and so adore, love or hate), but it is most likely from Plato,
for he, relying wholly on Socrates, *quem mori potius quam mentiri
voluisse scribit* [who, he says, would rather die than tell a false-
hood], out of Socrates' authority alone, made nine kinds of them;
which opinion, belike, Socrates took from Pythagoras, and he
from Trismegistus, he from Zoroaster: 1, God; 2, Ideæ; 3, Intelligences; 4, Archangels; 5, Angels; 6, Devils; 7, Heroes; 8, Principalities; 9, Princes: of which some were absolutely good, as
gods, some bad, some indifferent *inter deos et homines* [between
gods and men], as heroes and dæmons, which ruled men, and
were called genii, or as Proclus[2] and Iamblichus will, the
middle betwixt God and men, principalities and princes, which
commanded and swayed kings and countries, and had several
places in the spheres perhaps, for as every sphere is higher, so
hath it more excellent inhabitants: which, belike, is that Galilæus
à Galilæo and Kepler aims at in his *Nuncio Sidereo*, when he
will have Saturnine and Jovial inhabitants:[3] and which Tycho
Brahe doth in some sort touch or insinuate in one of his epistles:
but these things Zanchius justly explodes, *cap. 3, lib.* 4;[4] P.
Martyr *in* 1 *Sam.* 28.
  So that according to these men the number of ætherial spirits
must needs be infinite; for if that be true that some of our
mathematicians say: if a stone could fall from the starry heaven,
or eighth sphere, and should pass every hour an hundred miles,
it would be 65 years, or more, before it would come to ground,
by reason of the great distance of heaven from earth, which
contains, as some say, 170 millions 803 miles, besides those other
heavens, whether they be crystalline or watery, which Maginus
adds, which peradventure holds as much more; how many such
spirits may it contain?   And yet for all this Thomas,[5] Albertus,
and most, hold that there be far more angels than devils.

But be they more or less, *Quod supra nos nihil ad nos* [what is beyond our comprehension does not concern us]. Howsoever, as Martianus foolishly supposeth, *Ætherii dæmones non curant res humanas*, they care not for us, do not attend our actions, or look for us, those ætherial spirits have other worlds to reign in, belike, or business to follow. We are only now to speak in brief of those sublunary spirits or devils: for the rest, our divines determine that the devil had no power over stars or heavens. *Carminibus cœlo possunt deducere lunam*[1] [by their charms (verses) they can seduce the moon from the heavens], etc.—those are poetical fictions; and that they can *sistere aquam fluviis, et vertere sidera retro*[2] [stop rivers and turn the stars backward in their courses], etc., as Canidia in Horace, 'tis all false. They are confined until the day of judgment to this sublunary world, and can work no farther than the four elements, and as God permits them.[3] Wherefore of these sublunary devils, though others divide them otherwise according to their several places and offices, Psellus makes six kinds, fiery, aerial, terrestrial, watery, and subterranean devils, besides those fairies, satyrs, nymphs, etc.

Fiery spirits or devils are such as commonly work by blazing stars, fire-drakes, or *ignes fatui*; which lead men often *in flumina aut præcipitia* [into rivers or over precipices], saith Bodine, *lib. 2 Theat. naturæ, fol. 221. Quos, inquit, arcere si volunt viatores, clara voce Deum appellare aut prona facie terram contingente adorare oportet, et hoc amuletum majoribus nostris acceptum ferre debemus* [whom if travellers wish to keep off they must pronounce the name of God with a clear voice, or adore Him with their faces in contact with the ground], etc.; likewise they counterfeit suns and moons, stars oftentimes, and sit on ship-masts: *in navigiorum summitatibus visuntur*; and are called *Dioscuri*, as Eusebius, *lib. contra Philosophos, cap.* 48, informeth us, out of the authority of Zenophanes; or little clouds, *ad motum nescio quem volantes* [scudding along all ways]; which never appear, saith Cardan, but they signify some mischief or other to come unto men, though some again will have them to pretend good, and victory to that side they come towards in sea fights; St. Elmo's fires they commonly call them, and they do likely appear after a sea storm; Radzivilius, the Polonian duke, calls this apparition *Sancti Germani sidus* [the star of St. Germanus]; and saith moreover that he saw the same after or in a storm, as he was sailing, 1582, from Alexandria to Rhodes.[4] Our stories are full of such apparitions in all kinds:

Some think they keep their residence in that Hecla, a mountain in Iceland, Ætna in Sicily, Lipari, Vesuvius, etc. These devils were worshipped heretofore by that superstitious Πυρομαντεία [divination by fire] and the like.

Aerial spirits or devils are such as keep quarter most part in the air,[1] cause many tempests, thunder, and lightnings, tear oaks, fire steeples, houses, strike men and beasts, make it rain stones, as in Livy's time, wool, frogs, etc., counterfeit armies in the air, strange noises, swords, etc., as at Vienna before the coming of the Turks, and many times in Rome, as Scheretzius, *lib. de spect. cap.* 1, *part.* 1; Lavater, *de spect. part.* 1, *cap.* 17; Julius Obsequens, an old Roman, in his book of prodigies, *ab urb. cond.* 505. Machiavel hath illustrated by many examples,[2] and Josephus, in his book *de bello Judaico*; before the destruction of Jerusalem. All which Guil. Postellus, in his first book, *cap.* 7, *de orbis concordia*, useth as an effectual argument (as indeed it is) to persuade them that will not believe there be spirits or devils. They cause whirlwinds on a sudden, and tempestuous storms; which though our meteorologists generally refer to natural causes, yet I am of Bodine's mind, *Theat. Nat. lib.* 2, they are more often caused by those aerial devils, in their several quarters; for *tempestatibus se ingerunt* [they ride on the storm], saith Rich. Argentine;[3] as when a desperate man makes away himself, which by hanging or drowning they frequently do, as Kornmannus observes, *de mirac. mort. part.* 7, *cap.* 76, *tripudium agentes*, dancing and rejoicing at the death of a sinner. These can corrupt the air, and cause plagues, sickness, storms, shipwrecks, fires, inundations. At Mons Draconis in Italy, there is a most memorable example in Jovianus Pontanus:[4] and nothing so familiar (if we may believe those relations of Saxo Grammaticus, Olaus Magnus, Damianus à Goes) as for witches and sorcerers, in Lapland, Lithuania, and all over Scandia, to sell winds to mariners, and cause tempests, which Marcus Paulus the Venetian relates likewise of the Tartars. These kind of devils are much delighted in sacrifices (saith Porphyry),[5] held all the world in awe, and had several names, idols, sacrifices, in Rome, Greece, Egypt, and at this day tyrannize over and deceive those ethnics and Indians, being adored and worshipped for gods.[6] For the Gentiles' gods were devils (as Trismegistus confesseth in his *Asclepius*[7]), and he himself could make them come to their images by magic spells: and are now as much "respected by our papists" (saith Pictorius) "under the name of saints."[8] These are they which Cardan thinks desire so much carnal copulation with witches (incubi and succubi), transform bodies, and are so very cold if they be touched; and that serve magicians. His father had one of them (as he is not ashamed to relate [1]), an aerial devil, bound to him for twenty and eight years. As Agrippa's dog had a devil tied to his collar; some think that Paracelsus (or else Erastus belies him) had one confined to his sword pummel; others wear them in rings, etc. Jannes and Jambres did many things of old by their help; Simon Magus, Cinops, Apollonius Tyanæus, Iamblichus, and Trithemius of late, that showed Maximilian the emperor his wife, after she was dead; *et verrucam in collo ejus* (saith Godelman) [2] so much as the wart on her neck. Delrio, *lib.* 2, hath divers examples of their feats; Cicogna, *lib.* 3, *cap.* 3, and Wierus in his book *de præstig. dæmonum*; Boissardus, *de magis et veneficis.*

Water-devils are those naiades or water-nymphs [3] which have been heretofore conversant about waters and rivers. The water (as Paracelsus thinks) is their chaos, wherein they live; some call them fairies, and say that Habundia is their queen; these cause inundations, many times shipwrecks, and deceive men divers ways, as succubæ, or otherwise, appearing most part (saith Trithemius) in women's shapes. Paracelsus [4] hath several stories of them that have lived and been married to mortal men, and so continued for certain years with them, and after, upon some dislike, have forsaken them. Such a one was Egeria, with whom Numa was so familiar, Diana, Ceres, etc. Olaus Magnus [5] hath a long narration of one Hotherus, a king of Sweden, that having lost his company, as he was hunting one day, met with these water-nymphs or fairies, and was feasted by them; and Hector Boethius, of Macbeth and Banquo, two Scottish lords, that, as they were wandering in the woods, had their fortunes told them by three strange women. To these, heretofore, they did use to sacrifice, by that ὑδρομαντεία or divination by waters.

Terrestrial devils are those lares, [6] genii, fauns, satyrs, wood-nymphs, [7] foliots, fairies, Robin Goodfellows, *trolli* [trolls], etc., which as they are most conversant with men, so they do them most harm. Some think it was they alone that kept the heathen people in awe of old, and had so many idols and temples erected to them. Of this range was Dagon amongst the Philistines, Bel amongst the Babylonians, Astarte amongst the Sidonians, Baal amongst the Samaritans, Isis and Osiris amongst the Egyptians, etc.; some put our fairies [8] into this rank, which have been in former times adored with much superstition, with sweeping their houses, and setting of a pail of clean water, good victuals, and the like, and then they should not be pinched, but find money in their shoes, and be fortunate in their enterprises. These are they that dance on heaths and greens, as Lavater thinks[1] with Trithemius, and, as Olaus Magnus adds,[2] leave that green circle, which we commonly find in plain fields, which others hold to proceed from a meteor falling, or some accidental rankness of the ground, so Nature sports herself; they are sometimes seen by old women and children. Hieronym. Pauli, in his description of the city of Barcino in Spain, relates how they have been familiarly seen near that town, about fountains and hills. *Nonnunquam* (saith Trithemius) *in sua latibula montium simpliciores homines ducunt, stupenda mirantibus ostendentes miracula, nolarum sonitus, spectacula,* [sometimes they lead simple-minded peasants into their hiding-places in the mountains, where they show them marvellous sights, make them hear bells, and astonish them in other ways], etc. Giraldus Cambrensis gives instance in a monk of Wales that was so deluded. Paracelsus reckons up many places in Germany, where they do usually walk in little coats, some two foot long.[3] A bigger kind there is of them called with us hobgoblins, and Robin Goodfellows, that would in those superstitious times grind corn for a mess of milk, cut wood, or do any manner of drudgery work. They would mend old irons in those Æolian isles of Lipari, in former ages, and have been often seen and heard. Tholosanus[4] calls them *trollos* and *getulos*, and saith that in his days they were common in many places of France. Dithmarus Bleskenius, in his description of Iceland, reports for a certainty, that almost in every family they have yet some such familiar spirits; and Felix Malleolus, in his book *de crudel. dæmon.*, affirms as much, that these *trolli* or *telchines* are very common in Norway, "and seen to do drudgery work";[5] to draw water, saith Wierus, *lib.* 1, *cap.* 22, dress meat, or any such thing. Another sort of these there are, which frequent forlorn houses,[6] which the Italians call foliots, most part innoxious, Cardan holds:[7] "They will make strange noises in the night, howl sometimes pitifully, and then laugh again, cause great flame and sudden lights, fling stones, rattle chains, shave men, open doors and shut them, fling down platters, stools, chests, sometimes appear in the likeness of hares, crows, black dogs, etc.,"[8] of which read Pet. Thyræus the Jesuit, in his tract *de locis infestis, part.* 1, *cap.* 1 *et cap.* 4, who will have them to be devils

or the souls of damned men that seek revenge, or else souls out
of purgatory that seek ease;[1] for such examples peruse Sigismundus Scheretzius, *lib. de spectris, part.* 1, *cap.* 1, which he
saith he took out of Luther most part; there be many instances.
Plinius Secundus[2] remembers such a house at Athens, which
Athenodorus the philosopher hired, which no man durst inhabit
for fear of devils. Austin, *de Civ. Dei, lib.* 22, *cap.* 8, relates
as much of Hesperius the tribune's house at Zubeda, near their
city of Hippo, vexed with evil spirits, to his great hindrance,
cum afflictione animalium et servorum suorum [and to the great
distress of his animals and slaves]. Many such instances are
to be read in Niderius, *Formicar. lib.* 5, *cap.* 12, 13, etc. Whether
I may call these Zim and Ochim, which Isaiah, chap. xiii, 21,
speaks of, I make a doubt. See more of these in the said
Scheretz., *lib.* 1 *de spect. cap.* 4; he is full of examples. These
kind of devils many times appear to men, and affright them out
of their wits, sometimes walking at noonday,[3] sometimes at
nights, counterfeiting dead men's ghosts, as that of Caligula,
which (saith Suetonius) was seen to walk in Lavinia's garden;
where his body was buried, spirits haunted, and [in] the house
where he died; *nulla nox sine terrore transacta, donec incendio con-
sumpta;*[4] every night this happened, there was no quietness
till the house was burned. About Hecla, in Iceland, ghosts
commonly walk, *animas mortuorum simulantes* [resembling
the dead], saith Joh. Anan., *lib.* 3 *de nat. dæm.,* Olaus, *lib.* 2,
cap. 2, Natal. Tallopid., *lib. de apparit. spir.,* Kornmannus, *de
mirac. mort. part.* 1, *cap.* 44. Such sights are frequently seen
circa sepulchra et monasteria, saith Lavater, *lib.* 1, *cap.* 19, in
monasteries and about churchyards, *loca paludinosa, ampla
ædificia, solitaria, et cæde hominum notata,* [marshes, great buildings, solitary places, or places remarkable as the scene of some
murder] etc. Thyræus adds, *ubi gravius peccatum est commissum,
impii pauperum oppressores et nequiter insignes habitant* [where
some very heinous crime was committed, there the impious
and infamous generally dwell]. These spirits often foretell
men's deaths by several signs, as knocking, groanings, etc.,[5]
though Rich. Argentine, *cap.* 18 *de præstigiis dæmonum,* will
ascribe these predictions to good angels, out of the authority of
Ficinus and others; *prodigia in obitu principum sæpius contingunt* [prodigies frequently occur at the deaths of illustrious
men], etc., as in the Lateran Church in Rome,[6] the Popes' deaths
are foretold by Sylvester's tomb. Near Rupes Nova in Finland,
in the kingdom of Sweden, there is a lake, in which, before the

governor of the castle dies, a spectrum, in the habit of Arion
with his harp, appears and makes excellent music; like those
blocks in Cheshire,[1] which (they say) presage death to the
master of the family; or that oak in Lanthadran Park in Cornwall,[2] which foreshows as much. Many families in Europe are
so put in mind of their last by such predictions, and many men
are forewarned (if we may believe Paracelsus) by familiar spirits
in divers shapes, as cocks, crows, owls, which often hover about
sick men's chambers, *vel quia morientium fœditatem sentiunt*
[either because they smell a corpse], as Baracellus conjectures,[3]
et ideo super tectum infirmorum crocitant [and therefore they
croak over a house where someone is lying ill], because they
smell a corse; or for that (as Bernardinus de Bustis thinketh[4])
God permits the devil to appear in the form of crows and such-
like creatures, to scare such as live wickedly here on earth. A
little before Tully's death (saith Plutarch) the crows made a
mighty noise about him, *tumultuose perstrepentes*, they pulled
the pillow from under his head. Rob. Gaguinus, *Hist. Franc.
lib.* 8, telleth such another wonderful story at the death of
Johannes de Monteforti, a French lord, *anno* 1345; *tanta corvorum multitudo ædibus morientis insedit, quantam esse in Gallia
nemo judicasset* [a multitude of crows alighted on the house of
the dying man, such as no one imagined existed in France].
Such prodigies are very frequent in authors. See more of these
in the said Lavater, Thyræus, *de locis infestis, part. 3, cap.* 58,
Pictorius, Delrio, Cicogna, *lib. 3, cap.* 9. Necromancers take
upon them to raise and lay them at their pleasures. And so likewise those which Mizaldus calls *ambulones*, that walk about
midnight on great heaths and desert places, which (saith
Lavater[5]) "draw men out of the way, and lead them all night a
by-way, or quite bar them of their way"; these have several
names in several places; we commonly call them Pucks. In the
deserts of Lop, in Asia, such illusions of walking spirits are
often perceived, as you may read in M. Paulus the Venetian,
his travels; if one lose his company by chance, these devils will
call him by his name, and counterfeit voices of his companions
to seduce him. Hieronym. Pauli, in his book of the hills of
Spain, relates of a great mount in Cantabria,[6] where such
spectrums are to be seen; Lavater and Cicogna have variety of
examples of spirits and walking devils in this kind. Sometimes
they sit by the highway side, to give men falls, and make their
horses stumble and start as they ride (if you will believe the
relation of that holy man Ketellus in Nubrigensis,[7] that had an

especial grace to see devils, *gratiam divinitus collatam*, and talk
with them, *et impavidus cum spiritibus sermonem miscere*, without offence); and if a man curse or spur his horse for stumbling
they do heartily rejoice at it; with many such pretty feats.

Subterranean devils are as common as the rest, and do as
much harm.   Olaus Magnus, *lib*. 6, *cap*. 19, makes six kinds of
them; some bigger, some less.   These (saith Munster[1]) are
commonly seen about mines of metals, and are some of them
noxious; some again do no harm.   The metal-men in many
places account it good luck, a sign of treasure and rich ore when
they see them.   Georgius Agricola, in his book *de subterraneis
animantibus, cap*. 37, reckons two more notable kinds of them,
which he calls *getuli* and *cobali*; both "are clothed after the
manner of metal-men, and will many times imitate their works."[2]
Their office, as Pictorius and Paracelsus think, is to keep treasure
in the earth, that it be not all at once revealed; and besides,
Cicogna avers that they are the frequent causes of those horrible
earthquakes "which often swallow up, not only houses, but
whole islands and cities";[3] in his third book, *cap*. 11, he gives
many instances.

The last are conversant about the centre of the earth, to torture
the souls of damned men to the day of judgment; their egress
and regress some suppose to be about Ætna, Lipari, Mons
Hecla in Iceland, Vesuvius, Terra del Fuego, etc., because many
shrieks and fearful cries are continually heard thereabouts, and
familiar apparitions of dead men, ghosts, and goblins.

Thus the devil reigns, and in a thousand several shapes, "as
a roaring lion still seeks whom he may devour" (1 Pet. v), by
earth, sea, land, air, as yet unconfined, though some will have
his proper place the air;[4] all that space between us and the
moon for them that transgressed least, and hell for the wickedest
of them; *Hic velut in carcere ad finem mundi, tunc in locum
funestiorum trudendi* [here they are confined as in a prison
till the end of the world; then they are to be thrust forth into
a still more dreadful place], as Austin holds, *de Civit. Dei, cap*. 22,
lib. 14, *cap*. 3 *et* 23; but be where he will, he rageth while he
may to comfort himself, as Lactantius thinks,[5] with other men's
falls, he labours all he can to bring them into the same pit of
perdition with him.   For "men's miseries, calamities, and ruins
are the devil's banqueting dishes."[6]   By many temptations and
several engines, he seeks to captivate our souls.   The Lord
of Lies, saith Austin,[7] "as he was deceived himself, he seeks
to deceive others"; the ringleader to all naughtiness, as he did

by Eve and Cain, Sodom and Gomorrah, so would he do by all the world. Sometimes he tempts by covetousness, drunkenness, pleasure, pride, etc., errs, dejects, saves, kills, protects, and rides some men as they do their horses. He studies our overthrow, and generally seeks our destruction; and although he pretend many times human good, and vindicate himself for a god by curing of several diseases, *ægris sanitatem, et cæcis luminis usum restituendo* [by restoring health to the sick and sight to the blind] as Austin declares, *lib.* 10 *de Civit. Dei, cap.* 6, as Apollo, Æsculapius, Isis, of old have done; divert plagues, assist them in wars, pretend their happiness, yet *nihil his impurius, scelestius, nihil humano generi infestius*, nothing so impure, nothing so pernicious, as may well appear by their tyrannical and bloody sacrifices of men to Saturn and Moloch, which are still in use among those barbarous Indians, their several deceits and cozenings to keep men in obedience, their false oracles, sacrifices, their superstitious impositions of fasts, penury, etc., heresies, superstitious observations of meats, times, etc., by which they crucify the souls of mortal men,[1] as shall be showed in our Treatise of Religious Melancholy. *Modico adhuc tempore sinitur malignari*, as Bernard expresseth it,[2] by God's permission he rageth awhile, hereafter to be confined to hell and darkness, "which is prepared for him and his angels" (Matt. xxv).

How far their power doth extend it is hard to determine; what the ancients held of their effects, force, and operations I will briefly show you. Plato in *Critias*, and after him his followers, gave out that these spirits or devils "were men's governors and keepers, our lords and masters, as we are of our cattle. They govern provinces and kingdoms by oracles, auguries, dreams, rewards and punishments,"[3] prophecies, inspirations, sacrifices, and religious superstitions, varied in as many forms as there be diversity of spirits; they send wars, plagues, peace, sickness, health, dearth, plenty, *adstantes hic jam nobis, spectantes, et arbitrantes*[4] [standing by us here and now, watching and judging us], etc., as appears by those histories of Thucydides, Livius, Dionysius Halicarnasseus, with many others that are full of their wonderful stratagems, and were therefore by those Roman and Greek commonwealths adored and worshipped for gods with prayers and sacrifices, etc. In a word, *nihil magis quærunt quam metum et admirationem hominum*[5] [they seek nothing more eagerly than the fear and admiration of men]; and as another hath it, *dici non potest, quam impotenti ardore in homines dominium, et divinos cultus maligni spiritus affectent* [it is impossible to describe the ardour with which evil spirits seek to obtain dominion over men and the honours of divine worship]. Trithemius, in his book *de septem secundis*, assigns names to such angels as are governors of particular provinces, by what authority I know not, and gives them several jurisdictions. Asclepiades a Grecian, Rabbi Achiba the Jew, Abraham Avenezra and Rabbi Azariel, Arabians (as I find them cited by Cicogna[1]), farther add, that they are not our governors only, *sed ex eorum concordia et discordia, boni et mali affectus promanant*, but as they agree, so do we and our princes, or disagree; stand or fall. Juno was a bitter enemy to Troy, Apollo a good friend, Jupiter indifferent, *Æqua Venus Teucris, Pallas iniqua fuit* [Venus was for the Trojans, Pallas against]; some are for us still, some against us, *Premente deo, fert deus alter opem* [when one god threatens, another comes to the rescue]. Religion, policy, public and private quarrels, wars are procured by them, and they are delighted perhaps to see men fight, as men are with cocks, bulls and dogs, bears, etc.[2] Plagues, dearths depend on them, our *bene* and *male esse*, and almost all our other peculiar actions (for as Anthony Rusca contends, *lib.* 5, *cap.* 18, every man hath a good and a bad angel attending on him in particular all his life long, which Iamblichus calls *dæmonem*), preferments, losses, weddings, deaths, rewards and punishments, and as Proclus will,[3] all offices whatsoever, *alii genetricem, alii opificem potestatem habent* [some help in childbirth, others in manual labours], etc., and several names they give them according to their offices, as *Lares, Indigetes, Præstites*, etc. When the Arcades in that battle at Chæronea, which was fought against King Philip for the liberty of Greece, had deceitfully carried themselves, long after, in the very same place, *diis Græciæ ultoribus* [through the avenging gods of Greece] (saith mine author) they were miserably slain by Metellus the Roman: so likewise, in smaller matters, they will have things fall out, as these *boni* and *mali genii* favour or dislike us. *Saturnini non conveniunt Jovialibus*, etc. He that is *Saturninus* shall never likely be preferred. That base fellows are often advanced, undeserving Gnathos, and vicious parasites, whereas discreet, wise, virtuous and worthy men are neglected and unrewarded,[4] they refer to those domineering spirits, or subordinate genii; as they are inclined, or favour men, so they thrive, are ruled and overcome; for, as Libanius supposeth, in our ordinary conflicts and

contentions, *Genius genio cedit et obtemperat*,[1] one genius yields
and is overcome by another. All particular events almost they
refer to these private spirits; and (as Paracelsus adds) they
direct, teach, inspire, and instruct men. Never was any man
extraordinary famous in any art, action, or great commander,
that had not *familiarem dæmonem* [a familiar spirit] to inform
him, as Numa, Socrates, and many such (as Cardan illustrates,
cap. 128, *Arcanis prudentiæ civilis*); *speciali siquidem gratia se
a Deo donari asserunt magi, a geniis cælestibus instrui, ab iis
doceri* [2] [the Magians assert that they are vouchsafed from God
a special grace, that they are trained and instructed by the
heavenly spirits]. But these are most erroneous paradoxes,
ineptæ et fabulosæ nugæ, rejected by our divines and Christian
Churches. 'Tis true they have, by God's permission, power
over us, and we find by experience that they can hurt not our
fields only, cattle, goods, but our bodies and minds.[3] At
Hammel in Saxony, *ann.* 1484, 20 *Junii*, the devil, in likeness
of a pied piper, carried away 130 children that were never
after seen. Many times men are affrighted out of their wits,
carried away quite, as Scheretzius illustrates, *lib.* 1, *cap.* 4, and
severally molested by his means. Plotinus the Platonist, *lib.* 14
advers. Gnost., laughs them to scorn that hold the devil or
spirits can cause any such diseases.[4] Many think he can
work upon the body, but not upon the mind. But experience
pronounceth otherwise, that he can work both upon body and
mind. Tertullian is of this opinion, *cap.* 22, "that he can cause
both sickness and health," [5] and that secretly. Taurellus adds,
"By clancular poisons he can infect the bodies, and hinder the
operations of the bowels, though we perceive it not," [6] "closely
creeping into them," saith Lipsius,[7] and so crucify our souls:
et nociva melancholia furiosos efficit [and makes people mad from
noxious melancholy]. For being a spiritual body, he struggles
with our spirits, saith Rogers, and suggests (according to Cardan [8])
verba sine voce, species sine visu [words without speaking,
sights without showing anything], envy, lust, anger, etc., as
he sees men inclined.

The manner how he performs it, Biarmannus, in his Oration
against Bodine, sufficiently declares. "He begins first with the
phantasy, and moves that so strongly that no reason is able
to resist." [9] Now the phantasy he moves by mediation of
humours; although many physicians are of opinion that the devil
can alter the mind, and produce this disease of himself." *Quibusdam medicorum visum*, saith Avicenna, *quod melancholia*

contingat a dæmonio [1] [some doctors have held that melancholy is from the devil]. Of the same mind is Psellus, and Rhasis the Arab, *lib.* 1, *tract.* 9, *Cont.*, "that this disease proceeds especially from the devil, and from him alone." [2]   Arculanus, *cap.* 6, *in* 9 *Rhasis*; Ælianus Montaltus in his 9th *cap.*; Daniel Sennertus, *lib.* 1, *part.* 2, *cap.* 11, confirm as much, that the devil can cause this disease; by reason many times that the parties affected prophesy, speak strange language, but *non sine interventu humoris*, not without the humour, as he interprets himself; no more doth Avicenna: *Si contingat a dæmonio, sufficit nobis ut convertat complexionem ad choleram nigram, et sit causa ejus propinqua cholera nigra* [if it is from the devil, the sufficient sign is that it turns the humour to black bile and that its immediate cause is black bile]; the immediate cause is choler adust, which Pomponatius likewise labours to make good: [3] Galgerandus of Mantua, a famous physician, so cured a dæmoniacal woman in his time, that spake all languages, by purging black choler; and thereupon, belike, this humour of melancholy is called *balneum diaboli*, the devil's bath; the devil, spying his opportunity of such humours, drives them many times to despair, fury, rage, etc., mingling himself amongst these humours. This is that which Tertullian avers, *Corporibus infligunt acerbos casus, animæque repentinos, membra distorquent, occulte repentes* [they cause grievous bodily and mental harm; they distort the limbs, coming on stealthily], etc., and which Lemnius goes about to prove, *Immiscent se mali genii pravis humoribus, atque atræ bili* [evil spirits insert themselves in depraved humours and black bile], etc.   And Jason Pratensis, "that the devil, being a slender incomprehensible spirit, can easily insinuate and wind himself into human bodies, and, cunningly couched in our bowels, vitiate our healths, terrify our souls with fearful dreams, and shake our mind with furies." [4]   And in another place, "These unclean spirits settled in our bodies, and now mixed with our melancholy humours, do triumph as it were, and sport themselves as in another heaven." [5]   Thus he argues, and that they go in and out of our bodies, as bees do in a hive, and so provoke and tempt us as they perceive our temperature inclined of itself, and most apt to be deluded.   Agrippa [6] and Lavater [7] are persuaded that this humour invites the devil to it, wheresoever it is in extremity, and, of all other, melancholy persons are most subject to diabolical temptations and illusions, and most apt to entertain them, and the devil best able to work upon them.   But whether by obsession, or pos-

session, or otherwise, I will not determine; 'tis a difficult question.
Delrio the Jesuit, *tom.* 3, *lib.* 6; Sprenger and his colleague,
Mall. Malef.;[1] Pet. Thyræus the Jesuit, *lib. de dæmoniacis, de
locis infestis, de terrificationibus nocturnis*; Hieronymus Mengus,
Flagel. dæm., and others of that rank of pontifical writers, it
seems, by their exorcisms and conjurations approve of it, having
forged many stories to that purpose. A nun did eat a lettuce
without grace or signing it with the sign of the cross, and
was instantly possessed.[2] Durand, *lib.* 6 *Rational. cap.* 86,
num. 8, relates that he saw a wench possessed in Bononia with
two devils, by eating an unhallowed pomegranate, as she did
afterwards confess, when she was cured by exorcisms. And
therefore our papists do sign themselves so often with the sign
of the cross, *ne dæmon ingredi ausit* [that the demon may not dare
to enter], and exorcise all manner of meats, as being unclean or
accursed otherwise, as Bellarmine defends. Many such stories
I find amongst pontifical writers, to prove their assertions; let
them free their own credits; some few I will recite in this kind
out of most approved physicians. Cornelius Gemma, *lib.* 2
de nat. mirac. cap. 4, related of a young maid, called Katherine
Gualter, a cooper's daughter, *anno* 1571, that had such strange
passions and convulsions, three men could not sometimes hold
her; she purged a live eel, which he saw, a foot and a half long,
and touched himself; but the eel afterwards vanished; she
vomited some twenty-four pounds of fulsome stuff of all colours,
twice a day for fourteen days; and after that she voided great
balls of hair, pieces of wood, pigeon's dung, parchment, goose
dung, coals; and after them two pound of pure blood, and then
again coals and stones, of which some had inscriptions, bigger
than a walnut, some of them pieces of glass, brass, etc., besides
paroxysms of laughing, weeping and ecstasies, etc. *Et hoc
(inquit) cum horrore vidi*, "this I saw with horror." They could
do no good on her by physic, but left her to the clergy. Marcellus
Donatus, *lib.* 2, *cap.* 1, *de med. mirab.*, hath such another story of
a country fellow, that had four knives in his belly, *instar serræ
dentatos*, indented like a saw, every one a span long, and a
wreath of hair like a globe, with much baggage of like sort,
wonderful to behold: how it should come into his guts, he
concludes, *certo non alio quam dæmonis astutia et dolo* [could
assuredly only have been through the artifice of the devil].
Langius, *Epist. med. lib.* 1, *epist.* 38, hath many relations to
this effect, and so hath Christopherus à Vega: Wierus, Sckenkius,
Scribanius, all agree that they are done by the subtlety and

illusion of the devil. If you shall ask a reason of this, 'tis to exercise our patience; for as Tertullian holds,[1] *Virtus non est virtus, nisi comparem habet aliquem, in quo superando vim suam ostendat* [virtue is not worthy of the name till it has overcome an antagonist worthy of its steel]; 'tis to try us and our faith, 'tis for our offences, and for the punishment of our sins, by God's permission they do it, *carnifices vindictæ justæ Dei*, as Tholosanus styles them,[2] executioners of His will; or rather as David (Ps. lxxviii, 49), "He cast upon them the fierceness of his anger, indignation, wrath, and vexation, by sending out of evil angels"; so did He afflict Job, Saul, the lunatics and dæmoniacal persons whom Christ cured (Matt. iv, 8; Luke iv, 11; Luke xiii; Mark ix; Tobit viii, 3, etc.). This, I say, happeneth for a punishment of sin, for their want of faith, incredulity, weakness, distrust, etc.

SUBSECT. III.—*Of Witches and Magicians, how they cause Melancholy*

You have heard what the devil can do of himself, now you shall hear what he can perform by his instruments, who are many times worse (if it be possible) than he himself, and to satisfy their revenge and lust cause more mischief. *Multa enim mala non egisset dæmon, nisi provocatus a sagis*, as Erastus thinks;[3] much harm had never been done, had he not been provoked by witches to it. He had not appeared in Samuel's shape, if the Witch of Endor had let him alone; or represented those serpents in Pharaoh's presence, had not the magicians urged him unto it; *nec morbos vel hominibus vel brutis infligeret* (Erastus maintains) *si sagæ quiescerent:* men and cattle might go free, if the witches would let him alone. Many deny witches at all, or if there be any they can do no harm; of this opinion is Wierus, *lib. 3, cap. 53, de præstig. dæm.*, Austin Lerchemer, a Dutch writer, Biarmannus, Ewichius, Euwaldus, our countryman Scot;[4] with him in Horace,

> *Somnia, terrores magicos, miracula, sagas,*
> *Nocturnos lemures, portentaque Thessala risu*
> *Excipiunt.*

> [They laugh indignant at the schemes
> Of magic terrors, visionary dreams,
> Portentous wonders, witching imps of hell,
> The nightly goblin, and enchanting spell.]

They laugh at all such stories; but on the contrary are most lawyers, divines, physicians, philosophers, Austin, Hemingius, Danæus, Chytræus, Zanchius, Aretæus, etc., Delrio, Sprenger, Niderius, *lib. 5 Formicar.*,[1] Cujacius, Bartolus, *consil. 6, tom.* 1, Bodine, *Dæmoniant. lib. 2, cap.* 8, Godelman, Damhoderius, etc., Paracelsus, Erastus, Scribanius, Camerarius, etc. The parties by whom the devil deals may be reduced to these two: such as command him in show at least, as conjurors, and magicians, whose detestable and horrid mysteries are contained in their book called *Arbatell*;[2] *dæmones enim advocati præsto sunt, seque exorcismis et conjurationibus quasi cogi patiuntur, ut miserum magorum genus in impietate detineant* [the demons are always on the alert, and obey the call of incantations and charms, in order that they may confirm the accursed tribe of magicians in their impiety]; or such as are commanded, as witches, that deal *ex parte implicite*, or *explicite*, as the king hath well defined;[3] many subdivisions there are, and many several species of sorcerers, witches, enchanters, charmers, etc. They have been tolerated heretofore some of them; and magic hath been publicly professed in former times, in Salamanca,[4] Cracovia,[5] and other places, though after censured by several universities,[6] and now generally contradicted, though practised by some still, maintained and excused, *tanquam res secreta quæ non nisi viris magnis et peculiari beneficio de cælo instructis communicatur* [like a great secret, only to be communicated to notable men specially favoured by Heaven] (I use Boissardus his words[7]), and so far approved by some princes, *ut nihil ausi aggredi in politicis, in sacris, in consiliis, sine eorum arbitrio*; they consult still with them, and dare indeed do nothing without their advice. Nero and Heliogabalus, Maxentius and Julianus Apostata, were never so much addicted to magic of old as some of our modern princes and popes themselves are nowadays. Erricus, King of Sweden, had an enchanted cap,[8] by virtue of which, and some magical murmur or whispering terms, he could command spirits, trouble the air, and make the wind stand which way he would, insomuch that when there was any great wind or storm, the common people were wont to say, the king now had on his conjuring cap. But such examples are infinite. That which they can do, is as much almost as the devil himself, who is still ready to satisfy their desires, to oblige them the more unto him. They can cause tempests, storms, which is familiarly practised by witches in Norway, Iceland, as I have proved. They can make friends enemies, and enemies friends by philters; *turpes amores conciliare*,[9] enforce love, tell any man where his friends are, about what employed though in the most remote places; and if they will, "bring their sweethearts to them by night, upon a goat's back flying in the air"[1] (Sigismund Scheretzius, *part. 1, cap. 9, de spect.*, reports confidently that he conferred with sundry such, that had been so carried many miles, and that he heard witches themselves confess as much); hurt and infect men and beasts, vines, corn, cattle, plants, make women abortive, not to conceive, barren, men and women unapt and unable,[2] married and unmarried, fifty several ways, saith Bodine, *lib. 2, cap. 2*, fly in the air, meet when and where they will, as Cicogna proves, and Lavat. *de spec. part. 2, cap. 17*, "steal young children out of their cradles, *ministerio dæmonum* [with the help of the demons] and put deformed in their rooms, which we call changelings," saith Scheretzius, *part. 1, cap. 6*,[3] make men victorious, fortunate, eloquent; and therefore in those ancient monomachies and combats they were searched of old, they had no magical charms;[4] they can make stick frees,[5] such as shall endure a rapier's point, musket-shot, and never be wounded: of which read more in Boissardus, *cap. 6 de Magia*, the manner of the adjuration, and by whom 'tis made, where and how to be used *in expeditionibus bellicis, prœliis, duellis* [in military expeditions, battles, wars], etc., with many peculiar instances and examples; they can walk in fiery furnaces, make men feel no pain on the rack, *aut alias torturas sentire* [or feel other tortures]; they can stanch blood, represent dead men's shapes, alter and turn themselves and others into several forms, at their pleasures.[6] Agaberta, a famous witch in Lapland,[7] would do as much publicly to all spectators, *modo pusilla, modo anus, modo procera ut quercus, modo vacca, avis, coluber, etc.*, now young, now old, high, low, like a cow, like a bird, a snake, and what not? she could represent to others what forms they most desired to see, show them friends absent, reveal secrets, *maxima omnium admiratione* [to the great astonishment of all], etc. And yet for all this subtlety of theirs, as Lipsius well observes, *Physiolog. Stoicor. lib. 1, cap. 17*, neither these magicians nor devils themselves can take away gold or letters out of mine or Crassus' chest, *et clientelis suis largiri* [and make presents to their followers], for they are base, poor, contemptible fellows most part; as Bodine notes,[8] they can do nothing *in judicum decreta aut pœnas, in regum concilia vel arcana, nihil in rem nummariam aut thesauros*, they cannot give money to their clients, alter judges' decrees, or councils of kings, these *minuti genii* cannot do it, *altiores genii hoc sibi adservarunt*, the higher powers reserve these things to themselves. Now and then peradventure there may be some more famous magicians like Simon Magus, Apollonius Tyanæus,[1] Pases,[2] Iamblichus, Eudo de Stellis,[3] that for a time can build castles in the air, represent armies, etc., as they are said to have done,[4] command wealth and treasure, feed thousands with all variety of meats upon a sudden, protect themselves and their followers from all princes' persecutions, by removing from place to place in an instant, reveal secrets, future events, tell what is done in far countries, make them appear that died long since, etc., and do many such miracles, to the world's terror, admiration, and opinion of deity to themselves, yet the devil forsakes them at last, they come to wicked ends, and *raro aut nunquam* [rarely or never] such impostors are to be found. The vulgar sort of them can work no such feats. But to my purpose, they can, last of all, cure and cause most diseases to such as they love or hate, and this of melancholy amongst the rest.[5] Paracelsus, *tom. 4, de morbis amentium, tract.* 1, in express words affirms, *Multi fascinantur in melancholiam*, many are bewitched into melancholy, out of his experience. The same saith Danæus, *lib. 3 de sortiariis. Vidi, inquit, qui melancholicos morbos gravissimos induxerunt:* I have seen those that have caused melancholy in the most grievous manner, dried up women's' paps, cured gout, palsy; this and apoplexy, falling sickness, which no physic could help, *solo tactu*, by touch alone.[6] Ruland, in his 3rd *cent., cura* 91, gives an instance of one David Helde, a young man, who by eating cakes which a witch gave him, *mox delirare cœpit*, began to dote on a sudden, and was instantly mad:[7] F. H. D. in Hildesheim,[8] consulted about a melancholy man, thought his disease was partly magical, and partly natural, because he vomited pieces of iron and lead, and spake such languages as he had never been taught; but such examples are common in Scribanius, Hercules de Saxonia, and others. The means by which they work are usually charms, images, as that in Hector Boethius of King Duff; characters stamped of sundry metals, and at such and such constellations, knots, amulets, words, philters, etc., which generally make the parties affected melancholy;[9] as Monavius discourseth at large in an epistle of his to Acolsius, giving instance in a Bohemian baron that was so troubled by a philter taken. Not that there is any power at all in those spells, charms, characters, and barbarous words; but that the devil doth use such means to delude them, *Ut fideles inde magos* (saith Libanius[10]) *in officio retineat, tum in consortium malefactorum vocet* [that he may keep the Magi true to their allegiance, and then summon them to join the company of evil-doers].

Subsect. IV.—*Stars a Cause. Signs from Physiognomy, Metoposcopy, Chiromancy*

Natural causes are either primary and universal, or secondary and more particular. Primary causes are the heavens, planets, stars, etc., by their influence (as our astrologers hold) producing this and such-like effects. I will not here stand to discuss *obiter*, whether stars be causes, or signs; or to apologize for judicial astrology. If either Sextus Empiricus, Picus Mirandula, Sextus ab Heminga, Pererius, Erastus, Chambers, etc., have so far prevailed with any man, that he will attribute no virtue at all to the heavens, or to sun, or moon, more than he doth to their signs at an innkeeper's post, or tradesman's shop, or generally condemn all such astrological aphorisms approved by experience: I refer him to Bellantius, Pirovanus, Marascallerus, Goclenius, Sir Christopher Heydon, etc. If thou shalt ask me what I think, I must answer, *nam et doctis hisce erroribus versatus sum* [for I too am conversant with these learned errors], they do incline, but not compel; no necessity at all, *agunt non cogunt*:[1] and so gently incline, that a wise man may resist them; *sapiens dominabitur astris* [a wise man will rule the stars]; they rule us, but God rules them. All this (methinks) Joh. de Indagine hath comprised in brief:[2] *Quæris a me quantum in nobis operantur astra?* etc. "Wilt thou know how far the stars work upon us? I say they do but incline, and that so gently, that if we will be ruled by reason, they have no power over us; but if we follow our own nature, and be led by sense, they do as much in us as in brute beasts, and we are no better." So that, I hope, I may justly conclude with Cajetan,[3] *Cælum est vehiculum divinæ virtutis*, etc., that the heaven is God's instrument, by mediation of which He governs and disposeth these elementary bodies; or a great book, whose letters are the stars (as one calls it), wherein are written many strange things for such as can read, "or an excellent harp, made by an eminent workman, on which he that can but play will make most admirable music."[4] But to the purpose.

Paracelsus is of opinion "that a physician without the knowledge of stars can neither understand the cause or cure of any disease, either of this or gout, not so much as toothache; except

he see the peculiar geniture and scheme of the party affected." [1]
And for this proper malady, he will have the principal and
primary cause of it proceed from the heaven, ascribing more
to stars than humours, "and that the constellation alone many
times produceth melancholy, all other causes set apart." [2] He
gives instance in lunatic persons, that are deprived of their
wits by the moon's motion; and in another place refers all to
the ascendant, and will have the true and chief cause of it to
be sought from the stars. Neither is it his opinion only, but
of many Galenists and philosophers, though they [do] not so
peremptorily maintain as much. "This variety of melancholy
symptoms proceeds from the stars," saith Melancthon: [3] the
most generous melancholy, as that of Augustus, comes from the
conjunction of Saturn and Jupiter in Libra: the bad, as that
of Catiline's, from the meeting of Saturn and the Moon in Scorpio.
Jovianus Pontanus, in his tenth book and thirteenth chapter
de rebus cœlestibus, discourseth to this purpose at large: *Ex
atra bile varii generantur morbi,* etc., "many diseases proceed
from black choler, as it shall be hot or cold; and though it be
cold in its own nature, yet it is apt to be heated, as water may
be made to boil, and burn as bad as fire; or made cold as ice:
and thence proceed such variety of symptoms, some mad, some
solitary, some laugh, some rage," etc. [4] The cause of all which
intemperance he will have chiefly and primarily proceed from
the heavens, "from the position of Mars, Saturn, and Mercury." [5]
His aphorisms he these: "Mercury in any geniture, if he shall be
found in Virgo, or Pisces his opposite sign, and that in the horoscope, irradiated by those quartile aspects of Saturn or Mars,
the child shall be mad or melancholy." [6] Again, "He that
shall have Saturn and Mars, the one culminating, the other in
the fourth house, when he shall be born, shall be melancholy,
of which he shall be cured in time, if Mercury behold them. [7]
If the Moon be in conjunction or opposition at the birth time
with the Sun, Saturn or Mars, [8] or in a quartile aspect with
them" (*e malo cœli loco* [from a malign quarter of the heaven],
Leovitius adds), "many diseases are signified, especially the head
and brain is like to be misaffected with pernicious humours, to
be melancholy, lunatic, or mad"; Cardan adds, *quarta luna natos*
[those born on the fourth day after the new moon], [or in] eclipses,
earthquakes. Garcæus and Leovitius will have the chief judgment
to be taken from the lord of the geniture, or when there is an
aspect between the Moon and Mercury, and neither behold the
horoscope, or Saturn and Mars shall be lord of the present

conjunction or opposition in Sagittary or Pisces, of the Sun
or Moon, such persons are commonly epileptic, dote, dæmoniacal,
melancholy: but see more of these aphorisms in the above-named
Pontanus; Garcæus, *cap. 23 de Jud. genitur.*; Scheiner, *lib.* 1,
cap. 8, which he hath gathered out of Ptolemy;[1] Albubater,
and some other Arabians, Junctine, Ranzovius, Lindhout,
Origan, etc. But these men you will reject peradventure, as
astrologers, and therefore partial judges; then hear the testimony of physicians, Galenists themselves. Crato confesseth
the influence of stars to have a great hand to this peculiar
disease,[2] so doth Jason Pratensis, Lonicerus, *præfat. de Apoplexia,* Ficinus, Fernelius, etc. P. Cnemander acknowledgeth the
stars an universal cause, the particular from parents, and the
use of the six non-natural things.[3] Baptista Porta, *Mag. lib.* 1,
cap. 10, 12, 15, will have them causes to every particular *indi-
viduum.* Instances and examples, to evince the truth of those
aphorisms, are common amongst those astrologian treatises.
Cardan, in his thirty-seventh geniture, gives instance in Math.
Bolognius, Camerar., *Hor. natalit. centur.* 7, *genit.* 6 *et* 7, of Daniel
Gare, and others; but see Garcæus, *cap.* 33, Luc. Gauricus, *Tract.*
6, *de Azimenis,* etc. The time of this melancholy is, when the
significators of any geniture are directed according to art, as the
hor., moon, hylech, etc., to the hostile beams or terms of ♄
and ♂ especially, or any fixed star of their nature, or if ♄ by
his revolution, or *transitus,* shall offend any of those radical
promissors in the geniture.

Other signs there are taken from physiognomy, metoposcopy,
chiromancy, which because Joh. de Indagine, and Rotman, the
Landgrave of Hesse his mathematician, not long since in his
Chiromancy, Baptista Porta in his Celestial Physiognomy,
have proved to hold great affinity with astrology, to satisfy
the curious, I am the more willing to insert.

The general notions physiognomers[4] give, be these: "black
colour argues natural melancholy; so doth leanness, hirsuteness,
broad veins, much hair on the brows," saith Gratarolus,
cap. 7, and a little head, out of Aristotle; high, sanguine, red
colour, shows head melancholy ;[5] they that stutter and are bald
will be soonest melancholy (as Avicenna supposeth), by reason
of the dryness of their brains; but he that will know more of the
several signs of humour and wits out of physiognomy, let him
consult with old Adamantus and Polemus, that comment, or
rather paraphrase, upon Aristotle's Physiognomy, Baptista
Porta's four pleasant books, Michael Scot *de secretis naturæ,*

John de Indagine, Montaltus, Antony Zara, *Anat. ingeniorum, sect.* 1, *memb.* 13, *et lib.* 4.

Chiromancy hath these aphorisms to foretell melancholy. Taisnier, *lib.* 5, *cap.* 2, who hath comprehended the sum of John de Indagine, Tricassus, Corvinus, and others in his book, thus hath it: "The saturnine line going from the rascetta through the hand to Saturn's mount, and there intersected by certain little lines, argues melancholy;[1] so if the vital and natural make an acute angle" (Aphorism 100). "The saturnine, hepatic, and natural lines, making a gross triangle in the hand, argue as much"; which Goclenius, *cap.* 5 *Chiros.*, repeats verbatim out of him. In general they conclude all, that if Saturn's mount be full of many small lines and intersections, "such men are most part melancholy, miserable and full of disquietness, care and trouble, continually vexed with anxious and bitter thoughts, always sorrowful, fearful, suspicious; they delight in husbandry, buildings, pools, marshes, springs, woods, walks, etc."[2] Thaddæus Haggesius, in his *Metoposcopia*, hath certain aphorisms derived from Saturn's lines in the forehead, by which he collects a melancholy disposition; and Baptista Porta[3] makes observations from those other parts of the body, as if a spot be over the spleen; "or in the nails,[4] if it appear black, it signifieth much care, grief, contention, and melancholy"; the reason he refers to the humours, and gives instance in himself, that for seven years' space he had such black spots in his nails, and all that while was in perpetual lawsuits, controversies for his inheritance, fear, loss of honour, banishment, grief, care, etc., and when his miseries ended, the black spots vanished. Cardan, in his book *de libris propriis*, tells such a story of his own person, that a little before his son's death, he had a black spot, which appeared in one of his nails, and dilated itself as he came nearer to his end. But I am over-tedious in these toys, which howsoever, in some men's too severe censures, they may be held absurd and ridiculous, I am the bolder to insert, as not borrowed from circumforanean rogues and gipsies, but out of the writings of worthy philosophers and physicians, yet living some of them, and religious professors in famous universities, who are able to patronize that which they have said, and vindicate themselves from all cavillers and ignorant persons.

SUBSECT. V.—*Old Age a Cause*

Secondary peculiar causes efficient, so called in respect of the other precedent, are either *congenitæ, internæ, innatæ*, as they term them, inward, innate, inbred; or else outward and adventitious, which happen to us after we are born: congenite, or born with us, are either natural, as old age, or *præter naturam* [unnatural] (as Fernelius calls it [1]), that distemperature which we have from our parents' seed, it being an hereditary disease. The first of these, which is natural to all, and which no man living can avoid, is old age,[2] which being cold and dry, and of the same quality as melancholy is, must needs cause it, by diminution of spirits and substance, and increasing of adust humours; therefore Melancthon avers out of Aristotle,[3] as an undoubted truth, *senes plerumque delirasse in senecta*, that old men familiarly dote, *ob atram bilem,* for black choler, which is then superabundant in them: and Rhasis, that Arabian physician, in his *Cont. lib.* 1, *cap.* 9, calls it "a necessary and inseparable accident" [4] to all old and decrepit persons. After seventy years (as the Psalmist saith) "all is trouble and sorrow"; [5] and common experience confirms the truth of it in weak and old persons, especially such as have lived in action all their lives, had great employment, much business, much command, and many servants to oversee, and leave off *ex abrupto*, as Charles the Fifth did to King Philip, resign up all on a sudden; [6] they are overcome with melancholy in an instant: or if they do continue in such courses, they dote at last (*senex bis puer* [an old man is in his second boyhood]), and are not able to manage their estates through common infirmities incident in their age; full of ache, sorrow, and grief, children again, dizzards, they carle many times as they sit, and talk to themselves, they are angry, waspish, displeased with everything, "suspicious of all, wayward, covetous, hard" (saith Tully [7]), "self-willed, superstitious, self-conceited, braggers, and admirers of themselves," as Balthasar Castilio hath truly noted of them.[8]   This natural infirmity is most eminent in old women, and such as are poor, solitary, live in most base esteem and beggary, or such as are witches; insomuch that Wierus,[9] Baptista Porta, Ulricus Molitor, Edwicus, do refer all that witches are said to do, to imagination alone, and this humour of melancholy. And whereas it is controverted, whether they can bewitch cattle to death, ride in the air upon a cowl-staff out of a chimney-top, transform themselves into cats, dogs, etc., translate bodies from place to

place, meet in companies and dance, as they do, or have carnal
copulation with the devil, they ascribe all to this redundant
melancholy, which domineers in them, to somniferous potions,[1]
and natural causes, the devil's policy. *Non lædunt omnino*
(saith Wierus) *aut quid mirum faciunt* (*de Lamiis, lib. 3, cap. 36*),
ut putatur, solam vitiatam habent phantasiam; they do no such
wonders at all, only their brains are crazed.[2] "They think
they are witches, and can do hurt, but do not."[3] But this
opinion Bodine, Erastus, Danæus, Scribanius, Sebastian
Michaelis, Campanella, *de sensu rerum, lib. 4, cap. 9*, Dandinus
the Jesuit, *lib. 2 de Anima*,[4] explode; Cicogna confutes at large.[5]
That witches are melancholy they deny not, but not out of a
corrupt phantasy alone, so to delude themselves and others, or
to produce such effects.

Subsect. VI.—*Parents a Cause by Propagation*

That other inward, inbred cause of melancholy is our temperature, in whole or part, which we receive from our parents,
which Fernelius calls *præter naturam*,[6] or unnatural, it being
an hereditary disease; for as he justifies, *Quale parentum maxime
patris semen obtigerit, tales evadunt similares spermaticæque partes,
quocunque etiam morbo pater quum generat tenetur, cum semine
transfert in prolem;*[7] such as the temperature of the father is,
such is the son's, and look what disease the father had when he
begot him, his son will have after him;" and is as well inheritor of
his infirmities as of his lands."[8] "And where the complexion
and constitution of the father is corrupt, there" (saith Roger
Bacon) "the complexion and constitution of the son must needs
be corrupt, and so the corruption is derived from the father to
the son."[9] Now this doth not so much appear in the composition of the body, according to that of Hippocrates, "in habit,
proportion, scars, and other lineaments; but in manners and
conditions of the mind,"[10] *Et patrum in natos abeunt cum semine
mores* [the character of the parents is transmitted to the children
through the seed].

Seleucus had an anchor on his thigh, so had his posterity, as
Trogus records, *lib. 15*. Lepidus, in Pliny, *lib. 7, cap. 17*, was
purblind, so was his son. That famous family of Aenobarbi were
known of old, and so surnamed from their red beards; the
Austrian lip, and those Indians' flat noses are propagated, the
Bavarian chin, and goggle eyes amongst the Jews, as Buxtorfius
observes;[11] their voice, pace, gesture, looks, is likewise derived

with all the rest of their conditions and infirmities; such a mother, such a daughter; their very affections Lemnius contends "to follow their seed, and the malice and bad conditions of children are many times wholly to be imputed to their parents";[1] I need not therefore make any doubt of melancholy, but that it is an hereditary disease. Paracelsus in express words affirms it,[2] *lib. de morb. amentium, to.* 4, *tr.* 1; so doth Crato in an epistle of his to Monavius.[3] So doth Bruno Seidelius in his book *de morbo incurab.* Montaltus proves, *cap.* 11, out of Hippocrates and Plutarch, that such hereditary dispositions are frequent, *et hanc (inquit) fieri reor ob participatam melancholicam intemperantiam* (speaking of a patient), "I think he became so by participation of melancholy." Daniel Sennertus, *lib.* 1, *part.* 2, *cap.* 9, will have his melancholy constitution derived not only from the father to the son, but to the whole family sometimes: *quandoque totis familiis hæreditativam.* Forestus, in his medicinal observations,[4] illustrates this point, with an example of a merchant, his patient, that had this infirmity by inheritance; so doth Rodericus à Fonseca, *tom.* 1, *consul.* 69, by an instance of a young man that was so affected *ex matre melancholica*, had a melancholy mother, *et victu melancholico*, and bad diet together. Lodovicus Mercatus, a Spanish physician, in that excellent tract which he hath lately written of hereditary diseases, *tom.* 2 *oper. lib.* 5, reckons up leprosy, as those Galbots in Gascony,[5] hereditary lepers, pox, stone, gout, epilepsy, etc. Amongst the rest, this and madness after a set time comes to many, which he calls a miraculous thing in nature, and sticks for ever to them as an incurable habit. And that which is more to be wondered at, it skips in some families the father, and goes to the son, "or takes every other, and sometimes every third in a lineal descent, and doth not always produce the same, but some like, and a symbolizing disease."[6] These secondary causes hence derived are commonly so powerful, that (as Wolfius holds[7]) *sæpe mutant decreta siderum*, they do often alter the primary causes, and decrees of the heavens. For these reasons, belike, the Church and commonwealth, human and divine laws, have conspired to avoid hereditary diseases, forbidding such marriages as are any whit allied; and as Mercatus adviseth all families to take such, *si fieri possit, quæ maxime distant natura* [if possible, as are most distant in nature], and to make choice of those that are most differing in complexion from them, if they love their own, and respect the common good. And sure, I think, it hath been ordered by God's especial

providence, that in all ages there should be (as usually there is)
once in six hundred years, a transmigration of nations,[1] to
amend and purify their blood, as we alter seed upon our land,
and that there should be, as it were, an inundation of those
northern Goths and Vandals, and many such-like people which
came out of that continent of Scandia and Sarmatia (as some
suppose) and overran, as a deluge, most part of Europe and
Africa, to alter for our good our complexions, which were much
defaced with hereditary infirmities, which by our lust and intemperance we had contracted. A sound generation of strong
and able men were sent amongst us, as those northern men
usually are, innocuous, free from riot, and free from diseases;
to qualify and make us as those poor naked Indians are generally
at this day, and those about Brazil (as a late writer observes [2]),
in the Isle of Maragnan, free from all hereditary diseases or
other contagion, whereas without help of physic they live
commonly 120 years or more, as in the Orcades and many other
places. Such are the common effects of temperance and
intemperance; but I will descend to particulars, and show by
what means, and by whom especially, this infirmity is derived
unto us.

Filii ex senibus nati, raro sunt firmi temperamenti, old men's
children are seldom of a good temperament, as Scoltzius supposeth, *consult.* 177, and therefore most apt to this disease; and
as Levinus Lemnius farther adds, old men beget most part
wayward, peevish, sad, melancholy sons, and seldom merry.[3]
He that begets a child on a full stomach will either have a sick
child or a crazed son (as Cardan thinks,[4] *Contradict. med. lib.* 1,
contradict. 18), or if the parents be sick, or have any great pain
of the head, or megrim, headache (Hieronymus Wolfius doth
instance in a child of Sebastian Castalio's [5]), or if a drunken man
get a child, it will never likely have a good brain, as Gellius
argues, *lib.* 12, *cap.* 1. *Ebrii gignunt ebrios,* one drunkard begets
another, saith Plutarch,[6] *Symp. lib.* 1, *quest.* 5, whose sentence
Lemnius approves, *lib.* 1, *cap.* 4; [7] Alsarius Crucius Gen., *de
quæsit. med. cent.* 3, *fol.* 182; Macrobius, *lib.* 1; Avicenna, *lib.* 3,
fen. 21, *tract.* 1, *cap.* 8; and Aristotle himself, *sect.* 2, *prob.* 4.
Foolish, drunken, or hairbrain women most part bring forth
children like unto themselves, *morosos et languidos* [morose and
feeble], and so likewise he that lies with a menstruous woman.
*Intemperantia veneris, quam in nautis præsertim insectatur
Lemnius,[8] qui uxores ineunt, nulla menstrui decursus ratione
habita, nec observato interlunio, præcipua causa est, noxia,*

perniciosa (concubitum hunc exitialem ideo, et pestiferum vocat Rodericus a Castro, Lusitanus,[1] *detestantur ad unum omnes medici), tum et quarta luna concepti, infelices plerumque et amentes, deliri, stolidi, morbosi, impuri, invalidi, tetra lue sordidi, minime vitales, omnibus bonis corporis atque animi destituti: ad laborem nati, si seniores, inquit Eustathius, ut Hercules, et alii. Judæi maxime insectantur fœdum hunc et immundum apud Christianos concubitum, ut illicitum abhorrent, et apud suos prohibent; et quod Christiani toties leprosi, amentes, tot morbilli, impetigines, alphi, psoræ, cutis et faciei decolorationes, tam multi morbi epidemici, acerbi, et venenosi sint, in hunc immundum concubitum rejiciunt, et crudeles in pignora vocant, qui quarta luna profluente hac mensium illuvie concubitum hunc non perhorrescunt.*[2] *Damnavit olim divina lex et morte mulctavit hujusmodi homines* (Lev. xviii, xx), *et inde nati, si qui deformes aut mutili, pater dilapidatus, quod non contineret ab immunda muliere.*[3] *Gregorius Magnus, petenti Augustino numquid apud Britannos hujusmodi concubitum toleraret, severe prohibuit viris suis tum misceri feminas in consuetis suis menstruis, etc.*[4] I spare to English this which I have said. Another cause some give, inordinate diet, as if a man eat garlic, onions, fast overmuch, study too hard, be over-sorrowful, dull, heavy, dejected in mind, perplexed in his thoughts, fearful, etc., "their children" (saith Cardan, *Subtil. lib.* 18) "will be much subject to madness and melancholy; for if the spirits of the brain be fuzzled or misaffected by such means at such a time, their children will be fuzzled in the brain: they will be dull, heavy, timorous, discontented all their lives."[5] Some are of opinion, and maintain that paradox or problem, that wise men beget commonly fools; Suidas gives instance in Aristarchus the Grammarian, *duos reliquit filios, Aristarchum et Aristachorum, ambos stultos* [he left two sons, Aristarchus and Aristachorus, both stupid]; and which Erasmus urgeth in his *Moria*,[6] fools beget wise men. Cardan, *Subt. lib.* 12, gives this cause, *quoniam spiritus sapientum ob studium resolvuntur, et in cerebrum feruntur a corde:* because their natural spirits are resolved by study, and turned into animal; drawn from the heart, and those other parts, to the brain. Lemnius subscribes to that of Cardan, and assigns this reason, *quod persolvant debitum languide, et oscitanter, unde fœtus a parentum generositate desciscit:* they pay their debt (as Paul calls it) to their wives remissly, by which means their children are weaklings, and many times idiots and fools.

Some other causes are given, which properly pertain to, and do proceed from, the mother. If she be over-dull, heavy, angry, peevish, discontented, and melancholy, not only at the time of conception, but even all the while she carries the child in her womb (saith Fernelius, *Path. lib.* 1, 11), her son will be so likewise affected, and worse, as Lemnius adds,[1] *lib.* 4, *cap.* 7. If she grieve overmuch, be disquieted, or by any casualty be affrighted and terrified by some fearful object heard or seen, she endangers her child, and spoils the temperature of it; for the strange imagination of a woman works effectually upon her infant, that, as Baptista Porta proves, *Physiog. cœlestis, lib.* 5, *cap.* 2, she leaves a mark upon it, which is most especially seen in such as prodigiously long for such and such meats; the child will love those meats, saith Fernelius, and be addicted to like humours: "if a great-bellied woman see a hare, her child will often have an hare-lip," [2] as we call it. Garcæus, *de judiciis geniturarum, cap.* 33, hath a memorable example of one Thomas Nickell, born in the city of Brandenburg, 1551, "that went reeling and staggering all the days of his life, as if he would fall to the ground, because his mother being great with child saw a drunken man reeling in the street." [3] Such another I find in Martin Wenrichius, *Com. de ortu monstrorum, cap.* 17. "I saw" (saith he) "at Wittenberg, in Germany, a citizen that looked like a carcass; I asked him the cause, he replied, "His mother, when she bore him in her womb, saw a carcass by chance, and was so sore affrighted with it, that *ex eo fœtus ei assimilatus*, from a ghastly impression the child was like it." [4]

So many several ways are we plagued and punished for our fathers' defaults; insomuch that, as Fernelius truly saith, "It is the greatest part of our felicity to be well born, and it were happy for humankind, if only such parents as are sound of body and mind should be suffered to marry." [5] An husbandman will sow none but the best and choicest seed upon his land, he will not rear a bull or a horse, except he be right shapen in all parts, or permit him to cover a mare, except he be well assured of his breed; we make choice of the best rams for our sheep, rear the neatest kine, and keep the best dogs, *quanto id diligentius in procreandis liberis observandum !* and how careful then should we be in begetting of our children ! In former times some countries have been so chary in this behalf, so stern, that if a child were crooked or deformed in body or mind, they made him away: [6] so did the Indians of old by the relation of Curtius, and many other well-governed commonwealths, according to the discipline of those times. Heretofore in

Scotland, saith Hect. Boethius, "if any were visited with the
falling sickness, madness, gout, leprosy, or any such dangerous
disease, which was likely to be propagated from the father to
the son, he was instantly gelded; a woman kept from all company of men; and if by chance, having some such disease, she
were found to be with child, she with her brood were buried
alive:[1] and this was done for the common good, lest the whole
nation should be injured or corrupted." A severe doom, you
will say, and not to be used amongst Christians, yet more to
be looked into than it is. For now, by our too much facility
in this kind, in giving way for all to marry that will, too much
liberty and indulgence in tolerating all sorts, there is a vast
confusion of hereditary diseases, no family secure, no man,
almost, free from some grievous infirmity or other, when no
choice is had, but still the eldest must marry, as so many
stallions of the race; or if rich, be they fools or dizzards, lame
or maimed, unable, intemperate, dissolute, exhaust through
riot, as he said,[2] *jure hæreditario sapere jubentur*; they must be
wise and able by inheritance: it comes to pass that our generation is corrupt, we have many weak persons, both in body and
mind, many feral diseases raging amongst us, crazed families,
parentes peremptores [our parents are our ruin], our fathers
bad, and we are like to be worse.

MEMB. II

Subsect. I.—*Bad Diet a Cause. Substance. Quality of Meats*

According to my proposed method, having opened hitherto
these secondary causes, which are inbred with us, I must now
proceed to the outward and adventitious, which happen unto
us after we are born. And those are either evident, remote, or
inward, antecedent, and the nearest: continent causes some
call them. These outward, remote, precedent causes are subdivided again into necessary and not necessary. Necessary
(because we cannot avoid them, but they will alter us, as they
are used or abused) are those six non-natural things, so much
spoken of amongst physicians, which are principal causes of
this disease. For almost in every consultation, whereas they
shall come to speak of the causes, the fault is found, and this
most part objected to the patient: *Peccavit circa res sex non
naturales*, he hath still offended in one of those six. Montanus,
consil. 22, consulted about a melancholy Jew, gives that sentence,

so did Frisimelica in the same place; and in his 244th counsel,
censuring a melancholy soldier, assigns that reason of his
malady, "He offended in all those six non-natural things, which
were the outward causes, from which came those inward
obstructions";[1] and so in the rest.

These six non-natural things are diet, retention, and evacuation, which are more material than the other because they make
new matter, or else are conversant in keeping or expelling of it;
the other four are air, exercise, sleeping, waking, and perturbations of the mind, which only alter the matter. The first of
these is diet, which consists in meat and drink, and causeth
melancholy, as it offends in substance or accidents, that is
quantity, quality, or the like. And well it may be called a
material cause, since that, as Fernelius holds, "it hath such a
power in begetting of diseases, and yields the matter and
sustenance of them; for neither air, nor perturbations, nor any
of those other evident causes take place, or work this effect,
except the constitution of body and preparation of humours
do concur; that a man may say this diet is the mother of
diseases, let the father be what he will; and from this alone
melancholy and frequent other maladies arise."[2] Many
physicians, I confess, have written copious volumes of this one
subject, of the nature and qualities of all manner of meats; as
namely, Galen, Isaac the Jew; Halyabbas, Avicenna, Mesue,
also four[3] Arabians; Gordonius, Villanovanus, Wecker, Johannes
Bruerinus, *Sitologia de Esculentis et Poculentis*, Michael Savonarola, *tract. 2, cap. 8*, Anthony Fumanellus, *lib. de regimine senum*,
Curio in his Comment on Schola Salerna, Godefridus Stegius
Arte med., Marsilius Cognatus, Ficinus, Ranzovius, Fonseca,
Lessius, Magninus, *Regim. sanitatis*, Freitagius, Hugo Fridevallius, etc., besides many other in English;[4] and almost every
peculiar physician discourseth at large of all peculiar meats in
his chapter of melancholy: yet because these books are not at
hand to every man, I will briefly touch of what kind of meats
engender this humour, through their several species, and which
are to be avoided. How they alter and change the matter, spirits
first, and after humours, by which we are preserved, and the constitution of our body, Fernelius and others will show you. I hasten
to the thing itself: and first of such diet as offends in substance.

Beef, a strong and hearty meat (cold in the first degree, dry in
the second, saith Galen, *lib. 3, cap. 1, de alim. fac.*), is condemned
by him and all succeeding authors to breed gross melancholy
blood: good for such as are sound and of a strong constitution,

for labouring men if ordered aright, corned, young, of an ox (for all gelded meats in every species are held best), or if old, such as have been tired out with labour are preferred.[1] Aubanus and Sabellicus commend Portugal beef to be the most savoury, best and easiest of digestion; we commend ours: but all is rejected and unfit for such as lead a resty life, anyways inclined to melancholy, or dry of complexion; *Tales* (Galen thinks) *de facili melancholicis ægritudinibus capiuntur* [such easily fall a prey to the ailments of melancholy].

Pork, of all meats, is most nutritive in his own nature, but altogether unfit for such as live at ease, are anyways unsound of body or mind:[2] too moist, full of humours, and therefore *noxia delicatis*, saith Savonarola, *ex earum usu ut dubitetur an febris quartana generetur:* naught for queasy stomachs, insomuch that frequent use of it may breed a quartan ague.

Savonarola discommends goat's flesh, and so doth Bruerinus,[3] *lib.* 13, *cap.* 19, calling it a filthy beast, and rammish: and therefore supposeth it will breed rank and filthy substance; yet kid, such as are young and tender, Isaac accepts, Bruerinus, and Galen, *lib.* 1, *cap.* 1, *de alimentorum facultatibus.*

Hart and red deer hath an evil name: it yields gross nutriment:[4] a strong and great-grained meat, next unto a horse. Which, although some countries eat, as Tartars, and they of China, yet Galen condemns.[5] Young foals are as commonly eaten in Spain as red deer, and to furnish their navies, about Malaga especially, often used; but such meats ask long baking or seething to qualify them, and yet all will not serve.

All venison is melancholy, and begets bad blood; a pleasant meat: in great esteem with us (for we have more parks in England than there are in all Europe besides) in our solemn feasts. 'Tis somewhat better hunted than otherwise, and well prepared by cookery; but generally bad, and seldom to be used.

Hare, a black meat, melancholy, and hard of digestion; it breeds *incubus*, often eaten, and causeth fearful dreams, so doth all venison, and is condemned by a jury of physicians. Mizaldus and some others say that hare is a merry meat, and that it will make one fair, as Martial's epigram testifies to Gellia; but this is *per accidens*, because of the good sport it makes, merry company and good discourse that is commonly at the eating of it, and not otherwise to be understood.

Conies are of the nature of hares.[6] Magninus compares them to beef, pig, and goat, *Reg. sanit. part.* 3, *cap.* 17; yet young rabbits by all men are approved to be good.

Generally, all such meats as are hard of digestion breed melancholy. Aretæus, *lib.* 7, *cap.* 5, reckons up heads and feet, bowels, brains, entrails, marrow, fat, blood, skins, and those inward parts, as heart, lungs, liver, spleen, etc.[1] They are rejected by Isaac, *lib.* 2, *part.* 3; Magninus, *part.* 3, *cap.* 17; Bruerinus, *lib.* 12; Savonarola, *rub.* 32, *tract.* 2.

Milk, and all that comes of milk, as butter and cheese, curds, etc., increase melancholy (whey only excepted, which is most wholesome): some except asses' milk.[2]   The rest, to such as are sound, is nutritive and good, especially for young children, but because soon turned to corruption, not good for those that have unclean stomachs, are subject to headache, or have green wounds, stone, etc.[3]   Of all cheeses, I take that kind which we call Banbury cheese to be the best; *ex vetustis pessimus*, the older, stronger, and harder, the worst, as Langius discourseth in his epistle to Melancthon, cited by Mizaldus, Isaac, *part.* 5, Galen, *lib.* 3, *de cibis boni succi*, etc.

Amongst fowl, peacocks and pigeons, all fenny fowl are forbidden, as ducks, geese, swans, herons, cranes, coots, didappers, waterhens, with all those teals, currs, sheldrakes, and peckled fowls, that come hither in winter out of Scandia, Muscovy, Greenland, Friesland, which half the year are covered all over with snow and frozen up.[4]   Though these be fair in feathers, pleasant in taste, and have a good outside, like hypocrites, white in plumes, and soft, their flesh is hard, black, unwholesome, dangerous, melancholy meat; *Gravant et putrefaciunt stomachum* [they overload and spoil the stomach], saith Isaac, *part.* 5, *de vol.*; their young ones are more tolerable, but young pigeons he quite disapproves.

Rhasis and Magninus [5] discommend all fish, and say they breed viscosities, slimy nutriment, little and humorous nourishment. Savonarola adds cold; moist and phlegmatic, Isaac; and therefore unwholesome for all cold and melancholy complexions: others make a difference, rejecting only, amongst freshwater fish, eel, tench, lamprey, crawfish (which Bright approves, *cap.* 6), and such as are bred in muddy and standing waters, and have a taste of mud, as Franciscus Bonsuetus poetically defines, *lib. de aquatilibus*:

> *Nam pisces omnes, qui stagna lacusque frequentant,*
> *Semper plus succi deterioris habent.*

> All fish, that standing pools and lakes frequent,
> Do ever yield bad juice and nourishment.

Lampreys, Paulus Jovius, *cap.* 34, *de piscibus fluvial.*, highly magnifies, and saith, none speak against them, but *inepti* [fools] and *scrupulosi*, some scrupulous persons; but eels, *cap*. 33, "he abhorreth in all places, at all times, all physicians detest them, especially about the solstice." [1] Gomesius, *lib*. 1, *cap*. 22, *de sale*, doth immoderately extol sea-fish, which others as much vilify, and above the rest, dried, soused, indurate fish, as ling, fumadoes, red-herrings, sprats, stock-fish, haberdine, poor-john, all shell-fish. Tim. Bright excepts lobster and crab.[2] Messarius commends salmon, which Bruerinus contradicts, *lib*. 22, *cap*. 17. Magninus rejects conger, sturgeon, turbot, mackerel, skate.

Carp is a fish of which I know not what to determine. Franciscus Bonsuetus accounts it a muddy fish. Hippolytus Salvianus, in his book *de piscium natura et præparatione*, which was printed at Rome in folio, 1554, with most elegant pictures, esteems carp no better than a slimy, watery meat. Paulus Jovius, on the other side, disallowing tench, approves of it; so doth Dubravius in his books of Fish-ponds. Freitagius extols it for an excellent, wholesome meat, and puts it amongst the fishes of the best rank;[3] and so do most of our country gentlemen, that store their ponds almost with no other fish. But this controversy is easily decided, in my judgment, by Bruerinus, *lib*. 22, *cap*. 13. The difference riseth from the site and nature of pools, sometimes muddy, sometimes sweet;[4] they are in taste as the place is from whence they be taken. In like manner almost we may conclude of other fresh fish. But see more in Rondeletius, Bellonius, Oribasius, *lib*. 7, *cap*. 22, Isaac, *lib*. 1, especially Hippolytus Salvianus, who is *instar omnium solus*, etc. Howsoever they may be wholesome and approved, much use of them is not good; P. Forestus, in his Medicinal Observations, relates that Carthusian friars, whose living is most part fish, are more subject to melancholy than any other Order, and that he found by experience, being sometime their physician ordinary at Delft, in Holland.[5] He exemplifies it with an instance of one Buscodnese, a Carthusian of a ruddy colour, and well liking, that by solitary living and fish-eating became so misaffected.

Amongst herbs to be eaten I find gourds, cucumbers, coleworts, melons, disallowed, but especially cabbage. It causeth troublesome dreams, and sends up black vapours to the brain. Galen, *Loc. affect. lib*. 3, *cap*. 6, of all herbs condemns cabbage; and Isaac, *lib*. 2, *cap*. 1, *animæ gravitatem facit*, it brings heaviness to the soul. Some are of opinion that all raw herbs and sallets breed melancholy blood, except bugloss and lettuce.

Crato, *consil.* 21, *lib.* 2, speaks against all herbs and worts, except
borage, bugloss, fennel, parsley, dill, balm, succory; Magninus,
Regim. sanitatis, part. 3, *cap.* 31, *Omnes herbæ simpliciter malæ,
via cibi;* all herbs are simply evil to feed on (as he thinks). So
did that scoffing cook in Plautus hold: [1]

> *Non ego cœnam condio ut alii coqui solent,*
> *Qui mihi condita prata in patinis proferunt,*
> *Boves qui convivas faciunt, herbasque aggerunt.*

> Like other cooks I do not supper dress,
>   That put whole meadows into a platter,
> And make no better of their guests than beeves,
>   With herbs and grass to feed them fatter.

Our Italians and Spaniards do make a whole dinner of herbs
and sallets (which our said Plautus calls *cœnas terrestres* [earthy
meals], Horace, *cœnas sine sanguine* [bloodless meals]), by
which means, as he follows it:

> *Hic homines tam brevem vitam colunt . . .*
> *Qui herbas hujusmodi in alvum suum congerunt,*
> *Formidolosum dictu, non esu modo,*
> *Quas herbas pecudes non edunt, homines edunt.* [2]

> Their lives, that eat such herbs, must needs be short,
>   And 'tis a fearful thing for to report,
> That men should feed on such a kind of meat,
>   Which very juments would refuse to eat.

They are windy, and not fit, therefore, to be eaten of all men
raw, though qualified with oil, but in broths, or otherwise.[3]
See more of these in every husbandman and herbalist.[4]

Roots, *etsi quorundam gentium opes sint,* saith Bruerinus, the
wealth of some countries, and sole food, are windy and bad, or
troublesome to the head: as onions, garlic, scallions, turnips,
carrots, radishes, parsnips: Crato, *lib.* 2, *consil.* 11, disallows all
roots, though some approve of parsnips and potatoes.[5] Magninus is of Crato's opinion, "They trouble the mind, sending
gross fumes to the brain, make men mad,"[6] especially garlic,
onions, if a man liberally feed on them a year together.[7]
Guianerius, *tract.* 15, *cap.* 2, complains of all manner of roots,
and so doth Bruerinus, even parsnips themselves, which arc the
best, *lib.* 9, *cap.* 14, *Pastinacarum usus succos gignit improbos* [in-
dulgence in parsnips creates harmful juices]. Crato, *consil.* 21,
lib. 1, utterly forbids all manner of fruits, as pears, apples, plums,
cherries, strawberries, nuts, medlars, serves, etc. *Sanguinem
inficiunt,* saith Villanovanus, they infect the blood, and putrefy
it, Magninus holds, and must not therefore be taken *via cibi,
aut quantitate magna,* not to make a meal of, or in any great

quantity. Cardan makes that a cause of their continual sickness at Fez in Africa, "because they live so much on fruits,
eating them thrice a day." [1] Laurentius approves of many
fruits, in his Tract of Melancholy, which others disallow, and
amongst the rest apples, which some likewise commend, sweet-
ings, pearmains, pippins, as good against melancholy; but to
him that is any way inclined to, or touched with this malady,
Nicholas Piso, in his Practics,[2] forbids all fruits, as windy, or
to be sparingly eaten at least, and not raw. Amongst other
fruits, Bruerinus,[3] out of Galen, excepts grapes and figs, but
I find them likewise rejected.

All pulse are naught, beans, pease, fitches, etc., they fill the
brain (saith Isaac) with gross fumes, breed black, thick blood,
and cause troublesome dreams. And therefore, that which
Pythagoras said to his scholars of old may be for ever applied
to melancholy men, *A fabis abstinete*, eat no pease, nor beans;
yet to such as will needs eat them, I would give this counsel, to
prepare them according to those rules that Arnoldus Villanovanus and Freitagius prescribe, for eating, and dressing, fruits,
herbs, roots, pulse, etc.

Spices cause hot and head melancholy, and are for that cause
forbidden by our physicians to such men as are inclined to this
malady, as pepper, ginger, cinnamon, cloves, mace, dates, etc.,
honey, and sugar. Some except honey;[4] to those that are cold
it may be tolerable, but *Dulcia se in bilem vertunt* [5] [sweets turn
into bile], they are obstructive. Crato therefore forbids all
spice, in a consultation of his, for a melancholy schoolmaster,
omnia aromatica, et quicquid sanguinem adurit [all spices, and
whatever dries up the blood]: so doth Fernelius, *consil.* 45;
Guianerius, *tract.* 15, *cap.* 2; Mercurialis, *cons.* 189. To these
I may add all sharp and sour things, luscious and over-sweet,
or fat, as oil, vinegar, verjuice, mustard, salt; as sweet things
are obstructive, so these are corrosive. Gomesius, in his books
de sale, lib. 1, *cap.* 21, highly commends salt; so doth Codronchus
in his tract *de sale absinthii*, Lemn. *lib.* 3, *cap.* 9, *de occult. nat.
mir.*; yet common experience finds salt, and salt-meats, to be
great procurers of this disease. And for that cause belike those
Egyptian priests abstained from salt, even so much as in their
bread, *ut sine perturbatione anima esset*, saith mine author, that
their souls might be free from perturbations.

Bread that is made of baser grain, as pease, beans, oats, rye,
or over-hard baked, crusty,[6] and black, is often spoken against,
as causing melancholy juice and wind. Joh. Major, in the

first book of his History of Scotland, contends much for the
wholesomeness of oaten bread: it was objected to him, then
living at Paris in France, that his countrymen fed on oats and
base grain, as a disgrace; but he doth ingenuously confess,
Scotland, Wales, and a third part of England did most part
use that kind of bread, that it was as wholesome as any grain,
and yielded as good nourishment.   And yet Wecker, out of
Galen, calls it horse-meat, and fitter for juments than men to
feed on.   But read Galen himself, *lib.* 1 *de cibis boni et mali
succi,* more largely discoursing of corn and bread.

All black wines, over-hot, compound, strong, thick drinks, as
muscadine, malmsey, alicant, rumney, brown bastard, methe-
glin, and the like, of which they have thirty several kinds in
Muscovy, all such made drinks are hurtful in this case, to such
as are hot, or of a sanguine, choleric complexion, young, or
inclined to head-melancholy.   For many times the drinking of
wine alone causeth it.   Arculanus, *cap.* 16, *in* 9 *Rhasis,* puts in
wine for a great cause,[1] especially if it be immoderately used.
Guianerius, *tract.* 15, *cap.* 2, tells a story of two Dutchmen, to
whom he gave entertainment in his house, "that in one month's
space were both melancholy by drinking of wine, one did naught
but sing, the other sigh." [2]   Galen, *lib. de causis morb., cap.* 3;
Matthiolus on Dioscorides; and above all other Andreas Bachius,
lib. 3, *cap.* 18, 19, 20, have reckoned upon those inconveniences
that come by wine: yet notwithstanding all this, to such as are
cold, or sluggish melancholy, a cup of wine is good physic, and
so doth Mercurialis grant, *consil.* 25; in that case, if the temperature be cold, as to most melancholy men it is, wine is much
commended, if it be moderately used.

Cider and perry are both cold and windy drinks, and for
that cause to be neglected, and so are all those hot, spiced,
strong drinks.

Beer, if it be over-new, or over-stale, over-strong, or not
sod, smell of the cask, sharp, or sour, is most unwholesome,
frets, and galls, etc.   Henricus Ayrerus, in a consultation of
his,[3] for one that laboured of hypochondriacal melancholy,
discommends beer.   So doth Crato, in that excellent counsel
of his, *lib.* 2, *consil.* 21, as too windy, because of the hop.[4]
But he means, belike, that thick, black Bohemian beer used in
some other parts of Germany: [5]

Nil spissius illa
Dum bibitur, nil clarius est dum mingitur, unde
Constat, quod multas fæces in corpore linquat.

> Nothing comes in so thick,
> Nothing goes out so thin,
> It must needs follow then
> The dregs are left within.

As that old poet [1] scoffed, calling it *Stygiæ monstrum conforme paludi*, a monstrous drink, like the River Styx. But let them say as they list, to such as are accustomed unto it, "'tis a most wholesome" (so Polydore Virgil calleth it [2]) "and a pleasant drink," it is more subtile and better for the hop that rarefies it, hath an especial virtue against melancholy, as our herbalists confess, Fuchsius approves, *lib. 2, sec. 3, Instit. cap.* 11, and many others.

Standing waters, thick and ill-coloured, such as come forth of pools and moats where hemp hath been steeped or slimy fishes live, are most unwholesome, putrefied, and full of mites, creepers, slimy, muddy, unclean, corrupt, impure, by reason of the sun's heat and still standing; they cause foul distemperatures in the body and mind of man, are unfit to make drink of, to dress meat with, or to be used about men inwardly or outwardly.[3] They are good for many domestic uses, to wash horses, water cattle, etc., or in time of necessity, but not otherwise. Some are of opinion that such fat, standing waters make the best beer, and that seething doth defecate it, as Cardan holds, *lib. 13 Subtil.*, "It mends the substance and savour of it,"[4] but it is a paradox. Such beer may be stronger, but not so wholesome as the other, as Jobertus truly justifieth out of Galen, *Paradox. dec. 1, paradox.* 5, that the seething of such impure waters doth not purge or purify them; [5] Pliny, *lib.* 31, *cap.* 3, is of the same tenent, and P. Crescentius, *Agricult. lib.* 1 *et lib.* 4, *cap.* 11 *et cap.* 45. Pamphilius Herilachus, *lib.* 4 *de nat. aquarum*, such waters are naught, not to be used, and by the testimony of Galen, "breed agues, dropsies, pleurisies, splenetic and melancholy passions, hurt the eyes, cause a bad temperature and ill disposition of the whole body, with bad colour."[6] This Jobertus stiffly maintains, *Paradox. lib.* 1, *part.* 5, that it causeth blear eyes, bad colour, and many loathsome diseases to such as use it: this which they say, stands with good reason; for as geographers relate, the water of Astracan breeds worms in such as drink it. Axius, or as now called Verduri,[7] the fairest river in Macedonia, makes all cattle black that taste of it. [8] Aliacmon, now Peleca, another stream in Thessaly, turns cattle most part white, *si potui ducas* [if you take them to drink there]. J. Aubanus Bohemus refers that *struma* or poke of the Bava-

rians and Styrians to the nature of their waters,[1] as Munster
doth that of the Valesians in the Alps,[2] and Bodine supposeth
the stuttering of some families in Aquitania, about Labden, to
proceed from the same cause, "and that the filth is derived
from the water to their bodies."[3] So that they that use filthy,
standing, ill-coloured, thick, muddy water, must needs have
muddy, ill-coloured, impure, and infirm bodies. And because
the body works upon the mind, they shall have grosser understandings, dull, foggy, melancholy spirits, and be readily subject
to all manner of infirmities.

To these noxious simples we may reduce an infinite number
of compound, artificial, made dishes, of which our cooks afford
us a great variety, as tailors do fashions in our apparel. Such
are puddings stuffed with blood, or otherwise composed;[4] baked
meats, soused indurate meats, fried and broiled, buttered meats,
condite, powdered, and over-dried; all cakes, simnels, buns,
cracknels made with butter, spice, etc., fritters, pancakes, pies,
sausages, and those several sauces, sharp, or over-sweet,[5] of
which *scientia popinæ* [the learning of the cookshop], as Seneca
calls it, hath served those Apician tricks and perfumed dishes,
which Adrian the Sixth, Pope, so much admired in the accounts
of his predecessor Leo Decimus,[6] and which prodigious riot and
prodigality have invented in this age.[7] These do generally
engender gross humours, fill the stomach with crudities, and all
those inward parts with obstructions. Montanus, *consil.* 22,
gives instance in a melancholy Jew, that by eating such tart
sauces, made dishes, and salt meats, with which he was overmuch delighted, became melancholy, and was evil-affected.
Such examples are familiar and common.

SUBSECT. II.—*Quantity of Diet a Cause*

There is not so much harm proceeding from the substance
itself of meat, and quality of it, in ill dressing and preparing, as
there is from the quantity, disorder of time and place, unseasonable use of it, intemperance, overmuch or overlittle taking of
it.[8] A true saying it is, *Plures crapula quam gladius*, this
gluttony kills more than the sword, this *omnivorans et homicida
gula*, this all-devouring and murdering gut. And that of Pliny
is truer, "Simple diet is the best; heaping up of several meats
is pernicious, and sauces worse; many dishes bring many
diseases."[9] Avicen cries out, that "nothing is worse than to
feed on many dishes, or to protract the time of meats longer

than ordinary; from thence proceed our infirmities, and 'tis the
fountain of all diseases, which arise out of the repugnancy of
gross humours."[1]   Thence, saith Fernelius, come crudities,
wind, oppilations, cacochymia, plethora, cachexia, bradypepsia,[2]
Hinc subitæ mortes, atque intestata senectus,[3] sudden death, etc.,
and what not.

As a lamp is choked with a multitude of oil, or a little fire
with overmuch wood quite extinguished, so is the natural heat
with immoderate eating strangled in the body. *Perniciosa
sentina est abdomen insaturabile,* one saith, an insatiable paunch
is a pernicious sink, and the fountain of all diseases, both of
body and mind.   Mercurialis will have it a peculiar cause of
this private disease;[4] Solenander, *consil. 5, sect. 3,* illustrates
this of Mercurialis with an example of one so melancholy, *ab intempestivis commessationibus,* [from] unseasonable feasting. Crato
confirms as much, in that often cited counsel, *21, lib. 2,* putting
superfluous eating for a main cause.[5]   But what need I seek
farther for proofs?   Hear Hippocrates himself, *lib. 2, aphor. 10:*
"Impure bodies, the more they are nourished, the more they are
hurt, for the nourishment is putrefied with vicious humours."[6]

And yet for all this harm, which apparently follows surfeiting
and drunkenness, see how we luxuriate and rage in this kind;
read what Johannes Stuckius hath written lately of this subject,
in his great volume *de Antiquorum Conviviis,* and of our present
age; *Quam portentosæ cœnæ,*[7] [what] prodigious suppers, *Qui dum
invitant ad cœnam efferunt ad sepulchrum*[8] [who in inviting
us to supper conduct us to our graves], what Fagos, Epicures,
Apiciuses, Heliogables, our times afford! Lucullus' ghost walks
still, and every man desires to sup in Apollo; Æsop's costly dish
is ordinarily served up.   *Magis illa juvant, quæ pluris emunter*[9]
[the more they cost, the more we enjoy them].   The dearest
cates are best, and 'tis an ordinary thing to bestow twenty or
thirty pound on a dish, some thousand crowns upon a dinner:
Muley-Hamet, King of Fez and Morocco, spent three pounds
on the sauce of a capon:[10] it is nothing in our times, we scorn
all that is cheap.   "We loathe the very light" (some of us, as
Seneca notes) "because it comes free, and we are offended with
the sun's heat, and those cool blasts, because we buy them not."[11]
This air we breathe is so common, we care not for it; nothing
pleaseth but what is dear.   And if we be witty in anything, it
is *ad gulam;*[12] if we study at all, it is *erudito luxu* [the learning
of luxury], to please the palate, and to satisfy the gut.   "A
cook of old was a base knave" (as Livy complains), "but now a

great man in request; cookery is become an art, a noble science; cooks are gentlemen"; [1] *Venter Deus* [their belly is their god]. They wear "their brains in their bellies, and their guts in their heads," as Agrippa [2] taxed some parasites of his time, rushing on their own destruction, as if a man should run upon the point of a sword, *usque dum rumpantur comedunt* [they eat till they burst]: all day, all night, [3] let the physician say what he will, imminent danger and feral diseases are now ready to seize upon them, that will eat till they vomit, *Edunt ut vomant, vomunt ut edant* [they eat to vomit and vomit to eat], saith Seneca (which Dion relates of Vitellius, *Solo transitu ciborum nutriri judicatus*: his meat did pass through and away), or till they burst again. *Strage animantium ventrem onerant* [4] [they load their bellies with the spoil of the animal world], and rake over all the world, as so many slaves, [5] belly-gods, and land-serpents, *et totus orbis ventri nimis angustus*, the whole world cannot satisfy their appetite. "Sea, land, rivers, lakes, etc., may not give content to their raging guts." [6]   To make up the mess, what immoderate drinking in every place! *Senem potum pota trahebat anus* [old men, old women drunk go arm in arm], how they flock to the tavern! as if they were *fruges consumere nati*, born to no other end but to eat and drink, like Offellius Bibulus, that famous Roman parasite, *qui dum vixit, aut bibit aut minxit*; as so many casks to hold wine, yea worse than a cask, that mars wine, and itself is not marred by it, yet these are brave men, *Silenus ebrius* [drunken Silenus] was no braver. *Et quæ fuerunt vitia, mores sunt* [what once was vice is now highly moral]: 'tis now the fashion of our times, an honour: *Nunc vero res ista eo rediit* (as Chrysost., *serm.* 30 *in* 5 *Ephes.*, comments) *ut effeminatæ ridendæque ignaviæ loco habeatur, nolle inebriari;* 'tis now come to that pass that he is no gentleman, a very milksop, a clown, of no bringing-up, that will not drink; fit for no company; he is your only gallant that plays it off finest, no disparagement now to stagger in the streets, reel, rave, etc., but much to his fame and renown; as in like case Epidicus told Thesprio his fellow-servant, in the poet. [7] *Edepol facinus improbum* [in truth, a very wrong action], one urged; the other replied, *At jam alii fecere idem, erit illi illa res honori,* 'tis now no fault, there be so many brave examples to bear one out; 'tis a credit to have a strong brain, and carry his liquor well; the sole contention who can drink most, and fox his fellow the soonest. 'Tis the *summum bonum* of our tradesmen, their felicity, life, and soul (*Tanta dulcedine affectant*, saith Pliny, *lib.*

14, *cap.* 12, *ut magna pars non aliud vitæ præmium intelligat* [strong drink gives such pleasure that many people think there is nothing else worth living for]), their chief comfort, to be merry together in an alehouse or tavern, as our modern Muscovites do in their mead-inns, and Turks in their coffa-houses, which much resemble our taverns; they will labour hard all day long to be drunk at night, and spend *totius anni labores* [the earnings of a whole year], as St. Ambrose adds, in a tippling feast; convert day into night, as Seneca taxes some in his times, *Pervertunt officia noctis et lucis* [they turn day into night and night into day]; when we rise, they commonly go to bed, like our antipodes:

Nosque ubi primus equis oriens afflavit anhelis,
Illis sera rubens accendit lumina vesper.

[When dawn for us pants up the East on high,
For them the eve glows in the western sky.]

So did Petronius in Tacitus, Heliogabalus in Lampridius.

Noctes vigilabat ad ipsum
Mane, diem totum stertebat.[1]

[He drank the night away
Till rising dawn, then snor'd out all the day.]

Smindyrides the Sybarite never saw the sun rise or set so much as once in twenty years. Verres, against whom Tully so much inveighs, in winter he never was *extra tectum* [out of his house], *vix extra lectum,* never almost out of bed, still wenching and drinking;[2] so did he spend his time, and so do myriads in our days. They have *gymnasia bibonum* [training grounds for topers], schools and rendezvous; these Centaurs and Lapithæ toss pots and bowls as so many balls; invent new tricks, as sausages, anchovies, tobacco, caviare, pickled oysters, herrings, fumadoes, etc., innumerable salt meats to increase their appetite, and study how to hurt themselves by taking antidotes "to carry their drink the better";[3] "and when naught else serves, they will go forth, or be conveyed out, to empty their gorge, that they may return to drink afresh."[4] They make laws, *insanos leges, contra bibendi fallacias* [crazy laws against attempts to shirk drinking], and brag of it when they have done,[5] crowning that man that is soonest gone, as their drunken predecessors have done (*Quid ego video?* Ps. *Cum corona Pseudolum ebrium tuum.*[6] [What do I see? Your friend Pseudolus, drunk

and garlanded]), and when they are dead, will have a can of
wine with Maron's old woman[1] to be engraven on their tombs.
So they triumph in villainy, and justify their wickedness with
Rabelais, that French Lucian: drunkenness is better for the body
than physic, because there be more old drunkards than old
physicians. Many such frothy arguments they have, inviting
and encouraging others to do as they do,[2] and love them dearly
for it (no glue like to that of good fellowship). So did Alcibiades in Greece; Nero, Bonosus, Heliogabalus in Rome, or
Alegabalus rather, as he was styled of old (as Ignatius proves
out of some old coins[3]). So do many great men still, as Heres-
bachius observes.[4] When a prince drinks till his eyes stare,
like Bitias in the poet,

Ille impiger hausit
Spumantem vino pateram,[5]

[Eager he drained the bowl, brimming with wine,]

and comes off clearly, sound trumpets, fife and drums, the
spectators will applaud him, "the bishop himself" (if he belie
them not) "with his chaplain will stand by and do as much,"[6]
O dignum principe haustum, 'twas done like a prince. "Our
Dutchmen invite all comers with a pail and a dish, *velut
infundibula integras obbas exhauriunt, et in monstrosis poculis
ipsi monstrosi monstrosius epotant* [they take in whole beakers
like funnels, and swill hugely out of huge goblets], making
barrels of their bellies."[7] *Incredible dictu,* as one of their own
countrymen complains, *quantum liquoris immodestissima gens
capiat* [the amount of liquor these heavy drinkers can
consume is incredible], etc.; "how they love a man that will be
drunk, crown him and honour him for it, hate him that will
not pledge him, stab him, kill him":[8] a most intolerable offence,
and not to be forgiven. "He is a mortal enemy that will not
drink with him,"[9] as Munster relates of the Saxons. So in
Poland, he is the best servitor, and the honestest fellow, saith
Alexander Gaguinus, that drinketh most healths to the honour
of his master;[10] he shall be rewarded as a good servant, and held
the bravest fellow that carries his liquor best, whenas a brewer's
horse will bear much more than any sturdy drinker; yet for his
noble exploits in this kind he shall be accounted a most valiant
man, for *Tam inter epulas fortis vir esse potest ac in bello,*[11] as
much valour is to be found in feasting as in fighting, and some of
our city captains and carpet knights will make this good, and
prove it. Thus they many times wilfully pervert the good

temperature of their bodies, stifle their wits, strangle nature, and degenerate into beasts.

Some again are in the other extreme, and draw this mischief on their heads by too ceremonious and strict diet, being over-precise, cockney-like, and curious in their observation of meats, times, as that *medicina statica* [regimen of diet] prescribes, just so many ounces at dinner, which Lessius enjoins, so much at supper, not a little more, nor a little less, of such meat, and at such hours, a diet-drink in the morning, cock-broth, china-broth, at dinner plum-broth, a chicken, a rabbit, rib of a rack of mutton, wing of a capon, the merry-thought of a hen, etc.; to sounder bodies this is too nice and most absurd. Others offend in over-much fasting: pining adays, saith Guianerius,[1] and waking anights, as many Moors and Turks in these our times do. "Anchorites, monks, and the rest of that superstitious rank" (as the same Guianerius witnesseth, that he hath often seen to have happened in his time) "through immoderate fasting, have been frequently mad." Of such men belike Hippocrates speaks, 1 *Aphor.* 5, whenas he saith, "They more offend in too sparing diet, and are worse damnified, than they that feed liberally and are ready to surfeit." [2]

SUBSECT. III.—*Custom of Diet, Delight, Appetite, Necessity, how they cause or hinder*

No rule is so general, which admits not some exception; to this, therefore, which hath been hitherto said (for I shall otherwise put most men out of commons), and those inconveniences which proceed from the substance of meats, an intemperate or unseasonable use of them, custom somewhat detracts and qualifies, according to that of Hippocrates, 2 *Aphoris.* 50, "Such things as we have been long accustomed to, though they be evil in their own nature, yet they are less offensive." [3] Otherwise it might well be objected that it were a mere tyranny to live after those strict rules of physic; [4] for custom doth alter nature itself,[5] and to such as are used to them it makes bad meats wholesome, and unseasonable times to cause no disorder. Cider and perry are windy drinks, so are all fruits windy in themselves, cold most part, yet in some shires of England,[6] Normandy in France, Guipuscoa in Spain, 'tis their common drink, and they are no whit offended with it. In Spain, Italy, and Africa, they live most on roots, raw herbs, camel's milk,[7] and it agrees well with them: which to a stranger will cause much grievance. In Wales, *lacticiniis vescuntur*, as Humphrey Llwyd confesseth, a Cambro-Briton himself, in his elegant epistle to Abraham Ortelius, they live most on white meats; in Holland on fish, roots, butter;[1] and so at this day in Greece, as Bellonius observes, they had much rather feed on fish than flesh.[2]　With us, *maxima pars victus in carne consistit*, we feed on flesh most part, saith Polydore Virgil,[3] as all northern countries do; and it would be very offensive to us to live after their diet, or they to live after ours.　We drink beer, they wine; they use oil, we butter; we in the north are great eaters,[4] they most sparing in those hotter countries; and yet they and we following our own customs are well pleased.　An Ethiopian of old, seeing an European eat bread, wondered, *quomodo stercoribus vescentes viverimus*, how we could eat such kind of meats: so much differed his countrymen from ours in diet, that, as mine author infers,[5] *si quis illorum victum apud nos æmulari vellet*, if any man should so feed with us, it would be all one to nourish as cicuta, aconitum, or hellebore itself.　At this day in China the common people live in a manner altogether on roots and herbs, and to the wealthiest, horse, ass, mule, dog's, cat-flesh, is as delightsome as the rest, so Mat. Riccius the Jesuit relates,[6] who lived many years amongst them.　The Tartars eat raw meat, and most commonly horse-flesh, drink milk and blood, as the Nomades of old:[7] *Et lac concretum cum sanguine potat equino* [he drinks milk thickened with horse's blood].　They scoff at our Europeans for eating bread, which they call tops of weeds, and horse-meat, not fit for men; and yet Scaliger accounts them a sound and witty nation, living an hundred years; even in the civilest country of them they do thus, as Benedict the Jesuit observed in his travels from the Great Mogor's court by land to Paquin,[8] which Riccius contends to be the same with Cambalu in Cataia. In Scandia their bread is usually dried fish, and so likewise in the Shetland Isles; and their other fare, as in Iceland, saith Dithmarus Bleskenius,[9] "butter, cheese, and fish; their drink water, their lodging on the ground."　In America in many places their bread is roots, their meat palmitos, pinas, potatoes, etc., and such fruits.　There be of them too that familiarly drink salt sea-water all their lives,[10] eat raw meat, grass, and that with delight.[11]　With some, fish, serpents, spiders; and in divers places they eat man's flesh[12] raw and roasted, even the Emperor Metazuma himself.[13]　In some coasts, again, one tree yields them coco-nuts, meat and drink, fire, fuel, apparel with his leaves, oil, vinegar, cover for houses, etc.,[14] and yet these

men, going naked, feeding coarse, live commonly an hundred
years, are seldom or never sick; all which diet our physicians
forbid.   In Westphalia they feed most part on fat meats and
worts, knuckle-deep, and call it *cerebrum Jovis*[1] [Jupiter's
brain]; in the Low Countries with roots; in Italy frogs and snails
are used.   The Turks, saith Busbequius, delight most in fried
meats.   In Muscovy, garlic and onions are ordinary meat and
sauce, which would be pernicious to such as are unaccustomed
unto them, delightsome to others; and all is because they have
been brought up unto it.[2]   Husbandmen, and such as labour,
can eat fat bacon, salt gross meat, hard cheese, etc. (*O dura
messorum ilia !* [what tough insides have these mowers!]), coarse
bread at all times, go to bed and labour upon a full stomach,
which to some idle persons would be present death, and is
against the rules of physic, so that custom is all in all.   Our
travellers find this by common experience when they come in
far countries and use their diet; they are suddenly offended,[3]
as our Hollanders and Englishmen, when they touch upon the
coasts of Africa, those Indian capes and islands, are commonly
molested with calentures, fluxes, and much distempered by
reason of their fruits.   *Peregrina, etsi suavia, solent vescentibus
perturbationes insignes adferre ;*[4] strange meats, though pleasant,
cause notable alterations and distempers.   On the other side,
use or custom mitigates or makes all good again.   Mithridates
by often use, which Pliny wonders at, was able to drink poison;
and a maid, as Curtius records, sent to Alexander from King
Porus, was brought up with poison from her infancy.   The Turks,
saith Bellonius, *lib.* 3, *cap.* 15, eat opium familiarly, a dram
at once, which we dare not take in grains.   Garcias ab Horto
writes[5] of one whom he saw at Goa in the East Indies,
that took ten drams of opium in three days; and yet *consulto
loquebatur*, spake understandingly, so much can custom do.
Theophrastus speaks of a shepherd that could eat hellebore in
substance.[6]   And therefore Cardan concludes out of Galen,
Consuetudinem utcunque ferendam, nisi valde malam, custom is
howsoever to be kept, except it be extremely bad: he adviseth
all men to keep their old customs, and that by the authority of
Hippocrates himself,[7] *Dandum aliquid tempori, ætati, regioni,
consuetudini* [regard must be had to season, age, district, and
habit], and therefore to continue as they began, be it diet,
bath, exercise, etc., or whatsoever else.[8]

Another exception is delight, or appetite, to such and such
meats.   Though they be hard of digestion, melancholy, yet, as

Fuchsius excepts, *cap.* 6, *lib.* 2 *Instit. sect.* 2, "The stomach doth readily digest and willingly entertain such meats we love most and are pleasing to us, abhors on the other side such as we distaste." [1] Which Hippocrates confirms, *Aphoris.* 2, 38. Some cannot endure cheese, out of a secret antipathy; or to see a roasted duck, which to others is a delightsome meat.[2]

The last exception is necessity, poverty, want, hunger, which drives men many times to do that which otherwise they are loath, cannot endure, and thankfully to accept of it: as beverage in ships, and in sieges of great cities to feed on dogs, cats, rats, and men themselves.   Three outlaws in Hector Boethius,[3] being driven to their shifts, did eat raw flesh, and flesh of such fowl as they could catch, in one of the Hebrides for some few months. These things do mitigate or disannul that which hath been said of melancholy meats, and make it more tolerable; but to such as are wealthy, live plenteously, at ease, may take their choice, and refrain if they will, these viands are to be forborne, if they be inclined to, or suspect melancholy, as they tender their healths: otherwise if they be intemperate, or disordered in their diet, at their peril be it.   *Qui monet amat, Ave atque cave.*

[He who advises is your friend
Farewell, and to your health attend.]

SUBSECT. IV.—*Retention and Evacuation a Cause, and how*

Of retention and evacuation there be divers kinds, which are either concomitant, assisting, or sole causes many times of melancholy.   Galen reduceth defect and abundance to this head; [4] others, "all that is separated, or remains." [5]

In the first rank of these, I may well reckon up costiveness, and keeping in of our ordinary excrements, which as it often causeth other diseases, so this of melancholy in particular. Celsus, *lib.* 1, *cap.* 3, saith, "It produceth inflammation of the head, dullness, cloudiness, headache, etc." [6] Prosper Calenus, *lib. de atra bile*, will have it distemper not the organ only, "but the mind itself by troubling of it"; [7] and sometimes it is a sole cause of madness, as you may read in the first book of Sckenkius his Medicinal Observations.[8] A young merchant going to Nordeling Fair in Germany, for ten days' space never went to stool; at his return he was grievously melancholy,[9] thinking that he was robbed, and would not be persuaded but that all his money was gone; his friends thought he had some philtrum given him, but Cnelinus a physician being sent for, found his costiveness alone to be the cause,[1] and thereupon gave him a clyster, by which he was speedily recovered. Trincavellius, *consult.* 35, *lib.* 1, saith as much of a melancholy lawyer, to whom he administered physic, and Rodericus à Fonseca, *consult.* 85, *tom.* 2, of a patient of his, that for eight days was bound,[2] and therefore melancholy affected. Other retentions and evacuations there are, not simply necessary, but at some times, as Fernelius accounts them, *Path. lib.* 1, *cap.* 15; as suppression of hemrods, monthly issues in women, bleeding at nose,[3] immoderate or no use at all of Venus, or any other ordinary issues.

Detention of hemrods, or monthly issues, Villanovanus, *Breviar. lib.* 1, *cap.* 18; Arculanus, *cap.* 16, *in* 9 *Rhasis*; Victorius Faventinus, *Pract. mag. tract.* 2, *cap.* 15; Bruel, etc., put for ordinary causes. Fuchsius, *lib.* 2, *sect.* 5, *cap.* 30, goes farther, and saith that "many men unseasonably cured of the hemrods have been corrupted with melancholy; seeking to avoid Scylla, they fall into Charybdis."[4] Galen, *lib. de hum. commen.* 3, *ad text.* 26, illustrates this by an example of Lucius Martius, whom he cured of madness, contracted by this means: and Sckenkius hath two other instances of two melancholy and mad women, so caused from the suppression of their months.[5] The same may be said of bleeding at the nose, if it be suddenly stopped, and have been formerly used, as Villanovanus urgeth:[6] and Fuchsius, *lib.* 2, *sect.* 5, *cap.* 33, stiffly maintains "that without great danger such an issue may not be stayed."[7]

Venus omitted produceth like effects. Matthiolus, *epist.* 5, *lib. penult.*, avoucheth of his knowledge, "that some through bashfulness abstained from venery, and thereupon became very heavy and dull; and some others that were very timorous, melancholy, and beyond all measure sad."[8] Oribasius, *Med. collect. lib.* 6, *cap.* 37, speaks of some, "that if they do not use carnal copulation, are continually troubled with heaviness and headache; and some in the same case by intermission of it."[9] Not use of it hurts many; Arculanus, *cap.* 6, *in* 9 *Rhasis*, and Magninus, *part.* 3, *cap.* 5, think, because it "sends up poisoned vapours to the brain and heart."[10] And so doth Galen himself hold, "that if this natural seed be over-long kept (in some parties) it turns to poison."[11] Hieronymus Mercurialis, in his chapter of Melancholy, cites it for an especial cause of this malady, priapismus, satyriasis, etc.[12] Halyabbas, 5 *Theor. cap.* 36, reckons up this and many other diseases. Villanovanus, *Breviar. lib.* 1, *cap.* 18, saith, he "knew many monks and widows grievously

troubled with melancholy, and that from this sole cause." [1]
Lodovicus Mercatus, *lib. 2 de mulierum affect. cap.* 4, and
Rodericus à Castro, *de morbis mulier. lib.* 2, *cap.* 3, treat largely of
this subject, and will have it produce a peculiar kind of melancholy in stale maids, nuns, and widows; [2] *Ob suppressionem mensium et venerem omissam, timidæ, anxiæ, verecundæ, suspiciosæ,
languentes, consilii inopes, cum summa vitæ et rerum meliorum
desperatione,* etc., they are melancholy in the highest degree,
and all for want of husbands. Ælianus Montaltus, *cap.* 37 *de
melanchol.,* confirms as much out of Galen; so doth Wierus.
Christopherus à Vega, *de art. med. lib.* 3, *cap.* 14, relates many such
examples of men and women, that he had seen so melancholy.
Felix Plater, in the first book of his Observations, tells a
story of an ancient gentleman in Alsatia, that "married a young
wife, and was not able to pay his debts in that kind for a long
time together, by reason of his several infirmities: but she,
because of this inhibition of Venus, fell into a horrible fury,
and desired every one that came to see her, by words, looks,
and gestures, to have to do with her," etc. [3] Bernardus
Paternus, a physician, saith, he knew "a good honest godly
priest, that because he would neither willingly marry, nor
make use of the stews, fell into grievous melancholy fits." [4]
Hildesheim, *Spicil.* 2, hath such another example of an Italian
melancholy priest, in a consultation had *anno* 1580. Jason
Pratensis gives instance in a married man, that, from his wife's
death "abstaining after marriage, became exceedingly melancholy"; [5] Rodericus à Fonseca in a young man so misaffected,
tom. 2, *consult.* 85. To these you may add, if you please,
that conceited tale of a Jew, so visited in like sort, and so
cured, out of Poggius Florentinus.

Intemperate Venus is all out as bad in the other extreme.
Galen, *lib.* 6 *de morbis popular. sect.* 5, *text.* 26, reckons up
melancholy amongst those diseases which are "exasperated by
venery": [6] so doth Avicenna, 2, 3, *cap.* 11; Oribasius, *loc. citat.;*
Ficinus, *lib.* 2 *de sanitate tuenda;* Marsilius Cognatus; Montaltus, *cap.* 27; Guianerius, *tract.* 3, *cap.* 2. [7] Magninus, *cap.* 5,
part. 3, gives the reason, because "it infrigidates and dries up
the body, consumes the spirits"; and would therefore have all
such as are cold and dry to take heed of and to avoid it as a
mortal enemy. [8] Jacchinus, *in* 9 *Rhasis, cap.* 15, ascribes
the same cause, and instanceth in a patient of his, that
married a young wife in a hot summer, "and so dried himself
with chamber-work, that he became in short space, from

melancholy, mad": he cured him by moistening remedies.[1]
The like example I find in Lælius à Fonte Eugubinus, *consult.*
129, of a gentleman of Venice, that upon the same occasion
was first melancholy, afterwards mad. Read in him the story
at large.

Any other evacuation stopped will cause it, as well as these
above named, be it bile, ulcer,[2] issue, etc. Hercules de Saxonia,
lib. 1, *cap.* 16, and Gordonius, verify this out of their experience.
They saw one wounded in the head who, as long as the sore was
open, *lucida habuit mentis intervalla,* was well; but when it
was stopped, *rediit melancholia,* his melancholy fit seized on
him again.

Artificial evacuations are much like in effect, as hot-houses,
baths, blood-letting, purging, unseasonably and immoderately
used.   Baths dry too much, if used in excess, be they natural
or artificial, and offend extreme hot, or cold;[3] one dries,[4] the
other refrigerates overmuch. Montanus, *consil.* 137, saith they
over-heat the liver. Joh. Struthius, *Stigmat. artis, lib.* 4, *cap.* 9,
contends, "that if one stay longer than ordinary at the bath,
go in too oft, or at unseasonable times, he putrefies the humours
in his body."[5]   To this purpose writes Magninus, *lib.* 3, *cap.* 5.
Guianerius, *tract.* 15, *cap.* 21, utterly disallows all hot baths in
melancholy adust. "I saw" (saith he) "a man that laboured
of the gout, who to be freed of his malady came to the bath, and
was instantly cured of his disease, but got another worse, and
that was madness."[6]   But this judgment varies as the humour
doth, in hot or cold: baths may be good for one melancholy
man, bad for another; that which will cure it in this party
may cause it in a second.

Phlebotomy, many times neglected, may do much harm to
the body, when there is a manifest redundance of bad humours
and melancholy blood; and when these humours heat and boil,
if this be not used in time, the parties affected, so inflamed, are
in great danger to be mad; but if it be unadvisedly, importunely,
immoderately used, it doth as much harm by refrigerating the
body, dulling the spirits, and consuming them.   As Joh. Curio
in his 10th chapter[7] well reprehends, such kind of letting blood
doth more hurt than good; "the humours rage much more
than they did before; and is so far from avoiding melancholy,
that it increaseth it, and weakeneth the sight."[8]   Prosper
Calenus[9] observes as much of all phlebotomy, except they keep
a very good diet after it; yea, and as Leonartus Jacchinus
speaks out of his own experience,[10] "the blood is much blacker

to many men after their letting blood than it was at first."[1]
For this cause belike Sallust. Salvianus, *lib.* 2, *cap.* 1, will admit
or hear of no blood-letting at all in this disease, except it be
manifest it proceed from blood: he was (it appears) by his own
words in that place, master of an hospital of madmen, "and
found by long experience that this kind of evacuation, either
in head, arm, or any other part, did more harm than good."[2]
To this opinion of his Felix Plater[3] is quite opposite: "Though
some wink at, disallow and quite contradict all phlebotomy in
melancholy, yet by long experience I have found innumerable
so saved, after they had been twenty, nay, sixty times let
blood, and to live happily after it. It was an ordinary thing of
old, in Galen's time, to take at once from such men six pound
of blood, which now we dare scarce take in ounces." *Sed viderint
medici* [but this is a matter for the doctors]; great books are
written of this subject.

Purging upward and downward, in abundance of bad humours
omitted, may be for the worst; so likewise as in the precedent,
if overmuch, too frequent or violent, it weakeneth their strength,[4]
saith Fuchsius, *lib.* 2, *sect.* 2, *cap.* 17, or if they be strong or able
to endure physic, yet it brings them to an ill habit, they make
their bodies no better than apothecaries' shops; this and such-
like infirmities must needs follow.

SUBSECT. V.—*Bad Air a Cause of Melancholy*

Air is a cause of great moment in producing this or any
other disease, being that it is still taken into our bodies by
respiration, and our more inner parts. "If it be impure and
foggy, it dejects the spirits, and causeth diseases by infection
of the heart."[5] as Paulus hath it, *lib.* 1, *cap.* 49; Avicenna,
lib. 1; Gal. *de san. tuenda*; Mercurialis, Montaltus, etc. Fernelius
saith, "A thick air thickeneth the blood and humours."[6]
Lemnius[7] reckons up two main things most profitable and most
pernicious to our bodies: air and diet; and this peculiar disease
nothing sooner causeth (Jobertus holds[8]) than the air wherein
we breathe and live. Such as is the air, such be our spirits;
and as our spirits, such are our humours.[9] It offends commonly
if it be too hot and dry,[10] thick, fuliginous, cloudy, blustering,
or a tempestuous air. Bodine, in his fifth book, *De repub.*
cap. 1 and 5, of his Method of History, proves that hot countries
are most troubled with melancholy, and that there are therefore in Spain, Africa, and Asia Minor, great numbers of

madmen, insomuch that they are compelled in all cities of note, to build peculiar hospitals for them. Leo Afer, *lib.* 3, *de Fessa urbe*,[1] Ortelius, and Zuinger confirm as much: they are ordinarily so choleric in their speeches, that scarce two words pass without railing or chiding in common talk, and often quarrelling in their streets. Gordonius will have every man take notice of it:[2] "Note this" (saith he) "that in hot countries it is far more familiar than in cold." Although this we have now said be not continually so, for, as Acosta truly saith,[3] under the Equator itself is a most temperate habitation, wholesome air, a paradise of pleasure: the leaves ever green, cooling showers. But it holds in such as are intemperately hot, as Johannes à Meggen found in Cyprus,[4] others in Malta, Apulia,[5] and the Holy Land, where at some seasons of the year is nothing but dust, their rivers dried up, the air scorching hot, and earth inflamed; insomuch that many pilgrims, going barefoot for devotion sake from Joppa to Jerusalem upon the hot sands, often run mad; or else quite overwhelmed with sand, *profundis arenis*, as in many parts of Africa, Arabia Deserta, Bactriana, now Chorassan, when the west wind blows, *involuti arenis transeuntes necantur*[6] [travellers are sometimes buried by clouds of sand]. Hercules de Saxonia,[7] a professor in Venice, gives this cause why so many Venetian women are melancholy, *quod diu sub sole degant*, they tarry too long in the sun. Montanus, *consil.* 21, amongst other causes assigns this, why that Jew his patient was mad, *quod tam multum exposuit se calori et frigori:* he exposed himself so much to heat and cold. And for that reason in Venice there is little stirring in those brick-paved streets in summer about noon, they are most part then asleep: as they are likewise in the Great Mogor's countries, and all over the East Indies. At Aden in Arabia, as Lodovicus Vertomannus relates in his travels,[8] they keep their markets in the night, to avoid extremity of heat; and in Ormus, like cattle in a pasture, people of all sorts lie up to the chin in water all day long. At Braga in Portugal, Burgos in Castile, Messina in Sicily, all over Spain and Italy, their streets are most part narrow, to avoid the sunbeams. The Turks wear great turbans *ad fugandos solis radios*, to refract the sunbeams; and much inconvenience that hot air of Bantam in Java yields to our men that sojourn there for traffic; where it is so hot, "that they that are sick of the pox lie commonly bleaching in the sun, to dry up their sores."[9] Such a complaint I read of those isles of Cape Verde, fourteen degrees from the Equator, they do *male audire* [have a bad name];

one [1] calls them the unhealthiest clime of the world, for fluxes, fevers, frenzies, calentures, which commonly seize on seafaring men that touch at them, and all by reason of a hot distemperature of the air. The hardiest men are offended with this heat, and stiffest clowns cannot resist it, as Constantine affirms, *Agricult. lib.* 2, *cap.* 45. They that are naturally born in such air, may not endure it,[2] as Niger records of some part of Mesopotamia, now called Diarbecha:[3] *Quibusdam in locis sævienti æstui adeo subjecta est, ut pleraque animalia fervore solis et cœli extinguantur,* 'tis so hot there in some places, that men of the country and cattle are killed with it; and Adricomius of Arabia Felix,[4] by reason of myrrh, frankincense, and hot spices there growing, the air is so obnoxious to their brains, that the very inhabitants at some times cannot abide it, much less weaklings and strangers.[5] Amatus Lusitanus, *cent.* 1, *curat.* 45, reports of a young maid, that was one Vincent a currier's daughter, some thirteen years of age, that would wash her hair in the heat of the day (in July) and so let it dry in the sun, "to make it yellow, but by that means tarrying too long in the heat, she inflamed her head, and made herself mad." [6]

Cold air in the other extreme is almost as bad as hot, and so doth Montaltus esteem of it, *cap.* 11, if it be dry withal. In those northern countries, the people are therefore generally dull, heavy, and many witches, which (as I have before quoted) Saxo Grammaticus, Olaus, Baptista Porta ascribe to melancholy. But these cold climes are more subject to natural melancholy (not this artificial) which is cold and dry: for which cause Mercurius Britannicus [7] belike puts melancholy men to inhabit just under the Pole. The worst of the three is a thick, cloudy, misty, foggy air,[8] or such as come from fens, moorish grounds, lakes, muckhills, draughts, sinks, where any carcasses or carrion lies, or from whence any stinking fulsome smell comes: Galen, Avicenna, Mercurialis, new and old physicians, hold that such air is unwholesome, and engenders melancholy, plagues, and what not? Alexandretta, an haven-town in the Mediterranean Sea,[9] Saint John de Ulloa, an haven in Nova Hispania, are much condemned for a bad air, so are Durazzo in Albania, Lithuania, Ditmarsh, Pomptinæ Paludes [10] in Italy, the territories about Pisa, Ferrara, etc., Romney Marsh with us, the Hundreds in Essex, the fens in Lincolnshire. Cardan, *de rerum varietate, lib.* 17, *cap.* 96, finds fault with the site of those rich and most populous cities in the Low Countries, as Bruges, Ghent, Amsterdam, Leyden, Utrecht, etc., the air is bad; and so at

Stockholm in Sweden, Rhegium in Italy, Salisbury with us, Hull
and Lynn; they may be commodious for navigation, this new
kind of fortification, and many other good necessary uses; but
are they so wholesome? Old Rome hath descended from the
hills to the valley, 'tis the site of most of our new cities, and
held best to build in plains, to take the opportunity of rivers.
Leander Albertus pleads hard for the air and site of Venice,
though the black moorish lands appear at every low water:
the sea, fire, and smoke (as he thinks) qualify the air; and some
suppose that a thick foggy air helps the memory, as in them
of Pisa in Italy;[1] and our Camden, out of Plato, commends
the site of Cambridge, because it is so near the fens. But let
the site of such places be as it may, how can they be excused
that have a delicious seat, a pleasant air, and all that nature
can afford, and yet through their own nastiness and sluttish-
ness, immund and sordid manner of life, suffer their air to
putrefy, and themselves to be choked up? Many cities in
Turkey do *male audire* [have a bad name] in this kind: Constantinople itself, where commonly carrion lies in the street.
Some find the same fault in Spain, even in Madrid, the king's
seat; a most excellent air, a pleasant site, but the inhabitants
are slovens, and the streets uncleanly kept.

A troublesome tempestuous air is as bad as impure, rough
and foul weather, impetuous winds, cloudy dark days, as it is
commonly with us, *cœlum visu fœdum*, Polydore calls it,[2] a
filthy sky, *et in quo facile generantur nubes* [where the clouds
rapidly collect]; as Tully's brother Quintus wrote to him in
Rome, being then Quæstor in Britain. "In a thick and cloudy
air" (saith Lemnius[3]) "men are tetric, sad, and peevish: and if
the western winds blow, and that there be a calm, or a fair sunshine day, there is a kind of alacrity in men's minds; it cheers
up men and beasts: but if it be a turbulent, rough, cloudy,
stormy weather, men are sad, lumpish, and much dejected,
angry, waspish, dull, and melancholy." This was Virgil's
experiment of old:[4]

> *Verum ubi tempestas, et cœli mobilis humor*
> *Mutavere vices, et Jupiter humidus Austro,*
> *Vertuntur species animorum, et pectore motus*
> *Concipiunt alios.*

> But when the face of heaven changed is
> To tempests, rain, from season fair:
> Our minds are altered, and in our breasts
> Forthwith some new conceits appear.

And who is not weather-wise against such and such conjunctions of planets, moved in foul weather, dull and heavy in such
tempestuous seasons? *Gelidum contristat Aquarius annum* [1]
[chill, cheerless days Aquarius brings]: the time requires, and the
autumn breeds it; winter is like unto it, ugly, foul, squalid; the
air works on all men, more or less, but especially on such as are
melancholy, or inclined to it, as Lemnius holds: "They are
most moved with it, and those which are already mad rave
downright, either in or against a tempest. Besides, the devil
many times takes his opportunity of such storms, and when
the humours by the air be stirred, he goes in with them, exagi-
tates our spirits, and vexeth our souls; as the sea-waves, so
are the spirits and humours in our bodies tossed with tempestuous winds and storms." [2] To such as are melancholy,
therefore, Montanus, *consil.* 24, will have tempestuous and rough
air to be avoided, and, *consil.* 27, all night air, and would not
have them to walk abroad but in a pleasant day. Lemnius,
lib. 3, *cap.* 3, discommends the south and eastern winds, commends the north. Montanus, *consil.* 31, will not any windows
to be opened in the night.[3] *Consil.* 229, *et consil.* 230, he discommends especially the south wind, and nocturnal air: so
doth Plutarch.[4] The night and darkness makes men sad, the
like do all subterranean vaults, dark houses in caves and rocks;
desert places cause melancholy in an instant, especially such
as have not been used to it, or otherwise accustomed. Read
more of air in Hippocrates; Aetius, *lib.* 3, *a cap.* 171 *ad* 175;
Oribasius, *a cap.* 1 *ad* 21; Avicen, *lib.* 1, *can. fen.* 2, *doc.* 2,
fen. 1, *cap.* 123, to the 12, etc.

SUBSECT. VI.—*Immoderate Exercise a Cause, and how.*
Solitariness, Idleness

Nothing so good but it may be abused: nothing better than
exercise (if opportunely used) for the preservation of the body;
nothing so bad if it be unseasonable, violent, or overmuch.
Fernelius, out of Galen, *Path. lib.* 1, *cap.* 16, saith, "that much
exercise and weariness consumes the spirits and substance,
refrigerates the body; and such humours which nature would
have otherwise concocted and expelled, it stirs up and makes
them rage: which being so enraged, diversely affect and trouble
the body and mind." [5] So doth it, if it be unseasonably used,
upon a full stomach, or when the body is full of crudities, which
Fuchsius so much inveighs against, *lib.* 2 *Instit. sect.* 2, *cap.* 4,

giving that for a cause why schoolboys in Germany are so often scabbed, because they use exercise presently after meats. Bayerus puts in a caveat against such exercise,[1] because "it corrupts the meat in the stomach, and carries the same juice raw, and as yet undigested, into the veins" (saith Lemnius), "which there putrefies and confounds the animal spirits." [2] Crato, *consil.* 21, *lib.* 2, protests against all such exercise after meat, as being the greatest enemy to concoction that may be, and cause of corruption of humours, which produce this, and many other diseases.[3] Not without good reason then doth Sallust. Salvianus, *lib.* 2, *cap.* 1, and Leonartus Jacchinus *in* 9 *Rhasis*, Mercurialis, Arculanus, and many other, set down immoderate exercise[4] as a most forcible cause of melancholy.

Opposite to exercise is idleness (the badge of gentry) or want of exercise, the bane of body and mind, the nurse of naughtiness, stepmother of discipline, the chief author of all mischief, one of the seven deadly sins, and a sole cause of this and many other maladies, the devil's cushion, as Gualter calls it,[5] his pillow and chief reposal. "For the mind can never rest, but still meditates on one thing or other; except it be occupied about some honest business, of his own accord it rusheth into melancholy." "As too much and violent exercise offends on the one side, so doth an idle life on the other" (saith Crato), "it fills the body full of phlegm, gross humours, and all manner of obstructions, rheums, catarrhs, etc." [6] Rhasis, *Cont. lib.* 1, *tract.* 9, accounts of it as the greatest cause of melancholy. "I have often seen" (saith he) "that idleness begets this humour more than anything else." [7] Montaltus, *cap.* 1, seconds him out of his experience: "They that are idle are far more subject to melancholy than such as are conversant or employed about any office or business." [8] Plutarch reckons up idleness for a sole cause of the sickness of the soul: "There are they" (saith he) "troubled in mind, that have no other cause but this." [9] Homer, Iliad 1, brings in Achilles eating of his own heart in his idleness, because he might not fight. Mercurialis, *consil.* 86, for a melancholy young man, urgeth it is a chief cause; why was he melancholy? because idle.[10] Nothing begets it sooner, increaseth and continueth it oftener, than idleness;[11] a disease familiar to all idle persons, an inseparable companion to such as live at ease, *pingui otio desidiose agentes*, a life out of action, and have no calling or ordinary employment to busy themselves about, that have small occasions; and though they have, such is their laziness, dullness, they will not compose themselves to do aught;

they cannot abide work, though it be necessary, easy, as to dress
themselves, write a letter, or the like; yet, as he that is benumbed
with cold sits still shaking, that might relieve himself with a little
exercise or stirring, do they complain, but will not use the
facile and ready means to do themselves good; and so are still
tormented with melancholy. Especially if they have been
formerly brought up to business, or to keep much company,
and upon a sudden come to lead a sedentary life, it crucifies
their souls, and seizeth on them in an instant; for whilst they
are anyways employed, in action, discourse, about any business,
sport or recreation, or in company to their liking, they are
very well; but if alone or idle, tormented instantly again; one
day's solitariness, one hour's sometimes, doth them more harm
than a week's physic, labour, and company can do good. Melancholy seizeth on them forthwith being alone, and is such a torture that, as wise Seneca well saith, *Malo mihi male quam
molliter esse*, I had rather be sick than idle. This idleness is
either of body or mind. That of body is nothing but a kind
of benumbing laziness, intermitting exercise, which, if we may
believe Fernelius, "causeth crudities, obstructions, excremental
humours, quencheth the natural heat, dulls the spirits, and
makes them unapt to do anything whatsoever." [1]

Neglectis urenda filix innascitur agris. [2]

[Neglected fields yield bracken for burning.]

As fern grows in untilled grounds, and all manner of weeds, so
do gross humours in an idle body, *Ignavum corrumpunt otia
corpus*. A horse in a stable that never travels, a hawk in a mew
that seldom flies, are both subject to diseases; which, left unto
themselves, are most free from any such encumbrances. An
idle dog will be mangy, and how shall an idle person think to
escape? Idleness of the mind is much worse than this of the
body; wit without employment is a disease, *ærugo animi, rubigo
ingenii*: [3] the rust of the soul, a plague, a hell itself,[4] *maximum
animi nocumentum*,[5] Galen calls it. "As in a standing pool
worms and filthy creepers increase" (*et vitium capiunt ni move-
antur aquæ*, the water itself putrefies, and air likewise, if it be
not continually stirred by the wind), "so do evil and corrupt
thoughts in an idle person," [6] the soul is contaminated. In a
commonwealth, where is no public enemy, there is, likely, civil
wars, and they rage upon themselves: this body of ours, when
it is idle and knows not how to bestow itself, macerates and
vexeth itself with cares, griefs, false fears, discontents, and

suspicions; it tortures and preys upon his own bowels, and is
never at rest. Thus much I dare boldly say: he or she that
is idle, be they of what condition they will, never so rich, so
well allied, fortunate, happy, let them have all things in abundance and felicity that heart can wish and desire, all contentment,
so long as he or she or they are idle, they shall never be pleased,
never well in body and mind, but weary still, sickly still, vexed
still, loathing still, weeping, sighing, grieving, suspecting,
offended with the world, with every object, wishing themselves
gone or dead, or else carried away with some foolish phantasy
or other. And this is the true cause that so many great men,
ladies, and gentlewomen, labour of this disease in country and
city; for idleness is an appendix to nobility; they count it a
disgrace to work, and spend all their days in sports, recreations,
and pastimes, and will therefore take no pains, be of no vocation: they feed liberally, fare well, want exercise, action, employment (for to work, I say, they may not abide), and company
to their desires, and thence their bodies become full of gross
humours, wind, crudities, their minds disquieted, dull, heavy,
etc.; care, jealousy, fear of some diseases, sullen fits, weeping
fits, seize too familiarly on them.[1] For what will not fear and
phantasy work in an idle body? what distempers will they not
cause? When the children of Israel murmured against Pharaoh
in Egypt,[2] he commanded his officers to double their task, and
let them get straw themselves, and yet make their full number
of bricks; for the sole cause why they mutiny, and are evil at
ease, is, "they are idle." When you shall hear and see so many
discontented persons in all places where you come, so many
several grievances, unnecessary complaints, fear, suspicions,[3]
the best means to redress it is to set them awork, so to busy
their minds; for the truth is, they are idle. Well they may
build castles in the air for a time, and soothe up themselves with
phantastical and pleasant humours, but in the end they will
prove as bitter as gall, they shall be still, I say, discontent,
suspicious, fearful, jealous, sad, fretting and vexing of themselves;[4] so long as they be idle, it is impossible to please them.
*Otio qui nescit uti, plus habet negotii quam qui negotium in ne-
gotio,* as that A. Gellius could observe:[5] he that knows not how
to spend his time, hath more business, care, grief, anguish of mind
than he that is most busy in the midst of all his business. *Otiosus
animus nescit quid volet:* an idle person (as he follows it) knows
not when he is well, what he would have, or whither he would
go; *quum illuc ventum est, [ire] illinc lubet* [as soon as he comes

to a place, he wants to leave it], he is tired out with everything, displeased with all, weary of his life; *nec bene domi, nec
militiæ,* [happy] neither at home nor abroad, *errat, et præter
vitam vivitur,* he wanders and lives besides himself. In a word,
what the mischievous effects of laziness and idleness are, I
do not find anywhere more accurately expressed, than in these
verses of Philolaches in the comical poet,[1] which for their
elegancy I will in part insert.

> *Novarum ædium esse arbitror similem ego hominem,*
> *Quando hic natus est. Ei rei argumenta dicam.*
> *Ædes quando sunt ad amussim expolitæ,*
> *Quisque laudat fabrum, atque exemplum expetit,* etc.
> *At ubi illo migrat nequam homo indiligensque,* etc.
> *Tempestas venit, confringit tegulas, imbricesque,*
> *Putrefacit aer operam fabri,* etc.
> *Dicam ut homines similes esse ædium arbitremini,*
> *Fabri parentes fundamentum substruunt liberorum,*
> *Expoliunt, docent literas, nec parcunt sumptui,*
> *Ego autem sub fabrorum potestate frugi fui,*
> *Postquam autem migravi in ingenium meum,*
> *Perdidi operam fabrorum illico, oppido,*
> *Venit ignavia, ea mihi tempestas fuit,*
> *Adventuque suo grandinem et imbrem attulit,*
> *Illa mihi virtutem deturbavit,* etc.

A young man is like a fair new house; the carpenter leaves it
well built, in good repair, of solid stuff; but a bad tenant lets it
rain in, and for want of reparation fall to decay, etc. Our
parents, tutors, friends, spare no cost to bring us up in our
youth in all manner of virtuous education; but when we are
left to ourselves, idleness as a tempest drives all virtuous motions
out of our minds, *et nihili sumus*; on a sudden, by sloth and such
bad ways, we come to naught.

Cousin-german to idleness, and a concomitant cause which goes
hand in hand with it, is *nimia solitudo*, too much solitariness, by
the testimony of all physicians,[2] cause and symptom both; but
as it is here put for a cause, it is either coact, enforced, or else
voluntary. Enforced solitariness is commonly seen in students,
monks, friars, anchorites, that by their order and course of life
must abandon all company, society of other men, and betake
themselves to a private cell: *Otio superstitioso seclusi* [recluses
through superstition], as Bale and Hospinian well term it, such as
are the Carthusians of our time, that eat no flesh (by their order),
keep perpetual silence, never go abroad; such as live in prison, or
some desert place, and cannot have company, as many of our
country gentlemen do in solitary houses, they must either be alone

without companions, or live beyond their means, and entertain all comers as so many hosts, or else converse with their servants and hinds, such as are unequal, inferior to them, and of a contrary disposition: or else, as some do to avoid solitariness, spend their time with lewd fellows in taverns and in alehouses, and thence addict themselves to some unlawful disports, or dissolute courses. Divers again are cast upon this rock of solitariness for want of means, or out of a strong apprehension of some infirmity, disgrace, or through bashfulness, rudeness, simplicity, they cannot apply themselves to others' company. *Nullum solum infelici gratius solitudine, ubi nullus sit qui miseriam exprobret* [to the wretched no spot is more welcome than one where there is no one to upbraid his misery]. This enforced solitariness takes place, and produceth his effect soonest, in such as have spent their time jovially, peradventure in all honest recreations, in good company, in some great family or populous city, and are upon a sudden confined to a desert country cottage far off, restrained of their liberty, and barred from their ordinary associates; solitariness is very irksome to such, most tedious, and a sudden cause of great inconvenience.

Voluntary solitariness is that which is familiar with melancholy, and gently brings on like a siren, a shoeing-horn, or some sphinx to this irrevocable gulf; a primary cause, Piso calls it.[1] Most pleasant it is at first, to such as are melancholy given, to lie in bed whole days, and keep their chambers, to walk alone in some solitary grove, betwixt wood and water, by a brook side, to meditate upon some delightsome and pleasant subject, which shall affect them most; *amabilis insania* [a pleasing dotage], and *mentis gratissimus error* [a most flattering delusion]. A most incomparable delight it is so to melancholize, and build castles in the air, to go smiling to themselves, acting an infinite variety of parts, which they suppose and strongly imagine they represent, or that they see acted or done. *Blandum quidem ab initio* [it is delightful at first], saith Lemnius, to conceive and meditate of such pleasant things sometimes, "present, past, or to come,"[2] as Rhasis speaks. So delightsome these toys are at first, they could spend whole days and nights without sleep, even whole years alone in such contemplations and phantastical meditations, which are like unto dreams, and they will hardly be drawn from them, or willingly interrupt; so pleasant their vain conceits are, that they hinder their ordinary tasks and necessary business, they cannot address themselves to them, or almost to any study or employment, these phantastical and bewitching thoughts so covertly, so feelingly, so urgently, so continually set upon, creep in, insinuate, possess, overcome, distract, and detain them, they cannot, I say, go about their more necessary business, stave off or extricate themselves, but are ever musing, melancholizing, and carried along; as he (they say) that is led round about a heath with a Puck in the night, they run earnestly on in this labyrinth of anxious and solicitous melancholy meditations, and cannot well or willingly refrain, or easily leave off, winding and unwinding themselves as so many clocks, and still pleasing their humours, until at last the scene is turned upon a sudden by some bad object, and they, being now habituated to such vain meditations and solitary places, can endure no company, can ruminate of nothing but harsh and distasteful subjects. Fear, sorrow, suspicion, *subrusticus pudor* [a rustic bashfulness], discontent, cares, and weariness of life surprise them in a moment, and they can think of nothing else, continually suspecting; no sooner are their eyes open, but this infernal plague of melancholy seizeth on them, and terrifies their souls, representing some dismal object to their minds, which now by no means, no labour, no persuasions they can avoid, *hæret lateri lethalis arundo* [the deadly arrow still remains in their side], they may not be rid of it, they cannot resist.[1]   I may not deny but that there is some profitable meditation, contemplation, and kind of solitariness to be embraced, which the Fathers so highly commended, Hierome,[2] Chrysostom, Cyprian, Austin, in whole tracts, which Petrarch, Erasmus, Stella, and others so much magnify in their books; a paradise, a heaven on earth, if it be used aright, good for the body, and better for the soul: as many of those old monks used it, to divine contemplations; as Simulus, a courtier in Hadrian's time, Dioclesian the emperor, retired themselves, etc., in that sense, *Vatia solus scit vivere*, Vatia lives alone, which the Romans were wont to say when they commended a country life. Or to the bettering of their knowledge, as Democritus, Cleanthes, and those excellent philosophers have ever done, to sequester themselves from the tumultuous world, or as in Pliny's Villa Laurentana, Tully's Tusculan, Jovius' study, that they might better *vacare studiis et Deo*, serve God and follow their studies. Methinks, therefore, our too zealous innovators were not so well advised in that general subversion of abbeys and religious houses, promiscuously to fling down all; they might have taken away those gross abuses crept in

amongst them, rectified such inconveniences, and not so far to
have raved and raged against those fair buildings and everlasting monuments of our forefathers' devotion, consecrated to
pious uses; some monasteries and collegiate cells might have
been well spared, and their revenues otherwise employed, here
and there one, in good towns or cities at least, for men and
women of all sorts and conditions to live in, to sequester themselves from the cares and tumults of the world, that were not
desirous or fit to marry, or otherwise willing to be troubled
with common affairs, and know not well where to bestow themselves, to live apart in, for more conveniency, good education,
better company sake, to follow their studies (I say), to the
perfection of arts and sciences, common good, and, as some
truly devoted monks of old had done, freely and truly to serve
God.   For these men are neither solitary nor idle, as the poet
made answer to the husbandman in Æsop that objected idleness to him: he was never so idle as in his company; or that
Scipio Africanus in Tully,[1] *Nunquam minus solus, quam cum
solus; nunquam minus otiosus, quam quum esset otiosus :* never
less solitary than when he was alone, never more busy than
when he seemed to be most idle.   It is reported by Plato in
his dialogue *de Amore,* in that prodigious commendation of
Socrates, how a deep meditation coming into Socrates' mind
by chance, he stood still musing, *eodem vestigio cogitabundus,*
from morning to noon, and whenas then he had not yet finished
his meditation, *perstabat cogitans,* he so continued till the
evening; the soldiers (for he then followed the camp) observed
him with admiration, and on set purpose watched all night,
but he persevered immovable *ad exortum solis,* till the sun
rose in the morning, and then, saluting the sun, went his ways.
In what humour constant Socrates did thus, I know not, or
how he might be affected, but this would be pernicious to
another man; what intricate business might so really possess
him, I cannot easily guess.   But this is *otiosum otium* [a vacant
idleness], it is far otherwise with these men, according to
Seneca, *Omnia nobis mala solitudo persuadet* [solitude leads us
into all sorts of evil]; this solitude undoeth us, *pugnat cum
vita sociali* [it is the foe of the social life]; 'tis a destructive
solitariness.   These men are devils alone, as the saying is, *Homo
solus aut deus, aut dæmon :* a man alone is either a saint or a
devil; *mens ejus aut languescit, aut tumescit* [he becomes either
slow-witted or conceited]; and *Væ soli*[2] in this sense, woe
be to him that is so alone.   These wretches do frequently

degenerate from men, and of sociable creatures become beasts, monsters, inhuman, ugly to behold, *misanthropi*; they do even loathe themselves, and hate the company of men, as so many Timons, Nebuchadnezzars, by too much indulging to these pleasing humours, and through their own default. So that which Mercurialis, *consil.* 11, sometime expostulated with his melancholy patient, may be justly applied to every solitary and idle person in particular. *Natura de te videtur conqueri posse,* etc.[1] "Nature may justly complain of thee, that whereas she gave thee a good wholesome temperature, a sound body, and God hath given thee so divine and excellent a soul, so many good parts and profitable gifts, thou hast not only contemned and rejected, but hast corrupted them, polluted them, overthrown their temperature, and perverted those gifts with riot, idleness, solitariness, and many other ways; thou art a traitor to God and nature, an enemy to thyself and to the world. *Perditio tua ex te:* thou hast lost thyself wilfully, cast away thyself, thou thyself art the efficient cause of thine own misery, by not resisting such vain cogitations, but giving way unto them."

Subsect. VII.—*Sleeping and Waking, Causes*

What I have formerly said of exercise, I may now repeat of sleep. Nothing better than moderate sleep, nothing worse than it, if it be in extremes or unseasonably used. It is a received opinion, that a melancholy man cannot sleep overmuch; *somnus supra modum prodest* [extra sleep is beneficial], as an only antidote, and nothing offends them more, or causeth this malady sooner, than waking; yet in some cases sleep may do more harm than good, in that phlegmatic, swinish, cold, and sluggish melancholy which Melancthon speaks of, that thinks of waters, sighing most part, etc. It dulls the spirits, if overmuch, and senses;[2] fills the head full of gross humours; causeth distillations, rheums, great store of excrements in the brain, and all the other parts, as Fuchsius speaks of them,[3] that sleep like so many dormice. Or if it be used in the daytime, upon a full stomach, the body ill-composed to rest, or after hard meats, it increaseth fearful dreams, *incubus*, night-walking, crying out, and much unquietness; "such sleep prepares the body," as one observes,[4] "to many perilous diseases." But, as I have said, waking overmuch is both a symptom and an ordinary cause. "It causeth dryness of the brain, frenzy, dotage, and makes the body dry, lean, hard, and ugly to behold," as Lemnius hath it;[1] "the temperature of the brain is corrupted by it, the humours adust, the eyes made to sink into the head, choler increased, and the whole body inflamed": and, as may be added out of Galen, 3 *de sanitate tuenda,* Avicenna, 3, 1, "it overthrows the natural heat, it causeth crudities, hurts concoction," [2] and what not? Not without good cause therefore Crato, *consil.* 21, *lib.* 2, Hildesheim, *Spicil.* 2, *de delir. et mania,* Jacchinus, Arculanus on Rhasis, Guianerius, and Mercurialis reckon up this overmuch waking as a principal cause.

MEMB. III

Subsect. I.—*Passions and Perturbations of the Mind, how they cause Melancholy*

As that gymnosophist in Plutarch [3] made answer to Alexander (demanding which spake best), Every one of his fellows did speak better than the other: so may I say of these causes to him that shall require which is the greatest, every one is more grievous than other, and this of passion the greatest of all. A most frequent and ordinary cause of melancholy, *fulmen pertur-bationum* (Piccolomineus calls it [4]), this thunder and lightning of perturbation, which causeth such violent and speedy altera-tions in this our microcosm, and many times subverts the good estate and temperature of it. For as the body works upon the mind by his bad humours, troubling the spirits, sending gross fumes into the brain, and so *per consequens* [consequently] disturbing the soul, and all the faculties of it,

Corpus onustum
Hesternis vitiis animum quoque prægravat una,[5]

[By yesterday's excesses still oppressed,
The body suffers not the mind to rest,]

with fear, sorrow, etc., which are ordinary symptoms of this disease: so, on the other side, the mind most effectually works upon the body, producing by his passions and perturbations miraculous alterations, as melancholy, despair, cruel diseases, and sometimes death itself; insomuch that it is most true which Plato saith in his *Charmides, omnia corporis mala ab anima procedere,* all the mischiefs of the body proceed from the soul: [6] and Democritus in Plutarch urgeth,[7] *Damnatam iri animam a corpore,* if the body should in this behalf bring an action against the soul, surely the soul would be cast and convicted, that by her supine negligence had caused such inconveniences, having authority over the body, and using it for an instrument as a smith doth his hammer (saith Cyprian[1]), imputing all those vices and maladies to the mind. Even so doth Philostratus, *Non coinquinatur corpus, nisi consensu animæ:*[2] the body is not corrupted but by the soul. Lodovicus Vives will have such turbulent commotions proceed from ignorance and indiscretion.[3] All philosophers impute the miseries of the body to the soul, that should have governed it better, by command of reason, and hath not done it. The Stoics are altogether of opinion (as Lipsius[4] and Piccolomineus[5] record), that a wise man should be ἀπαθής, without all manner of passions and perturbations whatsoever, as Seneca reports of Cato,[6] the Greeks of Socrates,[7] and Jo. Aubanus of a nation in Africa,[8] so free from passion, or rather so stupid, that if they be wounded with a sword, they will only look back. Lactantius, 2 *Instit.*, will exclude fear from a wise man;[9] others except all, some the greatest passions. But let them dispute how they will, set down *in thesi* [in a thesis], give precepts to the contrary; we find that of Lemnius true by common experience: "No mortal man is free from these perturbations: or if he be so, sure he is either a god or a block."[10] They are born and bred with us, we have them from our parents by inheritance, *A parentibus habemus malum hunc assem,* saith Pelezius,[11] *nascitur una nobiscum, aliturque* [it is born and grows with us], 'tis propagated from Adam; Cain was melancholy, as Austin[12] hath it, and who is not? Good discipline, education, philosophy, divinity (I cannot deny), may mitigate and restrain these passions in some few men at some times, but most part they domineer, and are so violent, that as a torrent (*torrens velut aggere rupto*) bears down all before, and overflows his banks, *sternit agros, sternit sata* [lays waste the fields, prostrates the crops], they overwhelm reason, judgment, and pervert the temperature of the body;[13] *Fertur equis auriga, nec audit currus habenas*[14] [the driver is whirled along, the steeds obey not the rein]. Now such a man (saith Austin) "that is so led, in a wise man's eye is no better than he that stands upon his head."[15] It is doubted by some, *gravioresne morbi a perturbationibus, an ab humoribus,* whether humours or perturbations cause the more grievous maladies. But we find that of our Saviour (Matt. xxvi, 41) most true, "The spirit is willing, the flesh is weak," we cannot resist; and this of

Philo Judæus, "Perturbations often offend the body, and are
most frequent causes of melancholy, turning it out of the hinges
of his health." [1] Vives compares them to "winds upon the
sea, some only move as those great gales, but others turbulent
quite overturn the ship." [2] Those which are light, easy, and
more seldom, to our thinking do us little harm, and are therefore
contemned of us: yet if they be reiterated, "as the rain" (saith
Austin "doth a stone, so do these perturbations penetrate the
mind": [3] and (as one observes) "produce a habit of melancholy
at the last, which, having gotten the mastery in our souls, may
well be called diseases." [4]

How these passions produce this effect, Agrippa hath handled
at large, *Occult. Philos. lib.* 11, *cap.* 63; [5] Cardan, *lib.* 14 *Subtil.*;
Lemnius, *lib.* 1, *cap.* 12, *de occult. nat. mir., et lib.* 1, *cap.* 16; Suarez,
Met. disput. 18, *sect.* 1, *art.* 25; T. Bright, *cap.* 12 of his Melancholy Treatise; Wright the Jesuit, in his Book of the Passions of
the Mind, etc. Thus, in brief, to our imagination cometh, by
the outward sense of memory, some object to be known (residing
in the foremost part of the brain), which he, misconceiving or
amplifying, presently communicates to the heart, the seat of
all affections. The pure spirits forthwith flock from the brain
to the heart by certain secret channels, and signify what good
or bad object was presented; which immediately bends itself to
prosecute or avoid it, [6] and, withal, draweth with it other
humours to help it: so in pleasure, concur great store of purer
spirits; in sadness, much melancholy blood; in ire, choler. If
the imagination be very apprehensive, intent, and violent, it
sends great store of spirits to or from the heart, and makes a
deeper impression and greater tumult; as the humours in the
body be likewise prepared, and the temperature itself ill or well
disposed, the passions are longer and stronger; so that the first
step and fountain of all our grievances in this kind is *læsa
imaginatio* [7] [a disordered imagination], which, misinforming
the heart, causeth all these distemperatures, alteration and
confusion of spirits and humours; by means of which, so
disturbed, concoction is hindered, and the principal parts are
much debilitated; as Dr. Navarra well declared, being consulted
by Montanus about a melancholy Jew. [8] The spirits so confounded, the nourishment must needs be abated, bad humours
increased, crudities and thick spirits engendered, with melancholy
blood. The other parts cannot perform their functions, having
the spirits drawn from them by vehement passion, but fail in
sense and motion; so we look upon a thing, and see it not; hear,

and observe not; which otherwise would much affect us, had we been free. I may therefore conclude with Arnoldus,[1] *Maxima vis est phantasiæ, et huic uni fere, non autem corporis intemperiei, omnis melancholiæ causa est ascribenda*: great is the force of imagination, and much more ought the cause of melancholy to be ascribed to this alone, than to the distemperature of the body. Of which imagination, because it hath so great a stroke in producing this malady, and is so powerful of itself, it will not be improper to my discourse to make a brief digression, and speak of the force of it, and how it causeth this alteration. Which manner of digression howsoever some dislike, as frivolous and impertinent, yet I am of Beroaldus his opinion, "Such digressions do mightily delight and refresh a weary reader, they are like sauce to a bad stomach, and I do therefore most willingly use them." [2]

Subsect. II.—*Of the Force of Imagination*

What imagination is I have sufficiently declared in my digression of the anatomy of the soul. I will only now point at the wonderful effects and power of it; which, as it is eminent in all, so most especially it rageth in melancholy persons, in keeping the species of objects so long, mistaking, amplifying them by continual and strong meditation,[3] until at length it produceth in some parties real effects, causeth this and many other maladies. And although this phantasy of ours be a subordinate faculty to reason, and should be ruled by it, yet in many men, through inward or outward distemperature, defect of organs, which are unapt or hindered, or otherwise contaminated, it is likewise unapt, hindered, and hurt. This we see verified in sleepers, which by reason of humours and concourse of vapours troubling the phantasy, imagine many times absurd and prodigious things, and in such as are troubled with *incubus*, or witch-ridden (as we call it); if they lie on their backs, they suppose an old woman rides and sits so hard upon them that they are almost stifled for want of breath; when there is nothing offends but a concourse of bad humours, which trouble the phantasy. This is likewise evident in such as walk in the night in their sleep, and do strange feats: these vapours move the phantasy, the phantasy the appetite, which moving the animal spirits causeth the body to walk up and down as if they were awake.[4] Fracastorius, *lib. 3 de intellect.*, refers all ecstasies to this force of imagination, such as lie whole days together in a trance: as that priest whom Celsus speaks of, that could separate himself from his senses when he list, and lie like a dead man, void of life and sense.[1] Cardan brags of himself that he could do as much, and that when he list. Many times such men, when they come to themselves, tell strange things of heaven and hell, what visions they have seen; as that St. Owen, in Matthew Paris, that went into St. Patrick's Purgatory, and the monk of Evesham in the same author. Those common apparitions in Bede and Gregory, St. Bridget's revelations, Wier., *lib. 3 de lamiis, cap.* 11, Cæsar Vaninus in his Dialogues, etc., reduceth (as I have formerly said), with all these tales of witches' progresses, dancing, riding, transformations, operations, etc., to the force of imagination,[2] and the devil's illusions.[3] The like effects almost are to be seen in such as are awake: how many chimeras, antics, golden mountains, and castles in the air do they build unto themselves! I appeal to painters, mechanicians, mathematicians. Some ascribe all vices to a false and corrupt imagination, anger, revenge, lust, ambition, covetousness, which prefers falsehood before that which is right and good, deluding the soul with false shows and suppositions. Bernardus Penottus [4] will have heresy and superstition to proceed from this fountain; as he falsely imagineth, so he believeth; and as he conceiveth of it, so it must be, and it shall be, *contra gentes* [against the world], he will have it so. But most especially in passions and affections it shows strange and evident effects: what will not a fearful man conceive in the dark? what strange forms of bugbears, devils, witches, goblins? Lavater imputes the greatest cause of spectrums, and the like apparitions, to fear, which above all other passions begets the strongest imagination (saith Wierus [5]), and so likewise love, sorrow, joy, etc. Some die suddenly, as she that saw her son come from the battle at Cannæ, etc. Jacob the patriarch, by force of imagination, made peckled lambs, laying peckled rods before his sheep. Persina, that Ethiopian queen in Heliodorus, by seeing the picture of Perseus and Andromeda, instead of a blackamoor, was brought to bed of a fair, white child. In imitation of whom, belike, an hard-favoured fellow in Greece, because he and his wife were both deformed, to get a good brood of children, *elegantissimas imagines in thalamo collocavit*, etc., hung the fairest pictures he could buy for money in his chamber, "that his wife, by frequent sight of them, might conceive and bear such children." And if we may believe Bale, one of Pope Nicholas the Third's concubines, by seeing of a bear, was brought to bed of a monster.[6] "If a

woman" (saith Lemnius), "at the time of her conception think of
another man present or absent, the child will be like him." [1]
Great-bellied women, when they long, yield prodigious examples
in this kind, as moles, warts, scars, harelips, monsters, especially
caused in their children by force of a depraved phantasy in them.
Ipsam speciem quam animo effigiat, fœtui inducit: she imprints
that stamp upon her child which she conceives unto herself.[2]
And therefore, Lodovicus Vives, *lib. 2 de Christ. fem.*, gives a
special caution to great-bellied women, "that they do not admit
such absurd conceits and cogitations, but by all means avoid
those horrible objects, heard or seen, or filthy spectacles." [3]
Some will laugh, weep, sigh, groan, blush, tremble, sweat, at
such things as are suggested unto them by their imagination.
Avicenna speaks of one that could cast himself into a palsy when
he list; and some can imitate the tunes of birds and beasts, that
they can hardly be discerned. Dagobertus' and St. Francis'
scars and wounds, like those of Christ's (if at the least any such
were), Agrippa supposeth to have happened by force of imagination: [4] that some are turned to wolves, from men to women,
and women again to men (which is constantly believed) to the
same imagination; or from men to asses, dogs, or any other
shapes. Wierus [5] ascribes all those famous transformations to
imagination; that in hydrophobia they seem to see the picture
of a dog still in their water, that melancholy men and sick men
conceive so many phantastical visions, apparitions to themselves,
and have such absurd suppositions, as that they are kings, lords,
cocks, bears, apes, owls; [6] that they are heavy, light, transparent, great and little, senseless and dead (as shall be showed
more at large in our section of symptoms [7]), can be imputed
to naught else but to a corrupt, false, and violent imagination.
It works not in sick and melancholy men only, but even most
forcibly sometimes in such as are sound: it makes them suddenly
sick, and alters their temperature in an instant.[8] And sometimes a strong conceit or apprehension, as Valesius proves, will
take away diseases: [9] in both kinds it will produce real effects.
Men, if they see but another man tremble, giddy, or sick of
some fearful disease, their apprehension and fear is so strong
in this kind that they will have the same disease. Or if by
some soothsayer, wise man, fortune-teller, or physician they be
told they shall have such a disease, they will so seriously apprehend it that they will instantly labour of it. A thing familiar
in China (saith Riccius the Jesuit): "If it be told them they
shall be sick on such a day, when that day comes they will

surely be sick, and will be so terribly afflicted that sometimes
they die upon it." [1]   Dr. Cotta, in his Discovery of Ignorant
Practitioners of Physic, *cap*. 8, hath two strange stories to this
purpose, what fancy is able to do: the one of a parson's wife
in Northamptonshire, *anno* 1607, that, coming to a physician,
and told by him that she was troubled with the sciatica, as he
conjectured (a disease she was free from), the same night after
her return, upon his words, fell into a grievous fit of a sciatica;
and such another example he hath of another goodwife, that was
so troubled with the cramp, after the same manner she came by
it, because her physician did but name it.   Sometimes death
itself is caused by force of phantasy.   I have heard of one that,
coming by chance in company of him that was thought to be
sick of the plague (which was not so), fell down suddenly dead.
Another was sick of the plague with conceit.   One, seeing his
fellow let blood, falls down in a swoon.   Another (saith Cardan
out of Aristotle) fell down dead (which is familiar to women at
any ghastly sight), seeing but a man hanged.[2]   A Jew in
France (saith Lodovicus Vives) came by chance over a dangerous passage or plank that lay over a brook, in the dark,
without harm, the next day, perceiving what danger he was in,
fell down dead.[3]   Many will not believe such stories to be true,
but laugh commonly, and deride when they hear of them; but
let these men consider with themselves, as Peter Byarus illustrates it,[4] if they were set to walk upon a plank on high, they
would be giddy, upon which they dare securely walk upon the
ground.   Many (saith Agrippa), "strong-hearted men otherwise,.
tremble at such sights, dazzle, and are sick, if they look but down
from a high place, and what moves them but conceit?" [5]   As
some are so molested by phantasy; so some again, by fancy alone,
and a good conceit, are as easily recovered.   We see commonly
the toothache, gout, falling sickness, biting of a mad dog, and
many such maladies cured by spells, words, characters, and
charms, and many green wounds by that now so much used
unguentum armarium [weapon-salve] magnetically cured, which
Crollius and Goclenius in a book of late hath defended, Libavius in
a just tract as stiffly contradicts, and most men controvert.   All
the world knows there is no virtue in such charms or cures, but a
strong conceit and opinion alone, as Pomponatius holds, "which
forceth a motion of the humours, spirits, and blood, which
takes away the cause of the malady from the parts affected." [6]
The like we may say of our magical effects, superstitious cures,
and such as are done by mountebanks and wizards.   "As by

wicked incredulity many men are hurt" (so saith Wierus of
charms, spells, etc.), "we find in our experience, by the same
means many are relieved." [1]   An empiric oftentimes, and a
silly chirurgeon, doth more strange cures than a rational physician. Nymannus gives a reason, because the patient puts his
confidence in him, which Avicenna prefers before art, precepts, and all remedies whatsoever.[2] 'Tis opinion alone (saith
Cardan) that makes or mars physicians,[3] and he doth the best
cures, according to Hippocrates, in whom most trust. So
diversely doth this phantasy of ours affect, turn, and wind, so
imperiously command our bodies, which "as another Proteus, or
a chameleon, can take all shapes; and is of such force" (as Ficinus
adds), "that it can work upon others as well as ourselves." [4]
How can otherwise blear eyes in one man cause the like affection
in another? Why doth one man's yawning make another
yawn? [5] one man's pissing provoke a second many times to do
the like? Why doth scraping of trenchers offend a third, or
hacking of files? Why doth a carcass bleed when the murderer
is brought before it, some weeks after the murder hath been
done? Why do witches and old women fascinate and bewitch
children? but as Wierus, Paracelsus, Cardan, Mizaldus, Valleriola, Cæsar Vaninus, Campanella, and many philosophers
think, the forcible imagination of the one party moves and alters
the spirits of the other. Nay more, they can cause and cure
not only diseases, maladies, and several infirmities by this
means, as Avicenna, *de anim. lib. 4, sect.* 4, supposeth, in parties
remote, but move bodies from their places, cause thunder,
lightning, tempests, which opinion Alkindus, Paracelsus, and
some others approve of. So that I may certainly conclude this
strong conceit or imagination is *astrum hominis* [a man's
guiding star], and the rudder of this our ship, which reason
should steer, but, overborne by phantasy, cannot manage, and so
suffers itself and this whole vessel of ours to be overruled, and
often overturned. Read more of this in Wierus, *lib.* 3 *de lamiis,
cap.* 8, 9, 10; Franciscus Valesius, *Med. controv, lib.* 5, *cont.* 6;
Marcellus Donatus, *lib.* 2, *cap.* 1, *de hist. med. mirabil.*; Levinus
Lemnius, *de occult. nat. mir. lib.* 1, *cap.* 12; Cardan, *lib.* 18 *de
rerum var.*; Corn. Agrippa, *de occult. philos. cap.* 64, 65; Camerarius, *cent.* 1, *cap.* 54, *Horarum subcis.*; Nymannus, *in orat. de
Imag.*; Laurentius; and him that is *instar omnium* [the pick of
the bunch], Fienus, a famous physician of Antwerp, that wrote
three books *de viribus imaginationis* [on the force of imagina-
tion]. I have thus far digressed, because this imagination is

the *medium deferens* [instrument] of passions, by whose means they work and produce many times prodigious effects: and as the phantasy is more or less intended or remitted, and their humours disposed, so do perturbations move, more or less, and take deeper impression.

Subsect. III.—*Division of Perturbations*

Perturbations and passions which trouble the phantasy, though they dwell between the confines of sense and reason, yet they rather follow sense than reason, because they are drowned in corporeal organs of sense. They are commonly reduced into two inclinations, irascible and concupiscible.[1] The Thomists subdivide them into eleven, six in the coveting, and five in the invading. Aristotle reduceth all to pleasure and pain, Plato to love and hatred, Vives[2] to good and bad. If good, it is present, and then we absolutely joy and love; or to come, and then we desire and hope for it. If evil, we absolutely hate it; if present, it is sorrow; if to come, fear. These four passions Bernard compares to the wheels of a chariot, by which we are carried in this world.[3] All other passions are subordinate unto these four, or six, as some will: love, joy, desire, hatred, sorrow, fear; the rest, as anger, envy, emulation, pride, jealousy, anxiety, mercy, shame, discontent, despair, ambition, avarice, etc., are reducible unto the first; and if they be immoderate, they consume the spirits, and melancholy is especially caused by them.[4] Some few discreet men there are, that can govern themselves, and curb in these inordinate affections, by religion, philosophy, and such divine precepts, of meekness, patience, and the like; but most part, for want of government, out of indiscretion, ignorance, they suffer themselves wholly to be led by sense, and are so far from repressing rebellious inclinations, that they give all encouragement unto them, leaving the reins, and using all provocations to further them: bad by nature, worse by art, discipline, custom, education, and a perverse will of their own, they follow on, wheresoever their unbridled affections will transport them, and do more out of custom, self-will, than out of reason.[5] *Contumax voluntas*, as Melancthon calls it, *malum facit:* this stubborn will of ours perverts judgment, which sees and knows what should and ought to be done, and yet will not do it. *Mancipia gulæ*, slaves to their several lusts and appetite, they precipitate and plunge themselves into a labyrinth of cares, blinded with lust, blinded with ambition;[1] "They seek that at God's hands which they may give unto themselves, if they could but refrain from those cares and perturbations wherewith they continually macerate their minds."[2] But giving way to these violent passions of fear, grief, shame, revenge, hatred, malice, etc., they are torn in pieces, as Actæon was with his dogs, and crucify their own souls.[3]

SUBSECT. IV.—*Sorrow a Cause of Melancholy*

In this catalogue of passions which so much torment the soul of man and cause this malady (for I will briefly speak of them all, and in their order), the first place in this irascible appetite may justly be challenged by sorrow; an inseparable companion, "the mother and daughter of melancholy, her epitome, symptom, and chief cause"; as Hippocrates hath it, they beget one another, and tread in a ring, for sorrow is both cause and symptom of this disease.[4] How it is a symptom shall be showed in his place. That it is a cause all the world acknowledgeth; *Dolor nonnullis insaniæ causa fuit, et aliorum morborum insanabilium*, saith Plutarch to Apollonius; a cause of madness, a cause of many other diseases, a sole cause of this mischief, Lemnius calls it.[5] So doth Rhasis, *Cont. lib.* 1, *tract.* 9; Guianerius, *tract.* 15, *cap.* 5. And if it take root once, it ends in despair, as Felix Plater observes,[6] and as in Cebes' Table,[7] may well be coupled with it. Chrysostom, in his seventeenth epistle to Olympia, describes it to be "a cruel torture of the soul, a most inexplicable grief, poisoned worm, consuming body and soul and gnawing the very heart, a perpetual executioner, continual night, profound darkness, a whirlwind, a tempest, an ague not appearing, heating worse than any fire, and a battle that hath no end. It crucifies worse than any tyrant; no torture, no strappado, no bodily punishment is like unto it."[8] 'Tis the eagle without question which the poets feigned to gnaw Prometheus' heart,[9] and "no heaviness is like unto the heaviness of the heart" (Ecclus. xxxviii, 18). "Every perturbation is a misery, but grief a cruel torment,"[10] a domineering passion: as in old Rome, when the Dictator was created, all inferior magistracies ceased; when grief appears, all other passions vanish. "It dries up the bones," saith Solomon (Prov. xvii), makes them hollow-eyed, pale, and lean, furrow-faced, to have dead looks, wrinkled brows, rivelled cheeks, dry bodies,

and quite perverts their temperature that are misaffected with
it. As Elenora, that exiled mournful duchess (in our English
Ovid [1]), laments to her noble husband, Humphrey, Duke of
Gloucester:

> Sawest thou those eyes in whose sweet cheerful look
> Duke Humphry once such joy and pleasure took,
> Sorrow hath so despoil'd me of all grace,
> Thou couldst not say, This was my El'nor's face.
> Like a foul Gorgon, etc.

It hinders concoction, refrigerates the heart, takes away
stomach, colour, and sleep; [2] thickens the blood (Fernelius,
lib. 1, cap. 18, de morb. causis); [3] contaminates the spirits"
(Piso); [4] overthrows the natural heat, perverts the good estate of
body and mind, and makes them weary of their lives, cry out,
howl and roar for the very anguish of their souls.   David confessed as much, Psalm xxxviii, 8: "I have roared for the very
disquietness of my heart."   And Psalm cxix, part 4, v. 4: "My
soul melteth away for very heaviness"; v. 38: "I am like a
bottle in the smoke."   Antiochus complained that he could
not sleep, and that his heart fainted for grief; Christ Himself,
vir dolorum [a man of sorrows], out of an apprehension of
grief, did sweat blood; [5] Mark xiv: "His soul was heavy to the
death, and no sorrow was like unto his."   Crato, *consil. 21, lib. 2,*
gives instance in one that was so melancholy by reason of grief; [6]
and Montanus, *consil.* 30, in a noble matron, "that had no other
cause of this mischief." [7]   I. S. D., in Hildesheim, fully cured
a patient of his that was much troubled with melancholy, and
for many years, "but afterwards, by a little occasion of sorrow,
he fell into his former fits, and was tormented as before." [8]
Examples are common, how it causeth melancholy, desperation,
and sometimes death itself; [9] for (Ecclus. xxxviii, 18) "Of
heaviness comes death."   "Worldly sorrow causeth death" (2 Cor.
vii, 10); Psalm xxxi, 10: "My life is wasted with heaviness, and
my years with mourning."   Why was Hecuba said to be turned
to a dog?   Niobe into a stone? but that for grief she was
senseless and stupid.   Severus the emperor died for grief; [10]
and how many myriads besides! [11]   *Tanta illi est feritas, tanta
est insania luctus* [such wildness, such madness, is there in
grief].   Melancthon gives a reason of it, "the gathering of much
melancholy blood about the heart, which collection extinguisheth
the good spirits, or at least dulleth them; sorrow strikes the
heart, makes it tremble and pine away, with great pain; and
the black blood drawn from the spleen, and diffused under the

ribs on the left side, makes those perilous hypochondriacal convulsions which happen to them that are troubled with sorrow." [1]

Subsect. V.—*Fear a Cause*

Cousin-german to sorrow is fear, or rather a sister, *fidus Achates* [trusty squire], and continual companion, an assistant and a principal agent in procuring of this mischief; a cause and symptom as the other. In a word, as Virgil of the Harpies,[2] I may justly say of them both:

> *Tristius haud illis monstrum, nec sævior ulla*
> *Pestis et ira deum Stygiis sese extulit undis.*

A sadder monster, or more cruel plague so fell,
Or vengeance of the gods, ne'er came from Styx or hell.

This foul fiend of fear was worshipped heretofore as a god by the Lacedæmonians, and most of those other torturing affections,[3] and so was sorrow amongst the rest, under the name of Angerona Dea; they stood in such awe of them, as Austin, *de Civitat. Dei, lib.* 4, *cap.* 8, noteth out of Varro. Fear was commonly adored and painted in their temples with a lion's head;[4] and as Macrobius records, 1, 10 *Saturnalium*: "In the calends of January, Angerona had her holy day, to whom in the temple of Volupia, or goddess of pleasure, their augurs and bishops did yearly sacrifice; that, being propitious to them, she might expel all cares, anguish, and vexation of the mind for the year following." [5] Many lamentable effects this fear causeth in men, as to be red, pale, tremble, sweat; it makes sudden cold and heat to come over all the body, palpitation of the heart, syncope, etc.[6] It amazeth many men that are to speak or show themselves in public assemblies, or before some great personages; as Tully confessed of himself, that he trembled still at the beginning of his speech; and Demosthenes, that great orator of Greece, before Philippus. It confounds voice and memory, as Lucian wittily brings in Jupiter Tragœdus [7] so much afraid of his auditory, when he was to make a speech to the rest of the gods, that he could not utter a ready word, but was compelled to use Mercury's help in prompting. Many men are so amazed and astonished with fear, they know not where they are, what they say, what they do,[8] and that which is worst, it tortures them many days before with continual affrights and suspicion. It hinders most honourable attempts, and makes

their hearts ache, sad and heavy. They that live in fear are
never free, resolute, secure, never merry, but in continual
pain:[1] that, as Vives truly said, *Nulla est miseria major quam
metus*, no greater misery, no rack, nor torture like unto it; ever
suspicious, anxious, solicitous, they are childishly drooping
without reason, without judgment, "especially if some terrible
object be offered," as Plutarch hath it.[2]   It causeth oftentimes sudden madness, and almost all manner of diseases, as
I have sufficiently illustrated in my digression of the Force of
Imagination,[3] and shall do more at large in my section of
Terrors.[4] Fear makes our imagination conceive what it list,
invites the devil to come to us, as Agrippa and Cardan [5] avouch,
and tyrannizeth over our phantasy more than all other affections,
especially in the dark.   We see this verified in most men, as
Lavater saith,[6] *Quæ metuunt, fingunt:* what they fear they
conceive, and feign unto themselves; they think they see
goblins, hags, devils, and many times become melancholy
thereby.   Cardan, *Subtil. lib.* 18, hath an example of such an
one, so caused to be melancholy (by sight of a bugbear) all his
life after.   Augustus Cæsar durst not sit in the dark; *Nisi aliquo
assidente*, saith Suetonius,[7] *nunquam tenebris evigilavit* [unless
someone was with him, he never sat up in the dark].   And 'tis
strange what women and children will conceive unto themselves,
if they go over a churchyard in the night, lie or be alone in a
dark room, how they sweat and tremble on a sudden.   Many
men are troubled with future events, foreknowledge of their
fortunes, destinies, as Severus the Emperor, Hadrian, and Domitian, *quod sciret ultimum vitæ diem*, saith Suetonius, *valde
sollicitus*, much tortured in mind because he foreknew his end;
with many such, of which I shall speak more opportunely in
another place.[8] Anxiety, mercy, pity, indignation, etc., and
such fearful branches derived from these two stems of fear and
sorrow, I voluntarily omit; read more of them in Carolus
Pascalius,[9] Dandinus,[10] etc.

SUBSECT. VI.—*Shame and Disgrace, Causes*

Shame and disgrace cause most violent passions and bitter
pangs. *Ob pudorem et dedecus publicum, ob errorem commissum,
sæpe moventur generosi animi* (Felix Plater, *lib. 3 de alienat.
mentis*): generous minds are often moved with shame to despair
for some public disgrace.   And "he," saith Philo, *lib. 2 de provid.
Dei*, "that subjects himself to fear, grief, ambition, shame, is

not happy, but altogether miserable, tortured with continual
labour, care, and misery." [1] It is as forcible a batterer as any
of the rest. "Many men neglect the tumults of the world, and
care not for glory,[2] and yet they are afraid of infamy, repulse,
disgrace (Tully, *Offic. lib.* 1); they can severely contemn pleasure,
bear grief indifferently, but they are quite battered and broken
with reproach and obloquy" [3] (*siquidem vita et fama pari passu
ambulant* [seeing that life goes hand in hand with repute]),
and are so dejected many times for some public injury, disgrace,
as a box on the ear by their inferior, to be overcome of their
adversary, foiled in the field, to be out in a speech, some
foul fact committed or disclosed, etc., that they dare not
come abroad all their lives after, but melancholize in corners,
and keep in holes.   The most generous spirits are most subject
to it; *Spiritus altos frangit et generosos* [it breaks noble and lofty
spirits] (Hieronymus).   Aristotle, because he could not understand the motion of Euripus, for grief and shame drowned
himself (Cælius Rhodiginus, *Antiquar. lec. lib.* 29, *cap.* 8). *Homerus
pudore consumptus,* [Homer] was swallowed up with this passion of
shame "because he could not unfold the fisherman's riddle." [4]
Sophocles killed himself, "for that a tragedy of his was hissed
off the stage" [5] (Valer. Max., *lib.* 9, *cap.* 12).   Lucretia stabbed
herself, and so did Cleopatra, "when she saw that she was
reserved for a triumph, to avoid the infamy." [6] Antonius the
Roman, "after he was overcome of his enemy, for three days'
space sat solitary in the fore-part of the ship, abstaining from
all company, even of Cleopatra herself, and afterwards for very
shame butchered himself" [7] (Plutarch, *vita ejus*).   Apollonius
Rhodius "wilfully banished himself, forsaking his country, and
all his dear friends, because he was out in reciting his poems," [8]
(Plinius, *lib.* 7, *cap.* 23).   Ajax ran mad, because his arms were
adjudged to Ulysses.   In China 'tis an ordinary thing for such
as are excluded in those famous trials of theirs, or should take
degrees, for shame and grief to lose their wits (Mat. Riccius,
Expedit. ad Sinas, lib. 3, *cap.* 9).[9] Hostratus the friar took that book
which Reuchlin had writ against him, under the name of *Epist.
obscurorum virorum,* so to heart, that for shame and grief he
made away himself (Jovius, *in Elogiis*).[10] A grave and learned
minister, and an ordinary preacher at Alkmaar in Holland, was
(one day as he walked in the fields for his recreation) suddenly
taken with a lask or looseness, and thereupon compelled to retire
to the next ditch; but being surprised at unawares by some
gentlewomen of his parish wandering that way, was so abashed,

that he did never after show his head in public, or come into the
pulpit, but pined away with melancholy [1] (Pet. Forestus, *Med.
observat. lib.* 10, *observat.* 12).   So shame amongst other passions
can play his prize.

I know there be many base, impudent, brazen-faced rogues,
that will *nulla pallescere culpa* [2] [feel shame for no crime], be
moved with nothing, take no infamy or disgrace to heart, laugh
at all; let them be proved perjured, stigmatized, convict rogues,
thieves, traitors, lose their ears, be whipped, branded, carted,
pointed at, hissed, reviled, and derided with Ballio the bawd
in Plautus, [3] they rejoice at it: *Cantores probos!* [bravo!],
babæ! [whe-ew!] and *bombax!* [well, I never!], what care
they?   We have too many such in our times:

> *Exclamat Melicerta perisse
> Frontem de rebus.* [4]

[Men, cries Melicerta, have lost the power to blush.]

Yet a modest man, one that hath grace, a generous spirit, tender
of his reputation, will be deeply wounded, and so grievously
affected with it, that he had rather give myriads of crowns,
lose his life, than suffer the least defamation of honour or blot
in his good name.   And if so be that he cannot avoid it,
as a nightingale, *quæ cantando victa moritur* (saith Mizaldus [5]),
[which] dies for shame if another bird sing better, he languisheth
and pineth away in the anguish of his spirit.

Subsect. VII.—*Envy, Malice, Hatred, Causes*

Envy and malice are two links of this chain, and both, as
Guianerius, *tract.* 15, *cap.* 2, proves out of Galen, 3 *Aphorism.
com.* 22, "cause this malady by themselves, especially if their
bodies be otherwise disposed to melancholy." [6]   'Tis Valescus
de Taranta and Felix Plateus' observation, "Envy so gnaws
many men's hearts, that they become altogether melancholy." [7]
And therefore belike Solomon (Prov. xiv, 13) calls it "the rotting
of the bones"; Cyprian, *vulnus occultum* [a hidden wound]:

> *Siculi non invenere tyranni
> Majus tormentum,* [8]

the Sicilian tyrants never invented the like torment.   It
crucifies their souls, withers their bodies, makes them hollow-
eyed, pale, lean, and ghastly to behold [9] (Cyprian, *ser.* 2, *de zelo
et livore*).   "As a moth gnaws a garment, so," saith Chrysostom,

"doth envy consume a man"; [1] to be a living anatomy, a skeleton, to be "a lean and pale carcass,[2] quickened with a fiend"[3] (Hall, in Characters); for so often as an envious wretch sees another man prosper, to be enriched, to thrive, and be fortunate in the world, to get honours, offices, or the like, he repines and grieves.

Intabescitque videndo
Successus hominum . . . suppliciumque suum est.[4]

[When he beholds another doing well,
He wastes away, he suffers tortures fell.]

He tortures himself if his equal, friend, neighbour, be preferred, commended, do well; if he understand of it, it galls him afresh; and no greater pain can come to him than to hear of another man's well-doing; 'tis a dagger at his heart, every such object. He looks at him, as they that fell down in Lucian's rock of honour, with an envious eye, and will damage himself to do another a mischief: *Atque cadet subito, dum super hoste cadat* [ready to fall at once, so on a foe he fall]. As he did in Æsop, lose one eye willingly, that his fellow might lose both, or that rich man in Quintilian [5] that poisoned the flowers in his garden, because his neighbour's bees should get no more honey from them. His whole life is sorrow, and every word he speaks a satire: nothing fats him but other men's ruins. For to speak in a word, envy is naught else but *tristitia de bonis alienis*, sorrow for other men's good, be it present, past, or to come, *et gaudium de adversis,* and joy at their harms,[6] opposite to mercy, which grieves at other men's mischances, and misaffects the body in another kind;[7] so Damascene defines it, *lib. 2 de orthod. fid.*; Thomas, 2, 2, *quæst.* 36, *art.* 1; Aristotle, *lib. 2 Rhet. cap.* 4 *et* 10; Plato, *Philebo*; Tully, 3 *Tusc.*; Greg. Nic., *lib. de virt. animæ, cap.* 12; Basil *de Invidia*; Pindarus, *Od.* 1, *ser.* 5; and we find it true. 'Tis a common disease, and almost natural to us, as Tacitus holds,[8] to envy another man's prosperity. And 'tis in most men an incurable disease. "I have read," saith Marcus Aurelius, "Greek, Hebrew, Chaldee authors, I have consulted with many wise men for a remedy for envy; I could find none, but to renounce all happiness, and to be a wretch and miserable for ever."[9] 'Tis the beginning of hell in this life, and a passion not to be excused. "Every other sin hath some pleasure annexed to it, or will admit of an excuse; envy alone wants both. Other sins last but for a while; the gut may be satisfied, anger remits, hatred hath an end, envy never ceaseth"[10] (Cardan, *lib. 2 de sap.*). Divine and human examples are very familiar;

you may run and read them, as that of Saul and David, Cain
and Abel, *Angebat illum non proprium peccatum, sed fratris
prosperitas*, saith Theodoret, it was his brother's good fortune
galled him. Rachel envied her sister, being barren (Gen.
xxx); Joseph's brethren him (Gen. xxxvii); David had a touch of this
vice, as he confesseth[1] (Ps. lxxiii); Jeremy[2] and Habbakuk,[3]
they repined at others' good, but in the end they corrected themselves. Ps. lxxv: "Fret not thyself," etc. Domitian spited
Agricola for his worth, "that a private man should be so much
glorified."[4] Cæcina was envied of his fellow-citizens, because he
was more richly adorned.[5] But of all others, women are most
weak,[6] *Ob pulchritudinem invidæ sunt feminæ* [women are jealous
of other women's beauty] (Musæus); *Aut amat, aut odit, nihil
est tertium* (Granatensis): they love or hate, no medium amongst
them. *Implacabiles plerumque læsæ mulieres* [women as a rule
never forgive an injury]. Agrippina-like, "A woman, if she see
her neighbour more neat or elegant, richer in tires, jewels, or
apparel, is enraged, and like a lioness sets upon her husband,
rails at her, scoffs at her, and cannot abide her";[7] so the
Roman ladies in Tacitus did at Salonina, Cæcina's wife, "because
she had a better horse, and better furniture, as if she had hurt
them with it; they were much offended."[8] In like sort our
gentlewomen do at their usual meetings, one repines or scoffs
at another's bravery and happiness. Myrsine, an Attic wench,
was murdered of her fellows, "because she did excel the rest in
beauty"[9] (Constantine, *Agricult. lib.* ii, *cap.* 7). Every village
will yield such examples.

SUBSECT. VIII.—*Emulation, Hatred, Faction, Desire of Revenge, Causes*

Out of this root of envy spring those feral branches of faction,
hatred, livor, emulation,[10] which cause the like grievances, and
are *serræ animæ*, the saws of the soul, *consternationis pleni
affectus*,[11] affections full of desperate amazement; or as Cyprian
describes emulation, it is "a moth of the soul, a consumption,
to make another man's happiness his misery, to torture, crucify,
and execute himself, to eat his own heart. Meat and drink
can do such men no good, they do always grieve, sigh, and
groan, day and night without intermission, their breast is torn
asunder":[12] and a little after, "Whosoever he is whom thou
dost emulate and envy, he may avoid thee, but thou canst
neither avoid him nor thyself; wheresoever thou art, he is with

thee, thine enemy is ever in thy breast, thy destruction is
within thee, thou art a captive, bound hand and foot, as long
as thou art malicious and envious, and canst not be comforted.
It was the devil's overthrow";[1] and whensoever thou art
throughly affected with this passion, it will be thine. Yet no
perturbation so frequent, no passion so common.

Καὶ κεραμεὺς κεραμεῖ κοτέει, καὶ τέκτονι τέκτων,
Καὶ πτωχὸς πτωχῷ φθονέει, καὶ ἀοιδὸς ἀοιδῷ.[2]

A potter emulates a potter;
One smith envies another:
A beggar emulates a beggar;
A singing-man his brother.

Every society, corporation, and private family is full of it,
it takes hold almost of all sorts of men, from the prince to the
ploughman, even amongst gossips it is to be seen; scarce three
in a company but there is siding, faction, emulation betwixt
two of them, some *simultas*, jar, private grudge, heart-burning
in the midst of them.   Scarce two gentlemen dwell together in
the country (if they be not near kin or linked in marriage), but
there is emulation betwixt them and their servants, some
quarrel or some grudge betwixt their wives or children, friends
and followers, some contention about wealth, gentry, precedency,
etc., by means of which, like the frog in Æsop, "that would
swell till she was as big as an ox, burst herself at last,"[3]
they will stretch beyond their fortunes, callings, and strive so
long that they consume their substance in lawsuits, or otherwise in hospitality, feasting, fine clothes, to get a few bombast
titles, for *ambitiosa paupertate laboramus omnes* [though poor,
we all kill ourselves to make a show]; to outbrave one another,
they will tire their bodies, macerate their souls, and through
contentions or mutual invitations beggar themselves.   Scarce
two great scholars in an age, but with bitter invectives they
fall foul one on the other, and their adherents; Scotists, Thomists,
Reals, Nominals, Plato and Aristotle, Galenists and Paracelsians,
etc., it holds in all professions.

Honest emulation in studies, in all callings, is not to be disliked,[4] 'tis *ingeniorum cos*, as one calls it, the whetstone of wit,
the nurse of wit and valour, and those noble Romans out of this
spirit did brave exploits.   There is a modest ambition, as
Themistocles was roused up with the glory of Miltiades, Achilles'
trophies moved Alexander.

Ambire semper stulta confidentia est,
Ambire nunquam deses arrogantia est.[5]

[With all in all things constantly to vie
Shows foolish overweening confidence.
But for advancement never once to try
Shows slothful self-conceit and arrogance.]

'Tis a sluggish humour not to emulate or to sue at all, to with-draw himself, neglect, refrain from such places, honours, offices, through sloth, niggardliness, fear, bashfulness, or otherwise, to which by his birth, place, fortunes, education, he is called, apt, fit, and well able to undergo; but when it is immoderate, it is a plague and a miserable pain. What a deal of money did Henry VIII and Francis I, King of France, spend at that famous interview![1] and how many vain courtiers, seeking each to outbrave other, spent themselves, their livelihood and fortunes, and died beggars! Hadrian the emperor was so galled with it that he killed all his equals;[2] so did Nero. This passion made Dionysius the tyrant banish Plato and Philoxenus the poet, because they did excel and eclipse his glory, as he thought;[3] the Romans exile Coriolanus, confine Camillus, murder Scipio; the Greeks by ostracism to expel Aristides, Nicias, Alcibiades, imprison Theseus, make away Phocion, etc. When Richard I and Philip of France were fellow-soldiers together at the siege of Acre in the Holy Land, and Richard had approved himself to be the more valiant man, insomuch that all men's eyes were upon him, it so galled Philip (*Francum urebat regis victoria*, saith mine author,[4] *tam ægre ferebat Richardi gloriam, ut carpere dicta, calumniari facta*), that he cavilled at all his proceedings, and fell at length to open defiance; he could contain no longer, but hasting home, invaded his territories and professed open war. "Hatred stirs up contention" (Prov. x, 12), and they break out at last into immortal enmity, into virulency, and more than Vatinian hate[5] and rage; they persecute each other, their friends, followers, and all their posterity, with bitter taunts, hostile wars, scurrile invectives, libels, calumnies, fire, sword, and the like, and will not be reconciled.[6] Witness that Guelph and Ghibelline faction in Italy; that of the Adurni and Fregosi in Genoa; that of Cnæus Papirius and Quintus Fabius in Rome; Cæsar and Pompey; Orleans and Burgundy in France; York and Lancaster in England: yea, this passion so rageth many times, that it subverts not men only, and families, but even populous cities; Carthage[7] and Corinth can witness as much; nay, flourishing kingdoms are brought into a wilderness by it.[8] This hatred, malice, faction, and desire of revenge, invented first all those racks and wheels, strappadoes, brazen

bulls, feral engines, prisons, inquisitions, severe laws to macerate
and torment one another.   How happy, might we be, and end
our time with blessed days and sweet content, if we could contain ourselves, and, as we ought to do, put up injuries, learn
humility, meekness, patience, forget and forgive, as in God's
Word we are enjoined,[1] compose such small controversies amongst
ourselves, moderate our passions in this kind, "and think
better of others," as Paul would have us,[2] "than of ourselves:
be of like affection one towards another, and not avenge ourselves, but have peace with all men."   But being that we are
so peevish and perverse, insolent and proud, so factious and
seditious, so malicious and envious, we do *invicem angariare*
[by turns constrain], maul and vex one another, torture,
disquiet, and precipitate ourselves into that gulf of
woes and cares, aggravate our misery and melancholy, heap
upon us hell and eternal damnation.

Subsect. IX.—*Anger a Cause*

Anger, a perturbation, which carries the spirits outwards,
preparing the body to melancholy, and madness itself: *Ira
furor brevis est* [anger is temporary madness], and, as Piccolomineus accounts it,[3] one of the three most violent passions.
Aretæus sets it down for an especial cause (so doth Seneca,
ep. 18, lib. 1) of this malady.[4]   Magninus gives the reason, *Ex
frequenti ira supra modum calefiunt*,[5] it overheats their bodies,
and if it be too frequent, it breaks out into manifest madness,
saith St. Ambrose.   'Tis a known saying, *Furor fit læsa sæpius
patientia*, the most patient spirit that is, if he be often provoked, will be incensed to madness; it will make a devil of a
saint: and therefore Basil (belike) in his homily *de Ira*, calls it
tenebras rationis, morbum animæ, et dæmonem pessimum, the
darkening of our understanding, and a bad angel.   Lucian, *in
Abdicato, tom. 1*,[6] will have this passion to work this effect,
especially in old men and women.   "Anger and calumny"
(saith he) "trouble them at first, and after a while break out
into madness: many things cause fury in women, especially if
they love or hate overmuch, or envy, be much grieved or angry;
these things by little and little lead them on to this malady."
From a disposition they proceed to an habit, for there is no
difference between a madman and an angry man in the time
of his fit; anger, as Lactantius describes it, *lib. de Ira Dei, ad
Donatum, cap. 5*, is *sæva animi tempestas*, etc.,[7] a cruel tempest

of the mind, "making his eyes sparkle fire, and stare, teeth gnash in his head, his tongue stutter, his face pale or red, and what more filthy imitation can be of a madman?"

Ora tument ira, fervescunt sanguine venæ,
Lumina Gorgonio sævius angue micant.[1]

[Their faces swell, their blood boils up with ire,
Their eyes flash savagely with Gorgon fire.]

They are void of reason, inexorable, blind, like beasts and monsters for the time, say and do they know not what, curse, swear, rail, fight, and what not?   How can a madman do more? as he said in the comedy, *Iracundia non sum apud me*,[2] I am not mine own man [for anger]. If these fits be immoderate, continue long, or be frequent, without doubt they provoke madness. Montanus, *consil.* 21, had a melancholy Jew to his patient; he ascribes this for a principal cause: *Irascebatur levibus de causis*, he was easily moved to anger.   Ajax had no other beginning of his madness; and Charles the Sixth, that lunatic French king, fell into this misery, out of the extremity of his passion, desire of revenge and malice; incensed against the Duke of Britain,[3] he could neither eat, drink, nor sleep for some days together, and in the end, about the Calends of July, 1392, he became mad upon his horseback, drawing his sword, striking such as came near him promiscuously, and so continued all the days of his life (Æmilius, *lib.* 10 *Gal. hist.*).   Hegesippus, *de excid. urbis Hieros. lib.* 1, *cap.* 37, hath such a story of Herod, that out of an angry fit became mad; leaping out of his bed, he killed Josippus, and played many such bedlam pranks; the whole court could not rule him for a long time after:[4] sometimes he was sorry and repented, much grieved for that he had done, *postquam deferbuit ira* [when his rage had cooled down], by and by outrageous again.   In hot choleric bodies, nothing so soon causeth madness as this passion of anger, besides many other diseases, as Pelezius observes, *cap.* 21, *lib.* 1, *de hum. affect. causis*: *Sanguinem imminuit, fel auget* [it diminishes blood, it increases bile], and, as Valesius controverts, *Med. controv. lib.* 5, *contro.* 8,[5] many times kills them quite out.   If this were the worst of this passion, it were more tolerable, "but it ruins and subverts whole towns, cities,[6] families and kingdoms."[7] *Nulla pestis humano generi pluris stetit*, saith Seneca, *de Ira, lib.* 1, no plague hath done mankind so much harm.   Look into our histories, and you shall almost meet with no other subject but what a company of hare-brains have done in their rage.[8]

We may do well therefore to put this in our procession amongst the rest: "From all blindness of heart, from pride, vainglory, and hypocrisy, from envy, hatred, and malice, anger, and all such pestiferous perturbations, good Lord, deliver us."

SUBSECT. X.—*Discontents, Cares, Miseries, etc., Causes*

Discontents, cares, crosses, miseries, or whatsoever it is that shall cause any molestation of spirits, grief, anguish, and perplexity, may well be reduced to this head; preposterously placed here in some men's judgments they may seem, yet in that Aristotle in his Rhetoric [1] defines these cares, as he doth envy, emulation, etc., still by grief, I think I may well rank them in this irascible row; being that they are as the rest, both causes and symptoms of this disease, producing the like inconveniences, and are most part accompanied with anguish and pain. The common etymology will evince it, *cura quasi cor uro* [*cura* (care)=*cor uro* (I burn my heart)]; *dementes curæ, insomnes curæ, damnosæ curæ, tristes, mordaces, carnifices* etc., biting, eating, gnawing, cruel, bitter, sick, sad, unquiet, pale, tetric, miserable, intolerable cares, as the poets call them,[2] worldly cares, and are as many in number as the sea sands. Galen,[3] Fernelius, Felix Plater, Valescus de Taranta, etc., reckon afflictions, miseries, even all these contentions and vexations of the mind, as principal causes, in that they take away sleep, hinder concoction, dry up the body, and consume the substance of it. They are not so many in number, but their causes be as diverse, and not one of a thousand free from them, or that can vindicate himself, whom that *Ate dea*,

> *Per hominum capita molliter ambulans,*
> *Plantas pedum teneras habens :* [4]
>
> Over men's heads walking aloft,
> With tender feet treading so soft:

Homer's Goddess Ate, hath not involved into this discontented rank, or plagued with some misery or other.[5] Hyginus, *Fab. 220*, to this purpose hath a pleasant tale. Dame Cura [Care] by chance went over a brook, and taking up some of the dirty slime, made an image of it; Jupiter, eftsoons coming by, put life to it, but Cura and Jupiter could not agree what name to give him, or who should own him. The matter was referred to Saturn as judge; he gave this arbitrament: His name shall be *Homo* [Man], *ab humo* [from *humus* (earth)].

Cura eum possideat quamdiu vivat, Care shall have him whilst
he lives, Jupiter his soul, and Tellus [Earth] his body when he
dies. But to leave tales. A general cause, a continuate cause,
an inseparable accident to all men, is discontent, care, misery;
were there no other particular affliction (which who is free
from?) to molest a man in this life, the very cogitation of that
common misery were enough to macerate, and make him weary
of his life; to think that he can never be secure, but still in
danger, sorrow, grief, and persecution. For to begin at the
hour of his birth, as Pliny doth elegantly describe it,[1] "he is
born naked, and falls a-whining at the very first,[2] he is swaddled
and bound up like a prisoner, cannot help himself, and so he
continues to his life's end"; *cujusque feræ pabulum* [a prey
to every wild beast], saith Seneca,[3] impatient of heat and cold,
impatient of labour, impatient of idleness, exposed to fortune's
contumelies. To a naked mariner Lucretius compares him,
cast on shore by shipwreck, cold and comfortless in an unknown land. No estate, age, sex, can secure himself from this
common misery.[4] "A man that is born of a woman is of short
continuance, and full of trouble" (Job xiv, 1). "And while his
flesh is upon him he shall be sorrowful, and while his soul is in
him it shall mourn" (v. 22). "All his days are sorrow and his
travails griefs: his heart also taketh not rest in the night"
(Eccles. ii, 23); and (ii, 11), "All that is in it is sorrow and vexation of spirit." "Ingress, progress, regress, egress, much alike:
blindness seizeth on us in the beginning, labour in the middle,
grief in the end, error in all. What day ariseth to us without
some grief, care, or anguish? Or what so secure and pleasing
a morning have we seen, that hath not been overcast before
evening?"[5] One is miserable, another ridiculous, a third odious.
One complains of this grievance, another of that. *Aliquando
nervi, aliquando pedes vexant* (Seneca), *nunc distillatio, nunc
hepatis morbus; nunc deest, nunc superest sanguis* [sometimes his
sinews, sometimes his feet trouble him; now it is a catarrh,
now liver complaint; sometimes he has too much blood, sometimes too little]; now the head aches, then the feet, now the
lungs, then the liver, etc. *Huic census exuberat, sed est pudori
degener sanguis*, etc.; he is rich, but base-born; he is noble,
but poor; a third hath means, but he wants health peradventure,
or wit to manage his estate; children vex one, wife a second,
etc. *Nemo facile cum conditione sua concordat*, no man is
pleased with his fortune, a pound of sorrow is familiarly mixed
with a dram of content, little or no joy, little comfort, but

everywhere danger, contention, anxiety, in all places;[1] go where thou wilt, and thou shalt find discontents, cares, woes, complaints, sickness, diseases, encumbrances, exclamations. "If thou look into the market, there" (saith Chrysostom[2]) "is brawling and contention; if to the court, there knavery and flattery, etc.; if to a private man's house, there's cark and care, heaviness, etc." As he said of old, *Nil homine in terra spirat miserum magis alma:*[3] no creature so miserable as man, so generally molested, "in miseries of body, in miseries of mind, miseries of heart, in miseries asleep, in miseries awake, in miseries wheresoever he turns,"[4] as Bernard found. *Numquid tentatio est vita humana super terram?* A mere temptation is our life (Austin, *Confess., lib.* 10, *cap.* 28), *catena perpetuorum malorum* [a chain of perpetual ills]; *et quis potet molestias et difficultates pati?* who can endure the miseries of it? "In prosperity we are insolent and intolerable, dejected in adversity, in all fortunes foolish and miserable.[5] In adversity I wish for prosperity, and in prosperity I am afraid of adversity. What mediocrity may be found? Where is no temptation? What condition of life is free?"[6] "Wisdom hath labour annexed to it, glory envy; riches and cares, children and encumbrances, pleasure and diseases, rest and beggary, go together: as if a man were therefore born (as the Platonists hold) to be punished in this life for some precedent sins."[7] Or that, as Pliny complains, "Nature may be rather accounted a stepmother than a mother unto us, all things considered: no creature's life so brittle, so full of fear, so mad, so furious; only man is plagued with envy, discontent, griefs, covetousness, ambition, superstition."[8] Our whole life is an Irish Sea, wherein there is naught to be expected but tempestuous storms and troublesome waves, and those infinite:

Tantum malorum pelagus aspicio,
Ut non sit inde enatandi copia;[9]

[I behold a sea of ills so vast that to swim clear seems
   impossible;]

no halcyonian times, wherein a man can hold himself secure, or agree with his present estate; but, as Boethius infers, "There is something in every one of us which before trial we seek, and having tried abhor:[10] we earnestly wish, and eagerly covet, and are eftsoons weary of it."[11] Thus betwixt hope and fear, suspicions, angers, *Inter spemque metumque, timores inter et iras,*[12] betwixt falling in, falling out, etc., we bangle away our best days, befool out our times, we lead a contentious, discontent, tumultuous, melancholy, miserable life; insomuch, that if we could foretell what was to come, and it put to our choice, we should rather refuse than accept of this painful life. In a word, the world itself is a maze, a labyrinth of errors, a desert, a wilderness, a den of thieves, cheaters, etc., full of filthy puddles, horrid rocks, precipitiums, an ocean of adversity, an heavy yoke, wherein infirmities and calamities overtake and follow one another, as the sea-waves; and if we scape Scylla, we fall foul on Charybdis, and so in perpetual fear, labour, anguish, we run from one plague, one mischief, one burden to another, *duram servientes servitutem* [undergoing a hard bondage], and you may as soon separate weight from lead, heat from fire, moistness from water, brightness from the sun, as misery, discontent, care, calamity, danger, from a man. Our towns and cities are but so many dwellings of human misery, "in which grief and sorrow " (as he[1] right well observes out of Solon), "innumerable troubles, labours of mortal men, and all manner of vices are included, as in so many pens." Our villages are like mole-hills, and men as so many emmets, busy, busy still, going to and fro, in and out, and crossing one another's projects, as the lines of several sea-cards cut each other in a globe or map. "Now light and merry," but (as one follows it[2]) "by and by sorrowful and heavy; now hoping, then distrusting; now patient, to-morrow crying out; now pale, then red; running, sitting, sweating, trembling, halting," etc. Some few amongst the rest, or perhaps one of a thousand, may be *pullus Jovis* in the world's esteem, *gallinæ filius albæ*,[3] an happy and fortunate man, *ad invidiam felix* [prosperous enough to be envied], because rich, fair, well allied, in honour and office; yet peradventure ask himself, and he will say that of all others he is most miserable and unhappy.[4] A fair shoe, *Hic soccus novus, elegans*, as he said,[5] *sed nescis ubi urat*, but thou knowest not where it pincheth. It is not another man's opinion can make me happy but, as Seneca well hath it, "He is a miserable wretch that doth not account himself happy; though he be sovereign lord of a world, he is not happy if he think himself not to be so; for what availeth it what thine estate is, or seem to others, if thou thyself dislike it?"[6] A common humour it is of all men to think well of other men's fortunes, and dislike their own:

Cui placet alterius, sua nimirum est odio sors;[7]

[When he beholds another doing well,
He wastes away, he suffers tortures fell;]

but *Qui fit, Mæcenas,* etc.,[1] how comes it to pass, what's the cause of it? Many men are of such a perverse nature, they are well pleased with nothing (saith Theodoret[2]), "neither with riches nor poverty, they complain when they are well and when they are sick, grumble at all fortunes, prosperity and adversity; they are troubled in a cheap year, in a barren; plenty or not plenty, nothing pleaseth them, war nor peace, with children nor without." This for the most part is the humour of us all, to be discontent, miserable, and most unhappy, as we think at least; and show me him that is not so, or that ever was otherwise. Quintus Metellus his felicity is infinitely admired amongst the Romans, insomuch that, as Paterculus mentioneth of him, you can scarce find of any nation, order, age, sex, one for happiness to be compared unto him:[3] he had, in a word, *bona animi, corporis, et fortunæ,* goods of mind, body, and fortune; so had P. Mutianus Crassus.[4] Lampito, that Lacædemonian lady, was such another in Pliny's conceit, a king's wife, a king's mother, a king's daughter:[5] and all the world esteemed as much of Polycrates of Samos. The Greeks brag of their Socrates, Phocion, Aristides; the Psophidians in particular of their Aglaus, *omni vita felix, ab omni periculo immunis* [fortunate throughout life, escaping every danger] (which by the way Pausanias held impossible); the Romans of their Cato,[6] Curius, Fabricius, for their composed fortunes and retired estates, government of passions and contempt of the world: yet none of all these were happy, or free from discontent, neither Metellus, Crassus, nor Polycrates, for he died a violent death, and so did Cato; and how much evil doth Lactantius and Theodoret speak of Socrates, a weak man, and so of the rest. There is no content in this life, but as he[7] said, "All is vanity and vexation of spirit"; lame and imperfect. Hadst thou Sampson's hair, Milo's strength, Scanderbeg's arm, Solomon's wisdom, Absalom's beauty, Crœsus his wealth, *Pasetis obolum* [the obol of Pases], Cæsar's valour, Alexander's spirit, Tully's or Demosthenes' eloquence, Gyges' ring, Perseus' Pegasus and Gorgon's head, Nestor's years to come, all this would not make thee absolute, give thee content and true happiness in this life, or so continue it. Even in the midst of all our mirth, jollity, and laughter, is sorrow and grief, or if there be true happiness amongst us, 'tis but for a time:

Desinit in piscem mulier formosa superne,[8]

[A handsome maid above ends in a fish below.]

a fair morning turns to a lowering afternoon. Brutus and Cassius, once renowned, both eminently happy, yet you shall scarce find two (saith Paterculus) *quos fortuna maturius destituerit,* whom fortune sooner forsook. Hannibal, a conqueror all his life, met with his match, and was subdued at last. *Occurrit forti, qui mage fortis erit* [the strong at length meets one even stronger]. One is brought in triumph, as Cæsar into Rome, Alcibiades into Athens, *coronis aureis donatus,* crowned, honoured, admired; by and by his statues demolished, he hissed out, massacred, etc. Magnus Gonsalvo,[1] that famous Spaniard, was of the prince and people at first honoured, approved; forthwith confined and banished. *Admirandas actiones graves plerumque sequuntur invidiæ, et acres calumniæ:* 'tis Polybius his observation; grievous enmities and bitter calumnies commonly follow renowned actions. One is born rich, dies a beggar; sound to-day, sick to-morrow; now in most flourishing estate, fortunate and happy, by and by deprived of his goods by foreign enemies, robbed by thieves, spoiled, captivated, impoverished, as they of Rabbah, "put under iron saws, and under iron harrows, and under axes of iron, and cast into the tile-kiln." [2]

> *Quid me felicem toties jactastis, amici,*
> *Qui cecidit, stabili non erat ille gradu.* [3]

[My friends, why have you so often extolled me as happy? He that has fallen was never secure.]

He that erst marched like Xerxes with innumerable armies, as rich as Crœsus, now shifts for himself in a poor cock-boat, is bound in iron chains with Bajazet the Turk, and a footstool with Aurelian, for a tyrannizing conqueror to trample on. So many casualties there are, that, as Seneca said of a city consumed with fire, *Una dies interest inter maximam civitatem et nullam,* one day [lies] betwixt a great city and none: so many grievances from outward accidents, and from ourselves, our own indiscretion, inordinate appetite, one day betwixt a man and no man. And which is worse, as if discontents and miseries would not come fast enough upon us, *homo homini dæmon* [man is a devil to man]; we maul, persecute, and study how to sting, gall, and vex one another with mutual hatred, abuses, injuries; preying upon and devouring as so many ravenous birds;[4] and as jugglers, panders, bawds, cozening one another; or raging as wolves, tigers, and devils, we take a delight to torment one another;[5] men are evil, wicked, malicious, treacherous, and naught, not loving one another, or loving themselves, not hospitable, charitable, nor sociable as they ought to be, but counterfeit, dissemblers, ambidexters, all for their own ends, hard-hearted, merciless, pitiless, and, to benefit themselves, they care not what mischief they procure to others.[1] Praxinoe and Gorgo in the poet,[2] when they had got in to see those costly sights, they then cried *bene est* [we are all right], and would thrust out all the rest: when they are rich themselves, in honour, preferred, full, and have even that they would, they debar others of those pleasures which youth requires, and they formerly have enjoyed. He sits at table in a soft chair at ease, but he doth not remember in the meantime that a tired waiter stands behind him, "an hungry fellow ministers to him full; he is athirst that gives him drink" (saith Epictetus [3]), "and is silent whilst he speaks his pleasure; pensive, sad, when he laughs." *Pleno se proluit auro* [he drinks from a brimming golden goblet]; he feasts, revels, and profusely spends, hath variety of robes, sweet music, ease, and all the pleasure the world can afford, whilst many an hunger-starved poor creature pines in the street, wants clothes to cover him, labours hard all day long, runs, rides for a trifle, fights peradventure from sun to sun, sick and ill, weary, full of pain and grief, is in great distress and sorrow of heart. He loathes and scorns his inferior, hates or emulates his equal, envies his superior, insults over all such as are under him, as if he were of another species, a demi-god, not subject to any fall, or human infirmities. Generally they love not, are not beloved again: they tire out others' bodies with continual labour, they themselves living at ease, caring for none else, *sibi nati* [existing only for themselves]; and are so far many times from putting to their helping hand, that they seek all means to depress, even most worthy and well-deserving, better than themselves, those whom they are by the laws of nature bound to relieve and help as much as in them lies; they will let them caterwaul, starve, beg, and hang, before they will anyways (though it be in their power) assist or ease: so unnatural are they for the most part, so unregardful; so hard-hearted, so churlish, proud, insolent, so dogged, of so bad a disposition.[4] And being so brutish, so devilishly bent one towards another, how is it possible but that we should be discontent of all sides, full of cares, woes, and miseries?

If this be not a sufficient proof of their discontent and misery, examine every condition and calling apart. Kings, princes, monarchs, and magistrates seem to be most happy, but look into their estate, you shall find them to be most encumbered with cares, in perpetual fear, agony, suspicion, jealousy:[1] that, as he said of a crown, if they knew but the discontents that accompany it, they would not stoop to take it up.[2] *Quem mihi regem dabis* (saith Chrysostom) *non curis plenum?* What king canst thou show me, not full of cares? "Look not on his crown, but consider his afflictions; attend not his number of servants, but multitude of crosses."[3] *Nihil aliud potestas culminis, quam tempestas mentis*, as Gregory seconds him; sovereignty is a tempest of the soul: Sylla-like, they have brave titles, but terrible fits: *splendorem titulo, cruciatum animo;* which made Demosthenes vow,[4] *si vel ad tribunal, vel ad interitum duceretur*, if to be a judge, or to be condemned, were put to his choice, he would be condemned. Rich men are in the same predicament; what their pains are, *stulti nesciunt, ipsi sentiunt*, they feel, fools perceive not, as I shall prove elsewhere, and their wealth is brittle, like children's rattles: they come and go, there is no certainty in them: those whom they elevate, they do as suddenly depress, and leave in a vale of misery. The middle sort of men are as so many asses to bear burdens; or if they be free, and live at ease, they spend themselves, and consume their bodies and fortunes with luxury and riot, contention, emulation, etc. The poor I reserve for another place, and their discontents.[5]

For particular professions, I hold as of the rest, there's no content or security in any. On what course will you pitch, how resolve? To be a divine, 'tis contemptible in the world's esteem; to be a lawyer, 'tis to be a wrangler; to be a physician, *pudet lotii*,[6] 'tis loathed; a philosopher, a madman; an alchymist, a beggar; a poet, *esurit*, an hungry jack; a musician, a player; a schoolmaster, a drudge; an husbandman, an emmet; a merchant, his gains are uncertain; a mechanician, base; a chirurgeon, fulsome; a tradesman, a liar;[7] a tailor, a thief; a serving-man, a slave; a soldier, a butcher; a smith, or a metalman, the pot's never from 's nose; a courtier, a parasite; as he could find no tree in the wood to hang himself, I can show no state of life to give content. The like you may say of all ages; children live in a perpetual slavery, still under that tyrannical government of masters; young men, and of riper years, subject to labour and a thousand cares of the world, to treachery, falsehood, and cozenage:

> *Incedit per ignes,*
> *Suppositos cineri doloso;*[8]

> [You incautious tread
> On fires with faithless embers overspread;]

old are full of aches in their bones,[1] cramps and convulsions, *silicernia* [a funeral feast], dull of hearing, weak-sighted, hoary, wrinkled, harsh, so much altered as that they cannot know their own face in a glass, a burden to themselves and others; after seventy years, "all is sorrow" (as David hath it), they do not live, but linger. If they be sound, they fear diseases; if sick, weary of their lives: *Non est vivere, sed valere vita* [life is no life that is not lived in health]. One complains of want, a second of servitude, another of a secret or incurable disease; [2] of some deformity of body, of some loss, danger, death of friends, shipwreck, persecution, imprisonment, disgrace, repulse, contumely,[3] calumny, abuse, injury, contempt, ingratitude, unkindness, scoffs, flouts, unfortunate marriage, single life, too many children, no children, false servants, unhappy children, barrenness, banishment, oppression, frustrate hopes and ill success, etc.

> *Talia de genere hoc adeo sunt multa, loquacem ut*
> *Delassare valent Fabium:* [4]

talking Fabius will be tired before he can tell half of them; they are the subject of whole volumes, and shall (some of them) be more opportunely dilated elsewhere. In the meantime thus much I may say of them, that generally they crucify the soul of man, attenuate our bodies,[5] dry them, wither them, rivel them up like old apples, make them as so many anatomies (*Ossa atque pellis est totus, ita curis macet* [6] [he is nothing but skin and bone, he is so worn with care]), they cause *tempus fœdum et squalidum*, cumbersome days, *ingrataque tempora*, slow, dull, and heavy times: make us howl, roar, and tear our hairs, as Sorrow did in Cebes' Table,[7] and groan for the very anguish of our souls. Our hearts fail us as David's did (Ps. xl, 12), "for innumerable troubles that compassed him"; and we are ready to confess with Hezekiah (Is. xxxviii, 17), "Behold, for felicity I had bitter grief"; to weep with Heraclitus, to curse the day of our birth with Jeremy (xx, 14), and our stars with Job: to hold that axiom of Silenus, "Better never to have been born, and the best next of all, to die quickly": [8] or if we must live, to abandon the world, as Timon did; creep into caves and holes, as our anchorites; cast all into the sea, as Crates Thebanus; or as Cleombrotus Ambraciotes' four hundred auditors, precipitate ourselves to be rid of these miseries.

Subsect. XI.—*Concupiscible Appetite, as Desires, Ambition, Causes*

These concupiscible and irascible appetites are as the two twists of a rope, mutually mixed one with the other, and both twining about the heart: both good, as Austin holds, *lib.* 14, *cap.* 9, *de Civ. Dei*, "if they be moderate; both pernicious if they be exorbitant."[1] This concupiscible appetite, howsoever it may seem to carry with it a show of pleasure and delight, and our concupiscences most part affect us with content and a pleasing object, yet, if they be in extremes, they rack and wring us on the other side. A true saying it is, "Desire hath no rest," is infinite in itself, endless, and, as one[2] calls it, a perpetual rack, or horse-mill,[3] according to Austin, still going round as in a ring. They are not so continual as diverse; *Facilius atomos denumerare possem*, saith Bernard,[4] *quam motus cordis; nunc hæc, nunc illa cogito*, you may as well reckon up the motes in the sun as them. "It extends itself to everything," as Guianerius will have it, "that is superfluously sought after";[5] or to any fervent desire,[6] as Fernelius interprets it; be it in what kind soever, it tortures if immoderate, and is (according to Plater[7] and others) an especial cause of melancholy. *Multuosis concupiscentiis dilaniantur cogitationes meæ*, Austin confessed,[8] that he was torn a-pieces with his manifold desires: and so doth Bernard complain that he could not rest for them a minute of an hour: "this I would have, and that, and then I desire to be such and such."[9] 'Tis a hard matter therefore to confine them, being they are so various and many, unpossible to apprehend all. I will only insist upon some few of the chief, and most noxious in their kind, as that exorbitant appetite and desire of honour, which we commonly call ambition; love of money, which is covetousness, and that greedy desire of gain; self-love, pride, and inordinate desire of vain glory or applause; love of study in excess; love of women (which will require a just volume of itself). Of the other I will briefly speak, and in their order.

Ambition, a proud covetousness, or a dry thirst of honour, a great torture of the mind, composed of envy, pride, and covetousness, a gallant madness, one defines it a pleasant poison; Ambrose, "a canker of the soul,[10] an hidden plague"; Bernard, "a secret poison, the father of livor, and mother of hypocrisy, the moth of holiness, and cause of madness, crucifying and disquieting all that it takes hold of."[11] Seneca[12] calls it *rem sollicitam, timidam, vanam, ventosam,* a windy thing, a vain, solicitous, and fearful thing. For commonly they that, like Sisyphus, roll this restless stone of ambition, are in a perpetual agony, still perplexed,[1] *semper taciti, tristesque recedunt* [they fall back continually, silent and sorrowful] (Lucretius), doubtful, timorous, suspicious, loath to offend in word or deed, still cogging and colloguing, embracing, capping, cringing, applauding, flattering, fleering, visiting, waiting at men's doors, with all affability, counterfeit honesty, and humility.[2] If that will not serve, if once this humour (as Cyprian describes it [3]) possess his thirsty soul, *ambitionis salsugo ubi bibulam animam possidet,* by hook and by crook he will obtain it, "and from his hole he will climb to all honours and offices, if it be possible for him to get up; flattering one, bribing another, he will leave no means unassayed to win all." It is a wonder to see how slavishly these kind of men subject themselves, when they are about a suit, to every inferior person; [4] what pains they will take, run, ride, cast, plot, countermine, protest and swear, vow, promise, what labours undergo, early up, down late; how obsequious and affable they are, how popular and courteous, how they grin and fleer upon every man they meet; with what feasting and inviting, how they spend themselves and their fortunes, in seeking that, many times, which they had much better be without; as Cineas the orator told Pyrrhus: [5] with what waking nights, painful hours, anxious thoughts, and bitterness of mind, *inter spemque metumque* [oscillating between hope and fear], distracted and tired, they consume the interim of their time. There can be no greater plague for the present. If they do obtain their suit, which with such cost and solicitude they have sought, they are not so freed, their anxiety is anew to begin, for they are never satisfied, *nihil aliud nisi imperium spirant,* their thoughts, actions, endeavours are all for sovereignty and honour, like Lues Sforza, that huffing Duke of Milan, "a man of singular wisdom, but profound ambition, born to his own, and to the destruction of Italy," [6] though it be to their own ruin, and friends' undoing, they will contend, they may not cease, but as a dog in a wheel, a bird in a cage, or a squirrel in a chain (so Budæus compares them [7]), they climb and climb still, with much labour, but never make an end, never at the top.[8] A knight would be a baronet, and then a lord, and then a viscount, and then an earl, etc.; a doctor, a dean, and then a bishop; from tribune to prætor, from bailiff to mayor; first this office, and then that; as Pyrrhus in Plutarch,[9] they will first have Greece, then Africa, and then

Asia, and swell with Æsop's frog so long, till in the end
they burst, or come down with Sejanus *ad Gemonias scalas*
[to the Gemonian steps] [1] and break their own necks; or as
Evangelus, the piper in Lucian, that blew his pipe so long,
till he fell down dead.   If he chance to miss, and have a
canvas, he is in a hell on the other side; so dejected, that he
is ready to hang himself, turn heretic, Turk, or traitor in an
instant.   Enraged against his enemies, he rails, swears, fights,
slanders, detracts, envies, murders: and for his own part, *si
appetitum explere non potest, furor corripitur*: if he cannot
satisfy his desire (as Bodine writes [2]) he runs mad.[3]   So that
both ways, hit or miss, he is distracted so long as his ambition
lasts, he can look for no other but anxiety and care, discontent
and grief in the meantime, madness itself or violent death in
the end.[4]   The event of this is common to be seen in populous
cities, or in princes' courts, for a courtier's life (as Budæus
describes it) "is a gallimaufry of ambition, lust, fraud, imposture, dissimulation, detraction, envy, pride; the court, a common conventicle of flatterers, time-servers, politicians, etc.";[5]
or, as Anthony Perez will,[6] "the suburbs of hell itself."   If you
will see such discontented persons, there you shall likely find
them.   And, which he observed of the markets of old Rome:[7]

Qui perjurum convenire vult hominem, mitto in Comitium;
Qui mendacem et gloriosum, apud Cluacinæ sacrum;
Dites, damnosos maritos, sub Basilica quærito, etc.,

[If any one wants to find a perjurer, I send him to
the Comitium; a liar or a braggart, to the shrine of
Cluacina; rich and prodigal husbands can be found
under the Basilica,]

perjured knaves, knights of the post, liars, crackers, bad
husbands, etc., keep their several stations; they do still, and
always did in every commonwealth.

SUBSECT. XII.—Φιλαργυρία, *Covetousness, a Cause*

Plutarch, in his book whether the diseases of the body be
more grievous than those of the soul, is of opinion, "if you will
examine all the causes of our miseries in this life, you shall find
them most part to have had their beginning from stubborn
anger, that furious desire of contention, or some unjust or
immoderate affection, as covetousness," etc.[8]   "From whence

are wars and contentions amongst you?" St. James asks.[1]
I will add usury, fraud, rapine, simony, oppression, lying,
swearing, bearing false witness, etc.; are they not from this
fountain of covetousness, that greediness in getting, tenacity in
keeping, sordidity in spending? that they are so wicked, "unjust
against God, their neighbour, themselves," [2] all comes hence.
"The desire of money is the root of all evil, and they that lust
after it, pierce themselves through with many sorrows" (1 Tim.
vi, 10). Hippocrates therefore, in his Epistle to Crateva, an
herbalist, gives him this good counsel, that if it were possible,
"amongst other herbs, he should cut up that weed of covetousness by the roots, that there be no remainder left; and then
know this for a certainty, that together with their bodies thou
mayest quickly cure all the diseases of their minds." [3] For it
is indeed the pattern, image, epitome of all melancholy, the
fountain of many miseries, much discontent, care and woe;
this "inordinate, or immoderate desire of gain, to get or keep
money," as Bonaventura defines it: [4] or, as Austin describes
it, a madness of the soul; Gregory, a torture; Chrysostom,
an insatiable drunkenness; Cyprian, blindness, *speciosum
supplicium* [a splendid torment], a plague subverting kingdoms, families, an incurable disease; [5] Budæus, an ill habit,
"yielding to no remedies": [6] neither Æsculapius nor Plutus
can cure them: a continual plague, saith Solomon, and vexation
of spirit, another hell. I know there be some of opinion that
covetous men are happy and wordly-wise, that there is more
pleasure in getting of wealth than in spending, and no delight
in the world like unto it. 'Twas Bias' problem of old· "With
what art thou not weary? with getting money. What is most
delectable? to gain." [7] What is it, trow you, that makes a
poor man labour all his lifetime, carry such great burdens, fare
so hardly, macerate himself, and endure so much misery, undergo
such base offices with so great patience, to rise up early, and lie
down late, if there were not an extraordinary delight in getting
and keeping of money? What makes a merchant that hath no
need, *satis superque domi* [enough and to spare at home], to
range all over the world, through all those intemperate zones
of heat and cold; [8] voluntarily to venture his life, and be content
with such miserable famine, nasty usage, in a stinking ship; if
there were not a pleasure and hope to get money, which doth
season the rest, and mitigate his indefatigable pains? What
makes them go into the bowels of the earth, an hundred fathom
deep, endangering their dearest lives, enduring damps and filthy

smells, when they have enough already if they could be content, and no such cause to labour, but an extraordinary delight they take in riches? This may seem plausible at first show, a popular and strong argument; but let him that so thinks consider better of it, and he shall soon perceive that it is far otherwise than he supposeth; it may be haply pleasing at the first, as most part all melancholy is. For such men likely have some *lucida intervalla* [lucid intervals], pleasant symptoms intermixed; but you must note that of Chrysostom, "'Tis one thing to be rich, another to be covetous": [1] generally they are all fools, dizzards, madmen, miserable wretches, living besides themselves, *sine arte fruendi* [having no notion of enjoyment], in perpetual slavery, fear, suspicion, sorrow, and discontent; [2] *plus aloes quam mellis habent* [they have more aloes than honey], and are indeed "rather possessed by their money, than possessors," as Cyprian hath it; [3] *mancipati pecuniis*, bound prentice to their goods, as Pliny; [4] or as Chrysostom, *servi divitiarum*, slaves and drudges to their substance; and we may conclude of them all, as Valerius doth of Ptolemæus, King of Cyprus, "He was in title a king of that island, but in his mind a miserable drudge of money": [5]

> *potiore metallis*
> *Libertate carens,* [6]

wanting his liberty, which is better than gold. Damasippus the Stoic, in Horace, proves that all mortal men dote by fits, some one way, some another, but that covetous men are madder than the rest; [7] and he that shall truly look into their estates, and examine their symptoms, shall find no better of them but that they are all fools, [8] as Nabal was, *re et nomine* [by name and nature] (1 Sam. xxv). For what greater folly can there be, or madness, than to macerate himself when he need not? [9] and when, as Cyprian notes, "he may be freed from his burden and eased of his pains, will go on still, his wealth increasing, when he hath enough, to get more, to live besides himself," [10] to starve his genius, keep back from his wife and children, neither letting them nor other friends use or enjoy that which is theirs by right, and which they much need perhaps (like a hog, or dog in the manger, he doth only keep it because it shall do nobody else good, hurting himself and others), and, for a little momentary pelf, damn his own soul? [11] They are commonly sad and tetric by nature, as Ahab's spirit was because he could not get Naboth's vineyard (1 Kings xxii), and if he lay out his money at any time, though it be to necessary uses, to his own children's good, he brawls and scolds, his heart is heavy, much disquieted he is, and loath to part from it: *Miser abstinet ac timet uti* [the wretch does not touch it and is afraid to use it] (Hor.). He is of a wearish, dry, pale constitution, and cannot sleep for cares and worldly business; his riches, saith Solomon, will not let him sleep, and unnecessary business which he heapeth on himself; or if he do sleep, 'tis a very unquiet, interrupt, unpleasing sleep, with his bags in his arms:

> *Congestis undique saccis*
> *Indormit inhians.*

[He sleeps open-mouthed upon his money-bags.]

And though he be at a banquet, or at some merry feast, "he sighs for grief of heart" (as Cyprian hath it [1]) "and cannot sleep though it be upon a down bed"; his wearish body takes no rest, "troubled in his abundance, and sorrowful in plenty, unhappy for the present, and more unhappy in the life to come" [2] (Basil). He is a perpetual drudge, restless in his thoughts, and never satisfied,[3] a slave, a wretch, a dust-worm, *semper quod idolo suo immolet, sedulus observat* (Cypr., *prolog. ad sermon.*), still seeking what sacrifice he may offer to his golden god, *per fas et nefas*, he cares not how, his trouble is endless, *crescunt divitiæ, tamen curtæ nescio quid semper abest rei:* [4] his wealth increaseth, and the more he hath, the more he wants: [5] like Pharaoh's lean kine, which devoured the fat, and were not satisfied. Austin therefore defines covetousness,[6] *quarumlibet rerum inhonestam et insatiabilem cupiditatem,* a dishonest and insatiable desire of gain; and in one of his epistles compares it to hell, "which devours all, and yet never hath enough, a bottomless pit," [7] an endless misery; *in quem scopulum avaritiæ cadaverosi senes ut plurimum impingunt* [avarice is the rock on which gaunt old men mostly come to grief], and that which is their greatest corrosive, they are in continual suspicion, fear, and distrust. He thinks his own wife and children are so many thieves, and go about to cozen him, his servants are all false:

> *Rem suam periisse, sequo eradicarier,*
> *Et divum atque hominum clamat continuo fidem,*
> *De suo tigillo si qua exit foras.*

> If his doors creak, then out he cries anon,
> His goods are gone, and he is quite undone.

Timidus Plutus, an old proverb, "As fearful as Plutus": so doth Aristophanes and Lucian bring him in fearful still, pale, anxious, suspicious, and trusting no man. "They are afraid of tempests for their corn: they are afraid of their friends lest they should ask something of them, beg or borrow; they are afraid of their enemies lest they hurt them, thieves lest they rob them; they are afraid of war and afraid of peace, afraid of rich and afraid of poor; afraid of all." [1] Last of all, they are afraid of want, that they shall die beggars, which makes they lay up still, and dare not use that they have: what if a dear year come, or dearth, or some loss? and were it not that they are loath to lay out money on a rope, they would be hanged forthwith,[2] and sometimes die to save charges, and make away themselves, if their corn and cattle miscarry; though they have abundance left, as A. Gellius notes.[3] Valerius [4] makes mention of one that in a famine sold a mouse for two hundred pence, and famished himself: such are their cares, griefs, and perpetual fears.[5] These symptoms are elegantly expressed by Theophrastus in his character of a covetous man: "Lying in bed, he asked his wife whether she shut the trunks and chests fast, the capcase be sealed, and whether the hall door be bolted; and though she say all is well, he riseth out of his bed in his shirt, barefoot and bare-legged, to see whether it be so, with a dark lanthorn searching every corner, scarce sleeping a wink all night." [6] Lucian, in that pleasant and witty dialogue called *Gallus*, brings in Micyllus the cobbler disputing with his cock, sometime Pythagoras; where after much speech pro and con, to prove the happiness of a mean estate and discontents of a rich man, Pythagoras' cock in the end, to illustrate by examples that which he had said, brings him to Gnipho the usurer's house at midnight, and after that to Eucrates; whom they found both awake, casting up their accounts, and telling of their money, lean, dry, pale, and anxious,[7] still suspecting lest somebody should make a hole through the wall, and so get in; or if a rat or mouse did but stir, starting upon a sudden, and running to the door to see whether all were fast. Plautus, in his *Aulularia*, makes old Euclio commanding Staphyla his wife to shut the doors fast, and the fire to be put out, lest anybody should make that an errand to come to his house; [8] when he washed his hands, he was loath to fling away the foul water; complaining that he was undone, because the smoke got out of his roof.[9] And as he went from home, seeing a crow scrat upon the muck-hill, returned in all haste, taking it for *malum omen*, an ill sign, his money was digged up; with many such. He that will but observe their actions shall find these and many such passages not feigned for sport, but really performed, verified indeed by such covetous and miserable wretches, and that it is

manifesta phrenesis
Ut locuples moriaris egenti vivere fato,[1]

a mere madness, to live like a wretch, and die rich.

SUBSECT. XIII.—*Love of Gaming, etc., and Pleasures Immoderate, Causes*

It is a wonder to see, how many poor, distressed, miserable wretches one shall meet almost in every path and street, begging for an alms, that have been well descended, and sometime in flourishing estate, now ragged, tattered, and ready to be starved, lingering out a painful life, in discontent and grief of body and mind, and all through immoderate lust, gaming, pleasure, and riot. 'Tis the common end of all sensual epicures and brutish prodigals, that are stupefied and carried away headlong with their several pleasures and lusts. Cebes in his Table, St. Ambrose in his second book of Abel and Cain, and amongst the rest, Lucian, in his tract *de Mercede conductis*, hath excellent well deciphered such men's proceedings in his picture of Opulentia, whom he feigns to dwell on the top of a high mount, much sought after by many suitors; at their first coming they are generally entertained by Pleasure and Dalliance, and have all the content that possibly may be given, so long as their money lasts: but when their means fail, they are contemptibly thrust out at a backdoor, headlong, and there left to Shame, Reproach, Despair. And he at first that had so many attendants, parasites, and followers, young and lusty, richly arrayed, and all the dainty fare that might be had, with all kind of welcome and good respect, is now upon a sudden stript of all, pale, naked, old, diseased, and forsaken, cursing his stars, and ready to strangle himself; having no other company but Repentance, Sorrow, Grief, Derision, Beggary, and Contempt, which are his daily attendants to his life's end.[2] As the prodigal son [3] had exquisite music, merry company, dainty fare at first, but a sorrowful reckoning in the end; so have all such vain delights and their followers. *Tristes voluptatum exitus, et quisquis voluptatum suarum reminisci volet, intelliget* [4] [pleasures bring sadness in their train, as any one will perceive who recalls his own pleasures], as bitter as gall and wormwood is their last; grief of mind, madness itself. The ordinary rocks upon which such men do impinge and precipitate themselves, are cards, dice, hawks, and hounds (*insanum venandi studium* [the mad craze for hunting], one calls it), *insanæ substructiones*, their mad structures, disports, plays, etc., when they·are unseasonably used, imprudently handled, and beyond their fortunes. Some men are consumed by mad phantastical buildings, by making galleries, cloisters, terraces, walks, orchards, gardens, pools, rillets, bowers, and such-like places of pleasure; *inutiles domos* [useless buildings], Xenophon calls them,[1] which, howsoever they be delightsome things in themselves, and acceptable to all beholders, an ornament, and befitting some great men, yet unprofitable to others, and the sole overthrow of their estates. Forestus in his Observations hath an example of such a one that became melancholy upon the like occasion, having consumed his substance in an unprofitable building, which would afterward yield him no advantage. Others, I say, are overthrown by those mad sports of hawking and hunting;[2] honest recreations, and fit for some great men, but not for every base, inferior person; whilst they will maintain their falconers, dogs, and hunting nags, their wealth, saith Salmuth, "runs away with hounds, and their fortunes fly away with hawks."[3] They persecute beasts so long, till in the end they themselves degenerate into beasts, as Agrippa taxeth them,[4] Actæon-like,[5] for as he was eaten to death by his own dogs, so do they devour themselves and their patrimonies in such idle and unnecessary disports, neglecting in the meantime their more necessary business, and to follow their vocations. Over-mad, too, sometimes are our great men in delighting and doting too much on it, "when they drive poor husbandmen from their tillage,"[6] as Sarisburiensis objects, *Polycrat.*, *lib.* 1, *cap.* 4,[7] "fling down country farms and whole towns, to make parks and forests, starving men to feed beasts, and punishing in the meantime such a man that shall molest their game, more severely than him that is otherwise a common hacker, or a notorious thief."[8] But great men are some ways to be excused, the meaner sort have no evasion why they should not be counted mad. Poggius the Florentine tells a merry story to this purpose, condemning the folly and impertinent business of such kind of persons. A physician of Milan, saith he, that cured madmen, had a pit of water in his house, in which he kept his patients, some up to the knees, some to the girdle, some to the chin, *pro modo insaniæ*, as they were more or less affected. One of them by chance, that was well recovered, stood in the door, and seeing a gallant ride by with a hawk on his fist, well mounted, with his spaniels after him, would needs know to what use all this preparation served; he made answer, to kill certain fowls; the patient

demanded again, what his fowl might be worth which he killed
in a year; he replied, five or ten crowns; and when he urged him
farther what his dogs, horse, and hawks stood him in, he told
him four hundred crowns; with that the patient bade begone, as
he loved his life and welfare, "for if our master come and find
thee here, he will put thee in the pit amongst madmen up to
the chin": taxing the madness and folly of such vain men that
spend themselves in those idle sports, neglecting their business
and necessary affairs. Leo Decimus, that hunting pope, is
much discommended by Jovius in his life,[1] for his immoderate
desire of hawking and hunting,[2] insomuch that (as he saith) he
would sometimes live about Ostia weeks and months together,
leave suitors unrespected, bulls and pardons unsigned, to his
own prejudice and many private men's loss. "And if he had
been by chance crossed in his sport, or his game not so good,
he was so impatient, that he would revile and miscall many
times men of great worth with most bitter taunts, look so sour,
be so angry and waspish, so grieved and molested, that it is
incredible to relate it." [3] But if he had good sport, and been
well pleased on the other side, *incredibili munificentia*, with
unspeakable bounty and munificence he would reward all his
fellow-hunters, and deny nothing to any suitor when he was in
that mood. To say truth, 'tis the common humour of all
gamesters, as Galatæus observes; if they win, no men living are
so jovial and merry, but if they lose, though it be but a trifle,
two or three games at tables, or a dealing at cards for twopence
a game, they are so choleric and testy that no man may speak
with them, and break many times into violent passions, oaths,
imprecations, and unbeseeming speeches, little differing from
madmen for the time.[4] Generally of all gamesters and gaming,
if it be excessive, thus much we may conclude, that whether
they win or lose for the present, their winnings are not *munera
fortunæ, sed insidiæ*, as that wise Seneca determines, not fortune's gifts, but baits, the common catastrophe is beggary;[5]
Ut pestis vitam, sic adimit alea pecuniam,[6] as the plague takes
away life, doth gaming goods, for *omnes nudi, inopes et egeni* [7]
[they are all stripped, penniless, and in want];

> *Alea Scylla vorax, species certissima furti,*
> *Non contenta bonis, animum quoque perfida mergit,*
> *Fœda, furax, infamis, iners, furiosa, ruina.*[8]

> [Gaming is a whirlpool, the surest form of robbery;
> not content with one's goods, it crushes the mind
> as well; it is foul, thievish, infamous, slothful,
> mad, ruinous.]

For a little pleasure they take, and some small gains and gettings now and then, their wives and children are wringed in the meantime, and they themselves with loss of body and soul rue it in the end.   I will say nothing of those prodigious prodigals, *perdendæ pecuniæ genitos* [people born to waste money], as he[1] taxed Anthony, *qui patrimonium sine ulla fori calumnia amittunt* [who squander their patrimony without any public disgrace], saith Cyprian,[2] and mad sybaritical spendthrifts,[3] *quique una comedunt patrimonia cœna,* that eat up all at a break-fast, at a supper, or amongst bawds, parasites, and players, consume themselves in an instant, as if they had flung it into Tiber,[4] with great wagers, vain and idle expenses, etc., not them-selves only, but even all their friends; as a man desperately swimming drowns him that comes to help him, by suretyship and borrowing they will willingly undo all their associates and allies; *irati pecuniis,* as he saith,[5] angry with their money. What with "a wanton eye, a liquorish tongue, and a gamesome hand,"[6] when they have indiscreetly impoverished themselves, mortgaged their wits together with their lands, and entombed their ancestors' fair possessions in their bowels, they may lead the rest of their days in prison, as many times they do; they repent at leisure, and when all is gone begin to be thrifty: but *sera est in fundo parsimonia,* 'tis then too late to look about; their end is misery, sorrow, shame, and discontent.[7]   And well they deserve to be infamous and discontent, *catomidiari in Amphi-theatro*[8] [to be thrashed in the Amphitheatre], as by Hadrian the emperor's edict they were of old, *decoctores bonorum suorum,* so he calls them, prodigal fools, to be publicly shamed and hissed out of all societies, rather than to be pitied or relieved.[9]   The Tuscans and Bœotians brought their bankrupts into the market-place in a bier with an empty purse carried before them, all the boys following, where they sat all day *circumstante plebe* [in pre-sence of the crowd], to be infamous and ridiculous.   At Padua in Italy[10] they have a stone called the stone of turpitude, near the senate house, where spendthrifts, and such as disclaim non-payment of debts, do sit with their hinder parts bare, that by that note of disgrace others may be terrified from all such vain expense, or borrowing more than they can tell how to pay.   The civilians of old set guardians over such brain-sick prodigals,[11] as they did over madmen, to moderate their expenses, that they should not so loosely consume their fortunes, to the utter undoing of their families.

I may not here omit those two main plagues and common

dotages of human kind, wine and women, which have infatuated and besotted myriads of people: they go commonly
together.

> *Qui vino indulget, quemque alea decoquit, ille*
> *In Venerem putris.*[1]

> [Who wastes his health with drink, his wealth with play,
> The same with womenfolk shall rot away.]

To whom is sorrow, saith Solomon (Prov. xxiii, 29), to whom
is woe, but to such a one as loves drink? it causeth torture
(*vino tortus et ira* [tortured with drunken rage]) and bitterness of
mind (Sirac. xxxiv, 29). *Vinum furoris*, Jeremy calls it (xxv, 15),
wine of madness, as well he may, for *insanire facit sanos*, it
makes sound men sick and sad, and wise men mad,[2] to say
and do they know not what. *Accidit hodie terribilis casus*
(saith St. Austin[3]), hear a miserable accident; Cyrillus' son this
day in his drink *matrem prægnantem nequiter oppressit, sororem
violare voluit, patrem occidit fere, et duas alias sorores ad mortem
vulneravit*, would have violated his sister, killed his father, etc.
A true saying it was of him, *vino dari lætitiam et dolorem*, drink
causeth mirth, and drink causeth sorrow, drink causeth "poverty
and want" (Prov. xxi), shame and disgrace. *Multi ignobiles
evasere ob vini potum, et* (Austin) *amissis honoribus profugi
aberrarunt:* many men have made shipwreck of their fortunes,
and go like rogues and beggars, having turned all their
substance into *aurum potabile* [potable gold], that otherwise might have lived in good worship and happy estate, and
for a few hours' pleasure (for their Hilary term 's but short[4]), or
free madness, as Seneca calls it, purchase unto themselves
eternal tediousness and trouble.[5]

   That other madness is on women. *Apostatare facit cor* [it
maketh the heart go astray] saith the wise man, *atque homini
cerebrum minuit*[6] [and minishes the mind of man]. Pleasant
at first she is, like Dioscorides' rhododaphne, that fair plant to
the eye, but poison to the taste, the rest as bitter as wormwood in the end (Prov. v, 4), and sharp as a two-edged sword.
"Her house is the way to hell, and goes down to the chambers
of death" (Prov. vii, 27). What more sorrowful can be said?
they are miserable in this life, mad, beasts, led like "oxen to
the slaughter":[7] and that which is worse, whoremasters and
drunkards shall be judged; *Amittunt gratiam*, saith Austin, *perdunt gloriam, incurrunt damnationem æternam:* they lose grace
and glory:

Brevis illa voluptas
Abrogat æternum cœli decus; [1]

[That pleasure of a moment
Deprives him of eternal bliss above;]

they gain hell and eternal damnation.

SUBSECT. XIV. — *Philautia, or Self-love, Vainglory, Praise,
Honour, Immoderate Applause, Pride, overmuch Joy, etc.,
Causes*

Self-love, pride, and vainglory, *cæcus amor sui* [2] [blind love of
self], which Chrysostom calls one of the devil's three great nets;
Bernard, "an arrow which pierceth the soul through, and slays
it; a sly, insensible enemy, not perceived," [3] are main causes.
Where neither anger, lust, covetousness, fear, sorrow, etc., nor
any other perturbation can lay hold, this will slyly and insensibly
pervert us. *Quem non gula vicit, philautia superavit* (saith
Cyprian), whom surfeiting could not overtake, self-love hath
overcome. "He that hath scorned all money, bribes, gifts, upright
otherwise and sincere, hath inserted himself to no fond imagination, and sustained all those tyrannical concupiscences of the
body, hath lost all his honour, captivated by vainglory" [4]
(Chrysostom, *sup. Jo.*).

Tu sola animum mentemque peruris,
Gloria.

[By this one passion is my mind consumed,
By love of fame.]

A great assault and cause of our present malady, although we
do most part neglect, take no notice of it, yet this is a violent
batterer of our souls, causeth melancholy and dotage. This
pleasing humour, this soft and whispering popular air, *amabilis
insania*, this delectable frenzy, most irrefragable passion, *mentis
gratissimus error*, this acceptable disease, which so sweetly sets
upon us, ravisheth our senses, lulls our souls asleep, puffs up
our hearts as so many bladders, and that without all feeling,
insomuch as "those that are misaffected with it never so much
as once perceive it, or think of any cure." [5] We commonly
love him best in this malady [6] that doth us most harm, and
are very willing to be hurt; *adulationibus nostris libentur favemus*
[we lend a willing ear to flattery] (saith Jerome [7]), we love him,
we love him for it: *O Bonciari, suave, suave fuit a te tali hæc
tribui* [8] [ah, Bonciarius, 'twas sweet indeed to hear such praise

from such a man as thou]; 'twas sweet to hear it. And as
Pliny [1] doth ingenuously confess to his dear friend Augurinus,
"All thy writings are most acceptable, but those especially that
speak of us." Again, a little after to Maximus, "I cannot
express how pleasing it is to me to hear myself commended." [2]
Though we smile to ourselves, at least ironically, when parasites
bedaub us with false encomiums, as many princes cannot
choose but do, *quum tale quid nihil intra se repererint*, when they
know they come as far short as a mouse to an elephant of
any such virtues; yet it doth us good. Though we seem many
times to be angry, "and blush at our own praises, yet our souls
inwardly rejoice, it puffs us up"; [3] 'tis *fallax suavitas, blandus
dæmon* [a deceptive sweetness, a tickling devil], "makes us
swell beyond our bounds, and forget ourselves." Her two
daughters are lightness of mind, immoderate joy and pride,
not excluding those other concomitant vices, which Jodocus
Lorichius [4] reckons up; bragging, hypocrisy, peevishness, and
curiosity.

Now the common cause of this mischief ariseth from ourselves
or others; we are active and passive.[5] It proceeds inwardly
from ourselves, as we are active causes, from an overweening
conceit we have of our good parts, own worth (which indeed is
no worth), our bounty, favour, grace, valour, strength, wealth,
patience, meekness, hospitality, beauty, temperance, gentry,
knowledge, wit, science, art, learning, our excellent gifts and
fortunes,[6] for which, Narcissus-like, we admire, flatter, and
applaud ourselves, and think all the world esteems so of us;
and as deformed women easily believe those that tell them they
be fair, we are too credulous of our own good parts and praises,
too well persuaded of ourselves. We brag and venditate our
own works,[7] and scorn all others in respect of us; *inflati scientia*
(saith Paul), [puffed up with] our wisdom, our learning; all
our geese are swans, and we as basely esteem and vilify other
men's, as we do over-highly prize and value our own.[8] We
will not suffer them to be *in secundis* [in the second rank],
no, not *in tertiis* [in the third rank]; what? *mecum confertur
Ulysses?* [is Ulysses to be compared with me?]; they are *mures,
muscæ, culices præ se*, nits and flies compared to his inexorable
and supercilious, eminent and arrogant worship: though indeed
they be far before him. Only wise, only rich, only fortunate,
valorous, and fair, puffed up with this tympany of self-conceit;
as that proud Pharisee,[9] they are "not" (as they suppose)
"like other men," of a purer and more precious metal:[10] *soli rei*

gerendi sunt efficaces [they alone are competent], which that wise Periander held of such: *meditantur omne qui prius negotium,* [who first think over every undertaking], etc. *Novi quendam*[1] (saith Erasmus[2]), I knew one so arrogant that he thought himself inferior to no man living, like Callisthenes the philosopher, that neither held Alexander's acts, or any other subject, worthy of his pen, such was his insolency;[3] or Seleucus, King of Syria, who thought none fit to contend with him but the Romans: *Eos solos dignos ratus quibuscum de imperio certaret.*[4] That which Tully writ to Atticus long since, is still in force: "There was never yet true poet nor orator, that thought any other better than himself."[5] And such for the most part are your princes, potentates, great philosophers, historiographers, authors of sects or heresies, and all our great scholars, as Hierome defines:[6] "A natural philosopher is glory's creature, and a very slave of rumour, fame, and popular opinion," and though they write *de contemptu gloriæ* [on the contempt of fame], yet, as he observes, they will put their names to their books. *Vobis et famæ me semper dedi,* saith Trebellius Pollio, I have wholly consecrated myself to you and fame. "'Tis all my desire, night and day, 'tis all my study to raise my name." Proud Pliny[7] seconds him: *Quamquam O!* etc.; and that vainglorious orator[8] is not ashamed to confess in an epistle of his to Marcus Lucceius, *Ardeo incredibili cupiditate,* etc., "I burn with an incredible desire to have my name registered in thy book."[9] Out of this fountain proceed all those cracks and brags: *Speramus carmina fingi Posse linenda cedro, et leni servanda cupresso*[10] [we cherish hopes of composing poems worthy to be preserved by cedar oil, and to be stored in cypress chests]. *Non usitata nec tenui ferar penna . . . nec in terra morabor longius* [I am borne on no common or slender wing. . . . I shall not tarry long upon earth]. *Nil parvum aut humili modo, nil mortale loquor* [no mean or humble strain is mine, nor soon to be forgot]. *Dicar qua violens obstrepit Aufidus* [where Aufidus rolls noisily my name shall be known]. *Exegi monumentum ære perennius* [I have carved a monument more durable than brass]. *Jamque opus exegi, quod nec Jovis ira, nec ignis, etc.*[11] [I have achieved a work which neither the wrath of heaven nor fire, etc.]. *Cum venit ille dies, etc.; Parte tamen meliore mei super alta perennis Astra ferar, nomenque erit indelebile nostrum.* (This of Ovid I have paraphrased in English:

And when I am dead and gone,
My corpse laid under a stone,

> My fame shall yet survive,
> And I shall be alive,
> In these my works for ever,
> My glory shall persever, etc.)

And that of Ennius,

> *Nemo me lacrimis decoret, neque funera fletu*
> *Faxit; cur? volito docta per ora virum.*

[Let none shed tears over me, or grace my grave with
weeping, because I am eternally in the mouths
of men;]

with many such proud strains, and foolish flashes too common
with writers. Not so much as Demochares on the Topics,[1] but
he will be immortal. Typotius *de fama* shall be famous, and
well he deserves, because he writ of fame; and every trivial poet
must be renowned: *Plausuque petit clarescere vulgi* [he seeks
the applause of the mob]. This puffing humour it is, that
hath produced so many great tomes, built such famous monuments, strong castles, and Mausolean tombs, to have their acts
eternized, *Digito monstrari, et dicier hic est* [to be pointed at
with the finger, and to have it said, "There he goes"]; to see
their names inscribed, as Phryne on the walls of Thebes, *Phryne
fecit.* This causeth so many bloody battles, *Et noctes cogit
vigilare serenas* [and forces us to watch during calm nights];
long journeys—*Magnum iter intendo, sed dat mihi gloria vires*
[I contemplate a monstrous journey, but the love of glory
strengthens me for it]; gaining honour, a little applause, pride,
self-love, vainglory. This is it which makes them take such
pains, and break out into those ridiculous strains, this high
conceit of themselves, to scorn all others;[2] *ridiculo fastu et
intolerando contemptu,* as Palæmon the grammarian contemned
Varro, *secum et natas et morituras literas jactans*[3] [boasting that
literature had been born with him and would die with him],
and brings them to that height of insolency, that they cannot
endure to be contradicted, "or hear of anything but their own
commendation,"[4] which Hierome notes of such kind of men;
and, as Austin well seconds him,[5] "'tis their sole study day and
night to be commended and applauded." Whenas indeed, in
all wise men's judgments, *quibus cor capit* [who are blessed
with sense], they are mad,[6] empty vessels, fungos, beside themselves, derided, *et ut camelus in proverbio quærens cornua, etiam
quas habebat aures amisit* [and like the camel in the proverb,
who asked for horns and lost his ears], their works are toys, as
an almanac out of date, *Auctoris pereunt garrulitate sui*[7] [they

fall flat because their authors talk too much of them], they
seek fame and immortality, but reap dishonour and infamy,
they are a common obloquy, *insensati*, and come far short of
that which they suppose or expect.

> *O puer, ut sis vitalis metuo.*[1]
> [O boy, I fear thou art short-lived.]

Of so many myriads of poets, rhetoricians, philosophers,
sophisters, as Eusebius well observes,[2] which have written in
former ages, scarce one of a thousand's works remains, *nomina
et libri cum corporibus interierunt,* their books and bodies are
perished together.   It is not as they vainly think, they shall
surely be admired and immortal; as one told Philip of Macedon,
insulting after a victory, that his shadow was no longer than
before, we may say to them:

> *Nos demiramur, sed non cum deside vulgo,*
> *Sed velut Harpyas, Gorgonas, et Furias.*

> We marvel too, not as the vulgar we,
> But as we Gorgons, Harpies, or Furies see.

Or if we do applaud, honour and admire, *quota pars,* how
small a part, in respect of the whole world, never so much as
hears our names! how few take notice of us! how slender a
tract, as scant as Alcibiades his land in a map!   And yet every
many must and will be immortal, as he hopes, and extend his
fame to our antipodes, whenas half, no, not a quarter, of his
own province or city neither knows nor hears of him: but say
they did, what's a city to a kingdom, a kingdom to Europe,
Europe to the world, the world itself that must have an end,
if compared to the least visible star in the firmament, eighteen
times bigger than it? and then if those stars be infinite, and
every star there be a sun, as some will, and, as this sun of ours,
hath his planets about him, all inhabited, what proportion bear
we to them, and where's our glory?   *Orbem terrarum victor
Romanus habebat,* as he cracked in Petronius, all the world was
under Augustus; and so in Constantine's time, Eusebius brags
he governed all the world, *universum mundum præclare admodum
administravit, . . . et omnes orbis gentes imperatori subjecti*
[he governed the whole world with great distinction, and all
nations were subject to the emperor]: so of Alexander it is
given out, the four monarchies, etc., whenas neither Greeks
nor Romans ever had the fifteenth part of the now known world,
nor half of that which was then described.   What braggadocians

are they and we then! *quam brevis hic de nobis sermo*, as he said,[1]
pudebit aucti nominis,[2] how short a time, how little a while
doth this fame of ours continue! Every private province, every
small territory and city, when we have all done, will yield as
generous spirits, as brave examples in all respects, as famous as
ourselves; Cadwallader in Wales, Rollo in Normandy, Robin
Hood and Little John are as much renowned in Sherwood, as
Cæsar in Rome, Alexander in Greece, or his Hephæstion. *Omnis
ætas omnisque populus in exemplum et admirationem veniet*[3] [every
age, every people can furnish examples to excite our wonder],
every town, city, book, is full of brave soldiers, senators, scholars;
and though Brasidas[4] was a worthy captain, a good man, and,
as they thought, not to be matched in Lacedæmon, yet, as his
mother truly said, *plures habet Sparta Brasida meliores*, Sparta
had many better men than ever he was; and howsoever thou
admirest thyself, thy friend, many an obscure fellow the world
never took notice of, had he been in place or action, would
have done much better than he or he, or thou thyself.

Another kind of madmen there is opposite to these, that are
insensibly mad, and know not of it, such as contemn all praise
and glory, think themselves most free whenas indeed they are
most mad: *calcant sed alio fastu* [these also trample upon
others, but with another kind of pride]: a company of cynics,
such as are monks, hermits, anachorites, that contemn the
world, contemn themselves, contemn all titles, honours, offices,
and yet in that contempt are more proud than any man living
whatsoever. They are proud in humility, proud in that they are
not proud; *sæpe homo de vanæ gloriæ contemptu vanius gloriatur*
[a man can be most boastful in expressing his contempt of
fame], as Austin hath it, *Confess. lib.* 10, *cap.* 38; like Diogenes,
intus gloriantur, they brag inwardly, and feed themselves fat
with a self-conceit of sanctity, which is no better than hypocrisy.
They go in sheep's russet, many great men that might maintain
themselves in cloth of gold, and seem to be dejected, humble
by their outward carriage, whenas inwardly they are swollen
full of pride, arrogancy, and self-conceit. And therefore Seneca
adviseth his friend Lucilius,[5] "in his attire and gesture, outward
actions, especially to avoid all such things as are more notable
in themselves: as a rugged attire, hirsute head, horrid beard,
contempt of money, coarse lodging, and whatsoever leads to
fame that opposite way."

All this madness yet proceeds from ourselves, the main engine
which batters us is from others, we are merely passive in this

business: from a company of parasites and flatterers, that with
immoderate praise and bombast epithets, glozing titles, false
elogiums, so bedaub and applaud, gild over many a silly and undeserving man, that they clap him quite out of his wits. *Res
imprimis violenta est*, as Hierome notes, this common applause
is a most violent thing, *laudum placenta* [a cake of praises], a
drum, fife, and trumpet cannot so animate; that fattens men,
erects and dejects them in an instant. *Palma negata macrum,
donata reducit opimum.*[1] It makes them fat and lean, as frost
doth conies. "And who is that mortal man that can so contain himself, that, if he be immoderately commended and
applauded, will not be moved?"[2] Let him be what he will,
those parasites will overturn him: if he be a king, he is one
of the Nine Worthies, more than a man, a god forthwith
(*Edictum Domini Deique nostri*[3] [the edict of our Lord and
God]), and they will sacrifice unto him:

> *Divinos si tu patiaris honores,*
> *Ultro ipsi dabimus meritasque sacrabimus aras.*[4]

> [If you will accept divine honours, we will willingly pay them
> to you, and raise to you well-deserved altars.]

If he be a soldier, then Themistocles, Epaminondas, Hector,
Achilles, *duo fulmina belli* [two thunderbolts of war], *triumviri
terrarum* [the triumvirs of the universe[5]], etc., and the valour of
both Scipios is too little for him, he is *invictissimus, serenissimus,
multis trophæis ornatissimus, naturæ dominus* [invincible; most
serene, adorned with numerous trophies, lord of nature], although he be *lepus galeatus* [a helmeted hare], indeed a very
coward, a milksop, and as he[6] said of Xerxes, *postremus in
pugna, primus in fuga* [last in fight, first in flight], and such
a one as never durst look his enemy in the face. If he be a
big man, then is he a Samson, another Hercules; if he pronounce a speech, another Tully or Demosthenes (as of Herod.
in the Acts, "the voice of God and not of man"); if he can
make a verse, Homer, Virgil, etc. And then my silly weak
patient takes all these elogiums to himself; if he be a scholar
so commended for his much reading, excellent style, method,
etc., he will eviscerate himself like a spider, study to death;
Laudatas ostendit avis Junonia pennas, peacock-like he will
display all his feathers. If he be a soldier, and so applauded,
his valour extolled, though it be *impar congressus* [an unequal
match], as that of Troilus and Achilles, *infelix puer* [luckless
youth], he will combat with a giant, run first upon a breach;

as another Philippus,[1] he will ride into the thickest of his
enemies. Commend his housekeeping, and he will beggar himself; commend his temperance, he will starve himself.

> *Laudataque virtus*
> *Crescit, et immensum gloria calcar habet.*

> [Praise gives to virtue welcome nourishment,
> And glory spurs it on to high intent]

He is mad, mad, mad, no whoa with him;[2] *impatiens consortis
erit* [he will be impatient of a colleague], he will over the Alps
to be talked of, or to maintain his credit.[3] Commend an ambitious man, some proud prince or potentate, *si plus laudetur* (saith
Erasmus) *cristas erigit, exuit hominem, Deum se putat,*[4] he sets
up his crest, and will be no longer a man but a god.

> *Nihil est quod credere de se*
> *Non audet quum laudatur dis æqua potestas.*[5]

> [For princes think, when lauded to the skies,
> There is no height to which they cannot rise.]

How did this work with Alexander, that would needs be Jupiter's
son, and go like Hercules in a lion's skin! Domitian a god
(*Dominus Deus noster sic fieri jubet*[6] [the Master, our God, so
orders]), like the Persian kings, whose image was adored by
all that came into the city of Babylon.[7] Commodus the
emperor was so gulled by his flattering parasites that he must
be called Hercules. Antonius the Roman would be crowned
with ivy, carried in a chariot, and adored for Bacchus.[8] Cotys,
King of Thrace, was married to Minerva, and sent three several
messengers, one after another, to see if she were come to his
bed-chamber.[9] Such a one was Jupiter Menecrates,[10] Maximinus
Jovianus, Dioclesianus Herculeus, Sapor the Persian king,
brother of the sun and moon, and our modern Turks, that will
be gods on earth, kings of kings, God's shadow, commanders of
all that may be commanded, our kings of China and Tartary in
this present age. Such a one was Xerxes, that would whip the
sea, fetter Neptune, *stulta jactantia* [in his stupid pride], and
send a challenge to Mount Athos; and such are many sottish
princes, brought into a fool's paradise by their parasites. 'Tis a
common humour, incident to all men, when they are in great
places or come to the solstice of honour, have done or deserved
well, to applaud and flatter themselves. *Stultitiam suam
produnt* [they betray their folly], etc. (saith Platerus[11]); your
very tradesmen, if they be excellent, will crack and brag, and

show their folly in excess. They have good parts, and they
know it, you need not tell them of it; out of a conceit of their
worth, they go smiling to themselves, a perpetual meditation
of their trophies and plaudits; they run at last quite mad, and
lose their wits.[1] Petrarch, *lib.* 1 *de contemptu mundi*, confessed
as much of himself, and Cardan, in his fifth book of Wisdom,
gives an instance in a smith of Milan, a fellow-citizen of his, one
Galeus de Rubeis, that being commended for refinding of an instrument of Archimedes, for joy ran mad.[2] Plutarch, in the life
of Artaxerxes, hath such a like story of one Carius, a soldier,
that wounded King Cyrus in battle, and "grew thereupon so
arrogant, that in a short space after he lost his wits."[3] So
many men, if any new honour, office, preferment, booty, treasure,
possession, or patrimony *ex insperato* [unexpectedly] fall unto
them, for immoderate joy, and continual meditation of it,
cannot sleep or tell what they say or do;[4] they are so ravished
on a sudden, and with vain conceits transported, there is no
rule with them. Epaminondas, therefore, the next day after
his Leuctrian victory, "came abroad all squalid and submiss,"[5]
and gave no other reason to his friends of so doing, than that
he perceived himself the day before, by reason of his good
fortune, to be too insolent, overmuch joyed. That wise and
virtuous lady, Queen Katherine, Dowager of England,[6] in
private talk upon like occasion, said that "she would not
willingly endure the extremity of either fortune; but if it were
so, that of necessity she must undergo the one, she would be
in adversity, because comfort was never wanting in it, but still
counsel and government were defective in the other":[7] they
could not moderate themselves.

SUBSECT. XV.—*Love of Learning, or overmuch Study. With a
Digression of the Misery of Scholars, and why the Muses are
Melancholy*

Leonartus Fuchsius, *Instit. lib.* 3, *sect.* 1, *cap.* 1; Felix
Plater, *lib.* 3 *de mentis alienat.*; Herc. de Saxonia, *tract. post.
de melanch. cap.* 3, speak of a peculiar fury which comes by
overmuch study.[8] Fernelius, *lib.* 1, *cap.* 18, puts study, contemplation, and continual meditation as an especial cause of
madness:[9] and in his 86th *consul.* cites the same words. Jo.
Arculanus, *in lib.* 9 *Rhasis ad Almansorem, cap.* 16, amongst
other causes reckons up *studium vehemens* [passionate study]:
so doth Levinus Lemnius, *lib. de occul. nat. mirac. lib.* 1, *cap.* 16.

"Many men" (saith he) "come to this malady by continual study,[1] and night-waking, and of all other men, scholars are most subject to it";[2] and such, Rhasis adds, "that have commonly the finest wits"[3] (*Cont. lib.* 1, *tract.* 9). Marsilius Ficinus, *de sanit. tuenda, lib.* 1, *cap.* 7, puts melancholy amongst one of those five principal plagues of students, 'tis a common moll unto them all, and almost in some measure an inseparable companion. Varro belike for that cause calls *tristes philosophos et severos* [philosophers sad and austere]; severe, sad, dry, tetric, are common epithets to scholars: and Patricius therefore,[4] in the institution of princes, would not have them to be great students. For (as Machiavel holds) study weakens their bodies, dulls the spirits, abates their strength and courage; and good scholars are never good soldiers, which a certain Goth well perceived, for when his countrymen came into Greece, and would have burned all their books, he cried out against it, by all means they should not do it; "Leave them that plague, which in time will consume all their vigour, and martial spirits."[5] The Turks abdicated Corcutus, the next heir, from the empire, because he was so much given to his book:[6] and 'tis the common tenent of the world, that learning dulls and diminisheth the spirits, and so *per consequens* produceth melancholy.

Two main reasons may be given of it, why students should be more subject to this malady than others. The one is, they live a sedentary, solitary life, *sibi et musis* [for themselves and their studies], free from bodily exercise, and those ordinary disports which other men use; and many times if discontent and idleness concur with it, which is too frequent, they are precipitated into this gulf on a sudden; but the common cause is overmuch study: "Too much learning" (as Festus told Paul[7]) "hath made thee mad"; 'tis, that other extreme which effects it. So did Trincavellius, *lib.* 1, *consil.* 12 and 13, find by his experience, in two of his patients, a young baron and another, that contracted this malady by too vehement study. So Forestus, *Observat. lib.* 10, *observ.* 13, in a young divine in Louvain, that was mad, and said "he had a Bible in his head."[8] Marsilius Ficinus, *de sanit. tuend., lib.* 1, *cap.* 1, 3, 4, and *lib.* 2, *cap.* 16, gives many reasons "why students dote more often than others."[9] The first is their negligence: "Other men look to their tools; a painter will wash his pencils; a smith will look to his hammer, anvil, forge; a husbandman will mend his plough-irons, and grind his hatchet if it be dull; a falconer or huntsman will have an especial care of his hawks, hounds, horses, dogs, etc.; a musician will string and unstring his lute, etc.; only scholars neglect that instrument (their brain and spirits I mean) which they daily use, and by which they range over all the world, which by much study is consumed." [1] *Vide* (saith Lucian) *ne funiculum nimis intendendo, aliquando abrumpas:* "See thou twist not the rope so hard, till at length it break." [2] Facinus, in his fourth chap., gives some other reasons; Saturn and Mercury, the patrons of learning, are both dry planets: and Origanus [3] assigns the same cause why Mercurialists are so poor, and most part beggars; for that their president Mercury had no better fortune himself. The Destinies of old put poverty upon him as a punishment; since when, poetry and beggary are *gemelli*, twin-born brats, inseparable companions;

> And to this day is every scholar poor;
> Gross gold from them runs headlong to the boor: [4]

Mercury can help them to knowledge, but not to money. The second is contemplation, "which dries the brain and extinguisheth natural heat; for whilst the spirits are intent to meditation above in the head, the stomach and liver are left destitute, and thence come black blood and crudities by defect of concoction, and for want of exercise the superfluous vapours cannot exhale," [5] etc. The same reasons are repeated by Gomesius, *lib. 4, cap. 1, de sale*; Nymannus, *orat. de Imag.*; [6] Jo. Voschius, *lib. 2, cap. 5, de peste*; and something more they add, that hard students are commonly troubled with gouts, catarrhs, rheums, cachexia, bradypepsia, bad eyes, stone, and colic, crudities, oppilations, vertigo, winds, consumptions, and all such diseases as come by overmuch sitting; [7] they are most part lean, dry, ill-coloured, spend their fortunes, lose their wits, and many times their lives, and all through immoderate pains and extraordinary studies. If you will not believe the truth of this, look upon great Tostatus' and Thomas Aquinas' works, and tell me whether those men took pains? peruse Austin, Hierome, etc., and many thousands besides.

> *Qui cupit optatam cursu contingere metam,*
> *Multa tulit, fecitque puer, sudavit et alsit.*

> He that desires this wished goal to gain,
> Must sweat and freeze before he can attain,

and labour hard for it. So did Seneca, by his own confession, *ep.* 8; "Not a day that I spend idle, part of the night I keep mine eyes open, tired with waking, and now slumbering to their continual task." [8] Hear Tully, *pro Archia Poeta*: "Whilst others loitered, and took their pleasures, he was continually at his book"; so they do that will be scholars, and that to the hazard (I say) of their healths, fortunes, wits, and lives. How much did Aristotle and Ptolemy spend? *unius regni pretium* they say, more than a king's ransom; how many crowns per annum, to perfect arts, the one about his History of Creatures, the other on his Almagest? How much time did Thebet Benchorat employ, to find out the motion of the eighth sphere? forty years and more, some write. How many poor scholars have lost their wits, or become dizzards, neglecting all worldly affairs and their own health, *esse* and *bene esse* [being and well-being], to gain knowledge for which, after all their pains, in this world's esteem they are accounted ridiculous and silly fools, idiots, asses, and (as oft they are) rejected, contemned, derided, doting, and mad! Look for examples in Hildesheim, *Spicil. 2, de mania et delirio*; read Trincavellius, *lib. 3, consil. 36, et c. 17*; Montanus, *consil. 233*; Garcæus, *de Judic. genit. cap. 33*; [1] Mercurialis, *consil. 86, cap. 25*; Prosper Calenius in his book *de atra bile*.[2] Go to Bedlam and ask. Or if they keep their wits, yet they are esteemed scrubs and fools by reason of their carriage: "after seven years' study," [3]

> *statua taciturnius exit,*
> *Plerumque et risu populum quatit.*

> [Dumb as a statue, slow he stalks along,
> And shakes with laughter loud the gazing throng.]

Because they cannot ride an horse, which every clown can do; salute and court a gentlewoman, carve at table, cringe and make congees, which every common swasher can do, *his populus ridet*,[4] etc., they are laughed to scorn, and accounted silly fools by our gallants. Yea, many times, such is their misery, they deserve it: a mere scholar, a mere ass.

> *Obstipo capite, et figentes lumine terram,*
> *Murmura cum secum, et rabiosa silentia rodunt,*
> *Atque exporrecto trutinantur verba labello,*
> *Ægroti veteris meditantes somnia, gigni*
> *De nihilo nihilum ; in nihilum nil posse reverti.*[5]

> Who do lean awry
> Their heads, piercing the earth with a fixt eye;
> When, by themselves, they gnaw their murmuring,
> And furious silence, as 'twere balancing
> Each word upon their outstretched lip, and when
> They meditate the dreams of old sick men,
> As, "Out of nothing, nothing can be brought;
> And that which is, can ne'er be turn'd to nought." [6]

Thus they go commonly meditating unto themselves, thus they

sit, such is their action and gesture. Fulgosus, *lib.* 8, *cap.* 7, makes
mention how Th. Aquinas, supping with King Louis of France,
upon a sudden knocked his fist upon the table, and cried,
Conclusum est contra Manichæos [This proves the Manichæans
were wrong]; his wits were a-woolgathering, as they say, and
his head busied about other matters; when he perceived his
error, he was much abashed.[1] Such a story there is of Archimedes in Vitruvius, that having found out the means to know
how much gold was mingled with the silver in King Hiero's
crown, ran naked forth of the bath and cried Εὕρηκα, I have
found; "and was commonly so intent to his studies, that he
never perceived what was done about him: when the city was
taken, and the soldiers now ready to rifle his house, he took no
notice of it." [2] St. Bernard rode all day long by the Lemnian
lake,[3] and asked at last where he was (Marullus, *lib.* 2, *cap.* 4).
It was Democritus' carriage alone that made the Abderites
suppose him to have been mad, and send for Hippocrates to
cure him: if he had been in any solemn company, he would
upon all occasions fall a-laughing. Theophrastus saith as much
of Heraclitus, for that he continually wept, and Laertius of
Menedemus Lampsacus, because he ran like a madman, "saying
he came from hell as a spy, to tell the devils what mortal men
did." [4] Your greatest students are commonly no better, silly,
soft fellows in their outward behaviour, absurd, ridiculous to
others, and no whit experienced in worldly business; they can
measure the heavens, range over the world, teach others wisdom,
and yet in bargains and contracts they are circumvented by
every base tradesman. Are not these men fools? and how
should they be otherwise, "but as so many sots in schools,
when" (as he well observed [5]) "they neither hear nor see such
things as are commonly practised abroad"? how should they
get experience, by what means? "I knew in my time many
scholars," saith Æneas Sylvius (in an epistle of his to Gaspar
Schlick, chancellor to the emperor), "excellent well learned, but
so rude, so silly, that they had no common civility, nor knew
how to manage their domestic or public affairs. Paglarensis
was amazed, and said his farmer had surely cozened him, when
he heard him tell that his sow had eleven pigs, and his ass had
but one foal." [6] To say the best of this profession, I can give
no other testimony of them in general, than that of Pliny of
Isæus: "He is yet a scholar, than which kind of men there is
nothing so simple, so sincere, none better"; [7] they are most part
harmless, honest, upright, innocent, plain-dealing men.

Now because they are commonly subject to such hazards and inconveniences as dotage, madness, simplicity, etc., Jo. Voschius would have good scholars to be highly rewarded, and had in some extraordinary respect above other men, "to have greater privileges than the rest, that adventure themselves and abbreviate their lives for the public good." [1] But our patrons of learning are so far nowadays from respecting the Muses, and giving that honour to scholars, or reward, which they deserve and are allowed by those indulgent privileges of many noble princes, that after all their pains taken in the universities, cost and charge, expenses, irksome hours, laborious tasks, wearisome days, dangers, hazards (barred interim from all pleasures which other men have, mewed up like hawks all their lives), if they chance to wade through them, they shall in the end be rejected, contemned, and, which is their greatest misery, driven to their shifts, exposed to want, poverty, and beggary. Their familiar attendants are:

Pallentes morbi, luctus, curæque laborque,
Et metus, et malesuada fames, et turpis egestas,
Terribiles visu formæ. [2]

Grief, labour, care, pale sickness, miseries,
Fear, filthy poverty, hunger that cries,
Terrible monsters to be seen with eyes.

If there were nothing else to trouble them, the conceit of this alone were enough to make them all melancholy. Most other trades and professions, after some seven years' apprenticeship, are enabled by their craft to live of themselves. A merchant adventures his goods at sea, and though his hazard be great, yet if one ship return of four, he likely makes a saving voyage. An husbandman's gains are almost certain, *quibus ipse Jupiter nocere non potest* [whom Jove himself can't harm] ('tis Cato's hyperbole, a great husband himself [3]); only scholars methinks are most uncertain, unrespected, subject to all casualties, and hazards. For first, not one of a many proves to be a scholar, all are not capable and docile, *ex omni ligno non fit Mercurius* [4] [a figure of Mercury is not made out of every log]: we can make mayors and officers every year, but not scholars: kings can invest knights and barons, as Sigismund the emperor confessed; universities can give degrees; and *Tu quod es, e populo quilibet esse potest* [what you are any one can be]; but he, nor they, nor all the world, can give learning, make philosophers, artists, orators, poets. We can soon say, as Seneca well notes *O virum*

bonum! o divitem! point at a rich man, a good, a happy
man, a prosperous man, *sumptuose vestitum, calamistratum, bene
olentem* [a splendidly dressed man, a well-groomed man]; *magno
temporis impendio constat hæc laudatio, O virum literatum!*
but 'tis not so easily performed to find out a learned man.
Learning is not so quickly got; though they may be willing to
take pains, to that end sufficiently informed, and liberally
maintained by their patrons and parents, yet few can compass
it. Or if they be docile, yet all men's wills are not answerable
to their wits; they can apprehend, but will not take pains; they
are either seduced by bad companions, *vel in puellam impingunt,
vel in poculum* [or come to grief over women or wine], and so
spend their time to their friends' grief and their own undoings.
Or put case they be studious, industrious, of ripe wits, and
perhaps good capacities, then how many diseases of body and
mind must they encounter! No labour in the world like unto
study. It may be their temperature will not endure it, but
striving to be excellent, to know all, they lose health, wealth,
wit, life, and all. Let him yet happily escape all these hazards,
æreis intestinis, with a body of brass, and is now consummate and
ripe, he hath profited in his studies, and proceeded with all
applause: after many expenses, he is fit for preferment; where
shall he have it? he is as far to seek it as he was (after twenty
years' standing) at the first day of his coming to the university.
For what course shall he take, being now capable and ready?
The most parable and easy, and about which many are employed, is to teach a school, turn lecturer or curate, and for that
he shall have falconer's wages, ten pound per annum and his
diet, or some small stipend, so long as he can please his patron
or the parish; if they approve him not (for usually they do but
a year or two, as inconstant as they that cried "Hosanna" one
day, and "Crucify Him" the other[1]), serving-man-like, he must
go look a new master; if they do, what is his reward?

> *Hoc quoque te manet ut pueros elementa docentem
> Occupet extremis in vicis balba senectus.*[2]

> [At last thy stammering age in suburb schools,
> Shall toil in teaching boys their grammar rules.]

Like an ass, he wears out his time for provender, and can show
a stump rod, *togam tritam et laceram*, saith Hædus,[3] an old torn
gown, an ensign of his infelicity; he hath his labour for his
pain, a modicum to keep him till he be decrepit, and that is all.
Grammaticus non est felix [the schoolmaster is not a happy

man], etc. If he be a trencher-chaplain in a gentleman's house, as it befell Euphormio,[1] after some seven years' service, he may perchance have a living to the halves, or some small rectory with the mother of the maids at length, a poor kinswoman, or a cracked chambermaid, to have and to hold during the time of his life. But if he offend his good patron, or displease his lady mistress in the meantime,

> *Ducetur planta velut ictus ab Hercule Cacus,*
> *Poneturque foras, si quid tentaverit unquam*
> *Hiscere,*[2]

as Hercules did by Cacus, he shall be dragged forth of doors by the heels, away with him! If he bend his forces to some other studies, with an intent to be *a secretis* [private secretary] to some nobleman, or in such a place with an ambassador, he shall find that these persons rise like prentices one under another, and in so many tradesmen's shops, when the master is dead, the foreman of the shop commonly steps in his place. Now for poets, rhetoricians, historians, philosophers, mathematicians, sophisters, etc.,[3] they are like grasshoppers, sing they must in summer, and pine in the winter, for there is no preferment for them. Even so they were at first, if you will believe that pleasant tale of Socrates, which he told fair Phædrus under a plane-tree, at the banks of the river Ilissus. About noon, when it was hot, and the grasshoppers made a noise, he took that sweet occasion to tell him a tale, how grasshoppers were once scholars, musicians, poets, etc., before the Muses were born, and lived without meat and drink, and for that cause were turned by Jupiter into grasshoppers. And may be turned again, *in Tithoni cicadas, aut Lyciorum ranas* [into the grasshoppers of Tithonus or the frogs of the Lycians], for any reward I see they are like to have: or else, in the meantime, I would they could live, as they did, without any viaticum, like so many *manucodiatæ,*[4] those Indian birds of paradise, as we commonly call them, those, I mean, that live with the air and dew of heaven, and need no other food; for being as they are, their "rhetoric only serves them to curse their bad fortunes," [5] and many of them, for want of means, are driven to hard shifts; from grasshoppers they turn humble-bees and wasps, plain parasites, and make the Muses mules, to satisfy their hunger-starved paunches and get a meal's meat. To say truth, 'tis the common fortune of most scholars to be servile and poor, to complain pitifully, and lay open their wants to their respectless

patrons, as Cardan doth,[1] as Xylander[2] and many others; and,
which is too common in these dedicatory epistles, for hope of
gain to lie, flatter, and with hyperbolical elogiums and com-
mendations to magnify and extol an illiterate unworthy idiot
for his excellent virtues, whom they should rather, as Machiavel
observes, vilify and rail at downright for his most notorious
villainies and vices.[3] So they prostitute themselves, as fiddlers
or mercenary tradesmen, to serve great men's turns for a small
reward.   They are like Indians, they have store of gold, but
know not the worth of it:[4] for I am of Synesius' opinion, "King
Hiero got more by Simonides' acquaintance than Simonides
did by his";[5] they have their best education, good institution,
sole qualification from us, and when they have done well, their
honour and immortality from us; we are the living tombs,
registers, and as so many trumpeters of their fames: what
was Achilles without Homer? Alexander without Arrian and
Curtius? who had known the Cæsars, but for Suetonius and
Dion?

> *Vixerunt fortes ante Agamemnona*
> *Multi : sed omnes illacrimabiles*
> *Urgentur, ignotique longa*
> *Nocte, carent quia vate sacro.*[6]

> [Before great Agamemnon reign'd,
>   Reign'd kings as great as he, and brave,
> Whose huge ambition 's now contain'd
>   In the small compass of a grave:
> In endless night they sleep, unwept, unknown,
> No bard they had to make all time their own.]

They are more beholden to scholars, than scholars to them; but
they undervalue themselves, and so by those great men are kept
down.   Let them have that encyclopædian, all the learning in
the world; they must keep it to themselves, "live in base esteem,
and starve, except they will submit," as Budæus well hath it,
"so many good parts, so many ensigns of arts, virtues, be
slavishly obnoxious to some illiterate potentate, and live under
his insolent worship, or honour, like parasites,"[7] *qui tanquam
mures alienum panem comedunt* [who like mice eat other persons'
bread].   For to say truth, *artes hæ non sunt lucrativæ*, as
Guido Bonat, that great astrologer, could foresee, they be not
gainful arts these, *sed esurientes et famelicæ*, but poor and hungry.

> *Dat Galenus opes, dat Justinianus honores,*
> *Sed genus et species cogitur ire pedes.*[8]

> The rich physician, honour'd lawyers ride,
> Whilst the poor scholar foots it by their side.

Poverty is the Muses' patrimony, and as that poetical divinity
teacheth us, when Jupiter's daughters were each of them married
to the gods, the Muses alone were left solitary, Helicon forsaken
of all suitors, and I believe it was because they had no portion.

> *Calliope longum cælebs cur vixit in ævum?*
> *Nempe nihil dotis, quod numeraret, erat.*

> Why did Calliope live so long a maid?
> Because she had no dowry to be paid.

Ever since all their followers are poor, forsaken, and left unto
themselves; insomuch that, as Petronius argues, you shall
likely know them by their clothes. "There came," saith he,
"by chance into my company, a fellow not very spruce to look
on, that I could perceive by that note alone he was a scholar,
whom commonly rich men hate. I asked him what he was; he
answered, a poet. I demanded again why he was so ragged; he
told me this kind of learning never made any man rich." [1]

> *Qui pelago credit, magno se fænore tollit,*
> *Qui pugnas et rostra petit, præcingitur auro:*
> *Vilis adulator picto jacet ebrius ostro,*
> *Sola pruinosis horret facundia pannis.*

> A merchant's gain is great, that goes to sea;
> A soldier embossed all in gold;
> A flatterer lies fox'd in brave array;
> A scholar only ragged to behold.

All which our ordinary students, right well perceiving in the
universities, how unprofitable these poetical, mathematical, and
philosophical studies are, how little respected, how few patrons,
apply themselves in all haste to those three commodious professions of law, physic, and divinity, sharing themselves between
them, rejecting these arts in the meantime, history, philosophy,
philology, or lightly passing them over, as pleasant toys fitting
only table-talk, and to furnish them with discourse. [3] They
are not so behoveful: he that can tell his money hath arithmetic
enough: he is a true geometrician, can measure out a good fortune to himself; a perfect astrologer, that can cast the rise and
fall of others, and mark their errant motions to his own use.
The best optics are, to reflect the beams of some great men's
favour and grace to shine upon him. He is a good engineer
that alone can make an instrument to get preferment. This
was the common tenent and practice of Poland, as Cromerus
observed not long since, in the first book of his history; their

universities were generally base, not a philosopher, a mathematician, an antiquary, etc., to be found of any note amongst them, because they had no set reward or stipend, but every man betook himself to divinity, *hoc solum in votis habens, opimum sacerdotium*, a good parsonage was their aim. This was the practice of some of our near neighbours, as Lipsius inveighs;[1] "they thrust their children to the study of law and divinity, before they be informed aright, or capable of such studies." *Scilicet omnibus artibus antistat spes lucri, et formosior est cumulus auri, quam quicquid Græci Latinique delirantes scripserunt. Ex hoc numero deinde veniunt ad gubernacula reipub., intersunt et præsunt consiliis regum. O pater, o patria!* [The prospect of gain outweighs all studies, and a heap of money is more attractive than all the stuff written by the Greek and Latin authors. From this class we draw the leaders of the State, the counsellors and guides of kings. What a world!] So he complained, and so may others. For even so we find, to serve a great man, to get an office in some bishop's court (to practise in some good town), or compass a benefice, is the mark we shoot at, as being so advantageous, the highway to preferment.

Although many times, for aught I can see, these men fail as often as the rest in their projects, and are as usually frustrate of their hopes. For let him be a doctor of the law, an excellent civilian of good worth, where shall he practise and expatiate? Their fields are so scant, the civil law with us so contracted with prohibitions, so few causes, by reason of those all-devouring municipal laws, *quibus nihil illiteratius*, saith Erasmus,[2] an illiterate and a barbarous study (for though they be never so well learned in it, I can hardly vouchsafe them the name of scholars, except they be otherwise qualified), and so few courts are left to the profession, such slender offices, and those commonly to be compassed at such dear rates, that I know not how an ingenuous man should thrive amongst them. Now for physicians, there are in every village so many mountebanks, empirics, quacksalvers, Paracelsians, as they call themselves, *causifici et sanicidæ* [makers of pretexts and killers of healthy people], so Clenard terms them,[3] wizards, alchemists, poor vicars, cast apothecaries, physicians' men, barbers, and goodwives, professing great skill, that I make great doubt how they shall be maintained, or who shall be their patients. Besides, there are so many of both sorts, and some of them such harpies, so covetous, so clamorous, so impudent; and as he said,[4] litigious idiots,

Quibus loquacis affatim arrogantiæ est,
  Peritiæ parum aut nihil,
Nec ulla mica literarii salis,
  Crumenimulga natio :
Loquuteleia turba, litium strophæ,
  Maligna litigantium
Cohors, togati vultures,
  Lavernæ alumni, agyrtæ, etc.

Which have no skill but prating arrogance,
  No learning, such a purse-milking nation:
Gown'd vultures, thieves, and a litigious rout
  Of cozeners, that haunt this occupation, etc.

that they cannot well tell how to live one by another, but (as he jested in the comedy of clocks, they were so many), *major pars populi arida reptant fame,*[1] they are almost starved a great part of them, and ready to devour their fellows, *et noxia calliditate se corrupere*[2] [and become addicted to a mischievous cunning], such a multitude of pettifoggers and empirics, such impostors, that an honest man knows not in what sort to compose and behave himself in their society, to carry himself with credit in so vile a rout, *scientiæ nomen, tot sumptibus partum et vigiliis, profiteri dispudeat, postquam* [he is ashamed to lay claim to learning, which he has acquired with so much expense and trouble, now that], etc.

Last of all to come to our divines, the most noble profession and worthy of double honour, but of all others the most distressed and miserable. If you will not believe me, hear a brief of it, as it was not many years since publicly preached at Paul's Cross, by a grave minister then, and now a reverend bishop of this land:[3] "We that are bred up in learning, and destined by our parents to this end, we suffer our childhood in the grammar-school, which Austin calls *magnum tyrannidem, et grave malum* [a great despotism, a terrible evil], and compares it to the torments of martyrdom; when we come to the university, if we live of the college allowance, as Phalaris objected to the Leontines, παντῶν ἐνδεεῖς πλὴν λιμοῦ καὶ φόβου, needy of all things but hunger and fear, or if we be maintained but partly by our parents' cost, do expend in unnecessary maintenance, books, and degrees, before we come to any perfection, five hundred pounds, or a thousand marks. If by this price of the expense of time, our bodies and spirits, our substance and patrimonies, we cannot purchase those small rewards which are ours by law, and the right of inheritance, a poor parsonage, or a vicarage of £50 per annum, but we must pay to the patron

for the lease of a life (a spent and outworn life) either in annual
pension, or above the rate of a copyhold, and that with the
hazard and loss of our souls, by simony and perjury, and the
forfeiture of all our spiritual preferments, in *esse* and *posse*,
both present and to come. What father after a while will be
so improvident to bring up his son, to his great charge, to this
necessary beggary? What Christian will be so irreligious to
bring up his son in that course of life, which by all probability
and necessity *coget ad turpia*, enforcing to sin, will entangle
him in simony and perjury, when, as the poet said, *Invitatus
ad hæc aliquis de ponte negabit:* a beggar's brat taken from the
bridge where he sits a-begging, if he knew the inconvenience,
had cause to refuse it." This being thus, have not we fished
fair all this while, that are initiate divines, to find no better
fruits of our labours? *Hoc est cur palles? cur quis non prandeat
hoc est?* [1] [Is it for this we have pale faces and do without our
breakfasts?] Do we macerate ourselves for this? Is it for this
we rise so early all the year long, "leaping" (as he saith) "out of
our beds, when we hear the bell ring, as if we had heard a
thunderclap?" [2] If this be all the respect, reward and honour
we shall have, *Frange leves calamos, et scinde, Thalia, libellos* [3]
[break your pens, Thalia, and tear up your books], let us give
over our books, and betake ourselves to some other course of
life. To what end should we study? *Quid me litterulas stulti
docuere parentes?* [4] What did our parents mean to make us
scholars, to be as far to seek of preferment after twenty years'
study, as we were at first? Why do we take such pains? *Quid
tantum insanis juvant impallescere chartis?* [Why lose the colour
of our youthful age By constant bending o'er the stupid page?]
If there be no more hope of reward, no better encouragement,
I say again, *Frange leves calamos, et scinde, Thalia, libellos;* let 's
turn soldiers, sell our books and buy swords, guns, and pikes,
or stop bottles with them, turn our philosophers' gowns, as
Cleanthes once did, into millers' coats, leave all, and rather
betake ourselves to any other course of life than to continue
longer in this misery. *Præstat dentiscalpia radere, quam literariis
monumentis magnatum favorem emendicare* [5] [it is better to sharpen
toothpicks than to beg the favour of the great with literary
productions].

Yea, but methinks I hear some man except at these words,
that though this be true which I have said of the estate of
scholars, and especially of divines, that it is miserable and
distressed at this time, that the Church suffers shipwreck of

her goods, and that they have just cause to complain; there is a fault, but whence proceeds it? If the cause were justly examined, it would be retorted upon ourselves; if we were cited at that tribunal of truth, we should be found guilty, and not able to excuse it. That there is a fault among us, I confess, and were there not a buyer, there would not be a seller: but to him that will consider better of it, it will more than manifestly appear that the fountain of these miseries proceeds from these griping patrons. In accusing them, I do not altogether excuse us; both are faulty, they and we: yet in my judgment, theirs is the greater fault, more apparent causes, and much to be condemned. For my part, if it be not with me as I would, or as it should, I do ascribe the cause, as Cardan did in the like case,[1] *meo infortunio potius quam illorum sceleri*, to mine own infelicity rather than their naughtiness:[2] although I have been baffled in my time by some of them, and have as just cause to complain as another: or rather indeed to mine own negligence; for I was ever like that Alexander in Plutarch,[3] Crassus his tutor in philosophy, who, though he lived many years familiarly with rich Crassus, was even as poor when from (which many wondered at), as when he came first to him; he never asked, the other never gave anything; when he travelled with Crassus he borrowed a hat of him, at his return restored it again. I have had some such noble friends' acquaintance, and scholars', but most part (common courtesies and ordinary respects excepted), they and I parted as we met, they gave me as much as I requested, and that was—— And as Alexander ab Alexandro, *Genial. dier. lib.* 6, *cap.* 16, made answer to Hieronymus Massianus, that wondered, *quum plures ignavos et ignobiles ad dignitates et sacerdotia promotos quotidie videret* [when he saw many indolent and unworthy persons daily promoted to high posts in the State and the Church], when the other men rose, still he was in the same state, *eodem tenore et fortuna, cui mercedem laborum studiorumque deberi putaret*, whom he thought to deserve as well as the rest; he made answer that he was content with his present estate, was not ambitious, and although *objurgabundus suam segnitiem accusaret, cum obscuræ sortis homines ad sacerdotia et pontificatus evectos*, etc., he chid him for his backwardness, yet he was still the same: and for my part, though I be not worthy perhaps to carry Alexander's books, yet by some overweening and well-wishing friends the like speeches have been used to me; but I replied still with Alexander, that I had enough, and more peradventure than I deserved; and with Libanius Sophista, that rather chose (when honours and offices by the emperor were offered unto him) to be *talis sophista, quam talis magistratus* [such a sophist as he was than such a magistrate as others were], I had as lief be still Democritus Junior, and *privus privatus, si mihi jam daretur optio, quam talis fortasse doctor, talis dominus* [an obscure individual, if I had the choice, than a doctor of divinity or a bishop]. *Sed quorsum hæc?* [But why do I say all this?] For the rest 'tis on both sides *facinus detestandum* [a detestable crime] to buy and sell livings, to detain from the Church that which God's and men's laws have bestowed on it; but in them most, and that from the covetousness and ignorance of such as are interested in this business; I name covetousness in the first place, as the root of all these mischiefs, which, Achan-like, compels them to commit sacrilege, and to make simoniacal compacts (and what not), to their own ends, that kindles God's wrath,[1] brings a plague, vengeance, and an heavy visitation upon themselves and others. Some, out of that insatiable desire of filthy lucre, to be enriched, care not how they come by it, *per fas et nefas*, hook or crook, so they have it. And others, when they have with riot and prodigality embezzled their estates, to recover themselves, make a prey of the Church, robbing it, as Julian the Apostate did,[2] spoil parsons of their revenues (in keeping half back, as a great man amongst us observes [3]), "and that maintenance on which they should live": by means whereof, barbarism is increased, and a great decay of Christian professors: for who will apply himself to these divine studies, his son, or friend, when, after great pains taken, they shall have nothing whereupon to live? But with what event do they these things?

> *Opesque totis viribus venamini,*
> *At inde messis accidit miserrima.*[4]

[You hunt for wealth with all your might, but reap a most wretched reward.]

They toil and moil, but what reap they? They are commonly unfortunate families that use it, accursed in their progeny, and, as common experience evinceth, accursed themselves in all their proceedings. "With what face" (as he [5] quotes out of Austin) "can they expect a blessing or inheritance from Christ in heaven, that defraud Christ of His inheritance here on earth?" I would all our simoniacal patrons, and such as detain tithes, would read those judicious tracts of Sir Henry Spelman and Sir James Sempill, knights; those late elaborate and learned treatises of

Dr. Tillesley, and Mr. Montague, which they have written of that subject. But though they should read, it would be to small purpose, *clames licet et mare cœlo confundas*; thunder, lighten, preach hell and damnation, tell them 'tis a sin, they will not believe it; denounce and terrify, "they have cauterized consciences,"[1] they do not attend; as the enchanted adder, they stop their ears. Call them base, irreligious, profane, barbarous, pagans, atheists, epicures (as some of them surely are), with the bawd in Plautus, *Euge! optime!* [Bravo! excellent!] they cry, and applaud themselves with that miser, *Simul ac nummos contemplor in arca*[2] [As soon as I see the money in the strong-box . . .]; say what you will, *quocunque modo rem* [however you get it, money]; as a dog barks at the moon, to no purpose are your sayings: take your heaven, let them have money. A base, profane, epicurean, hypocritical rout: for my part, let them pretend what zeal they will, counterfeit religion, blear the world's eyes, bombast themselves, and stuff out their greatness with church spoils, shine like so many peacocks; so cold is my charity, so defective in this behalf, that I shall never think better of them, than that they are rotten at core, their bones are full of epicurean hypocrisy, and atheistical marrow, they are worse than heathens. For, as Dionysius Halicarnasseus observes, *Antiq. Rom. lib. 7, Primum locum*, etc.,[3] "Greeks and barbarians observe all religious rites, and dare not break them for fear of offending their gods"; but our simoniacal contractors, our senseless Achans, our stupefied patrons, fear neither God nor devil, they have evasions for it, it is no sin, or not due *jure divino* [by divine law], or if a sin, no great sin, etc. And though they be daily punished for it, and they do manifestly perceive that, as he said, frost and fraud come to foul ends, yet, as Chrysostom[4] follows it, *Nulla ex pœna sit correctio, et quasi adversis malitia hominum provocetur, crescit quotidie quod puniatur* [correction brings no improvement, and, as if to spite the lawgiver, the crime which is punished becomes more common]: they are rather worse than better, *iram atque animos a crimine sumunt* [the very commission of the crime makes them more daring], and the more they are corrected, the more they offend: but let them take their course, *Rode, caper, vites*[5] [nibble away, goat, at the vines], go on still as they begin, 'tis no sin, let them rejoice secure, God's vengeance will overtake them in the end, and these ill-gotten goods, as an eagle's feathers, will consume the rest of their substance;[6] it is *aurum Tholosanum*[7] [gold of Toulouse (i.e. plundered)], and will

produce no better effects. "Let them lay it up safe, and make
their conveyances never so close, lock and shut door," saith
Chrysostom, "yet fraud and covetousness, two most violent
thieves, are still included, and a little gain evil-gotten will
subvert the rest of their goods."[1]   The eagle in Æsop, seeing a
piece of flesh, now ready to be sacrificed, swept it away with
her claws, and carried it to her nest; but there was a burning
coal stuck to it by chance, which unawares consumed her young
ones, nest, and all together.   Let our simoniacal church-chopping
patrons and sacrilegious harpies look for no better success.

A second cause is ignorance, and from thence contempt;
successit odium in literas ab ignorantia vulgi [learning has become
odious through the ignorance of the public], which Junius
well perceived:[2] this hatred and contempt of learning proceeds
out of ignorance;[3] as they are themselves barbarous, idiots,
dull, illiterate, and proud, so they esteem of others. *Sint
Mæcenates, non deerunt, Flacce, Marones:* let there be bountiful
patrons, and there will be painful scholars in all sciences.   But
when they contemn learning, and think themselves sufficiently
qualified, if they can write and read, scramble at a piece of
evidence, or have so much Latin as that emperor[4] had: *Qui
nescit dissimulare, nescit vivere* [he who cannot dissemble cannot
live], they are unfit to do their country service, to perform or
undertake any action or employment which may tend to the
good of a commonwealth, except it be to fight, or to do country
justice with common sense, which every yeoman can likewise
do.   And so they bring up their children, rude as they are
themselves, unqualified, untaught, uncivil most part. *Quis e
nostra juventute legitime instituitur literis? Quis oratores aut
philosophos tangit? Quis historiam legit, illam rerum agendarum
quasi animam? Præcipitant parentes vota sua*[5] [Which of our
youths is properly trained in literature?   Which of them knows
anything of the orators or philosophers?   Who reads history,
the inspiration of public activity?   Parents are in too great a
hurry], etc., 'twas Lipsius' complaint to his illiterate countrymen, it may be ours.   Now shall these men judge of a scholar's
worth, that have no worth, that know not what belongs to a
student's labours, that cannot distinguish between a true
scholar and a drone? or him that by reason of a voluble tongue,
a strong voice, a pleasing tone, and some trivantly polyanthean
helps, steals and gleans a few notes from other men's harvests,
and so makes a fairer show than he that is truly learned indeed:
that thinks it no more to preach than to speak, "or to run away

with an empty cart," as a grave man said: [1] and thereupon vilify
us and our pains; scorn us and all learning. Because they
are rich, and have other means to live, they think it concerns
them not to know, or to trouble themselves with it; [2] a fitter
task for younger brothers, or poor men's sons, to be pen and
inkhorn men, pedantical slaves, and no whit beseeming the
calling of a gentleman; as Frenchmen and Germans commonly
do, neglect therefore all human learning, what have they to do
with it? Let mariners learn astronomy; merchants' factors
study arithmetic; surveyors get them geometry; spectacle-
makers optic; landleapers geography; town-clerks rhetoric;
what should he do with a spade, that hath no ground to dig;
or they with learning, that have no use of it? Thus they reason,
and are not ashamed to let mariners, prentices, and the
basest servants be better qualified than themselves. In former
times, kings, princes, and emperors were the only scholars,
excellent in all faculties.

Julius Cæsar mended the year, and writ his own Commentaries:

Media inter prælia semper,
Stellarum cœlique plagis, superisque vacavit.[3]

[In the midst of warfare he found time to study the
stars, the heavens, and the upper world.]

Antonius, Hadrian, Nero, Severus, Julian, etc.,[4] Michael the
emperor, and Isacius [5] were so much given to their studies that no
base fellow would take so much pains; Orion, Perseus, Alphonsus,
Ptolemæus, famous astronomers; Sabor, Mithridates, Lysimachus,
admired physicians; Plato's kings all; Evax, that Arabian
prince, a most expert jeweller and an exquisite philosopher;
the kings of Egypt were priests of old, and chosen from thence
—*Idem rex hominum Phœbique sacerdos* [both king he was of
men and priest to Phœbus]; but those heroical times are past;
the Muses are now banished in this bastard age *ad sordida
tuguriola* [to mean hovels], to meaner persons, and confined
alone almost to universities. In those days, scholars were
highly beloved, honoured,[6] esteemed; as old Ennius by Scipio
Africanus, Virgil by Augustus, Horace by Mæcenas: princes'
companions; dear to them, as Anacreon to Polycrates, Philoxenus to Dionysius, and highly rewarded. Alexander sent Xenocrates the philosopher fifty talents, because he was poor; *visu
rerum, aut eruditione præstantes viri, mensis olim regum adhibiti*
[men notable for foresight or learning formerly sat at table
with kings], as Philostratus relates of Hadrian and Lampridius

of Alexander Severus: famous clerks came to these princes'
courts, *velut in Lyceum*, as to an university, and were admitted
to their tables, *quasi divum epulis accumbentes* [as though being
entertained at feasts of the gods]; Archelaus, that Macedonian
king, would not willingly sup without Euripides (amongst the
rest he drank to him at supper one night and gave him a cup
of gold for his pains), *delectatus poetæ suavi sermone* [charmed
with the poet's delightful conversation]; and it was fit it should
be so, because, as Plato in his *Protagoras* well saith, a good
philosopher as much excels other men as a great king doth the
commons of his country;[1] and again, *quoniam illis nihil deest,
et minime egere solent, et disciplinas quas profitentur, soli a contemptu vindicare possunt*[2] [since they lack nothing and have
few wants, and alone are able to inspire respect for the arts
which they profess], they needed not to beg so basely, as they
compel scholars in our times to complain of poverty,[3] or crouch
to a rich chuff for a meal's meat, but could vindicate themselves, and those arts which they professed.   Now they would
and cannot: for it is held by some of them as an axiom, that
to keep them poor will make them study; they must be dieted,
as horses to a race, not pampered, *alendos volunt, non saginandos,
ne melioris mentis flammula extinguatur*[4] [they want them to
be fed, not stuffed, lest the spark of genius in them should be
extinguished]; a fat bird will not sing, a fat dog cannot hunt,
and so by this depression of theirs, some want means,[5] others
will, all want encouragement,[6] as being forsaken almost; and
generally contemned.   'Tis an old saying, *Sint Mæcenates, non
deerunt, Flacce, Marones* [let there be patrons like Mæcenas,
there will be poets like Virgil], and 'tis a true saying still.
Yet oftentimes, I may not deny it, the main fault is in ourselves.   Our academics too frequently offend in neglecting
patrons, as Erasmus well taxeth,[7] or making ill choice of them;
negligimus oblatos aut amplectimur parum aptos [we neglect
them when they offer themselves, or we cling to those that
are unsuitable], or if we get a good one, *non studemus mutuis
officiis favorem ejus alere*, we do not ply and follow him as we
should.   *Idem mihi accidit adolescenti* [this happened to me
when I was a young man] (saith Erasmus, acknowledging his
fault), *et gravissime peccavi*, and I made a very serious mistake,
and so may I say myself,[8] I have offended in this, and so
peradventure have many others.   We did not *respondere magnatum favoribus, qui cœperunt nos amplecti* [respond to the
favours of the great, who began to take us up], apply ourselves

with that readiness we should: idleness, love of liberty (*Immo-dicus amor libertatis effecit ut diu cum perfidis amicis*, as he con-fesseth, *et pertinaci paupertate colluctarer* [through an excessive love of liberty, I had for a long time to struggle with false friends and poverty]), bashfulness, melancholy, timorousness, cause many of us to be too backward and remiss. So some offend in one extreme, but too many on the other, we are most part too forward, too solicitous, too ambitious, too impudent; we commonly complain *deesse Mæcenates*, of want of encourage-ment, want of means, whenas the true defect is in our want of worth, our insufficiency. Did Mæcenas take notice of Horace or Virgil till they had shown themselves first? or had Bavius and Mævius any patrons? *Egregium specimen dent*, saith Erasmus, let them approve themselves worthy first, sufficiently qualified for learning and manners, before they presume or impudently intrude and put themselves on great men as too many do; with such base flattery, parasitical colloguing, such hyperbolical elogies they do usually insinuate, that it is a shame to hear and see. *Immodicæ laudes conciliant invidiam, potius quam laudem* [excessive praise brings envy rather than fame], and vain com-mendations derogate from truth, and we think in conclusion *non melius de laudato, pejus de laudante*, ill of both, the com-mender and commended. So we offend, but the main fault is in their harshness, defect of patrons. How beloved of old, and how much respected was Plato to Dionysius! How dear to Alexander was Aristotle, Demaratus to Philip, Solon to Crœsus, Anaxarchus and Trebatius to Augustus, Cassius to Vespasian, Plutarch to Trajan, Seneca to Nero, Simonides to Hiero! how honoured!

> *Sed hæc prius fuere, nunc recondita*
> *Senent quiete,*[1]

[But all this was in the past, now it is gone and forgotten,]

those days are gone;

> *Et spes et ratio studiorum in Cæsare tantum:*[2]

> [Nor hope have we or any cause to study,
> Save in great Cæsar:]

as he said of old, we may truly say now; he is our amulet, our sun,[3] our sole comfort and refuge, our Ptolemy, our common Mæcenas, *Jacobus munificus, Jacobus pacificus, mysta Musarum, rex Platonicus* [James the munificent, James the pacific, the votary of the Muses, the Platonic king], *Grande decus, columenque nostrum* [our great and crowning glory], a famous scholar himself, and the sole patron, pillar, and sustainer of learning: but his worth in this kind is so well known, that as Paterculus of Cato, *Jam ipsum laudare nefas sit* [praise itself would be impiety]: and which Pliny to Trajan,[1] *Seria te carmina, honorque æternus annalium, non hæc brevis et pudenda prædicatio colet* [Your glory will be enshrined in solemn epics and immortal histories, not in this fleeting and worthless oration]. But he is now gone, the sun of ours set, and yet no night follows, *Sol occubuit, nox nulla secuta est.* We have such another in his room, *aureus alter. Avulsus, simili frondescit virga metallo* [2] [when the first is plucked, another bough appears likewise of gold], and long may he reign and flourish amongst us.

Let me not be malicious, and lie against my genius; I may not deny but that we have a sprinkling of our gentry, here and there one, excellently well learned, like those Fuggeri in Germany; Du Bartas, Du Plessis, Sadael, in France; Picus Mirandula, Schottus, Barocius, in Italy; *Apparent rari nantes in gurgite vasto* [Some scattered swimmers in the vasty deep]. But they are but few in respect of the multitude, the major part (and some again excepted, that are indifferent) are wholly bent for hawks and hounds, and carried away many times with intemperate lust, gaming, and drinking. If they read a book at any time (*si quod est interim otii a venatu, poculis, alea, scortis* [if there is any time which they can spare from hunting, drinking, gambling, and women]) 'tis an English Chronicle, Sir Huon of Bordeaux, Amadis de Gaul, etc., a play-book, or some pamphlet of news, and that at such seasons only, when they cannot stir abroad, to drive away time, their sole discourse is dogs, hawks, horses, and what news? [3] If someone have been a traveller in Italy, or as far as the emperor's court, wintered in Orleans, and can court his mistress in broken French, wear his clothes neatly in the newest fashion, sing some choice outlandish tunes, discourse of lords, ladies, towns, palaces, and cities, he is complete and to be admired: otherwise he and they are much at one; [4] no difference between the master and the man, but worshipful titles: wink and choose betwixt him that sits down (clothes excepted) and him that holds the trencher behind him: yet these men must be our patrons, our governors too sometimes, statesmen, magistrates, noble, great, and wise by inheritance.

Mistake me not (I say again), *Vos, o patricius sanguis*, you that are worthy senators, gentlemen, I honour your names and persons, and with all submissiveness prostrate myself to your

censure and service. There are amongst you, I do ingenuously
confess, many well-deserving patrons and true patriots of my
knowledge, besides many hundreds which I never saw, no
doubt, or heard of, pillars of our commonwealth, whose worth,
bounty, learning, forwardness, true zeal in religion, and good
esteem of all scholars ought to be consecrated to all posterity; [1]
but of your rank, there are a debauched, corrupt, covetous,
illiterate crew again, no better than stocks, *merum pecus (testor
Deum, non mihi videri dignos ingenui hominis appellatione*)
[mere animals (as God lives, I do not think them worthy to
be called real human beings)], barbarous Thracians, *et quis ille
Thrax qui hoc neget?* [and what Thracian would deny this?],
a sordid, profane, pernicious company, irreligious, impudent,
and stupid, I know not what epithets to give them, enemies to
learning, confounders of the Church, and the ruin of a commonwealth; patrons they are by right of inheritance, and put in
trust freely to dispose of such livings to the Church's good; but
(hard taskmasters they prove) they take away their straw, and
compel them to make their number of brick; they commonly
respect their own ends, commodity is the steer of all their
actions, and him they present in conclusion as a man of greatest
gifts, that will give most; no penny, no paternoster,[2] as the
saying is. *Nisi preces auro fulcias, amplius irritas* [unless you
support your suit with gold, you merely vex them]; *ut Cerberus
offa*, their attendants and officers must be bribed, fee'd, and
made, as Cerberus is with a sop by him that goes to hell. It
was an old saying, *Omnia Romæ venalia* [all things are for sale at
Rome], 'tis a rag of Popery, which will never be rooted out,
there is no hope, no good to be done without money. A clerk
may offer himself, approve his worth, learning, honesty, religion,
zeal,[3] they will commend him for it; but *probitas laudatur et
alget*[4] [virtue is praised and left to freeze]. If he be a man of
extraordinary parts, they will flock afar off to hear him, as they
did in Apuleius, to see Psyche: *Multi mortales confluebant ad
videndum sæculi decus, speculum gloriosum; laudatur ab omnibus,
spectatur ob omnibus, nec quisquam non rex, non regius, cupidus
ejus nuptiarum, petitor accedit; mirantur quidem divinam formam
omnes, sed ut similacrum fabre politum mirantur:* many mortal
men came to see fair Psyche, the glory of her age, they did admire
her, commend, desire her for her divine beauty, and gaze upon
her; but as on a picture; none would marry her, *quod indotata*
[because she had no dowry]; fair Psyche had no money. So
they do by learning: [5]

Didicit jam dives avarus
Tantum admirari, tantum laudare disertos,
Ut pueri Junonis avem [1]

Your rich men have now learn'd of latter days
    T' admire, commend, and come together
To hear and see a worthy scholar speak,
    As children do a peacock's feather.

He shall have all the good words that may be given, "a proper man, and 'tis pity he hath no preferment," [2] all good wishes, but inexorable, indurate as he is, he will not prefer him, though it be in his power, because he is *indotatus*, he hath no money. Or if he do give him entertainment, let him be never so well qualified, plead affinity, consanguinity, sufficiency, he shall serve seven years, as Jacob did for Rachel, before he shall have it. If he will enter at first, he must yet in at that simoniacal gate, come off soundly, and put in good security to perform all covenants, else he will not deal with, or admit him. [3] But if some poor scholar, some parson chaff, will offer himself; some trencher-chaplain, that will take it to the halves, thirds, or accept of what he will give, he is welcome; be conformable, preach as he will have him, he likes him before a million of others; for the best is always best cheap: and then, as Hierome said to Chromatius, *patella dignum operculum* [the lid is worthy of the pan], such a patron, such a clerk; the cure is well supplied, and all parties pleased. So that is still verified in our age, which Chrysostom complained of in his time: *Qui opulentiores sunt, in ordinem parasitorum cogunt eos, et ipsos tanquam canes ad mensas suas enutriunt, corumque impudentes ventres iniquarum cœnarum reliquiis differciunt, iisdem pro arbitrio abutentes:* [4] rich men keep these lecturers and fawning parasites like so many dogs at their tables, and filling their hungry guts with the offals of their meat, they abuse tham at their pleasure, and make them say what they propose. "As children do by a bird or a butterfly in a string, pull in and let him out as they list, do they by their trencher-chaplains, prescribe, command their wits, let in and out as to them it seems best." [5] If the patron be precise, so must his chaplain be; if he be papistical, his clerk must be so, or else be turned out. These are those clerks which serve the turn, whom they commonly entertain and present to church livings, whilst in the meantime we that are university men, like so many hide-bound calves in a pasture, tarry out our time, wither away as a flower ungathered in a garden, and are never used; or, as so many candles, illuminate ourselves alone, obscuring one another's light, and are not discerned here at all, the least of which, translated to a dark room, or to some country benefice, where it might shine apart, would give a fair light and be seen over all. Whilst we lie waiting here, as those sick men did at the Pool of Bethesda,[1] till the angel stirred the water, expecting a good hour, they step between, and beguile us of our preferment. I have not yet said. If after long expectation, much expense, travel, earnest suit of ourselves and friends, we obtain a small benefice at last, our misery begins afresh; we are suddenly encountered with the flesh, world, and devil, with a new onset; we change a quiet life for an ocean of troubles, we come to a ruinous house, which, before it be habitable, must be necessarily to our great damage repaired; we are compelled to sue for dilapidations, or else sued ourselves, and scarce yet settled, we are called upon for our predecessors' arrearages; first-fruits, tenths, subsidies, are instantly to be paid, benevolence, procurations, etc., and, which is most to be feared, we light upon a cracked title, as it befell Clenard of Brabant, for his rectory and charge of his Beginæ; he was no sooner inducted, but instantly sued, *cœpimusque* (saith he[2]) *strenue litigare, et implacabili bello confligere* [we were at once involved in a tough lawsuit, and had to fight tooth and nail]; at length, after ten years' suit, as long as Troy's siege, when he had tired himself and spent his money, he was fain to leave all for quietness' sake, and give it up to his adversary. Or else we are insulted over and trampled on by domineering officers, fleeced by those greedy harpies to get more fees; we stand in fear of some precedent lapse; we fall amongst refractory, seditious sectaries, peevish puritans, perverse papists, a lascivious rout of atheistical epicures, that will not be reformed, or some litigious people (those wild beasts of Ephesus must be fought with) that will not pay their dues without much repining, or compelled by long suit; for *Laici clericis oppido infesti* [the laity hate the clergy], an old axiom; all they think well gotten that is had from the Church, and by such uncivil, harsh dealings they make their poor minister weary of his place, if not his life; and put case they be quiet, honest men, make the best of it, as often it falls out, from a polite and terse academic he must turn rustic, rude, melancholize alone, learn to forget, or else, as many do, become maltsters, graziers, chapmen, etc. (now banished from the academy, all commerce of the Muses, and confined to a country village, as Ovid was from Rome to Pontus), and daily converse with a company of idiots and clowns.

*Nos interim quod attinet (nec enim immunes ab hac noxa sumus)
idem reatus manet, idem nobis, et si non multo gravius, crimen
objici potest: nostra enim culpa sit, nostra incuria, nostra avaritia,
quod tam frequentes fœdæque fiant* in *Ecclesia nundinationes*
(templum est venale, deusque), *tot sordes invehantur, tanta
grassetur impietas, tanta nequitia, tam insanus miseriarum
euripus, et turbarum æstuarium, nostro, inquam, omnium
(academicorum imprimis) vitio sit. Quod tot respublica malis
afficiatur, a nobis seminarium; ultro malum hoc accersimus, et
quavis contumelia, quavis interim miseria digni, qui pro virili non
occurrimus. Quid enim fieri posse speramus, quum tot indies
sine delectu pauperes alumni, terræ filii, et cujuscunque ordinis
homunciones, ad gradus certatim admittantur? qui si definitionem,
distinctionemque unam aut alteram memoriter edidicerint, et
pro more tot annos in dialectica posuerint, non refert quo pro-
fectu, quales demum sint, idiotæ, nugatores, otiatores, aleatores,
compotores, indigni, libidinis voluptatumque administri,* Sponsi
Penelopes, nebulones, Alcinoique, *modo tot annos in academia
insumpserint, et se pro togatis venditarint; lucri causa, et amicorum
intercessu præsentantur: addo etiam et magnificis nonnunquam
elogiis morum et scientiæ; et jam valedicturi testimonialibus hisce
literis, amplissime conscriptis in eorum gratiam honorantur, ab
iis qui fidei suæ et existimationis jacturam proculdubio faciunt.*
Doctores enim et professores (*quod ait ille* [1]) id unum curant, ut
ex professionibus frequentibus, et tumultuariis potius quam
legitimis, commoda sua promoveant, et ex dispendio publico
suum faciant incrementum. *Id solum in votis habent annui
plerumque magistratus, ut ab incipientium numero pecunias
emungant,* [2] *nec multum interest qui sint, literatores an literati,
modo pingues, nitidi, ad aspectum speciosi, et quod verbo dicam,
pecuniosi sint. Philosophastri licentiantur in artibus, artem qui
non habent,* [3] eosque sapientes esse jubent, qui nulla prædити
sunt sapientia, et nihil ad gradum præterquam velle adferunt. [4]
*Theologastri (solvant modo), satis superque docti, per omnes
honorum gradus evehuntur et ascendunt. Atque hinc fit quod tam
viles scurræ, tot passim idiotæ, literarum crepusculo positi, larvæ
pastorum, circumforanei, vagi, barbi, fungi, crassi, asini, merum
pecus, in sacrosanctos theologiæ aditus illotis pedibus irrumpant,
præter inverecundam frontem adferentes nihil, vulgares quasdam
quisquilias, et scholarium quædam nugamenta, indigna quæ vel
recipiantur in triviis. Hoc illud indignum genus hominum et
famelicum, indigum, vagum, ventris mancipium, ad stivam potius
relegandum, ad haras aptius quam ad aras, quod divinas hasce*

literas turpiter prostituit; hi sunt qui pulpita complent, in ædes nobilium irrepunt, et quum reliquis vitæ destituantur subsidiis, ob corporis et animi egestatem, aliarum in repub. partium minime capaces sint; ad sacram hanc ancoram confugiunt, sacerdotium quovismodo captantes, non ex sinceritate, quod Paulus ait,[1] sed cauponantes verbum Dei. *Ne quis interim viris bonis detractum quid putet, quos habet Ecclesia Anglicana quamplurimos, egregie doctos, illustres, intactæ famæ homines, et plures forsan quam quævis Europæ provincia; ne quis a florentissimis Academiis, quæ viros undiquaque doctissimos, omni virtutum genere suspiciendos, abunde producunt. Et multo plures utraque habitura, multo splendidior futura, si non hæ sordes splendidum lumen ejus obfuscarent, obstaret corruptio, et cauponantes quædam harpyæ proletariique bonum hoc nobis non inviderent. Nemo enim tam cæca mente, qui non hoc ipsum videat: nemo tam stolido ingenio, qui non intelligat, tam pertinaci judicio, qui non agnoscat, ab his idiotis circumforaneis sacram pollui Theologiam, ac cælestes Musas quasi profanum quiddam prostitui.* Viles animæ et effrontes (*sic enim Lutherus alicubi vocat* [2]) lucelli causa, ut muscæ ad mulctra, ad nobilium et heroum mensas advolant, in spem sacerdotii, *cujuslibet honoris, officii, in quamvis aulam, urbem se ingerunt, ad quodvis se ministerium componunt:*

> *Ut nervis alienis mobile lignum*
> *Ducitur,*

offam sequentes, psittacorum more, in prædæ spem quidvis effutiunt: [3] *obsecundantes parasiti* (*Erasmus ait* [4]) quidvis docent, dicunt, scribunt, suadent, et contra conscientiam probant, non ut salutarem reddant gregem, sed ut magnificam sibi parent fortunam. Opiniones quasvis et decreta contra verbum Dei astruunt, ne non offendant patronum, sed ut retineant favorem procerum, et populi plausum, sibique ipsis opes accumulent.[5] *Eo etenim plerumque animo ad Theologiam accedunt, non ut rem divinam, sed ut suam facient; non ad Ecclesiæ bonum promovendum, sed expilandum; quærentes, quod Paulus ait,* non quæ Jesu Christi, sed quæ sua, *non Domini thesaurum, sed ut sibi, suisque thesaurizent. Nec tantum iis, qui vilioris fortunæ, et abjectæ sortis sunt, hoc in usu est: sed et medios, summos, elatos, ne dicam episcopos, hoc malum invasit.* Dicite, pontifices, in sacris quid facit aurum? [6] Summos sæpe viros transversos agit avaritia,[7] *et qui reliquis morum probitate prælucerent; hi facem præferunt ad simoniam, et in corruptionis hunc scopulum impingentes, non tondent pecus, sed deglubunt, et quocunque se conferunt, expilant, exhauriunt, abradunt, magnum famæ suæ, si non animæ, nau-*

fragium facientes; ut non ab infimis ad summos, sed a summis ad infimos malum promanasse videatur, et illud verum sit quod ille olim lusit, Emerat ille prius, vendere jure potest. Simoniacus enim *(quod cum Leone dicam)* gratiam non accepit; si non accipit, non habet, et si non habet, nec gratus potest esse. *Tantum enim absunt istorum nonnulli, qui ad clavum sedent a promovendo reliquos, ut penitus impediant, probe sibi conscii, quibus artibus illic pervenerint.* Nam qui ob literas emersisse illos credat, desipit; qui vero ingenii, eruditionis, experientiæ, probitatis, pietatis, et Musarum id esse pretium putat (*quod olim revera fuit, hodie promittitur*), planissime insanit.[1] *Utcunque vel undecunque malum hoc originem ducat, non ultra quæram, ex his primordiis cœpit vitiorum colluvies, omnis calamitas, omne miseriarum agmen in Ecclesiam invehitur. Hinc tam frequens simonia, hinc ortæ querelæ, fraudes, imposturæ, ab hoc fonte se derivarunt omnes nequitiæ. Ne quid obiter dicam de ambitione, adulatione plusquam aulica, ne tristi domicœnio laborent, de luxu, de fœdo nonnunquam vitæ exemplo, quo nonnullos offendunt, de compotatione Sybaritica, etc. Hinc ille squalor academicus,* tristes hac tempestate Camenæ, *quum quivis homunculus artium ignarus, his artibus assurgat, hunc in modum promoveatur et ditescat, ambitiosis appellationibus insignis, et multis dignitatibus augustus, vulgi oculos. perstringat, bene se habeat, et grandia gradiens majestatem quandam ac amplitudinem præ se ferens, miramque sollicitudinem, barba reverendos, toga nitidus, purpura coruscus, supellectilis splendore et famulorum numero maxime conspicuus.* Quales statuæ (*quod ait ille* [2]) quæ sacris in ædibus columnis imponuntur, velut oneri cedentes videntur, ac si insuderent, quum revera sensu sint carentes, et nihil saxeam adjuvent firmitatem: *Atlantes videri volunt, quum sint statuæ lapideæ, umbratiles revera homunciones, fungi forsan et bardi, nihil a saxo differentes. Quum interim docti viti, et vitæ sanctioris ornamentis præditi, qui æstum diei sustinent, his iniqua sorte serviant, minimo forsan salario contenti, puris nominibus nuncupati, humiles, obscuri, multoque digniores licet, egentes, inhonorati vitam privam privatam agant, tenuique sepulti sacerdotio, vel in collegiis suis in æternum incarcerati, inglorie delitescant. Sed nolo diutius hanc movere sentinam. Hinc illæ lacrimæ, lugubris Musarum habitus, hinc ipsa religio (quod cum Sesellio dicam) in* ludibrium et contemptum adducitur,[3] *abjectum sacerdotium (atque hæc ubi fiunt, ausim dicere, et putidum putidi dicterium de clero* [4] *usurpare)* putidum vulgus, *inops, rude, sordidum, melancholicum, miserum, despicabile, contemnendum.*

[As for ourselves (for we also are tarred with this brush), the same reproach applies to us, and the same charge can be brought against us even more forcibly. It is through our fault, our laxity, our greed, that there is so much disgraceful trafficking in the Church ("The temple is for sale, and eke its god"), that corruption, impiety, and wickedness are rampant in it, that it is a mad welter of misery, a seething mass of trouble. I say this is the fault of all of us, and especially those of us who belong to a university. It is we who are the ultimate cause of the evils under which the State is labouring. We have actually introduced these evils ourselves, though there is no reproach and no suffering we do not deserve for not having used all our might to oppose them. What can we expect when we vie with one another every day in admitting to degrees any and every impecunious student drawn from the dregs of the people who applies for one? They need only to have learnt by heart one or two definitions and distinctions, and to have spent the usual number of years in chopping logic—it matters not what progress they have made or of what character they are; they can be idiots, wasters, idlers, gamesters, boon companions, utterly worthless and abandoned, squanderers and profligates; let them only have spent so many years at the university in the capacity, real or supposed, of gownsmen, and they will find those who for the sake of profit or friendship will get them presented, and, what is more, in many cases with splendid testimonials to their character and learning. These they procure on leaving from persons who unquestionably jeopardize their own reputation by writing them. For (as one saith) doctors and professors think of nothing save how from their various professions, and especially those which are irregular, they may further their own advantage, and benefit themselves at the expense of the State. Our annual university heads as a rule pray only for the greatest possible number of freshmen to squeeze money from, and do not care whether they are educated or not, provided they are sleek, well groomed, and good-looking, and in one word, men of means. Philophasters innocent of the arts become Masters of Arts, and those are made wise by order who are endowed with no wisdom, and have no qualifications for a degree save a desire for it. Theologasters, if they can but pay, have enough learning and to spare, and proceed to the very highest degrees. Hence it comes that such a pack of vile buffoons, ignoramuses wandering in the twilight of learning, ghosts of clergymen, itinerant quacks, dolts, clods, asses, mere cattle, intrude with unwashed feet

upon the sacred precincts of Theology, bringing with them
nothing save brazen impudence, and some hackneyed quillets
and scholastic trifles not good enough for a crowd at a street
corner. This is that base and starveling class, needy, vagabond,
slaves of their bellies, worthy to be sent back to the plough-tail,
fitter for the pigsty than the altar, which has basely prostituted
the study of divinity. These it is who fill the pulpits and creep
into noblemen's houses. Having no other means of livelihood,
and being incapable both mentally and physically of filling any
other post, they find here an anchorage, and clutch at the
priesthood, not from religious motives, but, as Paul says,
"huckstering the word of God."

Let no one, however, think that I intend any disparagement
of the many excellent men who are to be found in the Church
of England, men eminent for their learning and of spotless
reputation, of whom perhaps we can show more than any
country in Europe; nor of our noble universities, which send out
in abundance men of the highest learning and endowed with
every virtue. Yet each of them would have many more such
and would rise to much greater eminence, were its lustre not
dimmed by these blots, and its purity corrupted by these
huckstering harpies and beggars who envy it this boon. No
one can be so blind as not to see, so stupid as not to perceive, so
obstinate as not to admit that sacred Theology is defiled and
the heavenly Muses prostituted by these ignorant mountebanks.
Vile and shameless souls (as Luther calls them somewhere), in
search of gain they fly to the tables of the nobility like flies to
the milk-pail, in the hope of getting a church living or any other
post or honour, they betake themselves to any hall or town, they
will accept any employment, like marionettes pulled by strings,
always on the scent, and like parrots babbling anything for the
sake of a morsel: complaisant parasites (as Erasmus calls them),
who will teach, write, say, recommend, approve anything, even
against their own consciences, not to edify their flocks, but to
improve their own fortunes. They subscribe to any opinions
and tenets contrary to the word of God, only so as not to offend
their patrons and to retain the favour of the nobles and the
applause of the masses, and thereby acquire riches for themselves. Their object in taking up theology is to serve not God
but themselves, not to promote the interests of the Church, but
to plunder it, "seeking," as Paul says, "not the things of Jesus
Christ but their own things"; not the treasure of the Lord, but
the enrichment of themselves and their families. Nor is this

the practice only of those of meaner fortune and humbler station, but also of the middle and higher ranks, even of the bishops. "Tell us, ye pontiffs, what doth gold among the sacraments?" Avarice often leads astray men of the highest position, and those who ought to outshine all others in virtue. These show the way to simony, and, falling foul of this stumbling-block, do not merely shear but fleece the flock, and wherever they turn they plunder, drain, and fleece, making shipwreck of their reputations, if not of their souls, so that the evil seems to proceed not from the bottom to the top, but from the top to the bottom. They provide an illustration of the old gibe, "What he had purchased he could rightly sell." For the simoniac (to use the words of Leo) has not received a favour; if he has not received it, he has it not; if he has it not, he cannot confer it. Indeed, some of those who sit at the helm are so far from promoting others that they do their best to hinder them, being conscious of the arts by which they themselves attained to their positions. For he who imagines that they rose to eminence on account of their learning is no more than a simpleton; and any one who thinks that their position has been the reward of talent, erudition, experience, virtue, piety, and love of letters (once this was actually the case, but nowadays only promises are secured by these means) is absolutely mad. How or where this evil originated, I shall not further inquire; these, however, are the beginnings of the foul stream of vice and the host of miseries that have invaded the Church. Hence the frequency of simony; here is the fount of complaints, frauds, impostures, and all villainies. I say nothing of their ambition, their flattery, grosser than that of the Court, whereby they seek to escape cheerless fare at home, their luxury, the scandal given by the bad example of their lives, their sybaritic drinking-bouts. Hence the degradation of the universities, "the sadness of the Muses in these times," when any contemptible ignoramus can rise by these arts, obtain promotion and wealth by these methods, with imposing titles and distinctions, in virtue of which he can dazzle the eyes of the multitude, give himself airs, and strut about with great pomp and dignity, paying great attention to his person, cultivating a flowing beard, wearing a robe glittering with purple, and further attracting attention by the splendour of his furniture and the number of his servants. Just as the statues (as he says) which are set on pillars in sacred buildings seem to be giving way under their load, and almost to sweat, though they are devoid of feeling and add nothing to the strength of the building; so these people wish to be thought Atlases, though they are merely stone statues, effeminate manikins, perhaps dizzards and dolts, differing in no way from stone. Meanwhile learned men, graced with all the distinctions of a holy life, and who bear the heat of the day, are condemned by a hard fate to serve these men, content perhaps with a scanty salary, without any titles to their names, humble and obscure, though eminently worthy, and so, needy and unhonoured, they lead a retired life, buried in some poor benefice or imprisoned for ever in their college chambers, where they languish in obscurity. But I will stir up these foul waters no more. Hence our tears, hence it is that the Muses are in mourning, and that religion itself, as Sesellius says, is brought into ridicule and contempt, and the clerical calling is rendered vile. And in view of these facts, I venture to repeat the abusive expressions which some vulgar fellow has applied to the clergy, that they are a rotten crowd, beggarly, uncouth, filthy, melancholy, miserable, despicable, and contemptible.]

MEMB. IV.

SUBSECT. I.—*Non-necessary, remote, outward, adventitious, or accidental Causes: as first from the Nurse*

OF those remote, outward, ambient, necessary causes, I have sufficiently discoursed in the precedent member. The non-necessary follow; of which, saith Fuchsius, no art can be made, by reason of their uncertainty, casualty, and multitude;[1] so called "not necessary" because, according to Fernelius, "they may be avoided, and used without necessity."[2] Many of these accidental causes, which I shall entreat of here, might have well been reduced to the former, because they cannot be avoided, but fatally happen to us, though accidentally and unawares, at some time or other: the rest are contingent and inevitable, and more properly inserted in this rank of causes. To reckon up all is a thing unpossible; of some, therefore, most remarkable of these contingent causes which produce melancholy, I will briefly speak, and in their order.

From a child's nativity, the first ill accident that can likely befall him in this kind is a bad nurse, by whose means alone he

may be tainted with this malady from his cradle.[1] Aulus
Gellius, *lib.* 12, *cap.* 1, brings in Favorinus, that eloquent philosopher, proving this at large, "that there is the same virtue
and property in the milk as in the seed, and not in men alone,
but in all other creatures." He gives instance in a kid and lamb:
"if either of them suck of the other's milk, the lamb of the
goat's, or the kid of the ewe's, the wool of the one will be hard,
and the hair of the other soft." [2] Giraldus Cambrensis, *Itinerar.*
Cambriæ, lib. 1, *cap.* 2, confirms this by a notable example which
happened in his time. A sow-pig by chance sucked a brach,
and when she was grown, "would miraculously hunt all manner of
deer, and that as well, or rather better than any ordinary
hound." [3] His conclusion is, "that men and beasts participate
of her nature and conditions by whose milk they are fed." [4]
Favorinus urgeth it farther, and demonstrates it more evidently,
that if a nurse be "misshapen, unchaste, unhonest, impudent,
drunk," [5] cruel,[6] or the like, the child that sucks upon her breast
will be so too"; all other affections of the mind and diseases are
almost engrafted, as it were, and imprinted into the temperature
of the infant, by the nurse's milk, as pox, leprosy, melancholy, etc.
Cato for some such reason would make his servants' children
suck upon his wife's breast, because by that means they would
love him and his the better, and in all likelihood agree with
them. A more evident example that the minds are altered by
milk cannot be given, than that of Dion, which he relates of
Caligula's cruelty; [7] it could neither be imputed to father nor
mother, but to his cruel nurse alone, that anointed her paps
with blood still when he sucked, which made him such a murderer, and to express her cruelty to a hair: and that of Tiberius,
who was a common drunkard, because his nurse was such a
one. *Et si delira fuerit* (one observes [8]), *infantulum delirum*
faciet, if she be a fool or dolt, the child she nurseth will take
after her, or otherwise be misaffected; which Franciscus Barbarus, *lib.* 2, *cap. ult. de re uxoria*, proves at full, and Ant. Guevara,
lib. 2, *de Marco Aurelio*: the child will surely participate. For
bodily sickness there is no doubt to be made. Titus, Vespasian's son, was therefore sickly, because the nurse was so
(Lampridius). And if we may believe physicians, many times
children catch the pox from a bad nurse (Botaldus, *cap.* 61 *de*
lue vener.). Besides evil attendance, negligence, and many gross
inconveniences which are incident to nurses, much danger may
so come to the child. For these causes [9] Aristotle, *Polit. lib.* 7,
cap. 17, Favorinus, and Marcus Aurelius would not have a

child put to nurse at all, but every mother to bring up her
own, of what condition soever she be; for a sound and able
mother to put out her child to nurse, is *naturæ intemperies* [an
outrage on Nature], so Guazzo calls it,[1] 'tis fit therefore she
should be nurse herself; the mother will be more careful, loving,
and attendant, than any servile woman, or such hired creatures;
this all the world acknowledgeth; *convenientissimum est* (as Rod.
à Castro, *de nat. mulierum, lib.* 4, *cap.* 12, in many words confesseth) *matrem ipsam lactare infantem* [it is most fit that the
mother should suckle her own infant]—who denies that it
should be so?—and which some women most curiously observe;
amongst the rest, that Queen of France, a Spaniard by birth,
that was so precise and zealous in this behalf, that when in her
absence a strange nurse had suckled her child, she was never
quiet till she had made the infant vomit it up again.[2]   But she
was too jealous.   If it be so, as many times it is, they must be
put forth, the mother be not fit or well able to be a nurse, I
would then advise such mothers (as Plutarch doth in his book
de liberis educandis,[3] and St. Hierome, *lib.* 2, *epist.* 27, *Lætæ de
institut. fil.,* Magninus, *part.* 2 *Reg. sanit. cap.* 7,[4] and the said
Rodericus), that they make choice of a sound woman, of a good
complexion, honest, free from bodily diseases, if it be possible,
all passions and perturbations of the mind, as sorrow, fear,
grief, folly,[5] melancholy.   For such passions corrupt the milk,
and alter the temperature of the child, which now being *udum
et molle lutum*[6] [moist and soft clay], is easily seasoned and
perverted.   And if such a nurse may be found out, that will be
diligent and careful withal, let Favorinus and M. Aurelius plead
how they can against it, I had rather accept of her in some
cases than the mother herself, and which Bonaciolus the physician, Nic. Biesius the politician, *lib.* 4 *de repub. cap.* 8, approves,
"some nurses are much to be preferred to some mothers."[7]
For why may not the mother be naught, a peevish, drunken
flirt, a waspish, choleric slut, a crazed piece, a fool (as many
mothers are), unsound, as soon as the nurse?   There is more
choice of nurses than mothers; and therefore, except the mother
be most virtuous, staid, a woman of excellent good parts, and
of a sound complexion, I would have all children in such cases
committed to discreet strangers.   And 'tis the only way; as by
marriage they are engrafted to other families to alter the breed,
or if anything be amiss in the mother, as Lodovicus Mercatus
contends, *tom.* 2, *lib. de morb. hæred.,* to prevent diseases and
future maladies, to correct and qualify the child's ill-disposed

temperature, which he had from his parents. This is an excellent remedy, if good choice be made of such a nurse.

SUBSECT. II.—*Education a Cause of Melancholy*

Education, of these accidental causes of melancholy, may justly challenge the next place, for if a man escape a bad nurse, he may be undone by evil bringing up.   Jason Pratensis [1] puts this of education for a principal cause; bad parents, stepmothers, tutors, masters, teachers, too rigorous, too severe, too remiss or indulgent on the other side, are often fountains and furtherers of this disease.   Parents, and such as have the tuition and over-sight of children, offend many times in that they are too stern, always threatening, chiding, brawling, whipping, or striking; by means of which their poor children are so disheartened and cowed, that they never after have any courage, a merry hour in their lives, or take pleasure in anything.   There is a great moderation to be had in such things, as matters of so great moment to the making or marring of a child.   Some fright their children with beggars, bugbears, and hobgoblins, if they cry, or be otherwise unruly; but they are much to blame in it, many times, saith Lavater, *de spectris, part.* 1, *cap.* 5, *ex metu in morbos graves incidunt et noctu dormientes clamant,* for fear they fall into many diseases, and cry out in their sleep, and are much the worse for it all their lives: these things ought not at all, or to be sparingly done, and upon just occasion.   Tyrannical, impatient, hair-brain schoolmasters, *aridi magistri* [dry masters], as Fabius terms them,[2] *Ajaces flagelliferi* [flogging bullies], are in this kind as bad as hangmen and executioners; they make many children endure a martyrdom all the while they are at school; with bad diet, if they board in their houses, too much severity and ill-usage, they quite pervert their temperature of body and mind: still chiding, railing, frowning, lashing, tasking, keeping, that they are *fracti animis,* moped many times, weary of their lives, *nimia severitate deficiunt et desperant* [3] [through harsh treatment they become dull and dispirited], and think no slavery in the world (as once I did myself) like to that of a grammar scholar.   *Praceptorum ineptiis discruciantur ingenia puerorum* [the teachers through their stupidities make the pupils suffer agonies of mind], saith Erasmus, they tremble at his voice, looks, coming in.   St. Austin, in the first book of his Confessions and 9th *cap.,* calls this schooling *meticulosam necessitatem* [a dreadful compulsion], and elsewhere a martyrdom, and confesseth of

himself, how cruelly he was tortured in mind for learning Greek:
*Nulla verba noveram, et sævis terroribus et pœnis, ut nossem,
instabatur mihi vehementer*, I knew nothing, and with cruel
terrors and punishment I was daily compelled. Beza [1] complains in like case of a rigorous schoolmaster in Paris, that made
him by his continual thunder and threats once in a mind to
drown himself, had he not met by the way with an uncle of his
that vindicated him from that misery for the time, by taking
him to his house. Trincavellius, *lib.* 1, *consil.* 16, had a patient
nineteen years of age, extremely melancholy, *ob nimium studium,
Tarvitii et præceptoris minas*, by reason of overmuch study, and
his tutor's threats.[2] Many masters are hard-hearted, and
bitter to their servants, and by that means do so deject, with
terrible speeches and hard usage so crucify them, that they
become desperate, and can never be recalled.

Others again, in that opposite extreme, do as great harm by
their too much remissness; they give them no bringing up, no
calling to busy themselves about, or to live in, teach them no
trade, or set them in any good course; by means of which their
servants, children, scholars, are carried away with that stream
of drunkenness, idleness, gaming, and many such irregular
courses, that in the end they rue it, curse their parents, and
mischief themselves. Too much indulgence causeth the like,
inepta patris lenitas et facilitas prava [3] [the father's gentleness
can be misplaced and his indulgence corrupting], whenas,
Micio-like, with too much liberty and too great allowance, they
feed their children's humours, let them revel, wench, riot,
swagger, and do what they will themselves, and then punish
them with a noise of musicians.

> *Obsonet, potet, oleat unguenta de meo;*
> *Amat? dabitur a me argentum ubi erit commodum.*
> *Fores effregit? restituentur; discidit*
> *Vestem? resarcietur. . . . Faciat quod lubet,*
> *Sumat, consumat, perdat, decretum est pati.* [4]

He wants to eat, drink, perfume? I will pay.
Money for his sweetheart? He shall have it.
He has broken doors? Rebuild them. Torn his coat?
Repair it. Let him do just what he likes.
He's free to take, to spend, to waste my all.
I will not murmur.

But, as Demea told him, *Tu illum corrumpi sinis*, your lenity will
be his undoing, *prævidere videor jam diem illum, quum hic egens
profugiet aliquo militatum* [methinks I foresee the day when he
will run away and join the army], I foresee his ruin. So parents

often err, many fond mothers especially, doat so much upon their children, like Æsop's ape,[1] till in the end they crush them to death, *Corporum nutrices animarum novercæ*, pampering up their bodies to the undoing of their souls: they will not let them be corrected or controlled,[2] but still soothed up in everything they do, that in conclusion "they bring sorrow, shame, heaviness to their parents" (Eccles. xxx, 8, 9), "become wanton, stubborn, wilful, and disobedient"; rude, untaught, headstrong, incorrigible, and graceless. "They love them so foolishly," saith Cardan, "that they rather seem to hate them, bringing them not up to virtue but to injury, not to learning but to riot, not to sober life and conversation but to all pleasure and licentious behaviour."[3] Who is he of so little experience that knows not this of Fabius to be true? "Education is another nature, altering the mind and will, and I would to God" (saith he) "we ourselves did not spoil our children's manners by our overmuch cockering and nice education, and weaken the strength of their bodies and minds; that causeth custom, custom nature,"[4] etc. For these causes Plutarch, in his book *de lib. educ.*, and Hierome, *Epist. lib.* 1, *epist.* 17, to Læta, *de institut. filiæ*, gives a most especial charge to all parents, and many good cautions about bringing up of children, that they be not committed to undiscreet, passionate, bedlam tutors, light, giddy-headed, or covetous persons, and spare for no cost, that they may be well nurtured and taught, it being a matter of so great consequence. For such parents as do otherwise, Plutarch esteems of them "that [they] are more careful of their shoes than of their feet,"[5] that rate their wealth above their children. And he, saith Cardan, "that leaves his son to a covetous schoolmaster to be informed, or to a close abbey to fast and learn wisdom together, doth no other, than that he be a learned fool, or a sickly wise man."[6]

SUBSECT. III.—*Terrors and Affrights, Causes of Melancholy*

Tully, in the fourth of his Tusculans, distinguishes these terrors which arise from the apprehension of some terrible object heard or seen, from other fears, and so doth Patricius, *lib.* 5, *tit.* 4, *de regis institut.* Of all fears they are most pernicious and violent, and so suddenly alter the whole temperature of the body, move the soul and spirits, strike such a deep impression, that the parties can never be recovered, causing more grievous and fiercer melancholy, as Felix Plater, *cap.* 3 *de mentis alienat.*, speaks out of his experience, than any inward cause whatsoever; "and imprints itself so forcibly in the spirits, brain, humours, that if all the mass of blood were let out of the body, it could hardly be extracted. This horrible kind of melancholy" (for so he terms it) "had been often brought before him, and troubles and affrights commonly men and women, young and old of all sorts."[1] Hercules de Saxonia calls this kind of melancholy (*ab agitatione spirituum*) by a peculiar name; it comes from the agitation, motion, contraction, dilatation of spirits,[2] not from any distemperature of humours, and produceth strong effects. This terror is most usually caused, as Plutarch will have, "from some imminent danger, when a terrible object is at hand,"[3] heard, seen, or conceived, "truly appearing,[4] or in a dream":[5] and many times the more sudden the accident, it is the more violent.

> *Stat terror animis, et cor attonitum salit,*
> *Pavidumque trepidis palpitat venis jecur.*[6]

> Their soul's affright, their heart amazed quakes,
> The trembling liver pants i' th' veins, and aches.

Artemidorus the grammarian lost his wits by the unexpected sight of a crocodile (Laurentius, 7 *de melan.*). The massacre at Lyons, 1572, in the reign of Charles IX, was so terrible and fearful, that many ran mad, some died, great-bellied women were brought to bed before their time, generally all affrighted and aghast.[7] Many lose their wits "by the sudden sight of some spectrum or devil, a thing very common in all ages,"[8] saith Lavater, *part.* 1, *cap.* 9, as Orestes did at the sight of the Furies which appeared to him in black (as Pausanias records[9]). The Greeks call them μορμολυκεῖα [bogies], which so terrify their souls, or if they be but affrighted by some counterfeit devils in jest,

> *Ut pueri trepidant, atque omina cæcis*
> *In tenebris metuunt,*[10]

as children in the dark conceive hobgoblins, and are so afraid, they are the worse for all their lives; some by sudden fires, earthquakes, inundations, or any such dismal objects—Themison the physician fell into an hydrophobia, by seeing one sick of that disease (Diosorides, *lib.* 6, *cap.* 33)—or by the sight of a monster, a carcass, they are disquieted many months following, and cannot endure the room where a corse hath been, for a world would not be alone with a dead man, or lie in that bed many years after in which a man hath died. At Basil many little children in the springtime went to gather flowers in a meadow at the

town's end, where a malefactor hung in gibbets; all gazing at
it, one by chance flung a stone, and made it stir, by which
accident the children affrighted ran away; one slower than the
rest, looking back, and seeing the stirred carcass wag towards
her, cried out it came after, and was so terribly affrighted that
for many days she could not rest, eat, or sleep, she could not
be pacified, but melancholy, died.[1]   In the same town another
child, beyond the Rhine, saw a grave opened, and upon the sight
of a carcass, was so troubled in mind that she could not be
comforted, but a little after departed, and was buried by it [2]
(Platerus, *Observat. lib.* 1). A gentlewoman of the same city saw a
fat hog cut up; when the entrails were opened, and a noisome
savour offended her nose, she much misliked, and would not
longer abide; a physician in presence told her, as that hog, so
was she, full of filthy excrements, and aggravated the matter
by some other loathsome instances, insomuch this nice gentlewoman apprehended it so deeply that she fell forthwith a-
vomiting, was so mightily distempered in mind and body, that
with all his art and persuasions, for some months after, he could
not restore her to herself again; she could not forget it, or
remove the object out of her sight (*Idem*).   Many cannot endure
to see a wound opened, but they are offended: a man executed,
or labour of any fearful disease, as possession, apoplexies, one
bewitched; or if they read by chance of some terrible thing,[3]
the symptoms alone of such a disease, or that which they
dislike, they are instantly troubled in mind, aghast, ready to
apply it to themselves, they are as much disquieted as if they
had seen it, or were so affected themselves. *Hecatas sibi
videntur somniare*, they dream and continually think of it.   As
lamentable effects are caused by such terrible objects heard,
read, or seen; *auditus maximos motus in corpore facit* [the body
is greatly affected through the sense of hearing], as Plutarch
holds,[4] no sense makes greater alteration of body and mind:
sudden speech sometimes, unexpected news, be they good or
bad, *prævisa minus oratio*, will move as much, *animum obruere,
et de sede sua dejicere*, as a philosopher observes,[5] will take away
our sleep and appetite, disturb and quite overturn us.   Let
them bear witness that have heard those tragical alarums,
outcries, hideous noises, which are many times suddenly heard
in the dead of night by irruption of enemies and accidental
fires, etc., those panic fears,[6] which often drive men out of
their wits, bereave them of sense, understanding, and all, some
for a time, some for their whole lives, they never recover it.

The Midianites were so affrighted by Gideon's soldiers, they
breaking but every one a pitcher;[1] and Hannibal's army by
such a panic fear was discomfited at the walls of Rome.[2]
Augusta Livia, hearing a few tragical verses recited out of
Virgil, *Tu Marcellus eris*, etc., fell down dead in a swoon.
Edinus, King of Denmark, by a sudden sound which he heard,
"was turned into fury with all his men"[3] (Cranzius, *lib.* 5 *Dan.
hist.* and Alexander ab Alexandro, *lib.* 3, *cap.* 5). Amatus
Lusitanus had a patient, that by reason of bad tidings became
epilepticus (*cen.* 2, *cura* 90). Cardan, *Subtil. lib.* 18, saw one that
lost his wits by mistaking of an echo. If one sense alone can cause
such violent commotions of the mind, what may we think when
hearing, sight, and those other senses are all troubled at once,
as by some earthquakes, thunder, lightning, tempests, etc.? At
Bologna in Italy, *anno* 1504, there was such a fearful earthquake about eleven o'clock in the night (as Beroaldus, in his
book *de terræ motu*, hath commended to posterity[4]) that all
the city trembled, the people thought the world was at an end,
actum de mortalibus; such a fearful noise it made, such a detestable smell, the inhabitants were infinitely affrighted, and some
ran mad. *Audi rem atrocem, et annalibus memorandum* (mine
author adds), hear a strange story, and worthy to be chronicled:
I had a servant at the same time called Fulco Argelanus, a bold
and proper man, so grievously terrified with it, that he was first
melancholy, after doted, at last mad, and made away himself.[5]
At Fuscinum in Japan "there was such an earthquake, and
darkness on a sudden, that many men were offended with
headache, many overwhelmed with sorrow and melancholy. At
Meacum whole streets and goodly palaces were overturned at
the same time, and there was such a hideous noise withal, like
thunder, and filthy smell, that their hair stared for fear, and
their hearts quaked, men and beasts were incredibly terrified.
In Sacai, another city, the same earthquake was so terrible
unto them, that many were bereft of their senses; and others
by that horrible spectacle so much amazed, that they knew
not what they did."[6] Blasius, a Christian, the reporter of
the news, was so affrighted for his part, that, though it were
two months after, he was scarce his own man, neither could he
drive the remembrance of it out of his mind. Many times,
some years following, they will tremble afresh at the remembrance or conceit of such a terrible object,[7] even all their lives
long, if mention be made of it. Cornelius Agrippa relates, out
of Gulielmus Parisiensis, a story of one that, after a distasteful

purge which a physician had prescribed unto him, was so much moved, "that at the very sight of physic he would be distempered";[1] though he never so much as smelled to it, the box of physic long after would give him a purge; nay, the very remembrance of it did effect it; "like travellers and seamen," saith Plutarch, "that when they have been sanded, or dashed on a rock, for ever after fear not that mischance only, but all such dangers whatsoever."[2]

SUBSECT. IV.—*Scoffs, Calumnies, bitter Jests, how they cause Melancholy*

It is an old saying, "A blow with a word strikes deeper than a blow with a sword";[3] and many men are as much galled with a calumny, a scurrile and bitter jest, a libel, a pasquil, satire, apologue, epigram, stage-plays, or the like, as with any misfortune whatsoever. Princes and potentates, that are otherwise happy and have all at command, secure and free, *quibus potentia sceleris impunitatem fecit* [who are able to commit crimes with impunity], are grievously vexed with these pasquilling libels and satires; they fear a railing Aretine more than an enemy in the field,[4] which made most princes of his time (as some relate) "allow him a liberal pension, that he should not tax them in his satires."[5] The gods had their Momus, Homer his Zoilus, Achilles his Thersites, Philip his Demades: the Cæsars themselves in Rome were commonly taunted. There was never wanting a Petronius, a Lucian in those times, nor will be a Rabelais, an Euphormio, a Boccalinus in ours. Adrian the sixth Pope[6] was so highly offended, and grievously vexed with pasquillers at Rome, he gave command that statue[7] should be demolished and burned, the ashes flung into the River Tiber, and had done it forthwith, had not Lodovicus Suessanus, a facete companion, dissuaded him to the contrary, by telling him that Pasquil's ashes would turn to frogs in the bottom of the river, and croak worse and louder than before.[8] *Genus irritabile vatum* [poets are a quick-tempered tribe], and therefore Socrates in Plato adviseth all his friends, "that respect their credits, to stand in awe of poets, for they are terrible fellows, can praise and dispraise as they see cause."[9] *Hinc quam sit calamus sævior ense patet* [Hence you may see, the written word Can be more cruel than the sword]. The prophet David complains (Ps. cxxiii, 4), "that his soul was full of the mocking of the wealthy, and of the despitefulness of the proud," and

(Ps. lv, 3, 4) "for the voice of the wicked, etc., and their hate; his heart trembled within him, and the terrors of death came upon him; fear and horrible fear," etc., and (Ps. lxix, 20) "Rebuke hath broken my heart, and I am full of heaviness." Who hath not like cause to complain, and is not so troubled, that shall fall into the mouths of such men? for many are of so petulant a spleen,[1] and have that figure *sarcasmus* so often in their mouths, so bitter, so foolish, as Balthasar Castilio notes of them, that "they cannot speak, but they must bite";[2] they had rather lose a friend than a jest; and what company soever they come in, they will be scoffing, insulting over their inferiors, especially over such as anyway depend upon them, humouring, misusing, or putting gulleries on some or other till they have made by their humouring or gulling *ex stulto insanum*[3] [a fool into a madman], a mope or a noddy, and all to make themselves merry:

Dummodo risum
Excutiat sibi, non hic cuiquam parcit amico.[4]

[To raise a laugh he will not spare a friend.]

Friends, neuters, enemies, all are as one, to make a fool a madman is their sport, and they have no greater felicity than to scoff and deride others; they must sacrifice to the god of laughter, with them in Apuleius,[5] once a day, or else they shall be melancholy themselves; they care not how they grind and misuse others, so they may exhilarate their own persons. Their wits indeed serve them to that sole purpose, to make sport, to break a scurrile jest, which is *levissimus ingenii fructus*, the froth of wit, as Tully holds,[6] and for this they are often applauded; in all other discourse, dry, barren, stramineous, dull and heavy, here lies their genius, in this they alone excel, please themselves and others. Leo Decimus, that scoffing pope, as Jovius hath registered in the fourth book of his life, took an extraordinary delight in humouring of silly fellows, and to put gulleries upon them; by commending some, persuading others to this or that,[7] he made *ex stolidis stultissimos et maxime ridiculos, ex stultis insanos*, soft fellows stark noddies, and such as were foolish quite mad before he left them. One memorable example he recites there, of Tarascomus of Parma, a musician that was so humoured by Leo Decimus and Bibbiena his second in this business, that he thought himself to be a man of most excellent skill (who was indeed a ninny); they "made him set foolish songs, and invent new ridiculous precepts, which they did highly commend,"[8] as to tie his arm that played on the

lute, to make him strike a sweeter stroke, "and to pull down
the arras hangings, because the voice would be clearer, by
reason of the reverberation of the wall." [1]   In the like manner
they persuaded one Baraballius, of Caieta, that he was as good
a poet as Petrarch; would have him to be made a laureate
poet, and invite all his friends to his instalment; and had so
possessed the poor man with a conceit of his excellent poetry,
that, when some of his more discreet friends told him of his
folly, he was very angry with them, and said "they envied his
honour, and prosperity": [2] it was strange (saith Jovius) to see
an old man of sixty years, a venerable and grave old man, so
gulled.   But what cannot such scoffers do, especially if they
find a soft creature on whom they may work?   Nay, to say
truth, who is so wise, or so discreet, that may not be humoured
in this kind, especially if some excellent wits shall set upon
him.   He that mads others, if he were so humoured, would be as
mad himself, as much grieved and tormented; he might cry
with him in the comedy, *Pro Jupiter, tu homo me adigis ad
insaniam* [Man alive, you are driving me mad].   For all is in
these things as they are taken; if he be a silly soul, and do
not perceive it, 'tis well, he may haply make others sport, and
be no whit troubled himself; but if he be apprehensive of his
folly, and take it to heart, then it torments him worse than
any lash.   A bitter jest, a slander, a calumny, pierceth deeper
than any loss, danger, bodily pain, or injury whatsoever; *leviter
enim volat* [it flies swiftly], as Bernard of an arrow, *sed graviter
vulnerat* [but wounds deeply], especially if it shall proceed from
a virulent tongue, "it cuts" (saith David) "like a two-edged sword.
They shoot bitter words as arrows" (Ps. lxiv, 3); "And they
smote with their tongues" (Jer. xviii, 18), and that so hard,
that they leave an incurable wound behind them   Many men
are undone by this means, moped, and so dejected, that they
are never to be recovered; and of all other men living, those
which are actually melancholy, or inclined to it, are most
sensible (as being suspicious, choleric, apt to mistake) and
impatient of an injury in that kind: they aggravate, and so
meditate continually of it, that it is a perpetual corrosive, not
to be removed till time wear it out.   Although they peradventure that so scoff do it alone in mirth and merriment, and
hold it *optimum aliena frui insania*, an excellent thing to enjoy
another man's madness; yet they must know that it is a mortal
sin (as Thomas holds [3]) and, as the prophet David denounceth,
"they that use it shall never dwell in God's tabernacle." [4]

I—*M[886]

Such scurrile jests, flouts, and sarcasms, therefore, ought
not at all to be used; especially to our betters, to those that are
in misery, or anyway distressed: for to such *ærumnarum incre-
menta sunt,* they multiply grief, and as he perceived,[1] *In multis
pudor, in multis iracundia,* etc., many are ashamed, many
vexed, angered, and there is no greater cause or furtherer of
melancholy. Martin Cromerus, in the sixth book of his history,
hath a pretty story to this purpose, of Uladislaus the Second,
King of Poland, and Peter Dunnius, Earl of Shrine; they had
been hunting late, and were enforced to lodge in a poor cottage.
When they went to bed, Uladislaus told the earl in jest, that
his wife lay softer with the Abbot of Shrine; he, not able to
contain, replied, *Et tua cum Dabesso,* And yours with Dabessus,
a gallant young gentleman in the court, whom Christina the
queen loved. *Tetigit id dictum principis animum,* these words
of his so galled the prince, that he was long after *tristis et cogitabundus,* very sad and melancholy for many months; but they
were the earl's utter undoing: for when Christina heard of it,
she persecuted him to death. Sophia the empress, Justinian's
wife, broke a bitter jest upon Narses the eunuch, a famous
captain, then disquieted for an overthrow which he lately had:
that he was fitter for a distaff, and to keep women company,
than to wield a sword, or to be general of an army; but it cost
her dear, for he so far distasted it, that he went forthwith to
the adverse part, much troubled in his thoughts, caused the
Lombards to rebel, and thence procured many miseries to the
commonwealth. Tiberius the emperor withheld a legacy from
the people of Rome, which his predecessor Augustus had lately
given, and perceiving a fellow round a dead corse in the ear,
would needs know wherefore he did so; the fellow replied, that
he wished the departed soul to signify to Augustus, the commons
of Rome were yet unpaid: for this bitter jest the emperor caused
him forthwith to be slain, and carry the news himself. For
this reason, all those that otherwise approve of jests in some
cases, and facete companions (as who doth not?), let them laugh
and be merry, *rumpantur et ilia Codro* [though Codrus should
burst], 'tis laudable and fit; those yet will by no means admit
them in their companies, that are anyway inclined to this
malady; *non jocandum cum iis qui miseri sunt et ærumnosi,* no
jesting with a discontented person: 'tis Castilio's caveat, Jo.
Pontanus',[2] and Galateus',[3] and every good man's.

> Play with me, but hurt me not:
> Jest with me, but shame me not.

Comitas. is a virtue between rusticity and scurrility, two extremes; as affability is between flattery and contention, it must not exceed, but be still accompanied with that ἀβλάβεια [1] or innocency, *quæ nemini nocet, omnem injuriæ oblationem abhorrens,* [which] hurts no man, abhors all offer of injury. Though a man be liable to such a jest or obloquy, have been overseen, or committed a foul fact, yet it is no good manners or humanity to upbraid, to hit him in the teeth with his offence, or to scoff at such a one; 'tis an old axiom, *turpis in reum omnis exprobratio* [it is unseemly to upbraid a prisoner with his crime]. I speak not of such as generally tax vice, Barclay, Gentilis, Erasmus, Agrippa, Fischartus, etc., the Varronists and Lucians of our time, satirists, epigrammatists, comedians, apologists, etc., but such as personate, rail, scoff, calumniate, perstringe by name, or in presence offend.

> *Ludit qui stolida procacitate,*
> *Non est Sestius ille, sed caballus.* [2]

> [He who goes jesting with stupid talkativeness is not Sestius but a horse.]

'Tis horse-play this, and those jests (as he saith [3]) "are no better than injuries," biting jests, *mordentes et aculeati,* they are poisoned jests, leave a sting behind them, and ought not to be used.

> Set not thy foot to make the blind to fall;
> Nor wilfully offend thy weaker brother:
> Nor wound the dead with thy tongue's bitter gall,
> Neither rejoice thou in the fall of other. [4]

If these rules could be kept, we should have much more ease and quietness than we have, less melancholy: whereas, on the contrary, we study to misuse each other, how to sting and gall, like two fighting boars, bending all our force and wit, friends, fortune, to crucify one another's souls; [5] by means of which there is little content and charity, much virulency, hatred, malice, and disquietness among us.

SUBSECT. V.—*Loss of Liberty, Servitude, Imprisonment, how they cause Melancholy*

To this catalogue of causes I may well annex loss of liberty, servitude, or imprisonment, which to some persons is as great a torture as any of the rest. Though they have all things convenient, sumptuous houses to their use, fair walks and

gardens, delicious bowers, galleries, good fare and diet, and all
things correspondent, yet they are not content, because they
are confined, may not come and go at their pleasure, have
and do what they will, but live *aliena quadra*,[1] at another man's
table and command. As it is in meats, so it is in all other
things,[2] places, societies, sports; let them be never so pleasant,
commodious, wholesome, so good; yet *omnium rerum est satietas,*
there is a loathing satiety of all things. The children of Israel
were tired with manna; it is irksome to them so to live, as to a
bird in a cage, or a dog in his kennel, they are weary of it.
They are happy, it is true, and have all things, to another
man's judgment, that heart can wish, or that they themselves
can desire, *bona si sua norint* [did they but know the blessings
they enjoy]; yet they loathe it, and are tired with the present.
Est natura hominum novitatis avida; men's nature is still desirous
of news, variety, delights; and our wandering affections are so
irregular in this kind, that they must change, though it must
be to the worst. Bachelors must be married, and married men
would be bachelors; they do not love their own wives, though
otherwise fair, wise, virtuous, and well qualified, because they
are theirs; our present estate is still the worst, we cannot endure
one course of life long, *et quod modo voverat, odit* [he hates what
he just now prayed for]; one calling long, *esse in honore juvat,*
mox displicet [honour at first delights him, in a while it likes
him not]; one place long, *Romæ Tibur amo, ventosus Tibure*
Romam[3] [As changeful as the wind, nowhere at home; At
Rome I Tibur miss, at Tibur Rome]; that which we earnestly
sought, we now contemn. *Hoc quosdam agit ad mortem* (saith
Seneca[4]) *quod proposita sæpe mutando in eadem revolvuntur, et*
non relinquunt novitati locum. Fastidio cœpit esse vita, et ipse
mundus, et subit illud rapidissimarum deliciarum, Quousque
eadem? This alone kills many a man, that they are tied to the
same still; as a horse in a mill, a dog in a wheel, they run round,
without alteration or news; their life groweth odious, the world
loathsome, and that which crosseth their furious delights, "What?
still the same?" Marcus Aurelius and Solomon, that had experience of all worldly delights and pleasure, confessed as much
of themselves; what they most desired was tedious at last,
and that their lust could never be satisfied, all was vanity and
affliction of mind.

Now if it be death itself, another hell, to be glutted with
one kind of sport, dieted with one dish, tied to one place;
though they have all things otherwise as they can desire, and

are in heaven to another man's opinion, what misery and
discontent shall they have, that live in slavery, or in prison
itself! *Quod tristius morte, in servitute vivendum,* as Hermolaus
told Alexander in Curtius,[1] worse than death is bondage: *hoc
animo scito omnes fortes, ut mortem servituti anteponant,*[2] all
brave men at arms (Tully holds) are so affected. *Equidem ego
is sum, qui servitutem extremum omnium malorum esse arbitror:*[3]
I am he (saith Boterus) that account servitude the extremity
of misery.   And what calamity do they endure, that live with
those hard taskmasters, in gold mines (like those 30,000 Indian
slaves at Potosi,[4] in Peru), tin-mines, lead-mines, stone-quarries,
coal-pits, like so many mouldwarps underground, condemned
to the galleys, to perpetual drudgery, hunger, thirst, and stripes,
without all hope of delivery!   How are those women in Turkey
affected, that most part of the year come not abroad; those
Italian and Spanish dames, that are mewed up like hawks,
and locked up by their jealous husbands! how tedious is it to
them that live in stones and caves half a year together! as in
Iceland, Muscovy, or under the Pole itself,[5] where they have
six months' perpetual night.   Nay, what misery and discontent
do they endure, that are in prison!   They want all those six
non-natural things at once, good air, good diet, exercise, company, sleep, rest, ease, etc., that are bound in chains all day
long, suffer hunger, and (as Lucian describes it[6]) "must abide
that filthy stink, and rattling of chains, howlings, pitiful outcries, that prisoners usually make; these things are not only
troublesome, but intolerable."   They lie nastily among toads
and frogs in a dark dungeon, in their own dung, in pain of
body, in pain of soul, as Joseph did (Ps. cv. 18): "They hurt
his feet in his stocks, the iron entered his soul."   They live
solitary, alone, sequestered from all company but heart-eating
melancholy; and, for want of meat, must eat that bread of
affliction, prey upon themselves.   Well might Arculanus put
long imprisonment for a cause,[7] especially to such as have lived
jovially, in all sensuality and lust, upon a sudden are estranged
and debarred from all manner of pleasures: as were Huniades,
Edward and Richard II, Valerian the Emperor, Bajazet the
Turk.   If it be irksome to miss our ordinary companions and
repast for once a day, or an hour, what shall it be to lose them
for ever?   If it be so great a delight to live at liberty, and to
enjoy that variety of objects the world affords, what misery
and discontent must it needs bring to him, that shall now be
cast headlong into that Spanish Inquisition, to fall from heaven

to hell, to be cubbed up upon a sudden, how shall he be perplexed, what shall become of him? Robert, Duke of Normandy,[1] being imprisoned by his youngest brother Henry I, *ab illo die inconsolabili dolore in carcere contabuit*, saith Matthew Paris, from that day forward pined away with grief. Jugurtha,[2] that generous captain, "brought to Rome in triumph, and after imprisoned, through anguish of his soul and melancholy, died." Roger, Bishop of Salisbury,[3] the second man from King Stephen (he that built that famous castle of Devizes[4] in Wiltshire), was so tortured in prison with hunger, and all those calamities accompanying such men, *ut vivere noluerit, mori nescierit*,[5] he would not live and could not die, betwixt fear of death and torments of life. Francis, King of France, was taken prisoner by Charles V, *ad mortem fere melancholicus*, saith Guicciardine, melancholy almost to death, and that in an instant. But this is as clear as the sun, and needs no further illustration.

Subsect. VI.—*Poverty and Want, Causes of Melancholy*

Poverty and want are so violent oppugners, so unwelcome guests, so much abhorred of all men, that I may not omit to speak of them apart. Poverty, although (if considered aright, to a wise, understanding, truly regenerate, and contented man) it be *donum Dei* [a gift of God], a blessed estate, the way to heaven, as Chrysostom calls it,[6] God's gift, the mother of modesty, and much to be preferred before riches (as shall be showed in his place[7]), yet as it is esteemed in the world's censure, it is a most odious calling, vile and base, a severe torture, *summum scelus*, a most intolerable burden; we shun it all,[8] *cane pejus et angue* [worse than a dog or a snake], we abhor the name of it — *Paupertas fugitur, totoque arcessitur orbe*[9] [poverty is shunned and barred from all the world]—as being the fountain of all other miseries, cares, woes, labours, and grievances whatsoever. To avoid which, we will take any pains —*extremos currit mercator ad Indos* [the merchant dashes to the farthest Ind]—we will leave no haven, no coast, no creek of the world unsearched, though it be to the hazard of our lives; we will dive to the bottom of the sea, to the bowels of the earth, five, six, seven, eight, nine hundred fathom deep,[10] through all five zones, and both extremes of heat and cold; we will turn parasites and slaves, prostitute ourselves, swear and lie, damn our bodies and souls, forsake God, abjure religion, steal, rob,

murder, rather than endure this unsufferable yoke of poverty,
which doth so tyrannize, crucify, and generally depress us.

For look into the world, and you shall see men most part
esteemed according to their means, and happy as they are
rich: *Ubique tanti quisque quantum habuit fuit* [1] [everywhere a
man is worth as much as he has]. If he be likely to thrive,
and in the way of preferment, who but he? In the vulgar
opinion, if a man be wealthy, no matter how he gets it, of what
parentage, how qualified, how virtuously endowed or villain-
ously inclined; let him be a bawd, a gripe, an usurer, a villain,
a pagan, a barbarian, a wretch, Lucian's tyrant,[2] "on whom
you may look with less security than on the sun"; so that he
be rich (and liberal withal) he shall be honoured, admired,
adored, reverenced, and highly magnified.[3] "The rich is had
in reputation because of his goods" (Ecclus. x, 30). He shall
be befriended, "for riches gather many friends" (Prov. xix, 4);
multos numerabit amicos, all happiness ebbs and flows
with his money.[4] He shall be accounted a gracious lord, a
Mæcenas, a benefactor, a wise, discreet, a proper, a valiant, a
fortunate man, of a generous spirit, *pullus Jovis, et gallinæ
filius albæ* [Jove's offspring, a chick of a white hen], a hopeful,
a good man, a virtuous, honest man. *Quando ego te Junonium
puerum, et matris partum vere aureum?* [When shall I see you,
my Junonian youth, your mother's golden boy?] as Tully [5]
said of Octavianus; while he was adopted Cæsar, and an heir
apparent of so great a monarchy, he was a golden child.[6] All
honour,[7] offices, applause, grand titles, and turgent epithets
are put upon him, *omnes omnia bona dicere* [all praises from all
men]; all men's eyes are upon him, God bless his good worship,
his honour! every man speaks well of him,[8] every man presents
him, seeks and sues to him for his love, favour, and protection,
to serve him, belong unto him; every man riseth to him, as to
Themistocles in the Olympics; if he speak, as of Herod, *Vox
Dei, non hominis*, [it is] the voice of God, not of man. All the
graces, veneres, pleasures, elegances attend him, golden Fortune
accompanies and lodgeth with him, and, as to those Roman
emperors, is placed in his chamber.[9]

> *Secura naviget aura,
> Fortunamque suo temperet arbitrio:* [10]

he may sail as he will himself, and temper his estate at his
pleasure; jovial days, splendour and magnificence, sweet music,
dainty fare, the good things and fat of the land, fine clothes,

rich attires, soft beds, down pillows are at his command; all
the world labours for him, thousands of artificers are his slaves
to drudge for him, run, ride, and post for him; divines (for
Pythia Philippizat [the oracle is on the side of Philip]), lawyers,
physicians, philosophers, scholars are his, wholly devote to his
service.[1]   Every man seeks his acquaintance,[2] his kindred, to
match with him, though he be an oaf, a ninny, a monster, a
goosecap, *uxorem ducat Danaen*, [he may have Danae for wife],
when and whom he will, *hunc optant generum rex et regina*
[the lord and lady want him for a son-in-law], he is an excellent
match for my son, my daughter, my niece, etc.[3] *Quicquid
calcaverit hic, rosa fiet* [the ground shall become roses under
his feet], let him go whither he will, trumpets sound, bells ring,
etc., all happiness attends him, every man is willing to entertain him, he sups in Apollo [4] wheresoever he comes; what
preparation is made for his entertainment![5] fish and fowl,
spices and perfumes, all that sea and land affords. What
cookery, masking, mirth to exhilarate his person!

> *Da Trebio, pone ad Trebium. Vis, frater, ab illis
> Ilibus?* [6]

[Give Trebius some, pass to Trebius.   Would you like
   some of the flank, brother?]

What dish will your good worship eat of?

> *Dulcia poma,
> Et quoscunque feret cultus tibi fundus honores,
> Ante Larem, gustet venerabilior Lare dives.*[7]

Sweet apples, and whate'er thy fields afford,
Before thy gods be serv'd, let serve thy lord.

What sport will your honour have? hawking, hunting, fishing,
fowling, bulls, bears, cards, dice, cocks, players, tumblers,
fiddlers, jesters, etc., they are at your good worship's command.
Fair houses, gardens, orchards, terraces, galleries, cabinets,
pleasant walks, delightsome places, they are at hand; *in aureis
lac, vinum in argenteis, adolescentulæ ad nutum speciosæ* [8] [milk
in gold cups, wine in silver, beautiful maidens at his beck],
wine, wenches, etc., a Turkey paradise, an heaven upon earth.
Though he be a silly soft fellow, and scarce have common
sense, yet if he be born to fortunes (as I have said) *jure hæreditario sapere jubetur* [9] [he is bidden to be wise by hereditary
right], he must have honour and office in his course: *Nemo nisi
dives honore dignus* [10] (Ambros. *Offic.* 21) none so worthy as
himself: he shall have it, *atque esto quicquid Servius aut Labeo*

[let him be whatever Servius or Labeo was]. Get money
enough and command kingdoms,[1] provinces, armies, hearts,
hands, and affections; thou shalt have popes, patriarchs to be
thy chaplains and parasites: thou shalt have (Tamerlane-like)
kings to draw thy coach, queens to be thy laundresses, emperors thy footstools, build more towns and cities than great
Alexander, Babel towers, pyramids and mausolean tombs, etc.,
command heaven and earth, and tell the world it is thy vassal;
*auro emitur diadema, argento cœlum panditur, denarius philo-
sophum conducit, nummus jus cogit, obolus literatum pascit,
metallum sanitatem conciliat, œs amicos conglutinat* [a diadem
is bought for gold, the gates of heaven are opened to silver, a
penny buys the philosopher, money controls the course of
justice, a farthing feeds the man of letters, cash procures health,
wealth attaches friends]. And therefore not without good
cause, John Medices, that rich Florentine, when he lay upon
his death-bed, calling his sons, Cosmus and Laurence, before
him, amongst other sober saying, repeated this, *Animo quieto
digredior, quod vos sanos et divites post me delinquam,* "It doth
me good to think yet, though I be dying, that I shall leave you,
my children, sound and rich"; for wealth sways all. It is not
with us, as amongst those Lacedæmonian senators of Lycurgus
in Plutarch, "he preferred that deserved best, was most virtuous
and worthy of the place; not swiftness, or strength, or wealth,
or friends carried it in those days"; [2] but *inter optimos optimus,
inter temperantes temperantissimus,* the most temperate and best.
We have no aristocracies but in contemplation, all oligarchies,
wherein a few rich men domineer, do what they list, and are
privileged by their greatness. They may freely trespass,[3] and
do as they please, no man dare accuse them, no, not so much as
mutter against them, there is no notice taken of it, they may
securely do it, live after their own laws, and for their money
get pardons, indulgences, redeem their souls from purgatory
and hell itself; *clausum possidet arca Jovem* [Jupiter is shut
up in the money-box]. Let them be epicures, or atheists,
libertines, Machiavellians (as they often are), *Et quamvis
perjurus erit, sine gente, cruentus* [4] [though perjured, base-
born, blood-stained], they may go to heaven through the eye
of a needle, if they will themselves, they may be canonized for
saints, they shall be honourably interred in mausolean tombs,[5]
commended by poets, registered in histories, have temples and
statues erected to their names: *E manibus illis . . . nascentur
violæ* [from his remains violets shall spring]. If he be

bountiful in his life and liberal at his death, he shall have one
to swear, as he did by Claudius the emperor in Tacitus, he saw
his soul go to heaven, and be miserably lamented at his funeral.
Ambubaiarum collegia, etc.[1]   *Trimalchionis tapanta* [Trimalchio's
all-in-all (i.e. his wife Fortunata)] in Petronius *recta in
cælum abiit,* went right to heaven: a base quean, "thou
wouldst have scorned once in thy misery to have a penny
from her";[2] and why? *modio nummos metiit,* she measured
her money by the bushel.   These prerogatives do not usually
belong to rich men, but to such as are most part seeming rich;
let him have but a good outside,[3] he carries it, and shall be
adored for a god, as Cyrus was amongst the Persians,[4] *ob
splendidum apparatum,* for his gay tires; now most men are
esteemed according to their clothes.   In our gullish times, whom
you peradventure in modesty would give place to, as being
deceived by his habit, and presuming him some great worshipful
man, believe it, if you shall examine his estate, he will likely
be proved a serving-man of no great note, my lady's tailor, his
lordship's barber, or some such gull, a Fastidious Brisk, Sir
Petronel Flash,[5] a mere outside.   Only this respect is given
him, that wheresoever he comes, he may call for what he will,
and take place by reason of his outward habit.

   But on the contrary, if he be poor (Prov. xv, 15), "all his
days are miserable," he is under hatches, dejected, rejected, and
forsaken, poor in purse, poor in spirit; *prout res nobis fluit, ita
et animus se habet;*[6] money gives life and soul.[7]   Though he
be honest, wise, learned, well-deserving, noble by birth, and of
excellent good parts; yet, in that he is poor, unlikely to rise,
come to honour, office, or good means, he is contemned, neglected, *frustra sapit, inter literas esurit, amicus molestus* [his
wisdom is worthless, he starves for all his learning, he is a
troublesome friend].   "If he speak, what babbler is this?"[8]
(Ecclus.), his nobility without wealth is *projecta vilior alga*[9]
[more worthless than the seaweed on the beach], and he not
esteemed.   *Nos viles pulli nati infelicibus ovis* [we are worthless
chicks of luckless fowls], if once poor, we are metamorphosed
in an instant, base slaves, villains, and vile drudges; for to be
poor is to be a knave, a fool, a wretch, a wicked, an odious
fellow, a common eye-sore, say poor and say all:[10] they are born
to labour, to misery, to carry burdens like juments, *pistum
stercus comedere* [to eat dung] with Ulysses' companions, and
as Chremylus objected in Aristophanes, *salem lingere,*[11] [to] lick
salt, to empty jakes, fay channels, carry out dirt and dunghills,

sweep chimneys, rub horse-heels, etc.[1] (I say nothing of Turks'
galley-slaves, which are bought and sold like juments,[2] or those
African negroes, or poor Indian drudges,[3] *qui indies hinc inde
deferendis oneribus occumbunt, nam quod apud nos boves et asini
vehunt, trahunt* [who daily succumb on the roadside under their
burdens, for they do the work of oxen and asses among us], etc.
Id omne misellis Indis, etc.). They are ugly to behold, and though
erst spruce, now rusty and squalid, because poor, *immundas
fortunas æquum est squalorem sequi*[4] [dirty luck naturally brings
on dirty living], it is ordinarily so.   "Others eat to live, but
they live to drudge,"[5] *servilis et misera gens nihil recusare audet,*[6]
a servile generation, that dare refuse no task.   *Heus tu,
Dromo, cape hoc flabellum, ventulum hinc facito dum lavamur,*[7]
Sirrah, blow wind upon us while we wash, and bid your fellow
get him up betimes in the morning; be it fair or foul, he shall
run fifty miles afoot to-morrow, to carry me a letter to my
mistress; *Sosia ad pistrinam*, Sosia shall tarry at home and
grind malt all day long, Tristan thresh.   Thus are they commanded, being indeed some of them as so many footstools for
rich men to tread on, blocks for them to get on horseback, or
as "walls for them to piss on."[8]   They are commonly such
people, rude, silly, superstitious idiots, nasty, unclean, lousy,
poor, dejected, slavishly humble, and, as Leo Afer observes of
the commonalty of Africa,[9] *natura viliores sunt, nec apud suos
duces majore in pretio quam si canes assent:* base by nature,
and no more esteemed than dogs,[10] *miseram, laboriosam, cala-
mitosam vitam agunt, et inopem, infelicem, rudiores asinis, ut e
brutis plane natos dicas* [their life is full of misery, toil and
suffering, want and misfortune; they are more ignorant than
asses, and you would say they were the offspring of brutes]: no
learning, no knowledge, no civility, scarce common sense,
naught but barbarism amongst them; *belluino more vivunt,
neque calceos gestant, neque vestes*, like rogues and vagabonds,
they go barefooted and barelegged, the soles of their feet being
as hard as horse-hoofs, as Radzivilius observed at Damietta in
Egypt,[11] leading a laborious, miserable, wretched, unhappy life,
"like beasts and juments, if not worse"[12] (for a Spaniard in
Yucatan[13] sold three Indian boys for a cheese, and an hundred
negro slaves for a horse); their discourse is scurrility, their
summum bonum a pot of ale.   There is not any slavery which
these villains will not undergo, *inter illos plerique latrinas evacu-
ant, alii culinariam curant, alii stabularios agunt, urinatores, et
id genus similia exercent*, etc., like those people that dwell in the

Alps,[1] "chimney-sweepers, jakes-farmers, dirt-daubers, vagrant
rogues," they labour hard, some, and yet cannot get clothes to
put on, or bread to eat. For what can filthy poverty give else,
but beggary, fulsome nastiness, squalor, contempt, drudgery,
labour, ugliness, hunger and thirst,[2] *pediculorum et pulicum
numerum*, as he[3] well followed it in Aristophanes, fleas and
lice, *pro pallio vestem laceram, et pro pulvinari lapidem bene
magnum ad caput*, rags for his raiment, and a stone for his
pillow, *pro cathedra ruptæ caput urnæ*, he sits in a broken pitcher,
or on a block for a chair, *et malvæ ramos pro panibus comedit*,
he drinks water, and lives on wort-leaves, pulse, like a hog, or
scraps like a dog; *ut nunc nobis vita afficitur, quis non putabit
insaniam esse, infelicitatemque?* as Chremylus concludes his
speech, as we poor men live nowadays, who will not take our
life to be infelicity, misery, and madness?[4]

If they be of [a] little better condition than those base villains,
hunger - starved beggars, wandering rogues, those ordinary
slaves and day-labouring drudges, yet they are commonly so
preyed upon by polling officers for breaking the laws,[5] by
their tyrannizing landlords, so flayed and fleeced by perpetual
exactions,[6] that though they do drudge, fare hard, and starve
their genius, they cannot live in some countries;[7] but what
they have is instantly taken from them; the very care they take to
live, to be drudges, to maintain their poor families, their trouble
and anxiety, "takes away their sleep" (Sirac. xxxi, 1), it makes
them weary of their lives: when they have taken all pains,
done their utmost and honest endeavours, if they be cast behind
by sickness, or overtaken with years, no man pities them; hard-
hearted and merciless, uncharitable as they are, they leave them
so distressed, to beg, steal, murmur, and rebel, or else starve.[8]
The feeling and fear of this misery compelled those old Romans,
whom Menenius Agrippa pacified, to resist their governors;
outlaws and rebels in most places, to take up seditious arms;
and in all ages hath caused uproars, murmurings, seditions,
rebellions, thefts, mutinies, jars and contentions in every
commonwealth: grudging, repining, complaining, discontent in
each private family, because they want means to live according
to their callings, bring up their children; it breaks their hearts,
they cannot do as they would. No greater misery than for a
lord to have a knight's living, a gentleman a yeoman's, not to
be able to live as his birth and place require. Poverty and want
are generally corsives to all kind of men, especially to such
as have been in good and flourishing estate, are suddenly

distressed, nobly born, liberally brought up, and by some
disaster and casualty miserably dejected.[1] For the rest, as they
have base fortunes, so have they base minds correspondent,
like beetles, *e stercore orti, e stercore victus, in stercore delicium,*
as they were obscurely[2] born and bred, so they delight in
obscenity; they are not so throughly touched with it. *Angustas
animas angusto in pectore versant* [narrow in soul, narrow in
spirit]. Yea, that which is no small cause of their torments,
if once they come to be in distress, they are forsaken of their
fellows, most part neglected, and left unto themselves; as poor
Terence[3] in Rome was by Scipio, Lælius, and Furius, his
great and noble friends.

> *Nil Publius Scipio profuit, nil ei Lælius, nil Furius,*
> *Tres per idem tempus qui agitabant nobiles facillime,*
> *Horum ille opera ne domum quidem habuit conductitiam.*

> [They were of so little use to him that he had not even
> money to pay for a lodging.]

'Tis generally so, *Tempora si fuerint nubila, solus eris* [should
the sky of your fortunes be overcast, you will be alone], he is
left cold and comfortless, *nullus ad amissas ibit amicus opes*
[to him that has lost his wealth no friend will go], all flee from
him as from a rotten wall, now ready to fall on their heads.
Prov. xix, 4: "Poverty separates them from their neighbours."[4]

> *Dum fortuna favet, vultum servatis, amici,*
> *Cum cecidit, turpi vertitis ora fuga.*[5]

> Whilst fortune favour'd, friends, you smil'd on me,
> But when she fled, a friend I could not see.

Which is worse yet, if he be poor every man contemns him,[6]
insults over him, oppresseth him, scoffs at, aggravates his
misery.

> *Quum cœpit quassata domus subsidere, partes*
> *In proclinatas omne recumbit onus.*[7]

> When once the tottering house begins to shrink,
> Thither comes all the weight by an instinct.

Nay, they are odious to their own brethren and dearest friends.
Prov. xix, 7: "His brethren hate him if he be poor"; *omnes
vicini oderunt,*[8] "his neighbours hate him" (Prov. xiv, 20);
Omnes me noti ac ignoti deserunt,[9] as he complained in the
comedy, Friends and strangers, all forsake me. Which is most
grievous, poverty makes men ridiculous, *Nil habet infelix*

paupertas durius in se, Quam quod ridiculos homines facit, they must endure jests,[1] taunts, flouts, blows of their betters, and take all in good part to get a meal's meat: *Magnum pauperies opprobrium, jubet quidvis et facere et pati* [2] [poverty is a great source of shame; it makes a man do and suffer anything]. He must turn parasite, jester, fool (*cum desipientibus desipere* [play the fool when others do so], saith Euripides[3]), slave, villain, drudge to get a poor living, apply himself to each man's humours, to win and please, etc., and be buffeted when he hath all done, as Ulysses was by Melanthius in Homer,[4] be reviled, baffled, insulted over, for *potentiorum stultitia perferenda est* [5] [the folly of the great has to be endured], and may not so much as mutter against it. He must turn rogue and villain; for, as the saying is, *Necessitas cogit ad turpia*, poverty alone makes men thieves, rebels, murderers, traitors, assassinates ("because of poverty we have sinned," Ecclus. xxvii, 1), swear and forswear, bear false witness, lie, dissemble, anything, as I say, to advantage themselves and to relieve their necessities; *culpæ scelerisque magistra est* [6] [it teaches guilt and crime]; when a man is driven to his shifts, what will he not do?

> *Si miserum fortuna Sinonem*
> *Finxit, vanum etiam mendacemque improba finget;*
>
> [The fate that brought Sinon to poverty
> A lying knave will make him eke to be;]

he will betray his father, prince, and country, turn Turk, forsake religion, abjure God and all; *nulla tam horrenda proditio, quam illi lucri causa* (saith Leo Afer[7]) *perpetrare nolint* [there is no reason so abominable that they will not commit it for the sake of gain]. Plato therefore calls poverty "thievish, sacrilegious, filthy, wicked, and mischievous"; [8] and well he might. For it makes many an upright man otherwise, had he not been in want, to take bribes, to be corrupt, to do against his conscience, to sell his tongue, heart, hand, etc., to be churlish, hard, unmerciful, uncivil, to use indirect means to help his present estate. It makes princes to exact upon their subjects, great men tyrannize, landlords oppress, justice mercenary, lawyers vultures, physicians harpies, friends importunate, tradesmen liars, honest men thieves, devout assassinates, great men to prostitute their wives, daughters, and themselves, middle sort to repine, commons to mutiny, all to grudge, murmur, and complain. A great temptation to all mischief, it compels some miserable wretches to counterfeit several diseases,

to dismember, make themselves blind, lame, to have a more
plausible cause to beg, and lose their limbs to recover their
present wants. Jodocus Damhoderius, a lawyer of Bruges,
Praxi rerum criminal. cap. 112, hath some notable examples of
such counterfeit cranks, and every village almost will yield
abundant testimonies amongst us; we have dummerers, Abraham-men, etc. And, that which is the extent of misery, it
enforceth them, through anguish and wearisomeness of their
lives, to make away themselves: they had rather be hanged,
drowned, etc., than to live without means.

> *In mare cetiferum, ne te premat aspera egestas,*
> *Desili, et a celsis corrue, Cyrne, jugis.*[1]

> Much better 'tis to break thy neck,
> Or drown thyself i' th' sea,
> Than suffer irksome poverty;
> Go make thyself away.

A Sybarite of old, as I find it registered in Athenæus,[2] supping
in *phiditiis* [at the public tables] in Sparta, and observing their
hard fare, said it was no marvel if the Lacedæmonians were
valiant men; "for his part, he would rather run upon a
sword-point (and so would any man in his wits), than live
with such base diet, or lead so wretched a life." In Japonia [3]
'tis a common thing to stifle their children if they be
poor, or to make an abort, which Aristotle commends. In
that civil commonwealth of China, the mother strangles her
child, if she be not able to bring it up, and had rather
lose than sell it, or have it endure such misery as poor
men do.[4] Arnobius, *lib.* 7 *adversus gentes*, Lactantius,
lib. 5, *cap.* 9, objects as much to those ancient Greeks and
Romans; "they did expose their children to wild beasts, strangle,
or knock out their brains against a stone [5] in such cases." If
we may give credit to Munster,[6] amongst us Christians in
Lithuania they voluntarily mancipate and sell themselves, their
wives and children to rich men, to avoid hunger and beggary;
many make away themselves in this extremity.[7] Apicius the
Roman, when he cast up his accounts and found but 100,000
crowns left, murdered himself for fear he should be famished to
death. P. Forestus, in his Medicinal Observations, hath a
memorable example of two brothers of Louvain that, being
destitute of means, became both melancholy, and in a discontented humour massacred themselves; another of a merchant, learned, wise otherwise and discreet, but, out of a deep

apprehension he had of a loss at seas, would not be persuaded but, as Ummidius in the poet,[1] he should die a beggar.   In a word, thus much I may conclude of poor men, that though they have good parts they cannot show or make use of them:[2] *ab inopia ad virtutem obsepta est via*[3] [poverty bars the way to the advance of merit], 'tis hard for a poor man to rise:

> *Haud facile emergunt, quorum virtutibus obstat*
> *Res angusta domi.*[4]

> ['Tis hard to rise to eminence for one
> Who by his poverty is still undone.]

"The wisdom of the poor is despised, and his words are not heard" (Eccles. ix, 16).   His works are rejected, contemned, for the baseness and obscurity of the author; though laudable and good in themselves, they will not likely take.

> *Nulla placere diu, neque vivere carmina possunt,*
> *Quæ scribuntur aquæ potoribus.*

> [No verses can please or live long that are
> written by water-drinkers.]

Poor men cannot please, their actions, counsels, consultations, projects, are vilified in the world's esteem, *amittunt consilium in re* [their counsel perishes with their money], which Gnatho long since observed.   *Sapiens crepidas sibi nunquam nec soleas fecit*, a wise man never cobbled shoes, as he[5] said of old, but how doth he prove it?   I am sure we find it otherwise in our days, *pruinosis horret facundia pannis*[6] [eloquence shivers in miserable rags].   Homer himself must beg if he want means, and, as by report sometimes he did, "go from door to door, and sing ballads, with a company of boys about him."[7]   This common misery of theirs must needs distract, make them discontent and melancholy, as ordinarily they are, wayward, peevish, like a weary traveller, for *Fames et mora bilem in nares conciunt* [hunger and waiting cause terrible impatience], still murmuring and repining.   *Ob inopiam morosi sunt, quibus est male* [want makes people ill-tempered], as Plutarch quotes out of Euripides, and that comical poet well seconds:

> *Omnes quibus res sunt minus secundæ, nescio quomodo*
> *Suspiciosi, ad contumeliam omnia accipiunt magis,*
> *Propter suam impotentiam se credunt negligi;*[8]

if they be in adversity, they are more suspicious and apt to mistake: they think themselves scorned by reason of their

misery; and therefore many generous spirits in such cases
withdraw themselves from all company, as that comedian
Terence [1] is said to have done; when he perceived himself to be
forsaken and poor, he voluntarily banished himself to Stym-
phalus, a base town in Arcadia, and there miserably died.

Ad summam inopiam redactus,
Itaque e conspectu omnium abiit Græciæ in terram ultimam.

[Being reduced to poverty, he withdrew out of sight of
all men to the extreme confines of Greece.]

Neither is it without cause, for we see men commonly respected
according to their means (*an dives sit omnes quærunt, nemo an
bonus* [2] [every one asks if a man is rich, no one if he is good]),
and vilified if they be in bad clothes. Philopœmen the orator
was set to cut wood, because he was so homely attired.[3] Terentius
was placed at the lower end of Cæcilius' table, because of his
homely outside.[4] Dante, that famous Italian poet, by reason
his clothes were but mean, could not be admitted to sit down
at a feast.[5] Gnatho scorned his old familiar friend because of
his apparel: *Hominem video pannis annisque obsitum, hic ego
illum contempsi præ me.*[6] King Persius, overcome, sent a letter
to Paulus Æmilius, the Roman general: *Perseus P. Consuli S.*
[Perseus to the Consul Publius, greeting]; but he scorned him
any answer, *tacite exprobrans fortunam suam* (saith mine author)
[silently] upbraiding him with his present fortune.[7] Carolus
Pugnax, that great Duke of Burgundy, made H. Holland, late
Duke of Exeter, exiled, run after his horse like a lackey, and
would take no notice of him:[8] 'tis the common fashion of the
world.[9] So that such men as are poor may justly be discontent,
melancholy, and complain of their present misery, and all
may pray with Solomon,[10] "Give me, O Lord, neither riches
nor poverty; feed me with food convenient for me."

SUBSECT. VII.—*An heap of other Accidents causing Melancholy,
Death of Friends, Losses, etc.*

In this labyrinth of accidental causes, the farther I wander,
the more intricate I find the passage; *multæ ambages* [there
are many windings], and new causes as so many by-paths offer
themselves to be discussed. To search out all, were an Herculean
work, and fitter for Theseus; I will follow mine intended thread,
and point only at some few of the chiefest.

Amongst which, loss and death of friends may challenge a

first place. *Multi tristantur*, as Vives [1] well observes, *post delicias, convivia, dies festos*, many are melancholy after a feast, holiday, merry meeting, or some pleasing sport, if they be solitary by chance, left alone to themselves, without employment, sport, or want their ordinary companions; some at the departure of friends only whom they shall shortly see again, weep and howl, and look after them as a cow lows after her calf, or a child takes on that goes to school after holidays. *Ut me levarat tuus adventus, sic discessus afflixit* (which Tully [2] writ to Atticus), "Thy coming was not so welcome to me as thy departure was harsh." Montanus, *consil.* 132, makes mention of a country-woman that, parting with her friends and native place, became grievously melancholy for many years; and Trallianus of another, so caused for the absence of her husband: which is an ordinary passion amongst our goodwives; if their husband tarry out a day longer than his appointed time, or break his hour, they take on presently with sighs and tears, "he is either robbed, or dead, some mischance or other is surely befallen him," they cannot eat, drink, sleep, or be quiet in mind till they see him again. If parting of friends, absence alone, can work such violent effects, what shall death do, when they must eternally be separated, never in this world to meet again? This is so grievous a torment for the time, that it takes away their appetite, desire of life, extinguisheth all delights, it causeth deep sighs and groans, tears, exclamations:

> *O dulce germen matris! o sanguis meus!*
> *Eheu! tepentes*, etc. . . . *o flos tener!*

[O sweet offspring of mine! my very blood! O tender flower!]

howling, roaring, many bitter pangs (*Lamentis gemituque et femineo ululatu Tecta fremunt* [3] [With groans and female lamentation loud The house resounds]), and by frequent medita-tion extends so far sometimes, "they think they see their dead friends continually in their eyes," [4] *observantes imagines* [per-ceiving their images], as Conciliator confesseth he saw his mother's ghost presenting herself still before him. *Quod nimis miseri volunt, hoc facile credunt* [in the excess of their misery, they easily believe what they wish]; still, still, still, that good father, that good son, that good wife, that dear friend runs in their minds; *totus animus hac una cogitatione defixus est* [their mind is absorbed by this one thought], all the year long, as Pliny complains to Romanus,[5] "Methinks I see Virginius, I hear Virginius, I talk with Virginius," etc.

Te sine, væ misero mihi, lilia nigra videntur,
Pallentesque rosæ, nec dulce rubens hyacinthus,
Nullos nec myrtus, nec laurus spirat odores.[1]

[Without thee, alas, the lilies seem black, the roses pale,
the hyacinth forgets to blush, the myrtle and the
laurel lose their scent.]

They that are most staid and patient are so furiously carried
headlong by the passion of sorrow in this case, that brave
discreet men otherwise oftentimes forget themselves, and weep
like children many months together,"as if that they to water
would,"[2] and will not be comforted.   They are gone, they are
gone!

Abstulit atra dies et funere mersit acerbo.

[In an ill-omened hour bitter death has overwhelmed them.]

What shall I do?

Quis dabit in lacrimas fontem mihi? quis satis altos
Accendet gemitus, et acerbo verba dolori?
Exhaurit pietas oculos, et hiantia frangit
Pectora, nec plenos avido sinit edere questus,
Magna adeo jactura premit, etc.

Fountains of tears who gives? who lends me groans,
Deep sighs sufficient to express my moans?
Mine eyes are dry, my breast in pieces torn,
My loss so great, I cannot enough mourn.

So Stroza *filius* [the younger], that elegant Italian poet, in his
Epicedium bewails his father's death; he could moderate his
passions in other matters (as he confesseth), but not in this,
he yields wholly to sorrow:

Nunç fateor do terga malis, mens illa fatiscit,
Indomitus quondam vigor et constantia mentis.

[No more can I bear up, my spirit quails,
My strength of mind is gone, my courage fails.]

How doth Quintilian[3] complain for the loss of his son, to
despair almost! Cardan lament his only child in his book *de
libris propriis,* and elsewhere in many other of his tracts! St.
Ambrose his brother's death![4] (*An ego possum non cogitare de te,
aut sine lacrimis cogitare? O amari dies! o flebiles noctes!* [Can
I ever cease to think of thee, or to think of thee without tears?
O bitter days! O nights of sorrow!] etc.);   Gregory Nazianzen
that noble Pulcheria! (*O decorem,* etc., *flos recens, pullulans*
[How beauteous, like a new blossoming flower], etc.).   Alexander,
a man of most invincible courage, after Hephæstion's death, as

Curtius relates, *triduum jacuit ad moriendum obstinatus*, lay
three days together upon the ground, obstinate to die with
him, and would neither eat, drink, nor sleep. The woman
that communed with Esdras (*lib.* 2, *cap.* 10), when her son fell
down dead, "fled into the field, and would not return into the
city, but there resolved to remain, neither to eat nor drink, but
mourn and fast until she died." "Rachel wept for her children,
and would not be comforted because they were not" (Matt. ii, 18).
So did Hadrian the emperor bewail his Antinous; Hercules,
Hylas; Orpheus, Eurydice; David, Absalom (O my dear son
Absalom!); Austin his mother Monica, Niobe her children, insomuch that the poets feigned her to be turned into a stone, as
being stupefied through the extremity of grief.[1] Ægeus, *signo
lugubri filii consternatus, in mare se præcipitem dedit*,[2] impatient
of sorrow for his son's death, drowned himself. Our late
physicians are full of such examples. Montanus, *consil.* 242,
had a patient troubled with this infirmity, by reason of
her husband's death, many years together.[3] Trincavellius, *lib.* 1,
cap. 14, hath such another, almost in despair, after his mother's
departure,[4] *ut se ferme præcipitem daret*, and ready through
distraction to make away himself; and, in his fifteenth counsel,
tells a story of one fifty years of age, "that grew desperate
upon his mother's death"; and, cured by Fallopius, fell many
years after into a relapse, by the sudden death of a daughter
which he had, and could never after be recovered. The fury
of this passion is so violent sometimes, that it daunts whole
kingdoms and cities. Vespasian's death was pitifully lamented
all over the Roman Empire, *totus orbis lugebat*, saith Aurelius
Victor. Alexander commanded the battlements of houses to
be pulled down, mules and horses to have their manes shorn
off, and many common soldiers to be slain, to accompany his
dear Hephæstion's death; which is now practised amongst the
Tartars, when a great Cham dieth,[5] ten or twelve thousand
must be slain, men and horses, all they meet; and among those
pagan Indians, their wives and servants voluntarily die with
them.[6] Leo Decimus was so much bewailed in Rome after
his departure, that, as Jovius gives out,[7] *communis salus,
publica hilaritas*, the common safety, all good fellowship, peace,
mirth, and plenty died with him, *tanquam eodem sepulchro cum
Leone condita lugebantur* [as though buried in the same grave
with Leo]; for it was a golden age whilst he lived, but after his
decease an iron season succeeded,[8] *barbara vis et fœda vastitas,
et dira malorum omnium incommoda*, wars, plagues, vastity,

discontent.   When Augustus Cæsar died, saith Paterculus, *orbis
ruinam timueramus*, we were all afraid, as if heaven had fallen
upon our heads.   Budæus records [1] how that, at Louis the
Twelfth his death, *tam subita mutatio, ut qui prius digito cœlum
attingere videbantur, nunc humi derepente serpere, sideratos esse
diceres*, they that were erst in heaven, upon a sudden, as if
they had been planet-strucken, lay grovelling on the ground:

> *Concussis cecidere animis, ceu frondibus ingens
> Silva dolet lapsis;* [2]

> [Nerveless they crashed, as when the forest moans
> Its fallen leaves;]

they looked like cropped trees.   At Nancy in Lorraine, when
Claudia Valesia, Henry the second French king's sister and the
duke's wife, deceased, the temples for forty days were all shut
up, no prayers nor masses but in that room where she was;
the senators all seen in black, "and for a twelvemonth's space
throughout the city they were forbid to sing or dance." [3]

> *Non ulli pastos illis egere diebus
> Frigida, Daphni, boves ad flumina, nulla nec amnem
> Libavit quadrupes, nec graminis attigit herbam.* [4]

> [The swains forgot their sheep, nor near the brink
> Of running waters brought their herds to drink;
> The thirsty cattle, of themselves, abstained
> From water, and their grassy fare disdained.]

How were we affected here in England for our Titus, *deliciæ
humani generis* [the darling of the human race], Prince Henry's
immature death, as if all our dearest friends' lives had exhaled
with his!   Scanderbeg's death was not so much lamented in
Epirus. [5]   In a word, as he [6] saith of Edward the First at the
news of Edward of Carnarvon his son's birth, *immortaliter gavisus*,
he was immortally glad, may we say on the contrary of friends'
deaths, *immortaliter gementes*, we are divers of us, as so many
turtles, eternally dejected with it.

There is another sorrow, which arises from the loss of temporal goods and fortunes, which equally afflicts, and may go
hand in hand with the precedent; loss of time, loss of honour,
office, of good name, of labour, frustrate hopes, will much
torment; but in my judgment, there is no torture like unto it,
or that sooner procureth this malady and mischief:

> *Ploratur lacrimis amissa pecunia veris:* [7]

> [Lost money is bewailed with grief sincere:]

it wrings true tears from our eyes, many sighs, much sorrow

from our hearts, and often causes habitual melancholy itself.
Guianerius, *tract*. 15, 5, repeats this for an especial cause: "Loss
of friends, and loss of goods, make many men melancholy, as
I have often seen by continual meditation of such things." [1]
The same causes Arnoldus Villanovanus inculcates, *Breviar. lib.* 1,
cap. 18, *ex rerum amissione, damno, amicorum morte* [from loss of
property, damage, death of friends], etc.   Want alone will make
a man mad, to be *sans argent* will cause a deep and grievous
melancholy.   Many persons are affected like Irishmen [2] in this
behalf, who if they have a good scimitar, had rather have a
blow on their arm than their weapon hurt: they will sooner
lose their life than their goods: and the grief that cometh
hence continueth long (saith Plater [3]) "and out of many dispositions, procureth an habit."   Montanus [4] and Frisimelica
cured a young man of twenty-two years of age, that so became
melancholy, *ob amissam pecuniam*, for a sum of money which
he had unhappily lost.   Sckenkius hath such another story of
one melancholy, because he overshot himself and spent his
stock in unnecessary building.   Roger, that rich Bishop of
Salisbury,[5] *exutus opibus et castris a Rege Stephano*, spoiled of
his goods by King Stephen, *vi doloris absorptus, atque in amen-
tiam versus, indecentia fecit*, through grief ran mad, spoke and
did he knew not what.   Nothing so familiar as for men in such
cases through anguish of mind to make away themselves.   A
poor fellow went to hang himself (which Ausonius hath elegantly
expressed in a neat epigram [6]), but finding by chance a pot of
money, flung away the rope and went merrily home; but he
that hid the gold, when he missed it, hanged himself with that
rope which the other man had left, in a discontented humour.

> *At qui condiderat, postquam non repperit aurum,*
> *Aptavit collo, quem reperit laqueum.*

Such feral accidents can want and penury produce.   Be it by
suretyship, shipwreck, fire, spoil and pillage of soldiers, or what
loss soever, it boots not, it will work the like effect, the same
desolation in provinces and cities, as well as private persons.
The Romans were miserably dejected after the battle of Cannæ,
the men amazed for fear, the stupid women tore their hair and
cried.   The Hungarians, when their King Ladislaus and bravest
soldiers were slain by the Turks, *Luctus publicus* [a public
mourning], etc.   The Venetians, when their forces were overcome by the French king Louis, the French and Spanish kings,
pope, emperor, all conspired against them at Cambrai, the

French herald denounced open war in the senate: *Lauredane,
Venetorum dux* [Loredano, Doge of Venice], etc., and they
had lost Padua, Brixia, Verona, Forum Julii, their territories
in the continent, and had now nothing left, but the city
of Venice itself, *et urbi quoque ipsi* (saith Bembus[1]) *timendum
putarent*, and the loss of that was likewise to be feared, *tantus
repente dolor omnes tenuit, ut nunquam alias*, etc., they were
pitifully plunged, never before in such lamentable distress.
Anno 1527, when Rome was sacked by Burbonius,[2] the common
soldiers made such spoil, that fair churches were turned to
stables, old monuments and books made horse-litter, or burned
like straw; relics, costly pictures defaced; altars demolished,
rich hangings, carpets, etc., trampled in the dirt;[3] their wives
and loveliest daughters constuprated by every base cullion,[4] as
Sejanus' daughter was by the hangman in public, before their
fathers' and husbands' faces; noblemen's children, and of the
wealthiest citizens, reserved for princes' beds, were prostitute
to every common soldier, and kept for concubines; senators and
cardinals themselves dragged along the streets, and put to
exquisite torments, to confess where their money was hid; the
rest, murdered on heaps, lay stinking in the streets; infants'
brains dashed out before their mothers' eyes. A lamentable
sight it was to see a goodly a city so suddenly defaced, rich
citizens sent a-begging to Venice, Naples, Ancona, etc., that
erst lived in all manner of delights. "Those proud palaces,
that even now vaunted their tops up to heaven, were dejected
as low as hell in an instant."[5] Whom will not such misery
make discontent? Terence the poet drowned himself (some
say) for the loss of his comedies, which suffered shipwreck.
When a poor man hath made many hungry meals, got together
a small sum, which he loseth in an instant; a scholar spent many
an hour's study to no purpose, his labours lost, etc., how should
it otherwise be? I may conclude with Gregory, *Temporalium
amor, quantum afficit, cum hæret possessio, tantum, quum sub-
trahitur, urit dolor;* riches do not so much exhilarate us with
their possession, as they torment us with their loss.

Next to sorrow still I may annex such accidents as procure
fear; for besides those terrors which I have before touched,[6]
and many other fears (which are infinite), there is a superstitious
fear, one of the three great causes of fear in Aristotle, commonly
caused by prodigies and dismal accidents, which much trouble
many of us. (*Nescio quid animus mihi præsagit mali* [my mind
has a presentiment of some evil]). As if a hare cross the way

at our going forth, or a mouse gnaw our clothes; if they bleed
three drops at nose, the salt falls towards them, a black spot
appear in their nails, etc., with many such, which Delrio,
tom. 2, *lib.* 3, *sect.* 4; Austin Niphus in his book *de auguriis*;
Polydore Virgil, *lib.* 3 *de prodigiis*; Sarisburiensis, *Polycrat. lib.* 1,
cap. 13, discuss at large.   They are so much affected that, with
the very strength of imagination, fear, and the devil's craft,
"they pull those misfortunes they suspect upon their own
heads, and that which they fear shall come upon them," [1] as
Solomon foretelleth (Prov. x, 24) and Isaiah denounceth (lxvi, 4),
which, "if they could neglect and contemn, would not come to
pass." [2]   *Eorum vires nostra resident opinione, ut morbi gravitas
ægrotantium cogitatione* [their force lies in our own fancy, as
the virulence of a disease depends on the mind of the patient],
they are intended and remitted as our opinion is fixed, more
or less.   *N. N. dat pœnas*, saith Crato of such a one,[3] *utinam non
attraheret !* he is punished, and is the cause of it himself.[4]   *Dum
fata fugimus fata stulti incurrimus* [5] [in fleeing from our destiny
we run into its arms].   "The thing that I feared," saith Job, "is
fallen upon me."

As much we may say of them that are troubled with their
fortunes, or ill destinies foreseen; *multos angit præscientia
malorum:* the foreknowledge of what shall come to pass
crucifies many men: foretold by astrologers, or wizards, *iratum
ob cœlum* [because of the anger of the heavens], be it ill accident,
or death itself: which often falls out by God's permission;
Quia dæmonem timent (saith Chrysostom), *Deus ideo permittit
accidere* [because they fear the devil, therefore God suffers it to
happen].   Severus, Hadrian, Domitian, can testify as much, of
whose fear and suspicion Suetonius, Herodian, and the rest of
those writers tell strange stories in this behalf.   Montanus,
consil. 31, hath one example of a young man, exceeding melancholy upon this occasion.[6]   Such fears have still tormented
mortal men in all ages, by reason of those lying oracles and
juggling priests.   There was a fountain in Greece, near Ceres'
temple in Achaia, where the event of such diseases was to be
known. "A glass let down by a thread," etc.[7]   Amongst those
Cyanean rocks at the springs of Lycia, was the oracle of
Thryxeus Apollo, "where all fortunes were foretold, sickness,
health, or what they would besides": so common people have
been always deluded with future events.   At this day, *metus
futurorum maxime torquet Sinas*, this foolish fear mightily
crucifies them in China; as Matthew Riccius the Jesuit in-

formeth us, in his commentaries of those countries,[1] of all
nations they are most superstitious, and much tormented in
this kind, attributing so much to their divinators, *ut ipse metus
fidem faciat*, that fear itself and conceit cause it to fall out;[2]
if he foretell sickness such a day, that very time they will be
sick, *vi metus afflicti in ægritudinem cadunt*, and many times
die as it is foretold.   A true saying, *Timor mortis, morte pejor*,
the fear of death is worse than death itself, and the memory
of that sad hour, to some fortunate and rich men, "is as bitter
as gall" (Ecclus. xli, 1).   *Inquietam nobis vitam facit mortis
metus* [the fear of death disturbs our life]; a worse plague
cannot happen to a man than to be so troubled in his mind;
'tis *triste divortium*, a heavy separation, to leave their goods,
with so much labour got, pleasures of the world which they
have so deliciously enjoyed, friends and companions whom they
so dearly loved, all at once.   Axiochus the philosopher was
bold and courageous all his life, and gave good precepts *de
contemnenda morte* [for contemning death], and against the
vanity of the world, to others; but being now ready to die
himself he was mightily dejected: *Hac luce privabor? his orbabor
bonis?* [Am I to be banished from light, to be deprived of so
many good things?] he lamented like a child, etc.   And though
Socrates himself was there to comfort him: *Ubi pristina virtutum
jactatio, o Axioche?* [Where is all your boasted virtue now, my
friend?] yet he was very timorous and impatient of death,
much troubled in his mind, *imbellis pavor et impatientia* [craven
fear and weakness], etc.   "O Clotho," Megapenthes, the tyrant in
Lucian, exclaims, now ready to depart, "let me live awhile
longer.   I will give thee a thousand talents of gold, and two
bowls besides, which I took from Cleocritus, worth an hundred
talents apiece."[3]   "Woe's me!" saith another,[4] "what goodly
manors shall I leave! what fertile fields! what a fine house!
what pretty children! how many servants! who shall gather
my grapes, my corn?   Must I now die so well settled? leave
all, so richly and well provided?   Woe's me, what shall I do?"
Animula vagula, blandula, quæ nunc abibis in loca?[5] [Poor
fluttering, coaxing soul of mine, What new abode shall now be
thine?]

   To these tortures of fear and sorrow may well be annexed
curiosity, that irksome, that tyrannizing care, *nimia sollicitudo*,
"superfluous industry about unprofitable things and their
qualities,"[6] as Thomas defines it: an itching humour or a
kind of longing to see that which is not to be seen, to do that

which ought not to be done, to know that secret which should
not be known, to eat of the forbidden fruit.[1] We commonly
molest and tire ourselves about things unfit and unnecessary,
as Martha troubled herself to little purpose. Be it in religion,
humanity, magic, philosophy, policy, any action or study, 'tis
a needless trouble, a mere torment. For what else is school
divinity? How many doth it puzzle! what fruitless questions
about the Trinity, resurrection, election, predestination, reprobation, hell-fire, etc., how many shall be saved, damned! What
else is all superstition, but an endless observation of idle ceremonies, traditions? What is most of our philosophy but a
labyrinth of opinions, idle questions, propositions, metaphysical
terms? Socrates therefore held all philosophers cavillers and
madmen, *circa subtilia cavillatores pro insanis habuit, palam
eos arguens*, saith Eusebius,[2] because they commonly sought
after such things *quæ nec percipi a nobis neque comprehendi
possent* [which can be neither perceived nor understood by us],
or put case they did understand, yet they were altogether
unprofitable. For what matter is it for us to know how high
the Pleiades are, how far distant Perseus and Cassiopea from
us, how deep the sea, etc.? We are neither wiser, as he follows
it, nor modester, nor better, nor richer, nor stronger for the
knowledge of it. *Quod supra nos nihil ad nos* [what is above
us does not concern us]. I may say the same of those genethliacal studies: what is astrology but vain elections, predictions?
all magic, but a troublesome error, a pernicious foppery?
physic, but intricate rules and prescriptions? philology, but
vain criticisms? logic, needless sophisms? metaphysics themselves, but intricate subtleties and fruitless abstractions?
alchemy, but a bundle or errors? To what end are such great
tomes? why do we spend so many years in their studies?
Much better to know nothing at all, as those barbarous Indians
are wholly ignorant, than, as some of us, to be so sore vexed
about unprofitable toys: *stultus labor est ineptiarum* [it is foolish
to labour at trifles], to build a house without pins, make a rope
of sand, to what end? *cui bono?* He studies on, but, as the boy
told St. Austin, when I have laved the sea dry, thou shalt
understand the mystery of the Trinity. He makes observations, keeps times and seasons; and as Conradus the emperor
would not touch his new bride till an astrologer had told him
a masculine hour;[3] but with what success? He travels into
Europe, Africa, Asia, searcheth every creek, sea, city, mountain,
gulf, to what end? See one promontory (said Socrates of old),

one mountain, one sea, one river, and see all. An alchemist spends his fortunes to find out the philosopher's stone forsooth, cure all diseases, make men long-lived, victorious, fortunate, invisible, and beggars himself, misled by those seducing impostors, (which he shall never attain) to make gold; an antiquary consumes his treasure and time to scrape up a company of old coins, statues, rolls, edicts, manuscripts, etc.; he must know what was done of old in Athens, Rome, what lodging, diet, houses they had, and have all the present news at first, though never so remote, before all others, what projects, counsels, consultations, etc., *quid Juno in aurem insusurraret Jovi* [what Juno whispered in Jupiter's ear], what's now decreed in France, what in Italy: who was he, whence comes he, which way, whither goes he, etc. Aristotle must find out the motion of Euripus; Pliny must needs see Vesuvius; but how sped they? One loseth goods, another his life. Pyrrhus will conquer Africa first, and then Asia. He will be a sole monarch, a second immortal, a third rich, a fourth commands. *Turbine magno spes sollicitæ in urbibus errant*[1] [one finds in cities a great turmoil of anxious hopes]; we run, ride, take indefatigable pains, all up early, down late, striving to get that which we had better be without (Ardelios,[2] busybodies as we are), it were much fitter for us to be quiet, sit still, and take our ease. His sole study is for words, that they be *lepide lexeis compostæ ut tesserulæ omnes* [elegant expressions put together like a mosaic], not a syllable misplaced, to set out a stramineous subject; as thine is about apparel, to follow the fashion, to be terse and polite, 'tis thy sole business; both with like profit. His only delight is building, he spends himself to get curious pictures, intricate models and plots; another is wholly ceremonious about titles, degrees, inscriptions; a third is oversolicitous about his diet, he must have such and such exquisite sauces, meat so dressed, so far-fetched, *peregrini aeris volucres* [birds from a foreign clime], so cooked, etc., something to provoke thirst, something anon to quench his thirst. Thus he redeems his appetite with extraordinary charge to his purse, is seldom pleased with any meal, whilst a trivial stomach useth all with delight and is never offended. Another must have roses in winter, *alieni temporis flores* [flowers out of season] snow-water in summer, fruits before they can be or are usually ripe, artificial gardens and fish-ponds on the tops of houses, all things opposite to the vulgar sort, intricate and rare, or else they are nothing worth. So busy, nice, curious wits make that unsupportable in all vocations, trades, actions, employments, which to duller apprehensions is not offensive, earnestly seeking that which others as scornfully neglect. Thus through our foolish curiosity do we macerate ourselves, tire our souls, and run headlong, through our indiscretion, perverse will, and want of government, into many needless cares and troubles, vain expenses, tedious journeys, painful hours; and when all is done, *quorsum hæc? cui bono?* to what end?

> *Nescire velle quæ Magister maximus*
> *Docere non vult, erudita inscitia est.*[1]

> [Humbly to be contented not to know
> What the Great Master hath not deigned to show,
> Though ignorance, is learning quite enow.]

Amongst these passions and irksome accidents, unfortunate marriage may be ranked: a condition of life appointed by God Himself in Paradise, an honourable and happy estate, and as great a felicity as can befall a man in this world, if the parties can agree as they ought,[2] and live as Seneca lived with his Paulina;[3] but if they be unequally matched, or at discord, a greater misery cannot be expected, to have a scold, a slut, an harlot, a fool, a fury or a fiend, there can be no such plague. "He that hath her is as if he held a scorpion," etc. (Ecclus. xxvi, 14), and "a wicked wife makes a sorry countenance, an heavy heart, and he had rather dwell with a lion than keep house with such a wife" (xxv, 23, 16). Her properties Jovianus Pontanus hath described at large, *Ant. dial. tom. 2*, under the name of Euphorbia.[4] Or if they be not equal in years, the like mischief happens; Cæcilius, in A. Gellius, *lib. 2, cap. 23*, complains much of an old wife: *Dum ejus morti inhio, egomet mortuus vivo inter vivos*, Whilst I gape after her death, I live a dead man amongst the living; or if they dislike upon any occasion:

> Judge who that are unfortunately wed
> What 'tis to come into a loathed bed.[5]

The same inconvenience befalls women.

> *At vos, o duri, miseram lugete parentes,*
> *Si ferro aut laqueo læva hac me exsolvere sorte*
> *Sustineo :*[6]

> Hard-hearted parents, both lament my fate,
> If self I kill or hang, to ease my state.

A young gentlewoman in Basil was married,[7] saith Felix Plater, *Observat. lib. 1*, to an ancient man against her will, whom

she could not affect; she was continually melancholy, and pined
away for grief; and though her husband did all he could possibly
to give her content, in a discontented humour at length she
hanged herself. Many other stories he relates in this kind.
Thus men are plagued with women, they again with men, when
they are of diverse humours and conditions; he a spendthrift,
she sparing; one honest, the other dishonest, etc. Parents
many times disquiet their children, and they their parents.
"A foolish son is an heaviness to his mother." [1] *Injusta noverca:*
a stepmother often vexeth a whole family, is matter of repentance, exercise of patience, fuel of dissension, which made Cato's
son expostulate with his father, why he should offer to marry
his client Salonius' daughter, a young wench, *cujus causa novercam induceret?* what offence had he done, that he should marry
again?

Unkind, unnatural friends, evil neighbours, bad servants,
debts and debates, etc.; 'twas Chilo's sentence, *comes æris
alieni et litis est miseria,* misery and usury do commonly together;
suretyship is the bane of many families, *Sponde, præsto noxa
est* [go surety, and ruin is near at hand]: "he shall be sore
vexed that is surety for a stranger" (Prov. xi, 15), "and he
that hateth suretyship is sure." Contention, brawling, lawsuits, falling out of neighbours and friends, *discordia demens*
[frantic discord] (Virg. Æn. 6), are equal to the first, grieve
many a man, and vex his soul. *Nihil sane miserabilius eorum
mentibus* (as Boter holds [2]) "nothing so miserable as such men,
full of cares, griefs, anxieties, as if they were stabbed with a
sharp sword; fear, suspicion, desperation, sorrow, are their
ordinary companions." Our Welshmen are noted by some of
their own writers,[3] to consume one another in this kind; but
whosoever they are that use it, these are their common symptoms, especially if they be convict or overcome, cast in a suit.
Arius, put out of a bishopric by Eustathius, turned heretic, and
lived after discontented all his life. Every repulse is of like
nature;[4] *Heu quanta de spe decidi!* [Alas, what prospects have
I lost!]. Disgrace, infamy, detraction, will almost effect as
much, and that a long time after. Hipponax, a satirical poet,
so vilified and lashed two painters in his iambics, *ut ambo
laqueo se suffocarent,* Pliny saith,[5] both hanged themselves. All
oppositions, dangers, perplexities, discontents, to live in any
suspense, are of the same rank: [6] *Potes hoc sub casu ducere somnos?*
[Can you sleep with such trouble impending?] Who can be
secure in such cases? Ill-bestowed benefits, ingratitude,

unthankful friends, much disquiet and molest some. Unkind speeches trouble as many, uncivil carriage or dogged answers, weak women above the rest; if they proceed from their surly husbands, are as bitter as gall, and not to be digested.[1] A glassman's wife in Basil became melancholy because her husband said he would marry again if she died. "No cut to unkindness," as the saying is; a frown and hard speech, ill respect, a brow-beating, or bad look, especially to courtiers, or such as attend upon great persons, is present death: *Ingenium vultu statque caditque suo*, they ebb and flow with their masters' favours. Some persons are at their wits' ends, if by chance they overshoot themselves in their ordinary speeches or actions, which may after turn to their disadvantage or disgrace, or have any secret disclosed. Ronseus, *Epist. miscel.* 3, reports of a gentlewoman twenty-five years old, that, falling foul with one of her gossips, was upbraided with a secret infirmity (no matter what) in public, and so much grieved with it, that she did thereupon *solitudines quærere, omnes ab se ablegare, ac tandem, in gravissimam incidens melancholiam, contabescere*, forsake all company, quite moped, and in a melancholy humour pine away. Others are as much tortured to see themselves rejected, contemned, scorned, disabled, diffamed, detracted, undervalued, or "left behind their fellows." [2] Lucian brings in Hetœmocles, a philosopher, in his *Lapith. convivio*, much discontented that he was not invited amongst the rest, expostulating the matter, in a long epistle, with Aristænetus their host. *Prætextatus*, a robed gentleman in Plutarch, would not sit down at a feast, because he might not sit highest, but went his ways all in a chafe. We see the common quarrellings that are ordinary with us, for taking of the wall, precedency, and the like, which though toys in themselves, and things of no moment, yet they cause many distempers, much heart-burning amongst us. Nothing pierceth deeper than a contempt or disgrace, especially if they be generous spirits,[3] scarce anything affects them more than to be despised or vilified. Crato, *consil.* 16, *lib.* 2, exemplifies it, and common experience confirms it. Of the same nature is oppression: "Surely oppression makes a man mad" (Eccles. vii, 7); loss of liberty, which made Brutus venture his life, Cato kill himself, and Tully complain,[4] *Omnem hilaritatem in perpetuum amisi*,[5] Mine heart's broken, I shall never look up, or be merry again; *hæc jactura intolerabilis*, to some parties 'tis a most intolerable loss. Banishment, a great misery, as Tyrtæus describes it in an epigram of his:

*Nam miserum est patria amissa, laribusque, vagari
Mendicum, et timida voce rogare cibos :
Omnibus invisus, quocunque accesserit, exul
Semper erit, semper spretus egensque jacet,* etc.

A miserable thing 'tis so to wander,
And like a beggar for to whine at door,
Contemn'd of all the world an exile is,
Hated, rejected, needy still and poor.

Polynices, in his conference with Jocasta in Euripides,[1] reckons
up five miseries of a banished man, the least of which alone
were enough to deject some pusillanimous creatures. Oftentimes a too great feeling of our own infirmities or imperfections
of body or mind will rivel us up; as if we be long sick:

*O beata sanitas! te præsente, amœnum
Ver floret gratiis, absque te nemo beatus.*

[O blessed health! when thou art with us the spring is
full of charms, without thee no one is happy.]

O blessed health! "thou art above all gold and treasure"
(Ecclus. xxx, 15), the poor man's riches, the rich man's bliss,
without thee there can be no happiness: or visited with some
loathsome disease, offensive to others, or troublesome to ourselves; as a stinking breath, deformity of our limbs, crookedness,
loss of an eye, leg, hand, paleness, leanness, redness, baldness,
loss or want of hair, etc., *hic ubi fluere cœpit, diros ictus cordi
infert,* saith Synesius [2] (he himself troubled not a little *ob comœ
defectum*), the loss of hair alone strikes a cruel stroke to the heart.
Acco, an old woman, seeing by chance her face in a true glass
(for she used false flattering glasses belike at other times, as most
gentlewomen do), *animi dolore in insaniam delapsa est* (Cælius
Rhodiginus, *lib.* 17, *cap.* 2), ran mad. Broteas, the son of
Vulcan, because he was ridiculous for his imperfections, flung
himself into the fire.[3] Lais of Corinth, now grown old, gave
up her glass to Venus, for she could not abide to look upon it.
Qualis sum nolo, qualis eram nequeo [what I am I fain would not
be, what I was I cannot be].[4] Generally to fair nice pieces, old
age and foul linen are two most odious things, a torment of
torments, they may not abide the thought of it.

*O deorum
Quisquis hæc audis, utinam inter errem
Nuda leones,
Antequam turpis macies decentes
Occupet malas, teneræque succus
Defluat prædæ, speciosa quæro
Pascere tigres.*[5]

[Hear me, some gracious heavenly power,
Let lions this naked corse devour.
My cheeks ere hollow wrinkles seize,
Ere yet their rosy bloom decays;
While youth yet rolls its vital flood,
Let tigers fiercely riot in my blood.]

To be foul, ugly, and deformed! much better be buried alive.
Some are fair but barren, and that galls them: "Hannah wept
sore, did not eat, and was troubled in spirit, and all for her
barrenness" (1 Sam. 1); and (Gen. 30), Rachel said "in the
anguish of her soul, Give me a child, or I shall die"; another
hath too many: one was never married, and that's his hell,
another is, and that's his plague. Some are troubled in that they
are obscure; others by being traduced, slandered, abused, disgraced, vilified, or anyway injured: *minime miror eos* (as he said)
qui insanire occipiunt ex injuria, I marvel not at all if offences
make men mad. Seventeen particular causes of anger and
offence Aristotle reckons them up, which for brevity's sake I
must omit. No tidings troubles one; ill reports, rumours, bad
tidings or news, hard hap, ill success, cast in a suit, vain hopes,
or hope deferred, another: expectation, *adeo omnibus in rebus
molesta semper est expectatio* [expectation in all circumstances
brings annoyance] as Polybius observes; [1] one is too eminent,
another too base-born, and that alone tortures him as much as
the rest: one is out of action, company, employment; another
overcome and tormented with worldly cares and onerous business. But what tongue can suffice to speak of all? [2]

Many men catch this malady by eating certain meats, herbs,
roots, at unawares; as henbane, nightshade, cicuta, mandrakes,
etc. A company of young men at Agrigentum, in Sicily, came
into a tavern; [3] where after they had freely taken their liquor,
whether it were the wine itself, or something mixed with it 'tis
not yet known, but upon a sudden they began to be so troubled
in their brains, and their phantasy so crazed, that they thought
they were in a ship at sea, and now ready to be cast away by
reason of a tempest. [4] Wherefore, to avoid shipwreck and
present drowning, they flung all the goods in the house out at
the windows into the street, or into the sea, as they supposed;
thus they continued mad a pretty season, and being brought
before the magistrate to give an account of this their fact, they
told him (not yet recovered of their madness) that what was
done they did for fear of death, and to avoid imminent danger.
The spectators were all amazed at this their stupidity, and gazed

on them still, whilst one of the ancientest of the company, in a grave tone, excused himself to the magistrate upon his knees, *O viri Tritones, ego in imo jacui,* I beseech your deities, etc., for I was in the bottom of the ship all the while: another besought them, as so many sea-gods, to be good unto them, and if ever he and his fellows came to land again, he would build an altar to their service.[1] The magistrate could not sufficiently laugh at this their madness, bid them sleep it out, and so went his ways. Many such accidents frequently happen upon these unknown occasions. Some are so caused by philters, wandering in the sun, biting of a mad dog, a blow on the head, stinging with that kind of spider called tarantula, an ordinary thing, if we may believe Sckenkius, *lib.* 6 *de venenis,* in Calabria and Apulia in Italy, Cardan, *Subtil. lib.* 9, Scaliger, *exercitat.* 185. Their symptoms are merrily described by Jovianus Pontanus, *Ant. dial.,* how they dance altogether, and are cured by music. Cardan[2] speaks of certain stones, if they be carried about one, which will cause melancholy and madness; he calls them unhappy, as an adamant, selenites, etc. "which dry up the body, increase cares, diminish sleep":[3] Ctesias, *in Persicis,* makes mention of a well in those parts, of which if any man drink, "he is mad for twenty-four hours."[4] Some lose their wits by terrible objects (as elsewhere I have more copiously dilated,[5] and life itself many times, as Hippolytus affrighted by Neptune's sea-horses, Athamas by Juno's Furies: but these relations are common in all writers.

> *Hic alias poteram, et plures subnectere causas,*
> *Sed jumenta vocant, et sol inclinat, eundum est.*[6]

> Many such causes, much more could I say,
> But that for provender my cattle stay:
> The sun declines, and I must needs away.

These causes, if they be considered and come alone, I do easily yield, can do little of themselves, seldom, or apart (an old oak is not felled at a blow), though many times they are all-sufficient every one: yet if they concur, as often they do, *vis unita fortior; et quæ non absunt singula, multa nocent* [union gives strength; things which singly hurt not can do injury when in a mass], they may batter a strong constitution; as Austin said, "many grains and small sands sink a ship, many small drops make a flood," etc.,[7] often reiterated; many dispositions produce an habit.

MEMB. V.

Subsect. I.—*Continent, inward, antecedent, next Causes, and how the Body works on the Mind*

As a purly hunter, I have hitherto beaten about the circuit of the forest of this microcosm, and followed only those outward adventitious causes. I will now break into the inner rooms, and rip up the antecedent immediate causes which are there to be found. For as the distraction of the mind, amongst other outward causes and perturbations, alters the temperature of the body, so the distraction and distemper of the body will cause a distemperature of the soul, and 'tis hard to decide which of these two do more harm to the other. Plato, Cyprian, and some others, as I have formerly said, lay the greatest fault upon the soul, excusing the body; others again, accusing the body, excuse the soul, as a principal agent. Their reasons are, because "the manners do follow the temperature of the body," [1] as Galen proves in his book of that subject, Prosper Calenius, *de atra bile*, Jason Pratensis, *cap. de mania*, Lemnius, *lib.* 4, *cap.* 16, and many others. And that which Gualter hath commented, *Hom.* 10 *in epist. Johannis*, is most true, concupiscence and original sin, inclinations, and bad humours are radical [2] in every one of us, causing these perturbations, affections, and several distempers, offering many times violence unto the soul. "Every man is tempted by his own concupiscence" (James i, 14), "the spirit is willing but the flesh is weak, and rebelleth against the spirit," as our apostle teacheth us: [3] that methinks the soul hath the better plea against the body, which so forcibly inclines us, that we cannot resist, *Nec nos obniti contra, nec tendere tantum Sufficimus* [To make a stand, and manfully resist, Our strength avails not]. How the body, being material, worketh upon the immaterial soul, by mediation of humours and spirits, which participate of both, and ill-disposed organs, Cornelius Agrippa hath discoursed, *lib.* 1 *de occult. Philos., cap.* 63, 64, 65; Levinus Lemnius, *lib.* 1 *de occult. nat. mir. cap.* 12 *et* 16 *et* 21, *Institut. ad opt. vit.*; Perkins, *lib.* 1, Cases of Conscience, *cap.* 12; T. Bright, *capp.* 10, 11, 12, in his Treatise of Melancholy. For as anger,[4] fear, sorrow, obtrectation, emulation, etc., *si mentis intimos recessus occuparint*, saith Lemnius,[5] *corpori quoque infesta sunt, et illi teterrimos morbos inferunt,* cause grievous diseases in the body, so bodily diseases affect the soul by consent. Now the

chiefest causes proceed from the heart, humours, spirits:[1] as they
are purer, or impurer, so is the mind, and equally suffers, as a lute
out of tune; if one string or one organ be distempered, all the
rest miscarry, *Corpus onustum Hesternis vitiis, animum quoque
prægravat una*[2] [By yesterday's éxcesses still oppressed, The body
suffers not the mind to rest].   The body is *domicilium animæ* [the
dwelling of the soul], her house, abode, and stay; and as a torch
gives a better light, a sweeter smell, according to the matter it
is made of, so doth our soul perform all her actions, better or
worse, as her organs are disposed; or as wine savours of the cask
wherein it is kept, the soul receives a tincture from the body,
through which it works.   We see this in old men, children,
Europeans, Asians, hot and cold climes; sanguine are merry,
melancholy sad, phlegmatic dull, by reason of abundance of
those humours, and they cannot resist such passions which are
inflicted by them.   For in this infirmity of human nature, as
Melancthon declares, the understanding is so tied to and captivated by his inferior senses, that without their help he cannot
exercise his functions, and the will, being weakened, hath but a
small power to restrain those outward parts, but suffers herself
to be overruled by them; that I must needs conclude with
Lemnius, *spiritus et humores maximum nocumentum obtinent,*
spirits and humours do most harm in troubling the soul.[3]   How
should a man choose but be choleric and angry, that hath his
body so clogged with abundance of gross humours? or melancholy, that is so inwardly disposed?   That thence comes then
this malady, madness, apoplexies, lethargies, etc. it may not
be denied.

Now this body of ours is most part distempered by some
precedent diseases, which molest his inward organs and instruments, and so *per consequens* [consequently] cause melancholy,
according to the consent of the most approved physicians.
"This humour"[4] (as Avicenna, *lib.* 3, *fen.* 1, *tract.* 4, *cap.* 18,
Arnoldus, *Breviar. lib.* 1, *cap.* 18, Jacchinus, *Comment. in* 9
Rhasis, cap. 15, Montaltus, *cap.* 10, Nicholas Piso, *cap. de melan.*,
etc., suppose) "is begotten by the distemperature of some inward
part, innate, or left after some inflammation, or else included in
the blood after an ague,[5] or some other malignant disease."
This opinion of theirs concurs with that of Galen, *lib.* 3, *cap.* 6,
de locis affect.   Guianerius gives an instance in one so caused by
a quartan ague, and Montanus, *consil.* 32, in a young man of
twenty-eight years of age, so distempered after a quartan, which
had molested him five years together; Hildesheim, *Spicil.* 2 *de*

mania, relates of a Dutch baron, grievously tormented with
melancholy after a long ague: [1] Galen, *lib. de atra bile, cap.* 4,
puts the plague a cause; Botaldus, in his book *de lue vener.
cap.* 2, the French pox for a cause; others frenzy, epilepsy,
apoplexy, because those diseases do often degenerate into this.
Of suppression of hemrods, hæmorrhagia, or bleeding at the nose,
menstruous retentions (although they deserve a larger explication, as being the sole cause of a proper kind of melancholy,
in more ancient maids, nuns and widows, handled apart by
Rodericus à Castro and Mercatus, as I have elsewhere signified),
or any other evacuation stopped, I have already spoken. Only
this I will add, that this melancholy, which shall be caused by
such infirmities, deserves to be pitied of all men, and to be
respected with a more tender compassion, according to Laurentius, as coming from a more inevitable cause.

Subsect. II.—*Distemperature of particular Parts, Causes*

There is almost no part of the body which, being distempered,
doth not cause this malady, as the brain and his parts, heart,
liver, spleen, stomach, matrix or womb, pylorus, myrach,
mesentery, hypochondries, meseraic veins; and in a word, saith
Arculanus,[2] "there is no part which causeth not melancholy,
either because it is adust, or doth not expel the superfluity of the
nutriment." Savonarola, *Pract. major, rubric.* 11, *tract.* 6, *cap.* 1,
is of the same opinion, that melancholy is engendered in each
particular part, and Crato [3] *in consil.* 17, *lib.* 2. Gordonius,
who is *instar omnium* [the pick of the bunch], *lib. med. partic.* 2,
cap. 19, confirms as much, putting the "matter of melancholy
sometimes in the stomach, liver, heart, brain, spleen, myrach,
hypochondries, whenas the melancholy humour resides there,
or the liver is not well cleansed from melancholy blood." [4]
The brain is a familiar and frequent cause, too hot, or too
cold, "through adust blood so caused," as Mercurialis will
have it, "within or without the head," [5] the brain itself being
distempered. Those are most apt to this disease, "that have a
hot heart and moist brain," [6] which Montaltus, *cap.* 11 *de
melanch.*, approves out of Halyabbas, Rhasis, and Avicenna.
Mercurialis, *consil.* 11, assigns the coldness of the brain a cause,
and Sallustius Salvianus, *Med. lect. lib.* 2, *cap.* 1, will have it
arise from a "cold and dry distemperature of the brain." [7]
Piso, Benedictus Victorius Faventinus, will have it proceed
from a "hot distemperature of the brain"; [8] and Montaltus,

cap. 10, from the brain's heat, scorching the blood.[1]   The brain
is still distempered by himself, or by consent: by himself or his
proper affection, as Faventinus calls it, "or by vapours which
arise from the other parts, and fume up into the head, altering
the animal faculties." [2]

Hildesheim, *Spicil.* 2, *de mania*, thinks it may be caused from
a "distemperature of the heart; sometimes hot; sometimes
cold." [3]   A hot liver, and a cold stomach, are put for usual
causes of melancholy: Mercurialis, *consil.* 11, *et consil.* 6,
consil. 86, assigns a hot liver and cold stomach for ordinary
causes.   Monavius, in an epistle of his to Crato, in Scoltzius,[4]
is of opinion that hypochondriacal melancholy may proceed
from a cold liver; the question is there discussed.   Most agree
that a hot liver is in fault.   "The liver is the shop of humours,
and especially causeth melancholy by his hot and dry distemperature.[5]   The stomach and meseraic veins do often concur,
by reason of their obstructions, and thence their heat cannot
be avoided, and many times the matter is so adust and inflamed
in those parts, that it degenerates into hypochondriacal melancholy." [6]   Guianerius, *cap.* 2, *tract.* 15, holds the meseraic
veins to be a sufficient cause alone.[7]   The spleen concurs to this
malady, by all their consents, and suppression of hemrods, *dum
non expurget altera causa lien*, saith Montaltus, if it be "too cold
and dry,[8] and do not purge the other parts as it ought," *consil.* 23.
Montanus puts the "spleen stopped" [9] for a great cause.
Christopherus à Vega reports,[10] of his knowledge, that he hath
known melancholy caused from putrefied blood in those seed-
veins and womb; Arculanus, "from that menstruous blood
turned into melancholy, and seed too long detained" (as I have
already declared) "by putrefaction or adustion." [11]

The mesenterium, or midriff, diaphragma, is a cause, which
the Greeks called φρένες, because by his inflammation the mind
is much troubled with convulsions and dotage.[12]   All these,
most part, offend by inflammation, corrupting humours and
spirits, in this non-natural melancholy: for from these are
engendered fuliginous and black spirits.   And for that reason
Montaltus, *cap.* 10 *de causis melan.*, will have "the efficient
cause of melancholy to be hot and dry, not a cold and dry distemperature, as some hold, from the heat of the brain roasting
the blood, immoderate heat of the liver and bowels, and inflammation of the pylorus.   And so much the rather, because that,"
as Galen holds, "all spices inflame the blood, solitariness, waking,
agues, study, meditation, all which heat: and therefore he

concludes that this distemperature causing adventitious melancholy is not cold and dry, but hot and dry." [1]　But of this I have sufficiently treated in the matter of melancholy, and hold that this may be true in non-natural melancholy, which produceth madness, but not in that natural, which is more cold, and being immoderate, produceth a gentle dotage.　Which opinion Geraldus de Solo maintains in his comment upon Rhasis.[2]

SUBSECT. III.—*Causes of Head-Melancholy*

After a tedious discourse of the general causes of melancholy, I am now returned at last to treat in brief of the three particular species, and such causes as properly appertain unto them. Although these causes promiscuously concur to each and every particular kind, and commonly produce their effects in that part which is most weak, ill-disposed, and least able to resist, and so cause all three species, yet many of them are proper to some one kind, and seldom found in the rest.　As for example, head-melancholy is commonly caused by a cold or hot distemperature of the brain, according to Laurentius, *cap. 5 de melan.*, but, as Hercules de Saxonia contends,[3] from that agitation or distemperature of the animal spirits alone.　Sallust. Salvianus, before mentioned, *lib. 2, cap. 3, de re med.*, will have it proceed from cold: but that I take of natural melancholy, such as are fools and dote: for as Galen writes, *lib. 4 de puls.* 8, and Avicenna, "a cold and moist brain is an inseparable companion of folly." [4] But this adventitious melancholy which is here meant, is caused of a hot and dry distemperature, as Damascen the Arabian, *lib. 3, cap. 22,*[5] thinks, and most writers; Altomarus and Piso call it "an innate burning untemperateness, turning blood and choler into melancholy." [6]　Both these opinions may stand good, as Bruel maintains, and Capivaccius, *si cerebrum sit calidius*: "if the brain be hot, the animal spirits will be hot, and thence comes madness; if cold, folly." [7]　David Crusius, *Theat. morb. Hermet. lib. 2, cap. 6, de atra bile*, grants melancholy to be a disease of an inflamed brain, but cold notwithstanding of itself: *calida per accidens, frigida per se,* hot by accident only; I am of Capivaccius' mind for my part.　Now this humour, according to Salvianus, is sometimes in the substance of the brain, sometimes contained in the membranes and tunicles that cover the brain, sometimes in the passages of the ventricles of the brain, or veins of those ventricles.　It follows many times "frenzy, long diseases, agues, long abode in hot places, or under the sun,

a blow on the head," as Rhasis informeth us:[1] Piso adds solitariness, waking, inflammations of the head, proceeding most part
from much use of spices, hot wines, hot meats:[2] all which Montanus reckons up, *consil.* 22, for a melancholy Jew; and Heurnius
repeats, *cap.* 12 *de mania*: hot baths, garlic, onions, saith Guianerius, bad air, corrupt, much waking, etc.,[3] retention of seed or
abundance, stopping of hæmorrhagia, the midriff misaffected;
and according to Trallianus, *lib.* 1, 16, immoderate cares,
troubles, griefs, discontent, study, meditation, and, in a word,
the abuse of all those six non-natural things. Hercules de
Saxonia, *cap.* 16, *lib.* 1, will have it caused from a cautery, or
boil dried up, or any issue.[4] Amatus Lusitanus, *cent.* 2, *cura* 67,
gives instance in a fellow that had a hole in his arm, "after that
was healed, ran mad, and when the wound was open, he was
cured again."[5] Trincavellius, *consil.* 13, *lib.* 1, hath an example
of a melancholy man so caused by overmuch continuance in the
sun, frequent use of venery, and immoderate exercise: and, in
his *cons.* 49, *lib.* 3, from an headpiece overheated,[6] which caused
head-melancholy. Prosper Calenus brings in Cardinal Cæsius
for a pattern of such as are so melancholy by long study; but
examples are infinite.

SUBSECT. IV.—*Causes of Hypochondriacal or Windy Melancholy*

In repeating of these causes, I must *cramben bis coctam
apponere*, say that again which I have formerly said, in applying
them to their proper species. Hypochondriacal or flatuous
melancholy is that which the Arabians call myrachial, and is in
my judgment the most grievous and frequent, though Bruel and
Laurentius make it least dangerous, and not so hard to be known
or cured. His causes are inward or outward. Inward from
divers parts or organs, as midriff, spleen, stomach, liver, pylorus,
womb, diaphragma, meseraic veins, stopping of issues, etc.
Montaltus, *cap.* 15, out of Galen, recites, "heat and obstruction
of those meseraic veins, as an immediate cause, by which means
the passage of the chylus to the liver is detained, stopped, or
corrupted, and turned into rumbling and wind."[7] Montanus,
consil. 233, hath an evident demonstration, Trincavellius
another, *lib.* 1, *cap.* 12, and Plater a third, *Observat. lib.* 1, for a
doctor of the law visited with this infirmity, from the said
obstruction and heat of these meseraic veins, and bowels:
quoniam inter ventriculum et jecur venæ effervescunt, the veins
are inflamed about the liver and stomach. Sometimes those

other parts are together misaffected, and concur to the produc-
tion of this malady: a hot liver and cold stomach, or cold belly;
look for instances in Hollerius, Victor Trincavellius, *consil.* 35,
lib. 3, Hildesheim, *Spicil.* 2, *fol.* 132, Solenander, *consil.* 9, *pro
cive Lugdunensi*, Montanus, *consil.* 229, for the Earl of Montfort
in Germany, 1549, and Frisimelica in the 233rd consultation of
the said Montanus. J. Cæsar Claudinus gives instance of a
cold stomach and over-hot liver, almost in every consultation,
cons. 89, for a certain count, and *cons.* 106, for a Polonian baron;
by reason of heat the blood is inflamed, and gross vapours sent
to the heart and brain. Mercurialis subscribes to them, *cons.* 89,
"the stomach being misaffected," [1] which he calls the king of the
belly, because if he be distempered, all the rest suffer with him,
as being deprived of their nutriment, or fed with bad nourishment, by means of which come crudities, obstructions, wind,
rumbling, griping, etc. Hercules de Saxonia, besides heat,
will have the weakness of the liver and his obstruction a cause,
facultatem debilem jecinoris, which he calls the mineral of melancholy. Laurentius assigns this reason, because the liver over-
hot draws the meat undigested out of the stomach, and burneth
the humours. Montanus, *cons.* 244, proves that sometimes a
cold liver may be a cause. Laurentius, *cap.* 12, Trincavellius,
lib. 12 *consil.*, and Gualter Bruel, seem to lay the greatest fault
upon the spleen, that doth not his duty in purging the liver as
he ought, being too great, or too little, in drawing too much blood
sometimes to it, and not expelling it, as P. Cnemander in a
consultation of his noted; [2] *tumorem lienis* [swelling of the
spleen], he names it, and the fountain of melancholy. Diocles
supposed the ground of this kind of melancholy to proceed from
the inflammation of the pylorus, which is the nether mouth of
the ventricle. Others assign the mesenterium or midriff distempered by heat, the womb misaffected, stopping of hemrods,
with many such. All which Laurentius, *cap.* 12, reduceth to
three, mesentery, liver, and spleen, from whence he denominates
hepatic, splenetic, and meseraic melancholy. Outward causes
are bad diet, care, griefs, discontents, and in a word all those
six non-natural things, as Montanus found by his experience,
consil. 244. Solenander, *consil.* 9, for a citizen of Lyons in
France, gives his reader to understand that he knew this mischief
procured by a medicine of cantharides, which an unskilful
physician ministered his patient to drink *ad venerem excitandam*
[to excite desire]. But most commonly fear, grief, and some
sudden commotion or perturbation of the mind begin it, in

such bodies especially as are ill disposed. Melancthon, *tract.* 14, *cap.* 2, *de anima,* will have it as common to men, as the mother to women, upon some grievous trouble, dislike, passion, or discontent. For as Camerarius records in his life, Melancthon himself was much troubled with it, and therefore could speak out of experience. Montanus, *consil.* 22, *pro delirante Judæo,* confirms it, grievous symptoms of the mind brought him to it.[1] Rondeletius relates of himself, that being one day very intent to write out a physician's notes, molested by an occasion, he fell into a hypochondriacal fit, to avoid which he drank the decoction of wormwood, and was freed. Melancthon ("being the disease is so troublesome and frequent") holds it "a most necessary and profitable study for every man to know the accidents of it, and a dangerous thing to be ignorant," [2] and would therefore have all men in some sort to understand the causes, symptoms, and cures of it.

SUBSECT. V.—*Causes of Melancholy from the whole Body*

As before, the cause of this kind of melancholy is inward or outward. Inward, "when the liver is apt to engender such a humour, or the spleen weak by nature, and not able to discharge his office." [3] A melancholy temperature, retention of hemrods, monthly issues, bleeding at nose, long diseases, agues, and all those six non-natural things increase it; but especially bad diet, as Piso thinks,[4] pulse, salt meat, shell-fish, cheese, black wine, etc. Mercurialis, out of Averroes and Avicenna, condemns all herbs; Galen, *lib.* 3 *de loc. affect. cap.* 7, especially cabbage. So likewise fear, sorrow, discontents, etc., but of these before. And thus in brief you have had the general and particular causes of melancholy.

Now go and brag of thy present happiness, whosoever thou art, brag of thy temperature, of thy good parts, insult, triumph, and boast; thou seest in what a brittle state thou art, how soon thou mayest be dejected, how many several ways, by bad diet, bad air, a small loss, a little sorrow or discontent, an ague, etc.; how many sudden accidents may procure thy ruin, what a small tenure of happiness thou hast in this life, how weak and silly a creature thou art. "Humble thyself therefore under the mighty hand of God" (1 Peter, v, 6), know thyself, acknowledge thy present misery, and make right use of it. *Qui stat videat ne cadat* [let him that is upright see that he fall not]. Thou dost

now flourish, and hast *bona animi, corporis, et fortunæ,* goods of
body, mind, and fortune, *nescis quid serus secum vesper ferat,*
thou knowest not what storms and tempests the late evening
may bring with it.   Be not secure then, "be sober and watch,"
fortunam reverenter habe [1] [be not puffed up by good fortune], if
fortunate and rich; if sick and poor, moderate thyself.   I
have said.

SECT. III.   MEMB. I.

Subsect. I.—*Symptoms, or Signs of Melancholy in the Body*

Parrhasius, a painter of Athens, amongst those Olynthian
captives Philip of Macedon brought home to sell, bought one
very old man; and when he had him at Athens, put him to
extreme torture and torment, the better by his example to
express the pains and passions of his Prometheus, whom he
was then about to paint.[2]   I need not be so barbarous, inhuman,
curious, or cruel, for this purpose to torture any poor melancholy man; their symptoms are plain, obvious and familiar, there
needs no such accurate observation or far-fetched object, they
delineate themselves, they voluntarily bewray themselves, they
are too frequent in all places, I meet them still as I go, they cannot conceal it, their grievances are too well known, I need not
seek far to describe them.

Symptoms therefore are either universal or particular, saith
Gordonius, *lib. med. cap.* 19, *part.* 2, to persons, to species; [3]
"some signs are secret, some manifest, some in the body, some
in the mind, and diversely vary, according to the inward or
outward causes" (Capivaccius); or from stars, according to
Jovianus Pontanus, *de reb. cœlest. lib.* 10, *cap.* 13, and celestial
influences, or from the humours diversely mixed (Ficinus, *lib.* 1,
cap. 4, *de sanit. tuenda*).   As they are hot, cold, natural, unnatural, intended or remitted, so will Aetius have *melancholica
deliria multiformia,* diversity of melancholy signs.   Laurentius
ascribes them to their several temperatures, delights, natures,
inclinations, continuance of time, as they are simple or mixed
with other diseases, as the causes are divers, so must the signs
be almost infinite (Altomarus, *cap.* 7 *art. med.*).   And as wine
produceth divers effects, or that herb Tortocolla in Laurentius,[4]
"which makes some laugh, some weep, some sleep, some dance,

some sing, some howl, some drink, etc.," so doth this our melancholy humour work several signs in several parties.

But to confine them, these general symptoms may be reduced to those of the body or the mind. Those usual signs appearing in the bodies of such as are melancholy be these, cold and dry, or they are hot and dry, as the humour is more or less adust. From these first qualities arise many other second,[1] as that of colour,[2] black, swarthy, pale, ruddy, etc., some are *impense rubri*, as Montaltus, *cap.* 16, observes out of Galen, *lib. 3 de locis affectis*, very red and high coloured. Hippocrates in his book *de insania et melan.*[3] reckons up these signs, that they are "lean, withered, hollow-eyed, look old, wrinkled, harsh, much troubled with wind and a griping in their bellies, or belly-ache, belch often, dry bellies and hard, dejected looks, flaggy beards, singing of the ears, vertigo, light-headed, little or no sleep, and that interrupt, terrible and fearful dreams."[4]

> *Anna soror, quae me suspensum insomnia terrent!*[5]
>
> [O sister Anna, terrifying dreams
> My sleep have troubled.]

The same symptoms are repeated by Melanelius (in his book of Melancholy, collected out of Galen), Ruffus, Aetius, by Rhasis, Gordonius, and all the juniors, "continual, sharp, and stinking belchings, as if their meat in their stomachs were putrefied, or that they had eaten fish, dry bellies, absurd and interrupt dreams, and many phantastical visions about their eyes, vertiginous, apt to tremble, and prone to venery."[6] Some[7] add palpitation of the heart, cold sweat, as usual symptoms, and a leaping in many parts of the body, *saltum in multis corporis partibus*, a kind of itching, saith Laurentius, on the superficies of the skin, like a flea-biting sometimes. Montaltus, *cap.* 21, puts fixed eyes and much twinkling of their eyes for a sign,[8] and so doth Avicenna, *oculos habentes palpitantes, trauli, vehementer rubicundi, etc., lib. 3, fen. 1, tract. 4, cap.* 18. They stut most part, which he took out of Hippocrates' Aphorisms. Rhasis[9] makes "headache and a binding heaviness" for a principal token, "much leaping of wind about the skin, as well as stutting, or tripping in speech, etc., hollow eyes, gross veins, and broad lips." To some too, if they be far gone, mimical gestures are too familiar, laughing, grinning, fleering, murmuring, talking to themselves, with strange mouths and faces, inarticulate voices, exclamations, etc. And although they be commonly lean, hirsute, uncheerful in countenance,

withered, and not so pleasant to behold, by reason of those
continual fears, griefs, and vexations, dull, heavy, lazy, restless,
unapt to go about any business; yet their memories are most
part good, they have happy wits, and excellent apprehensions.
Their hot and dry brains make them they cannot sleep, *Ingentes
habent et crebras vigilias* (Aretæus), mighty and often watchings,
sometimes waking for a month, a year together. Hercules de
Saxonia [1] faithfully averreth, that he hath heard his mother
swear, she slept not for seven months together: Trincavellius,
tom. 2, cons. 16, speaks of one that waked fifty days, and
Sckenkius hath examples of two years, and all without offence.
In natural actions their appetite is greater than their concoction,
multa appetunt, pauca digerunt, as Rhasis hath it, they covet to
eat, but cannot digest. And although they "do eat much, yet
they are lean, ill-liking," saith Aretæus, "withered and hard,
much troubled with costiveness," [2] crudities, oppilations, spitting,
belching, etc. Their pulse is rare and slow, except it be of the
carotides, which is very strong; [3] but that varies according to
their intended passions or perturbations, as Struthius hath
proved at large, *Sphygmaticæ artis lib.* 4, *cap.* 13. To say truth,
in such chronic diseases the pulse is not much to be respected,
there being so much superstition in it, as Crato [4] notes, and so
many differences in Galen, that he dares say thay may not be
observed or understood of any man.

Their urine is most part pale, and low coloured, *urina pauca,
acris, biliosa* (Aretæus), not much in quantity; but this, in my
judgment, is all out as uncertain as the other, varying so often
according to several persons, habits, and other occasions not
to be respected in chronic diseases. "Their melancholy excrements in some very much, in others little, as the spleen plays
his part," [5] and thence proceeds wind, palpitation of the heart,
short breath, plenty of humidity in the stomach, heaviness of
heart and heartache, and intolerable stupidity and dullness of
spirits. Their excrements or stool hard, black to some, and
little. If the heart, brain, liver, spleen, be misaffected, as
usually they are, many inconveniences proceed from them,
many diseases accompany, as incubus, apoplexy,[6] epilepsy,
vertigo, those frequent wakings and terrible dreams, intempestive
laughing, weeping, sighing, sobbing, bashfulness, blushing,
trembling, sweating, swooning, etc.[7] All their senses are
troubled,[8] they think they see, hear, smell, and touch that which
they do not, as shall be proved in the following discourse.

SUBSECT. II.—*Symptoms or Signs in the Mind*

Arculanus, *in* 9 *Rhasis ad Almansor. cap.* 16, will have these symptoms to be infinite, as indeed they are, varying according to the parties, "for scarce is there one of a thousand that dotes alike" (Laurentius, *cap.* 16).[1] Some few of greater note I will point at; and amongst the rest, fear and sorrow, which, as they are frequent causes, so if they persevere long, according to Hippocrates' and Galen's [2] aphorisms, they are most assured signs, inseparable companions, and characters of melancholy; of present melancholy and habituated, said Montaltus, *cap.* 11, and common to them all, as the said Hippocrates, Galen, Avicenna, and all neoterics hold. But as hounds many times run away with a false cry, never perceiving themselves to be at a fault, so do they. For Diocles of old (whom Galen confutes), and, amongst the juniors, Hercules de Saxonia,[3] with Lod. Mercatus, *cap.* 17, *lib.* 1 *de melan.*, take just exceptions at this aphorism of Hippocrates; 'tis not always true, or so generally to be understood. Fear and sorrow are no common symptoms to all melancholy; "Upon more serious consideration, I find some" (saith he) "that are not so at all. Some indeed are sad, and not fearful; some fearful, and not sad; some neither fearful nor sad; some both." Four kinds he excepts: fanatical persons, such as were Cassandra, Manto, Nicostrata, Mopsus, Proteus, the Sibyls, whom Aristotle [4] confesseth to have been deeply melancholy. Baptista Porta seconds him, *Physiog. lib.* 1, *cap.* 8, they were *atra bile perciti*. Demoniacal persons, and such as speak strange languages, are of this rank: some poets; such as laugh always, and think themselves kings, cardinals, etc.; sanguine they are, pleasantly disposed most part, and so continue. Baptista Porta [5] confines fear and sorrow to them that are cold; but lovers, sibyls, enthusiasts, he wholly excludes. So that I think I may truly conclude, they are not always sad and fearful, but usually so: and that without a cause,[6] *timent de non timendis* (Gordonius), *quæque momenti non sunt* [they fear where there is no ground for fear, they are alarmed about trifles]; "although not all alike" (saith Altomarus), "yet all likely fear,[7] some with an extraordinary and a mighty fear" [8] (Aretæus). "Many fear death, and yet, in a contrary humour, make away themselves" [9] (Galen, *lib.* 3 *de loc. affec. cap.* 7) Some are afraid that heaven will fall on their heads: some they are damned, or shall be. "They are troubled with scruples of conscience, distrusting God's mercies, think they shall go

certainly to hell, the devil will have them, and make great
lamentation"[1] (Jason Pratensis). Fear of devils, death, that
they shall be so sick, of some such or such disease, ready to
tremble at every object, they shall die themselves forthwith,
or that some of their dear friends or near allies are certainly
dead; imminent danger, loss, disgrace still torment others, etc.;
that they are all glass, and therefore will suffer no man to come
near them: that they are all cork, as light as feathers; others
as heavy as lead; some are afraid their heads will fall off their
shoulders, that they have frogs in their bellies, etc. Montanus,
consil. 23, speaks of one "that durst not walk alone from home,
for fear he should swoon or die."[2] A second "fears every man
he meets will rob him, quarrel with him, or kill him."[3] A
third dares not venture to walk alone, for fear he should meet
the devil, a thief, be sick; fears all old women as witches, and
every black dog or cat he sees he suspecteth to be a devil, every
person comes near him is maleficiated, every creature, all
intend to hurt him, seek his ruin; another dares not go over a
bridge, come near a pool, rock, steep hill, lie in a chamber where
cross-beams are, for fear he be tempted to hang, drown, or
precipitate himself. If he be in a silent auditory, as at a sermon,
he is afraid he shall speak aloud at unawares, something undecent,
unfit to be said. If he be locked in a close room, he is afraid of
being stifled for want of air, and still carries biscuit, aquavitæ,
or some strong waters about him, for fear of deliquiums, or being
sick; or if he be in a throng, middle of a church, multitude, where
he may not well get out, though he sit at ease, he is so
misaffected. He will freely promise, undertake any business
beforehand, but when it comes to be performed, he dare not
adventure, but fears an infinite number of dangers, disasters,
etc. Some are "afraid to be burned,[4] or that the ground will
sink under them,[5] or swallow them quick,[6] or that the king will
call them in question for some fact they never did" (Rhasis,
Cont.), "and that they shall surely be executed." The terror of
such a death troubles them, and they fear as much, and are
equally tormented in mind, "as they that have committed a
murder, and are pensive without a cause, as if they were now
presently to be put to death"[7] (Plater, *cap.* 3 *de mentis alienat.*).
They are afraid of some loss, danger, that they shall surely lose
their lives, goods, and all they have, but why they know not.
Trincavellius, *consil.* 13, *lib.* 1, had a patient that would needs
make away himself, for fear of being hanged, and could not be
persuaded for three years together, but that he had killed a

man. Plater, *Observat. lib.* 1, have two other examples of such
as feared to be executed without a cause. If they come in a
place where a robbery, theft, or any such offence hath been
done, they presently fear they are suspected, and many times
betray themselves without a cause. Louis the Eleventh, the
French king, suspected every man a traitor that came about
him, durst trust no officer. *Alii formidolosi omnium, alii
quorundam* (Fracastorius, *lib. 2 de intellect.*), "some fear all
alike, some certain men," [1] and cannot endure their companies,
are sick in them, or if they be from home. Some suspect
treason [2] still, others "are afraid of their dearest and nearest
friends" [3] (Melanelius, *e Galeno, Ruffo, Aetio*), and dare not be
alone in the dark for fear of hobgoblins and devils: he suspects
everything he hears or sees to be a devil, or enchanted, and
imagineth a thousand chimeras and visions, which to his thinking he certainly sees, bugbears, talks with black men, ghosts,
goblins, etc.,

> *Omnes se terrent auræ, sonus excitat omnis.* [4]
>
> [At every rustle of the breeze he quakes,
> He starts at every sound.]

Another through bashfulness, suspicion, and timorousness will
not be seen abroad, "loves darkness as life, and cannot endure
the light," [5] or to sit in lightsome places, his hat still in his eyes,
he will neither see nor be seen by his good will (Hippocrates,
lib. de insania et melancholia). He dare not come in company for
fear he should be misused, disgraced, overshoot himself in
gesture or speeches, or be sick; he thinks every man observes
him, aims at him, derides him, owes him malice. Most part
"they are afraid they are bewitched, possessed, or poisoned by
their enemies," and sometimes they suspect their nearest friends:
"he thinks something speaks or talks within him, or to him, and
he belcheth of the poison." [6] Christopherus à Vega, *lib. 2,
cap.* 1, had a patient so troubled, that by no persuasion or physic
he could be reclaimed. Some are afraid that they shall have
every fearful disease they see others have, hear of, or read, and
dare not therefore hear or read of any such subject, no, not of
melancholy itself, lest by applying to themselves that which
they hear or read, they should aggravate and increase it. If they
see one possessed, bewitched, an epileptic paroxysm, a man
shaking with the palsy, or giddy-headed, reeling or standing in
a dangerous place, etc., for many days after it runs in their minds,
they are afraid they shall be so too, they are in like danger, as

Perkins, *cap.* 12, *sect.* 2, well observes in his Cases of Conscience,
and many times by violence of imagination they produce it.
They cannot endure to see any terrible object, as a monster, a
man executed, a carcass, hear the devil named, or any tragical
relation seen, but they quake for fear, *Hecatas somniare sibi
videntur* (Lucian), they dream of hobgoblins, and may not get
it out of their minds a long time after: they apply (as I have
said) all they hear, see, read, to themselves; as Felix Plater
notes [1] of some young physicians, that studying to cure diseases,
catch them themselves, will be sick, and appropriate all symptoms
they find related of others to their own persons.   And therefore
(*quod iterum moneo, licet nauseam paret lectori, malo decem potius
verba, decies repetita licet, abundare, quam unum desiderari*)
[I repeat my warning, though it be *ad nauseam*; I had rather say
a hundred words too much than one too little] I would advise
him that is actually melancholy not to read this tract of
Symptoms, lest he disquiet or make himself for a time worse,
and more melancholy than he was before.   Generally of them all
take this, *de inanibus semper conqueruntur et timent,* saith
Aretæus; they complain of toys, and fear without a cause,[2]
and still think their melancholy to be most grievous, none so
bad as they are, though it be nothing in respect, yet never any
man sure was so troubled, or in this sort: as really tormented
and perplexed, in as great an agony for toys and trifles (such
things as they will after laugh at themselves) as if they were
most material and essential matters indeed, worthy to be feared,
and will not be satisfied.   Pacify them for one, they are instantly
troubled with some other fear; always afraid of something which
they foolishly imagine or conceive to themselves, which never
peradventure was, never can be, never likely will be; troubled
in mind upon every small occasion, unquiet, still complaining,
grieving, vexing, suspecting, grudging, discontent, and cannot
be freed so long as melancholy continues.   Or if their minds
be more quiet for the present, and they free from foreign fears,
outward accidents, yet their bodies are out of tune, they suspect
some part or other to be amiss; now their head aches, heart,
stomach, spleen, etc., is misaffected, they shall surely have this
or that disease; still troubled in body, mind, or both, and through
wind, corrupt phantasy, some accidental distemper, continually
molested.   Yet for all this, as Jacchinus notes,[3] "in all other
things they are wise, staid, discreet, and do nothing unbeseeming their dignity, person, or place, this foolish, ridiculous, and
childish fear excepted"; which so much, so continually tortures

and crucifies their souls, like a barking dog that always bawls,
but seldom bites, this fear ever molesteth, and, so long as
melancholy lasteth, cannot be avoided.

Sorrow is that other character, and inseparable companion,
as individual as Saint Cosmus and Damian, *fidus Achates*, as all
writers witness, a common symptom, a continual, and still
without any evident cause, *mœrent omnes, et si roges eos reddere
causam, non possunt*:[1] grieving still, but why they cannot tell:
agelasti, mœsti, cogitabundi [never smiling, gloomy, wrapt in
thought], they look as if they had newly come forth of Trophonius' den.   And though they laugh many times, and seem
to be extraordinary merry (as they will by fits), yet extreme
lumpish again in an instant, dull and heavy, *semel et simul*
[both at once], merry and sad, but most part sad: *Si qua placent,
abeunt; inimica tenacius hærent*[2] [that which pleases soon departs, that which hurts clings fast]: sorrow sticks by them still
continually, gnawing as the vulture did Tityus' bowels,[3] and
they cannot avoid it.   No sooner are their eyes open, but after
terrible and troublesome dreams their heavy hearts begin to
sigh: they are still fretting, chafing, sighing, grieving, complaining, finding faults, repining, grudging, weeping, *Heautonti-
morumenoi*, vexing themselves, disquieted in mind,[4] with restless, unquiet thoughts, discontent, either for their own, other
men's or public affairs, such as concern them not; things past,
present, or to come, the remembrance of some disgrace, loss,
injury, abuse, etc. troubles them now being idle afresh, as if it
were new done; they are afflicted otherwise for some danger,
loss, want, shame, misery, that will certainly come, as they
suspect and mistrust.   *Lugubris Ate* [mournful Ate] frowns upon
them, insomuch that Aretæus well calls it *angorem animi*, a
vexation of the mind, a perpetual agony.   They can hardly be
pleased or eased, though in other men's opinion most happy;
go, tarry, run, ride, *post equitem sedet atra cura*[5] [close behind the
rider sits black care]: they cannot avoid this feral plague; let
them come in what company they will, *hæret lateri lethalis
arundo*[6] [the deadly arrow in his side is fixed], as to a deer that
is struck, whether he run, go, rest with the herd, or alone, this
grief remains: irresolution, inconstancy, vanity of mind, their
fear, torture, care, jealousy, suspicion, etc., continues, and they
cannot be relieved.   So he complained[7] in the poet:

Domum revortor mœstus, atque animo fere
Perturbato, atque incerto præ ægritudine,
Assido: accurrunt servi, soccos detrahunt:

Video alios festinare, lectos sternere,
Cœnam apparare, pro se quisque sedulo
Faciebant, quo illam mihi lenirent miseriam.

He came home sorrowful and troubled in his mind; his
servants did all they possibly could to please him; one pulled
off his socks, another made ready his bed, a third his supper,
all did their utmost endeavours to ease his grief and exhilarate
his person; he was profoundly melancholy, he had lost his son,
illud angebat [that was torturing him], that was his *cordolium*
[heart-sorrow], his pain, his agony which could not be removed.
Hence it proceeds many times that they are weary of their
lives, and feral thoughts to offer violence to their own persons
come into their minds; *tædium vitæ* [weariness of life] is a common
symptom, *tarda fluunt, ingrataque tempora* [time passes slowly
and without enjoyment], they are soon tired with all things;
they will now tarry, now be gone; now in bed they will rise,
now up, then go to bed, now pleased, then again displeased;
now they like, by and by dislike all, weary of all, *sequitur nunc
vivendi, nunc moriendi cupido* [at one time they want to live,
at another to die], saith Aurelianus, *lib. 1, cap.* 6, but most part
vitam damnant [1] [they declare life not worth living], discontent,
disquieted, perplexed upon every light or no occasion, object:
often tempted, I say, to make away themselves: *Vivere nolunt,
mori nesciunt:* [2] they cannot die, they will not live: they complain, weep, lament, and think they lead a most miserable life,
never was any man so bad, or so before, every poor man they see
is most fortunate in respect of them, every beggar that comes to
the door is happier than they are, they could be contented to
change lives with them, especially if they be alone, idle, and
parted from their ordinary company, molested, displeased, or
provoked: grief, fear, agony, discontent, wearisomeness, laziness, suspicion, or some such passion, forcibly seizeth on them.
Yet by and by, when they come in company again which they
like, or be pleased, *suam sententiam rursus damnant, et vitæ
solatio delectantur,* as Octavius Horatianus observes, *lib. 2, cap.* 5,
they condemn their former mislike, and are well pleased to live.
And so they continue, till with some fresh discontent they be
molested again, and then they are weary of their lives, weary of
all, they will die, and show rather a necessity to live than a
desire.   Claudius the emperor, as Suetonius describes him, [3] had
a spice of this disease, for when he was tormented with the pain
of his stomach, he had a conceit to make away himself.   Julius
Cæsar Claudinus, *consil.* 84, had a Polonian to his patient so

affected, that through fear and sorrow, with which he was still disquieted, hated his own life, wished for death every moment, and to be freed of his misery; [1] Mercurialis another, and another that was often minded to dispatch himself, and so continued for many years.

Suspicion and jealousy are general symptoms: they are commonly distrustful, apt to mistake, and amplify, *facile irascibiles*, testy,[2] pettish, peevish, and ready to snarl upon every small occasion,[3] *cum amicissimis* [with their dearest friends], and without a cause, *datum vel non datum*, it will be *scandalum acceptum* [they will take offence, whether it is given or not]. If they speak in jest, he takes it in good earnest. If they be not saluted, invited, consulted with, called to counsel, etc., or that any respect, small compliment, or ceremony be omitted, they think themselves neglected and contemned; for a time that tortures them. If two talk together, discourse, whisper, jest, or tell a tale in general, he thinks presently they mean him, applies all to himself, *de se putat omnia dici*. Or if they talk with him, he is ready to misconster every word they speak, and interpret it to the worst; he cannot endure any man to look steadily on him, speak to him almost, laugh, jest, or be familiar, or hem, or point, cough, or spit, or make a noise sometimes, etc. He thinks they laugh or point at him, or do it in disgrace of him, circumvent him, contemn him;[4] every man looks at him, he is pale, red, sweats for fear and anger, lest somebody should observe him. He works upon it, and long after this false conceit of an abuse troubles him. Montanus, *consil. 22*, gives instance in a melancholy Jew, that was *iracundior Adria* [more tempestuous than the Adriatic Sea], so waspish and suspicious, *tam facile iratus* [so quick to anger], that no man could tell how to carry himself in his company.

Inconstant they are in all their actions, vertiginous, restless, unapt to resolve of any business, they will and will not, persuaded to and fro upon every small occasion, or word spoken: and yet if once they be resolved, obstinate, hard to be reconciled. If they abhor, dislike, or distaste, once settled, though to the better by odds, by no counsel or persuasion to be removed; yet in most things wavering, irresolute, unable to deliberate, through fear, *faciunt, et mox facti pœnitent* (Aretæus), *avari, et paulo post prodigi*: now prodigal, and then covetous, they do, and by and by repent them of that which they have done, so that both ways they are troubled, whether they do or do not, want or have, hit or miss, disquieted of all hands, soon weary, and still seeking

change, restless, I say, fickle, fugitive, they may not abide to
tarry in one place long:

> *Romæ rus optans, absentem rusticus urbem*
> *Tollit ad astra ;* [1]

[At Rome, he fain would to the country fly;
When there, he lauds the city to the sky;]

no company long, or to persevere in any action or business:

> *Et similis regum pueris, pappare minutum*
> *Poscit, et iratus mammæ lallare recusat ;* [2]

[Like the children of the rich, he wants his food cut up
small, and being cross with his nurse will not let
her sing him to sleep;]

eftsoons pleased, and anon displeased; as a man that's bitten
with fleas, or that cannot sleep, turns to and fro in his bed,
their restless minds are tossed and vary, they have no patience
to read out a book, to play out a game or two, walk a mile, sit
an hour, etc.; erected and dejected in an instant; animated to
undertake, and upon a word spoken again discouraged.

Extreme passionate, *Quicquid volunt valde volunt*; and what
they desire, they do most furiously seek: anxious ever and very
solicitous, distrustful and timorous, envious, malicious, profuse
one while, sparing another, but most part covetous, muttering,
repining, discontent, and still complaining, grudging, peevish,
injuriarum tenaces, prone to revenge, soon troubled, and most
violent in all their imaginations, not affable in speech, or apt to
vulgar compliment, but surly, dull, sad, austere; *cogitabundi* still,
very intent, and as Albertus Durer paints Melancholy,[3] like a
sad woman leaning on her arm with fixed looks, neglected habit,
etc.; held therefore by some proud, soft, sottish, or half-mad,
as the Abderites esteemed of Democritus, and yet of a deep
reach, excellent apprehension, judicious, wise and witty: for
I am of that nobleman's mind,[4] "Melancholy advanceth men's
conceits more than any humour whatsoever," improves their
meditations more than any strong drink or sack.   They are of
profound judgment in some things, although in others *non recte
judicant inquieti* [people in a passion do not judge correctly],
saith Fracastorius, *lib. 2 de intell.*   And as Arculanus, *cap.* 16
in 9 *Rhasis*, terms it, *Judicium plerumque perversum, corruptum,
cum judicant honesta inhonesta, et amicitiam habent pro inimicitia,*
[their judgment is generally perverse and corrupt, since] they
count honesty dishonesty, friends as enemies, they will abuse
their best friends, and dare not offend their enemies.   Cowards

most part, *et ad inferendam injuriam timidissimi*, saith Cardan,
lib. 8, cap. 4, de rerum varietate : loath to offend; and if they
chance to overshoot themselves in word or deed, or any small
business or circumstance be omitted, forgotten, they are miserably tormented, and frame a thousand dangers and inconveniences to themselves, *ex musca elephantem* [make a fly into
an elephant], if once they conceit it: overjoyed with every
good rumour, tale, or prosperous event, transported beyond
themselves: with every small cross again, bad news, misconceived injury, loss, danger, afflicted beyond measure, in great
agony, perplexed, dejected, astonished, impatient, utterly
undone: fearful, suspicious of all. Yet again, many of them
desperate hairbrains, rash, careless, fit to be assassinates, as being
void of all fear and sorrow, according to Hercules de Saxonia,[1]
"most audacious, and such as dare walk alone in the night,
through deserts and dangerous places, fearing none."

They are prone to love, and easy to be taken:[2] *propensi
ad amorem et excandescentiam* (Montaltus, *cap.* 21), quickly
enamoured, and dote upon all, love one dearly, till they see
another, and then dote on her, *et hanc, et hanc, et illam, et omnes*
[this one, and that one, and all of them]; the present moves most,
and the last commonly they love best. Yet some again *anterotes*
[enemies of love], cannot endure the sight of a woman, abhor the
sex, as that same melancholy duke of Muscovy, that was instantly
sick if he came but in sight of them;[3] and that anchorite, that
fell into a cold palsy when a woman was brought before him.[4]

Humorous they are beyond all measure, sometimes profusely
laughing, extraordinarily merry, and then again weeping without a cause (which is familiar with many gentlewomen) groaning,
sighing, pensive, sad, almost distracted, *multa absurda fingunt,
et a ratione aliena* (saith Frambesarius[5]), they feign many
absurdities, vain, void of reason. One supposeth himself to be
a dog, cock, bear, horse, glass, butter, etc. He is a giant, a
dwarf, as strong as an hundred men, a lord, duke, prince, etc.
And if he be told he hath a stinking breath, a great nose, that
he is sick, or inclined to such or such a disease, he believes it
eftsoons, and peradventure by force of imagination will work it
out. Many of them are immovable, and fixed in their conceits,
others vary upon every object, heard or seen. If they see a
stage-play, they run upon that a week after; if they hear music,
or see dancing, they have naught but bagpipes in their brain;
if they see a combat, they are all for arms. If abused, an abuse
troubles them long after; if crossed, that cross, etc.[6] Restless in

their thoughts and actions, continually meditating, *velut ægri
somnia, vanæ finguntur species*, more like dreams than men awake,
they feign a company of antic, phantastical conceits, they have
most frivolous thoughts, impossible to be effected; and sometimes think verily they hear and see present before their eyes
such phantasms or goblins, they fear, suspect, or conceive, they
still talk with, and follow them. In fine, *cogitationes somni-
antibus similes, id vigilant, quod alii somniant cogitabundi*: still,
saith Avicenna, they wake, as others dream, and such for the
most part are their imaginations and conceits, absurd, vain,
foolish toys,[1] yet they are most curious [2] and solicitous, continual,
et supra modum (Rhasis, *Cont. lib.* 1, *cap.* 9) *præmeditantur de
aliqua re* [and are excessively engrossed in one thing or other];
as serious in a toy, as if it were a most necessary business, of great
moment, importance, and still, still, still thinking of it: *sæviunt
in se*, macerating themselves. Though they do talk with you,
and seem to be otherwise employed, and to your thinking very
intent and busy, still that toy runs in their mind, that fear,
that suspicion, that abuse, that jealousy, that agony, that
vexation, that cross, that castle in the air, that crotchet, that
whimsy, that fiction, that pleasant waking dream, whatsoever
it is. *Nec interrogant* (saith Fracastorius [3]) *nec interrogatis
recte respondent* [they do not ask questions themselves nor
answer properly the questions put to them]; they do not much
heed what you say, their mind is on another matter; ask what
you will, they do not attend, or much intend that business they
are about, but forget themselves what they are saying, doing,
or should otherwise say or do, whither they are going, distracted
with their own melancholy thoughts. One laughs upon a
sudden, another smiles to himself, a third frowns, calls, his lips
go still, he acts with his hand as he walks, etc. "'Tis proper to
all melancholy men," saith Mercurialis, *consil.* 11, "what
conceit they have once entertained, to be most intent, violent,
and continually about it." [4] *Invitis occurrit*, do what they may,
they cannot be rid of it, against their wills they must think of
it a thousand times over, *perpetuo molestantur, nec oblivisci
possunt*, they are continually troubled with it, in company, out
of company; at meat, at exercise, at all times and places, *non
desinunt ea, quæ minime volunt, cogitare* [5] [they cannot put out of
their minds the matters they least wish to think of]; if it be
offensive especially, they cannot forget it, they may not rest or
sleep for it, but still tormenting themselves, *Sisyphi saxum
volvunt sibi ipsis* [they endure the torments of Sisyphus],

as Brunner observes,[1] *perpetua calamitas et miserabile flagellum* [perpetually in suffering and under the lash].

Crato,[2] Laurentius,[3] and Fernelius put bashfulness for an ordinary symptom; *subrusticus pudor*, or *vitiosus pudor* [*mauvaise honte*], is a thing which much haunts and torments them. If they have been misused, derided, disgraced, chidden, etc., or by any perturbation of mind misaffected, it so far troubles them, that they become quite moped many times, and so disheartened, dejected, they dare not come abroad, into strange companies especially, or manage their ordinary affairs, so childish, timorous, and bashful, they can look no man in the face; some are more disquieted in this kind, some less, longer some, others shorter, by fits, etc., though some on the other side (according to Fracastorius [4]) be *inverecundi et pertinaces*, impudent and peevish. But most part they are very shamefaced, and that makes them with Pet. Blesensis, Christopher Urswick, and many such, to refuse honours, offices, and preferments, which sometimes fall into their mouths; they cannot speak, or put forth themselves as others can, *timor hos, pudor impedit illos*, timorousness and bashfulness hinder their proceedings, they are contented with their present estate, unwilling to undertake any office, and therefore never likely to rise. For that cause they seldom visit their friends, except some familiars: *pauciloqui*, of few words, and oftentimes wholly silent. Frambesarius, a Frenchman,[5] had two such patients, *omnino taciturnos* [completely taciturn], their friends could not get them to speak: Rodericus à Fonseca, *Consult. tom. 2, 85 consil.* gives instance in a young man, of twenty-seven years of age, that was frequently silent, bashful, moped, solitary, that would not eat his meat, or sleep, and yet again by fits apt to be angry, etc.

Most part they are, as Plater notes, *desides, taciturni, ægre impulsi* [indolent, taciturn, sluggish], *nec nisi coacti procedunt*, etc., they will scarce be compelled to do that which concerns them, though it be for their good, so diffident, so dull, of small or no compliment, unsociable, hard to be acquainted with, especially of strangers; they had rather write their minds than speak, and above all things love solitariness. *Ob voluptatem, an ob timorem soli sunt?* Are they so solitary for pleasure (one asks) or pain? for both; yet I rather think for fear and sorrow, etc.

Hinc metuunt cupiuntque, dolent fugiuntque, nec auras
Respiciunt, clausi tenebris, et carcere cæco.[6]

Hence 'tis they grieve and fear, avoiding light,
And shut themselves in prison dark from sight.

As Bellerophon in Homer,[1]

Qui miser in silvis mœrens errabat opacis,
Ipse suum cor edens, hominum vestigia vitans:

That wandered in the woods sad all alone,
Forsaking men's society, making great moan;

they delight in floods and waters, desert places, to walk alone
in orchards, gardens, private walks, back lanes; averse from
company, as Diogenes in his tub, or Timon Misanthropus, they
abhor all companions at last,[2] even their nearest acquaintances
and most familiar friends, for they have a conceit (I say) every
man observes them, will deride, laugh to scorn, or misuse them,
confining themselves therefore wholly to their private houses
or chambers, *fugiunt homines sine causa* (saith Rhasis) *et odio
habent* [they shun people for no reason, and hate them], *Cont.
lib.* 1, *cap.* 9, they will diet themselves, feed and live alone.
It was one of the chiefest reasons why the citizens of Abdera
suspected Democritus to be melancholy and mad, because that,
as Hippocrates related in his epistle to Philopœmen, "he forsook the city, lived in groves and hollow trees, upon a green
bank by a brook side, or confluence of waters all day long, and
all night." [3] *Quæ quidem* (saith he) *plurimum atra bile vexatis
et melancholicis eveniunt, deserta frequentant, hominumque congressum aversantur;* which is an ordinary thing with melancholy
men.[4]   The Egyptians therefore in their hieroglyphics expressed
a melancholy man by a hare sitting in her form, as being a
most timorous and solitary creature (Pierius, *Hieroglyph. lib.* 12).
But this and all precedent symptoms are more or less apparent,
as the humour is intended or remitted, hardly perceived in
some, or not at all, most manifest in others.   Childish in some,
terrible in others; to be derided in one, pitied or admired in
another; to him by fits, to a second continuate: and howsoever
these symptoms be common and incident to all persons, yet
they are the more remarkable, frequent, furious, and violent in
melancholy men.   To speak in a word, there is nothing so vain,
absurd, ridiculous, extravagant, impossible, incredible, so
monstrous a chimera, so prodigious and strange, such as painters
and poets durst not attempt,[5] which they will not really fear,
feign, suspect and imagine unto themselves: and that which
Lod. Vives [6] said in a jest of a silly country fellow, that killed
his ass for drinking up the moon, *ut lunam mundo redderet* [that

he might restore the moon to the world], you may truly say of them in earnest; they will act, conceive all extremes, contrarieties, and contradictions, and that in infinite varieties. *Melancholici plane incredibilia sibi persuadent, ut vix omnibus sæculis duo reperti sint, qui idem imaginati sint* (Erastus, *de lamiis*), scarce two of two thousand that concur in the same symptoms. The tower of Babel never yielded such confusion of tongues, as the chaos of melancholy doth variety of symptoms. There is in all melancholy *similitudo dissimilis*, like men's faces, a disagreeing likeness still; and as in a river we swim in the same place, though not in the same numerical water; as the same instrument affords several lessons, so the same disease yields diversity of symptoms. Which howsoever they be diverse, intricate, and hard to be confined, I will adventure yet in such a vast confusion and generality to bring them into some order; and so descend to particulars.

Subsect. III.—*Particular Symptoms from the influence of Stars, parts of the Body, and Humours*

Some men have peculiar symptoms, according to their temperament and *crasis* [constitution], which they had from the stars and those celestial influences, variety of wits and dispositions, as Anthony Zara contends, *Anat. ingen. sect.* 1, *memb.* 11, 12, 13, 14, *Plurimum irritant influentiæ cœlestes, unde cientur animi ægritudines et morbi corporum.* One saith,[1] diverse diseases of the body and mind proceed from their influences, as I have already proved [2] out of Ptolemy, Pontanus, Lemnius, Cardan, and others, as they are principal significators of manners, diseases, mutually irradiated, or lords of the geniture, etc. Ptolemæus in his Centiloquy, Hermes, or whosoever else the author of that tract, attributes all these symptoms which are in melancholy men to celestial influences: which opinion Mercurialis, *de affect. lib.* 1, *cap.* 10, rejects; but, as I say, Jovianus Pontanus [3] and others stiffly defend. That some are solitary, dull, heavy, churlish, some again blithe, buxom, light, and merry, they ascribe wholly to the stars. As if Saturn be predominant in his nativity, and cause melancholy in his temperature, then he shall be very austere, sullen, churlish, black of colour, profound in his cogitations, full of cares, miseries, and discontents, sad and fearful, always silent, solitary, still delighting in husbandry, in woods, orchards, gardens, rivers,

I—o 886

ponds, pools, dark walks and close: [1] *cogitationes sunt velle
ædificare, velle arbores plantare, agros colere* [their thoughts
turn on plans of building, planting trees, tilling fields], etc.,
to catch birds, fishes, etc., still contriving and musing of such
matters. If Jupiter domineers, they are more ambitious, still
meditating of kingdoms, magistracies, offices, honours, or that
they are princes, potentates, and how they would carry themselves, etc. If Mars, they are all for wars, brave combats,
monomachies, testy, choleric, harebrain, rash, furious, and
violent in their actions. They will feign themselves victors,
commanders, are passionate and satirical in their speeches,
great braggers, ruddy of colour. And though they be poor in
show, vile and base, yet like Telephus and Peleus in the poet,[2]
ampullas jactant et sesquipedalia verba [they fling about their
swelling and gigantic words], their mouths are full of myriads,
and tetrarchs at their tongues' end. If the Sun, they will be
lords, emperors, in conceit at least, and monarchs, give offices,
honours, etc. If Venus, they are still courting of their mistresses,
and most apt to love, amorously given, they seem to hear
music, plays, see fine pictures, dancers, merriments, and the
like; ever in love, and dote on all they see. Mercurialists are
solitary, much in contemplation, subtle, poets, philosophers,
and musing most part about such matters. If the Moon have
a hand, they are all for peregrinations, sea voyages, much
affected with travels, to discourse, read, meditate of such things;
wandering in their thoughts, diverse, much delighting in waters,
to fish, fowl, etc.

But the most immediate symptoms proceed from the temperature itself and the organical parts, as head, liver, spleen,
meseraic veins, heart, womb, stomach, etc., and most especially
from distemperature of spirits (which, as Hercules de Saxonia
contends,[3] are wholly immaterial), or from the four humours in
those seats, whether they be hot or cold, natural, unnatural,
innate or adventitious, intended or remitted, simple or mixed,
their diverse mixtures and several adustions, combinations,
which may be as diversely varied as those four first qualities [4]
in Clavius,[5] and produce as many several symptoms and monstrous fictions as wine doth effects, which, as Andreas Bachius
observes, *lib.* 3 *de vino, cap.* 20, are infinite. Of greater note
be these.

If it be natural melancholy, as Lod. Mercatus, *lib.* 1, *cap.* 17,
de melan., T. Bright, *cap.* 16, hath largely described, either of
the spleen or of the veins, faulty by excess of quantity or

thickness of substance, it is a cold and dry humour, as Montanus affirms, *consil.* 26, the parties are sad, timorous and fearful. Prosper Calenus, in his book *de atra bile,* will have them to be more stupid' than ordinary, cold, heavy, dull, solitary, sluggish, *si multam atram bilem et frigidam habent* [if they have a quantity of black and cold bile]. Hercules de Saxonia, *cap.* 19, *lib.* 7, holds these that are naturally melancholy to be of a leaden colour or black,[1] and so doth Guianerius, *cap.* 3, *tract.* 15, and such as think themselves dead many times, or that they see, talk with black men, dead men, spirits and goblins frequently, if it be in excess. These symptoms vary according to the mixture of those four humours adust, which is unnatural melancholy. For, as Trallianus hath written, *cap.* 16, *lib.* 7, "There is not one cause of this melancholy, nor one humour which begets, but divers diversely intermixed, from whence proceeds this variety of symptoms": [2] and those varying again as they are hot or cold. "Cold melancholy" (saith Benedictus Victorius Faventinus, *Pract. Mag.*) "is a cause of dotage, and more mild symptoms; if hot or more adust, of more violent passions and furies." [3] Fracastorius, *lib.* 2 *de intellect.*, will have us to consider well of it, "with what kind of melancholy every one is troubled, for it much avails to know it; one is enraged by fervent heat, another is possessed by sad and cold; one is fearful, shamefaced; the other impudent and bold"; [4] as Ajax, *Arma rapit superosque furens in prælia poscit* [snatches his arms and challenges the gods], quite mad or tending to madness: *nunc hos, nunc impetit illos* [now these he rushes at, now those]. Bellerophon, on the other side, *solis errat male sanus in agris,* wanders alone in the woods; one despairs, weeps, and is weary of his life, another laughs, etc. All which variety is produced from the several degrees of heat and cold, which Hercules de Saxonia [5] will have wholly proceed from the distemperature of spirits alone, animal especially, and those immaterial, the next and immediate causes of melancholy, as they are hot, cold, dry, moist, and from their agitation proceeds that diversity of symptoms which he reckons up in the thirteenth chapter of his Tract of Melancholy, and that largely through every part.[6] Others will have them come from the diverse adustion of the four humours, which in this unnatural melancholy, by corruption of blood, adust choler, or melancholy natural, "by excessive distemper of heat turned, in comparison of the natural, into a sharp lye by force of adustion, cause, according to the diversity of their matter, diverse and strange symptoms," [7] which T. Bright reckons up in his following

chapter. So doth Arculanus,[1] according to the four principal
humours adust, and many others.

For example, if it proceed from phlegm (which is seldom and
not so frequently as the rest), it stirs up dull symptoms, and a
kind of stupidity, or impassionate hurt:[2] they are sleepy, saith
Savonarola,[3] dull, slow, cold, blockish, ass-like, *asininam
melancholiam*, Melancthon[4] calls it; "they are much given to
weeping, and delight in waters, ponds, pools, rivers, fishing,
fowling, etc." (Arnoldus, *Breviar.* I, *cap.* 18). They are pale
of colour,[5] slothful, apt to sleep, heavy; "much troubled with
headache,"[6] continual meditation, and muttering to themselves;
they dream of waters, that they are in danger of drowning,
and fear such things (Rhasis).[7] They are fatter than others
that are melancholy, of a muddy complexion, apter to spit,
sleep,[8] more troubled with rheum than the rest, and have their
eyes still fixed on the ground. Such a patient had Hercules de
Saxonia, a widow in Venice, that was fat and very sleepy still;
Christophorus à Vega another affected in the same sort. If it
be inveterate or violent, the symptoms are more evident, they
plainly dote and are ridiculous to others, in all their gestures,
actions, speeches; imagining impossibilities, as he in Christophorus à Vega, that thought he was a tun of wine, and that
Siennois, that resolved within himself not to piss, for fear he
should drown all the town.[9]

If it proceed from blood adust, or that there be a mixture of
blood in it, "such are commonly ruddy of complexion, and
high-coloured,"[10] according to Sallust. Salvianus and Hercules
de Saxonia; and as Savonarola, Victorius Faventinus Empir.,
farther add, "the veins of their eyes be red, as well as their
faces."[11] They are much inclined to laughter, witty and merry,
conceited in discourse, pleasant, if they be not far gone, much
given to music, dancing, and to be in women's company. They
meditate wholly on such things, and think "they see or hear
plays, dancing, and such-like sports"[12] (free from all fear and
sorrow, as Hercules de Saxonia supposeth[13]), if they be more
strongly possessed with this kind of melancholy, Arnoldus adds,
Breviar. lib. I, *cap.* 18, like him of Argos in the poet, that
sat laughing all day long, as if he had been at a theatre.[14] Such
another is mentioned by Aristotle,[15] living at Abydos, a town of
Asia Minor, that would sit after the same fashion, as if he had
been upon a stage, and sometimes act himself; now clap his
hands, and laugh, as if he had been well pleased with the sight.
Wolfius relates of a country fellow called Brunsellius, subject

to this humour, "that being by chance at a sermon, saw a woman fall off from a form half asleep, at which object most of the company laughed, but he for his part was so much moved, that for three whole days after he did nothing but laugh, by which means he was much weakened, and worse a long time following."[1]   Such a one was old Sophocles, and Democritus himself had *hilare delirium* [a merry madness], much in this vein.   Laurentius, *cap. 3 de melan.*, thinks this kind of melancholy, which is a little adust with some mixture of blood, to be that which Aristotle meant, when he said melancholy men of all others are most witty, which causeth many times a divine ravishment, and a kind of *enthusiasmus*, which stirreth them up to be excellent philosophers, poets, prophets, etc.   Mercurialis, *consil.* 110, gives instance in a young man his patient, sanguine melancholy, "of a great wit, and excellently learned."[2]

If it arise from choler adust, they are bold and impudent, and of a more hairbrain disposition, apt to quarrel and think of such things, battles, combats, and their manhood; furious, impatient in discourse, stiff, irrefragable and prodigious in their tenents; and if they be moved, most violent, outrageous, ready to disgrace, provoke any, to kill themselves and others;[3] Arnoldus adds, stark mad by fits, "they sleep little, their urine is subtile and fiery."[4]   Guianerius: "In their fits you shall hear them speak all manner of languages, Hebrew, Greek, and Latin, that never were taught or knew them before."   Apponensis, *in com. in Pro. sec.* 30, speaks of a mad woman that spake excellent good Latin: and Rhasis knew another, that could prophesy in her fit, and foretell things truly to come.   Guianerius[5] had a patient could make Latin verses when the moon was combust, otherwise illiterate.   Avicenna and some of his adherents will have these symptoms, when they happen, to proceed from the devil, and that they are rather *demoniaci*, possessed, than mad or melancholy, or both together, as Jason Pratensis thinks, *immiscent se mali genii* [evil spirits insinuate themselves], etc., but most ascribe it to the humour, which opinion Montaltus, *cap.* 21, stiffly maintains, confuting Avicenna and the rest, referring it wholly to the quality and disposition of the humour and subject.   Cardan, *de rerum var. lib. 8, cap.* 10, holds these men of all others fit to be assassinates, bold, hardy, fierce, and adventurous, to undertake anything by reason of their choler adust.   "This humour," saith he, "prepares them to endure death itself, and all manner of torments, with invincible courage, and 'tis a wonder to see with what alacrity they will

undergo such tortures," [1] *ut supra naturam res videatur* [so that
it seems to be unnatural]: he ascribes this generosity, fury, or
rather stupidity, to this adustion of choler and melancholy: but
I take these rather to be mad or desperate than properly
melancholy; for commonly this humour, so adust and hot,
degenerates into madness.

If it come from melancholy itself adust, "those men," saith
Avicenna, "are usually sad and solitary, and that continually,
and in excess, more than ordinarily suspicious, more fearful,
and have long, sore, and most corrupt imaginations"; [2] cold
and black, bashful, and so solitary, that as Arnoldus writes,
"they will endure no company, they dream of graves still, and
dead men, and think themselves bewitched or dead": [3] if it be
extreme, they think they hear hideous noises, see and talk
"with black men, and converse familiarly with devils, and such
strange chimeras and visions" [4] (Gordonius), or that they are
possessed by them, that somebody talks to them, or within
them. *Tales melancholici plerumque dæmoniaci* [melancholy
persons of this kind are usually possessed with a spirit] (Montaltus, *consil.* 26, *ex Avicenna*).   Valescus de Taranta had such
a woman in cure, "that thought she had to do with the devil": [5]
and Gentilis Fulgosus, *quæst.* 55, writes that he had a melancholy
friend, that "had a black man in the likeness of a soldier" still
following him wheresoever he was.[6]   Laurentius, *cap.* 7, hath
many stories of such as have thought themselves bewitched by
their enemies; and some that would eat no meat as being dead.
Anno 1550, an advocate of Paris fell into such a melancholy
fit, that he believed verily he was dead; he could not be persuaded otherwise, or to eat or drink, till a kinsman of his, a
scholar of Bourges, did eat before him dressed like a corse.[7]
The story, saith Serres, was acted in a comedy before Charles
the Ninth.   Some think they are beasts, wolves, hogs, and cry
like dogs, foxes, bray like asses, and low like kine, as King
Prœtus' daughters.[8]   Hildesheim, *Spicil.* 2 *de mania*, hath an
example of a Dutch baron so affected, and Trincavellius, *lib.* 1,
consil. 11, another of a nobleman in his country, "that thought
he was certainly a beast, and would imitate most of their voices,"[9]
with many such symptoms, which may properly be reduced to
this kind.

If it proceed from the several combinations of these four
humours, or spirits (Hercules de Saxonia adds hot, cold, dry,
moist, dark, confused, settled, constringed, as it participates of
matter, or is without matter), the symptoms are likewise mixed.

One thinks himself a giant, another a dwarf; one is heavy as lead, another is as light as a feather. Marcellus Donatus, *lib.* 2, *cap.* 41, makes mention out of Seneca, of one Senecio, a rich man, that "thought himself and everything else he had great—great wife, great horses; could not abide little things, but would have great pots to drink in, great hose, and great shoes bigger than his feet." [1] Like her in Trallianus, that "supposed she could shake all the world with her finger," [2] and was afraid to clinch her hand together, lest she should crush the world like an apple in pieces: or him in Galen, that thought he was Atlas, and sustained heaven with his shoulders. [3] Another thinks himself so little, that he can creep into a mouse-hole: one fears heaven will fall on his head; a second is a cock; and such a one Guianerius [4] saith he saw at Padua, that would clap his hands together and crow. Another thinks he is a nightingale, and therefore sings all the night long; [5] another he is all glass, a pitcher, and will therefore let nobody come near him, and such a one Laurentius gives out upon his credit, that he knew in France. [6] Christophorus à Vega, *cap.* 3, *lib.* 14, Sckenkius, and Marcellus Donatus, *lib.* 2, *cap.* 1, have many such examples, and one amongst the rest of a baker in Ferrara, that thought he was composed of butter, and durst not sit in the sun or come near the fire for fear of being melted: of another that thought he was a case of leather, stuffed with wind. Some laugh, weep; some are mad, some dejected, moped, in much agony, some by fits, others continuate, etc. Some have a corrupt ear—they think they hear music, or some hideous noise as their phantasy conceives—corrupt eyes; some smelling, some one sense, some another. Louis the Eleventh had a conceit everything did stink about him; all the odoriferous perfumes they could get would not ease him, but still he smelled a filthy stink. [7] A melancholy French poet in Laurentius, [8] being sick of a fever, and troubled with waking, by his physicians was appointed to use *unguentum populeum* [an ointment made of poplar] to anoint his temples; but he so distasted the smell of it, that for many years after, all that came near him he imagined to scent of it, and would let no man talk with him but aloof off, or wear any new clothes, because he thought still they smelled of it; in all other things wise and discreet, he would talk sensibly, save only in this. A gentleman in Limousin, saith Anthony de Verdeur, was persuaded he had but one leg, affrighted by a wild boar that by chance struck him on the leg; he could not be satisfied his leg was sound (in all other things well) until two

Franciscans, by chance coming that way, fully removed him from the conceit. *Sed abunde fabularum audivimus* [but we have heard enough tales].

SUBSECT. IV.—*Symptoms from Education, Custom, Continuance of Time, our Condition, mixed with other Diseases, by Fits, Inclination, etc.*

Another great occasion of the variety of these symptoms proceeds from custom, discipline, education, and several inclinations "This humour will imprint in melancholy men the objects most answerable to their condition of life, and ordinary actions, and dispose men according to their several studies and callings." [1] If an ambitious man become melancholy, he forthwith thinks he is a king, an emperor, a monarch, and walks alone, pleasing himself with a vain hope of some future preferment, or present as he supposeth, and withal acts a lord's part, takes upon him to be some statesman or magnifico, makes congees, gives entertainment, looks big, etc. Francisco Sansovino records of a melancholy man in Cremona, that would not be induced to believe but that he was pope, gave pardons, made cardinals, etc. Christophorus à Vega makes mention of another of his acquaintance, that thought he was a king, driven from his kingdom,[2] and was very anxious to recover his estate. A covetous person is still conversant about purchasing of lands and tenements, plotting in his mind how to compass such and such manors, as if he were already lord of, and able to go through with it; all he sees is his, *re* or *spe*, he hath devoured it in hope, or else in conceit esteems it his own; like him in Athenæus,[3] that thought all the ships in the haven to be his own. A lascivious *inamorato* plots all the day long to please his mistress, acts and struts, and carries himself as if she were in presence, still dreaming of her, as Pamphilus of his Glycerium, or as some do in their morning sleep. Marcellus Donatus [4] knew such a gentlewoman in Mantua, called Elionora Meliorina, that constantly believed she was married to a king, and "would kneel down and talk with him, as if he had been there present with his associates; and if she had found by chance a piece of glass in a muck-hill or in the street, she would say that it was a jewel sent from her lord and husband." [5] If devout and religious, he is all for fasting, prayer, ceremonies, alms, interpretations, visions, prophecies, revelations, he is inspired by the Holy Ghost, full of the spirit: [6] one while he is saved, another while damned, or still troubled in mind for his sins, the devil will surely have him, etc. More of these in the third Partition, of Love-melancholy. A scholar's mind is busied about his studies, he applauds himself for that he hath done, or hopes to do, one while fearing to be out in his next exercise, another while contemning all censures; envies one, emulates another; or else with indefatigable pains and meditation consumes himself.[1] So of the rest, all which vary according to the more remiss and violent impression of the object, or as the humour itself is intended or remitted. For some are so gently melancholy, that in all their carriage, and to the outward apprehension of others, it can hardly be discerned, yet to them an intolerable burden, and not to be endured. *Quædam occulta, quædam manifesta*,[2] some signs are manifest and obvious to all at all times, some to few, or seldom, or hardly perceived; let them keep their own counsel, none will take notice or suspect them. "They do not express in outward show their depraved imaginations," as Hercules de Saxonia observes, "but conceal them wholly to themselves, and are very wise men, as I have often seen; some fear, some do not fear at all, as such as think themselves kings or dead, some have more signs, some fewer, some great, some less,"[3] some vex, fret, still fear, grieve, lament, suspect, laugh, sing, weep, chafe, etc., by fits (as I have said) or more during and permanent. Some dote in one thing, are most childish and ridiculous and to be wondered at in that, and yet for all other matters most discreet and wise. To some it is in disposition, to another in habit; and as they write of heat and cold, we may say of this humour, one is *melancholicus ad octo* [eight degrees melancholy], a second two degrees less, a third half-way. 'Tis superparticular, *sesquialtera, sesquitertia,* and *superbipartiens tertias, quintas melancholiæ*,[4] etc.; all those geometrical proportions are too little to express it. "It comes to many by fits, and goes; to others it is continuate":[5] many (saith Faventinus[6]) "in spring and fall only are molested," some once a year, as that Roman Galen speaks of;[7] one, at the conjunction of the moon alone, or some unfortunate aspects, at such and such set hours and times, like the sea-tides;[8] to some women when they be with child, as Plater notes,[9] never otherwise: to others 'tis settled and fixed. To one, led about and variable still by that *ignis fatuus* of phantasy, like an *arthritis* or running gout, 'tis here and there, and in every joint, always molesting some part or other; or if the body be free, in a myriad of forms exercising the mind. A second once peradventure in his life hath a most

grievous fit, once in seven years, once in five years, even to the
extremity of madness, death, or dotage, and that upon some feral
accident or perturbation, terrible object, and that for a time,
never perhaps so before, never after. A third is moved upon all
such troublesome objects, cross fortune, disaster, and violent
passions, otherwise free, once troubled in three or four years.
A fourth, if things be to his mind, or he in action, well pleased,
in good company, is most jocund, and of a good complexion: if
idle, or alone, all amort, or carried away wholly with pleasant
dreams and phantasies, but if once crossed and displeased,

> *Pectore concipiet nil nisi triste suo ;*
> [He will imagine naught save sadness in his heart;]

his countenance is altered on a sudden, his heart heavy, irksome
thoughts crucify his soul, and in an instant he is moped or
weary of his life, he will kill himself. A fifth complains in his
youth, a sixth in his middle age, the last in his old age.

Generally thus much we may conclude of melancholy: that it
is most pleasant at first,[1] I say, *mentis gratissimus error* [a most
pleasing delusion], a most delightsome humour, to be alone,
dwell alone, walk alone, meditate, lie in bed whole days, dreaming awake as it were, and frame a thousand phantastical imaginations unto themselves. They are never better pleased than
when they are so doing, they are in paradise for the time, and
cannot well endure to be interrupt; with him in the poet, *Pol,
me occidistis, amici, non servastis, ait* [2] ["In sooth, good friends,
you have killed, not cured me," says he]; you have undone him,
he complains, if you trouble him: tell him what inconvenience
will follow, what will be the event, all is one, *canis ad vomitum*
[like a dog to his vomit], 'tis so pleasant he cannot refrain.[3]
He may thus continue peradventure many years by reason of a
strong temperature, or some mixture of business, which may
divert his cogitations: but at the last *læsa imaginatio*, his
phantasy is crazed, and, now habituated to such toys, cannot
but work still like a fate; the scene alters upon a sudden, fear
and sorrow supplant those pleasing thoughts, suspicion, discontent, and perpetual anxiety succeed in their places; so by
little and little, by that shoeing-horn of idleness, and voluntary
solitariness, melancholy, this feral fiend, is drawn on, *et quantum
vertice ad auras Æthereas, tantum radice in Tartara tendit* [4] [High
as his topmost boughs to heaven ascend, So low his roots to
hell's dominions tend]; it was not so delicious at first, as now it
is bitter and harsh; a cankered soul macerated with cares and

discontents, *tædium vitæ*, impatience, agony, inconstancy, irresolution, precipitate them unto unspeakable miseries. They cannot endure company, light, or life itself; some unfit for action, and the like. Their bodies are lean and dried up,[1] withered, ugly, their looks harsh, very dull, and their souls tormented, as they are more or less entangled, as the humour hath been intended, or according to the continuance of time they have been troubled.

To discern all which symptoms the better, Rhasis the Arabian [2] makes three degrees of them. The first is *falsa cogitatio*, false conceits and idle thoughts: to misconster and amplify, aggravating everything they conceive or fear; the second is *falso cogitata loqui*, to talk to themselves, or to use inarticulate, incondite voices, speeches, obsolete gestures, and plainly to utter their minds and conceits of their hearts by their words and actions, as to laugh, weep, to be silent, not to sleep, eat their meat, etc.; the third is to put in practice that which they think or speak.[3] Savonarola, *rub.* 11, *tract.* 8, *cap.* 1, *de ægritudine*, confirms as much: "when he begins to express that in words, which he conceives in his heart, or talks idly, or goes from one thing to another," [4] which Gordonius [5] calls *nec caput habentia, nec caudam* [having neither head nor tail], he is in the middle way: "but when he begins to act it likewise, and to put his fopperies in execution, he is then in the extent of melancholy, or madness itself." [6] This progress of melancholy you shall easily observe in them that have been so affected; they go smiling to themselves at first, at length they laugh out; at first solitary, at last they can endure no company: or if they do, they are now dizzards, past sense and shame, quite moped, they care not what they say or do, all their actions, words, gestures, are furious or ridiculous. At first his mind is troubled, he doth not attend what is said, if you tell him a tale, he cries at last, "What said you?" but in the end he mutters to himself, as old women do many times, or old men when they sit alone, upon a sudden they laugh, whoop, halloo, or run away, and swear they see or hear players, devils,[7] hobgoblins, ghosts, strike or strut, etc., grow humorous in the end: like him in the poet, *sæpe ducentos, sæpe decem servos* [often he keeps two hundred servants, often only ten], he will dress himself, and undress, careless at last, grows insensible, stupid, or mad. He howls like a wolf, barks like a dog, and raves like Ajax and Orestes, hears music and outcries which no man else hears.[8] As he [9] did whom Amatus Lusitanus mentioneth, *cent.* 3, *cura* 55, or that woman in Sprenger,[1] that spake many languages, and said she was possessed: that farmer in Prosper Calenius,[2] that disputed and discoursed learnedly in philosophy and astronomy with Alexander Achilles, his master, at Bologna in Italy. But of these I have already spoken.

Who can sufficiently speak of these symptoms, or prescribe rules to comprehend them? as Echo to the painter in Ausonius, *Vane, quid affectus*, etc., Foolish fellow, what wilt? if you must needs paint me, paint a voice, *et similem si vis pingere, pinge sonum;* if you will describe melancholy, describe a phantastical conceit, a corrupt imagination, vain thoughts and different, which who can do? The four-and-twenty letters make no more variety of words in divers languages than melancholy conceits produce diversity of symptoms in several persons. They are irregular, obscure, various, so infinite, Proteus himself is not so diverse; you may as well make the moon a new coat as a true character of a melancholy man; as soon find the motion of a bird in the air as the heart of man, a melancholy man. They are so confused, I say, diverse, intermixed with other diseases. As the species be confounded (which I have showed[3]), so are the symptoms; sometimes with headache, cachexia, dropsy, stone, as you may perceive by those several examples and illustrations collected by Hildesheim, *Spicil.* 2:[4] Mercurialis, *consil.* 118, *cap.* 6 *et* 11, with headache, epilepsy, priapismus; Trincavellius, *consil.* 12, *lib.* 1, *consil.* 49, with gout, *caninus appetitus*; Montanus, *consil.* 26, etc., 23, 234, 249, with falling sickness, headache, vertigo, lycanthropia, etc.; J. Cæsar Claudinus, *consult.* 4 *consult.* 89 *et* 116, with gout, agues, hemrods, stone, etc. Who can distinguish these melancholy symptoms so intermixed with others, or apply them to their several kinds, confine them into method? 'Tis hard, I confess; yet I have disposed of them as I could, and will descend to particularize them according to their species. For hitherto I have expatiated in more general lists or terms, speaking promiscuously of such ordinary signs, which occur amongst writers. Not that they are all to be found in one man, for that were to paint a monster or chimera, not a man; but some in one, some in another, and that successively or at several times.

Which I have been the more curious to express and report, not to upbraid any miserable man, or by way of derision (I rather pity them), but the better to discern, to apply remedies unto them; and to show that the best and soundest of us all is in great danger, how much we ought to fear our own fickle

estates, remember our miseries and vanities, examine and
humiliate ourselves, seek to God, and call to Him for mercy;
that needs not look for any rods to scourge ourselves, since we
carry them in our bowels, and that our souls are in a miserable
captivity, if the light of grace and heavenly truth doth not shine
continually upon us: and by our discretion to moderate ourselves,
to be more circumspect and wary in the midst of these dangers.

MEMB. II.

SUBSECT. I.—*Symptoms of Head-Melancholy*

"IF no symptoms appear about the stomach, nor the blood be
misaffected, and fear and sorrow continue, it is to be thought
the brain itself is troubled, by reason of a melancholy juice
bred in it, or otherwise conveyed into it, and that evil juice is
from the distemperature of the part, or left after some inflammation." [1] Thus far Piso. But this is not always true, for
blood and hypochondries both are often affected even in head-
melancholy. Hercules de Saxonia differs here from the common
current of writers, putting peculiar signs of head-melancholy
from the sole distemperature of spirits in the brain, as they are
hot, cold, dry, moist, "all without matter, from the motion
alone, and tenebrosity of spirits"; [2] of melancholy which proceeds from humours by adustion he treats apart, with their
several symptoms and cures. The common signs, if it be by
essence in the head, are ruddiness of face, high sanguine complexion, most part *rubore saturato* [with a flushed red colour] (one
calls it a bluish, and sometimes full of pimples), with red eyes [3]
(Avicenna, *lib.* 3, *fen.* 2, *tract.* 4, *cap.* 18, Duretus and others
out of Galen, *de affect. lib.* 3, *cap.* 6). Hercules de Saxonia to
this of redness of face adds "heaviness of the head, fixed and
hollow eyes." [4] "If it proceed from dryness of the brain,
then their heads will be light, vertiginous, and they most apt
to wake, and to continue whole months together without sleep.
Few excrements in their eyes and nostrils," [5] "and often bald
by reason of excess of dryness," Montaltus adds, *cap.* 17. If
it proceed from moisture, dullness, drowsiness, headache
follows; and as Sallust. Salvianus, *cap.* 2, *lib.* 2, out of his own
experience found, epileptical, with a multitude of humours in
the head. They are very bashful; if ruddy, apt to blush, and

to be red upon all occasions, *præsertim si metus accesserit*
[especially if any fear troubles them].   But the chiefest symptom
to discern this species, as I have said, is this, that there be no
notable signs in the stomach, hypochondries, or elsewhere, *digna*,
as Montaltus terms them,[1] or of greater note, because oftentimes
the passions of the stomach concur with them.   Wind is common
to all three species, and is not excluded, only that of the hypochondries is more windy than the rest,[2] saith Hollerius. Aetius,
Tetrab. lib. 2, sec. 2, cap. 9 *et* 10, maintains the same; if there
be more signs, and more evident in the head than elsewhere,
the brain is primarily affected; and prescribes head-melancholy
to be cured by meats amongst the rest, void of wind, and good
juice, not excluding wind, or corrupt blood, even in head-
melancholy itself: [3] but these species are often confounded, and
so are their symptoms, as I have already proved.   The symptoms
of the mind are superfluous and continual cogitations: "for
when the head is heated, it scorcheth the blood, and from thence
proceed melancholy fumes, which trouble the mind" [4] (Avicenna).
They are very choleric, and soon hot, solitary, sad, often silent,
watchful, discontent (Montaltus, *cap.* 24).   If anything trouble
them, they cannot sleep, but fret themselves still, till another
object mitigate, or time wear it out.   They have grievous
passions, and immoderate perturbations of the mind, fear,
sorrow, etc., yet not so continuate but that they are sometimes
merry, apt to profuse laughter, which is more to be wondered
at, and that by the authority of Galen himself,[5] by reason of
mixture of blood, *prærubri jocosis delectantur et irrisores plerumque
sunt*, if they be ruddy, they are delighted in jests, and oftentimes scoffers themselves, conceited, and, as Rodericus à Vega
comments on that place of Galen, merry, witty, of a pleasant
disposition, and yet grievously melancholy anon after.   *Omnia
discunt sine doctore*, saith Aretæus, they learn without a teacher:
and, as Laurentius [6] supposeth, those feral passions and symptoms of such as think themselves glass, pitchers, feathers, etc.,
speak strange languages, proceed *a calore cerebri* (if it be in
excess), from the brain's distempered heat.

Subsect. II.—*Symptoms of Windy Hypochondriacal Melancholy*

"In this hypochondrical or flatuous melancholy, the symptoms
are so ambiguous," saith Crato in a counsel of his for a noblewoman,[7] "that the most exquisite physicians cannot determine

of the part affected." Matthew Flaccius, consulted about a
noble matron, confessed as much, that in this malady he with
Hollerius, Fracastorius, Fallopius, and others, being to give
their sentence of a party labouring of hypochondriacal melancholy, could not find out by the symptoms which part was most
especially affected; some said the womb, some heart, some
stomach, etc., and therefore Crato, *consil*. 24, *lib*. 1, boldly avers
that, in this diversity of symptoms which commonly accompany
this disease, "no physician can truly say what part is affected." [1]
Galen, *lib. 3 de loc. affect*., reckons up these ordinary symptoms,
which all the neoterics repeat, of Diocles; only this fault he
finds with him, that he puts not fear and sorrow amongst the
other signs. Trincavellius excuseth Diocles, *lib. 3, consil*. 35,
because that oftentimes in a strong head and constitution, a
generous spirit, and a valiant, these symptoms appear not, by
reason of his valour and courage. Hercules de Saxonia [2] (to
whom I subscribe) is of the same mind (which I have before
touched) that fear and sorrow are not general symptoms; some
fear and are not sad; some be sad and fear not; some neither
fear nor grieve. The rest are these, beside fear and sorrow,
"sharp belchings, fulsome crudities, heat in the bowels, wind and
rumbling in the guts, vehement gripings, pain in the belly and
stomach sometimes after meat that is hard of concoction, much
watering of the stomach, and moist spittle, cold sweat," [3]
importunus sudor, unseasonable sweat all over the body, as
Octavius Horatianus, *lib. 2, cap*. 5, calls it; "cold joints, indigestion, they cannot endure their own fulsome belchings, continual
wind about their hypochondries, heat and griping in their
bowels, *præcordia sursum convelluntur*, midriff and bowels are
pulled up, the veins about their eyes look red, and swell from
vapours and wind." [4] Their ears sing now and then, vertigo
and giddiness come by fits, turbulent dreams, dryness, leanness;
apt they are to sweat upon all occasions, of all colours and
complexions. Many of them are high-coloured, especially after
meals, which symptom Cardinal Cæsius was much troubled with,
and of which he complained to Prosper Calenus his physician;
he could not eat, or drink a cup of wine, but he was as red in
the face as if he had been at a mayor's feast. That symptom
alone vexeth many. Some again are black, pale, ruddy, sometimes their shoulders, and shoulder-blades ache, there is a
leaping all over their bodies, sudden trembling, a palpitation of
the heart, and that *cardiaca passio*, grief in the mouth of the
stomach, which maketh the patient think his heart itself acheth,

and sometimes suffocation, *difficultas anhelitus*, short breath, hard wind, strong pulse, swooning.[1] Montanus, *consil.* 55; Trincavellius, *lib.* 3, *consil.* 36 *et* 37; Fernelius, *cons.* 43; Frambesarius, *Consult. lib.* 1, *consil.* 17; Hildesheim, Claudinus, etc., give instance of every particular. The peculiar symptoms which properly belong to each part be these. If it proceed from the stomach, saith Savonarola,[2] 'tis full of pain, wind. Guianerius adds vertigo, nausea, much spitting, etc. If from the myrach, a swelling and wind in the hypochondries, a loathing, and appetite to vomit, pulling upward. If from the heart, aching and trembling of it, much heaviness. If from the liver, there is usually a pain in the right hypochondry. If from the spleen, hardness and grief in the left hypochondry, a rumbling, much appetite and small digestion (Avicenna). If from the meseraic veins and liver on the other side, little or no appetite (Hercules de Saxonia). If from the hypochondries, a rumbling inflation, concoction is hindered, often belching, etc. And from these crudities, windy vapours ascend up to the brain, which trouble the imagination, and cause fear, sorrow, dullness, heaviness, many terrible conceits and chimeras, as Lemnius well observes, *lib.* 1, *cap.* 16: "As a black and thick cloud covers the sun, and intercepts his beams and light, so doth this melancholy vapour obnubilate the mind, enforce it to many absurd thoughts and imaginations,"[3] and compel good, wise, honest, discreet men (arising to the brain from the lower parts, "as smoke out of a chimney"[4]) to dote, speak and do that which becomes them not, their persons, callings, wisdoms. One, by reason of those ascending vapours and gripings rumbling beneath, will not be persuaded but that he hath a serpent in his guts, a viper; another frogs. Trallianus relates a story of a woman that imagined she had swallowed an eel or a serpent; and Felix Platerus, *Observat. lib.* 1, hath a most memorable example of a countryman of his, that by chance falling into a pit where frogs and frogs' spawn was, and a little of that water swallowed, began to suspect that he had likewise swallowed frogs' spawn, and with that conceit and fear, his phantasy wrought so far, that he verily thought he had young live frogs in his belly, *qui vivebant ex alimento suo*, that lived by his nourishment, and was so certainly persuaded of it, that for many years following he could not be rectified in his conceit. He studied physic seven years together to cure himself, travelled into Italy, France and Germany to confer with the best physicians about it, and, *anno* 1609, asked his counsel amongst the rest; he told

him it was wind, his conceit, etc., but *mordicus contradicere, et
ore et scriptis probare nitebatur* [he obstinately contradicted him,
and maintained his view both in speech and writing]: no saying
would serve, it was no wind, but real frogs: "and do you not hear
them croak?" Platerus would have deceived him by putting
live frogs into his excrements; but he, being a physician himself,
would not be deceived, *vir prudens alias, et doctus*, a wise and
learned man otherwise, a doctor of physic, and after seven
years' dotage in this kind, *a phantasia liberatus est*, he was cured.
Laurentius and Goulart have many such examples, if you be
desirous to read them. One commodity, above the rest which
are melancholy, these windy flatuous have, *lucida intervalla*
[lucid intervals], their symptoms and pains are not usually so
continuate as the rest, but come by fits, fear and sorrow and
the rest: yet in another they exceed all others; and that is,
they are luxurious, incontinent, and prone to venery, by reason
of wind,[1] *et facile amant, et quamlibet fere amant* [and easily fall
in love, and with any woman almost] (Jason Pratensis). Rhasis [2]
is of opinion that Venus doth many of them much good. The
other symptoms of the mind be common with the rest.

SUBSECT. III.—*Symptoms of Melancholy abounding in the
whole Body*

Their bodies that are affected with this universal melancholy
are most part black, "the melancholy juice is redundant all
over," [3] hirsute they are, and lean, they have broad veins, their
blood is gross and thick. "Their spleen is weak," [4] and liver
apt to engender the humour; they have kept bad diet, or have
had some evacuation stopped, as hemrods, or months in women,
which Trallianus,[5] in the cure, would have carefully to be
inquired, and withal to observe of what complexion the party is
of, black or red. For, as Forestus and Hollerius contend, if
they be black,[6] it proceeds from abundance of natural melancholy; if it proceed from cares, agony, discontents, diet, exercise,
etc., they may be as well of any other colour, red, yellow, pale,
as black, and yet their whole blood corrupt: *prærubri colore
sæpe sunt tales, sæpe flavi* [such people are often ruddy, often
yellowish] (saith Montaltus, *cap.* 22). The best way to discern
this species is to let them bleed;[7] if the blood be corrupt, thick
and black, and they withal free from these hypochondriacal
symptoms, and not so grievously troubled with them or those of
the head, it argues they are melancholy *a toto corpore* [through-

out the whole body]. The fumes which arise from this corrupt blood disturb the mind, and make them fearful and sorrowful, heavy-hearted, as the rest, dejected, discontented, solitary, silent, weary of their lives, dull and heavy, or merry, etc., and if far gone, that which Apuleius wished to his enemy, by way of imprecation, is true in them: "Dead men's bones, hobgoblins, ghosts are ever in their minds, and meet them still in every turn; all the bugbears of the night, and terrors, fairybabes of tombs and graves are before their eyes and in their thoughts, as to women and children, if they be in the dark alone."[1] If they hear, or read, or see any tragical object, it sticks by them; they are afraid of death, and yet weary of their lives; in their discontented humours they quarrel with all the world, bitterly inveigh, tax satirically, and because they cannot otherwise vent their passions, or redress what is amiss as they mean, they will by violent death at last be revenged on themselves.

SUBSECT. IV.—*Symptoms of Maids', Nuns', and Widows' Melancholy*

Because Lodovicus Mercatus, in his second book *de mulier. affect. cap.* 4, and Rodericus à Castro, *de morb. mulier. cap.* 3, *lib.* 2, two famous physicians in Spain, Daniel Sennertus of Wittenberg, *lib.* 1, *part.* 2, *cap.* 13, with others, have vouchsafed, in their works not long since published, to write two just treatises *de melancholia virginum, monialium et viduarum* [of the melancholy of maids, nuns, and widows], as a particular species of melancholy (which I have already specified) distinct from the rest, for it much differs from that which commonly befalls men and other women, as having one only cause proper to women alone,[2] I may not omit, in this general survey of melancholy symptoms, to set down the particular signs of such parties so misaffected.

The causes are assigned out of Hippocrates, Cleopatra, Moschion, and those old *gynæciorum scriptores* [writers on women's diseases], of this feral malady, in more ancient maids, widows, and barren women, *ob septum transversum violatum,* saith Mercatus, by reason of the midriff or *diaphragma,* heart and brain offended with those vicious vapours which come from menstruous blood; *inflammationem arteriæ circa dorsum,* Rodericus adds, an inflammation of the back, which with the rest is offended by that fuliginous exhalation of corrupt seed, troubling the brain, heart and mind;[3] the brain, I say, not in essence, but by consent; *universa enim hujus affectus causa ab utero pendet, et a sanguinis menstrui malitia*, for, in a word, the whole malady proceeds from that inflammation, putridity, black smoky vapours, etc.; from thence comes care, sorrow, and anxiety, obfuscation of spirits, agony, desperation, and the like, which are intended or remitted, *si amatorius accesserit ardor* [should the amatory passion be aroused], or any other violent object or perturbation of mind. This melancholy may happen to widows, with much care and sorrow, as frequently it doth, by reason of a sudden alteration of their accustomed course of life, etc.; to such as lie in child-bed, *ob suppressam purgationem*; but to nuns and more ancient maids, and some barren women, for the causes abovesaid, 'tis more familiar, *crebrius his quam reliquis accidit, inquit Rodericus* [it happens to these more frequently than to the rest, saith Rodericus]; the rest are not altogether excluded.

Out of these causes Rodericus defines it, with Aretæus, to be *angorem animi*, a vexation of the mind, a sudden sorrow from a small, light, or no occasion, with a kind of still dotage and grief of some part or other, head, heart, breasts, sides, back, belly, etc., with much solitariness, weeping, distraction, etc., from which they are sometimes suddenly delivered, because it comes and goes by fits, and is not so permanent as other melancholy.[1]

But, to leave this brief description, the most ordinary symptoms be these: *pulsatio juxta dorsum*, a beating about the back, which is almost perpetual; the skin is many times rough, squalid, especially, as Aretæus observes, about the arms, knees, and knuckles. The midriff and heart-strings do burn and beat very fearfully, and when this vapour or fume is stirred, flieth upward, the heart itself beats, is sore grieved, and faints,[2] *fauces siccitate præcluduntur, ut difficulter possit ab uteri strangulatione decerni*, like fits of the mother; *alvus plerisque nil reddit, aliis exiguum, acre, biliosum, lotium flavum*. They complain many times, saith Mercatus, of a great pain in their heads, about their hearts and hypochondries, and so likewise in their breasts, which are often sore; sometimes ready to swoon, their faces are inflamed and red, they are dry, thirsty, suddenly hot, much troubled with wind, cannot sleep, etc. And from hence proceed *ferina deliramenta*, a brutish kind of dotage, troublesome sleep, terrible dreams in the night, *subrusticus pudor, et verecundia ignava*, a foolish kind of bashfulness to some, perverse conceits and opinions, dejection of mind, much discontent, preposterous judgment.[3] They are apt to loathe, dislike, disdain, to be weary

of every object, etc., each thing almost is tedious to them, they
pine away, void of counsel, apt to weep and tremble, timorous,
fearful, sad, and out of all hope of better fortunes.   They take
delight in nothing for the time, but love to be alone and solitary,
though that do them more harm: and thus they are affected
so long as this vapour lasteth; but by and by as pleasant and
merry as ever they were in their lives, they sing, discourse, and
laugh in any good company, upon all occasions; and so by fits it
takes them now and then, except the malady be inveterate,
and then 'tis more frequent, vehement, and continuate.   Many
of them cannot tell how to express themselves in words, or how
it holds them, what ails them; you cannot understand them, or
well tell what to make of their sayings; so far gone sometimes,
so stupefied and distracted, they think themselves bewitched,
they are in despair, *aptæ ad fletum, desperationem* [prone to
weeping, despondency]; *dolores mammis et hypochondriis*, Mercatus therefore adds, now their breasts, now their hypochondries,
belly and sides, then their heart and head aches; now heat, then
wind, now this, now that offends, they are weary of all; and
yet will not, cannot again tell how, where, or what offends
them,[1] though they be in great pain, agony, and frequently
complain, grieving, sighing, weeping, and discontented still,
sine causa manifesta [without apparent cause], most part; yet,
I say, they will complain, grudge, lament, and not be persuaded
but that they are troubled with an evil spirit, which is frequent
in Germany, saith Rodericus, amongst the common sort; and
to such as are most grievously affected (for he makes three
degrees of this disease in women), they are in despair, surely
forspoken or bewitched, and in extremity of their dotage (weary
of their lives), some of them will attempt to make away themselves.   Some think they see visions, confer with spirits and
devils, they shall surely be damned, are afraid of some treachery,
imminent danger, and the like, they will not speak, make answer
to any question, but are almost distracted, mad, or stupid for
the time, and by fits: and thus it holds them, as they are more or
less affected, and as the inner humour is intended or remitted,
or by outward objects and perturbations aggravated, solitariness,
idleness, etc.

Many other maladies there are incident to young women,
out of that one and only cause above specified, many feral
diseases.   I will not so much as mention their names; melancholy alone is the subject of my present discourse, from which
I will not swerve.   The several cures of this infirmity, concerning

diet, which must be very sparing, phlebotomy, physic, internal,
external remedies, are at large in great variety in Rodericus à
Castro,[1] Sennertus, and Mercatus, which whoso will, as occasion
serves, may make use of. But the best and surest remedy of
all, is to see them well placed, and married to good husbands
in due time; *hinc illæ lachrymæ* [hence those tears], that's the
primary cause, and this the ready cure, to give them content
to their desires. I write not this to patronize any wanton, idle
flirt, lascivious or light huswives, which are too forward many
times, unruly, and apt to cast away themselves on him that
comes next, without all care, counsel, circumspection, and
judgment. If religion, good discipline, honest education,
wholesome exhortation, fair promises, fame, and loss of good
name cannot inhibit and deter such (which to chaste and sober
maids cannot choose but avail much), labour and exercise,
strict diet, rigour, and threats may more opportunely be used,
and are able of themselves to qualify and divert an ill-disposed
temperament. For seldom should you see an hired servant,
a poor handmaid, though ancient, that is kept hard to her work
and bodily labour, a coarse country wench, troubled in this
kind, but noble virgins, nice gentlewomen, such as are solitary
and idle, live at ease, lead a life out of action and employment,
that fare well, in great houses and jovial companies, ill-disposed
peradventure of themselves, and not willing to make any
resistance, discontented otherwise, of weak judgment, able
bodies, and subject to passions (*grandiores virgines*, saith Mercatus, *steriles, et viduæ plerumque melancholicæ* [grown-up girls,
barren women, and widows are usually melancholy]); such for
the most part are misaffected, and prone to this disease. I do
not so much pity them that may otherwise be eased, but those
alone that out of a strong temperament, innate constitution,
are violently carried away with this torrent of inward humours,
and though very modest of themselves, sober, religious, virtuous,
and well given (as many so distressed maids are), yet cannot
make resistance; these grievances will appear, this malady will
take place, and now manifestly shows itself, and may not otherwise be helped. But where am I? Into what subject have I
rushed? What have I to do with nuns, maids, virgins, widows?
I am a bachelor myself, and lead a monastic life in a college,
næ ego sane ineptus qui hæc dixerim [it is certainly very foolish
of me to speak thus], I confess 'tis an indecorum, and as Pallas,
a virgin, blushed when Jupiter by chance spake of love matters
in her presence, and turned away her face, *me reprimam* [I will

check myself]; though my subject necessarily require it, I will say no more.

And yet I must and will say something more, add a word or two *in gratiam virginum et viduarum* [in favour of maids and widows], in favour of all such distressed parties, in commiseration of their present estate. And as I cannot choose but condole their mishap that labour of this infirmity and are destitute of help in this case, so must I needs inveigh against them that are in fault, more than manifest causes, and as bitterly tax those tyrannizing pseudo-politicians, superstitious orders, rash vows, hard-hearted parents, guardians, unnatural friends, allies (call them how you will), those careless and stupid overseers, that, out of worldly respects, covetousness, supine negligence, their own private ends (*cum sibi sit interim bene* [being themselves comfortably situated in the meanwhile]), can so severely reject, stubbornly neglect, and impiously contemn, without all remorse and pity, the tears, sighs, groans, and grievous miseries of such poor souls committed to their charge. How odious and abominable are those superstitious and rash vows of popish monasteries, so to bind and enforce men and women to vow virginity, to lead a single life, against the laws of nature, opposite to religion, policy, and humanity, so to starve, to offer violence, to suppress the vigour of youth! by rigorous statutes, severe laws, vain persuasions, to debar them of that to which by their innate temperature they are so furiously inclined, urgently carried, and sometimes precipitated, even irresistibly led, to the prejudice of their souls' health, and good estate of body and mind! and all for base and private respects, to maintain their gross superstition, to enrich themselves and their territories, as they falsely suppose, by hindering some marriages, that the world be not full of beggars, and their parishes pestered with orphans! Stupid politicians! *hæccine fieri flagitia?* ought these things so to be carried? Better marry than burn, saith the Apostle, but they are otherwise persuaded. They will by all means quench their neighbour's house if it be on fire, but that fire of lust, which breaks out into such lamentable flames, they will not take notice of; their own bowels oftentimes, flesh and blood, shall so rage and burn, and they will not see it: *Miserum est*, saith Austin, *seipsum non miserescere*, and they are miserable in the meantime that cannot pity themselves, the common good of all, and *per consequens* their own estates. For let them but consider what fearful maladies, feral diseases, gross inconveniences, come to both sexes by this enforced temperance;

it troubles me to think of, much more to relate, those frequent aborts and murdering of infants in their nunneries (read Kemnisius [1] and others), their notorious fornications, those *spintrias, tribadas, ambubaias,* etc., those rapes, incests, adulteries, mastuprations, sodomies, buggeries of monks and friars. See Bale's Visitation of Abbeys, Mercurialis,[2] Rodericus à Castro, Peter Forestus, and divers physicians; I know their ordinary apologies and excuses for these things, *sed viderint politici, medici, theologi* [but let the politicians, the physicians and the theologians look out]; I shall more opportunely meet with them elsewhere.[3]

> *Illius viduæ, aut patronum virginis hujus,*
> *Ne me forte putes, verbum non amplius addam.*

> [Lest you should think I am pleading the cause of
> this widow or that virgin, I will say no more.]

MEMB. III.

Immediate Cause of these precedent Symptoms

To give some satisfaction to melancholy men that are troubled with these symptoms, a better means in my judgment cannot be taken than to show them the causes whence they proceed; not from devils as they suppose, or that they are bewitched or forsaken of God, hear or see, etc., as many of them think, but from natural and inward causes; that so knowing them, they may better avoid the effects, or at least endure them with more patience. The most grievous and common symptoms are fear and sorrow, and that without a cause, to the wisest and discreetest men, in this malady not to be avoided. The reason why they are so Aetius discusseth at large, *Tetrabib,* 2, 2, in his first problem out of Galen, *lib. 2 de causis, sympt.* 1. For Galen imputeth all to the cold that is black, and thinks that the spirits being darkened, and the substance of the brain cloudy and dark, all the objects thereof appear terrible, and the mind itself, by those dark, obscure, gross fumes, ascending from black humours,[4] is in continual darkness, fear, and sorrow; divers terrible monstrous fictions in a thousand shapes and apparitions occur, with violent passions, by which the brain and phantasy are troubled and eclipsed. Fracastorius, *lib. 2 de intellect.,* will have cold to be the cause of fear and sorrow;

"for such as are cold are ill-disposed to mirth, dull, and heavy,
by nature solitary, silent; and not for any inward darkness (as
physicians think), for many melancholy men dare boldly be,
continue, and walk in the dark, and delight in it":[1] *solum
frigidi timidi* [only the cold are timid]: if they be hot, they are
merry; and the more hot, the more furious, and void of fear,
as we see in madmen: but this reason holds not, for then no
melancholy, proceeding from choler adust, should fear. Averroes
scoffs at Galen for his reasons, and brings five arguments to
refel them: so doth Hercules de Saxonia, *tract. de melanch.
cap.* 3, assigning other causes, which are copiously censured and
confuted by Ælianus Montaltus, *cap.* 5 *et* 6; Lod. Mercatus,
de inter. morb. cur. lib. 1, *cap.* 17; Altomarus, *cap.* 7 *de mel.*;
Guianerius, *tract.* 15, *cap.* 1; Bright, *cap.* 37; Laurentius,
cap. 5; Valesius, *Med. cont. lib.* 5, *cont.* 1. "Distemperature,"
they conclude, "makes black juice, blackness obscures the
spirits, the spirits obscured cause fear and sorrow."[2] Laurentius, *cap.* 13, supposeth these black fumes offend specially the
diaphragma or midriff, and so *per consequens* the mind, which is
obscured as the sun by a cloud.[3] To this opinion of Galen almost
all the Greeks and Arabians subscribe, the Latins new and old;
internæ tenebræ offuscant animum, ut externæ nocent pueris, as
children are affrighted in the dark, so are melancholy men at
all times, as having the inward cause with them, and still
carrying it about.[4] Which black vapours, whether they proceed
from the black blood about the heart, as T[homas] W[right],
Jes[uit], thinks in his Treatise of the Passions of the Mind, or
stomach, spleen, midriff, or all the misaffected parts together,
it boots not; they keep the mind in a perpetual dungeon, and
oppress it with continual fears, anxieties, sorrows, etc. It is
an ordinary thing for such as are sound to laugh at this dejected
pusillanimity and those other symptoms of melancholy, to make
themselves merry with them, and to wonder at such, as toys
and trifles, which may be resisted and withstood, if they will
themselves: but let him that so wonders consider with himself,
that if a man should tell him on a sudden some of his especial
friends were dead, could he choose but grieve? Or set him upon
a steep rock, where he should be in danger to be precipitated,
could he be secure? His heart would tremble for fear, and his
head be giddy. P. Byarus, *tract. de pest.*, gives instance (as
I have said): "And put case" (saith he) "in one that walks
upon a plank; if it lie on the ground, he can safely do it, but if
the same plank be laid over some deep water, instead of a

bridge, he is vehemently moved, and 'tis nothing but his imagination, *forma cadendi impressa* [the idea of falling], to which his other members and faculties obey." [1] Yea, but you infer that such men have a just cause to fear, a true object of fear; so have melancholy men .an inward cause, a perpetual fume and darkness, causing fear, grief, suspicion, which they carry with them, an object which cannot be removed, but sticks as close, and is as inseparable, as a shadow to a body, and who can expel or overrun his shadow? Remove heat of the liver, a cold stomach, weak spleen; remove those adust humours and vapours arising from them, black blood from the heart, all outward perturbations; take away the cause, and then bid them not grieve nor fear, or be heavy, dull, lumpish; otherwise counsel can do little good; you may as well bid him that is sick of an ague not to be adry, or him that is wounded not to feel pain.

Suspicion follows fear and sorrow at heels, arising out of the same fountain, so thinks Fracastorius,[2] "that fear is the cause of suspicion, and still they suspect some treachery, or some secret machination to be framed against them," still they distrust. Restlessness proceeds from the same spring, variety of fumes make them like and dislike. Solitariness, avoiding of light, that they are weary of their lives, hate the world, arise from the same causes, for their spirits and humours are opposite to light, fear makes them avoid company, and absent themselves, lest they should be misused, hissed at, or overshoot themselves, which still they suspect. They are prone to venery by reason of wind. Angry, waspish, and fretting still, out of abundance of choler, which causeth fearful dreams, and violent perturbations to them both sleeping and waking. That they suppose they have no heads, fly, sink, they are pots, glasses, etc., is wind in their heads. Hercules de Saxonia [3] doth ascribe this to the several motions in the animal spirits, "their dilation, contraction, confusion, alteration, tenebrosity, hot or cold distemperature," excluding all material humours. Fracastorius accounts it "a thing worthy of inquisition, why they should entertain such false conceits, as that they have horns, great noses, that they are birds, beasts," etc.,[4] why they should think themselves kings, lords, cardinals. For the first, Fracastorius gives two reasons: "One is the disposition of the body; the other the occasion of the phantasy," [5] as if their eyes be purblind, their ears sing, by reason of some cold and rheum, etc. To the second Laurentius answers, the imagination, inwardly or outwardly moved, represents to the understanding, not enticements only, to favour the passion or dislike, but a very intensive pleasure follows the passion or displeasure, and the will and reason are captivated by delighting in it.

Why students and lovers are so often melancholy and mad, the philosophers of Coimbra [1] assign this reason, "because by a vehement and continual meditation of that wherewith they are affected, they fetch up the spirits into the brain, and with the heat brought with them they incend it beyond measure: and the cells of the inner senses dissolve their temperature, which being dissolved, they cannot perform their offices as they ought."

Why melancholy men are witty, which Aristotle hath long since maintained in his Problems, and that all learned men, famous philosophers, and lawgivers, *ad unum fere omnes melancholici*, have still been melancholy,[2] is a problem much controverted. Jason Pratensis will have it understood of natural melancholy, which opinion Melancthon inclines to, in his book *de anima*, and Marsilius Ficinus, *de san. tuend. lib. 1, cap. 5*, but not simple, for that makes men stupid, heavy, dull, being cold and dry, fearful, fools, and solitary, but mixed with the other humours, phlegm only excepted; and they not adust, but so mixed as that blood be half,[3] with little or no adustion, that they be neither too hot nor too cold. Apponensis, cited by Melancthon, thinks it proceeds from melancholy adust, excluding all natural melancholy as too cold. Laurentius condemns his tenent, because adustion of humours makes men mad, as lime burns when water is cast on it. It must be mixed with blood, and somewhat adust, and so that old aphorism of Aristotle may be verified, *Nullum magnum ingenium sine mixtura dementiæ*, no excellent wit without a mixture of madness. Fracastorius shall decide the controversy:[4] "Phlegmatic are dull; sanguine lively, pleasant, acceptable, and merry, but not witty; choleric are too swift in motion, and furious, impatient of contemplation, deceitful wits; melancholy men have the most excellent wits, but not all; this humour may be hot or cold, thick, or thin; if too hot, they are furious and mad: if too cold, dull, stupid, timorous, and sad: if temperate, excellent, rather inclining to that extreme of heat than cold." This sentence of his will agree with that of Heraclitus, a dry light makes a wise mind; temperate heat and dryness are the chief causes of a good wit; therefore, saith Ælian, an elephant is the wisest of all brute beasts, because his brain is driest, *et ob atræ bilis copiam* [and on account of his abundance of black bile]: this reason Cardan approves, *Subtil. lib.* 12.   Jo. Baptista Silvaticus, a physician of Milan, in his first Controversy, hath copiously handled this question; Rulandus in his Problems; Cœlius Rhodiginus, *lib.* 17; Valleriola, 6*to narrat. med.*; Hercules de Saxonia, *tract. posth. de mel. cap.* 3; Lodovicus Mercatus, *de inter. morb. cur. lib. cap.* 17; Baptista Porta, *Physiog. lib.* 1, *cap.* 13; and many others.

Weeping, sighing, laughing, itching, trembling, sweating, blushing, hearing and seeing strange noises, visions, wind, crudity, are motions of the body, depending upon these precedent motions of the mind: neither are tears affections, but actions (as Scaliger holds): "The voice of such as are afraid trembles, because the heart is shaken" [1] (*Conimb. prob. 6, sec. 3, de som.*). Why they stut or falter in their speech, Mercurialis and Montaltus, *cap.* 17, give like reasons out of Hippocrates, "dryness, which makes the nerves of the tongue torpid." [2] Fast speaking (which is a symptom of some few) Aetius will have caused from abundance of wind, and swiftness of imagination: [3] baldness comes from excess of dryness,[4] hirsuteness from a dry temperature. The cause of much waking is a dry brain, continual meditation, discontent, fears, and cares, that suffer not the mind to be at rest; incontinency is from wind, and a hot liver (Montanus, *cons.* 26). Rumbling in the guts is caused from wind, and wind from ill concoction, weakness of natural heat, or a distempered heat and cold; palpitation of the heart from vapours, heaviness and aching from the same cause.[5] That the belly is hard, wind is a cause, and of that leaping in many parts. Redness of the face, and itching, as if they were flea-bitten, or stung with pismires, from a sharp subtile wind; cold sweat from vapours arising from the hypochondries, which pitch upon the skin;[6] leanness for want of good nourishment. Why their appetite is so great, Aetius answers: [7] *Os ventris frigescit*, cold in those inner parts, cold belly, and hot liver, causeth crudity, and intention proceeds from perturbations; our soul for want of spirits cannot attend exactly to so many intentive operations; being exhaust, and overswayed by passion, she cannot consider the reasons which may dissuade her from such affections.[8]

Bashfulness and blushing [9] is a passion proper to men alone, and is not only caused for some shame and ignominy, or that they are guilty unto themselves of some foul fact committed,[10] but, as Fracastorius well determines,[11] *ob defectum proprium, et timorem*, "from fear, and a conceit of our defects; the face

labours and is troubled at his presence that sees our defects,
and nature, willing to help, sends thither heat, heat draws the
subtilest blood, and so we blush.   They that are bold, arrogant,
and careless, seldom or never blush, but such as are fearful."
Anthonius Lodovicus, in his book *de pudore*, will have this subtile
blood to arise in the face, not so much for the reverence of our
betters in presence, "but for joy and pleasure, or if anything
at unawares shall pass from us, a sudden accident, occurse, or
meeting "[1] (which Disarius in Macrobius confirms), any object
heard or seen, for blind men never blush, as Dandinus observes,[2]
the night and darkness make men impudent.   Or that we be
stayed before our betters, or in company we like not, or if
anything molest and offend us, *erubescentia* turns to *rubor*,
blushing to a continuate redness.[3]   Sometimes the extremity of
the ears tingle, and are red, sometimes the whole face, *etsi
nihil vitiosum commiseris* [although you have done nothing
wrong] as Lodovicus holds: though Aristotle is of opinion,
omnis pudor ex vitio commisso, all shame [is] for some offence.
But we find otherwise; it may as well proceed from fear, from
force and inexperience (so Dandinus holds[4]), as vice; a hot
liver, saith Duretus (*notis in Hollerium*); "from a hot brain,
from wind, the lungs heated, or after drinking of wine, strong
drink, perturbations," etc.[5]

"Laughter, what it is," saith Tully,[6] "how caused, where,
and so suddenly breaks out that, desirous to stay it, we cannot,
how it comes to possess and stir our face, veins, eyes, countenance, mouth, sides, let Democritus determine."   The cause
that it often affects melancholy men so much, is given by
Gomesius, *lib. 3 de sale genial. cap.* 18, abundance of pleasant
vapours, which, in sanguine melancholy especially, break from
the heart, "and tickle the midriff, because it is transverse and
full of nerves: by which titillation the sense being moved, and
arteries distended, or pulled, the spirits from thence move and
possess the sides, veins, countenance, eyes." [7]   See more in
Jossius, *de risu et fletu*, Vives, *3 de anima*.   Tears, as Scaliger
defines, proceed from grief and pity, "or from the heating of a
moist brain, for a dry cannot weep." [8]

That they see and hear so many phantasms, chimeras, noises,
visions, etc., as Fienus hath discoursed at large in his book of
Imagination, and Lavater, *de spectris, part.* 1, *cap.* 2, 3, 4, their
corrupt phantasy makes them see and hear that which indeed
is neither heard nor seen.[9]   *Qui multum jejunant, aut noctes
ducunt insomnes*, they that much fast, or want sleep, as melan-

choly or sick men commonly do, see visions, or such as are weak-
sighted, very timorous by nature, mad, distracted, or earnestly
seek. *Sabini quod volunt somniant,* as the saying is, they dream
of that they desire. Like Sarmiento the Spaniard, who, when
he was sent to discover the Straits of Magellan and confine
places by the Prorex [Viceroy] of Peru, standing on the top of
a hill, *amœnissimam planitiem despicere sibi visus fuit, œdificia
magnifica, quamplurimos pagos, altas turres, splendida templa*
[imagined he was looking down on a most pleasant valley, with
splendid buildings, numerous villages, lofty towers, glittering
temples], and brave cities, built like ours in Europe, not, saith
mine author,[1] that there was any such thing, but that he was *vanis-
simus et nimis credulus* [very untrustworthy and credulous],
and would fain have had it so. Or as Lod. Mercatus proves,[2]
by reason of inward vapours, and humours from blood, choler,
etc., diversely mixed, they apprehend and see outwardly, as
they suppose, divers images, which indeed are not. As they
that drink wine think all runs round, when it is in their own
brain; so is it with these men, the fault and cause is inward,
as Galen affirms, madmen and such as are near death, *quas
extra se videre putant imagines, intra oculos habent* [3] [the figures
which they think they see before them are really in their own
eyes], 'tis in their brain, which seems to be before them; the
brain, as a concave glass, reflects solid bodies. *Senes etiam
decrepiti cerebrum habent concavum et aridum, ut imaginentur se
videre* (saith Boissardus[4]) *quæ non sunt* [old men have a concave
and dry brain which makes them think they see non-existent
objects], old men are too frequently mistaken and dote in like
case; or, as he that looketh through a piece of red glass judgeth
everything he sees to be red, corrupt vapours mounting from
the body to the head, and distilling again from thence to the
eyes, when they have mingled themselves with the watery
crystal which receiveth the shadows of things to be seen, make
all things appear of the same colour, which remains in the
humour that overspreads our sight, as to melancholy men all
is black, to phlegmatic all white, etc. Or else, as before, the
organs, corrupt by a corrupt phantasy, as Lemnius, *lib.* 1,
cap. 16, well quotes, "cause a great agitation of spirits and
humours, which wander to and fro in all the creeks of the
brain, and cause such apparitions before their eyes." [5] One
thinks he reads something written in the moon, as Pythagoras
is said to have done of old; another smells brimstone, hears
Cerberus bark; Orestes, now mad, supposed he saw the

Furies tormenting him, and his mother still ready to run
upon him:

> *O mater, obsecro noli me persequi*
> *His furiis, aspectu anguineis, horribilibus,*
> *Ecce ! ecce ! me invadunt, in me jam ruunt ;*

[Mother, I beseech thee, persecute me not with furies
of horrid, snaky aspect. Look, look how they
rush upon me and assail me;]

but Electra told him thus raving in his mad fit, he saw no such
sights at all, it was but his crazed imagination.

> *Quiesce, quiesce, miser, in linteis tuis,*
> *Non cernis etenim quæ videre te putas.*

[Lie quiet, poor soul, upon thy couch, for thou seest
these things but in fancy.]

So Pentheus (*in Bacchis Euripidis*) saw two suns, two Thebes,
his brain alone was troubled.   Sickness is an ordinary cause of
such sights.   Cardan, *Subtil. 8, Mens ægra laboribus et jejuniis
fracta, facit eos videre, audire*, etc. [over-exertion and want of
food affect their minds so that they see and hear, etc.].   And.
Osiander beheld strange visions, and Alexander ab Alexandro,
both in their sickness, which he relates, *de rerum varietat. lib. 8,
cap.* 44.   Albategnius, that noble Arabian, on his death-bed
saw a ship ascending and descending, which Fracastorius records
of his friend Baptista Turrianus.   Weak sight, and a vain
persuasion withal, may effect as much, and second causes concurring, as an oar in water makes a refraction, and seems bigger,
bended double, etc.   The thickness of the air may cause such
effects; or any object not well discerned in the dark, fear and
phantasy will suspect to be a ghost, a devil, etc.   *Quod nimis
miseri timent, hoc facile credunt* [1] [persons in great misery readily
believe what they fear], we are apt to believe, and mistake in
such cases.   Marcellus Donatus, *lib. 2, cap.* 1, brings in a story
out of Aristotle, of one Antipheron, which likely saw, wheresoever he was, his own image in the air, as in a glass.   Vitellio,
lib. 10 *Perspect.*, hath such another instance of a familiar
acquaintance of his, that after the want of three or four nights'
sleep, as he was riding by a river side, saw another riding with
him, and using all such gestures as he did, but when more
light appeared, it vanished.   Eremites and anachorites have
frequently such absurd visions, revelations by reason of much
fasting and bad diet; many are deceived by legerdemain, as Scot
hath well showed in his book of the Discovery of Witchcraft,

and Cardan, *Subtil.* 18. Suffites, perfumes, suffumigations, mixed candles, perspective glasses, and such natural causes, make men look as if they were dead, or with horse-heads, bull's horns, and such-like brutish shapes, the room full of snakes, adders, dark, light, green, red, of all colours, as you may perceive in Baptista Porta, Alexis, Albertus, and others; glow-worms, fire-drakes, meteors, *ignis fatuus*, which Plinius, *lib.* 2, *cap.* 37, calls Castor and Pollux, with many such that appear in moorish grounds, about churchyards, moist valleys, or where battles have been fought, the causes of which read in Goclenius, Velcurius, Finkius, etc. Such feats are often done, to frighten children with squibs, rotten wood, etc., to make folks look as if they were dead, *solito majores*,[1] bigger [than usual], lesser, fairer, fouler; *ut astantes sine capitibus videantur, aut toti igniti, aut forma dæmonum, accipe pilos canis nigri, etc.* [to make them appear headless, or on fire, or in the form of devils, take the hairs of a black dog, etc.], saith Albertus; and so 'tis ordinary to see strange uncouth sights by catoptrics; who knows not that if in a dark room the light be admitted at one only little hole, and a paper or glass put upon it, the sun shining will represent on the opposite wall all such objects as are illuminated by his rays? With concave and cylinder glasses, we may reflect any shape of men, devils, antics (as magicians most part do, to gull a silly spectator in a dark room), we will ourselves, and that hanging in the air, when 'tis nothing but such an horrible image as Agrippa demonstrates,[2] placed in another room. Roger Bacon of old is said to have represented his own image walking in the air by this art, though no such thing appear in his Perspectives. But most part it is in the brain that deceives them, although I may not deny but that oftentimes the devil deludes them, takes his opportunity to suggest, and represent vain objects to melancholy men, and such as are ill affected. To these you may add the knavish impostures of jugglers, exorcists, mass-priests, and mountebanks, of whom Roger Bacon speaks, etc., *de miraculis naturæ et artis*, [of the wonders of nature and art] *cap.* 1. They can counterfeit the voices of all birds and brute beasts almost, all tones and tunes of men, and speak within their throats, as if they spoke afar off, that they make their auditors believe they hear spirits, and are thence much astonished and affrighted with it.[3] Besides, those artificial devices to overhear their confessions, like that whispering place of Gloucester [4] with us, or like the duke's place at Mantua in Italy, where the sound is reverberated by a concave wall;

a reason of which Blancanus in his *Echometria* gives, and mathematically demonstrates.

So that the hearing is as frequently deluded as the sight, from the same causes almost, as he that hears bells will make them sound what he list. "As the fool thinketh, so the bell clinketh." Theophilus in Galen thought he heard music, from vapours which made his ears sound, etc. Some are deceived by echoes, some by roaring of waters, or concaves and reverberation of air in the ground, hollow places and walls. At Cadurcum, in Aquitaine, words and sentences are repeated by a strange echo to the full, or whatsoever you shall play upon a musical instrument, more distinctly and louder than they are spoken at first.[1] Some echoes repeat a thing spoken seven times, as at Olympus, in Macedonia, as Pliny relates, *lib*. 36, *cap*. 15; some twelve times, as at Charenton, a village near Paris, in France. At Delphi, in Greece, heretofore was a miraculous echo, and so in many other places. Cardan, *Subtil. lib*. 18, hath wonderful stories of such as have been deluded by these echoes. Blancanus the Jesuit, in his *Echometria*, hath variety of examples, and gives his reader full satisfaction of all such sounds by way of demonstration. At Barry, an isle in the Severn mouth, they seem to hear a smith's forge:[2] so at Lipari, and those sulphureous isles, and many such-like which Olaus speaks of in the continent of Scandia, and those northern countries. Cardan, *de rerum var. lib*. 15, *cap*. 84, mentioneth a woman that still supposed she heard the devil call her, and speaking to her; she was a painter's wife in Milan: and many such illusions and voices, which proceed most part from a corrupt imagination.

Whence it comes to pass that they prophesy, speak several languages, talk of astronomy, and other unknown sciences to them (of which they have been ever ignorant), I have in brief touched;[3] only this I will here add, that Arculanus,[4] Bodine, *lib*. 3, *cap*. 6, *Dæmon*., and some others, hold as a manifest token that such persons are possessed with the devil;[5] so doth Hercules de Saxonia,[6] and Apponensis, and fit only to be cured by a priest. But Guianerius,[7] Montaltus,[8] Pomponatius of Padua, and Lemnius, *lib*. 2, *cap*. 2, refer it wholly to the ill disposition of the humour,[9] and that out of the authority of Aristotle, *Prob*. 30, 1, because such symptoms are cured by purging; and as by the striking of a flint fire is enforced, so, by the vehement motion of spirits, they do *elicere voces inauditas*, compel strange speeches to be spoken: another argument he hath from Plato's *reminiscentia* [recollection], which is all out as likely as that which Marsilius Ficinus speaks of his friend Pierleonus;[1] by a divine kind of infusion he understood the secrets of nature, and tenents of Grecian and barbarian philosophers, before ever he heard of, saw, or read their works: but in this I should rather hold with Avicenna and his associates, that such symptoms proceed from evil spirits, which take all opportunities of humours decayed, or otherwise, to pervert the soul of man: and besides, the humour itself is *balneum diaboli*, the devil's bath, and, as Agrippa proves, doth entice him to seize upon them.

SECT. IV. MEMB. I.

Prognostics of Melancholy

PROGNOSTICS, or signs of things to come, are either good or bad. If this malady be not hereditary, and taken at the beginning, there is good hope of cure, *recens curationem non habet difficilem*, saith Avicenna, *lib.* 3, *fen.* 1, *tract.* 4, *cap.* 18. That which is with laughter, of all others is most secure, gentle, and remiss (Hercules de Saxonia). "If that evacuation of hemrods, or *varices*, which they call the water between the skin, shall happen to a melancholy man, his misery is ended"[2] (Hippocrates, *Aphor.* 6, 11). Galen, *lib.* 6, *de morbis vulgar. com.* 8, confirms the same; and to this aphorism of Hippocrates all the Arabians, new and old Latins subscribe: Montaltus, *cap.* 25, Hercules de Saxonia, Mercurialis, Victorius Faventinus, etc. . Sckenkius, *lib.* 1 *Observat. med. cap. de mania*, illustrates this aphorism with an example of one Daniel Federer, a coppersmith, that was long melancholy, and in the end mad about the twenty-seventh year of his age; these *varices* or water began to arise in his thighs, and he was freed from his madness. Marius the Roman was so cured, some say, though with great pain. Sckenkius hath some other instances of women that have been helped by flowing of their months, which before were stopped. That the opening of the hemrods will do as much for men, all physicians jointly signify. so they be voluntary, some say, and not by compulsion. All melancholy are better after a quartan; Jobertus saith,[3] scarce any man hath that ague twice; but whether it free him from this malady, 'tis a question;

I—P 886

for many physicians ascribe all long agues for especial causes, and a quartan ague amongst the rest. Rhasis, *Cont. lib.* 1, *tract.* 9: "When melancholy gets out at the superficies of the skin, or settles, breaking out in scabs, leprosy, morphew, or is purged by stools, or by the urine, or that the spleen is enlarged, and those *varices* appear, the disease is dissolved." [1] Guianerius, *cap.* 5, *tract.* 15, adds dropsy, jaundice, dysentery, leprosy, as good signs, to these scabs, morphews, and breaking out, and proves it out of the sixth of Hippocrates' Aphorisms.

Evil prognostics on the other part. *Inveterata melancholia incurabilis,* if it be inveterate, it is incurable,[2] a common axiom, *aut difficulter curabilis,* [or], as they say that make the best, hardly cured. This Galen witnesseth, *lib.* 3 *de loc. affect. cap.* 6: "Be it in whom it will, or from what cause soever, it is ever long, wayward, tedious, and hard to be cured, if once it be habituated." [3] As Lucian said of the gout, she was "the queen of diseases, and inexorable," [4] may we say of melancholy. Yet Paracelsus will have all diseases whatsoever curable, and laughs at them which think otherwise, as T. Erastus, *part.* 3, objects to him; although in another place, hereditary diseases he accounts incurable, and by no art to be removed.[5] Hildesheim, *Spicil.* 2 *de mel.,* holds it less dangerous if only "imagination be hurt, and not reason;[6] the gentlest is from blood, worse from choler adust, but the worst of all from melancholy putrefied." [7] Bruel esteems hypochondriacal least dangerous, and the other two species (opposite to Galen) hardest to be cured.[8] The cure is hard in man, but much more difficult in women.[9] And both men and women must take notice of that saying of Montanus, *consil.* 230, *pro Abbate Italo:* "This malady doth commonly accompany them to their grave; physicians may ease, and it may lie hid for a time, but they cannot quite cure it, but it will return again more violent and sharp than at first, and that upon every small occasion or error": [10] as in Mercury's weather-beaten statue, that was once all over gilt, the open parts were clean, yet there was *in fimbriis aurum,* in the chinks a remnant of gold: there will be some relics of melancholy left in the purest bodies (if once tainted), not so easily to be rooted out. Oftentimes it degenerates into epilepsy, apoplexy, convulsions, and blindness;[11] by the authority of Hippocrates and Galen, all aver,[12] if once it possess the ventricles of the brain, Frambesarius, and Sallust. Salvianus adds, if it get into the optic nerves, blindness. Mercurialis, *consil.* 20, had a woman to his patient, that from melancholy became

epileptic and blind.   If it come from a cold cause, or so continue cold, or increase, epilepsy, convulsions follow, and blindness, or else in the end they are moped, sottish, and in all their
actions, speeches, gestures ridiculous.[1]   If it come from a
hot cause, they are more furious and boisterous, and in conclusion mad.[2]   *Calescentem melancholiam sæpius sequitur mania.*
If it heat and increase, that is the common event,[3] *per circuitus,*
aut semper, insanit,[4] he is mad by fits, or altogether.   For, as
Sennertus contends out of Crato,[5] there is *seminarius ignis* in
this humour, the very seeds of fire.   If it come from melancholy
natural adust, and in excess, they are often demoniacal
(Montanus).

Seldom this malady procures death, except (which is the
greatest, most grievous calamity, and the misery of all miseries)
they make away themselves,[6] which is a frequent thing, and
familiar amongst them.   'Tis Hippocrates' observation,[7] Galen's
sentence, *Etsi mortem timent, tamen plerumque sibi ipsis mortem*
consciscunt [although they fear death, yet many of them commit
suicide], *lib. 3 de locis affect. cap. 7,* the doom of all physicians.
'Tis Rabbi Moses' aphorism,[8] the prognosticon of Avicenna,
Rhasis, Aetius, Gordonius, Valescus, Altomarus, Sallustius
Salvianus, Capivaccius, Mercatus, Hercules de Saxonia, Piso,
Bruel, Fuchsius, all, etc.

> *Et sæpe usque adeo mortis formidine vitæ*
> *Percipit infelix odium lucisque videndæ,*
> *Ut sibi consciscat mærenti pectore letum.*[9]

> And so far forth death's terror doth affright,
> He makes away himself, and hates the light:
> To make an end of fear and grief of heart,
> He voluntary dies to ease his smart.

In such sort doth the torture and extremity of his misery
torment him, that he can take no pleasure in his life, but is in
a manner enforced to offer violence unto himself, to be freed
from his present insufferable pains. So some (saith Fracastorius[10])
"in fury, but most in despair, sorrow, fear, and out of the
anguish and vexation of their souls, offer violence to themselves: for their life is unhappy and miserable.   They can take
no rest in the night, nor sleep, or if they do slumber, fearful
dreams astonish them."   In the day-time they are affrighted
still by some terrible object, and torn in pieces with suspicion,
fear, sorrow, discontents, cares, shame, anguish, etc., as so many
wild horses, that they cannot be quiet an hour, a minute of time,
but even against their wills they are intent, and still thinking

of it, they cannot forget it, it grinds their souls day and night, they are perpetually tormented, a burden to themselves, as Job was, they can neither eat, drink, nor sleep. Ps. cvii, 18: "Their soul abhorreth all meat, and they are brought to death's door," "being bound in misery and iron";[1] they curse their stars with Job, "and day of their birth,[2] and wish for death"[3] for, as Pineda and most interpreters hold, Job was even melancholy to despair, and almost madness itself;[4] they murmur many times against the world, friends, allies, all mankind, even against God Himself in the bitterness of their passion, *vivere nolunt, mori nesciunt*,[5] live they will not, die they cannot. And in the midst of these squalid, ugly, and such irksome days, they seek at last, finding no comfort, no remedy in this wretched life, to be eased of all by death.[6] *Omnia appetunt bonum*, all creatures seek the best, and for their good as they hope, *sub specie*, in show at least, *vel quia mori pulchrum putant* (saith Hippocrates[7]) *vel quia putant inde se majoribus malis liberari* [either because they count it best to die or because they think in this way to be freed from greater evils], to be freed as they wish. Though many times, as Æsop's fishes, they leap from the frying-pan into the fire itself, yet they hope to be eased by his means: and therefore (saith Felix Platerus[8]) "after many tedious days, at last, either by drowning, hanging, or some such fearful end, they precipitate or make away themselves; many lamentable examples are daily seen amongst us:" *alius ante fores se laqueo suspendit* (as Seneca notes), *alius se præcipitavit a tecto, ne dominum stomachantem audiret, alius ne reduceretur a fuga ferrum redegit in viscera* [one hanged himself before his own door; another threw himself from the house-top, to avoid his master's anger; a third, to escape return from exile, plunged a dagger into his heart], so many causes there are—*His amor exitio est, furor his*—love, grief, anger, madness, and shame, etc. 'Tis a common calamity, a fatal end to this disease,[9] they are condemned to a violent death by a jury of physicians, furiously disposed, carried headlong by their tyrannizing wills, enforced by miseries, and there remains no more to such persons, if that heavenly Physician, by His assisting grace and mercy alone, do not prevent (for no human persuasion or art can help), but to be their own butchers, and execute themselves. Socrates his *cicuta* [hemlock], Lucretia's dagger, Timon's halter, are yet to be had; Cato's knife and Nero's sword are left behind them, as so many fatal engines, bequeathed to posterity, and will be used to the world's end by such distressed souls: so intolerable, insufferable, grievous, and violent is their pain, so unspeakable and continuate.[1] One day of grief is an hundred years, as Cardan observes: 'tis *carnificina hominum* [a man-killer], *angor animi*, as well saith Aretæus, a plague of the soul, the cramp and convulsion of the soul, an epitome of hell; and if there be a hell upon earth, it is to be found in a melancholy man's heart.

> For that deep torture may be call'd an hell,
> When more is felt than one hath power to tell.

Yea, that which scoffing Lucian said of the gout in jest, I may truly affirm of melancholy in earnest.

> *O triste nomen ! o diis odibile!*
> *Melancholia lacrimosa,*[2] *Cocyti filia,*
> *Tu Tartari specubus opacis edita*
> *Erinnys, utero quam Megæra suo tulit,*
> *Et ab uberibus aluit, cuique parvulæ*
> *Amarulentum in os lac Alecto dedit,*
> *Omnes abominabilem te dæmones*
> *Produxere in lucem, exitio mortalium.*

Et paulo post.
> *Non Jupiter ferit tale telum fulminis,*
> *Non ulla sic procella sævit æquoris,*
> *Non impetuosi tanta vis est turbinis.*
> *An asperos sustineo morsus Cerberi ?*
> *Num virus echidnæ membra mea depascitur ?*
> *Aut tunica sanie tincta Nessi sanguinis ?*
> *Illacrimabile et immedicabile malum hoc.*

> O sad and odious name! a name so fell,
> Is this of melancholy, brat of hell.
> There born in hellish darkness doth it dwell.
> The Furies brought it up, Megæra's teat,
> Alecto gave it bitter milk to eat.
> And all conspired a bane to mortal men,
> To bring this devil out of that black den. . . . .
> Jupiter's thunderbolt, not storm at sea,
> Nor whirlwind doth our hearts so much dismay.
> What? am I bit by that fierce Cerberus?
> Or stung by serpent[3] so pestiferous?
> Or put on shirt that 's dipt in Nessus' blood?
> My pain 's past cure; physic can do no good.

No torture of body like unto it, *Siculi non invenere tyranni majus tormentum* [the Sicilian tyrants invented no worse torture], no strappadoes, hot irons, Phalaris' bulls,

> *Nec ira deum tantum, nec tela, nec hostis,*
> *Quantum sola noces animis illapsa.*[4]

> Jove's wrath, nor devils can
> Do so much harm to th' soul of man.

All fears, griefs, suspicions, discontents, imbonities, insuavities
are swallowed up and drowned in this Euripus, this Irish Sea,
this ocean of misery, as so many small brooks; 'tis *coagulum
omnium ærumnarum* [a banding together of all griefs], which
Ammianus [1] applied to his distressed Palladius.   I say of our
melancholy man, he is the cream of human adversity, the
quintessence,[2] and upshot; all other diseases whatsoever are
but flea-bitings to melancholy in extent: 'tis the pith of them all.

> *Hospitium est calamitatis; quid verbis opus est ?*
> *Quamcunque malam rem quæris, illic reperies :* [3]
>
> What need more words? 'tis calamity's inn,
> Where seek for any mischief, 'tis within;

and a melancholy man is that true Prometheus, which is bound
to Caucasus; the true Tityus, whose bowels are still by a vulture
devoured (as poets feign), for so doth Lilius Giraldus interpret
it,[4] of anxieties and those griping cares, and so ought it to be
understood.   In all other maladies we seek for help; if a leg or
an arm ache, through any distemperature or wound, or that
we have an ordinary disease, above all things whatsoever we
desire help and health, a present recovery, if by any means
possible it may be procured; we will freely part with all our
other fortunes, substance, endure any misery, drink bitter
potions, swallow those distasteful pills, suffer our joints to be
seared, to be cut off, anything for future health: so sweet, so
dear, so precious above all other things in this world is life;
'tis that we chiefly desire, long life and happy days, *Multos da,
Jupiter, annos*,[5] increase of years all men wish; but to a melancholy man, nothing so tedious, nothing so odious; that which
they so carefully seek to preserve he abhors, he alone;[6] so
intolerable are his pains.   Some make a question, *graviores
morbi corporis an animi*, whether the diseases of the body or
mind be more grievous, but there is no comparison, no doubt
to be made of it, *multo enim sævior longeque est atrocior animi,
quam corporis cruciatus* (Lemnius, *lib. 1, cap. 12*), the diseases
of the mind are far more grievous.   *Totum hic pro vulnere
corpus*, body and soul is misaffected here, but the soul especially.
So Cardan testifies, *de rerum var. lib. 8, 40.*   Maximus Tyrius,
a Platonist, and Plutarch [7] have made just volumes to prove it.
Dies adimit ægritudinem hominibus [8] [time cures men's sorrows];
in other diseases there is some hope likely, but these unhappy
men are born to misery, past all hope of recovery, incurably

sick, the longer they live the worse they are, and death alone must ease them.

Another doubt is made by some philosophers, whether it be lawful for a man, in such extremity of pain and grief, to make away himself: and how these men that so do are to be censured. The Platonists approve of it, that it is lawful in such cases, and upon a necessity (Plotinus, *lib. de beatitud. cap.* 7), and Socrates himself defends it in Plato's *Phædo*: "If any man labour of an incurable disease, he may dispatch himself, it it be to his good." Epicurus and his followers, the Cynics and Stoics in general affirm it, Epictetus and Seneca [1] amongst the rest, *quamcunque veram esse viam ad libertatem*, any way is allowable that leads to liberty; "Let us give God thanks, that no man is compelled to live against his will"; [2] *Quid ad hominem claustra, carcer, custodia? liberum ostium habet* [3] [What need a man care about bars or prison? The way of escape is at hand], death is always ready and at hand. *Vides illum præcipitem locum, illud flumen?* dost thou see that steep place, that river, that pit, that tree? there's liberty at hand, *effugia servitutis et doloris sunt* [there are ways of escape from servitude and pain], as that Laconian lad cast himself headlong (*non serviam, aiebat puer* [I will not be a slave, said the boy]) to be freed of his misery: every vein in thy body, if these be *nimis operosi exitus* [too troublesome means of egress], will set thee free; *quid tua refert finem facias an accipias?* [what matters whether you make or await your end?] there's no necessity for a man to live in misery. *Malum est in necessitate vivere; sed in necessitate vivere, necessitas nulla est* ['tis evil to live in need; but there is no need to live in need]. *Ignavus qui sine causa moritur, et stultus qui cum dolore vivit* [he is a coward who kills himself for nothing, and a fool who lives on in pain] (*idem, Epist.* 58). Wherefore hath our mother the earth brought out poisons, saith Pliny,[4] in so great a quantity, but that men in distress might make away themselves? which kings of old had ever in a readiness, *ad incerta fortunæ venenum sub custode promptum* [had poison ready to hand in case of emergency], Livy writes, and executioners always at hand. Speusippus being sick was met by Diogenes, and, carried on his slaves' shoulders, he made his moan to the philosopher; "But I pity thee not," quoth Diogenes, "*qui cum talis vivere sustines* [since being in such plight thou endurest to live]; thou mayst be freed when thou wilt," meaning by death. Seneca therefore [5] commends Cato, Dido, and Lucretia, for their generous courage in so doing, and others that voluntarily die, to avoid a greater mischief, to free themselves from misery, to save their honour, or vindicate their good name, as Cleopatra did, as Sophonisba, Syphax' wife, did, Hannibal did, as Junius Brutus, as Vibius Virius, and those Campanian senators in Livy (*Dec.* 3, *lib.* 6), to escape the Roman tyranny that poisoned themselves. Themistocles drank bull's blood, rather than he would fight against his country, and Demosthenes chose rather to drink poison, Publius *Crassi filius* [the son of Crassus], Censorius, and Plancus, those heroical Romans, to make away themselves, than to fall into their enemies' hands. How many myriads besides in all ages might I remember, *qui sibi letum Insontes peperere manu* [who though innocent committed suicide], etc. Razis in the Maccabees is magnified for it,[1] Samson's death approved. So did Saul and Jonas sin, and many worthy men and women, *quorum memoria celebratur in Ecclesia* [whose memory is celebrated in the Church], saith Leminchus,[2] for killing themselves to save their chastity and honour, when Rome was taken, as Austin instances, *lib.* 1 *de Civit. Dei, cap.* 16. Jerome vindicateth the same, *in Jonam*, and Ambrose, *lib.* 3 *de virginitate*, commendeth Pelagia for so doing. Eusebius, *lib.* 8, *cap.* 15, admires a Roman matron for the same fact to save herself from the lust of Maxentius the tyrant. Adelhelmus, Abbot of Malmesbury, calls them *beatas virgines quæ sic* [blessed virgins who], etc. Titus Pomponius Atticus, that wise, discreet, renowned Roman senator, Tully's dear friend, when he had been long sick, as he supposed of an incurable disease, *vitamque produceret ad augendos dolores, sine spe salutis* [by prolonging his life only increased his pain, without hope of cure], was resolved voluntarily by famine to dispatch himself to be rid of his pain; and whenas Agrippa and the rest of his weeping friends earnestly besought him, *osculantes obsecrarent, ne id quod natura cogeret ipse acceleraret*, not to offer violence to himself, "with a settled resolution he desired again they would approve of his good intent, and not seek to dehort him from it"; and so constantly died, *precesque eorum taciturna sua obstinatione depressit* [and silenced their prayers by his determined attitude]. Even so did Corellius Rufus, another grave senator, by the relation of Plinius Secundus, *Epist. lib.* 1, *epist.* 12, famish himself to death; *pedibus correptus cum incredibiles cruciatus et indignissima tormenta pateretur, a cibis omnino abstinuit* [being terribly tortured by the gout, he entirely abstained from food]; neither he nor Hispulla his wife could divert him, but *destinatus mori obstinate magis*, etc., die he would, and die he did. So did Lycurgus. Aristotle, Zeno, Chrysippus, Empedocles, with myriads, etc. In wars, for a man to run rashly upon imminent danger and present death is accounted valour and magnanimity, to be the cause of his own, and many a thousand's ruin besides, to commit wilful murder in a manner, of himself and others, is a glorious thing, and he shall be crowned for it.[1] The Massagetæ [2] in former times, Derbiccians,[3] and I know not what nations besides, did stifle their old men after seventy years, to free them from those grievances incident to that age. So did the inhabitants of the island of Choa; because their air was pure and good, and the people generally long-lived, *antevertebant fatum suum, priusquam manci forent, aut imbecillitas accederet, papavere vel cicuta*, with poppy or hemlock, [before they became infirm or imbecile], they prevented death. Sir Thomas More in his *Utopia* commends voluntary death, if he be *sibi aut aliis molestus*, troublesome to himself or others "(especially if to live be a torment to him), let him free himself with his own hands from this tedious life, as from a prison, or suffer himself to be freed by others." [4] And 'tis the same tenent which Laertius related of Zeno of old, *Juste sapiens sibi mortem consciscit, si in acerbis doloribus versetur, membrorun mutilatione aut morbis ægre curandis* [the wise man rightly commits suicide if through accident or disease he suffers acute pain], and which Plato, 9 *de legibus*, approves, if old age, poverty, ignominy, etc. oppress, and which Fabius expresseth in effect (*Præfat.* 7 *Institut.*), *nemo nisi sua culpa diu dolet* [5] [if any one suffers pain long, it is his own fault]. It is an ordinary thing in China (saith Mat. Riccius the Jesuit), "if they be in despair of better fortunes, or tired and tortured with misery, to bereave themselves of life, and many times, to spite their enemies the more, to hang at their door." [6] Tacitus the historian, Plutarch the philosopher, much approve a voluntary departure, and Austin, *de Civ. Dei, lib.* 1, *cap.* 29, defends a violent death, so that it be undertaken in a good cause: *Nemo sic mortuus, qui non fuerat aliquando moriturus; quid autem interest, quo mortis genere vita ista finiatur, quando ille cui finitur iterum mori non cogitur?* [No one dies in this way who would not have had to die at some time or other. What difference then does it make by what kind of death life is finished, seeing that he whose life is finished has not to die again?], etc. No man so voluntarily dies, but *volens nolens*, he must die at last, and our life is subject to innumerable casualties, who knows when they may happen? *utrum satius est unam perpeti moriendo, an omnes timere vivendo?*

I—*p 886

rather suffer one [death] than fear all.[1]   "Death is better than
a bitter life" (Eccl. xxx, 17), and a harder choice to live in fear
than by once dying to be freed from all.[2]   Cleombrotus Ambraciotes persuaded I know not how many hundreds of his
auditors, by a luculent oration he made of the miseries of this,
and happiness of that other life, to precipitate themselves; and,
having read Plato's divine tract *de anima*, for example's sake
led the way first.   That neat epigram of Callimachus will tell
you as much:

> *Jamque vale soli cum diceret Ambraciotes,*
>   *In Stygios fertur desiluisse lacus,*
> *Morte nihil dignum passus: sed forte Platonis*
> .   *Divini eximium de nece legit opus.*

> [To daylight having bid his last farewell,
>   The Ambraciot plunged into the Stygian hole,
> Although no crime or sorrow did compel—
>   He simply had read Plato on the Soul.]

Calenus and his Indians hated of old to die a natural death:[3]
the Circumcellions and Donatists, loathing life, compelled others
to make them away, with many such:[4] but these are false and
pagan positions, profane Stoical paradoxes, wicked examples;
it boots not what heathen philosophers determine in this kind,
they are impious, abominable, and upon a wrong ground.
"No evil is to be done that good may come of it"; *reclamat
Christus, reclamat Scriptura* [Christ and Scripture cry out against
it], God and all good men are against it.[5]   He that stabs another
can kill his body; but he that stabs himself kills his own soul.
*Male meretur, qui dat mendico quod edat; nam et illud quod dat,
perit; et illi producit vitam ad· miseriam:*[6] he that gives a beggar
an alms (as that comical poet said) doth ill, because he doth but
prolong his miseries.   But Lactantius, *lib. 6, cap. 7, de vero
cultu*, calls it a detestable opinion, and fully confutes it, *lib. 3
de sap. cap.* 18, and St. Austin, *Ep. 52 ad Macedonïum, cap.* 61,
ad Dulcitium Tribunum; so doth Hierome to Marcella of Blæsilla's
death, *Non recipio tales animas*, etc., he calls such men *martyres
stultæ philosophiæ* [the victims of a stupid philosophy]; so doth
Cyprian, *de duplici martyrio : Si qui sic moriantur, aut infirmitas,
aut ambitio, aut dementia cogit eos* [those who so die are driven
to it by illness or ambition or madness]; 'tis mere madness so
to do, *furor est ne moriare mori*[7] ['tis mad for fear of death to
kill oneself].   To this effect writes Arist., 3 *Ethic.*, Lipsius,
Manuduc. ad Stoicam philosophiam, lib. 3, *dissertat.* 23, but it

needs no confutation. This only let me add, that in some cases those hard censures of such as offer violence to their own persons,[1] or in some desperate fit to others, which sometimes they do, by stabbing, slashing, etc., are to be mitigated, as in such as are mad, beside themselves for the time, or found to have been long melancholy, and that in extremity; they know not what they do, deprived of reason, judgment, all, as a ship that is void of a pilot must needs impinge upon the next rock or sands, and suffer shipwreck.[2] P. Forestus [3] hath a story of two melancholy brethren that made away themselves, and for so foul a fact were accordingly censured to be infamously buried, as in such cases they use, to terrify others, as it did the Milesian virgins of old; but upon farther examination of their misery and madness, the censure was revoked,[4] and they were solemnly interred, as Saul was by David (2 Sam. ii, 4); and Seneca well adviseth, *Irascere interfectori, sed miserere interfecti:* be justly offended with him as he was a murderer, but pity him now as a dead man. Thus of their goods and bodies we can dispose; but what shall become of their souls, God alone can tell; His mercy may come *inter pontem et fontem, inter gladium et jugulum,* betwixt the bridge and the brook, the knife and the throat. *Quod cuiquam contigit, cuivis potest* [what happens to someone may happen to any one]. Who knows how he may be tempted? It is his case, it may be thine: *Quæ sua sors hodie est, cras fore vestra potest.*[5] We ought not to be so rash and rigorous in our censures as some are; charity will judge and hope the best; God be merciful unto us all!

NOTES

PAGE 3

[1] Hæc comice dicta cave ne male capias.

PAGE 7

[1] These verses refer to the frontispiece, which is divided into ten compartments that are here severally explained.

PAGE 15

[1] Seneca, in ludo in mortem Claudii Cæsaris.
[2] Lib. de Curiositate.
[3] Modo hæc tibi usui sint, quemvis auctorem fingito.—Wecker.
[4] Lib. 10, cap. 12. Multa a male feriatis in Democriti nomine commenta data, nobilitatis auctoritatisque ejus perfugio utentibus.
[5] Martialis, lib. 10, epigr. 4.

PAGE 16

[1] Juv. Sat. 1.
[2] Auth. Pet. Besseo, edit. Coloniæ, 1616.
[3] Hip. Epist. Damaget.   [4] Laert. lib. 9.
[5] Hortulo sibi cellulam seligens, ibique, seipsum includens, vixit solitarius.
[6] Floruit Olympiade 80; 700 annis post Troiam.
[7] Diacos. quod cunctis operibus facile excellit.—Laert.
[8] Col. lib. 1, cap. 1.   [9] Const. lib. de agric. passim.
[10] Volucrum voces et linguas intelligere se dicit Abderitani.—Ep. Hip.
[11] Sabellicus, Exempl. lib. 10. Oculis se privavit, ut melius contemplationi operam daret, sublimi vir ingenio, profundæ cogitationis, etc.
[12] Naturalia, moralia, mathematica, liberales disciplinas, artiumque omnium peritiam callebat.
[13] Veni Athenas, et nemo me novit.
[14] Idem contemptui et admirationi habitus.
[15] Solebat ad portam ambulare, et inde, etc.—Hip. Ep. Damag.
[16] Perpetuo risu pulmonem agitare solebat Democritus.—Juv., Sat. 10.

PAGE 17

[1] Non sum dignus præstare matellam.—Mart.
[2] Christ Church in Oxford.   [3] Præfat. Hist.
[4] Keeper of our college library, lately revived by Otho Nicolson, Esq.
[5] Scaliger.   [6] In Theæt.
[7] Phil. Stoic. li. diff. 8. Dogma cupidis et curiosis ingeniis imprimendum, ut sit talis qui nulli rei serviat, aut exacte unum aliquid elaboret, alia negligens, ut artifices, etc.
[8] Delibare gratum de quocunque cibo, et pittisare de quocunque dolio jucundum.
[9] Essays, lib. 3.   [10] Præfat. Bibliothec.

Page 18

[1] Ambo fortes et fortunati, Mars idem magisterii dominus juxta primam Leovitii regulam.

[2] Heinsius Primerio.

[3] Calide †ambientes, sollicite litigantes, aut misere excidentes, voces, strepitum, contentiones, etc.

[4] Cyp. ad Donat. Unice securus, ne excidam in foro, aut in mari Indico bonis eluam, de dote filiæ, patrimonio filii non sum sollicitus.

Page 19

[1] Hor.   [2] Per.   [3] Hor.

[4] Secundum mœnia locus erat frondosis populis opacus, vitibusque sponte natis, tenuis prope aqua defluebat, placide murmurans, ubi sedile et domus Democriti conspiciebatur.

[5] Ipse composite considebat, super genua volumen habens, et utrinque alia patentia parata, dissectaque animalia cumulatim strata, quorum viscera rimabatur.

Page 20

[1] Cum mundus extra se sit, et mente captus sit, et nesciat se languere, ut medelam adhibeat.

[2] Scaliger, Ep. ad Patissonem. Nihil magis lectorem invitat quam inopinatum argumentum, neque vendibilior merx est quam petulans liber.

[3] Lib. 20, cap. 11. Miras sequuntur inscriptionum festivitates.

[4] Præfat. Nat. Hist. Patri obstetricem parturienti filiæ accersenti moram injicere possunt.

[5] Anatomy of Popery, Anatomy of Immortality, Angelus Salas' Anatomy of Antimony, etc.

[6] Cont. lib. 4, cap. 9. Non est cura melior quam labor.

Page 21

[1] Hor. de Arte Poet.

[2] Non quod de novo quid addere, aut a veteribus prætermissum, sed propriæ exercitationis causa.

[3] Qui novit, neque id quod sentit exprimit, perinde est ac si nesciret.

[4] Jovius, Præf. Hist.   [5] Erasmus.

[6] Otium otio dolorem dolore sum solatus.   [7] Observat. lib. 1.

[8] Mr. Joh. Rouse, our Protobib. Oxon., Mr. Hopper, Mr. Guthridge, etc.

Page 22

[1] Quæ illi audire et legere solent, eorum partim vidi egomet, alia gessi, quæ illi literis, ego militando didici, nunc vos existimatê facta an dicta pluris sint.

[2] Dido Virg. [Taught by that Power that pities me, I learn to pity them.]

[3] Camden. Ipsa elephantiasi correpta elephantiasis hospitium construxit.

[4] Iliada post Homerum.   [5] [To bring twice-boiled cabbage to table.]

[6] Nihil prætermissum quod a quovis dici possit.   [7] Martialis.

[8] Magis impium mortuorum lucubrationes, quam vestes furari.

[9] [Many are possessed with an incurable itch for writing.]

[10] Eccles. ult.

[11] Libros eunuchi gignunt, steriles pariunt.

[12] D. King, præfat. lect. Jonas, the late Right Reverend Lord B. of London.

[13] Homines famelici gloriæ ad ostentationem eruditionis undique congerunt.—Buchananus.

[14] Effascinati etiam laudis amore, etc.—Justus Baronius.

[15] Ex ruinis alienæ existimationis sibi gradum ad famam struunt.

Page 23

[1] Exercit. 288.

[2] Omnes sibi famam quærunt et quovis modo in orbem spargi contendunt, ut novæ alicujus rei habeantur auctores.—Præf. Biblioth.

[3] Præfat. Hist.   [4] Plautus.   [Three-letter men (*f u r* = thief).]

[5] E Democriti puteo.   [6] Non tam refertæ bibliothecæ quam cloacæ.

[7] Et quicquid chartis amicitur ineptis.

[8] Epist. ad Patiss.   In regno Franciæ omnibus scribendi datur libertas, paucis facultas.

[9] Olim literæ ob homines in pretio, nunc sordent ob homines.

[10] Aus. Pacat.

[11] Inter tot mille volumina vix unus a cujus lectione quis melior evadat, immo potius non pejor.

Page 24

[1] Palingenius.

[2] Lib. 5 de sap.

[3] Sterile oportet esse ingenium quod in hoc scripturientum pruritu, etc.

[4] Cardan, præf. ad Consol.   [5] Hor. lib. 1, Sat. 4.

[6] Epist. lib. 1.   Magnum poetarum proventum annus hic attulit, mense Aprili nullus fere dies quo non aliquis recitavit.

[7] Idem.

[8] Principibus et doctoribus deliberandum relinquo, ut arguantur auctorum furta et millies repetita tollantur, et temere scribendi libido coerceatur, aliter in infinitum progressura.

[9] Onerabuntur ingenia, nemo legendis sufficit.

[10] Libris obruimur, oculi legendo, manus volutando dolent.—Fam. Strada, Momo.

Page 25

[1] Quicquid ubique bene dictum facio meum, et illud nunc meis ad compendium, nunc ad fidem et auctoritatem alienis exprimo verbis, omnes auctores meos clientes esse arbitror, etc.—Sarisburiensis ad Polycrat. prol.

[2] In Epitaph. Nep.   Illud Cyp. hoc Lact. illud Hilar. est, ita Victorinus, in hunc modum locutus est Arnobius, etc.

[3] Præf. ad Syntax. med.

[4] In Luc. 10, tom. 2.   Pigmæi gigantum humeris impositi plusquam ipsi gigantoo vident.

Page 26

[1] Nec aranearum textus ideo melior quia ex se fila gignuntur, nec noster ideo vilior, quia ex alienis libamus ut apes.—Lipsius adversus dialogist.

[2] Uno absurdo dato mille sequuntur.

[3] Non dubito multos lectores hic fore stultos.   [4] Martial, 13, 2.

Page 27

[1] Ut venatores feram e vestigio impresso, virum scriptiuncula.—Lips.

[2] Hor.   [3] Hor.   [4] Antwerp, fol. 1607.

[5] Muretus.   [6] Lipsius.

Page 28

[1] Hor.

[2] Fieri non potest, ut quod quisque cogitat, dicat unus.—Muretus.

[3] Lib. 1 de ord. cap. 11.   [4] Erasmus.

[5] Annal. tom. 3, ad annum 360.   Est porcus ille qui sacerdotem ex amplitudine redituum sordide demetitur.

[6] Erasm. Dial.

[7] Epist. lib. 6.   Cujusque ingenium non statim emergit, nisi materiæ fautor, occasio, commendatorque contingat.   [8] Præf. Hist.

PAGE 29

[1] Laudari a laudato laus est.   [2] Vit. Persii.   ["Which Probus" = what Probus said.]
[3] Minuit præsentia famam.   [4] Lipsius, Judic. de Seneca.
[5] Lib. 10. Plurimum studii, multam rerum cognitionem, omnem studiorum materiam, etc.; multa in eo probanda, multa admiranda.
[6] Suet. Arena sine calce.   [7] Introduct. ad Sen.
[8] Judic. de Sen. Vix aliquis tam absolutus, ut alteri per omnia satisfaciat, nisi longa temporis præscriptio, semota judicandi libertate, religione quadam animos occuparit.

PAGE 30

[1] Hor. Ep. lib. 1, 19.
[2] Æque turpe frigide laudari ac insectanter vituperari. Favorinus, A. Gel. lib. 19, cap. 2.
[3] Ovid. Trist. 1, eleg. 7.   [4] Juven. Sat. 9.
[5] Aut artis inscii aut quæstui magis quam literis student. Hab. Cantab. et Lond. excus. 1576.
[6] Ovid. de Pont. Eleg. 1, 5.

PAGE 31

[1] Hor.
[2] Tom. 3, Philopseud. Accepto pessulo, quum carmen quoddam dixisset, effecit ut ambularet, aquam hauriret, urnam pararet, etc.
[3] Eusebius, Eccles. Hist. lib. 6.
[4] Stans pede in uno [standing on one foot] as he [Lucilius] made verses.
[5] Virg.   [6] Non eadem a summo expectes, minimoque poeta.
[7] Stilus hic nullus, præter parrhesiam.

PAGE 32

[1] Qui rebus se exercet, verba negligit, et qui callet artem dicendi, nullam disciplinam habet recognitam.
[2] Palingenius.
[3] Cujuscunque orationem vides politam et sollicitam, scito animum in pusillis occupatum, in scriptis nil solidum.—Epist. lib. 1, 21.
[4] Philostratus, lib. 8, vit. Apol. Negligebat oratoriam facultatem, et penitus aspernabatur ejus professores, quod linguam duntaxat, non autem mentem redderent eruditiorem.
[5] Hic enim, quod Seneca de Ponto, bos herbam, ciconia lacertum, canis leporem, virgo florem legat.
[6] Pet. Nannius, not. in Hor.

PAGE 33

[1] Non hic colonus domicilium habeo, sed topiarii in morem, hinc inde florem vellico, ut canis Nilum lambens.
[2] Supra bis mille notabiles errores Laurentii demonstravi, etc.
[3] Philo de Con.   [4] Virg.

PAGE 34

[1] Frambesarius, Sennertus, Ferrandus, etc.   [2] Ter. Adelph.
[3] Heaut. Act. 1, sc. 1.   [4] Gellius, lib. 18, cap. 3.

PAGE 35

[1] Et inde catena quædam fit, quæ hæredes etiam ligat.—Cardan. Heinsius.
[2] Malle se bellum cum magno principe gerere, quam cum uno ex fratrum mendicantium ordine.
[3] Hor. Epod. lib. od. 7.   [4] Epist. 86, ad Casulam presb.
[5] Lib. 12, cap. 1. Mutos nasci, et omni scientia egere satius fuisset, quam sic in propriam perniciem insanire.

PAGE 36

[1] Infelix mortalitas! inutilibus quæstionibus ac disceptationibus vitam traducimus, naturæ principes thesauros, in quibus gravissimæ morborum medicinæ collocatæ sunt, interim intactos relinquimus. Nec ipsi solum relinquimus, sed et alios prohibemus, impedimus, condemnamus, ludibriisque afficimus.

[2] [Let the shoemaker stick to his last.]

[3] Quod in praxi minime fortunatus esset, medicinam reliquit, et ordinibus initiatus in theologia postmodum scripsit.—Gesner, Bibliotheca.

[4] P. Jovius.

[5] Mr. W. Burton, Preface to his Description of Leicestershire, printed at London by W. Jaggard for J. White, 1622.

PAGE 37

[1] In Hygiasticon. Neque enim hæc tractatio aliena videri debet a theologo, etc., agitur de morbo animæ.

[2] Dr. Clayton in comitiis, anno 1621.   [3] Hor.

[4] In Newark in Nottinghamshire. Cum duo edificasset castella, ad tollendam structionis invidiam, et expiandam maculam, duo instituit cœnobia, et collegis religiosis implevit.

PAGE 38

[1] Ferdinando de Quiros, anno 1612 Amstelodami impress.

[2] Præfat. ad Characteres. Spero enim (O Polycles) libros nostros meliores inde futuros, quod istiusmodi memoriæ mandata reliquerimus, ex preceptis et exemplis nostris ad vitam accommodatis, ut se inde corrigant.

[3] Part. 1, sect. 3.   [4] Præf. lectori.

PAGE 39

[1] Ep. 2, lib. 2, ad Donatum. Paulisper te crede subduci in ardui montis verticem celsiorem, speculare inde rerum jacentium facies, et oculis in diversa porrectis, fluctuantis mundi turbines intuere, jam simul aut ridebis aut misereberis, etc.

[2] Controv. lib. 2, cont. 7, and lib. 6, cont.   [3] Horatius.

[4] Idem Hor. lib. 2, Satira 3. Damasippus Stoicus probat omnes stultos insanire.

PAGE 40

[1] Tom. 2, Sympos. lib. 5, cap. 6. Animi affectiones, si diutius inhæreant, pravos generant habitus.

[2] Lib. 28, cap. 1, Synt. art. mir. Morbus nihil est aliud quam dissolutio quædam ac perturbatio fœderis in corpore existentis, sicut et sanitas est consentientis bene corporis consummatio quædam.

[3] Lib. 9 Geogr. Plures olim gentes navigabant illuc sanitatis causa.

[4] Eccles. ii, 26.

PAGE 41

[1] [Isaiah.]

[2] Jure hæreditario sapere jubentur.—Euphormio Satyr.

[3] Apud quos virtus, insania et furor esse dicitur.

[4] Calcagninus, Apol. Omnes mirabantur, putantes illisam iri stultitiam. Sed præter expectationem res evenit. Audax stultitia in eam irruit, etc., illa cedit irrisa, et plures hinc habet sectatores stultitia.

[5] Non est respondendum stulto secundum stultitiam.

[6] 2 Reg. vii.   [7] Lib. 10, ep. 97.   [8] Aug. Ep. 178.

PAGE 42

[1] Quis nisi mentis inops, etc.

[2] Quid insanius quam pro momentanea felicitate æternis te mancipare suppliciis?

[3] In fine Phædonis. Hic finis fuit amici nostri, o Echecrates, nostro quidem judicio omnium quos experti sumus optimi et apprime sapientissimi, et justissimi.

[4] Xenoph. lib. 4 de dictis Socratis, ad finem. Talis fuit Socrates, quem omnium optimum et felicissimum statuam.

[5] Lib. 25 Platonis Convivio.

PAGE 43

[1] Lucretius.   [2] Anaxagoras olim mens dictus ab antiquis.

[3] Regula naturæ, naturæ miraculum, ipsa eruditio dæmonium hominis, sol scientiarum, mare, sophia, antistes literarum et sapientiæ, ut Scioppius olim de Scal.; et Heinsius: Aquila in nubibus, Imperator literatorum, columen literarum, abyssus eruditionis, ocellus Europæ, Scaliger.

[4] Lib. 3 de sap. cap. 17 et 20. Omnes philosophi aut stulti aut insani; nulla anus, nullus æger ineptius deliravit.

[5] Democritus, a Leucippo doctus, hæreditatem stultitiæ reliquit Epicuro.

[6] Hor. Car. lib. 1, od. 34, in Epicur.

[7] Nihil interest inter hos et bestias nisi quod loquantur.—De sap. lib. 26, cap. 8.

[8] Cap. de virt.

PAGE 44

[1] Neb. et Ranis.

[2] Omnium disciplinarum ignarus.

[3] Pulchorum adolescentum causa frequenter gymnasium obibat, etc.

[4] Seneca. Scis rotunda metiri, sed non tuum animum.

[5] Ab uberibus sapientia lactati cæcutire non possunt.

[6] Cor Zenodoti et jecur Cratetis.

PAGE 45

[1] Lib. de nat. boni.

[2] Hic profundissimæ Sophiæ fodinæ.

[3] Panegyr. Trajano. Omnes actiones exprobrare stultitiam videntur.

[4] Ser. 4, in domi Pal. Mundus qui ob antiquitatem deberet esse sapiens, semper stultizat, et nullis flagellis alteratur, sed ut puer vult rosis et floribus coronari.

[5] [Apuleius was regarded as the hero as well as the author of the Golden Ass.]

[6] Insanum te omnes pueri, clamantque puellæ.—Hor.

[7] Plautus, Aulular.

PAGE 46

[1] Adelph. Act. 5, sc. 8.   [2] Tully, Tusc. 5.

[3] Plato, Apologia Socratis.   [4] Ant. Dial.

[5] Lib. 3 de sap. Pauci ut video sanæ mentis sunt.

[6] Stulte et incaute omnia agi video.

[7] Insania non omnibus eadem (Erasm. chil. 3, cent. 10). Nemo mortalium qui non aliqua in re desipit, licet alius alio morbo laboret, hic libidinis, ille avaritiæ, ambitionis, invidiæ.

[8] Hor. lib. 2, sat. 3.

[9] Lib. 1 de Aulico. Est in unoquoque nostrum seminarium aliquod stultitiæ, quod si quando excitetur, in infinitum facile excrescit.

PAGE 47

[1] Primaque lux vitæ prima erroris erat.

[2] Tibullus. Stulti prætereunt dies, their wits are a-woolgathering. So fools commonly dote.

[3] Dial. Contemplantes, tom. 2.   [4] Catullus.

Page 48

[1] Sub ramosa platano sedentem, solum, discalceatum, super lapidem, valde pallidum ac macilentum, promissa barba, librum super genibus habentem.

[2] De furore, mania, melancholia scribo, ut sciam quo pacto in hominibus gignatur, fiat, crescat, cumuletur, minuatur; hæc, inquit, animalia quæ vides propterea seco, non Dei opera perosus, sed fellis bilisque naturam disquirens.

[3] Aust. lib. 1 in Gen. Jumenti et servi tui obsequium rigide postulas, et tu nullum præstas aliis, nec ipsi Deo.

[4] Uxores ducunt, mox foras ejiciunt.   [5] Pueros amant, mox fastidiunt.

[6] Quid hoc ab insania deest?   [7] Reges eligunt, deponunt.

Page 49

[1] Contra parentes, frates, cives perpetuo rixantur, et inimicitias agunt.

[2] Credo equidem vivos ducent e marmore vultus.

[3] Idola inanimata amant, animata odio habent; sic pontificii.

[4] Suam stultitiam perspicit nemo, sed alter alterum deridet.

Page 50

[1] Denique sit finis quærendi, cumque habeas plus, Pauperiem metuas minus, et finire laborem Incipias, partis quod avebas, utere.—Hor.

[2] Astutam vapido servat sub pectore vulpem. Et cum vulpe positus pariter vulpinaricr. Cretizandum cum Crete.

[3] Qui fit, Mæcenas, ut nemo quam sibi sortem, Seu ratio dederit, seu sors objecerit, illa Contentus vivat, etc.—Hor.

[4] Diruit, ædificat, mutat quadrata rotundis. Trajanus pontem struxit super Danubium, quem successor ejus Adrianus statim demolitus.

[5] Qua quid in re ab infantibus differunt, quibus mens et sensus sine ratione inest, quicquid sese his offert volupe est? [Plut.]

Page 51

[1] Idem Plut.

[2] Ut insaniæ causam disquiram bruta macto et seco, cum hoc potius in hominibus investigandum esset.

[3] 'Totus a nativitate morbus est.

[4] In vigore furibundus, quum decrescit insanabilis.

[5] Cyprian. ad Donatum. Qui sedet crimina judicaturus, etc.

[6] Tu pessimus omnium latro es, as a thief told Alexander in Curtius. Damnat foras judex, quod intus operatur.—Cyprian.

[7] Vultus magna cura, magna animi incuria.—Am. Marcel.

[8] Horrenda res est, vix duo verba sine mendacio proferuntur: et quamvis solenniter homines ad veritatem dicendam invitentur, pejerare tamen non dubitant, ut ex decem testibus vix unus verum dicat.—Calv. in viii John, serm. 1.

[9] Sapientiam insaniam esse dicunt.

Page 52

[1] Siquidem sapientiæ suæ admiratione me complevit, offendi sapientissimum virum, qui salvos potest omnes homines reddere.

[2] E Græc. epig.

[3] Plures Democriti nunc non sufficiunt, opus Democrito qui Democritum rideat.—Eras. Moria.

[4] Polycrat. lib. 3, cap. 8, e Petron.

[5] Ubi omnes delirabant, omnes insani, etc.; hodie nauta, cras philosophus; hodie faber, cras pharmacopola; hic modo regem agebat multo satellitio, tiara, et sceptro ornatus, nunc vili amictus centiculo, asinum clitellarium impellit.

[6] Calcagninus, Apol. Chrysalus e cæteris auro dives, manicato peplo et tiara conspicuus, levis alioquin et nullius consilii, etc. Magno fastu ingredienti assurgunt dii, etc.

PAGE 53

[1] Sed hominis levitatem Jupiter perspiciens, At tu (inquit) esto bombilio, etc., protinusque vestis illa manicata in alas versa est, et mortales inde Chrysalides vocant hujusmodi homines.

[2] [Provinces of Moronia, or Foolsland, in Joseph Hall's Mundus Alter et Idem.]

[3] Hor.   [4] Juven.

[5] De bello Jud. l. 8, cap. 11. Iniquitates vestræ neminem latent, inque dies singulos certamen habetis quis pejor sit.

[6] Hor.   [7] Lib. 5, epist. 8.   [8] Hor.

PAGE 54

[1] Superstitio est insanus error.   [2] Lib. 8 Hist. Belg.

[3] Lucan.

[4] Father Angelo, the Duke of Joyeux, going barefoot over the Alps to Rome, etc.

[5] Si cui intueri vacet quæ patiuntur superstitiosi, invenies tam indecora honestis, tam indigna liberis, tam dissimilia sanis, ut nemo fuerit dubitaturus furere eos, si cum paucioribus furerent.—Senec.

[6] Quid dicam de eorum indulgentiis, oblationibus, votis, solutionibus, jejuniis, cœnobiis, somniis, horis, organis, cantilenis, campanis, simulacris, missis, purgatoriis, mitris, breviariis, bullis, lustralibus, aquis, rasuris, unctionibus, candelis, calicibus, crucibus, mappis, cereis, thuribulis, incantationibus, exorcismis, sputis, legendis, etc.—Baleus, de actis Rom. Pont.

[7] Th. Naogeor.

PAGE 55

[1] Dum simulant spernere, acquisiverunt sibi 30 annorum spatio bis centena millia librarum annua.—Arnold.

[2] Et quum interdiu de virtute locuti sunt, sero in latibulis clunes agitant labore nocturno.—Agrippa.

[3] 1 Tim. iii, 13. But they shall prevail no longer, their madness shall be known to all men.

[4] Benignitatis sinus solebat esse, nunc litium officina curia Romana.—Budæus.

[5] Quid tibi videtur facturus Democritus, si horum spectator contigisset?

PAGE 56

[1] Ob inanes ditionum titulos, ob præreptum locum, ob interceptam mulierculam, vel quod e stultitia natum, vel e malitia, quod cupido dominandi, libido nocendi, etc.

[2] Bellum rem plane belluinam vocat Morus, Utop. lib. 2.

[3] Munster, Cosmog. lib. 5, cap. 3, e Dict. Cretens.

[4] Jovius, vit. ejus.   [5] Comineus.   [6] Lib. 3.

PAGE 57

[1] Hist. of the Siege of Ostend, fol. 23.

[2] Erasmus de bello. Ut placidum illud animal benevolentiæ natum tam ferina vecordia in mutuam rueret perniciem.

[3] Rich. Dinoth. præfat. Belli civilis Gal.   [4] Jovius.

[5] Dolus, asperitas, injustitia propria bellorum negotia.—Tertul.

[6] Tully.   [7] Lucan.

[8] Pater in filium, affinis in affinem, amicus in amicum, etc. Regio cum regione, regnum regno colliditur. Populus populo in mutuam perniciem, belluarum instar sanguinolente ruentium.

Page 58

[1] Libanii Declam.

[2] Ira enim et furor Bellonæ consultores, etc., dementes sacerdotes sunt.

[3] Bellum quasi bellua et ad omnia scelera furor immissus.

[4] Gallorum decies centum millia ceciderunt. Ecclesiarum 20 millia fundamentis excisa.

[5] Belli civilis Gal. lib. 1. Hoc ferali bello et cædibus omnia repleverunt, et regnum amplissimum a fundamentis pene everterunt, plebis tot myriades gladio, bello, fame miserabiliter perierunt. [6] Pont. Heuterus.

[7] Comineus. Ut nullus non execretur et admiretur crudelitatem, et barbaram insaniam, quæ inter homines eodem sub cœlo natos, ejusdem linguæ, sanguinis, religionis, exercebatur.

[8] Lucan. [9] Virg. [10] Bishop of Cusco, an eye-witness.

Page 59

[1] Read Meteran of his stupend cruelties.

[2] Heinsius Austriaco. [3] Virg. Georg.

[4] Jansenius Gallobelgicus, 1596. Mundus furiosus, inscriptio libri.

[5] Exercitat. 250, serm. 4. [6] Fleat Heraclitus an rideat Democritus?

[7] Curæ leves loquuntur, ingentes stupent.

[8] Arma amens capio, nec sat rationis in armis. [9] Erasmus.

[10] Pro Murena. Omnes urbanæ res, omnia studia, omnis forensis laus et industria latet in tutela et præsidio bellicæ virtutis, et simul atque increpuit suspicio tumultus, artes illico nostræ conticescunt.

[11] Ser. 13.

[12] Eobanus Hessus. Quibus omnis in armis Vita placet, non ulla juvat nisi morte, nec ullam Esse putant vitam, quæ non assueverit armis.

Page 60

[1] Crudelissimos sævissimosque latrones, fortissimos haberi propugnatores, fidissimos duces habent, bruta persuasione donati.

[2] Lib 10 vit. Scanderbeg.

[3] De benef. lib. 2, cap. 16. [4] Nat. quæst. lib. 3.

[5] Nulli beatiores habiti, quam qui in prœliis cecidissent.—Brisonius, de rep. Persarum, lib. 3, fol. 3, 44. Idem Lactantius de Romanis et Græcis. Idem Ammianus, lib. 23, de Parthis. Judicatur is solus beatus apud eos, qui in prœlio fuderit animam.

Page 61

[1] Boterus, Amphitridion. Busbequius, Turc. Hist. Per cædes et sanguinem parare hominibus ascensum in cœlum putant.—Lactan. de falsa relig. lib. 1, cap. 8.

[2] Quoniam bella acerbissima Dei flagella sunt quibus hominum pertinaciam punit, ea perpetua oblivione sepelienda potius quam memoriæ mandanda plerique judicant.—Rich. Dinoth, præf. Hist. Gall.

[3] Cruentam humani generis pestem, et perniciem divinitatis nota insigniunt.

[4] Et quod dolendum, applausum habent et occursum viri tales.

[5] Herculi eadem porta ad cœlum patuit, qui magnam generis humani partem perdidit.

[6] Virg. Æneid 7.

[7] Homicidium quum committunt singuli, crimen est, quum publice geritur, virtus vocatur.—Cyprianus.

[8] Seneca. [9] Juven.

[10] De vanit. scient., de princip. nobilitatis.

Page 62

[1] Juven. Sat. 4.
[2] Pansa rapit, quod Natta reliquit. Tu pessimus omnium latro es, as Demetrius the pirate told Alexander in Curtius.
[3] Non ausi mutire, etc.—Æsop.
[4] Improbum et stultum, si divitem, multos bonos viros in servitutem habentem, ob id duntaxat quod ei contingat aureorum numismatum cumulus, ut appendices et additamenta numismatum.—Morus, Utopia.
[5] Eorumque detestantur Utopienses insaniam, qui divinos honores iis impendunt, quos sordidos et avaros agnoscunt; non alio respectu honorantes, quam quod dites sint.—Idem, lib. 2.

Page 63

[1] Cyp. 2 ad Donat. ep. Ut reus innocens pereat, fit nocens. Judex damnat foras, quod intus operatur.
[2] Sidonius, Apo. [3] Salvianus, lib. 3, de providen.
[4] Ergo judicium nihil est nisi publica merces.—Petronius. Quid faciant leges ubi sola pecunia regnat?—Idem.
[5] Hic arcentur hæreditatibus liberi, hic donatur bonis alienis, falsum consulit, alter testamentum corrumpit, etc.—Idem.
[6] Vexat censura columbas. [7] Plaut. Mostel.
[8] Idem. [9] Juven. Sat. 4.
[10] Quod tot sint fures et mendici, magistratuum culpa fit, qui malos imitantur præceptores, qui discipulos libentius verberant quam docent.—Morus, Utop. lib. 1.

Page 64

[1] Decernuntur furi gravia et horrenda supplicia, quum potius providendum multo foret ne fures sint, ne cuiquam tam dira furandi aut pereundi sit necessitas.—Idem.
[2] Boterus de augment. urb. lib. 3, cap. 3.
[3] E fraterno corde sanguinem eliciunt.
[4] [Go it, Socrates! go it, Xanthippe!]
[5] Milvus rapit ac deglubit. [6] Petronius de Crotone civit.
[7] Quid forum? locus quo alius alium circumvenit.
[8] Vastum chaos, larvarum emporium, theatrum hypocrisios, etc.
[9] Nemo cœlum, nemo jusjurandum, nemo Jovem pluris facit, sed omnes apertis oculis bona sua computant.—Petron.

Page 65

[1] Plutarch. vit. ejus. Indecorum animatis ut calceis uti aut vitris, quæ ubi fracta abjicimus, nam, ut de meipso dicam, nec bovem senem vendiderim, nedum hominem natu grandem laboris socium.
[2] Jovius. Cum innumera illius beneficia rependere non posset aliter, interfici jussit.
[3] Beneficia eo usque læta sunt, dum videntur solvi posse, ubi multum antevenere pro gratia odium redditur.—Tac.
[4] Paucis carior est fides quam pecunia.—Sallust.
[5] Prima fere vota et cunctis, etc.
[6] Et genus et formam regina pecunia donat. Quantum quisque sua nummorum servat in arca, Tantum habet et fidei.
[7] Non a peritia sed ab ornatu et vulgi vocibus habemur excellentes.—Cardan, lib. 2 de cons.
[8] Perjurata suo postponit numina lucro Mercator. Ut necessarium sit vel Deo displicere, vel ab hominibus contemni, vexari, negligi.
[9] Qui Curios simulant et Bacchanalia vivunt.
[10] Tragelapho similes vel centauris, sursum homines, deorsum equi.

PAGE 66

[1] Præceptis suis cœlum promittunt, ipsi interim pulveris terreni vilia mancipia.

[2] Æneas Sylv.

[3] Arridere homines ut sæviant, blandiri ut fallant.—Cyp. ad Donatum.

[4] Love and hate are like the two ends of a perspective glass, the one multiplies, the other makes less.

[5] Ministri locupletiores iis quibus ministratur, servus majores opes habens quam patronus.

[6] Qui terram colunt equi paleis pascuntur, qui otiantur caballi avena saginantur, discalceatus discurrit qui calces aliis facit.

[7] Juven.   [8] Bodine, lib. 4 de repub. cap. 6.

[9] Plinius, lib. 37, cap. 3. Capillos habuit succineos, exinde factum ut omnes puellæ Romanæ colorem illum affectarent.

[10] Odit damnatos.—Juv.

PAGE 67

[1] Agrippa, Ep. 28, lib. 7. Quorum cerebrum est in ventre, ingenium in patinis.

[2] Psal. [liii, 4]. They eat up my people as bread.

[3] Absumit hæres Cæcuba dignior Servata centum clavibus, et mero Tinguet pavimentis superbo, Pontificum potiore cœnis.—Hor.

[4] Qui Thaidem pingere, inflare tibiam, crispare crines.

[5] Doctus spectare lacunar.

[6] Tullius. Est enim proprium stultitiæ aliorum cernere vitia, oblivisci suorum. Idem Aristippus Charidemo apud Lucianum. Omnino stultitiæ cujusdam esse puto, etc.

[7] Execrari publice quod occulte agat. Salvianus, lib. de prov. Acres ulciscendis vitiis quibus ipsi vehementer indulgent.

PAGE 68

[1] Adamus, Eccl. Hist. cap. 212. Siquis damnatus fuerit, lætus esse gloria est; nam lacrimas et planctum cæteraque compunctionum genera quæ nos salubria censemus, ita abominantur Dani, ut nec pro peccatis nec pro defunctis amicis ulli flere liceat.

[2] Orbi dat leges foras, vix famulum regit sine strepitu domi.

[3] Quicquid ego volo hoc vult mater mea, et quod mater vult, facit pater.

[4] Oves, olim mite pecus, nunc tam indomitum et edax ut homines devorent, etc.—Morus, Utop. lib. 1.

[5] Diversos variis tribuit natura furores.

[6] Democrit. Ep. præd. Hos dejerantes et potantes deprehendet, hos vomentes, illos litigantes, insidias molientes, suffragantes, venena miscentes, in amicorum accusationem subscribentes, hos gloria, illos ambitione, cupiditate, mente captos, etc.

[7] Ad Donat. ep. 2, cap. 9. O si posses in specula sublimi constitutus, etc.

PAGE 69

[1] Lib. 1 de nup. Philol. In qua quid singuli nationum populi quotidianis motibus agitarent, relucebat.

[2] O Jupiter! contingat mihi aurum, hæreditas, etc. Multos da Jupiter annos! Dementia quanta est hominum, turpissima vota diis insusurrant, si quis admoverit aurem, conticescunt; et quod scire homines nolunt Deo narrant.—Senec. Ep. 10.

[3] Plautus, Menæch. Non potest hæc res hellebori jugere obtinerier.

[4] Eoque gravior morbus quo ignotior periclitanti.

[5] Quæ lædunt oculos, festinas demere; si quid Est animum, differs curandi tempus in annum.—Hor.

[6] Si caput, crus dolet, brachium, etc., medicum accersimus, recte et honeste, si par etiam industria in animi morbis poneretur.—Joh. Pelezius, Jesuita, lib. 2 de hum. affec. morborumque cura.

[7] Et quotusquisque tamen est qui contra tot pestes medicum requirat vel ægrotare se agnoscat? Ebullit ira, etc. Et nos tamen ægros esse negamus. Incolumes medicum recusant. Præsens ætas stultitiam priscis exprobrat.—Bud. de affec. lib. 5.

[8] Senes pro stultis habent juvenes.—Balth. Cast.

PAGE 70

[1] Clodius accusat mœchos.

[2] Omnium stultissimi qui auriculas studiose tegunt.—Sat. Menip.

[3] Hor. Epist. 2.   [4] Prosper.

[5] Statim sapiunt, statim sciunt, neminem reverentur, neminem imitantur, ipsi sibi exemplo.—Plin. Epist. lib. 8.

[6] Nulli alteri sapere concedit, ne desipere videatur.—Agrip.

[7] Omnis orbis percæcus a Persis ad Lusitaniam.   [8] Florid.

PAGE 71

[1] August. Qualis in oculis hominum qui inversis pedibus ambulat, talis in oculis sapientum et angelorum qui sibi placet, aut cui passiones dominantur.

[2] Plautus, Menæchmi.

[3] Governor of Africa by Cæsar's appointment.

[4] Nunc sanitatis patrocinium est insanientium turba.—Sen.

[5] Pro Roscio Amerino. Et quod inter omnes constat insanissimus, nisi inter eos, qui ipsi quoque insaniunt.

[6] Necesse est cum insanientibus furere, nisi solus relinqueris.—Petronius.

[7] Quoniam non est genus unum stultitiæ qua me insanire putas.

[8] Stultum me fateor, liceat concedere verum, Atque etiam insanum.—Hor.

[9] Odi, nec possum cupiens non esse quod odi.—Ovid. Errore grato libenter omnes insanimus.

PAGE 72

[1] Amator scortum vitæ præponit, iracundus vindictam, fur prædam, parasitus gulam, ambitiosus honores, avarus opes, etc., odimus hæc et accersimus.—Cardan. lib. 2 de consol.

[2] Prov. xxvi, 11.

[3] Plutarch. Gryllo. Suilli homines, sic Clem. Alex.

[4] Non persuadebis, etiamsi persuaseris.   [5] Tully.

[6] Malo cum illis insanire, quam cum aliis bene sentire.

[7] Qui inter hos enutriuntur, non magis sapere possunt, quam qui in culina bene olere.—Petron.

[8] Persius.   [9] Hor. Sat. 2.

[10] Vesanum exagitant pueri, innuptæque puellæ.   [11] Plautus.

PAGE 73

[1] Hor. Sat. 2, 3. Superbam stultitiam Plinius vocat, Epist. 7, 21, quod semel dixi, fixum ratumque sit.

[2] Multi sapientes proculdubio fuissent, si se non putassent ad sapientiæ summum pervenisse.

[3] Idem.   [4] Plutarchus, Solone. Detur sapientiori.

[5] Tam præsentibus plena est numinibus, ut facilius possis deum quam hominem invenire.

PAGE 74

[1] Pulchrum bis dicere non nocet.   [2] Malefactors.

[3] Who can find a faithful man?—Prov. xx, 6.

⁴ In Ps. xlix. Qui momentanea sempiternis, qui dilapidat heri absentis bona, mox in jus vocandus et damnandus.

⁵ Perquam ridiculum est homines ex animi sententia vivere, et quæ diis ingrata sunt exequi, et tamen a solis diis velle salvos heri, quum propriæ salutis curam abjecerint.—Theod. cap. 6, de provid. lib. de curat. Græc. affect.

⁶ Sapiens sibi qui imperiosus, etc.—Hor. Sat. 2, 7.

⁷ Conclus. lib. de vic. offer. Certum est animi morbis laborantes pro mortuis censendos.

⁸ Lib. de sap. Ubi timor adest, sapientia adesse nequit.

PAGE 75

¹ Quid insanius Xerxe Hellespontum verberante, etc.

² Eccles. xxi, 12. "Where is bitterness, there is no understanding." Prov. xii, 16. "An angry man is a fool."

³ 3 Tusc. Injuria in sapientem non cadit.

⁴ Hom. 6, in 2 Epist. ad Cor. Hominem te agnoscere nequeo, cum tanquam asinus recalcitres, lascivias ut taurus, hinnias ut equus post mulieres, ut ursus ventri indulgeas, quum rapias ut lupus, etc. At, inquis, formam hominis habeo. Id magis terret, quum feram humana specie videre me putem.

⁵ Epist. lib. 2, ep. 13. Stultus semper incipit vivere. Fœda hominum levitas, nova quotidie fundamenta vitæ ponere, novas spes, etc.

⁶ De curial. miser. Stultus, qui quærit quod nequit invenire, stultus qui quærit quod nocet inventum, stultus qui cum plures habet calles, deteriorem deligit. Mihi videntur omnes deliri, amentes, etc.

PAGE 76

¹ Ep. Damageto.

² Amicis nostris Rhodi dicito, ne nimium rideant, aut nimium tristes sint.

³ Per multum risum poteris cognoscere stultum.—Offic. 3, cap. 9.

⁴ Sapientes liberi, stulti servi, libertas est potestas, etc.

⁵ Hor. 2, ser. 7. ⁶ Juven.

⁷ [Charles the Wise (of France), Philip the Good (of Burgundy), Louis the Pious (St. Louis of France).]

PAGE 77

¹ Hypocrit. ² Ut mulier aulica nullius pudens.

³ Epist. 33. Quando fatuo delectari volo, non est longe quærendus, me video.

⁴ Primo Contradicentium. ⁵ Lib. de causis corrupt. artium.

⁶ Actione ad subtil. in Scal. fol. 1226. ⁷ Lib. 1 de sap.

⁸ Vide, miser homo, quia totum est vanitas, totum stultitia, totum dementia, quicquid facis in hoc mundo, præter hoc solum quod propter Deum facis.—Ser. de miser. hom.

⁹ In 2 Platonis dial. lib. de justo.

PAGE 78

¹ Dum iram et odium in Deo revera ponit. ² Virg. Ecl. 3.

³ Ps. Inebriabuntur ab ubertate domus. ⁴ In Ps. civ, Anstin.

⁵ In Platonis Tim. sacerdos Ægyptius. ⁶ Hor. Vulgus insanum.

⁷ Patet ea divisio probabilis, etc., ex Arist. Top. lib. 1, cap. 8. Rog. Bac. Epist. de secret. art. et nat., cap. 8. Non est judicium in vulgo.

⁸ [i.e. not a pin to choose between them. See Apperson's English Proverbs, p. 27.]

Page 79

[1] De occult. philosoph. lib. 1, cap. 25 et 19 ejusd. lib.; lib. 10, cap. 4.
[2] See Lipsius, Epist.
[3] De politia illustrium, lib. 1, cap. 4. Ut in humanis corporibus variæ accidunt mutationes corporis, animique, sic in republica, etc.
[4] Ubi reges philosophantur.—Plato. [5] Lib. de re rust.
[6] Vel publicam utilitatem: Salus publica suprema lex esto. Beata civitas non ubi pauci beati, sed tota civitas beata.—Plato, quinto de republica.

Page 80

[1] Mantua væ miseræ nimium vicina Cremonæ.
[2] Interdum a feris, ut olim Mauritania, etc.
[3] Deliciis Hispaniæ, anno 1604. Nemo malus, nemo pauper, optimus quisque atque ditissimus. Pie sancteque vivebant, summaque cum veneratione et timore, divino cultui, sacrisque rebus incumbebant.
[4] [Barcelona.] [5] Polit. lib. 5, cap. 3.

Page 81

[1] Boterus, Polit. lib. 1, cap. 1. Cum nempe princeps rerum gerendarum imperitus, segnis, oscitans, suique muneris immemor, aut fatuus est.
[2] Non viget respublica cujus caput infirmatur.—Sarisburiensis, cap. 22.
[3] See Dr. Fletcher's Relation, and Alexander Gaguinus' History.
[4] Abundans omni divitiarum affluentia, incolarum multitudine, splendore ac potentia.
[5] Not above two hundred miles in length, sixty in breadth, according to Adricomius.
[6] Romulus Amaseus.
[7] Sabellicus. Si quis incola vetus, non agnosceret, si quis peregrinus, ingemisceret.
[8] Polit. lib. 5, cap. 6. Crudelitas principum, impunitas scelerum, violatio legum, peculatus pecuniæ publicæ, etc.
[9] Epist.
[10] De increm. urb. cap. 20. Subditi miseri, rebelles, desperati, etc.
[11] R. Dallington, 1596, conclusio libri.

Page 82

[1] Boterus, lib. 9, cap. 4 Polit. Quo fit ut aut rebus desperatis exulent, aut conjuratione subditorum crudelissime tandem trucidentur.
[2] [Galeazzo Sforza, Duke of Milan.]
[3] Mutuis odiis et cædibus exhausti, etc.
[4] Lucra ex malis, sceleratisque causis. [5] Sallust.
[6] For most part we mistake the name of politicians, accounting such as read Machiavel and Tacitus great statesmen, that can dispute of political precepts, supplant and overthrow their adversaries, enrich themselves get honours, dissemble; but what is this to the *bene esse*, or preservation of a commonwealth?
[7] Imperium suapte sponte corruit.
[8] Apul. Prim. Flor. Ex innumerabilibus, pauci senatores genere nobiles, e consularibus pauci boni, e bonis adhuc pauci eruditi.
[9] Non solum vitia concipiunt ipsi principes, sed etiam infundunt in civitatem, plusque exemplo quam peccato nocent.—Cic. de legibus.
[10] Epist. ad Zen. Juven. Sat. 4. Paupertas seditionem gignit et maleficium.—Arist. Pol. 2, 3, 7.

Page 83

[1] Sallust. Semper in civitate quibus opes nullæ sunt bonis invident, vetera odere, nova exoptant, odio suarum rerum mutari omnia petunt.

² De legibus. Profligatæ in repub. disciplinæ est indicium juris-peritorum numerus, et medicorum copia.

³ In præf. Stud. juris. Multiplicantur nunc in terris ut locustæ, non patriæ parentes, sed pestes, pessimi homines, majore ex parte superciliosi, contentiosi, etc., licitum latrocinium exercent.

⁴ Dousa, Epod. Loquutuleia turba, vultures togati.

⁵ Barc. Argen.

⁶ Jurisconsulti domus oraculum civitatis.—Tully.   ⁷ Lib. 3.

⁸ Lib. 1 de rep. Gallorum. Incredibilem reipub. perniciem afferunt.

PAGE 84

¹ Polycrat. lib.

² Is stipe contentus, at hi asses integros sibi multiplicari jubent.

³ Plus accipiunt tacere, quam nos loqui.

⁴ Totius injustitiæ nulla capitalior, quam eorum qui cum maxime decipiunt, id agunt, ut boni viri esse videantur.

⁵ Nam quocunque modo causa procedat, hoc semper agitur, ut loculi impleantur, etsi avaritia nequit satiari.

⁶ Camden, in Norfolk. Qui si nihil sit litium e juris apicibus lites tamen serere callent.

⁷ Plutarch, Vit. Cat. Causas apud inferos quas in suam fidem receperunt, patrocinio suo tuebuntur.

⁸ Lib. 2 de Helvet. repub. Non explicandis, sed moliendis contro-versiis operam dant, ita ut lites in multos annos extrahantur summa cum molestia utriusque partis et dum interea patrimonia exhauriantur.

PAGE 85

¹ Lupum auribus tenent.   ² Hor.

³ Lib. de Helvet. repub. Judices quocunque pago constituunt qui amica aliqua transactione si fieri possit, lites tollant. Ego majorum nostrorum simplicitatem admiror, qui sic causas gravissimas composuerint, etc.

⁴ Clenard. Ep. lib. 1. Si quæ controversiæ utraque pars judicem adit, is semel et simul rem transigit, audit: nec quid sit appellatio, lacrimosæque moræ noscunt.

⁵ Camden.

⁶ [Lacedæmonian cylinder: a secret letter written on a slip of papyrus and rolled round a cylinder.]

⁷ Lib. 10 Epist. ad Atticum, epist. 10.

⁸ Biblioth. lib. 3.   ⁹ Lib. de Anim.

¹⁰ Lib. major morb. corp. an animi. Hi non conveniunt ut diis more majorum sacra faciant, non ut Jovi primitias offerant, aut Baccho com-missationes, sed anniversarius morbus exasperans Asiam huc eos coegit, ut contentiones hic peragant.

PAGE 86

¹ 1 Cor. vi, 5, 6.

² Stulti, quando demum sapietis?—Ps. xciv, 8.

³ Of which text read two learned sermons, so intituled [i.e. "Christ's Counsel," etc.] and preached by our Regius Professor, Dr. Prideaux; printed at London by Felix Kingston, 1621.

⁴ Sæpius bona materia cessat sine artifice. Sabellicus de Germania: Si quis videret Germaniam urbibus hodie excultam, non diceret ut olim tristem cultu, asperam cœlo, terram informem.

⁵ By his Majesty's Attorney-General there.

PAGE 87

¹ As Zeipland, Bemster in Holland, etc.

² From Gaunt [Ghent] to Sluce [Sluys], from Bruges to the sea, etc.

[3] Ortelius, Boterus, Mercator, Meteranus, etc.

[4] Jam inde non minus belli gloria, quam humanitatis cultu inter florentissimas orbis Christiani gentes imprimis floruit.—Camden, Brit., de Normannis.

[5] Geog. Kecker.

[6] Tam hieme quam æstate intrepide sulcant Oceanum, et duo illorum duces non minore audacia quam fortuna totius orbem terræ circumnavigarunt.—Amphitheatro Boterus.

[7] A fertile soil, good air, etc. Tin, lead, wool, saffron, etc.

[8] Tota Britannia unica velut arx.—Boter.

PAGE 88

[1] Lib. 1 Hist.   [2] Increment. urb. lib. 1, cap. 9.

[3] Angliæ, excepto Londinio, nulla est civitas memorabilis, licet ea natio rerum omnium copia abundet.

[4] Cosmog. lib. 3, cap. 119. Villarum non est numerus, nullus locus otiosus aut incultus.

[5] Chytræus, Orat. edit. Francof. 1583.

[6] [Thuringia.]   [7] Maginus, Geog.

[8] Ortelius, e Vaseo et Pet. de Medina.

[9] ["Portugal between two rivers," i.e. the province of Entre-Douro-e-Minho, or Minho.]

[10] An hundred families in each.

PAGE 89

[1] Populi multitudo diligente cultura fecundat solum.—Boter. lib. 8, cap. 3.

[2] Orat. 35. Terra ubi oves stabulantur optima agricolis ob stercus.

[3] De re rust. lib. 2, cap. 1.

[4] Hodie urbibus desolatur, et magna ex parte incolis destituitur.—Gerbelius, Desc. Græciæ, lib. 6.

PAGE 90

[1] Videbit eas fere omnes aut eversas, aut solo æquatas, aut in rudera fœdissime dejectas.—Gerbelius.

[2] Lib. 7. Septuaginta olim legiones scriptæ dicuntur; quas vires hodie, etc.

[3] [Lucca and Siena.]   [4] Polit. lib. 3, cap. 8.

[5] For dyeing of cloths, and dressing, etc.

[6] Valer. lib. 2, cap. 1.   [7] [i.e. the first of that name.]

PAGE 91

[1] Hist. Scot. lib. 10. Magnis propositis præmiis, ut Scoti ab iis edocerentur.

[2] Munst. Cosm. lib. 5, cap. 74. Agro omnium rerum infecundissimo, aqua indigente, inter saxeta, urbs tamen elegantissima, ob Orientis negotiationes et Occidentis.

[3] Lib. 8 Geogr.: ob asperum situm.

[4] Lib. edit. a Nic. Tregant. Belg. anno 1616, Expedit. in Sinas.

PAGE 92

[1] Ubi nobiles probri loco habent artem aliquam profiteri.—Cleonard. Ep. lib. 1.

[2] Lib. 13 Belg. Hist. Non tam laboriosi ut Belgæ, sed ut Hispani otiatores vitam ut plurimum otiosam agentes: artes manuariæ quæ plurimum habent in se laboris et difficultatis, majoremque requirunt industriam, a peregrinis et exteris exercentur; habitant in piscosissimo mari, interea tantum non piscantur quantum insulæ suffecerit, sed a vicinis emere coguntur.

³ Grotii liber.

⁴ Urbs animis numeroque potens, et robore gentis.—Scaliger.

⁵ Camden.   ⁶ York, Bristow, Norwich, Worcester, etc.

⁷ Mr. Gainsford's argument, "Because gentlemen dwell with us in the country villages, our cities are less," is nothing to the purpose: put three hundred or four hundred villages in a shire, and every village yield a gentleman, what is four hundred families to increase one of our cities, or to contend with theirs, which stand thicker? And whereas ours usually consist of seven thousand, theirs consist of forty thousand inhabitants.

⁸ Maxima pars victus in carne consistit.—Polyd. lib. 1 Hist.

PAGE 93

¹ Refrænate monopolii licentiam, pauciores alantur otio, redintegretur agricolatio, lanificium instauretur, ut sit honestum negotium quo se exerceat otiosa illa turba. Nisi his malis medentur, frustra exercent justitiam.—Mor. Utop. lib. 1.

² Mancipiis locuples eget æris Cappadocum rex.—Hor.

³ Regis dignitatis non est exercere imperium in mendicos sed in opulentos. Non est regni decus, sed carceris esse custos.—Mor. Utop. lib. 1.

⁴ Colluvies hominum mirabiles excocti sole, immundi veste, fœdi visu, furti imprimis acres, etc.

⁶ Cosmog. lib. 3, cap. 5.

⁸ Seneca. Haud minus turpia principi multa supplicia, quam medico multa funera.

⁷ Ac pituitam et bilem a corpore (8 de Rep.) omnes vult exterminari.

⁸ See Lipsius, Admiranda.

⁹ De quo Suet. in Claudio, et Plinius, cap. 36.

¹⁰ [The Baths of Diocletian at Salona.]

¹¹ [Lago Fucino, or di Celano, drained in 1862.]

¹² Ut egestati simul et ignaviæ occurratur, opificia condiscantur, tenues subleventur.—Bodin. lib. 6, cap. 2, num. 6, 7.

¹³ Amasis Ægypti rex legem promulgavit, ut omnes subditi quotannis rationem redderent unde viverent.

¹⁴ Buscoldus, Discursu polit. cap. 2.

¹⁵ Lib. 1 de increm. urb. cap. 6.

¹⁶ Cap. 5 de increm. urb. Quas flumen, lacus, aut mare alluit.

PAGE 94

¹ Incredibilem commoditatem, vectura mercium tres fluvii navigabiles, etc.—Boterus de Gallia.

² Ind. Orient. cap. 2. Rotam in medio flumine constituunt, cui ex pellibus animalium consutos uteres appendunt, hi dum rota movetur, aquam per canales, etc.

³ Herodotus.   ⁴ Centum pedes lata fossa, 30 alta.

⁶ Contrary to that of Archimedes, who holds the superficies of all waters even.   ⁶ Lib. 1, cap. 3.

⁷ Dion, Pausanias, et Nic. Gerbelius. Munster, Cosm. lib. 4, cap. 36. Ut brevior foret navigatio et minus periculosa.

⁸ Charles the Great went about to make a channel from the Rhine to the Danube (Bil. Pirckheimerus, Descript. Ger. The ruins are yet seen about Weissenburg from Rednich to Altimul [from the Rednitz to the Altmühl]), ut navigabilia inter se Occidentis et Septentrionis littora fierent.

PAGE 95

¹ Maginus, Geogr. Simlerus, de rep. Helvet. lib. 1, describit.

² [The Douro.]   ³ Camden, in Lincolnshire. Fossdyke.

⁴ Near St. Albans.

NOTES

458

PAGE 96

[1] [Rosicrucians.]
[2] Lilius Giraldus, Nat. Comes.
[3] Apuleius, lib. 4 Flor. Lar familiaris inter homines ætatis suæ cultus est, litium omnium et jurgiorum inter propinquos arbiter et disceptator. Adversus iracundiam, invidiam, avaritiam, libidinem, ceteraque animi humani vitia et monstra philosophus iste Hercules fuit. Pestes eas mentibus exegit omnes, etc.   [4] Votis Navig.

PAGE 97

[1] [The Unknown Southern Land, i.e. Australia.]
[2] Ragguaglios, part. 2, cap. 2, et part. 3, cap. 17.
[3] Valent. Andreæ Apolog. manip. 604.
[4] Qui sordidus est, sordescat adhuc.   [5] Hor.

PAGE 98

[1] Ferdinando de Quiros, 1612.
[2] [The South Sea, Pacific Ocean.]
[3] Vide Acosta et Laiet.
[4] Vide Patricium, lib. 8, tit. 10, de Instit. Reipub.
[5] Sic olim Hippodamus Milesius, Arist. Polit. cap. 11, et Vitruvius, lib. 1, cap. ult.

PAGE 99

[1] With walls of earth, etc.
[2] De his Plin. epist. 42, lib. 2, et Tacit. Annal. lib. 15.
[3] Vide Brisonium de regno Pers. lib. 3, de his, et Vegetium, lib. 2, cap. 3, de Annona.
[4] Not to make gold, but for matters of physic.
[5] Brisonius; Josephus, lib. 21 Antiquit. Jud. cap. 6; Herod. lib. 3.
[6] So Lod. Vives thinks best, Comineus, and others.

PAGE 100

[1] Plato de leg. lib. 6. Ædiles creari vult, qui fora, fontes, vias, portus, plateas, et id genus alia procurent. Vide Isaacum Pontanum de civ. Amstel. (hæc omnia, etc.), Gotardum et alios.
[2] De increm. urb. cap. 13. Ingenue fateor me non intelligere cur ignobilius sit urbes bene munitas colere nunc quam olim, aut casæ rusticæ præesse quam urbi. Idem Ubertus Foliot, de Neapoli.
[3] Ne tantillum quidem soli incultum relinquitur, ut verum sit ne pollicem quidem agri in his regionibus sterilem aut infecundum reperiri. —Marcus Hemingius Augustanus de regno Chinæ, lib. 1, cap. 3.
[4] Mr. Carew, in his Survey of Cornwall, saith that before that country was enclosed, the husbandmen drank water, did eat little or no bread (fol. 66, lib. 1), their apparel was coarse, they went bare-legged, their dwelling was correspondent; but since enclosure they live decently, and have money to spend (fol. 23); when their fields were common, their wool was coarse, Cornish hair; but since enclosure, it is almost as good as Cotswold, and their soil much mended. Tusser, cap. 52 of his Husbandry, is of his opinion, one acre enclosed is worth three common: "The country enclosed I praise; The other delighteth not me, For nothing of wealth it doth raise," etc.
[5] Incredibilis navigiorum copia, nihilo pauciores in aquis, quam in continenti commorantur.—M. Riccius, Expedit. in Sinas, lib. 1, cap. 3.
[6] To this purpose Aristotle (Polit. 2, cap. 6) allows a third part of their revenues, Hippodamus half.
[7] Ita lex Agraria olim Romæ.

PAGE 101

[1] Lucanus, lib. 6.   [2] Virg. Georg. 1.
[3] Joh. Valent. Andreas.   [4] Lord Verulam.
[5] So is it in the kingdom of Naples and France.
[6] See Contarenus, and Osorius de rebus gestis Emanuelis.
[7] Claudian.

PAGE 102

[1] Herodotus, Erato, lib. 6. Cum Ægyptiis Lacedæmonii in hoc congruunt, quod eorum præcones, tibicines, coqui, et reliqui artifices, in paterno artificio succedunt, et coquus a coquo gignitur et paterno opere perseverat. Idem Marcus Polus de Quinzay. Idem Osorius de Emanuele rege Lusitano, Riccius de Sinis.
[2] Hippol. à Collibus de increm. urb. cap. 20. Plato, 8 de legibus. Quæ ad vitam necessaria, et quibus carere non possumus, nullum dependi vectigal, etc.
[3] Plato, 12 de legibus, 40 annos natos vult, ut si quid memorabile viderent apud exteros, hoc ipsum in rempub. recipiatur.
[4] Simlerus, in Helvetia.

PAGE 103

[1] Utopienses causidicos excludunt, qui causas callide et vafre tractent et disputent. Iniquissimum censent hominem ullis obligari legibus, quæ aut numerosiores sunt, quam ut perlegi queant, aut obscuriores quam ut a quovis possint intelligi. Volunt ut suam quisque causam agat, eamque referat judici quam narraturus fuerat patrono, sic minus erit ambagum, et veritas facilius elicietur.—Mor. Utop. lib. 2.
[2] Medici ex publico victum sumunt.—Boter. lib. 1, cap. 5, de Ægyptiis.
[3] De his lege Patricium, lib. 3, tit. 8, de reip. instit.
[4] Nihil a clientibus patroni accipiant, priusquam lis finita est.—Barcl. Argen. lib. 3.
[5] It is so in most free cities in Germany.
[6] Mat. Riccius, Exped. in Sinas, lib. 1, cap. 5, de examinatione electionum copiose agit, etc.
[7] Contar. de repub. Venet. lib. 1. [The reference is to the elaborate system of lot and ballot by which the doges were chosen.]
[8] Osor. lib. 11 de reb. gest. Eman. Qui in literis maximos progressus fecerint maximis honoribus afficiuntur, secundus honoris gradus militibus assignatur, postremi ordinis mechanicis. Doctorum hominum judiciis in altiorem locum quisque præfertur, et qui a plurimis approbatur, ampliores in rep. dignitates consequitur. Qui in hoc examine primas habet, insigni per totam vitam dignitate insignitur, marchioni similis, aut duci apud nos.
[9] Cedant arma togæ.
[10] As in Berne, Lucerne, Freiburg in Switzerland, a vicious liver is uncapable of any office; if a senator, instantly deposed.—Simlerus.
[11] Not above three years.—Arist. Polit. 5, cap. 8.
[12] Nam quis custodiet ipsos custodes?
[13] Chytræus, in Creisgeia. Qui non ex sublimi despiciant inferiores, nec ut bestias conculcent sibi subditos, auctoritatis nomini confisi, etc.

PAGE 104

[1] Sesellius de rep. Gallorum, lib. 1 et 2.
[2] Si quis egregium aut bello aut pace perfecerit.—Sesel. lib. 1.
[3] Ad regendam rempub. soli literati admittuntur, nec ad eam rem gratia magistratuum aut regis indigent, omnia explorata cujusque scientia et virtute pendent.—Riccius, lib. 1, cap. 5.
[4] In defuncti locum eum jussit subrogari, qui inter majores virtute reliquis præiret; non fuit apud mortales ullum excellentius certamen, aut

cujus victoria magis esset expetenda, non enim inter celeres celerrimo, non inter robustos robustissimo, etc.

[5] Nullum videres vel in hac vel in vicinis regionibus pauperem, nullum obæratum, etc.

[6] Nullus mendicus apud Sinas, nemini sano quamvis oculis turbatus sit, mendicare permittitur, omnes pro viribus laborare coguntur, cæci molis trusatilibus versandis addicuntur, soli hospitiis gaudent, qui ad labores sunt inepti. Osor. lib. 11 de reb. gest. Eman. Heming. de reg. Chin. lib. 1, cap. 3. Gotard. Arth. Orient. Ind. descr.

[7] Alex. ab Alex. 3, cap. 12.

[8] Sic olim Romæ. Isaac. Pontan. de his optime, Amstel. lib. 2, cap. 9.

[9] Idem Aristot. Pol. 5, cap. 8. Vitiosum quum soli pauperum liberi educantur ad labores, nobilium et divitum in voluptatibus et deliciis.

PAGE 105

[1] Quæ hæc injustitia ut nobilis quispiam, aut fænerator qui nihil agat, lautam et splendidam vitam agat, otio et deliciis, quum interim auriga, faber, agricola, quo respub. carere non potest, vitam adeo miseram ducat, ut pejor quam jumentorum sit ejus conditio? Iniqua resp. quæ dat parasitis, adulatoribus, inanium voluptatum artificibus generosis et otiosis tanta munera prodigit, at contra agricolis, carbonariis, aurigis, fabris, etc., nihil prospicit, sed eorum abusa labore florentis ætatis fame penset et ærumnis.—Mor. Utop. lib. 2.

[2] In Segovia nemo otiosus, nemo mendicus nisi per ætatem aut morbum opus facere non potest: nulli deest unde victum quærat, aut quo se exerceat. —Cypr. Echovius, Delic. Hispan. Nullus Genevæ otiosus, ne septennis puer.—Paulus Heutzner, Itiner.

[3] Athenæus, lib. 14. [4] Simlerus de repub. Helvet.

[5] [Horsed and flogged in the Amphitheatre.] Spartian. Olim Romæ sic.

[6] He that provides not for his family is worse than a thief.—Paul.

[7] Alfredi lex. Utraque manus et lingua præcidatur, nisi eam capite redemerit.

[8] Si quis nuptam stuprarit, virga virilis ei præcidatur; si mulier, nasus et auricula præcidantur.—Alfredi lex. En leges ipsi Veneri Martique timendas.

[9] Pauperes non peccant, quum extrema necessitate coacti rem alienam capiunt.—Maldonat. Summula, quæst. 8, art. 3. Ego cum illis sentio qui licere putant a divite clam accipere, qui tenetur pauperi subvenire.—Emmanuel Sa, Aphor. confess.

[10] Lib. 2 de reg. Persarum. [11] Lib. 23.

[12] Aliter Aristoteles, a man at twenty-five, a woman at twenty.—Polit.

[13] Lex olim Lycurgi, hodie Chinensium ; vide Plutarchum, Riccium, Hemingium, Arnisæum, Nevisanum, et alios de hac quæstione.

[14] Alfredus.

[15] Apud Lacones olim virgines sine dote nubebant.—Boter. lib. 3, cap. 3.

[16] Lege cautum non ita pridem apud Venetos, ne quis patricius dotem excederet 1500 coron.

[17] Bux. Synag. Jud. Sic Judæi. Leo Afer, Africæ descript. Ne sint aliter incontinentes ob reipub. bonum. Ut August. Cæsar orat. ad cælibes Romanos olim edocuit.

[18] Speciosissimi juvenes liberis dabunt operam.—Plato de Rep. lib. 5.

[19] Morbo laborans, qui in prolem facile diffunditur, ne genus humanum fœda contagione lædatur, juventute castratur, mulieres tales procul a consortio virorum ablegantur, etc.—Hector Boethius, Hist. lib. 1, de vet. Scotorum moribus.

[20] The Saxons exclude dumb, blind, leprous, and such-like persons from all inheritance, as we do fools.

[21] Ut olim Romani, Hispani hodie, etc.

[22] Riccius, lib. 11, cap. 5, de Sinarum expedit. Sic Hispani cogunt Mauros arma deponere. So it is in most Italian cities.

PAGE 106

[1] Idem Plato, 12 de legibus. It hath ever been immoderate, vide Guil. Stuckium, Antiq. convival. lib. 1, cap. 26.

[2] Plato, 6 de legibus.

[3] As those Lombards beyond seas, though with some reformation, mons pietatis, or bank of charity, as Malines terms it (cap. 33, Lex mercat. part. 2), that lend money upon easy pawns, or take money upon adventure for men's lives.

[4] That proportion will make merchandise increase, land dearer, and better improved, as he [Malines] hath judicially proved in his tract of usury, exhibited to the Parliament *anno* 1621.

[5] Hoc fere Zanchius, Com. in 4 cap. ad Ephes. Æquissimam vocat usuram et caritati Christianæ consentaneam, modo non exigant, etc., nec omnes dent ad fœnus, sed ii qui in pecuniis bona habent, et ob ætatem, sexum, artis alicujus ignorantiam, non possunt uti. Nec omnibus, sed mercatoribus et iis qui honeste impendent, etc.

[6] Idem apud Persas olim; lege Brisonium.

[7] Idem Plato de Rep.

PAGE 107

[1] Lib. 30. Optimum quidem fuerat eam patribus nostris mentem a diis datam esse, ut vos Italiæ, nos Africæ imperio contenti essemus. Neque enim Sicilia aut Sardinia satis digna pretia sunt pro tot classibus, etc.

[2] Claudian. [3] Thucydides.

[4] A depopulatione, agrorum incendiis, et ejusmodi factis immanibus.—Plato.

[5] Hungar. dec. 1, lib. 9.

[6] Sesellius, lib. 2 de repub. Gal. Valde enim est indecorum, ubi quod præter opinionem accidit dicere, Non putaram, presertim si res præcaveri potuerit. Livius, lib. 1. Dion, lib. 2. Diodorus Siculus, lib. 2.

[7] Peragit tranquilla potestas, Quod violenta nequit.—Claudian.

[8] Bellum nec timendum nec provocandum.—Plin. Panegyr. Trajano.

[9] Lib. 3 Poet. cap. 19. [10] Lib. 4 de repub. cap. 2.

[11] Peucer, lib. 1 de divinat. [12] Camden, in Cheshire.

PAGE 108

[1] Iliad 6.

[2] Vide Puteani Comum, Goclenium de portentosis cœnis nostrorum temporum.

[3] Mirabile dictu est, quantum opsoniorum una domus singulis diebus absumat; sternuntur mensæ in omnes pene horas calentibus semper eduliis. —Descrip. Britan.

[4] Lib. 1 de rep. Gallorum. Quod tot lites et causæ forenses, aliæ ferantur ex aliis, in immensum producantur, et magnos sumptus requirant, unde fit ut juris administri plerumque nobilium possessiones adquirant, tum quod sumptuose vivant, et a mercatoribus absorbentur et splendissime vestiantur, etc.

PAGE 109

[1] Ter. [2] Plaut. Captivi. [3] Paling. Filius aut fur.

[4] Catus cum mure, duo galli simul in æde, Et glotes binæ nunquam vivunt sine lite.

[5] Res angusta domi.

[6] When pride and beggary meet in a family, they roar and howl, and cause as many flashes of discontents as fire and water, when they concur, make thunderclaps in the skies.

[7] Plautus, Aulular.

I—Q 886

PAGE 110

[1] Lib. 7, cap. 6.
[2] Pellitur in bellis sapientia, vi geritur res. Vetus proverbium, aut regem aut fatuum nasci oportere.
[3] Lib. 5 Hist. Rom. Similes tot bacculorum calculis, secundum computantis arbitrium, modo ærei sunt, modo aurei; ad nutum regis nunc beati sunt, nunc miseri.
[4] Ærumnosique Solones in Sa, 3 de miser. curialium.

PAGE 111

[1] Hoc cognomento cohonestati Romæ, qui cæteros mortales sapientia præstarent. Testis Plin. lib. 7, cap. 34.
[2] J. Dousæ Epod. lib. 1, cap. 13.
[3] Insanire parant certa ratione modoque; mad by the book they, etc.
[4] Juvenal.   [5] Solomon.
[6] Communis irrisor stultitiæ.   [7] [Objections and solutions.]
[8] Wit, whither wilt?   [9] Scaliger, exercitat. 324.   [10] Vit. ejus.

PAGE 112

[1] Ennius.
[2] Lucian. Ter mille drachmis olim empta; studens inde sapientiam adipiscetur.
[3] Epist. 21, lib. 1. Non oportet orationem sapientis esse politam aut sollicitam.
[4] Lib. 3, cap. 13. Multo anhelitu jactatione furentes pectus, frontem cædentes, etc.
[5] Lipsius. Voces sunt, præterea nihil.
[6] Lib. 30. Plus mali facere videtur qui oratione quam qui pretio quemvis corrumpit: nam, etc.
[7] In Gorg. Platonis.   [8] In Naugerio.
[9] Si furor sit Lyæus, etc., quoties furit, furit, furit, amans, bibens, et poeta, etc.

PAGE 113

[1] Morus, Utop. lib. 11.   [2] Macrob. Satur. 7, 16.
[3] Epist. 88.   [4] Lib. de causis corrup. artium.
[5] Lib. 2 in Ausonium, cap. 19 et 32.   [6] Edit. 7 volum. Jano Gutero.
[7] Aristophanis Ranis.   [8] Lib. de beneficiis.

PAGE 114

[1] Delirus et amens dicatur merito. Hor. Seneca.
[2] Ovid. Met.
[3] Plutarch. Amatorio est amor insanus.   [4] Epist. 39.
[5] Sylvæ nuptialis lib. 1, num. 11. Omnes mulieres ut plurimum stultæ.
[6] Aristotle.
[7] Dolere se dixit quod tum vita egrederetur.
[8] Lib. 1, num. 11. Sapientia et divitiæ vix simul possideri possunt.
[9] They get their wisdom by eating pie-crust, some. [An allusion to the proverb, "Pie-lid makes people wise"—i.e. its removal reveals what the pie is made of.]
[10] χρήματα τοῖς θνητοῖς γίγνεται ἀφροσύνη. Opes quidem mortalibus sunt amentia.—Theognis.
[11] Fortuna nimium quem fovet, stultum facit.   [12] Job xxviii.

PAGE 115

[1] Mag. moral. lib. 2.   [2] Hor. lib. 1, sat. 4.
[3] Insana gula, insanæ substructiones, insanum venandi studium; discordia demens (Virg. Æn.).

[4] Heliodorus Carthaginiensis ad extremum orbis sarcophago testamento me hic jussi condier, ut viderem an quis insanior ad me visendum usque ad hæc loca penetraret.—Ortelius, in Gad.

[5] If it be his work, which Gaspar Veretus suspects.

[6] Livy. Ingentes virtutes, ingentia vitia. [7] [Cosmo de' Medici.]

PAGE 116

[1] Hor. Quisquis Ambitione mala aut argenti pallet amore, Quisquis luxuria, tristique superstitione. Persius.

[2] Chronica Slavonica, ad annum 1257: de cujus pecunia jam incredibilia dixerunt.

[3] A fool and his money are soon parted.

[4] Orat. de imag. Ambitiosus et audax naviget Anticyras.

[5] Navis stulta, quæ continuo movetur, nautæ stulti qui se periculis exponunt, aqua insana quæ sic fremit, etc., aer jactatur, etc.; qui mari se committit stolidum unum terra fugiens, 40 mari invenit.—Gaspar Ens, Moros.

[6] Cap. de alien. mentis. [7] Deipnosophist. lib. 8.

[8] Tibicines mente capti.—Erasm. Chi. 14, cer. 7.

[9] Prov. xxxi. Insana libido. Hic rogo non furor est, non est hæc mentula demens?—Mart. ep. 76, lib. 3.

[10] Mille puellarum et puerorum mille furores.

[11] Uter est insanior horum?—Hor. Ovid, Virg., Plin.

[12] Plin. lib. 36.

PAGE 117

[1] Tacitus, 3 Annal.

[2] [The "good, doting citizen" in Jonson's Every Man out of His Humour.]

[3] Ovid. 7 Met. E fungis nati homines ut olim Corinthi primævi illius loci accolæ, quia stolidi et fatui fungis nati dicebantur, idem et alibi dicas.

[4] Famian. Strada de bajulis, de marmore semisculptis.

[5] Arrianus periplo maris Euxini portus ejus meminit, et Gillius, l. 3 de Bosphor. Thracio. Et laurus insana quæ allata in convivium convivas omnes insania affecit. Guliel. Stuckius, Comment., etc. [The "insane laurel" is probably Azalea pontica, the honey from which drove Xenophon's soldiers out of their wits (Anab. 4, 8, 20).]

[6] Lepidum poema sic inscriptum [a witty poem so entitled].

PAGE 118

[1] Stultitiam simulare non potes nisi taciturnitate.

[2] Extortus non cruciatur, ambustus non læditur, prostratus in lucta, non vincitur; non fit captivus ab hoste venundatus. Etsi rugosus, senex edentulus, luscus, deformis, formosus tamen, et deo similis, felix, dives, rex nullius egens, etsi denario non sit dignus.

[3] Illum contendunt non injuria affici, non insania, non inebriari, quia virtus non eripitur ob constantes comprehensiones.—Lips. Phys. Stoic. lib. 3, diffi. 18.

[4] Taraeus Hebius, epig. 102, lib. 8. [5] Hor.

[6] Fratres sancti Roseæ Crucis.

[7] An sint, quales sint, unde nomen illud asciverint.

[8] Turri Babel.

[9] Omnium artium et scientiarum instaurator.

[10] Divinus ille vir. Auctor notarum in Epist. Rog. Bacon. ed. Hambur. 1608.

[11] Sapientiæ desponsati.

PAGE 119

[1] Justus is the first name of Lipsius and the quotation refers to him.
[2] Solus hic est sapiens, alii volitant velut umbræ.
[3] In ep. ad Balthas. Moretum.
[4] Rejectiunculæ ad Patavium; Felinus cum reliquis.
[5] Magnum virum sequi est sapere, some think; others desipere.   Catul.
[6] Plaut. Menæchmi.   [7] Juv. Sat. 14.
[8] Or to send for a cook to the Anticyræ, to make hellebore pottage, settle-brain pottage.
[9] Aliquantulum tamen inde me solabor, quod una cum multis et sapientibus et celeberrimis viris ipse insipiens sim, quod se Menippus Luciani in Necyomantia.

PAGE 120

[1] Petronius, in Catalect.
[2] That I mean of Andr. Vale. Apolog. manip. lib. 1 et 26 apol.
[3] Hæc affectio nostris temporibus frequentissima.
[4] Cap. 15 de Mel.
[5] De anima.   Nostro hoc sæculo morbus frequentissimus.
[6] Consult. 98.   Adeo nostris temporibus frequenter ingruit ut nullus fere ab ejus labe immunis reperiatur et omnium fere morborum occasio existat.

PAGE 121

[1] Mor. Encom.   Si quis calumnietur levius esse quam decet theologum, aut mordacius quam deceat Christianum.
[2] Hor. Sat. 4, lib. 1.
[3] Epi. ad Dorpium de Moria.   Si quispiam offendatur et sibi vindicet, non habet quod expostulet cum eo qui scripsit; ipse si volet, secum agat injuriam, utpote sui proditor, qui declaravit hoc ad se proprie pertinere.
[4] Si quis se læsum clamabit, aut conscientiam prodit suam, aut certe metum.—Phædr. lib. 3 Æsop. Fab.

PAGE 122

[1] Hor.   [2] Mart. lib. 7, 25.
[3] Ut lubet feriat, abstergant hos ictus Democriti pharmaco.
[4] Rusticorum dea præesse vacantibus et otiosis putabatur, cui post labores agricola sacrificabat.—Plin. lib. 3, cap. 12.   Ovid. lib. 6. Fast. Jam quoque cum fiunt antiquæ sacra Vacunæ, Ante Vacunales stantque sedentque focos.   Rosinus.   [Vacuna was the goddess of rural leisure.]
[5] Ter. Prol. Eunuch.   [6] [A gesture of anger.]
[7] Ariost. lib. 39, staff 58.
[8] Ut enim ex studiis gaudium sic studia ex hilaritate proveniunt.—Plinius Maximo suo, Ep. lib. 8.

PAGE 123

[1] Annal. 15.
[2] Sir Francis Bacon in his Essays, now Viscount St. Albans.
[3] Quod Probus, Persii βιογράφος, virginali verecundia Persium fuisse dicit, ego, etc.
[4] Quas aut incuria fudit, Aut humana parum cavit natura.—Hor.
[5] Prol. quer. Plaut.

PAGE 124

[1] Si me commorit, melius non tangere clamo.—Hor.
[2] Hippoc. epist. Damageto.   Accersitus sum ut Democritum tanquam insanum curarem, sed postquam conveni, non per Jovem desipientiæ negotium, sed rerum omnium receptaculum deprehendi, ejusque ingenium

demiratus sum. Abderitanos vero tanquam non sanos accusavi, veratri potione ipsos potius eguisse dicens.
  [3] Mart.

PAGE 130

  [1] Magnum miraculum.
  [2] Mundi epitome, naturæ deliciæ.
  [3] Finis rerum omnium, cui sublunaria serviunt.—Scalig. exercit. 365, sec. 3.   Vales. de sacr. Phil. cap. 5.
  [4] Ut in numismate Cæsaris imago, sic in homine Dei.   [5] Gen. i.
  [6] Imago mundi in corpore, Dei in anima.   Exemplumque dei quisque est in imagine parva.
  [7] Eph. iv, 24.   [8] Palanterius.   [9] Ps. xlix, 20.
  [10] Lascivia superat equum, impudentia canem, astu vulpem, furore leonem.—Chrys. 23 Gen.
  [11] Gen. iii, 13.

PAGE 131

  [1] Ecclus. xl, 1, 2, 3, 4, 5, 8.   [2] Gen. iii, 17.
  [3] Illa cadens tegmen manibus decussit, et unà Perniciem immisit miseris mortalibus atram.—Hesiod. Oper.
  [4] Hom. 5 ad pop. Antioch.
  [5] Ps. cvii, 17.   [6] Prov. i, 27.
  [7] Quod autem crebrius bella concutiant, quod sterilitas et fames sollicitudinem cumulent, quod sævientibus morbis valitudo frangitur, quod humanum genus luis populatione vastatur; ob peccatum omnia. —Cypr.
  [8] Si raro desuper pluvia descendat, si terra situ pulveris squaleat, si vix jejunas et pallidas herbas sterilis gleba producat, si turbo vineam debilitet, etc.—Cypr.

PAGE 132

  [1] Mat. xiv, 3.
  [2] Philostratus, lib. 8 vit. Apollonii. Injustitiam ejus, et sceleratus nuptias, et cætera quæ præter rationem fecerat, morborum causas dixit.
  [3] 16.   [4] 18.   [5] 20.   [6] Verse 27.
  [7] 28.   Deus quos diligit, castigat.   [8] Isa. v, 13, 25.
  [9] Nostræ salutis avidus continenter aures vellicat, ac calamitate subinde nos exercet.—Levinus Lemn. lib. 2, cap. 29, de occult. nat. mir.
  [10] Vexatio dat intellectum. Isa. xxviii, 19.

PAGE 133

  [1] Lib. 7. Cum judicio mores et facta recognoscit et se intuetur. Dum fero languorem, fero religionis amorem. Expers languoris non sum memor hujus amoris.
  [2] Summum esse totius philosophiæ, ut tales esse sani perseveremus, quales nos futuros esse infirmi profitemur.
  [3] Petrarch.   [4] Prov. iii, 12.
  [5] Hor. Epist. lib. 1, 4.
  [6] Deut. viii, 11.   Qui stat videat ne cadat.
  [7] Quanto majoribus beneficiis a Deo cumulatur, tanto obligatiorem se debitorem fateri.

PAGE 134

  [1] Boterus de inst. urbium.
  [2] Lege hist. relationem Lod. Frois de rebus Japonicis ad annum 1596.
  [3] Guicciard. descript. Belg. anno 1421.
  [4] Giraldus Cambrensis.   [5] Janus Dousa, Ep. lib. 1, car. 10.
  [6] Munster, lib. 3, Cos. cap. 462.   [7] Buchanan. Baptist.

Page 135

[1] Homo homini lupus, homo homini dæmon.
[2] Ovid. Trist. lib. 5, eleg. 8. [3] Miscent aconita novercæ.
[4] Lib. 2, epist. 2, ad Donatum. [5] Ezech. xviii, 2.
[6] Hor. lib. 3, Od. 6. [7] 2 Tim. iii, 2.

Page 136

[1] Ezech. xviii, 31. [2] 1 Macc. iii, 12.
[3] Part. 1, sec. 2, memb. 2.
[4] Nequitia est quæ te non sinet esse senem. [5] Homer. Iliad.

Page 137

[1] Intemperantia, luxus, ingluvies, et infinita hujusmodi flagitia, quæ divinas pœnas merentur.—Crato.
[2] Fern. Path. lib. 1, cap. 1. Morbus est affectus contra naturam corporis insidens.
[3] Fuchs. Instit. lib. 3, sect. 1, cap. 3: a quo primum vitiatur actio.
[4] Dissolutio fœderis in corpore, ut sanitas est consummatio.
[5] Lib. 4, cap. 2. Morbus est habitus contra naturam, qui usum ejus, etc.
[6] Cap. 11, lib. 7. [7] Horat. lib. 1, ode 3.
[8] Cap. 50, lib. 7. Centum et quinque vixit annos sine ullo incommodo.
[9] Intus mulso, foras oleo.
[10] Exemplis genitur. præfixis Ephemer. cap. de infirmitat.

Page 138

[1] Qui, quoad pueritiæ ultimam memoriam recordari potest, non meminit se ægrotum decubuisse.
[2] Lib. de vita longa. [3] Opera et Dies.
[4] See Fernelius, Path. lib. 1, cap. 9, 10, 11, 12; Fuchsius, Instit. lib. 3, sect. 1, cap. 7; Wecker, Synt.
[5] Præfat. de morbis capitis. In capite ut variæ habitant partes, ita variæ querelæ ibi eveniunt.
[6] Of which read Heurnius, Montaltus, Hildesheim, Quercetan, Jason Pratensis, etc.

Page 139

[1] [?caros, torpor.]
[2] ["A distemper accompanied with a strong inclination to sleep, without being able to do so."—Bailey's Dictionary.]
[3] Cap. 2 de melanchol.
[4] Cap. 2 de physiologia sagarum. Quod alii minus recte fortasse dixerint, nos examinare, melius dijudicare, corrigere studeamus.
[5] Cap. 4 de mel. [6] Art. Med. cap. 7.

Page 140

[1] Plerique medici uno complexu perstringunt hos duos morbos, quod ex eadem causa oriantur, quodque magnitudine et modo solum distent, et alter gradus ad alterum existat.—Jason Pratens.
[2] Lib. Med. [3] Pars maniæ mihi videtur.
[4] Insanus est, qui ætate debita et tempore debito per se, non momentaneam et fugacem, ut vini, solani, hyoscyami, sed confirmatam habet impotentiam bene operandi circa intellectum.—Lib 2, de intellectione.
[5] Of which read Felix Plater, cap. 3 de mentis alienatione.

Page 141

[1] Lib. 6, cap. 11. [2] Lib. 3, cap. 16.
[3] Cap. 9, Art. med. [4] De præstig. dæmonum, lib. 3, cap. 21.
[5] Observat. lib. 10, de morbis cerebri, cap. 15.

[6] Hippocrates, lib. de insania.
[7] Lib. 8, cap. 22. Homines interdum lupos fieri; et contra.
[8] Met. lib. 1. [9] Cap. de mania.
[10] Ulcerata crura, sitis ipsis adest immodica, pallidi, lingua sicca.
[11] Cap, 9, art. Hydrophobia.

PAGE 142

[1] Lib. 3, cap. 9.   [2] Lib. 7, de venenis.
[3] Lib. 3, cap. 13, de morbis acutis.   [4] Spicil. 2.
[5] Sckenkius, 7 lib. de venenis.   [6] Lib. de hydrophobia.
[7] Observat. lib. 10, 25.
[8] Lascivam choream.—Tom. 4, de morbis amentium, tract. 1.
[9] Eventu, ut plurimum rem, ipsam comprobante.

PAGE 143

[1] Lib. 1, cap. de mania.   [2] Cap. 3 de mentis alienat.
[3] Cap. 4 de mel.   [4] Part. 3.

PAGE 144

[1] De quo homine securitas, de quo certum gaudium? Quocunque se convertit, in terrenis rebus amaritudinem animi inveniet.—Aug. in Psal. viii, 5.
[2] Job. xiv, 1.
[3] Omni tempore Socratem eodem vultu videri, sive domum rediret, sive domo egrederetur.
[4] Lib. 7, cap. 1. Natus in florentissima totius orbis civitate, nobilissimis parentibus, corporis vires habuit et rarissimas animi dotes, uxorem conspicuam, pudicam, felices liberos, consulare decus, sequentes triumphos, etc.
[5] Ælian. [6] Homer. Iliad.
[7] Lipsius, cent. 3, ep. 45. Ut cœlum, sic nos homines sumus: illud ex intervallo nubibus obducitur et obscuratur. In rosario flores spinis intermixti. Vita similis aeri, udum modo, sudum, tempestas, serenitas: ita vices rerum sunt, præmia gaudiis, et sequaces curæ.
[8] Lucretius, lib. 4, 1134.
[9] Prov. xiv, 13. Extremum gaudii luctus occupat.
[10] Natalitia, inquit, celebrantur, nuptiæ hic sunt; at ibi quid celebratur quod non dolet, quod non transit?

PAGE 145

[1] Apuleius, 4 Florid. Nihil quicquam homini tam prosperum divinitus datum, quin ei admixtum sit aliquid difficultatis ut etiam amplissima quaque lætitia, subsit quæpiam vel parva querimonia conjugatione quadam mellis et fellis.
[2] Caduca nimirum et fragilia, et puerilibus consentanea crepundiis, sunt ista quæ vires et opes humanæ vocantur; affluunt subito, repente dilabuntur, nullo in loco, nulla in persona, stabilibus nixa radicibus consistunt, sed incertissimo flatu fortunæ quos in sublime extulerunt improviso recursu destitutos in profundo miseriarum valle miserabiliter immergunt.—Valerius, lib. 6, cap. 11.
[3] Huic seculo parum aptus es, aut potius omnium nostrorum conditionem ignoras, quibus reciproco quodam nexu, etc.—Lorchanus Gallobelgicus, lib. 3, ad annum 1598.
[4] Horum omnia studia dirigi debent, ut humana fortiter feramus.
[5] 2 Tim. ii, 3.
[6] Epist. 96, lib. 10. Affectus frequentes contemptique morbum faciunt. Distillatio una nec adhuc in morem adaucta, tussim facit, assidua et violenta phthisim.

Page 146

[1] Calidum ad octo: frigidum ad octo.
[2] Una hirundo non facit æstatem.   [One swallow doesn't make a summer.]
[3] Lib. 1, cap. 6.
[4] Fuchsius, lib. 3, sec. 1, cap. 7.   Hildesheim, fol. 130.
[5] Psal. cxxxix, 14, 15.

Page 147

[1] De anima.   Turpe enim est homini ignorare sui corporis (ut ita dicam) ædificium, præsertim cum ad valetudinem et mores hæc cognitio plurimum conducat.

[2] De usu part.   [3] History of Man.
[4] Dr. Crooke.   [5] In Syntaxi.
[6] De anima.   [7] Instit. lib. 1.
[8] Physiol. lib. 1, 2.   [9] Anat. lib. 1, cap. 18.
[10] In Micro.   Succos, sine quibus animal sustentari non potest.
[11] Morbosos humores.

Page 148

[1] Spiritalis anima.

Page 149

[1] Laurentius, cap. 20, lib. 1, Anat.
[2] In these they observe the beating of the pulse.

Page 150

[1] Cujus est pars similaris a vi cutifica, ut interiora muniat.—Capivac. Anat. pag. 252.
[2] Anat. lib. 1, cap. 19.   Celebris est et pervulgata partium divisio in principes et ignobiles partes.

Page 151

[1] Dr. Crooke, out of Galen, and others.
[2] Vos vero veluti in templum ac sacrarium quoddam vos duci putetis, etc. Suavis et utilis cognitio.
[3] Lib. 1, cap. 12, sect. 5.

Page 153

[1] Hæc res est præcipue digna admiratione, quod tanta affectuum varietate cietur cor, quod omnes res tristes et lætæ statim corda feriunt et movent.
[2] Physio. lib. 1, cap. 8.
[3] Ut orator regi: sic pulmo vocis instrumentum annectitur cordi, etc.—Melancth.

Page 154

[1] De anima, cap. 1.
[2] Scalig. Exerc. 307; Tolet. in lib. de anima, cap. 1, etc.
[3] Lib. de anima, cap. 1.   [4] Tuscul. quæst.
[5] Lib. 6, Doct. Val. Gentil. cap. 13, pag. 1216.   [6] Aristot.
[7] Anima quæque intelligimus, et tamen quæ sit ipsa intelligere non valemus.
[8] Spiritualem animam a reliquis distinctam tuetur, etiam in cadavere inhærentem post mortem per aliquot menses.

Page 155

[1] Lib. 3, cap. 31.
[2] Cœlius, lib. 2, cap. 31; Plutarch in Gryllo; Lips. Cen. 1, ep. 50; Jossius de risu et fletu; Averroes, Campanella, etc.

³ Philip. de anima, cap. 1. Cœlius, 20 Antiq. cap. 3. Plutarch. de placit. philos.

⁴ De vit. et mort. part. 2, cap. 3, prop. 1; De vit. et mort. 2, cap. 22.

⁵ Nutritio est alimenti transmutatio, viro naturalis.—Scal. Exerc. 101, sec. 17.

⁶ See more of attraction in Scal. Exer. 343.

PAGE 156

¹ Vita consistit in calido et humido.

PAGE 158

¹ Lumen est actus perspicui. Lumen a luce provenit, lux est in corpore lucido.

² In Phædone.   ³ De pract. philos. 4.

⁴ Saturn. 7, cap. 14.   ⁵ Lac. cap. 8 de opif. Dei, 1.   ⁶ Lib. 19, cap. 2.

PAGE 159

¹ Phys. lib. 5, cap. 8.

PAGE 160

¹ Exercit. 280.

PAGE 161

¹ T[homas] W[right], Jesuit, in his Passions of the Mind.

² Velcurio.

PAGE 162

¹ Nervi a spiritu moventur, spiritus ab anima.—Melanct.

² Velcurio.   Jucundum et anceps subjectum.

³ Goclenius in Ψυχολ. pag. 302; Bright in Phys. Scrib. lib. 1; David Crusius, Melancthon, Hippius Heurnius, Levinus Lemnius, etc.

⁴ Lib, an mores sequantur, etc.

⁵ Cæsar, 6 Com.

⁶ Read Æneas Gazæus' dial. of the immortality of the soul.

PAGE 163

¹ Ovid. Met. 15.   ² In Gallo.

³ Ovid. Met. 15.   ⁴ Nicephorus, Hist. lib. 10, cap."35.

⁵ Phædo.   ⁶ Claudian, lib. 1. de rap. Proserp.

⁷ [Pliny the Elder; "Uncle Pliny," as Burton calls him elsewhere.]

⁸ Hæc quæstio multos per annos varie ac mirabiliter impugnata, etc.

⁹ Colerus, ibid.

PAGE 164

¹ De eccles. dog. cap. 16.   ² Ovid. 4 Met.

³ Bonorum lares, malorum vero larvas et lemures.

⁴ Some say at three days, some six weeks, others otherwise.

PAGE 165

¹ Melancthon.

² Nihil in intellectu, quod non prius fuerat in sensu.—Velcurio.

PAGE 166

¹ [=tabula rasa, a smooth tablet, "clean slate."]

² The pure part of the conscience.

³ Quod tibi fieri non vis, alteri ne feceris.

I—*Q 886

Page 167

[1] Res ab intellectu monstratas recipit, vel rejicit; approbat, vel improbat.—Philip. Ignoti nulla cupido.
[2] Melancthon. Operationes plerumque feræ, etsi libera sit illa in essentia sua.
[3] In civilibus libera, sed non in spiritualibus.—Osiander.
[4] Tota voluntas aversa a Deo. Omnis homo mendax.
[5] Virg.
[6] Vel propter ignorantiam, quod bonis studiis non sit instructa mens ut debuit, aut divinis præceptis exculta.

Page 168

[1] Medea, Ovid.   [2] Ovid.   [3] Seneca, Hipp.

Page 169

[1] Melancholicos vocamus, quos exuperantia vel pravitas melancholiæ ita male habet, ut inde insaniant vel in omnibus, vel in pluribus, iisque manifestis sive ad rectam rationem, voluntatem pertinent, vel electionem, vel intellectus operationes.
[2] Pessimum et pertinacissimum morbum qui homines in bruta degenerare cogit.
[3] Panth. Med.
[4] Angor animi in una contentione defixus, absque febre.

Page 170

[1] Cap. 16, lib. 1.
[2] Eorum definitio morbus quid non sit, potius quam quid sit, explicat.
[3] Animæ functiones imminuuntur in fatuitate, tolluntur in mania, depravantur solum in melancholia.—Herc. de Sax. cap. 1, tract. de Melanch.
[4] Cap. 4 de mel.
[5] Per consensum sive per essentiam.   [6] Cap. 4 de mel.

Page 171

[1] Sec. 7, de mor. vulgar. lib. 6.   [2] Spicil. de melancholia.
[3] Cap. 3 de mel. Pars affecta cerebrum sive per consensum, sive per cerebrum contingat, et procerum auctoritate et ratione stabilitur.
[4] Lib. de mel. Cor vero vicinitatis ratione una afficitur, ac septum transversum ac stomachus cum dorsali spina, etc.
[5] Lib. 1, cap. 10. Subjectum est cerebrum interius.
[6] Raro quisquam tumorem effugit lienis, qui hoc morbo afficitur.—Piso.
[7] See Donat. ab Altomar.
[8] Facultas imaginandi, non cogitandi, nec memorandi læsa hic.
[9] Lib. 3, fen. 1, tract. 4, cap. 8.   [10] Lib. 3, cap. 5.
[11] Lil. Med. cap. 19, part. 2. Tract. 15, cap. 2.
[12] Hildesheim, Spicil. 2 de melanc. fol. 207, et fol. 127. Quandoque etiam rationalis si affectus inveteratus sit.

Page 172

[1] Lib. posthumo de melanc. edit. 1620. Deprivatur fides, discursus, opinio, etc., per vitium imaginationis, ex accidenti.
[2] Qui parvum caput habent, insensati plerique sunt.—Arist. in Physiognomia.
[3] Aretæus, lib. 3, cap. 5.
[4] Qui prope statum sunt.—Aret. Mediis convenit ætatibus.—Piso.
[5] De quartano.   [6] Lib. 1, part. 2, cap. 11.
[7] Primus ad melancholiam non tam mœstus sed et hilares, jocosi, cachinnantes, irrisores, et qui plerumque prærubri sunt.

[8] Qui sunt subtilis ingenii, et multæ perspicacitatis, de facili incidunt in melancholiam.—Lib. 1 Cont. tract. 9.
[9] Nunquam sanitate mentis excidit aut dolore capitur.—Erasmus.
[10] In laud. calvit.
[11] Vacant conscientiæ carnificina, nec pudefiunt, nec verentur, nec dilacerantur millibus curarum, quibus tota vita obnoxia est.

PAGE 173

[1] Lib. 1, tract. 3, contradic. 18. [2] Lib. 1, cont. 21.
[3] Bright, cap. 16. [4] Lib. 1, cap. 6, de sanit. tuenda.
[5] Quisve aut qualis sit humor aut quæ istius differentiæ, et quomodo gignantur in corpore, scrutandum, hac enim re multi veterum laboraverunt, nec facile accipere ex Galeno sententiam ob loquendi varietatem.—Leon. Jacch. Com. in 9 Rhasis, cap. 15, cap. 16 in 9 Rhasis.
[6] Lib. postum. de melan. edit. Venetiis 1620, cap. 7 et 8. Ab intemperie calida, humida, etc.
[7] Secundum magis aut minus si in corpore fuerit, ad intemperiem plusquam corpus salubriter ferre poterit: inde corpus morbosum efficitur.
[8] Lib. 1 Controvers. cap. 21. [9] Lib. 1, sect. 4, cap. 4.
[10] Consil. 26. [11] Lib. 2 Contradic. cap. 11.
[12] De feb. tract. diff. 2, cap. 1. Non est negandum ex hac fieri melancholicos.

PAGE 174

[1] In Syntax.
[2] Varie aduritur, et miscetur, unde variæ amentium species.—Melanct.
[3] Humor frigidus delirii causa, furoris calidus, etc.
[4] Lib. i, cap. 10, de affect. cap.
[5] Nigrescit hic humor, aliquando supercalefactus, aliquando superfrigefactus, cap. 7.
[6] Humor hic niger aliquando præter modum calefactus, et alias refrigeratus evadit: nam recentibus carbonibus ei quid simile accidit, qui durante flamma pellucidissime candent, ea extincta prorsus nigrescunt.—Hippocrates.
[7] Guianerius, diff. 2, cap. 7.
[8] Non est mania, nisi extensa melancholia. [9] Cap. 6, lib. 1.

PAGE 175

[1] 2 Ser. 2, cap. 9. Morbus hic est omnifarius.
[2] Species indefinitæ sunt.
[3] Si aduratur naturalis melancholia, alia fit species, si sanguis alia, si flava bilis, alia, diversa a primis: maxima est inter has differentia, et tot doctorum sententiæ, quot ipsi numero sunt.
[4] Tract. de mel. cap. 7.
[5] Quædam incipiens, quædam consummata.
[6] Cap. de humor. lib. de anima. Varie aduritur et miscetur ipsa melancholia, unde variæ amentium species.
[7] Cap. 16, in 9 Rhasis.
[8] Laurentius, cap. 4 de mel. [9] Cap. 13.

PAGE 176

[1] 480 et 116 consult. consil. 12. [2] Hildesheim, Spicil. 2, fol. 166.
[3] Trincavellius, tom. 2, consil. 15 et 16.
[4] Cap. 13, tract. posth. de melan. [5] Guarion. Cons. med. 2.

PAGE 177

[1] Laboravit per essentiam et a toto corpore.
[2] Machiavel, etc. Smithus, de rep. Angl. cap. 8, lib. 1; Buscoldus, Discurs. Polit. discurs. 5, cap. 7; Arist. lib. 3 Polit. cap. ult; Keckerm., alii, etc.

³ Lib. 6.
⁴ Primo Artis curativæ.
⁵ Nostri primum sit propositi affectionum causas indagare; res ipsa hortari videtur, nam alioqui earum curatio manca et inutilis esset.
⁶ Path. lib. I, cap. II.   Rerum cognoscere causas, medicis imprimis necessarium, sine qua nec morbum curare, nec præcavere licet.
⁷ Tanta enim morbi varietas ac differentia ut non facile dignoscatur, unde initium morbus sumpserit.—Melanelius, e Galeno.
⁸ Felix qui potuit rerum cognoscere causas.

PAGE 178

¹ I Sam. xvi, 14.   ² Dan. v, 21.
³ Lactant. Instit. lib. 2, cap. 8.
⁴ Mente captus, et summo animi mœrore consumptus.
⁵ Munster. Cosmog. lib. 4, cap. 43. De cœlo substernebantur, tanquam insani de saxis præcipitati, etc.
⁶ Livius, lib. 38.
⁷ Gaguin. lib. 3, cap. 4. Quod Dionysii corpus discooperuerat, in insaniam incidit.
⁸ Idem, lib. 9, sub Carol. 6. Sacrorum contemptor, templi foribus effractis, dum s. Johannis argenteum simulacrum rapere contendit, simulacrum aversâ facie dorsum ei versat, nec mora sacrilegus mentis inops, atque in semet insaniens in proprios artus desævit.
⁹ Giraldus Cambrensis, lib. I, cap. I, Itinerar. Cambriæ.

PAGE 179

¹ Delrio, tom. 3 lib. 6, sect. 3, quæst. 3.   ² Psal. xliv, I.
³ Lib. 8, cap. de Hierar.   ⁴ Claudian.
⁵ [Thou hast conquered, O Galilean.]
⁶ De Babila Martyre.   ⁷ Lib. I, cap. 5, Prog.
⁸ Lib. I, de abditis rerum causis.
⁹ Respons. med. resp. 12.   ¹⁰ I Pet. v, 6.

PAGE 180

¹ Lib. I, cap. 7, de orbis concordia.   In nulla re major fuit altercatio, major obscuritas, minor opinionum concordia, quam de dæmonibus et substantiis separatis.
² Lib. 3 de Trinit. cap. I.
³ Pererius in Genesin, lib. 4, in cap. iii, v. 23.
⁴ See Strozzius Cicogna, Omnifariæ mag. lib. 2, cap. 15, Jo. Aubanus, Bredenbachius.

PAGE 181

¹ Angelus per superbiam separatus a Deo, qui in veritate non stetit.—Austin.
² Nihil aliud sunt dæmones quam nudæ animæ quæ corpore deposito priorem miserati vitam, cognatis succurrunt commoti misericordia, etc.
³ De Deo Socratis.
⁴ He lived five hundred years since.

PAGE 182

¹ Apuleius. Spiritus animalia sunt animo passibilia, mente rationalia, corpore aeria, tempore sempiterna.
² Nutriuntur, et excrementa habent; quod pulsata doleant solido percussa corpore.
³ Lib. 4 Theol. nat. fol. 535.

[4] Cyprianus, in Epist. Montes etiam et animalia transferri possunt: as the devil did Christ to the top of the pinnacle; and witches are often translated. See more in Strozzius Cicogna, lib. 3, cap. 4, Omnif. mag. Per aera subducere et in sublime corpora ferre possunt.—Biarmannus. Percussi dolent et uruntur in conspicuos cineres.—Agrippa, lib. 3, cap. 18, de occult. philos.
[5] [Bel and the Dragon, 36.]

PAGE 183

[1] Agrippa de occult. philos. lib. 3, cap. 18.
[2] Part. 3, sect. 2, mem. 1, subs. 1, Love Melancholy.
[3] Genial. dierum. Ita sibi visum et compertum quum prius an essent ambigeret. Fidem suam liberet.
[4] Lib. 1 de verit. fidei. Benzo, etc.

PAGE 184

[1] Lib. de divinatione et magia.
[2] Cap. 8. Transportavit in Livoniam cupiditate videndi, etc.
[3] Sic Hesiodus, de nymphis, vivere dicit 10 ætates phœnicum, vel 9720. [See Pantagruel's discourse on the subject of Rabelais, iv. 27.]
[4] Custodes hominum et provinciarum, etc., tanto meliores hominibus, quanto hi brutis animantibus.
[5] Præsides, pastores, gubernatores hominum, ut illi animalium.

PAGE 185

[1] Natura familiares ut canes hominibus; multi aversantur et abhorrent.
[2] Ab homine plus distant quam homo ab ignobilissimo verme, et tamen quidam ex his ab hominibus superantur ut homines a feris, etc.
[3] Cibo et potu uti et venere cum hominibus ac tandem mori.—Cicogna, part. 1, lib. 2, cap. 3.
[4] Plutarch. de defect. oraculorum.
[5] Lib. de Zilphis et Pigmæis.
[6] Dii gentium a Constantio profligati sunt, etc.
[7] Octavian. dial. Judæorum deum fuisse Romanorum numinibus una cum gente captivum.
[8] Omnia spiritibus plena, et ex eorum concordia et discordia omnes boni et mali effectus promanant, omnia humana reguntur: paradoxa veterum de quo Cicogna, Omnif. mag. lib. 2, cap. 3.

PAGE 186

[1] Oves quas abacturus erat in quascunque formas vertebat. Pausanias, Hyginus.
[2] Austin in lib. 2 de Gen. ad literam, cap. 17. Partim quia subtilioris sensus acumine, partim scientia callidiore vigent et experientia propter magnam longitudinem vitæ, partim ab angelis discunt, etc.
[3] Lib. 3 Omnif. mag. cap. 3.   [4] Lib. 18 Quest.
[5] Quum tanta sit et tam profunda spirituum scientia, mirum non est tot tantasque res visu admirabiles ab ipsis patrari, et quidem rerum naturalium ope quas multo melius intelligunt, multoque peritius suis locis et temporibus applicare norunt, quam homo.—Cicogna.
[6] Aventinus. Quicquid interdiu exhauriebatur, noctu explebatur. Inde pavefacti curatores, etc.
[7] In lib. 2 de anima, text. 29. Homerus discriminatim omnes spiritus dæmones vocat.

PAGE 187

[1] A Jove ad inferos pulsi, etc.

[2] De Deo Socratis. Adest mihi divina sorte dæmonium quoddam a prima pueritia me secutum; sæpe dissuadet, impellit nonnunquam instar vocis. —Plato.

[3] Agrippa, lib. 3 de occul. ph. cap. 18, Zanch., Pictorius, Pererius, Cicogna, lib. 3, cap. 1.

[4] Vasa iræ, cap. 13.

[5] Quibus datum est nocere terræ et mari, etc.

PAGE 188

[1] [Meririm, according to Cornelius Agrippa.]

[2] Physiol. Stoicorum e Senec. lib. 1, cap. 28.

[3] Usque ad lunam animas esse ætherias vocarique heroas, lares, genios.

[4] Mart. Capella.

[5] Nihil vacuum ab his ubi vel capillum in aerem vel aquam jacias.

[6] Lib. de Zilph.   [7] Palingenius.

[8] Lib. 7, cap. 34 et 35, Syntax. art. mirab.

PAGE 189

[1] Comment in dial. Plat. de amore, cap. 5. Ut sphæra quælibet super nos, ita præstantiores habent habitatores suæ sphæræ consortes, ut habet nostra.

[2] Lib. de anima. et dæmone. Med. inter deos et homines, diva ad nos et nostra æqualiter ad deos ferunt.

[3] Saturninas et Joviales accolas.   [The reference is to Kepler's *Dissertatio cum Nuncio Sidereo*, in which he discourses with a messenger from the stars concerning Galileo's discoveries.]

[4] In loca detrusi sunt infra cœlestes orbes in aerem scilicet et infra ubi Judicio generali reservantur.

[5] Q. 36, art. 9.

PAGE 190

[1] Virg. Ecl. 8.   [2] Æn. 4.

[3] Austin. Hoc dixi, ne quis existimet habitare ibi mala dæmonia ubi Solem et Lunam et Stellas Deus ordinavit, et alibi nemo arbitraretur Dæmonem cœlis habitare cum Angelis suis unde lapsum credimus.   Idem Zanch. lib. 4, cap. 3, de Angel. malis; Pererius in Gen. cap. 6, lib. 8, in ver. 2.

[4] Peregrin. Hierosol.

PAGE 191

[1] Domus diruunt, muros dejiciunt, immiscent se turbinibus et procellis, et pulverem instar columnæ evehunt.—Cicogna, lib. 5, cap. 5.

[2] Quæst. in Liv.

[3] De præstigiis dæmonum, cap. 16.   Convelli culmina videmus, prosterni sata, etc.

[4] De bello Neapolitano, lib. 5.

[5] Suffitibus gaudent.   Idem Just. Mart. Apol. pro Christianis.

[6] In Dei imitationem, saith Eusebius.

[7] Dii gentium dæmonia, etc.; ego in eorum statuas pellexi.

[8] Et nunc sub divorum nomine coluntur a pontificiis.

PAGE 192

[1] Lib. 11 de rerum var.

[2] Lib. 3, cap. 3, de magis et veneficis, etc.   [3] Nereides.

[4] Lib. de Zilphis.   [5] Lib. 3.

[6] Pro salute hominum excubare se simulant, sed in eorum perniciem omnia moliuntur.—Aust.

[7] Dryades, Oreades, Hamadryades.

[8] Elvas Olaus vocat [Olaus calls them elves], lib. 3.

PAGE 193

[1] Part 1, cap. 19.
[2] Lib. 3, cap. 11. Elvarum choreas Olaus, lib. 3, vocat. Saltum adeo profunde in terras imprimunt, ut locus insigni deinceps virore orbicularis sit, et gramen non pereat.
[3] Lib. de Zilph. et Pigmæis. Olaus, lib. 3.
[4] Lib. 7, cap. 14. Qui et in famulitio viris et feminis inserviunt, conclavia scopis purgant, patinas mundant, ligna portant, equos curant, etc.
[5] Ad ministeria utuntur.
[6] Where treasure is hid (as some think) or some murder, or such-like villainy committed.
[7] Lib. 16, de rerum varietat.
[8] Quidam lemures domesticis instrumentis noctu ludunt: patinas, ollas, cantharas, et alia vasa dejiciunt, et quidam voces emittunt, ejulant, risum emittunt, etc.; ut canes nigri, feles, variis formis, etc.

PAGE 194

[1] Vel spiritus sunt hujusmodi damnatorum, vel e purgatorio, vel ipsi dæmones.—Cap. 4.
[2] Epist. lib. 7.
[3] Meridionales dæmones Cicogna calls them, or Alastores, lib. 3, cap. 9.
[4] Sueton. cap. 59 in Caligula.
[5] Strozzius Cicogna, lib. 3 Mag. cap. 5.   [6] Idem, cap. 18.

PAGE 195

[1] [Logs of wood that appeared floating in a pool at Brereton in Cheshire.]
[2] Mr. Carew, Survey of Cornwall, lib. 2, folio 140. [The Lanhadron or Arundell oak, which usually bore white or variegated leaves; it foretold the death of the lord of the manor by leafing normally.]
[3] Horto Geniali, folio 137.
[4] Part. 1, cap. 19. Abducunt eos a recta via, et viam iter facientibus intercludunt.
[5] Lib. 1, cap. 44. Dæmonum cernuntur et audiuntur ibi frequentes illusiones, unde viatoribus cavendum ne se dissocient, aut a tergo maneant, voces enim fingunt sociorum, ut a recto itinere abducant, etc.
[6] Mons sterilis et nivosus, ubi intempesta nocte umbræ apparent.
[7] Lib. 2, cap. 21. Offendicula faciunt transeuntibus in via et petulanter rident cum vel hominem vel jumentum ejus pedes atterere faciant, et maxime si homo maledictis et calcaribus sæviat.

PAGE 196

[1] In Cosmogr.
[2] Vestiti more metallicorum, gestus et opera eorum imitantur.
[3] Immisso in terræ carceres vento horribiles terræ motus efficiunt, quibus sæpe non domus modo et turres, sed civitates integræ et insulæ haustæ sunt.
[4] Hierom. in 3 Ephes. Idem Michaelis, cap. 4 de spiritibus. Idem Thyræus de locis infestis.
[5] Lactantius, 2 de origine erroris, cap. 15. Hi maligni spiritus per omnem terram vagantur, et solatium perditionis suæ perdendis hominibus operantur.
[6] Mortalium calamitates epulæ sunt malorum dæmonum.—Synesius.
[7] Dominus mendacii a seipso deceptus, alios decipere cupit, adversarius humani generis, inventor mortis, superbiæ institutor, radix malitiæ, scelerum caput, princeps omnium vitiorum, furit inde in Dei contumeliam, hominum perniciem. De horum conatibus et operationibus lege Epiphanium, 2 tom. lib. 2; Dionysium, cap. 4; Ambros. Epistol. lib. 10, ep. 84; August. de Civ. Dei, lib. 5, cap. 9, lib. 8, cap. 22, lib. 9, 18, lib. 10, 21;

476 NOTES

Theophil. in 12 Mat.; Basil. ep. 141; Leonem, Ser.; Theodoret. in 11 Cor. ep. 22; Chrys. hom. 53 in 12 Gen.; Greg. in 1 cap. John; Barthol. de prop. lib. 2, cap. 20; Zanch. lib. 4 de malis angelis; Perer. in Gen. lib. 8, in cap. 6, 2; Origen. Sæpe præliis intersunt, itinera et negotia nostra quæcunque dirigunt, clandestinis subsidiis optatos sæpe præbent successus. Pet. Mar. in Sam. etc.; Ruscam de Inferno.

PAGE 197

[1] Et velut mancipia circumfert.—Psellus.   [2] Lib. de transmut. Malac. ep.

[3] Custodes sunt hominum, et eorum, ut nos animalium: tum et provinciis præpositi regunt auguriis, somniis, oraculis, præmiis, etc.

[4] Lipsius, Physiol. Stoic. lib. 1, cap. 19.

[5] Leo Suavius.   Idem et Trithemius.

PAGE 198

[1] Omnif. mag. lib. 2, cap. 23.

[2] Ludus deorum sumus.   [3] Lib. de anima et dæmone.

[4] Quoties fit, ut principes novitium aulicum divitiis et dignitatibus pene obruant, et multorum annorum ministrum, qui non semel pro hero periculum subiit, ne teruncio donent, etc. Idem. Quod philosophi non remunerentur, cum scurra et ineptus ob insulsum jocum sæpe præmium reportet, inde fit, etc.

PAGE 199

[1] Lib. de cruent. cadaver.   [2] Boissardus, cap. 6, Magia.

[3] Godelmannus, cap. 3, lib. 1, de magis. Idem Zanchius, lib. 4, cap. 10 et 11, de malis angelis.

[4] Nociva melancholia furiosos efficit, et quandoque penitus interficit.— G. Piccolomineus. Idemque Zanch. cap. 10, lib. 4. Si Deus permittat, corpora nostra movere possunt, alterare, quovis morborum et malorum genere afficere, imo et in ipsa penetrare et sævire.

[5] Inducere potest morbos et sanitates.

[6] Viscerum actiones potest inhibere latenter, et venenis nobis ignotis corpus inficere.

[7] Irrepentes corporibus occulto morbos fingunt, mentes terrent, membra distorquent.—Lips. Phys. Stoic. lib. 1, cap. 19.

[8] De rerum var. lib. 16, cap. 93.

[9] Quum mens immediate decipi nequit, primum movet phantasiam, et ita obfirmat vanis conceptibus ut ne quem facultati æstimativæ rationive locum relinquat. Spiritus malus invadit animam, turbat sensus, in furorem conjicit.—Austin, de vit. Beat.

PAGE 200

[1] Lib. 3, fen. 1, tract. 4, cap. 18.

[2] A Dæmone maxime proficisci, et sæpe solo.   [3] Lib. de incant.

[4] Cap. de mania, lib. de morbis cerebri. Dæmones, quum sint tenues et incomprehensibiles spiritus, se insinuare corporibus humanis possunt, et occulte in visceribus operti, valetudinem vitiare, somniis animas terrere et mentes furoribus quatere.

[5] Insinuant se melancholicorum penetralibus intus, ibique considunt et deliciantur tanquam in regione clarissimorum siderum, coguntque animum furere.

[6] Lib. 1, cap. 6, Occult. Philos.   [7] Part. 1, cap. 1, de spectris.

PAGE 201

[1] [*Malleus Maleficarum* or *Hexenhammer*, the standard textbook on witchcraft, by Jakob Sprenger and Heinrich Krämer.]

[2] Sine cruce et sanctificatione sic a dæmone obsessa.—Dial. Greg. Pag. cap. 9.

Page 202

[1] Penult. de opific. Dei.   [2] Lib. 28, cap. 26, tom. 2.   [3] De lamiis.
[4] [Reginald Scot, or Scott, author of the Discovery of Witchcraft.]

Page 203

[1] Et quomodo venefici fiant enarrat.
[2] De quo plura legas in Boissardo, lib. 1 de præstig.
[3] Rex Jacobus, Dæmonol. lib. 1, cap. 3.
[4] An university in Spain in Old Castile.   [5] The chief town in Poland.
[6] Oxford and Paris, see finem P. Lombardi.
[7] Præfat. de magis et veneficis.
[8] Rotatum pileum habebat, quo ventos violentos cieret, aerem turbaret, et in quam partem, etc.   [9] Erastus.

Page 204

[1] Ministerio hirci nocturni.
[2] Steriles nuptos et inhabiles. Vide Petrum de Palude, lib. 4, distinct. 34; Paulum Guiclandum.
[3] Infantes matribus suffurantur, aliis suppositivis in locum verorum conjectis.
[4] Milles.
[5] D. Luther, in primum præceptum, et Leon. Varius, lib. 1 de fascinat.
[6] Lavat., Cicog.   [7] Boissardus, de Magia.   [8] Dæmon. lib. 3, cap. 3.

Page 205

[1] Vide Philostratum, vita ejus; Boissardum de Magia.
[2] Vide Suidam de Pasete.   [3] Nubrigensem lege, lib. 1, cap. 19.
[4] Erastus. Adolphus Scribanius.
[5] Virg. Æneid. 4, incantatricem describens: Hæc se carminibus promittit solvere mentes, Quas velit, ast aliis duras immittere curas.
[6] Godelmannus, cap. 7, lib. 1. Nutricum mammas præsiccant, solo tactu podagram, apoplexiam, paralysin, et alios morbos, quos medicina curare non poterat.
[7] Factus inde maniacus.   [8] Epic. 2, fol. 147.
[9] Omnia philtra etsi inter se differant, hoc habent commune, quod hominem efficiant melancholicum.—Epist. 231 Scholtzii.
[10] De cruent. cadaver.

Page 206

[1] Astra regunt homines, et regit astra Deus.
[2] Chirom. lib. Quæris a me quantum operantur astra? dico, in nos nihil astra urgere, sed animos proclives trahere: qui sic tamen liberi sunt, ut si ducem sequantur rationem, nihil efficiant, sin vero naturam, id agere quod in brutis fere.
[3] Cœlum vehiculum divinæ virtutis, cujus mediante motu, lumine et influentia, Deus elementaria corpora ordinat et disponit.—Th. de Vio, Cajetanus, in Psa. civ.
[4] Mundus iste quasi lyra ab excellentissimo quodam artifice concinnata, quem qui norit mirabiles eliciet harmonias.—J. Dee, Aphorismo 11.

Page 207

[1] Medicus sine cœli peritia nihil est, etc., nisi genesim sciverit, ne tantillum poterit.—Lib. de podag.
[2] Constellatio in causa est; et influentia cœli morbum hunc movet, interdum omnibus aliis amotis. Et alibi: Origo ejus a cœlo petenda est.—Tr. de morbis amentium.
[3] Lib. de anima, cap. de humorib. Ea varietas in Melancholia habet cœlestes causas ♂ ♄ et ♃ in ♎ ♂ ♂ et ☾ in ♏.

⁴ Ex atra bile varii generantur morbi perinde ut ipse multum calidi aut frigidi in se habuerit, quum utrique suscipiendo quam aptissima sit, tametsi suapte natura frigida sit. Annon aqua sic afficitur a calore ut adreat; et a frigore, ut in glaciem concrescat? et hæc varietas distinctionum, alii fient, rident, etc.

⁵ Hanc ad intemperantiam gignendam plurimum confert ♂ et ♄ positus, etc.

⁶ ☿ quoties alicujus genitura in ♏ et ♓ adverso signo positus, horoscopum partiliter tenuerit atque etiam a ♂ vel ♄ □ radio percussus fuerit, natus ab insania vexabitur.

⁷ Qui ♄ et ♂ habet, alterum in culmine, alterum imo cœlo, cum in lucem venerit, melancholicus erit, à qua sanabitur, si ☿ illos irradiarit.

⁸ Hac configuratione natus, aut lunaticus, aut mente captus.

PAGE 208

¹ Ptolemæus centiloquio, et quadripartito tribuit omnium melancholicorum symptomata siderum influentiis.

² Arte Medica. Accedunt ad has causas affectiones siderum. Plurimum incitant et provocant influentiæ cælestes.—Velcurio, lib. 4, cap. 15.

³ Hildesheim, Spicil. 2, de mel.

⁴ Joh. de Indag. cap. 9; Montaltus, cap. 22.

⁵ Caput parvum qui habent cerebrum et spiritus plerumque angustos; facile incident in melancholiam rubicundi.—Aetius. Idem Montaltus, cap. 21, e Galeno.

PAGE 209

¹ Saturnina a rascetta per mediam manum decurrens, usque ad radicem montis Saturni, a parvis lineis intersecta, arguit melancholicos.—Aphoris.78.

² Agitantur miseriis, continuis inquietudinibus, neque unquam a sollicitudine liberi sunt, anxie affliguntur amarissimis intra cogitationibus, semper tristes, suspiciosi, meticulosi: cogitationes sunt, velle agrum colere, stagna amant et paludes, etc.—Jo. de Indagine, lib. 1.

³ Cælestis Physiognom. lib. 10.

⁴ Cap. 14, lib. 5, idem. Maculæ in ungulis nigræ, lites, rixas, melancholiam significant, ab humore in corde tali.

PAGE 210

¹ Lib. 1 Path. cap. 11.

² Venit enim properata malis inopina senectus: Et dolor ætatem jussit inesse meam.—Boethius, met. 1, de consol. Philos.

³ Cap. de humoribus, lib. de anima.

⁴ Necessarium accidens decrepitis, et inseparabile.

⁵ Ps. xc, 10.   ⁶ Meteran. Belg. hist. lib. 1.

⁷ Sunt morosi, et anxii, et iracundi, et difficiles senes, si quærimus, etiam avari.—Tull. de senectute.

⁸ Lib. 2 de Aulico. Senes avari, morosi, jactabundi, philauti, deliri, superstitiosi, suspiciosi, etc.

⁹ Lib. 3 de lamiis, cap. 17 et 18.

PAGE 211

¹ Solanum, opium, lupi adeps, lacr. asini, etc., sanguis infantum, etc.

² Corrupta est iis ab humore melancholico phantasia.—Nymannus.

³ Putant se lædere quando non lædunt.

⁴ Qui hæc in imaginationis vim referre conati sunt, aut atræ bilis, inanem prorsus laborem susceperunt.

⁵ Lib. 3, cap. 4, Omnif. mag.   ⁶ Lib. 1, cap. 11, Path.

⁷ Ut arthritici, epileptici, etc.

⁸ Ut filii non tam possessionum quam morborum hæredes sint.

[9] Epist. de secretis artis et naturæ, cap. 7. Nam in 'hoc'quod patres corrupti sunt, generant filios corruptæ complexionis, et compositionis, et filii eorum eadem de causa se corrumpunt, et sic derivatur corruptio a patribus ad filios.

[10] Non tam (inquit Hippocrates) gibbos et cicatrices oris et corporis habitum agnoscis ex iis, sed verum incessum gestus, mores, morbos, etc.

[11] Synagog. Jud.

Page 212

[1] Affectus parentum in fœtus transeunt, et puerorum malitia parentibus imputanda.—Lib. 4, cap. 3, de occult. nat. mirac.

[2] Ex pituitosis pituitosi, ex biliosis biliosi, ex lienosis et melancholicis melancholici.

[3] Epist. 174, in Scoltz. Nascitur nobiscum illa aliturque et una cum parentibus habemus malum hunc assem. Jo. Pelezius, lib. 2 de cura humanorum affectuum.

[4] Lib. 10, observat. 15.

[5] Maginus, Geog. [For Galbots, Southey and Shilleto suggest Cagots.]

[6] Sæpe non eundem, sed similem producit effectum, et illæso parente transit in nepotem.

[7] Dial. præfix. genituris Leovitii.

Page 213

[1] Bodin. de rep. cap. de periodis reip.

[2] Claudius Albaville, Capuchin, in his voyage to Maragnan, 1614, cap. 45. Nemo fere ægrotus, sano omnes et robusto corpore, vivunt annos 120, 140, sine medicina. Idem Hector Boethius de insulis Orcad. et Damianus à Goes de Scandia.

[3] Lib. 4, cap. 3, de occult. nat. mir. Tetricos plerumque filios senes progenerant et tristes, rarius exhilaratos.

[4] Coitus super repletionem pessimus, et filii qui tum gignuntur, aut morbosi sunt, aut stolidi.

[5] Dial. præfix. Leovitio.   [6] Lib. de ed. liberis.

[7] De occult. nat. mir. Temulentæ et stolidæ mulieres liberos plerumque producunt sibi similes.

[8] Lib. 2, cap, 8. de occult. nat. mir. Good Master Schoolmaster, do not English this.

Page 214

[1] De nat. mul. lib. 3, cap. 4.   [2] Buxtorfius, cap. 31 Synag. Jud. Ezek. xviii.

[3] Drusius, Obs. lib. 3, cap. 20.

[4] Beda, Eccl. hist. lib. 1, cap. 27, respons. 10.

[5] Nam spiritus cerebri si tum male afficiantur, tales procreant, et quales fuerint affectus, tales filiorum: ex tristibus tristes, ex jucundis jucundi nascuntur, etc.

[6] Fol. 129. Socrates' children were fools.—Sabel.

Page 215

[1] De occul. nat. mir.

[2] Baptista Porta, loco præd. Ex leporum intuitu plerique infantes edunt bifido superiore labello.

[3] Quasi mox in terram collapsurus, per omnem vitam incedebat, cum mater gravida ebrium hominem sic incedentem viderat.

[4] Civem facie cadaverosa, qui dixit, etc.

[5] Optimum bene nasci, maxima pars felicitatis nostræ bene nasci ; quamobrem præclare humano generi consultum videretur, si soli parentes bene habiti et sani, liberis operam darent.

[6] Infantes infirmi præcipitio necati. Bohemus, lib. 3, cap. 3. Apud Laconas olim. Lipsius, epist. 85, cent. ad Belgas, Dionysio Villerio. Si quos aliqua membrorum parte inutiles notaverint, necari jubent.

PAGE 216

[1] Lib. 1, de veterum Scotorum moribus. Morbo comitiali, dementia, mania, lepra, etc., aut simili labe, quæ facile in prolem transmittitur, laborantes inter eos, ingenti facta indagine, inventos, ne gens fæda contagione læderetur ex iis nata, castraverunt, mulieres hujusmodi procul a virorum consortio ablegarunt, quod si harum aliqua concepisse inveniebatur, simul cum fœtu nondum edito defodiebatur viva.
[2] Euphormio Satyr.

PAGE 217

[1] Fecit omnia delicta quæ fieri possunt circa res sex non naturales, et eæ fuerunt causæ extrinsecæ, ex quibus postea ortæ sunt obstructiones.
[2] Path. lib. 1, cap. 2. Maximam in gignendis morbis vim obtinet, pabulum, materiamque morbi suggerens: nam nec ab aere, nec a perturbationibus, vel aliis evidentibus causis morbi sunt, nisi consentiat corporis præparatio, et humorum constitutio. Ut semel dicam, una gula est omnium morborum mater, etiamsi alius est genitor. Ab hac morbi sponte sæpe emanant nulla alia cogente causa.
[3] Shilleto omits "also four." Perhaps some name should replace "also."
[4] Cogan, Elyot, Vaughan, Venner.

PAGE 218

[1] Freitagius.   [2] Isaac.
[3] Non laudatur quia melancholicum præbet alimentum.
[4] Male alit cervina (inquit Freitagius) crassissimum eb atribilarium suppeditat alimentum.
[5] Lib. de subtiliss. diæta. Equina caro et asinina equinis danda est hominibus et asininis.
[6] Parum absunt a natura leporum. Bruerinus, lib. 13, cap. 25. Pullorum tenera et optima.

PAGE 219

[1] Illaudabilis succi nauseam provocant.   [2] Piso, Altomarus.
[3] Curio. Freitagius, Magninus, part. 3, cap. 17. Mercurialis, de affect. lib. 1, cap. 10, excepts all milk meats in hypochondriacal melancholy.
[4] Wecker, Syntax. theor., p. 2; Isaac; Bruer. lib. 15, cap. 30 et 31.
[5] Cap. 18, part. 3.

PAGE 220

[1] Omni loco et omni tempore medici detestantur anguillas, præsertim circa solstitium. Damnantur tum sanis tum ægris.
[2] Cap. 6 in his Tract of Melancholy.
[3] Optime nutrit omnium judicio inter primæ notæ pisces gustu præstanti.
[4] Non est dubium, quin pro vivariorum situ, ac natura, magnas alimentorum sortiantur differentias, alibi suaviores, alibi lutulentiores.
[5] Observat. 16, lib. 10.

PAGE 221

[1] Pseudolus, Act. 3, sc. 2.   [2] Plautus, ibid.
[3] Quare rectius valetudini suæ quisque consulet, qui lapsus priorum parentum memor, eas plane vel omiserit vel parce degustarit.—Kersleius, cap. 4 de vero usu med.
[4] In Mizaldo de Horto, P. Crescent., Herbastein, etc.
[5] Cap. 13, part. 3, Bright in his Tract of Melancholy.
[6] Intellectum turbant, producunt insaniam.
[7] Audivi (inquit Magnin.) quod si quis ex iis per annum continue comedat, in insaniam caderet (cap. 13). Improbi succi sunt (cap. 12).

PAGE 222

[1] De rerum varietat. In Fessa plerumque morbosi, quod fructus comedant ter in die.
[2] Cap. de Mel. [3] Lib. 11, cap. 3.
[4] Bright, cap. 6, excepts honey. [5] Hor. apud Scoltzium, consil. 186.
[6] Ne comedas crustam, choleram quia gignit adustam.—Schol. Sal.

PAGE 223

[1] Vinum turbidum.
[2] Ex vini potentis bibitione, duo Alemanni in uno mense melancholici facti sunt.
[3] Hildesheim, Spicil. fol. 273. [4] Crassum generat sanguinem.
[5] About Dantzic in Spruce [Prussia], Hamburg, Leipsic.

PAGE 224

[1] Henricus Abrincensis.
[2] Potus tum salubris tum jucundus, l. 1.
[3] Galen, lib. 1 de san. tuend. Cavendæ sunt aquæ quæ ex stagnis hauriuntur, et quæ turbidæ et male olentes, etc.
[4] Innoxium reddit et bene olentem.
[5] Contendit hæc vitia coctione non emendari.
[6] Lib. de bonitate aquæ. Hydropem auget, febres putridas, splenem, tusses, nocet oculis, malum habitum corporis et colorem.
[7] [Vardar.] [8] Mag. Nigritatem inducit si pecora biberint.

PAGE 225

[1] Aquæ ex nivibus coactæ strumosos faciunt.
[2] Cosmog. lib. 3, cap. 36.
[3] Method. hist. cap. 5. Balbutiunt Labdoni in Aquitania ob aquas, atque hi morbi ab aquis in corpora derivantur.
[4] Edulia ex sanguine et suffocato parta.—Hildesheim.
[5] Cupedia vero, placentæ, bellaria, commentaque alia curiosa pistorum et coquorum gustui servientium, conciliant morbos tum corpori tum animo insanabiles.—Philo Judæus, lib. de victimis.
[6] P. Jov. vita ejus.
[7] As lettuce steeped in wine, birds fed with fennel and sugar, as a Pope's concubine used in Avignon.—Stephan.
[8] Animæ negotium illa facessit, et de templo Dei immundum stabulum facit.—Pelezius, cap. 10.
[9] Lib. 11, cap. 52. Homini cibus utilissimus simplex, acervatio ciborum pestifera, et condimenta perniciosa, multos morbos multa fercula ferunt.

PAGE 226

[1] Dec. 31, cap. 2. Nihil deterius quam si tempus justo longius comedendo protrahatur, et varia ciborum genera conjungantur: inde morborum scaturigo, quæ ex repugnantia humorum oritur.
[2] Path. lib. 1, cap. 14. [3] Juv. Sat. 1.
[4] Nimia repletio ciborum facit melancholicum.
[5] Comestio superflua cibi, et potus quantitas nimia.
[6] Impura corpora, quanto magis nutris, tanto magis lædis: putrefacit enim alimentum vitiosus humor.
[7] Vid. Goclen. de portentosis cœnis, etc., Puteani Com.
[8] Amb. lib. de jeju. cap. 14. [9] Juvenal. [10] Guicciardine.
[11] Nat. quæst. 4, cap. ult. Fastidio est lumen gratuitum, dolet quod sole, quod spiritum emere non possimus, quod hic aer non emptus ex facili, etc., adeo nihil placet, nisi quod carum est.
[12] Ingeniosi ad gulam.

Page 227

[1] Olim vile mancipium, nunc in omni æstimatione, nunc ars haberi cœpta, etc.
[2] Epist. 28, lib. 7. Quorum in ventre ingenium, in patinis, etc.
[3] In lucem cœnat Sertorius. [4] Seneca.
[5] Mancipia gulæ, dapes non sapore sed sumptu æstimantes.—Seneca, Consol. ad Helviam.
[6] Sævientia guttura satiare non possunt fluvii et maria.—Æneas Sylvius, de miser. curial. [7] Plautus.

Page 228

[1] Hor. lib. 1, sat. 3.
[2] Diei brevitas conviviis, noctis longitudo stupris conterebatur.
[3] Et quo plus capiant, irritamenta excogitantur.
[4] Foras portantur ut ad convivium reportentur, repleri ut exhauriant, et exhauriri ut bibant.—Ambros.
[5] Ingentia vasa velut ad ostentationem, etc. [6] Plautus.

Page 229

[1] Lib. 3 Anthol. cap. 20. [2] Gratiam conciliant potando.
[3] Notis ad Cæsares. [4] Lib. de educandis principum liberis.
[5] Virg. Æn. 1.
[6] Idem strenui potatoris episcopi sacellanus, cum ingentem pateram exhaurit princeps.
[7] Bohemus in Saxonia. Adeo immoderate et immodeste ab ipsis bibitur, ut in compotationibus suis non cyathis solum et cantharis sat infundere possint, sed impletum mulctrale apponant, et scutella injecta hortantur quemlibet ad libitum potare.
[8] Dictu incredibile, quantum hujusce liquoris immodesta gens capiat, plus potantem amicissimum habent, et serto coronant, inimicissimum e contra qui non vult, et cæde et fustibus expiant.
[9] Qui potare recusat, hostis habetur, et cæde nonnunquam res expiatur.
[10] Qui melius bibit pro salute domini, melior habetur minister.
[11] Græc. poeta apud Stobæum, ser. 18.

Page 230

[1] Qui de die jejunant, et nocte vigilant, facile cadunt in melancholiam; et qui naturæ modum excedunt, cap. 5, tract. 15; cap. 2: Longa famis tolerantia, ut iis sæpe accidit qui tanto cum fervore Deo servire cupiunt per jejunium, quod maniaci efficiantur, ipse vidi sæpe.
[2] In tenui victu ægri delinquunt, ex quo fit ut majori afficiantur detrimento, majorque fit error tenui quam pleniore victu.
[3] Quæ longo tempore consueta sunt, etiamsi deteriora, minus in assuetis molestare solent.
[4] Qui medice vivit, misere vivit. [5] Consuetudo altera natura.
[6] Herefordshire, Gloucestershire, Worcestershire.
[7] Leo Afer, lib. 1. Solo camelorum lacte contenti, nil præterea deliciarum ambiunt.

Page 231

[1] Flandri vinum butyro dilutum bibunt (nauseo referens), ubique butyrum, inter omnia fercula et bellaria locum obtinet.—Steph. præfat. Herod.
[2] Delectantur Græci piscibus magis quam carnibus.
[3] Lib. 1 Hist. Ang.
[4] P. Jovius, Descript. Britonum. They sit, eat and drink all day at dinner in Iceland, Muscovy, and those northern parts.
[5] Suidas, vit. Herod. Nihilo cum eo melius quam si quis cicutam, aconitum, etc.

⁶ Expedit. in Sinas, lib. 1, cap. 3. Hortensium herbarum et olerum apud Sinas quam apud nos longe frequentior usus, complures quippe de vulgo reperias nulla alia re vel tenuitatis, vel religionis causa vescentes. Equos, mulos, asellos, etc., æque fere vescuntur ac pabula omnia.—Mat. Riccius, lib. 5, cap. 12.

⁷ Tartari mulis, equis vescuntur et crudis carnibus, et fruges contemnunt, dicentes hoc jumentorum pabulum et boum, non hominum.

⁸ [Peking.]

⁹ Islandiæ descriptione. Victus eorum butyro, lacte, caseo consistit: pisces loco panis habent, potus aqua, aut serum, sic vivunt sine medicina multi ad annos 200.

¹⁰ Laet. occident. Ind. descrip. lib. 11, cap. 10. Aquam marinam bibere sueti absque noxa.

¹¹ Davies' second voyage.   ¹² Patagones.

¹³ Benzo et Fer. Cortesius, lib. Novus Orbis inscrip.

¹⁴ Linschoten, cap. 56. Palmæ instar totius orbis arboribus longe præstantior.

PAGE 232

¹ Lips. epist.   ² Teneris assuescere multum.

³ Repentinæ mutationes noxam pariunt.—Hippocrat. Aphorism. 21, Epist. 6, sect. 3.

⁴ Bruerinus, lib. 1, cap. 23.   ⁵ Simpl. med. cap. 4, lib. 1.

⁶ Heurnius, lib. 3, cap. 19, Prax. med.   ⁷ Aphoris. 17.

⁸ In dubiis consuetudinem sequatur adolescens, et inceptis perseveret.

PAGE 233

¹ Qui cum voluptate assumuntur cibi, ventriculus avidius complectitur, expeditiusque concoquit, et quæ displicent aversatur.

² Nothing against a good stomach, as the saying is.

³ Lib. 7 Hist. Scot.   ⁴ 30 Artis.

⁵ Quæ excernuntur aut subsistunt.

⁶ Ex ventre suppresso, inflammationes, capitis dolores, caligines crescunt.

⁷ Excrementa retenta mentis agitationem parere solent.

⁸ Cap. de mel.   ⁹ Tam delirus, ut vix se hominem agnosceret.

PAGE 234

¹ Alvus astrictus causa.

² Per octo dies alvum siccum habet, et nihil reddit.

³ Sive per nares, sive hæmorrhoides.

⁴ Multi intempestive ab hæmorrhoidibus curati, melancholia corrupti sunt. Incidit in Scyllam, etc.

⁵ Lib. 1 de mania.   ⁶ Breviar. lib. 7, cap. 18.

⁷ Non sine magno incommodo ejus, cui sanguis a naribus promanat, noxii sanguinis vacuatio impediri potest.

⁸ Novi quosdam præ pudore a coitu abstinentes, torpidos pigrosque factos; nonnullos etiam melancholicos, præter modum mœstos timidosque.

⁹ Nonnulli nisi coeant, assidue capitis gravitate infestantur. Dicit se novisse quosdam tristes et ita factos ex intermissione Veneris.

¹⁰ Vapores venenatos mittit sperma ad cor et cerebrum.

¹¹ Sperma plus diu retentum transit in venenum.

¹² Graves producit corporis et animi ægritudines.

PAGE 235

¹ Ex spermate supra modum retento monachos et viduas melancholicos sæpe fieri vidi.

² Melancholia orta a vasis seminariis in utero.

³ Nobilis senex Alsatus juvenem uxorem duxit, at ille, colico dolore et

multis morbis correptus, non potuit præstare officium mariti, vix inito matrimonio ægrotus. Illa in horrendum furorum incidit, ob Venerem cohibitam ut omnium eam invisentium congressum, voce, vultu, gestu expeteret, et quum non consentirent, molossos Anglicanos magno expetiit clamore.

[4] Vidi sacerdotem optimum et pium, qui, quod nollet uti Venere, in melancholica symptomata incidit.

[5] Ob abstinentiam a concubitu incidit in melancholiam.

[6] Quæ a coitu exacerbantur.

[7] Superfluum coitum causam ponunt.

[8] Exsiccat corpus, spiritus consumit, etc. Caveant ab hoc sicci, velut inimico mortali.

PAGE 236

[1] Ita exsiccatus ut e melancholico statim fuerit insanus; ab humectantibus curatus.

[2] Ex cauterio et ulcere exsiccato.

[3] Gord., cap. 10, lib. 1, discommends cold baths as noxious.

[4] Siccum reddunt corpus.

[5] Si quis longius moretur in iis, aut nimis frequenter, aut importune utatur, humores putrefacit.

[6] Ego anno superiore quendam guttosum vidi adustum, qui ut liberaretur de gutta, ad balnea accessit, et de gutta liberatus, maniacus factus est.

[7] On Schola Salernitana.

[8] Calefactio et ebullitio per venæ incisionem magis sæpe incitatur et augetur, majore impetu humores per corpus discurrunt.

[9] Lib. de flatulenta melancholia. Frequens sanguinis missio corpus extenuat.

[10] In 9 Rhasis. Atram bilem parit, et visum debilitat.

PAGE 237

[1] Multo nigrior spectatur sanguis post dies quosdam, quam fuit ab initio.

[2] Non laudo eos qui in desipientia docent secandam esse venam frontis, quia spiritus debilitatur inde, et ego longa experientia observavi in proprio xenodochio, quod desipientes ex phlebotomia magis læduntur, et magis desipiunt, et melancholici sæpe fiunt inde pejores.

[3] De mentis alienat. cap. 3. Etsi multos hoc improbasse sciam, innumeros hac ratione sanatos longa observatione cognovi, qui vigesies, sexagies venas tundendo, etc.

[4] Vires debilitat.

[5] Impurus aer spiritus dejicit, infecto corde gignit morbos.

[6] Sanguinem densat, et humores.—Path. lib. 1, cap. 13.

[7] Lib. 3, cap. 3.

[8] Lib. de quartana. Ex aere ambiente contrahitur humor melancholicus.

[9] Qualis aer, talis spiritus: et cujusmodi spiritus, humores.

[10] Ælianus Montaltus, cap. 11, Calidus et siccus, frigidus et siccus, paludinosus, crassus.

PAGE 238

[1] Multa hic in xenodochiis fanaticorum millia quæ strictissime catenata servantur.

[2] Lib. med. part. 2, cap. 19. Intellige quod in calidis regionibus frequenter accidit mania, in frigidis autem tarde.

[3] Lib. 2.   [4] Hodœporicon, cap. 7.

[5] Apulia æstivo calore maxime fervet, ita ut ante finem Maii pene exusta sit.   [6] Maginus, Pers.

[7] Pantheo seu Pract. med. lib. 1, cap. 16. Venetæ mulieres, quæ diu sub sole vivunt; aliquando melancholicæ evadunt.

⁸ Navig. lib. 2, cap. 4.   Commercia nocte, hora secunda, ob nimios qui sæviunt interdiu æstus, exercent.
⁹ Morbo Gallico laborantes exponunt ad solem ut morbos exsiccent.

PAGE 239

¹ Sir Richard Hawkins in his Observations, sect. 13.
² Hippocrates, 3 Aphorismorum, idem ait.
³ [Diarbekr.]   ⁴ Idem Maginus in Persia.   ⁵ Descrip. Ter. Sanctæ.
⁶ Quum ad solis radios in Leone longam moram traheret, ut capillos salvos redderet, in maniam incidit.
⁷ Mundus Alter et Idem, seu Terra Australis Incognita.   [Joseph Hall's satirical Utopia, published in 1607, under the name of Mercurius Britannicus.]
⁸ Crassus et turbidus aer tristem efficit animam.
⁹ Commonly called Scandaroon in Asia Minor.
¹⁰ [The Pontine Marshes.]

PAGE 240

¹ Atlas Geographicus.   Memoria valent Pisani, quod crassiore fruantur aere.
² Lib. 1 Hist.
³ Lib. 2, cap. 41: Aura densa ac caliginosa tetrici homines existunt, et subtristes. Et cap. 3: Flante subsolano et Zephyro, maxima in mentibus hominum alacritas existit, mentisque erecto ubi telum solis splendore nitescit.   Maxima dejectio mærorque si quando aura caliginosa est.
⁴ Geor.

PAGE 241

¹ Hor.
² Mens quibus vacillat, ab aere cito offenduntur, et multi insani apud Belgas ante tempestates sæviunt, aliter quieti.   Spiritus quoque aeris et mali genii aliquando se tempestatibus ingerunt, et menti humanæ se latenter insinuant, eamque vexant, exagitant, et ut fluctus marin humanum corpus ventis agitatur
³ Aer noctu densatur, et cogit mœstitiam.
⁴ Lib. de Iside et Osiride.
⁵ Multa defatigatio spiritus viriumque substantiam exhaurit, et corpus refrigerat.   Humores corruptos qui aliter a natura concoqui et domari possint, et demum blande excludi, irritat, et quasi in furorem agit, qui postea, mota Camarina, tetro vapore corpus varie lacessunt, animumque.

PAGE 242

¹ In Veni mecum, libro sic inscripto.
² Instit. ad vit. Christ. cap. 44. Cibos crudos in venas rapit, qui putrescentes illic spiritus animales inficiunt.
³ Crudi hæc humoris copia per venas aggreditur, unde morbi multiplices.
⁴ Immodicum exercitium.
⁵ Hom. 31, in 1 Cor. vi.   Nam qua mens hominis quiescere non possit, sed continuo circa varias cogitationes discurrat, nisi honesto aliquo negotio occupetur, ad melancholiam sponte delabitur.
⁶ Crato, consil. 21.   Ut immodica corporis exercitatio nocet corporibus, ita vita deses et otiosa: otium animal pituitosum reddit, viscerum obstructiones, et crebras fluxiones, et morbos concitat.
⁷ Et vidi quod una de rebus quæ magis generat melancholiam, est otiositas.
⁸ Reponitur otium ab aliis causa, et hoc a nobis observatum eos huic malo magis obnoxios qui plane otiosi sunt, quam eos qui aliquo munere versantur exsequendo.

[9] De tranquil. animæ. Sunt quos ipsum otium in animi conjicit ægritudinem.

[10] Nihil est quod æque melancholiam alat ac augeat, ac otium et abstinentia a corporis et animi exercitationibus.

[11] Nihil magis excæcat intellectum quam otium.—Gordonius, de observat. vit. hum. lib. 1.

PAGE 243

[1] Path. lib. 1, cap. 17. Exercitationis intermissio, inertem calorem, languidos spiritus, et ignavos, et ad omnes actiones segniores reddit; cruditates, obstructiones, et excrementorum proventus facit.

[2] Hor. Ser. 1, sat. 3.

[3] Seneca. [4] Mœrorem animi, et maciem, Plutarch calls it.

[5] [The greatest harm to the soul.]

[6] Sicut in stagno generantur vermes, sic et otioso malæ cogitationes.—Sen.

PAGE 244

[1] Now this leg, now that arm, now their head, heart, etc.

[2] Exod. v.

[3] (For they cannot well tell what aileth them, or what they would have themselves) my heart, my head, my husband, my son, etc.

[4] Prov. xviii. Pigrum dejiciet timor. Heautontimorumenos.

[5] Lib. 19, cap. 10.

PAGE 245

[1] Plautus, Prol. Mostel.

[2] Piso, Montaltus, Mercurialis, etc.

PAGE 246

[1] A quibus malum, velut a primaria causa, occasionem nactum est.

[2] Jucunda rerum præsentium, præteritarum, et futurarum meditatio.

PAGE 247

[1] Facilis descensus Averni: Sed revocare gradum, superasque evadere ad auras, Hic labor, hoc opus est.—Virg.

[2] Hieronymus, ep. 72, dixit oppida et urbes videri sibi tetros carceres, solitudinem Paradisum: solum scorpionibus infectum, sacco amictus, humi cubans, aqua et herbis victitans, Romanis prætulit deliciis.

PAGE 248

[1] Offic. 3. [2] Eccles. iv.

PAGE 249

[1] Natura de te videtur conqueri posse, quod cum ab ea temperatissimum corpus adeptus sis, tam præclarum a Deo ac utile donum, non contempsisti modo, verum corrupisti, fœdasti, prodidisti, optimam temperaturam otio, crapula, et aliis vitæ erroribus, etc.

[2] Path. lib. cap. 17 Fernel. Corpus infrigidat, omnes sensus, mentisque vires, torpore debilitat.

[3] Lib. 2, sect. 2, cap. 4. Magnam excrementorum vim cerebro et aliis partibus conservat.

[4] Jo. Ratzius, lib. de rebus 6 non naturalibus. Præparat corpus talis somnus ad multis periculosas ægritudines.

PAGE 250

[1] Instit. ad vitam optimam, cap. 26. Cerebro siccitatem adfert, phrenesin et delirium, corpus aridum facit, squalidum, strigosum, humores adurit, temperamentum cerebri corrumpit, maciem inducit: exsiccat corpus, bilem accendit, profundos reddit oculos, calorem auget.

² Naturalem calorem dissipat, læsa concoctione cruditates facit. Attenuant juvenum vigilatæ corpora noctes.

³ Vita Alexan. ⁴ Grad. 1, cap. 14. ⁵ Hor.

⁶ Perturbationes clavi sunt, quibus corpori animus seu patibulo affigitur. —Iambl. de myst.

⁷ Lib. de sanitat. tuend.

PAGE 251

¹ Prolog. de virtute Christi. Quæ utitur corpore, ut faber malleo.

² Vita Apollonii, lib. 1.

³ Lib. de anim. Ab inconsiderantia et ignorantia omnes animi motus.

⁴ De Physiol. Stoic. ⁵ Grad. 1, cap. 32.

⁶ Epist. 104. ⁷ Ælianus.

⁸ Lib. 1, cap. 6. Si quis ense percusserit eos, tantum respiciunt.

⁹ Terror in sapiente esse non debet.

¹⁰ De occult nat. mir. lib. 1, cap. 16. Nemo mortalium qui affectibus non ducatur: qui non movetur, aut saxum, aut deus est.

¹¹ Instit. lib. 2, de humanorum affect. morborumque curat.

¹² Epist. 105. ¹³ Granatensis. ¹⁴ Virg.

¹⁵ De Civit. Dei, lib. 14, cap. 9. Qualis in oculis hominum qui inversis pedibus ambulat, talis in oculis sapientum, cui passiones dominantur.

PAGE 252

¹ Lib. de Decal. Passiones maxime corpus offendunt et animam, et frequentissimæ causæ melancholiæ, dimoventes ab ingenio et sanitate pristina (lib. 3, de anima).

² Fræna et stimuli animi, velut in mari quædam auræ leves, quædam placidæ, quædam turbulentæ: sic in corpore quædam affectiones excitant tantum, quædam ita movent, ut de statu judicii depellant.

³ Ut gutta lapidem, sic paulatim hæ penetrant animum.

⁴ Usu valentes recte morbi animi vocantur.

⁵ Imaginatio movet corpus, ad cujus motum excitantur humores, et spiritus vitales, quibus alteratur.

⁶ Eccles. xiii, 26. "The heart alters the countenance to good or evil, and distraction of the mind causeth distemperature of the body."

⁷ Spiritus et sanguis a læsa imaginatione contaminantur, humores enim mutati actiones animi immutant.—Piso.

⁸ Montani consil. 22. Hæ vero quomodo causent melancholiam, clarum; et quod concoctionem impediant, et membra principalia debilitent.

PAGE 253

¹ Breviar. lib. 1, cap. 18.

² Solent hujusmodi egressiones favorabiliter oblectare, et lectorem lassum jucunde refovere, stomachumque neauseantem quodam quasi condimento reficere, et ego libenter excurro.

³ Ab imaginatione oriuntur affectiones, quibus anima componitur, aut turbata deturbatur.—Jo. Sarisbur. Metolog. lib. 4, cap. 10.

⁴ Scalig. exercit.

PAGE 254

¹ Qui, quoties volebat, mortuo similis jacebat, auferens se a sensibus, et quum pungeretur dolorem non sensit.

² Idem Nymannus, Orat. de imaginat.

³ Verbis et unctionibus se consecrant dæmoni pessimæ mulieres qui iis ad opus suum utitur, et earum phantasiam regit, ducitque ad loca ab ipsis desiderata, corpora vero earum sine sensu permanent, quæ umbra cooperit diabolus, ut nulli sint conspicua, et post, umbra sublata, propriis corporibus eas restituit.—Wier. lib. 3, cap. 11.

[4] Denario medico.

[5] Solet timor, præ omnibus affectibus, fortes imaginationes gignere; post amor, etc.—Lib. 2, cap. 8.

[6] Ex viso urso, talem peperit.

PAGE 255

[1] Lib. 1, cap. 4, de occult. nat. mir. Si inter amplexus et suavia cogitet de uno, aut alio absente, ejus effigies solet in fœtu elucere.

[2] Quid non fœtui adhuc matri unito, subita spirituum vibratione per nervos, quibus matrix cerebro conjuncta est, imprimit impregnatæ imaginatio? ut si imaginetur malum granatum, illius notas secum proferet fœtus : si leporem, infans editur supremo labello bifido et dissecto. Vehemens cogitatio movet rerum species.—Wier. lib. 3, cap. 8.

[3] Ne, dum uterum gestent, admittant absurdas cogitationes, sed et visu audituque fœda et horrenda devitent.

[4] Occult. Philos. lib. 1, cap. 64.

[5] Lib. 3 de lamiis, cap. 10.   [6] Agrippa, lib. 1, cap. 64.

[7] Sect. 3, memb. 1, subsect. 3.

[8] Malleus malefic. fol. 77. Corpus mutari potest in diversas ægritudines, ex forti apprehensione.

[9] Fr. Vales. lib. 5, cont. 6. Nonnunquam etiam morbi diuturnic onsequuntur, quandoque curantur.

PAGE 256

[1] Expedit. in Sinas, lib. 1, cap. 9. Tantum porro multi prædictoribus hisce tribuunt ut ipse metus fidem faciat: nam si prædictum iis fuerit tali die eos morbo corripiendos, ii ubi dies advenerit, in morbum incidunt, et vi metus afflicti, cum ægritudine, aliquando etiam cum morte, colluctantur.

[2] Subtil. 18.

[3] Lib. 3 de anima, cap. de mel.   [4] Lib. de peste.

[5] Lib. 1, cap. 63. Ex alto despicientes aliqui præ timore contremiscunt, caligant, infirmantur; sic singultus, febres, morbi comitiales quandoque sequuntur, quandoque recedunt.

[6] Lib. de incantatione. Imaginatio subitum humorum et spirituum motum infert, under vario affectu rapitur sanguis, ac una morbificas causas partibus affectis eripit.

PAGE 257

[1] Lib. 3, cap. 18, de præstig. Ut impia credulitate quis læditur, sic et levari eundem credibile est, usuque observatum.

[2] Ægri persuasio et fiducia omni arti et consilio et medicinæ præferenda. —Avicen.

[3] Plures sanat in quem plures confidunt.—Lib. de sapientia.

[4] Marsilius Ficinus, lib. 13, cap. 18, de theologia Platonica. Imaginatio est tanquam Proteus vel chamæleon, corpus proprium et alienum nonnunquam afficiens.

[5] Cur oscitantes oscitent?—Wierus.

PAGE 258

[1] T[homas] W[right], Jesuit.   [2] 3 de anima.

[3] Ser. 35. Hæ quatuor passiones sunt tanquam rotæ in curru, quibus vehimur hoc mundo.

[4] Harum quippe immoderatione spiritus marcescunt.—Fernel. lib. 1 Path. cap. 18.

[5] Mala consuetudine depravatur ingenium ne bene faciat.—Prosper Calenus, lib. de atra bile. Plura faciunt homines e consuetudine, quam e ratione. A teneris assuescere multum est. Video meliora proboque, deteriora sequor.—Ovid.

NOTES 489

Page 259

[1] Nemo læditur nisi a seipso.

[2] Multi se in inquietudinem præcipitant ambitione et cupiditatibus excæcati, non intelligunt se illud a diis petere, quod sibi ipsis si velint præstare possint, si curis et perturbationibus, quibus assidue se macerant, imperare vellent.

[3] Tanto studio miseriarum causas, et alimenta dolorum quærimus, vitamque secus felicissimam, tristem et miserabilem efficimus.—Petrarch. præfat. de Remediis, etc.

[4] Timor et mœstitia, si diu perseverent, causa et soboles atri humoris sunt, et in circulum se procreant.—Hip. Aphoris. 23, lib. 6. Idem Montaltus, cap. 19, Victorius Faventinus, Pract. imag.

[5] Multi ex mærore et metu huc delapsi sunt.—Lemn. lib. 1, cap. 16.

[6] Multa cura et tristitia facinnt accedere melancholiam (cap. 3 de mentis alien.); si altas radices agat, in veram fixamque degenerat melancholiam et in desperationem desinit.

[7] Ille luctus, ejus vero soror desperatio simul ponitur.

[8] Animarum crudele tormentum, dolor inexplicabilis, tinea, non solum ossa, sed corda pertingens, perpetuus carnifex, vires animæ consumens, jugis nox, et tenebræ profundæ, tempestas et turbo et febris non apparens, omni igne validius incendens; longior, et pugnæ finem non habens. . . . Crucem circumfert dolor, faciemque omni tyranno crudeliorem præ se fert.

[9] Nat. Comes, Mythol. lib. 4, cap. 6.

[10] Tully, 3 Tusc. Omnis perturbatio miseria, et carnificina est dolor.

Page 260

[1] Mr. Drayton, in his Heroical Epistles.

[2] Crato, consil. 21, lib. 2. Mœstitia universum infrigidat corpus, calorem innatum extinguit, appetitum destruit.

[3] Cor refrigerat tristitia, spiritus exsiccat, innatumque calorem obruit, vigilias inducit, concoctionem labefactat, sanguinem incrassat, exaggeratque melancholicum succum.

[4] Spiritus et sanguis hoc contaminatur.—Piso.

[5] Luke xxii, 44.

[6] Mærore maceror, marcesco et consenesco miser, ossa atque pellis sum misera macritudine.—Plaut.

[7] Malum inceptum et actum a tristitia sola.

[8] Hildesheim, Spicil. 2 de melancholia. Mærore animi postea accedente, in priora symptomata incidit.

[9] Vives, 3 de anima, cap. de mærore. Sabin. in Ovid.

[10] Herodian, lib. 3. Mærore magis quam morbo consumptus est.

[11] Bothwellius atrabilarius obiit.—Brizarrus Genuensis, hist., etc.

Page 261

[1] Mœstitia cor quasi percussum constringitur, tremit et languescit cum acri sensu doloris. In tristitia cor fugiens attrahit ex splene lentum humorem melancholicum, qui effusus sub costis in sinistro latere hypochondriacos flatus facit, quod sæpe accidit iis qui diuturna cura et mœstitia conflictantur.—Melancthon.

[2] Lib. 3 Æn.

[3] Et metum ideo deam sacrarunt ut bonam mentem concederet. Varro, Lactantius, Aug.

[4] Lilius Girald. Syntag. 1, de diis miscellaniis.

[5] Calendis Jan. feriæ sunt divæ Angeronæ, cui pontifices in sacello Volupiæ sacra faciunt, quod angores et animi sollicitudines propitiata propellat.

[6] Timor inducit frigus, cordis palpitationem, vocis defectum atque

pallorem.—Agrippa, lib. 1, cap. 63. Timidi semper spiritus habent frigidos.
—Mont.

[7] [Jupiter the Tragedian, in the dialogue of that name.]
[8] Effusas cernens fugientes agmine turmas, Quis mea nunc inflat cornua?
Faunus ait.—Alciat.

PAGE 262

[1] Metus non solum memoriam consternat, sed et institutum animi
omne et laudabilem conatum impedit.—Thucydides.
[2] Lib. de fortitudine et virtute Alexandri. Ubi prope res adfuit terribilis.
[3] Sect. 2. mem. 3, subs. 2.   [4] Sect. 2, memb. 4, subs. 3.
[5] Subtil. lib. 18.   Timor attrahit ad se dæmonas. Timor et error multum
in hominibus possunt.
[6] Lib. 2 de spectris, cap. 3.   Fortes raro spectra vident, quia minus timent.
[7] Vita ejus.   [8] Sect. 2, memb. 4, subs. 7.   [9] De virt. et vitiis.
[10] Com. in Arist. de anima.

PAGE 263

[1] Qui mentem subjecit timoris dominationi, cupiditatis, doloris, ambitionis, pudoris, felix non est, sed omnino miser, assiduis laboribus torquetur
et miseria.
[2] Multi contemnunt mundi strepitum, reputant pro nihilo gloriam
sed timent infamiam, offensionem, epulsam. Voluptatem severissime,
contemnunt, in dolore sunt molliores, gloriam negligunt, franguntur
infamia.
[3] Gravius contumeliam ferimus quam detrimentum, ni abjecto nimis
animo simus.—Plut. in Timol.
[4] Quod piscatoris ænigma solvere non posset.
[5] Ob tragœdiam explosam, mortem sibi gladio conscivit.
[6] Cum vidit in triumphum se servari, causa ejus ignominiæ mortem sibi
conscivit.—Plut.
[7] Bello victus, per tres dies sedit in prora navis, abstinens ab omni
consortio, etiam Cleopatræ; postea se interfecit.
[8] Cum male recitasset Argonautica, ob pudorem exulavit.
[9] Quidam præ verecundia simul et dolore in insaniam incidunt, eo
quod a literatorum gradu in examine excluduntur.
[10] Hostratus cucullatus adeo graviter ob Reuclini librum, qui inscribitur
Epistolæ obscurorum virorum, dolore simul et pudore sauciatus, ut seipsum
interfecerit.

PAGE 264

[1] Propter ruborem confusus, statim cœpit delirare, etc., ob suspicionem,
quod vili illum crimine accusarent.
[2] Horat.
[3] Ps. Impudice. B. Ita est. Ps. Sceleste. B. Dicis vera. Ps. Verbero. B.
Quippeni? Ps. Furcifer. B. Factum optime. Ps. Sociofraude. B. Sunt
mea istæc. Ps. Parricida. B. Perge tu. Ps. Sacrilege. B. Fateor. Ps.
Perjure. B. Vera dicis. Ps. Pernicies adolescentum. B. Acerrime. Ps.
Fur. B. Babæ. Ps. Fugitive. B. Bombax. Ps. Fraus populi. B.
Planissime. Ps. Impure leno, cœnum. B. Cantores probos.—Pseudolus,
Act. 1, sc. 3.
[4] Persius, Sat. 5.   [5] Cent. 7, e Plinio.
[6] Multos videmus propter invidiam et odium in melancholiam incidisse:
et illos potissimum quorum corpora ad hanc apta sunt.
[7] Invidia affligit homines adeo et corrodit, ut hi melancholici penitus
fiant.   [8] Hor.
[9] His vultus minax, torvus aspectus, pallor in facie, in labiis tremor,
stridor in dentibus, etc.

PAGE 265

[1] Ut tinea corrodit vestimentum, sic invidia eum qui zelatur consumit.

[2] Pallor in ore sedet, macies in corpore toto. Nusquam recta acies, livent rubigine dentes.

[3] Diaboli expressa imago, toxicum caritatis, venenum amicitiæ, abyssus mentis, non est eo monstrosius monstrum, damnosius damnum; urit, torret, discruciat macie et squalore conficit.—Austin, Domin. prim. Advent. [4] Ovid.

[5] Declam. 13. Linivit flores maleficis succis in venenum mella convertens.

[6] Statuis cereis Basilius eos comparat, qui liquefiunt ad præsentiam solis, qua alii gaudent et ornantur. Muscis alii, quæ ulceribus gaudent, amœna prætereunt, sistunt in fœtidis.

[7] Misericordia etiam quæ tristitia quædam est, sæpe miserantis corpus male afficit.—Agrippa, lib. 1, cap. 63.

[8] Insitum mortalibus a natura recentem aliorum felicitatem ægris oculis intueri.—Hist. lib. 2, Tacit.

[9] Legi Chaldæos, Græcos, Hebræos, consului sapientes pro remedio invidiæ; hoc enim inveni, renuntiare felicitati, et perpetuo miser esse.

[10] Omne peccatum aut excusationem secum habet, aut voluptatem, sola invidia utraque caret. Reliqua vitia finem habent, ira defervescit, gula satiatur, odium finem habet, invidia nunquam quiescit.

PAGE 266

[1] Urebat me æmulatio propter stultos.

[2] Jer. xii, 1. [3] Hab. i.

[4] Invidit privati nomen supra principis attolli.

[5] Tacit. Hist. lib. 2. part. 6.

[6] Perituræ dolore et invidia, si quem viderint ornatiorem se in publicum prodiisse.—Platina, Dial. amorum.

[7] Ant. Gulanorius, lib. 2, cap. 8, vit. M. Aurelii. Femina vicinam elegantius se vestitam videns, leænæ instar in virum insurgit, etc.

[8] Quod insigni equo et ostro veheretur, quanquam nullius cum injuria, ornatum illum tanquam læsæ gravabantur.

[9] Quod pulchritudine omnes excelleret, puellæ indignatæ occiderunt.

[10] Late patet invidiæ fecundæ pernicies, et livor radix omnium malorum, fons cladium, inde odium surgit, emulatio.—Cyprian, ser. 2, de livore.

[11] Valerius, lib. 3, cap. 9.

[12] Qualis est animi tinea, quæ tabes pectoris, zelare in altero vel aliorum felicitatem suam facere miseriam, et velut quosdam pectori suo admovere carnifices, cogitationibus et sensibus suis adhibere tortores, qui se intestinis cruciatibus lacerent! Non cibus talibus lætus, non potus potest esse jucundus; suspiratur semper et gemitur, et doletur dies et noctes; pectus sine intermissione laceratur.

PAGE 267

[1] Quisquis est ille quem æmularis, cui invides is te subterfugere potest, at tu non te; ubicunque fugeris, adversarius tuus tecum est, hostis tuus semper in pectore tuo est, pernicies intus inclusa, ligatus es, victus, zelo dominante captivus: nec solatia tibi ulla subveniunt; hinc diabolus inter initia statim mundi, et periit primus, et perdidit.—Cyprian, ser. 2, de zelo et livore.

[2] Hesiod, Op. et Dies.

[3] Rana, cupida æquandi bovem, se distendebat, etc.

[4] Æmulatio alit ingenia.—Paterculus, poster. vol.

[5] Grotius, Epig. lib. 1.

PAGE 268

[1] Anno 1519, between Ardres and Guisnes.
[2] Spartian.   [3] Plutarch.
[4] Johannes Heraldus, lib. 2, cap. 12 de bello sacro.
[5] [See Catullus, 14, 3.   The allusion is to Cicero's vehement denunciation of Publius Vatinius.]
[6] Nulla dies tantum poterit lenire furorem. Æterna bella pace sublata gerunt. Jurat odium, nec ante invisum esse desinit, quam esse desiit.—Paterculus, vol. i.
[7] Carthago æmula Romani imperii funditus interiit.—Sallust. Catil.
[8] Ita sævit hæc Stygia ministra ut urbes subvertat aliquando, deleat populos, provincias alioqui florentes redigat in solitudines, mortales vero miseros in profunda miseriarum valle miserabiliter immergat.

PAGE 269

[1] Paul, Col. iii.   [2] Rom. xii.   [3] Grad. 1, cap. 54.
[4] Ira et mœror et ingens animi consternatio melancholicos facit.—Aretæus.   Ira immodica gignit insaniam.
[5] Reg. sanit. parte 2, cap. 8.   In apertam insaniam mox ducitur iratus.
[6] Gilberto Cognato interprete.   Multis, et præsertim senibus ira; impotens insaniam facit, et importuna calumnia; hæc initio perturbat animum, paulatim vergit ad insaniam. Porro mulierum corpora multa infestant, et in hunc morbum adducunt, præcipue si quæ oderint aut invideant, etc.; hæc paulatim in insaniam tandem evadunt.
[7] Sæva animi tempestas, tantos excitans fluctus ut statim ardescant oculi, os tremat, lingua titubet, dentes concrepant, etc.

PAGE 270

[1] Ovid.   [2] Terence.
[3] Infensus Britanniæ Duci, et in ultionem versus, nec cibum cepit, nec quietem; ad Calendas Julias, 1392, comites occidit. [Britain = Brittany.]
[4] Indignatione nimia furens, animique impotens, exsiliit de lecto, furentem non capiebat aula, etc.
[5] An ira possit hominem interimere.
[6] As Troy: sævæ memorem Junonis ob iram.
[7] Abernethy.
[8] Stultorum regum et populorum continet æstus.

PAGE 271

[1] Lib. 2.   Invidia est dolor, et ambitio est dolor, etc.
[2] Insomnes, Claudianus; tristes, Virg.; mordaces, Luc.; edaces, Hor.; mœstæ, amaræ, Ovid.; damnosæ, inquietæ, Mart.; urentes, rodentes, Mant., etc.
[3] Galen, lib. 3, cap. 7, de locis affectis.   Homines sunt maxime melancholici, quando vigiliis multis, et sollicitudinibus, et laboribus, et curis fuerint circumventi.
[4] Lucian. Podag.
[5] Omnia imperfecta, confusa, et perturbatione plena.—Cardan.

PAGE 272

[1] Lib. 7 Nat. hist. cap. 1. Hominem nudum, et ad vagitum edit natura. Flens ab initio, devinctus jacet, etc.
[2] Δακρυχέων γενόμην καὶ δακρύσας ἀποθνήσκω, ὦ γένος ἀνθρώπων πολυδάκρυτον, ἀσθενές, οἰκτρόν. Lacrimans natus sum, et lacrimans morior, etc.
[3] Ad Marciam.   [4] Boethius.
[5] Initium cæcitas, progressus labor, exitus dolor, error omnia: quem tranquillum, quæso, quem non laboriosum aut anxium diem egimus?—Petrarch.

NOTES

[1] Ubique periculum, ubique dolor, ubique naufragium, in hoc ambitu quocunque me vertam.—Lipsius.

[2] Hom. 10. Si in forum iveris, ibi rixæ et pugnæ; si in curiam, ibi fraus, adulatio; si in domum privatam, etc.

[3] Homer.

[4] Multis repletur homo miseriis, corporis miseriis, animi miseriis, dum dormit, dum vigilat, quocunque se vertit. Lususque rerum temporumque nascimur.

[5] In blandiente fortuna intolerandi, in calamitatibus lugubres, semper stulti et miseri.—Cardan.

[6] Prospera in adversis desidero, et adversa prosperis timeo, quis inter hæc medius locus, ubi non fit humanæ vitæ tentatio?

[7] Cardan, Consol. Sapientiæ labor annexus, gloriæ invidia, divitiis curæ, soboli sollicitudo, voluptati morbi, quieti paupertas, ut quasi fruendorum scelerum causa nasci hominem possis cum Platonistis agnoscere.

[8] Lib. 7, cap. 1. Non satis æstimare, an melior parens natura homini, an tristior noverca fuerit: nulli fragilior vita, pavor, confusio, rabies major; uni animantium ambitio data, luctus, avaritia, uni superstitio.

[9] Euripides.

[10] De consol. lib. 2. Nemo facile cum conditione sua concordat; inest singulis quod imperiti petant, experti horreant.

[11] Esse in honore juvat, mox displicet. [12] Hor.

[1] Borrhæus, in 6 Job. Urbes et oppida nihil aliud sunt quam humanarum ærumnarum domicilia, quibus luctus et mœror, et mortalium varii infinitique labores, et omnis generis vitia, quasi septis includuntur.

[2] Nat. Chytræus, de lit. Europæ. Lætus nunc, mox tristis; nunc sperans, paulo post diffidens; patiens hodie, cras ejulans; nunc pallens, rubens, currens, sedens, claudicans, tremens, etc.

[3] See. p 347.

[4] Sua cuique calamitas præcipua. [5] Cn. Græcinus.

[6] Epist. 9, lib. 7. Miser est qui se beatissimum non judicat; licet imperet mundo non est beatus, qui se non putat: quid enim refert qualis status tuus sit, si tibi videtur malus?

[7] Hor. Ep. lib. 1, 14.

[1] Hor. Ser. 1, sat. 1.

[2] Lib. de curat. Græc. affect. cap. 6, de provident. Multis nihil placet; atque adeo et divitias damnant, et paupertatem; de morbis expostulant, bene valentes graviter ferunt, atque, ut semel dicam, nihil eos delectat, etc.

[3] Vix ullius gentis, ætatis, ordinis, hominem invenies cujus felicitatem fortunæ Metelli compares.—Vol. 1.

[4] P. Crassus Mutianus quinque habuisse dicitur rerum bonarum maxima, quod esset ditissimus, quod esset nobilissimus, eloquentissimus, jurisconsultissimus, pontifex maximus.

[5] Lib. 7. Regis filia, regis uxor, regis mater.

[6] Qui nihil unquam mali aut dixit, aut fecit, aut sensit, qui bene semper fecit, quod aliter facere non potuit.

[7] Solomon, Eccles. i, 14. [8] Hor. Art. Poet.

[1] Jovius, vita ejus. [Gonsalvo de Cordova, "The Great Captain' (1453–1515).]

[2] 2 Sam: xii, 31. [3] Boethius, lib. 1, Met. 1.

I—R 886

[4] Omnes hic aut captantur, aut captant: aut cadavera quæ lacerantur, aut corvi qui lacerant.—Petron.

[5] Homo omne monstrum est, ille nam superat feras, luposque et ursos pectore obscuro tegit.—Heins.

Page 277

[1] Quod Paterculus de populo Romano, durante bello Punico per annos 115, aut bellum inter eos, aut belli præparatio, aut infida pax, idem ego de mundi accolis.

[2] Theocritus, Idyll. 15.

[3] Qui sedet in mensa, non meminit sibi otioso ministrare negotiosos, edenti esurientes, bibenti sitientes, etc.

[4] Quando in adolescentia sua ipsi vixerint lautius, et liberius voluptates suas expleverint, illi gnatis imponunt duriores continentiæ leges.

Page 278

[1] Lugubris Ate luctusque ferus Regum tumidas obsidet arces. Res est inquieta felicitas.

[2] Plus aloes quam mellis habet.—Juv. Non humi jacentem tolleres.—Valer. lib. 7, cap. 3.

[3] Non diadema aspicias, sed vitam afflictione refertam, non catervas satellitum, sed curarum multitudinem.

[4] As Plutarch relateth.

[5] Sect. 2, memb. 4, subsect. 6.

[6] Stercus et urina, medicorum fercula prima.

[7] Nihil lucrantur, nisi admodum mentiendo.—Tull. Offic.

[8] Hor. lib. 2, Od. 1.

Page 279

[1] Rarus felix idemque senex.—Seneca, in Herc. Œtæo.

[2] Omitto ægros, exsules, mendicos, quos nemo audet felices dicere.—Card. lib. 8, cap. 46, de rer. var.

[3] Spretæque injuria formæ.

[4] Hor.

[5] Attenuant vigiles corpus miserabile curæ.

[6] Plautus.

[7] Hæc quæ crines evellit, Ærumna.

[8] Optimum non nasci, aut cito mori.

Page 280

[1] Bonæ si rectam rationem sequuntur, malæ si exorbitant.

[2] Tho. Buovie. Prob. 18.

[3] Molam asinariam.

[4] Tract. de Inter. cap. 92.

[5] Circa quamlibet rem mundi hæc passio fieri potest, quæ superflue diligatur.—Tract. 15, cap. 17.

[6] Ferventius desiderium.

[7] Imprimis vero appetitus, etc.—3 de alien. ment.

[8] Conf. lib. 1, cap. 29.

[9] Per diversa loca vagor, nullo temporis momento quiesco, talis et talis esse cupio, illud atque illud habere desidero.

[10] Ambros. lib. 3 super Lucam. Ærugo animæ.

[11] Nihil animum cruciat, nihil molestius inquietat, secretum virus, pestis occulta, etc.—Epist. 126.

[12] Ep. 88.

Page 281

[1] Nihil infelicius his; quantus iis timor, quanta dubitatio, quantus conatus, quanta sollicitudo! nulla illis a molestiis vacua hora.

[2] Semper attonitus, semper pavidus quid dicat, faciatve: ne displiceat humilitatem simulat, honestatem mentitur.

³ Cypr. Prolog. ad ser. to. 2.   Cunctos honorat, universis inclinat, subsequitur, obsequitur; frequentat curias, visitat optimates, amplexatur, applaudit, adulatur: per fas et nefas e latebris, in omnem gradum ubi aditus pater se ingerit, discurrit.

⁴ Turbæ cogit ambitio regem inservire, ut Homerus Agamemnonem querentem inducit.

⁵ Plutarchus.   Quin convivemur, et in otio nos oblectemur, quoniam in promptu id nobis sit, etc.

⁶ Jovius, Hist. lib. 1.   Vir singulari prudentia, sed profunda ambitione, ad exitium Italiæ natus.

⁷ Lib. 3, de contemptu rerum fortuitarum.   Magno conatu et impetu moventur, super eodem centro rotati, non proficiunt, nec ad finem perveniunt.

⁸ Ut hedera arbori adhæret, sic ambitio, etc.   ⁹ Vita Pyrrhi.

PAGE 282

¹ [Where the bodies of executed criminals were dragged to be thrown into the Tiber.]

² Lib. 5 de rep. cap. 1.

³ Ambitio in insaniam facile delabitur, si excedat.—Patricius, lib. 4, tit. 20, de regis instit.

⁴ Imprimis vero appetitus, seu concupiscentia nimia rei alicujus, honestæ vel inhonestæ, phantasiam lædunt; unde multi ambitiosi, philauti, irati, avari, insani, etc.—Felix Plater, lib. 3 de mentis alien.

⁵ Aulica vita colluvies ambitionis, cupiditatis, simulationis, imposturæ, fraudis, invidiæ, superbiæ Titaniacæ; diversosium aula, et commune conventiculum assentandi artificum, etc.—Budæus de asse. lib. 5.

⁶ In his Aphor.   ⁷ Plautus, Curcul. Act. 4, sc. 2.

⁸ Tom. 2. Si examines, omnes miseriæ causas vel a furioso contendendi studio, vel ab injusta cupiditate, originem traxisse scies.   Idem fere Chrysostomus, Com. in cap. 6 ad Romanos, ser. 11.

PAGE 283

¹ Cap. 4, 1.   ² Ut sit iniquus in Deum, in proximum, in seipsum.

³ Si vero, Crateva, inter cæteras herbarum radices, acaritiæ radicem secare posses amaram, ut nullæ reliquiæ essent, probe scito, etc.

⁴ Cap. 6 Dietæ salutis.   Avaritia est amor immoderatus pecuniæ vel acquirendæ vel retinendæ.

⁵ Malus est morbus maleque afficit avaritia, siquidem censeo, etc. Avaritia difficilius curatur quam insania: quoniam hac omnes fere medici laborant.—Hip. Ep. Abderit.

⁶ Ferum profecto dirumque ulcus animi, remediis non cedens medendo exasperatur.

⁷ Qua re non es lassus? lucrum faciendo: quid maxime delectabile? lucrari.

⁸ Extremos currit mercator ad Indos.—Hor.

PAGE 284

¹ Hom. 2.   Aliud avarus, aliud dives.

² Divitiæ ut spinæ animum hominis timoribus, sollicitudinibus, angoribus, mirifice pungunt, vexant, cruciant.—Greg. in Hom.

³ Epist. ad Donat. cap. 2.   ⁴ Lib. 9, ep. 30.

⁵ Lib. 9, cap. 4. Insulæ rex titulo, sed animo pecuniæ miserabile mancipium.   ⁶ Hor. 10, lib. 1.

⁷ Danda est hellebori multo pars maxima avaris.

⁸ Luke xii, 20. Stulte, hac nocte eripiam animam tuam.

⁹ Opes quidem mortalibus sunt dementia.—Theognis.

[10] Ed. 2, lib. 2. Exonerare cum se possit et relevare ponderibus, pergit magis fortunis augentibus pertinaciter incubare.

[11] Non amicis, non liberis, non ipsi sibi quidquam impertit; possidet ad hoc tantum, ne possidere alteri liceat, etc. Hieron. ad Paulin. Tam deest quod habet quam quod non habet.

PAGE 285

[1] Epist. 2, lib. 2. Suspirat in convivio, bibat licet gemmis et toro molliore marcidum corpus condiderit, vigilat in pluma.

[2] Angustatur ex abundantia, contristatur ex opulentia, infelix præsentibus bonis, infelicior in futuris.

[3] Illorum cogitatio nunquam cessat qui pecunias supplere diligunt.— Guianer. tract. 15, cap. 17.

[4] Hor. 3 Od. 24. Quo plus sunt potæ, plus sitiuntur aquæ.

[5] Hor. lib. 2, Sat. 6. O si angulus ille Proximus accedat, qui nunc deformat agellum.

[6] Lib. 3 de lib. arbit. Immoritur studiis, et amore senescit habendi.

[7] Avarus vir inferno est similis, etc.; modum non habet, hoc egentior quo plura habet.

PAGE 286

[1] Erasm. Adag. chil. 3, cent. 7, prov. 2. Nulli fidentes omnium formidant opes, ideo pavidum malum vocat Euripides: metuunt tempestates ob frumentum, amicos ne rogent, inimicos ne lædant, fures ne rapiant, bellum timent, pacem timent, summos, medios, infimos.

[2] Hall, Characters.

[3] A. Gellius, lib. 3, cap. 1. Interdum eo sceleris perveniunt ob lucrum, ut vitam propriam commutent.

[4] Lib. 7, cap. 6.

[5] Omnes perpetuo morbo agitantur, suspicatur omnes timidus sibique ob aurum insidiari putat, nunquam quiescens.—Plin. Prooem. lib. 14.

[6] Cap. 18. In lecto jacens interrogat uxorem an arcam probe clausit, an capsula, etc. E lecto surgens nudus et absque calceis, accensa lucerna omnia obiens et lustrans, et vix somno indulgens.

[7] Curis extenuatus, vigilans et secum supputans.

[8] Cave quemquam alienum in ædes intromiseris. Ignem extingui volo, ne causæ quidquam sit quod te quisquam quæritet. Si bona fortuna veniat, ne intromiseris. Occlude sis fores ambobus pessulis. Discrucior animi quia domo abeundum est mihi. Nimis hercule invitus abeo, nec quid agam scio.

[9] Plorat aquam profundere, etc. Periit dum fumus de tigillo exit foras.

PAGE 287

[1] Juv. Sat. 14.

[2] Ventricosus, nudus, pallidus, læva pudorem occultans, dextra seipsum strangulans. Occurrit autem exeunti Pœnitentia, his miserum conficiens, etc.

[3] Luke xv. [4] Boethius.

PAGE 288

[1] In Œconom. Quid si nunc ostendam eos qui magna vi argenti domus inutiles ædificant? inquit Socrates.

[2] Sarisburiensis Polycrat. lib. 1, cap. 14. Venatores omnes adhuc institutionem redolent centaurorum. Raro invenitur quisquam eorum modestus et gravis, raro continens, et ut credo sobrius nunquam.

[3] Pancirol. Tit. 23. Avolant opes cum accipitre.

[4] Insignis venatorum stultitia, et supervacanea cura eorum, qui dum nimium venationi insistunt, ipsi abjecta omni humanitate in feras degenerant, ut Actæon, etc.

[5] Sabin. in Ovid. Metamor.

⁶ Agrippa de vanit. scient. Insanum venandi studium, dum a novalibus arcentur agricolæ, subtrahunt prædia rusticis, agricolonis præcluduntur silvæ et prata pastoribus ut augeantur pascua feris. . . . Majestatis reus agricola si gustarit.

⁷ A novalibus suis arcentur agricolæ, dum feræ habeant vagandi libertatem: istis, ut pascua augeantur, prædia subtrahuntur,etc.—Sarisburiensis.

⁸ Feris quam hominibus æquiores. — Camden de Guil. Conq. qui 36 ecclesias matrices depopulatus est ad Forestam Novam (Mat. Paris).

PAGE 289

¹ Tom. 2 de vitis illustrium, lib. 4, de vit. Leon. 10.

² Venationibus adeo perdite studebat et aucupiis.

³ Aut infeliciter venatus tam impatiens inde, ut summos sæpe viro acerbissimis contumeliis oneraret, et incredibile est quali vultus animique habitu dolorem iracundiamque præferret, etc.

⁴ Unicuique autem hoc a natura insitum est, ut doleat sicubi erraverit aut deceptus sit.

⁵ Juven. Sat. 1. Nec enim loculis comitantibus itur Ad casum tabulæ, positased luditur arca. Lemnius, Instit. cap. 44. Mendaciorum quidem, et perjuriorum, et paupertatis mater est alea, nullam habens patrimonii reverentiam, quum illud effuderit, sensim in furta delabitur et rapinas. Saris. Polycrat. lib. 1, cap. 5.   ⁶ Damhoderius.

⁷ Dan. Souter.   ⁸ Petrar. dial. 27.

PAGE 290

¹ Sallust.   ² Tom. 3, Ser. de alea.

³ Plutus in Aristoph. calls all such gamesters madmen: Si in insanum hominem contigero. Spontaneum ad se trahunt, furorem, et os, et nares, et oculos rivos faciunt furoris et diversoria.—Chrys. Hom. 17.

⁴ Paschasius Justus, lib. 1 de alea.

⁵ Seneca.   ⁶ Hall.

⁷ Juv. Sat. 11. Sed deficiente crumena et crescente gula, quis te manet exitus . . . rebus in ventrem mersis?

⁸ Spartian. Adriano.

⁹ Alex. ab Alex. lib. 6, cap. 10. Idem Gerbelius, lib. 5 Græc. desc.

¹⁰ Fynes Moryson.   ¹¹ Justinian. in Digestis.

PAGE 291

¹ Persius, Sat. 5.

² Poculum quasi sinus in quo sæpe naufragium faciunt, jactura tum pecuniæ tum mentis.—Erasm. in Prov. Calicum remiges, chil. 4, cent. 7, prov. 41.

³ Ser. 33, ad frat. in Eremo.

⁴ [A play on words, "Hilary Term" standing for "season of merriment."

⁵ Liberæ unius horæ insaniam æterno temporis tædio pensant.

⁶ Menander.   ⁷ Prov. vii, 22.

PAGE 292

¹ Merlin. Cocc.   ² Hor.

³ Sagitta quæ animam penetrat, leviter penetrat, sed non leve infligit vulnus.—Sup. Cant.

⁴ Qui omnem pecuniarum contemptum habent, et nulli imaginationis totius mundi se immiscuerint, et tyrannicas corporis concupiscentias sustinuerint, hi multoties capti a vana gloria omnia perdiderunt.

⁵ Hac correpti non cogitant de medela.

⁶ Di talem a terris avertite pestem.

⁷ Ep. ad Eustochium, de custod. virgin.   ⁸ Lips. Ep. ad Bonciarium.

PAGE 293

[1] Ep. lib. 9. Omnia tua scripta pulcherrima existimo, maxime tamen illa quæ de nobis.

[2] Exprimere non possum quam sit jucundum, etc.

[3] Hierome. Et licet nos indignos dicimus et calidus rubor ora perfundat, attamen ad laudem suam intrinsecus animæ lætantur.

[4] Thesaur. Theo.

[5] Nec enim mihi cornea fibra est.—Pers.

[6] E manibus illis Nascentur violæ.—Pers. Sat. 1.

[7] Omnia enim nostra, supra modum placent.

[8] Fab. lib. 10, cap. 3. Ridentur mala qui componunt carmina, verum Gaudent scribentes, et se venerantur, et ultro, Si taceas laudant, quicquid scripsere beati.—Hor. Ep. 2, lib. 2.

[9] Luke xviii, 10. [10] De meliore luto finxit præcordia Titan.

PAGE 294

[1] Auson. Sap.

[2] Chil. 3, cent. 10, prov. 97. Qui se crederet neminem ulla in re præstantiorem.

[3] Tanto fastu scripsit, ut Alexandri gesta inferiora scriptis suis existimaret.—Jo. Voschius, lib. 1, cap. 9, de hist.

[4] Plutarch, vit. Catonis.

[5] Nemo unquam poeta aut orator, qui quemquam se meliorem arbitraretur.

[6] Consol. ad Pammachium. Mundi philosophus, gloriæ animal, et popularis auræ et rumorum venale mancipium.

[7] Epist. 5, Capitoni suo. Diebus ac noctibus hoc solum cogito si qua me possum levare humo. Id voto meo sufficit, etc.

[8] Tullius.

[9] Ut nomen meum scriptis tuis illustretur. Inquies animus studio æternitatis, noctes et dies angebatur.—Heinsius, Orat. funeb. de Scal.

[10] Hor. Art. Poet. [11] Vade, liber felix!—Palingen. lib. 18.

PAGE 295

[1] In lib. 8. [2] De ponte dejicere.

[3] Sueton. lib. de gram. [4] Nihil libenter audiunt nisi laudes suas.

[5] Epis. 56. Nihil aliud dies noctesque cogitant nisi ut in studiis suis audentur ab hominibus.

[6] Quæ major dementia aut dici, aut excogitari potest, quam sic ob gloriam cruciari? Insaniam istam, Domine, longe fac a me.—Austin, Conf. lib. 10, cap. 37.

[7] Mart. lib. 5, 52.

PAGE 296

[1] Hor. Sat. lib. 1, 2. [2] Lib. cont. philos. cap. 1.

PAGE 297

[1] Macrobius, Som. Scip. [2] Boethius.

[3] Putean. Cisalp. hist. lib. 1. [4] Plutarch, Lycurgo.

[5] Epist. 13. Illud te admoneo, ne eorum more facias, qui non proficere, sed conspici cupiunt, quæ in habitu tuo, aut genere vitæ notabilia sunt. Asperum cultum et vitiosum caput, negligentiorem barbam, indictum argento odium, cubile humi positum, et quicquid ad laudem perversa via sequitur, evita.

PAGE 298

[1] Hor.
[2] Quis vero tam bene modulo suo metiri se novit, ut eum assiduæ et immodicæ laudationes non moveant?—Hen. Steph.
[3] Mart.   [4] Stroza.
[5] Antony, Octavian, Lepidus.]   [6] Justin.

PAGE 299

[1] Livius. Gloria tantum elatus, non ira, in medios hostes irruere, quod completis muris conspici se pugnantem, a muro spectantibus, egregium ducebat.
[2] [No whoa, or ho, with him; i.e. there's no stopping him. Proverbial.]
[3] I demens, et sævas curre per Alpes. Aude aliquid, etc., Ut pueris placeas, et declamatio fias.—Juv. Sat. 10.
[4] In Moriæ Encom.   [5] Juvenal. Sat. 4.
[6] Sueton. cap. 12, in Domitiano.   [7] Brisonius.
[8] Antonius ab assentatoribus evectus Liberum se patrem appellari jussit, et pro deo se venditavit. Redimitus hedera, et corona velatus aurea, et thyrsum tenens, cothurnisque succinctus, curru velut Liber pater vectus est Alexandriæ.—Pater. vol. post.
[9] Minervæ nuptias ambit, tanto furore percitus, ut satellites mitteret ad videndum num dea in thalamis venisset, etc.
[10] Ælian, lib. 12.   [11] De mentis alienat. cap. 3.

PAGE 300

[1] Sequiturque superbia formam. Livius, lib. 11: Oraculum est, vivida sæpe ingenia luxuriare hac et evanescere, multosque sensum penitus amisisse. Homines intuentur, ac si ipsi non essent homines.
[2] Galeus de Rubeis, civis noster faber ferrarius, ob inventionem instrumenti, cochleæ olim Archimedis dicti, præ lætitia insanivit.
[3] Insania postmodum correptus, ob nimiam inde arrogantiam. ["One Carius, a soldier" = a Carian soldier.]
[4] Bene ferre magnam disce fortunam.—Hor. Fortunam reverenter habe, quicunque repente Dives ab exili progrediere loco.—Ausonius.
[5] Processit squalidus et submissus, ut hesterni diei gaudium intemperans hodie castigaret.   [6] Uxor Hen. 8.
[7] Neutrius se fortunæ extremum libenter experturam dixit: sed si necessitas alterius subinde imponeretur, optaro se difficilem et adversam: quod in hac nulli unquam defuit solatium, in altera multis consilium, etc. —Lod. Vives.
[8] Peculiaris furor, qui ex literis fit.
[9] Nihil magis auget, ac assidua studia, et profundæ cogitationes.

PAGE 301

[1] Study is a continual and earnest meditation, applied to something with great desire.—Tully.
[2] Non desunt, qui ex jugi studio, et intempestiva lucubratione, huc devenerunt, hi præ cæteris enim plerumque melancholia solent infestari.
[3] Et illi qui sunt subtilis ingenii, et multæ præmeditationis, de facili incidunt in melancholiam.
[4] Ob studiorum sollicitudinem, lib. 5, tit. 5.
[5] Gaspar Ens,Thesaur. Polit. Apoteles. 31. Græcis hanc pestem relinquite quæ dubium non est, quin brevi omnem iis vigorem ereptura Martiosque spiritus exhaustura sit, ut ad arma tractanda plane inhabiles futuri sint.
[6] Knolles, Turk. Hist.   [7] Acts xxvi, 24.
[8] Nimiis studiis melancholicus evasit, dicens se Biblium in capite habere.
[9] Cur melancholia assidua, crebrisque deliramentis, vexentur eorum animi ut desipere cogantur.

PAGE 302

[1] Sollers quilibet artifex instrumenta sua diligentissime curat; penicillos pictor; malleos incudesque faber ferrarius; miles equos, arma; venator, auceps, aves et canes; citharam citharædus, etc.; soli Musarum mystæ tam negligentes sunt, ut instrumentum illud quo mundum universum metiri solent, spiritum scilicet, penitus negligere videantur.

[2] Arcus et arma tibi non sunt imitanda Dianæ. Si nunquam cesses tendere mollis erit.—Ovid.

[3] Ephemer. [4] [Marlowe, Hero and Leander, First Sestiad.]

[5] Contemplatio cerebrum exsiccat et extinguit calorem naturalem, unde cerebrum frigidum et siccum evadit, quod est melancholicum. Accedit ad hoc, quod natura in contemplatione, cerebro prorsus cordique intenta, stomachum heparque destituit, unde ex alimentis male coctis, sanguis crassus et niger efficitur, dum nimio otio membrorum superflui vapores non exhalant.

[6] Cerebrum exsiccatur, corpora sensim gracilescunt.

[7] Studiosi sunt cachectici et nunquam bene colorati; propter debilitatem digestivæ facultatis, multiplicantur in iis superfluitates.—Jo. Voschius, parte 2, cap. 5, de peste.

[8] Nullus mihi per otium dies exit, partem noctis studiis dedico, non vero somno, sed oculos vigilia fatigatos cadentesque, in opere detineo.

PAGE 303

[1] Johannes Hanuschius Bohemus, nat. 1516, eruditus vir, nimiis studiis in phrenesin incidit. Montanus instances in a Frenchman of Tolosa.

[2] Cardinalis Cæsius; ob laborem, vigiliam, et diuturna studia factus melancholicus.

[3] Ingenium sibi quod vanas desumpsit Athenas, Et septem studiis annos dedit, insenuitque Libris et curis, statua taciturnius exit, Plerumque et risu populum quatit.—Hor. Ep. 1, lib. 2.

[4] Pers. Sat. 3. They cannot fiddle; but, as Themistocles said, he could make a small town become a great city.

[5] Pers. Sat. [6] Translated by Mr. B[arton] Holliday.

PAGE 304

[1] Thomas rubore confusus dixit se de argumento cogitasse.

[2] Plutarch, vita Marcelli. Nec sensit urbem captam, nec milites in domum irruentes, adeo intentus studiis, etc.

[3] [Lake Leman.]

[4] Sub furiæ larva circumivit urbem, dictitans se exploratorem ab inferis venisse, delaturum dæmonibus mortalium peccata.

[5] Petronius. Ego arbitror in scholis stultissimos fieri, quia nihil eorum quæ in usu habemus aut audiunt aut vident.

[6] Novi meis diebus, plerosque studiis literarum deditos, qui disciplinis admodum abundabant, sed si nihil civilitatis habent, nec rem publ. nec domesticam regere norant. Stupuit Paglarensis et furti villicum accusavit, qui suem fetam undecim porcellos, asinam unum duntaxat pullum enixam retulerat.

[7] Lib. 1, Epist. 3. Adhuc scholasticus tantum est; quo genere hominum, nihil aut est simplicius, aut sincerius, aut melius.

PAGE 305

[1] Jure privilegiandi, qui ob commune bonum abbreviant sibi vitam.

[2] Virg. 6 Æn.

[3] Plutarch. vita ejus. Certum agricolationis lucrum, etc.

[4] Quotannis fiunt consules et proconsules, rex et poeta quotannis non nascitur.

PAGE 306

[1] Matt. xxi.   [2] Hor. Epist. 20, lib. 1.
[3] Lib. 1 de contem. amor.

PAGE 307

[1] Satyricon.   [2] Juv. Sat. 5.
[3] Ars colit astra.   [4] Aldrovandus de avibus, lib. 12, Gesner, etc.
[5] Literas habent queis sibi et fortunæ suæ maledicant.—Sat. Menip.

PAGE 308

[1] Lib. de libris propriis, fol. 24.
[2] Præfat translat. Plutarch.
[3] Polit. disput.   Laudibus extollunt eos ac si virtutibus pollerent quos ob infinita scelera potius vituperare oporteret.
[4] Or as horses know not their strength, they consider not their own worth.
[5] Plura ex Simonidis familiaritate Hiero consecutus est, quam ex Hieronis Simonides.
[6] Hor. lib. 4, od. 9.
[7] Inter inertes et plebeios fere jacet, ultimum locum habens, nisi tot artis virtutisque insignia, turpiter, obnoxie, supparisitando fascibus subjecerit protervæ insolentisque potentiæ.—Lib. 1 de contempt. rerum fortuitarum.   [8] Buchanan, Eleg. lib.

PAGE 309

[1] In Satyricon.   Intrat senex, sed cultu non ita speciosus, ut facile appareret eum hac nota literatum esse, quos divites odisse solent. Ego, inquit, poeta sum. Quare ergo tam male vestitus es?   Propter hoc ipsum; amor ingenii neminem unquam divitem fecit.
[2] Petronius Arbiter.
[3] Oppressus paupertate animus nihil eximium, aut sublime cogitare potest, amœnitates literarum, aut elegantiam, quoniam nihil præsidii in his ad vitæ commodum videt, primo negligere, mox odisse incipit.—Heins.

PAGE 310

[1] Epistol. quæst. lib. 4, ep. 21.   [2] Ciceron. dial.
[3] Epist. lib. 2.   [4] Ja. Dousa, Epodon lib. 2, car. 2.

PAGE 311

[1] Plautus.   [2] Barcl. Argenis, lib. 3.
[3] Joh. Howson, 4 Novembris 1597.   The sermon was printed by Arnold Hartfield.

PAGE 312

[1] Pers. Sat. 3.
[2] E lecto exsilientes, ad subitum tintinnabuli plausum quasi fulmine territi.
[3] Mart.   [4] Mart.   [5] Sat. Menip.

PAGE 313

[1] Lib. 3 de cons.
[2] I had no money, I wanted impudence, I could not scramble, temporize, dissemble: non pranderet olus, etc.   Vis, dicam? ad palpandum et adulandum penitus insulsus, recudi non possum, jam senior ut sim talis, et fingi nolo, utcunque male cedat in rem meam et obscurus inde delitescam.
[3] Vit. Crassi. Nec facile judicare potest utrum pauperior cum primo ad Crassum, etc.

PAGE 314

[1] Deum habent iratum, sibique mortem æternam acquirunt, aliis miserabilem ruinam.—Serrarius in Josuam, 7.
[2] Nicephorus, lib. 10, cap. 5.
[3] Lord Cook, in his Reports, second part, fol. 44.   [4] Euripides.
[5] Sir Henry Spelman, de non temerandis ecclesiis.

PAGE 315

[1] 1 Tim. iv, 2.   [2] Hor.
[3] Primum locum apud omnes gentes habet patricius deorum cultus, et geniorum, nam hunc diutissime custodiunt, tam Græci quam Barbari, etc.
[4] Tom. 1, de steril. trium annorum sub Elia sermone.
[5] Ovid. Fast.
[6] De male quæsitis vix gaudet tertius hæres. [Ill-gotten goods thrive not to the third heir.]   [7] Strabo, lib. 4 Geog.

PAGE 316

[1] Nihil facilius opes evertet, quam avaritia et fraude parta. Etsi enim seram addas tali arcæ et exteriore janua et vecte eam communias, intus tamen fraudem et avaritiam, etc.—In 5 Corinth.
[2] Acad. cap. 7.
[3] Ars neminem habet inimicum præter ignorantem.
[4] [Frederick Barbarossa, whose favourite bit of Latin follows.]
[5] Lipsius, Epist. quest. lib. 4, epist. 21.

PAGE 317

[1] Dr. King, in his last lecture on Jonah, sometime Right Reverend Lord Bishop of London.
[2] Quibus opes et otium, hi barbaro fastu litteras contemnunt.
[3] Lucan. lib. 8.   [4] Spartian. Solliciti de rebus nimis.
[5] Nicet. 1. Anal. Fumis lucubrationum sordebant.
[6] Grammaticis olim et dialectices jurisque professoribus, qui specimen eruditionis dedissent, eadem dignitatis insignia decreverunt Imperatores, quibus ornabant heroas.—Erasm. ep. Jo. Fabio epis. Vien.

PAGE 318

[1] Probus vir et philosophus magis præstat inter alios homines, quam rex inclytus inter plebeios.   [2] Heinsius, præfat. Poematum.
[3] Servile nomen scholaris jam.   [4] Seneca.
[5] Haud facile emergunt, etc.
[6] Media quod noctis ab hora Sedisti qua nemo faber, qua nemo sedebat, Qui docet obliquo lanam deducere ferro: Rara tamen merces.—Juv. Sat. 7.
[7] Chil. 4, cent. 1, adag. 1.
[8] Had I done as others did, put myself forward, I might have haply been as great a man as many of my equals.

PAGE 319

[1] Catullus.   [2] Juven.
[3] Nemo est quem non Phœbus hic noster solo intuitu lubentiorem reddat.

PAGE 320

[1] Panegyr.   [2] Virgil.
[3] Rarus enim ferme sensus communis in illa Fortuna.—Juv. Sat. 8.
[4] Quis enim generosum dixerit hunc qui Indignus genere, et præclaro nomine tantum Insignis.—Juv. Sat. 8.

Page 321

[1] I have often met with myself, and conferred with, divers worthy gentlemen in the country, no whit inferior, if not to be preferred for divers kind of learning, to many of our academics.

[2] Ipse licet Musis venias comitatus Homere, Nil tamen attuleris, ibis, Homere, foras.

[3] Et legat historias, auctores noverit omnes Tanquam ungues digitosque suos.—Juv. Sat. 7.   [4] Juvenal.

[5] Tu vero licet Orpheus sis, saxa sono testudinis emolliens, nisi plumbea eorum corda auri vel argenti malleo emollias, etc.—Sarisburiensis, Polycrat. lib. 5, cap. 10.

Page 322

[1] Juven. Sat. 7.

[2] Euge! bene! no need. Dousa, Epod. lib. 2. Dos ipsa scientia sibique congiarium est.

[3] Quatuor ad portas Ecclesias itur ad omnes; Sanguinis aut Simonis, præsulis atque Dei.—Holcot.

[4] Lib. contra Gentiles de Babila martyre.

[5] Præscribunt, impèrant, in ordinem cogunt, ingenium nostrum prout ipsis videbitur, astringunt et relaxant ut papilionem pueri aut bruchum filo demittunt, aut attrahunt, nos a libidine sua pendere æquum censentes. —Heinsius.

Page 323

[1] John v.

[2] Epist. lib. 2. Jam suffectus in locum demortui, protinus exortus est adversarius, etc.; post multos labores, sumptus, etc.

Page 324

[1] Jun. Acad. cap. 6.

[2] Accipiamus pecuniam, demittamus asinum ut apud Patavinos, Italos.

[3] Hos non ita pridem perstrinxi, in Philosophastro, Comœdia Latina, in Æde Christi Oxon. publice habita, anno 1617, Feb. 16.

[4] Sat. Menip.

Page 325

[1] 2 Cor. ii, 17.   [2] Comment. in Gal.   [3] Heinsius.
[4] Ecclesiast.   [5] Luth. in Gal.
[6] Pers. Sat. 2.   [7] Sallust.

Page 326

[1] Sat. Menip.   [2] Budæus, de Asse, lib. 5.
[3] Lib. de rep. Gallorum.   [4] Campian.

Page 330

[1] Proem lib. 2. Nulla ars constitui potest.

[2] Lib. 1, cap. 19, de morborum causis. Quas declinare licet aut nulla necessitate utimur.

Page 331

[1] Quo semel est imbuta recens servabit odorem Testa diu.—Hor.

[2] Sicut valet ad fingendas corporis atque animi similitudines visĵet natura seminis, sic lactis proprietas. Neque id in hominibus solum, sed in pecudibus animadversum. Nam si ovium lacte hædi, aut caprarum agni alerentur, constat fieri in his lanam duriorem, in illis capillum gigni severiorem.

[3] Adulta in ferarum persecutione ad miraculum usque sagax.

[4] Tam animal quodlibet quam homo, ab illa cujus lacte nutritur, naturam contrahit.

[5] Improba, informis, impudica, temulenta nutrix, etc.; quoniam in moribus efformandis magnam sæpe partem ingenium altricis et natura lactis tenet.

[6] H'rcanæque admorunt ubera tigres.—Virg.

[7] Lib. 2 de Cæsaribus.

[8] Beda, cap. 27, lib. 1, Eccles. hist.

[9] Ne insitivo lactis alimento degeneret corpus, et animus corrumpatur.

Page 332

[1] Lib. 3 de civ. convers.   [2] Stephanus.

[3] To. 2.   Nutrices non quasvis, sed maxime probas deligamus.

[4] Nutrix non sit lasciva aut temulenta.—Hier.

[5] Prohibendum ne stolida lactet.   [6] Pers.

[7] Nutrices interdum matribus sunt meliores.

Page 333

[1] Lib. de morbis capitis, cap. de mania. Haud postrema causa supputatur educatio, inter has mentis abalienationis causas. Injusta noverca.

[2] Lib. 2, cap. 4.

[3] Idem. Et quod maxime nocet, dum in teneris ita timent nihil conantur.

Page 334

[1] Præfat. ad Testam.

[2] Plus mentis pædagogico supercilio abstulit, quam unquam præceptis suis sapientiæ instillavit.

[3] Ter. Adel. 3, 3.   [4] Idem, Act. 1, sc. 2.

Page 335

[1] Camerarius, Emb. 77, cent. 2, hath elegantly expressed it an emblem: Perdit amando, etc.

[2] Prov. xiii, 24. He that spareth the rod hates his son.

[3] Lib. 2 de consol. Tam stulte pueros diligimus ut odisse potius videamur; illos non ad virtutem sed ad injuriam, non ad eruditionem sed ad luxum, non ad virtutem sed voluptatem educantes.

[4] Lib. 1, cap. 3. Educatio altera natura, alterat animos et voluntatem, atque utinam (inquit) liberorum nostrorum mores non ipsi perderemus, quum infantiam statim deliciis solvimus: mollior ista educatio, quam indulgentiam vocamus, nervos omnes, et mentis et corporis frangit; fit ex his consuetudo, inde natura.

[5] Perinde agit ac siquis de calceo sit sollicitus, pedem nihil curet. Juven. Nil patri minus est quam filius.

[6] Lib. 3. de sapientia. Qui avaris pædagogis pueros alendos dant, vel clausos in cœnobiis jejunare simul et sapere, nihil aliud agunt, nisi ut sint vel non sine stultitia eruditi, vel non integra vita sapientes.

Page 336

[1] Terror et metus, maxime ex improviso accedentes, ita animum commovent, ut spiritus nunquam recuperent, gravioremque melancholiam terror facit, quam quæ ab interna causa fit. Impressio tam fortis in spiritibus humoribusque cerebri, ut extracta tota sanguinea massa, ægre exprimatur, et hæc horrenda species melancholiæ frequenter oblata mihi, omnes exercens, viros, juvenes, senes.

[2] Tract. de melan. cap. 7 et 8. Non ab intemperie, sed agitatione, dilatatione, contractione, motu spirituum.

[3] Lib. de fort. et virtut. Alex. Præsertim ineunte periculo, ubi res prope adsunt terribiles.

NOTES   505

⁴ Fit a visione horrenda, revera apparente, vel per insomnia.—Platerus.
⁵ A painter's wife in Basil, 1600, somniavit filium bello mortuum, inde melancholica consolari noluit.
⁶ Senec. Het.
⁷ Quarta pars comment. de statu religionis in Gallia sub Carolo 9, 1572.
⁸ Ex occursu dæmonium aliqui furore corripiuntur, ut experientia notum est.   ⁹ Lib. 8, in Arcad.   ¹⁰ Lucret.

PAGE 337

¹ Puellæ extra urbem in prato concurrentes, etc.; mæsta et melancholica domum rediit per dies aliquot vexata, dum mortua est.—Platerus.
² Altera trans-Rhenana ingressa sepulchrum recens apertum, vidit cadaver, et domum subito reversa putavit eam vocare; post paucos dies obiit, proximo sepulchro collocata. Altera patibulum sero præteriens, metuebat ne urbe exclusa illic pernoctaret, unde melancholica facta, per multos annos laboravit.—Platerus.
³ Subitus occursus, inopinata lectio.
⁴ Lib. de auditione.   ⁵ Theod. Prodromus, lib. 7 Amorum.
⁶ Effuso cernens fugientes agmine turmas, Quis mea nunc inflat cornua? Faunus ait.—Alciat. embl. 122.

PAGE 338

¹ Judges vii, 19.   ² Plutarchus, vita ejus.
³ In furorem cum sociis versus.   ⁴ Subitarius terræ motus.
⁵ Cœpit inde desipere cum dispendio sanitatis, inde adeo dementans, ut sibi ipsi mortem inferret.
⁶ Historica relatio de rebus Japonicis, tract 2, de legat. regis Chinensis, a Lodovico Frois Jesuita. A. 1596. Fuscini derepente tanta acris caligo et terræ motus, ut multi capite dolerent, plurimis cor mœrore et melancholia obrueretur. Tantum fremitum edebat, ut tonitru fragorem imitari videretur, tantamque, etc. In urbe Sacai tam horrificus fuit, ut homines vix sui compotes essent, a sensibus abalienati, mœrore oppressi tam horrendo spectaculo, etc. [Froe's narrative is in Hakluyt (Everyman ed. iv, 195–209).]
⁷ Quum subit illius tristissima noctis imago.

PAGE 339

¹ Qui solo aspectu medicinæ movebatur ad purgandum.
² Sicut viatores si ad saxum impegerint, aut nautæ, memores sui casus, non ista modo quæ offendunt, sed et similia horrent perpetuo et tremunt.
³ Leviter volant, graviter vulnerant.—Bernardus.
⁴ Ensis sauciat corpus, mentem sermo.
⁵ Sciatis eum esse qui a nemine fere ævi sui magnate non illustre stipendium habuit, ne mores ipsorum satiris suis notaret.—Gasp. Barthius, præfat. Pornoboscodid.
⁶ [i.e. Pope Adrian VI.]
⁷ [The statue popularly called Pasquino or Pasquillo, to which the pasquinades were affixed, and from which they got their name.]
⁸ Jovius, in vita ejus. Gravissime tulit famosis libellis nomen suum ad Pasquilli statuam fuisse laceratum, decrevitque ideo statuam demoliri, etc.
⁹ Plato, lib. 13 de legibus. Qui existimationem curant, poetas vereantur, quia magnam vim habent ad laudandum et vituperandum.

PAGE 340

¹ Petulanti splene cachinno.
² Curial. lib. 2. Ea quorundam est inscitia, ut quoties loqui, toties mordere licere sibi putent.
³ Ter. Eunuch.   ⁴ Hor. Ser. lib. 2, sat. 4.

[5] Lib. 2.   [6] De orat.
[7] Laudando, et mira iis persuadendo.
[8] Et vana inflatus opinione, incredibilia ac ridenda quædam musices præcepta commentaretur, etc.

PAGE 341

[1] Ut voces, nudis parietibus illisæ, suavius ac acutius resilirent.
[2] Immortalitati et gloriæ suæ prorsus invidentes.
[3] 2, 2dæ quæst. 75. Irrisio mortale peccatum.   [4] Ps. xv, 3.

PAGE 342

[1] Balthasar Castilio, lib. 2 de aulico.
[2] De sermone lib. 4, cap. 3.   [3] Fol. 55, Galateus.

PAGE 343

[1] Tully, Tusc. quæst.   [2] Mart. lib. 1, epig. 41.
[3] Tales joci ab injuriis non possint discerni.—Galateus, fol. 55.
[4] Pybrac, in his Quatrains, 37.
[5] Ego hujus misera fatuitate et dementia conflictor.—Tull. ad Attic. lib. 11.

PAGE 344

[1] Miserum est aliena vivere quadra.—Juv.
[2] Crambe bis cocta. Vitæ me redde priori.
[3] Hor.   [4] De tranquil. animæ.

PAGE 345

[1] Lib. 8.   [2] Tullius Lepido, Fam. 10, 27.
[3] Boterus, lib. 1 Polit. cap. 4.   [4] Laet. descrip. Americæ.
[5] If there be any inhabitants.
[6] In Toxari. Interdiu quidem collum vinctum est, et manus constricta, noctu vero totum corpus vincitur; ad has miserias accedit corporis fœtor, strepitus ejulantium, somni brevitas; hæc omnia plane molesta et intolerabilia.   [7] In 9 Rhasis.

PAGE 346

[1] William the Conqueror's eldest son.
[2] Sallust. Romam triumpho ductus tandemque in carcerem conjectus, animi dolore periit.
[3] Camden, in Wiltsh. Miserum senem ita fame et calamitatibus in carcere fregit, inter mortis metum et vitæ tormenta, etc.
[4] Vies hodie. ["The Vize" (Burton's "Vies") is the local name.]
[5] Seneca.   [6] Com. ad Hebræos.
[7] Part. 2, sect. 3, memb. 3.
[8] Quem ut difficilem morbum pueris tradere formidamus.—Plut.
[9] Lucan. lib. 1.
[10] As in the silver mines at Freiburg in Germany.—Fynes Moryson.

PAGE 347

[1] Euripides.
[2] Tom. 4 dial. Minore periculo solem quam hunc defixis oculis licet intueri.
[3] Omnis enim res, Virtus, fama, decus, divina humanaque, pulchris Divitiis parent.—Hor. Ser. lib. 2, sat. 3. Clarus eris, fortis justus, sapiens, etiam rex, Et quicquid volet.—Hor.
[4] Et genus, et formam, regina pecunia donat. Money adds spirits, courage, etc.   [5] Epist. ad Brutum.
[6] Our young master, a fine towardly gentleman (God bless him!) and

hopeful; why, he is heir apparent to the right worshipful, to the right honourable, etc.

⁷ O nummi, nummi! vobis hunc præstat honorem.

⁸ Exinde sapere eum omnes dicimus, ac quisque fortunam habet.—Plaut. Pseud.

⁹ Aurea fortuna, principum cubiculis reponi solita.—Julius Capitolinus, vita Antonini.   ¹⁰ Petronius.

PAGE 348

¹ Theologi opulentis adhærent, jurisperiti pecuniosis, literati nummosis, liberalibus artifices.

² Multi illum juvenes, multæ petiere puellæ.

³ Dummodo sit dives barbarus, ille placet.

⁴ Plut. in Lucullo, a rich chamber so called.

⁵ Panis pane melior.   ⁶ Juv. Sat. 5.   ⁷ Hor. Sat. 5, lib. 2.

⁸ Bohemus de Turcis, et Bredenbach.·   ⁹ Euphormio.

¹⁰ Qui pecuniam habent, elati sunt animis, [those who have money are] lofty spirits, brave men at arms; all rich men are generous, courageous, etc.

PAGE 349

¹ Nummus ait, Pro me nubat Cornubia Romæ.

² Non fuit apud mortales ullum excellentius certamen, non inter celeres celerrimo, non inter robustos robustissimo, etc.

³ Quicquid libet licet.   ⁴ Hor. Sat. 5, lib. 2.

⁵ Cum moritur dives concurrunt undique cives: Pauperis ad funus vix est ex millibus unus.

PAGE 350

¹ [See Horace, Sat. 1, 2, 1.]

² Et modo quid fuit? Ignoscet mihi genius tuus, noluisses de manu ejus nummos accipere.

³ He that wears silk, satin, velvet, and gold lace, must needs be a gentleman.

⁴ Xenophon, Cyropæd. lib. 8.

⁵ [Fastidious Brisk is a character in Jonson's Every Man out of his Humour; Sir Petronel Flash is in Eastward Ho! by Jonson, Chapman, and Marston.]

⁶ Euripides.   ⁷ Est sanguis atque spiritus pecunia mortalibus.

⁸ In tenui rare est facundia panno.—Juv.   ⁹ Hor.

¹⁰ Egere est offendere, et indigere scelestum esse.—Sat. Menip.

¹¹ Plautus [Curculio], Act. 4.

PAGE 351

¹ Nullum tam barbarum, tam vile munus est, quod non lubentissime obire velit gens vilissima.

² Lausius, orat. in Hispaniam.

³ Laet. descrip. Americæ.   ⁴ Plautus.

⁵ Leo Afer, cap. ult. lib. 1. Edunt non ut bene vivant, sed ut fortiter laborent.—Heinsius.

⁶ Munster de rusticis Germaniæ, Cosmog. cap. 27, lib. 3.

⁷ Ter. Eunuch.

⁸ Pauper paries factus, quem caniculæ commingant.

⁹ Lib. 1, cap. ult.

¹⁰ Deos omnes illis infensos diceres: tam pannosi, fame fracti, tot assidue malis afficiuntur, tanquam pecora quibus splendor rationis emortuus.

¹¹ Peregrin. Hieros.

¹² Nihil omnino meliorem vitam degunt, quam feræ in silvis, jumenta in terris.—Leo Afer.   ¹³ Bartholomæus à Casa.

PAGE 352

[1] Ortelius, in Helvetia. Qui habitant in Cæsia valle ut plurimum latomi, in Oscella valle cultrorum fabri fumarii, in Vigetia sordidum genus hominum, quod repurgandis caminis victum parat.

[2] I write not this anyways to upbraid, or scoff at, or misuse poor men, but rather to condole and pity them by expressing, etc.

[3] Chremylus, Act. 4 Plut.

[4] Paupertas durum onus miseris mortalibus.

[5] Vexat censura columbas.

[6] Deux-ace non possunt, et six-cinque solvere nolunt: Omnibus est notum quater-tre solvere totum.

[7] Scandia, Africa, Lithuania.

[8] Montaigne, in his Essays, speaks of certain Indians in France, that being asked how they liked the country, wondered how a few rich men could keep so many poor men in subjection, that they did not cut their throats.

PAGE 353

[1] Angustas animas animoso in pectore versant.

[2] [?obscenely.]   [3] Donatus, vit. ejus.

[4] Prov. xix, 7: "Though he be instant, yet they will not."

[5] Petronius.

[6] Non est qui doleat vicem; ut Petrus Christum, jurant se hominem non novisse.

[7] Ovid. in Trist.   [8] Horat.   [9] Ter. Eunuchus, Act. 2.

PAGE 354

[1] Quid quod materiam præbet causamque jocandi: Si toga sordida sit?—Juv. Sat. 3.

[2] Hor.   [3] In Phœniss.   [4] Odyss. 17.   [5] Idem.

[6] Mantuan.   [7] De Africa, lib. 1, cap. ult.

[8] Lib. 5 de legibus. Furacissima paupertas, sacrilega, turpis, flagitiosa, omnium malorum opifex.

PAGE 355

[1] Theognis.

[2] Deipnosophist, lib. 12. Millies potius moriturum (si quis sibi mente constaret) quam tam vilis et ærumnosi victus communionem habere.

[3] Gasper Vilela Jesuita, Epist. Japon. lib.

[4] Mat. Riccius, Expedit. in Sinas, lib. 1, cap. 3.

[5] Vos Romani procreatos filios feris et canibus exponitis, nunc strangulatis vel in saxum eliditis, etc.

[6] Cosmog. 4 lib. cap. 22. Vendunt liberos victu carentes tanquam pecora, interdum et seipsos; ut apud divites saturentur cibis.

[7] Vel bonorum desperatione vel malorum perpessione fracti et fatigati, plures violentas manus sibi inferunt.

PAGE 356

[1] Hor.

[2] Ingenio poteram superas volitare per arces: Ut me pluma levat, sic grave mergit onus.

[3] Terent.   [4] Hor. Sat. 3, lib. 1.   [5] Paschalius.   [6] Petronius.

[7] Herodotus, vita ejus. Scaliger in Poet. Potentiorum ædes ostiatim adiens, aliquid accipiebat, canens carmina sua, concomitante eum puerorum choro.

[8] Hegio, Ter. Adelph. Act. 4, sc. 3.

Page 357

[1] Donat. vita ejus.   [2] Euripides.   [3] Plutarch, vita ejus.
[4] Vita Ter.   [5] Gomesius, lib. 3, cap. 21, de sale.
[6] Ter. Eunuch. Act. 2, scen. 2.   [7] Liv. dec. 5, lib. 2.   [8] Comineus.
[9] He that hath £5 per annum coming in more than others, scorns him that hath less, and is a better man.   [10] Prov. xxx, 8.

Page 358

[1] De anima, cap. de mœrore.   [2] Lib. 12 Epist.   [3] Virg. Æn. 4.
[4] Patres mortuos coram astantes et filios, etc.—Marcellus Donatus.
[5] Epist. lib. 2.   Virginium video, audio defunctum, cogito, alloquor.

Page 359

[1] Calpurnius Græcus.   [2] Chaucer.   [3] Præfat. lib. 6.
[4] Lib. de obitu Satyri fratis.

Page 360

[1] Ovid. Met.   [2] Plut. vita ejus.
[3] Nobilis matrona melancholica ob mortem mariti.
[4] Ex matris obitu in desperationem incidit.
[5] Matthias à Michou. Boter. Amphitheat.
[6] Lo. Vertoman. M. Polus Venetus, lib. 1, cap. 54. Perimunt eos quos in via obvios habent, dicentes, Ite, et domino nostro regi servite in alia vita. Nec tam in homines insaniunt, sed in equos, etc.
[7] Vita ejus.
[8] Lib. 4 vitæ ejus. Auream ætatem condiderat ad humani generis salutem, quum nos, statim ab optimi principis excessu, vere ferream pateremur, famem, pestem, etc.

Page 361

[1] Lib. de asse.   [2] Maph.
[3] Ortelius, Itinerario. Ob annum integrum a cantu, tripudiis, et saltationibus tota civitas abstinere jubetur.
[4] Virg.   [5] See Barletius, de vita et ob. Scanderbeg. lib. 13 Hist.
[6] Matt. Paris.   [7] Juvenalis.

Page 362

[1] Multi qui res amatas perdiderant, ut filios, opes, non sperantes recuperare, propter assiduam talium considerationem melancholici fiunt, ut ipse vidi.
[2] Stanihurstus, Hib. hist.
[3] Cap. 3. Melancholia semper venit ob jacturam pecuniæ, victoriæ repulsam, mortem liberorum, quibus longo post tempore animus torquetur, et a dispositione sit habitus.
[4] Consil. 26.   [5] Nubrigensis.   [6] Epig. 22.

Page 363

[1] Lib. 8 Venet. hist.   [2] [Charles, the Constable de Bourbon.]
[3] Templa ornamentis nudata, spoliata, in stabula equorum et asinorum versa, etc. Infulæ humi conculcatæ pedibus, etc.
[4] In oculis maritorum dilectissimæ conjuges ab Hispanorum lixis constupratæ sunt. Filiæ magnatum toris destinatæ, etc.
[5] Ita fastu ante unum mensem turgida civitas, et cacuminibus cœlum pulsare visa, ad inferos usque paucis diebus dejecta.
[6] Sect. 2, memb. 4, subs. 3.

PAGE 364

[1] Accersunt sibi malum.
[2] Si non observemus, nihil valent.—Polydore.
[3] Consil. 26, lib. 2.　　　　　　[4] Harm watch, harm catch.
[5] Geor. Buchanan.
[6] Juvenis, sollicitus de futuris frustra, factus melancholicus.
[7] Pausanias in Achaicis, lib. 7.　Ubi omnium eventus dignoscuntur. Speculum tenui suspensum funiculo demittunt: et ad Cyaneas petras ad Lyciæ fontes, etc.

PAGE 365

[1] Expedit. in Sinas, lib. 1, cap. 3.
[2] Timendo præoccupat quod vitat ultro, provocatque quod fugit, gaudetque mærens et lubens miser fuit.—Heinsius Austriaco.
[3] Tom. 4, dial. 8, Cataplous.　Auri puri mille talenta, me hodie tibi daturum promitto, etc.
[4] Ibidem.　Hei mihi! quæ relinquenda prædia! quam fertiles agri! etc.
[5] Hadrian.　　　[6] Industria superflua circa res inutiles.

PAGE 366

[1] Flavæ secreta Minervæ ut viderat Aglauros.—Ov. Met. 2.
[2] Contra Philos. cap. 61.　　　　　　[3] Matt. Paris.

PAGE 367

[1] Seneca.　　[2] [Roman busybodies referred to by Phædrus and Martial.]

PAGE 368

[1] Jos. Scaliger, in Gnomis.
[2] "A virtuous woman is the crown of her husband" (Prov. xii, 4): "but she," etc.
[3] Lib. 17, epist. 105.　　　　[4] Titionatur, candelabratur, etc.
[5] Daniel, in Rosamund.　　　[6] Chalonerus, lib. 9 de repub.Angl.
[7] Elegans virgo invita cuidam e nostratibus nupsit, etc.

PAGE 369

[1] Prov. x, 1.
[2] De increm. urb. lib. 3, cap. 3.　Tanquam diro mucrone confossis, his nulla requies, nulla delectatio, sollicitudine, gemitu, furore, desperatione, timore, tanquam ad perpetuam ærumnam infeliciter rapti.
[3] Humfredus Lluyd, epist. ad Abrahamum Ortelium.　Mr. Vaughan in his Golden Fleece.　Litibus et controversiis usque ad omnium bonorum consumptionem contendunt.
[4] Quæque repulsa gravis.　　　[5] Lib. 36, cap. 5.
[6] Nihil æque amarum, quam diu pendere: quidam æquiore animo ferunt præcidi spem suam suam quam trahi. Seneca, cap. 3, lib. 2, de ben. Virg.　Plater. Observat. lib. 1.

PAGE 370

[1] Spretæque injuria formæ.　　　　　　[2] Turpe relinqui est.—Hor.
[3] Scimus enim generosas naturas nulla re citius moveri aut gravius affici quam contemptu ac despicientia.
[4] Ad Atticum epist. lib. 12.　　　　[5] Epist. ad Brutum.

PAGE 371

[1] In Phœniss.　　　　　[2] In laudem calvit.　　　[3] Ovid.
[4] E Cret.　　　　　[5] Hor. Car. lib. 3, ode 27.

[1] Hist. lib. 3.
[2] Non mihi si centum linguæ sint, oraque centum, Omnia causarum percurrere nomina possem.
[3] Cælius, lib. 17, cap. 2.
[4] Ita mente exagitati sunt, ut in triremi se constitutos putarent, marique vagabundo tempestate jactatos, proinde naufragium veriti, egestis undique rebus, vasa omnia in viam e fenestris, ceu in mare, præcipitarunt: postridie, etc.

PAGE 373

[1] Aram vobis servatoribus diis erigemus.
[2] Lib. de gemmis.
[3] Quæ gestatæ infelicem et tristem reddunt, curas augent, corpus siccant, somnum minuunt.
[4] Ad unum die mente alienatus.
[5] Part 1, sect. 2, subsect. 3.   [6] Juven. Sat. 3.
[7] Intus bestiæ minutæ multæ necant. Numquid minutissima sunt grana arenæ? sed si arena amplius in navem mittatur, mergit illam. Quam minutæ guttæ pluviæ! et tamen implent flumina, domus ejiciunt, timenda ergo ruina multitudinis, si non magnitudinis.

PAGE 374

[1] Mores sequuntur temperaturam corporis.
[2] Scintillæ latent in corporibus.   [3] Gal. v.
[4] Sicut ex animi affectionibus corpus languescit: sic ex corporis vitiis, et morborum plerisque cruciatibus animum videmus hebetari.—Galenus.
[5] Lib. 1, cap. 16.

PAGE 375

[1] Corporis itidem morbi animam per consensum, a lege consortii afficiunt, et quanquam objecta multos motus turbulentos in homine concitent, præcipua tamen causa in corde et humoribus spiritibusque consistit, etc.
[2] Hor.   [3] Humores pravi mentiem obnubilant.
[4] Hic humor vel a partis intemperie generatur, vel relinquitur post inflammationes, vel crassior in venis conclusus vel torpidus malignam qualitate contrahit.
[5] Sæpe constat in febre hominem melancholicum vel post febrem reddi, aut alium morbum. Calida intemperies innata, vel a febre contracta.

PAGE 376

[1] Raro quis diuturno morbo laborat, qui non sit melancholicus.—Mercurialis, de affect. capitis, lib. 1, cap. 10, de melanc.
[2] Ad nonum lib. Rhasis ad Almansor. cap. 16. Universaliter a quacunque parte potest fieri melancholicus, vel quia aduritur, vel quia non expellit superfluitatem excrementi.
[3] A liene, jecinore, utero, et aliis partibus oritur.
[4] Materia melancholiæ aliquando in corde, in stomacho, hepate, ab hypochondriis, myrache, splene, cum ibi remanet humor melancholicus.
[5] Ex sanguine adusto, intra vel extra caput.
[6] Qui calidum cor habent, cerebrum humidum, facile melancholici.
[7] Sequitur melancholia malam intemperiem frigidam et siccam ipsius cerebri.
[8] Sæpe fit ex calidiore cerebro, aut corpore colligente melancholiam.—Piso.

PAGE 377

[1] Vel per propriam affectionem, vel per consensum, cum vapores exhalant in cerebrum.—Montalt. cap. 14.

[2] Aut ibi gignitur melancholicus fumus, aut aliunde vehitur, alterando animales facultates.

[3] Ab intemperie cordis, modo calidiore, modo frigidiore.

[4] Epist. 209 Scoltzii.

[5] Officina humorum hepar concurrit, etc.

[6] Ventriculus et venæ meseraicae concurrunt, quod hæ partes obstructæ sunt, etc.

[7] Per se sanguinem adurentes.

[8] Lien frigidus et siccus, cap. 13.

[9] Splen obstructus.   [10] De arte med. lib. 3, cap. 24.

[11] A sanguinis putredine in vasis seminariis et utero, et quandoque a spermate diu retento, vel sanguine menstruo in melancholiam verso per putrefactionem, vel adustionem.

[12] Maginus.

PAGE 378

[1] Ergo efficiens causa melancholiæ est calida et sicca intemperies, non frigida et sicca, quod multi opinati sunt; oritur enim a calore cerebri assante sanguinem, etc., tum quod aromata sanguinem incendunt, solitudo, vigilæ, febris præcedens, meditatio, studium, et hæc omnia calefaciunt, ergo ratum sit, etc.

[2] Lib. 1, cap. 13, de melanch.

[3] Lib. 3 Tract. posthum. de melan.

[4] A fatuitate inseparabilis cerebri frigiditas.

[5] Ab interno calore assatur.

[6] Intemperies innata exurens, flavam bilem ac sanguinem in melancholiam convertens.

[7] Si cerebrum sit calidius, fiet spiritus animalis calidior, et delirium maniacum; si frigidior, fiet fatuitas.

PAGE 379

[1] Melancholia capitis accedit post phrenesim aut longam moram moram sub sole, aut persussionem in capite.—Cap. 13, lib. 1.

[2] Qui bibunt vina potentia, et sæpe sunt sub sole.

[3] Curæ validæ, largiores vini et aromatum usus.

[4] A cauterio aut ulcere exsiccato.

[5] Ab ulcere curato incidit in insaniam, aperto vulnere curatur.

[6] A galea nimis calefacta.

[7] Exuritur sanguis aut venæ obstruuntur, quibus obstructis prohibetur transitus chyli ad jecur, corrumpitur et in rugitus et flatus vertitur.

PAGE 380

[1] Stomacho læso robur corporis imminuitur, et reliqua membra alimento orbata, etc.   [2] Hildesheim.

PAGE 381

[1] Habuit sæva animi symptomata quæ impediunt concoctionem, etc.

[2] Usitatissimus morbus cum sit, utile est hujus visceris accidentia considerare, nec leve periculum hujus causas morbi ignorantibus.

[3] Jecur aptum ad generandum talem humorem, splen natura imbecillior. Piso, Altomarus, Guianerius.

[4] Melancholiam, quæ fit a redundantia humoris in toto corpore, victus imprimis generat qui eum humorem parit.

PAGE 382

[1] Ausonius.   [2] Seneca, Cont. lib. 10, cont. 5.

[3] Quædam universalia, particularia, quædam manifesta, quædam in corpore, quædam in cogitatione et animo; quædam a stellis, quædam ab humoribus, quæ ut vinum corpus varie disponit, etc. Diversa phantasmata pro varietate causæ externae, internæ.

[4] Lib. 1 de risu, fol. 17.   Ad ejus esum alii sudant, alii vomunt, stent, bibunt, saltant, alii rident, tremunt, dormiunt, etc.

PAGE 383

[1] T. Bright, cap. 20.

[2] Nigrescit hic humor aliquando supercalefactus, aliquando super-frigefactus.—Melanel. e Gal.

[3] Interprete F. Calvo.

[4] Oculi his excavantur, venti gignuntur circum præcordia et acidi ructus, sicci fere ventres, vertigo, tinnitus aurium, somni pusilli, somnia terribilia et interrupta.   [5] Virg. Æn.

[6] Assiduæ eæque acidæ ructationes quæ cibum virulentum pisculentumque nidorem, etsi nil tale ingestum sit, referant ob cruditatem. Ventres hisce aridi, somnus plerumque parcus et interruptus, somnia absurdissima, turbulenta, corporis tremor, capitis gravedo, strepitus circa aures et visiones ante oculos, ad venerem prodigi.

[7] Altomarus, Bruel, Piso, Montaltus.

[8] Frequentes habent oculorum nictationes, aliqui tamen fixis oculis plerumque sunt.

[9] Cent. lib. 1, tract. 9.   Signa hujus morbi sunt plurimus saltus, sonitus aurium, capitis gravedo; lingua titubat, oculi excavantur, etc.

PAGE 384

[1] In Pantheon, cap. de Melancholia.

[2] Alvus arida nihil dejiciens, cibi capaces, nihilominus tamen extenuati sunt.

[3] Nic. Piso. Inflatio carotidum, etc.

[4] Andreas Dudith, Rahamo ep. lib. 3 Crat. epist.   Multa in pulsibus superstitio, ausim etiam dicere, tot differentias quæ describuntur a Galeno, néque intelligi a quoquam nec observari posse.

[5] T. Bright, cap. 20.

[6] Post 40 ætat. annum, saith Jacchinus in 15, 9 Rhasis.   Idem Mercurialis, consil. 86; Trincavellius, tom. 2, cons. 17.

[7] Gordonius.   Modo rident, modo fient, silent, etc.

[8] Fernelius, consil. 43 et 45.   Montanus, consil. 230.   Galen de locis affectis, lib. 3, cap. 6.

PAGE 385

[1] Aphorism. et lib. de melan.

[2] Lib. 2, cap. 6, de locis affect.   Timor et mœstitia, si diutius perseverent, etc.

[3] Tract. posthumo de melan. edit. Venetiis 1620, per Bolzettam bibliop. Mihi diligentius hanc rem consideranti, patet quosdam esse, qui non laborant mœrore et timore.

[4] Prob. lib. 3.

[5] Physiog. lib. 1, cap. 8.   Quibus multa frigida bilis atra, stolidi et timidi, at qui calidi, ingeniosi, amasii, divinosi, spiritu instigati, etc.

[6] Omnes exercent metus et tristitia, et sine causa.

[7] Omnes timent, licent non omnibus idem timendi modus.—Aetius, Tetrab. lib. 2, sect. 2, cap. 9.

[8] Ingenti pavore trepidant.

[9] Multi mortem timent, et tamen sibi ipsis mortem consciscunt, alii cœli ruinam timent.

NOTES

514

PAGE 386

[1] Affligit eos plena scrupulis conscientia, divinæ misericordiæ diffidentes, Orco se destinant, fœda lamentatione deplorantes.
[2] Non ausus egredi domo, ne deficeret.
[3] Multi dæmones timent, latrones, insidias.—Avicenna.
[4] Alii comburi, alii de rege.—Rhasis.
[5] Ne terra absorbeantur.—Forestus.
[6] Ne terra dehiscat.—Gordon.
[7] Alii timore mortis timentur et mala gratia principum putant 'se aliquid commisisse, et ad supplicium requiri.

PAGE 387

[1] Alius domesticos timet, alius omnes.—Aetius.
[2] Alii timent insidias.—Aurel. lib. 1 de morb. chron. cap. 6.
[3] Ille carissimos, hic omnes homines citra discrimen timet.
[4] Virgil.
[5] Hic in lucem prodire timet, tenebrasque quærit; contra, ille caliginosa fugit.
[6] Quidam larvas, et malos spiritus ab inimicis veneficiis et incantationibus sibi putant objectari. Hippocrates. Potionem se veneficam sumpsisse putat, et de hac ructare sibi crebro videtur. Idem Montaltus, cap. 21, Aetius, lib. 2, et alii. Trallianus, lib. 1, cap. 16.

PAGE 388

[1] Observat. lib. 1. Quando iis nil nocet, nisi quod mulieribus melancholicis.
[2] Timeo tamen metusque causæ nescius, causa est metus.—Heinsius Austriaco.
[3] Cap. 15 in 9 Rhasis. In multis vidi, præter rationem semper aliquid timent, in cæteris tamen optime se gerunt, neque aliquid præter dignitatem committunt.

PAGE 389

[1] Altomarus, cap. 7. Aretæus. Tristes sunt.
[2] Mant. Egl. 1.
[3] Ovid. Met. 4.
[4] Inquies animus.
[5] Hor. lib. 3, od. 1.
[6] Virg.
[7] Menedemus, Heautont. Act. 1, sc. 1.

PAGE 390

[1] Altomarus.
[2] Seneca.
[3] Cap. 31. Quo stomachi dolore correptum se etiam de consciscenda morte cogitasse dixit.

PAGE 391

[1] Luget et semper tristatur, solitudinem amat, mortem sibi precatur, vitam propriam odio habet.
[2] Facile in iram incidunt.—Aret.
[3] Ira sine causa, velocitas iræ. — Savonarola, Pract. major. Velocitas iræ signum.—Avicenna, lib. 3, fen. 1, tract. 4, cap. 18.
[4] Suspicio, diffidentia, symptomata. — Crato, Ep. Julio Alexandrino, cons. 185 Scoltzii.

PAGE 392

[1] Hor.
[2] Pers. Sat. 3.
[3] In his Dutch-work picture.
[4] Howard, cap. 7 Differ.

Page 393

[1] Tract. de mel. cap. 2.   Noctu ambulant per silvas, et loca periculosa; neminem timent.

[2] Facile amant.—Altom.   [3] Bodine.

[4] Jo. Major, vitis patrum, fol. 202.   Paulus Abbas eremita tanta solitudine perseverat, ut nec vestem, nec nec vultum mulieris ferre possit, etc.

[5] Consult. lib. 1, cons. 17.

[6] Generally as they are pleased or displeased, so are their continual cogitations pleasing or displeasing.

Page 394

[1] Omnes exercent vanæ intensæque animi cogitationes (N. Piso, Bruel) et assiduæ.

[2] Curiosi de rebus minimis.—Aretæus.

[3] Lib. 2 de intell.

[4] Hoc melancholicis omnibus proprium, ut quas semel imaginationes valde receperint, non facile rejiciant, sed hæ etiam vel invitis semper occurrant.

[5] Tullius, de Sen.

Page 395

[1] Consil. med. pro hypochondriaco.   [2] Consil. 43.

[3] Cap. 5.   [4] Lib. 2 de intell.

[5] Consult. 15 et 16, lib. 1.   [6] Virg. Æn. 6.

Page 396

[1] Iliad 6.

[2] Si malum exasperetur, homines odio habent et solitaria petunt.

[3] Democritus solet noctes et dies apud se degere, plerumque autem in speluncis, sub amœnis arborum umbris vel in tenebris, et mollibus herbis, vel ad aquarum crebra et quieta fluenta, etc.

[4] Gaudet tenebris, aliturque dolor.   Ps. cii.   Vigilavi, et factus sum velut nycticorax in domicilio, passer solitarius in templo.

[5] Et quæ vix audet fabula, monstra parit.

[6] In cap. 18, lib. 10, de Civ. Dei.   Lunam ab asino epotam videns.

Page 397

[1] Velc. lib. 4, cap. 5.   [2] Sect. 2, memb. 1, subs. 4.

[3] De reb. cœlest. lib. 10, cap. 13.

Page 398

[1] J. de Indagine, Goclenius.   [2] Hor. de art. poet.

[3] Tract. 7, de Melan.   [4] Humidum, calidum, frigidum, siccum.

[5] Com. in 1 cap. Johannis de Sacrobosco.

Page 399

[1] Si residet melancholia naturalis, tales plumbei coloris aut nigri, stupidi, solitarii.

[2] Non una melancholiæ causa est, nec unus humor vitii parens, sed plures, et alius aliter mutatus, unde non omnes eadem sentiunt symptomata.

[3] Humor frigidus delirii causa, humor calidus furoris.

[4] Multum refert qua quisque melancholia teneatur, hunc fervens et accensa agitat, illum tristis et frigens occupat: hi timidi, illi inverecundi, intrepidi, etc.

[5] Cap. 7 et 8, Tract. de Mel.

[6] Signa melancholiæ ex intemperie et agitatione spirituum sine materia.

[7] T. Bright, cap. 16, Treat. Mel.

PAGE 400

[1] Cap. 16, in 9 Rhasis. [2] Bright, cap. 16.
[3] Pract. major. Somnians, piger, frigidus.
[4] De anima, cap. de humor. Si a phlegmate, semper in aquis fere sunt, et circa fluvios plorant multum, etc.
[5] Pigra nascitur ex colore pallido et albo.—Her. de Saxon.
[6] Savonarola.
[7] Muros cadere in se, aut submergi timent, cum torpore et segnitie, et fluvios amant tales.—Alexand. cap. 16, lib. 7.
[8] Semper fere dormit somnolenta, cap. 16, lib. 7.
[9] Laurentius.
[10] Cap. 6 de mel. Si a sanguine, venit rubedo oculorum et faciei, plurimus risus.
[11] Venæ oculorum sunt rubræ, vide an præcesserit vini et aromatum usus, et frequens balneum, Trallian. lib. 1, 16, an præcesserit mora sub sole.
[12] Ridet patiens si a sanguine, putat se videre choreas, musicam audire, ludos, etc.
[13] Cap. 2, tract. de melan.
[14] Hor. Ep. lib. 2. Quidam haud ignobilis Argis, etc.
[15] Lib. de reb. mir.

PAGE 401

[1] Cum inter concionandum mulier dormiens e subsellio caderet, et omnes reliqui qui id viderent, riderent, tribus post diebus, etc.
[2] Juvenis et non vulgaris eruditionis.
[3] Si a cholera, furibundi interficiunt se et alios, putant se videre pugnas.
[4] Urina subtilis et ignea, parum dormiunt.
[5] Tract. 15, cap. 4.

PAGE 402

[1] Ad hæc perpetranda furore rapti ducuntur, cruciatus quosvis tolerant, et mortem, et furore exacerbato audent et ad supplicia plus irritantur; mirum est quantum habeant in tormentis patientiam.
[2] Tales plus cæteris timent, et continue tristantur, valde suspiciosi, solitudinem diligunt, corruptissimas habent imaginationes, etc.
[3] Si a melancholia adusta, tristes, de sepulchris somniant, timent ne fascinentur, putant se mortuos, aspici nolunt.
[4] Videntur sibi videre monachos nigros et dæmones, et suspensos et mortuos.
[5] Quavis nocte se cum dæmone coire putavit.
[6] Semper fere vidisse militem nigrum præsentem.
[7] Anthony de Verdeur.
[8] Quidam mugitus boum æmulantur, et pecora se putant, ut Prœti filiæ.
[9] Baro quidam mugitus boum, et rugitus asinorum, et aliorum animalium voces effingit.

PAGE 403

[1] Omnia magna putabat, uxorem magnam, grandes equos; abhorruit omnia parva; magna pocula, et calceamenta pedibus majora.
[2] Lib. 1, cap. 16. Putavit se uno digito posse totum mundum conterere.
[3] Sustinet humeris cœlum cum Atlante. Alii cœli ruinam timent.
[4] Cap. 1, tract. 15. Alius se gallum putat, alius lusciniam.
[5] Trallianus. [6] Cap. 7 de mel.
[7] Anthony de Verdeur. [8] Cap. 7 de mel.

PAGE 404

[1] Laurentius, cap. 6.
[2] Lib. 3, cap. 14. Qui se regem putavit regno expulsum.
[3] Deipnosophist. lib. Thrasylaus putavit omnes naves in Piræum portum appellantes suas esse.

⁴ De hist. med. mirab. lib. 2, cap. 1.
⁵ Genibus flexis loqui cum illo voluit, et adstare jam tum putavit, etc.
⁶ Gordonius. Quod sit propheta, et inflatus a Spiritu Sancto.

PAGE 405

¹ Qui forensibus causis insudat, nil nisi arresta cogitat, et supplices libellos; alius non nisi versus facit.—P. Forestus.
² Gordonius.
³ Verbo non exprimunt, nec opere, sed alta mente recondunt, et sunt viri prudentissimi, quos ego saepe novi; cum multi sint sine timore, ut qui se reges et mortuos putant, plura signa quidam habent, pauciora, majora, minora.
⁴ [In the ratio of three to two, four to three, five to three, seven to five of melancholy.]
⁵ Trallianus, lib. 1, 16. Alii intervalla quaedam habent, ut etiam consueta administrent, alii in continuo delirio sunt, etc.
⁶ Prac. mag. Vere tantum et autumno.
⁷ Lib. de humoribus. ⁸ Guianerius.
⁹ De mentis alienat. cap. 3.

PAGE 406

¹ Levinus Lemnius, Jason Pratensis. Blanda ab initio. ² Hor.
³ Facilis descensus Averni. ⁴ Virg.

PAGE 407

¹ Corpus cadaverosum. Ps. lxvii: Cariosa est facies mea prae aegritudine animae.
² Lib. 9, ad Almansorem. ³ Practica majore.
⁴ Quum ore loquitur quae corde concepit, quum subito de una re ad aliud transit, neque rationem de aliquo reddit, tunc est in medio, at quum incipit operari quae loquitur, in summo gradu est.
⁵ Cap. 19, partic. 2. Loquitur secum et ad alios, ac si vere praesentes. Aug. cap. 11, lib. de cura pro mortuis gerenda. Rhasis.
⁶ Quum res ad hoc devenit, ut ea quae cogitare coeperit, ore promat, atque acta permisceat, tum perfecta melancholia est.
⁷ Melancholicus se videre et audire putat daemones.—Lavater, de spectris, part. 3, cap. 2.
⁸ Wierus, lib. 3, cap. 31. ⁹ Michael, a musician.

PAGE 408

¹ Malleo malef. ² Lib. de atra bile.
³ Part. 1, subs. 2, memb. 2. ⁴ De delirio, melancholia et mania.

PAGE 409

¹ Nicholas Piso. Si signa circa ventriculum non apparent, nec sanguis male affectus, et adsunt timor et moestitia, cerebrum ipsum existimandum est, etc.
² Tract. de mel. cap. 13, etc. Ex intemperie spirituum, et cerebri motu, tenebrositate.
³ Facie sunt rubente et livescente, quibus etiam aliquando adsunt pustulae.
⁴ Jo. Pantheon. cap. de mel. Si cerebrum primario afficiatur, adsunt capitis gravitas, fixi oculi, etc.
⁵ Laurent. cap. 5. Si a cerebro ex siccitate, tum capitis erit levitas, sitis, vigilia, paucitas superfluitatum in oculis et naribus.

[1] Si nulla digna læsio ventriculo, quoniam in hac melancholia capitis exigua nonnunquam ventriculi pathemata coeunt, duo enim hæc membra sibi invicem affectionem transmittunt.

[2] Postrema magis flatuosa.

[3] Si minus molestiæ circa ventriculum aut ventrem, in iis cerebrum primario afficitur, et curare oportet hunc affectum, per cibos flatus exsortes, et bonæ concoctionis, etc.; raro cerebrum afficitur sine ventriculo.

[4] Sanguinem adurit caput calidius, et inde fumi melancholici adusti, animum exagitant.

[5] Lib. de loc. affect. cap. 6.   [6] Cap. 6.

[7] Hildesheim, Spicil. 1 de mel. In hypochondriaca melancholia adeo ambigua sunt symptomata, ut etiam exercitatissimi medici de loco affecto statuere non possint.

[1] Medici de loco affecto nequeunt statuere.

[2] Tract. posthumo de mel., Patavii edit. 1620 per Bolzettam bibliop., cap. 2.

[3] Acidi ructus, cruditates, æstus in præcordiis, flatus, interdum ventriculi dolores vehementes, sumptoque cibo concoctu difficili, sputum humidum idque multum sequetur, etc. Hip. lib. de mel., Galenus, Melanelius e Ruffo et Aetio, Altomarus, Piso, Montaltus, Bruel, Wecker, etc.

[4] Circa præcordia de assidua inflatione queruntur, et cum sudore totius corporis importuno, frigidos articulos sæpe patiuntur, indigestione laborant, ructus suos insuaves perhorrescunt, viscerum dolores habent.

[1] Montaltus, cap. 13, Wecker, Fuchsius, cap. 13, Altomarus, cap. 7, Laurentius, cap. 73, Bruel, Gordon.

[2] Pract. major. Dolor in eo et ventositas, nausea.

[3] Ut atra densaque nubes soli effusa, radios et lumen ejus intercipit et offuscat; sic, etc.

[4] Ut fumus e camino.

[1] Hypochondriaci maxime affectant coire, et multiplicatur coitus in ipsis, eo quod ventositates multiplicantur in hypochondriis, et coitus sæpe allevat has ventositates.

[2] Cont. lib. 1, tract. 9.

[3] Wecker. Melancholicus succus toto corpore redundans.

[4] Splen natura imbecillior.—Montaltus, cap. 22.

[5] Lib. 1, cap. 16. Interrogare convenit, an aliqua evacuationis retentio obvenerit, viri in hæmorrhoid., mulierum menstruis, et vide faciem similiter an sit rubicunda.

[6] Naturales nigri acquisiti a toto corpore, sæpe rubicundi.

[7] Montaltus, cap. 22. Piso. Ex colore sanguinis si minuas venam, si fluat niger, etc.

[1] Apul. lib. 1. Semper obviæ species mortuorum; quicquid umbrarum est uspiam, quicquid lemurum et larvarum oculis suis aggerunt; sibi fingunt omnia noctium occursacula, omnia bustorum formidamina, omnia sepulchrorum terriculamenta.

[2] Differt enim ab ea quæ viris et reliquis feminis communiter contingit, propriam habens causam.

[3] Ex menstrui sanguinis tetra ad cor et cerebrum exhalatione, vitiatum

semen mentem perturbat, etc., non per essentiam, sed per consensum. Animus mœrens et anxius inde malum trahit, et spiritus cerebrum obfuscantur, quæ cuncta augentur, etc.

Page 415

[1] Cum tacito delirio ac dolore alicujus partis internæ, dorsi, hypochondrii, cordis regionem et universam mammam interdum occupantis, etc.
[2] Cutis aliquando squalida, aspera, rugosa, præcipue cubitis, genibus, et digitorum articulis; præcordia ingenti sæpe terrore æstuant et pulsant, cumque vapor excitatus sursum evolat, cor palpitat aut premitur, animus deficit, etc.
[3] Animi dejectio, perversa rerum existimatio, præposterum judicium. Fastidiosæ, languentes, tædiosæ, consilii inopes, lacrimosæ, timentes, mœstæ, cum summa rerum meliorum desperatione, nulla re delectantur, solitudinem amant, etc.

Page 416

[1] Nolunt aperire molestiam quam patiuntur, sed conqueruntur tamen de capite, corde, mammis, etc. In puteos fere maniaci prosilire, ac strangulari cupiunt, nulla orationis suavitate ad spem salutis recuperandam erigi, etc. Familiares non curant, non loquuntur, non respondent, etc., et hæc graviora, si, etc.

Page 417

[1] Clysteres et helleborismum Matthioli summe laudat.

Page 419

[1] Examen Conc. Trident. de cælibatu sacerd.
[2] Cap. de satyr. et priapis.   [3] Part. 3, sect. 2, memb. 5, subs. 5.
[4] Vapores crassi et nigri, a ventriculo in cerebrum exhalant.—Fel. Platerus.

Page 420

[1] Calidi hilares, frigidi indispositi ad lætitiam et ideo solitarii, taciturni, non ob tenebras internas, ut medici volunt, sed ob frigus: multi melancholici nocte ambulant intrepidi. Vapores melancholici, spiritibus misti, tenebrarum causæ sunt (cap. 1).
[2] Intemperies facit succum nigrum, nigrities obscurat spiritum, obscuratio spiritus facit metum et tristitiam.
[3] Ut nubecula solem offuscat. Constantinus, lib. de melanch.
[4] Altomarus, cap. 7. Causam timoris circumfert ater humor passionis materia, et atri spiritus perpetuam animæ domicilio offundunt noctem.

Page 421

[1] Pone exemplum, quod quis potest ambulare super trabem quæ est in via: sed si sit super aquam profundam, loco pontis, non ambulabit super eam, eo quod imaginatur in animo et timet vehementer, forma cadendi impressa, cui obediunt membra omnia, et facultates reliquæ.
[2] Lib. 2 de intellectione. Suspiciosi ob timorem et obliquum discursum, et semper inde putant sibi fieri insidias. Lauren. 5.
[3] Tract. de mel., cap. 7. Ex dilatione, contractione, confusione, tenebrositate spirituum, calida, frigida intemperie, etc.
[4] Illud inquisitione dignum, cur tam falsa recipiant, habere se cornua, esse mortuos, nasutos, esse aves, etc.
[5] 1. Dispositio corporis. 2. Occasio imaginationis.

Page 422

[1] In pro. lib. de cœlo. Vehemens et assidua cogitatio rei erga quam afficitur, spiritus in cerebrum evocat.

[2] Melancholici ingeniosi omnes, summi viri in artibus et disciplinis, sive circum imperatoriam aut reip. disciplinam omnes fere melancholici.—Aristoteles.

[3] Adeo miscentur, ut sit duplum sanguinis ad reliqua duo.

[4] Lib. 2 de intellectione. Pingui sunt Minerva phlegmatici: sanguinei amabiles, grati, hilares, at non ingeniosi; cholerici celeres motu, et ob id contemplationis impatientes: melancholici solum excellentes, etc.

Page 423

[1] Trepidantium vox tremula, quia cor quatitur.

[2] Ob ariditatem quæ reddit nervos linguæ torpidos.

[3] Incontinentia linguæ ex copia flatuum, et velocitate imaginationis.

[4] Calvities ob siccitatis excessum.   [5] Aetius.

[6] Lauren. cap. 13.   [7] Tetrab. 2, ser. 2, cap. 10.

[8] Ant. Lodovicus, Prob. lib. 1, sect. 5, de atrabilariis.

[9] Subrusticus pudor, vitiosus pudor.

[10] Ob ignominiam aut turpitudinem facti, etc.

[11] De symp. et antip. cap. 12. Laborat facies ob præsentiam ejus qui defectum nostrum videt, et natura quasi opem latura calorem illuc mittit, calor sanguinem trahit, unde rubor. Audaces non rubent, etc.

Page 424

[1] Ob gaudium et voluptatem foras exit sanguis, aut ob melioris reverentiam, aut ob subitum occursum, aut si quid incautius exciderit.

[2] Com. in Arist. de anima. Cæci ut plurimum impudentes, nox facit impudentes.

[3] Alexander Aphrodisiensis makes all bashfulness a virtue, eamque se refert in seipso experiri solitum, etsi esset admodum senex.

[4] Com. in Arist. de anima. Tam a vi et inexperientia quam a vitio.

[5] Sæpe post cibum apti ad ruborem, ex potu vini, ex timore sæpe et ab hepate calido, cerebro calido, etc.

[6] 2 De oratore. Quid ipse risus, quo pacto concitetur, ubi sit, etc.

[7] Diaphragma titillant, quia transversum et nervosum, quia titillatione moto sensu atque arteriis distentis, spiritus inde latera, venas, os, oculos occupant.

[8] Ex calefactione humidi cerebri: nam ex sicco lacrimæ non fluunt.

[9] Res mirandas imaginantur: et putant se videre quæ nec vident, nec audiunt.

Page 425

[1] Laet. lib. 13, cap. 2, descript. Indiæ Occident.

[2] Lib. 1, cap. 17, cap. de mel.

[3] Insani, et qui morti vicini sunt, res quas extra se videre putant, intra oculos habent.

[4] Cap. 10, de spirit. apparitione.   [5] De occult. nat. mirac.

Page 426

[1] Seneca. Quod metuunt nimis, nunquam amoveri posse, nec tolli putant.

Page 427

[1] Sanguis upupæ cum melle compositus et centaurea, etc.—Albertus.

[2] Lib. 1, Occult. philos. Imperiti homines dæmonum et umbrarum imagines videre se putant, quum nihil sint aliud quam simulacra animæ expertia.

³ Pythonissæ, vocum varietatem in ventre et gutture fingentes, formant voces humanas a longe vel prope, prout volunt, ac si spiritus cum homine loqueretur, et sonos brutorum fingunt, etc.
⁴ [Gloucester Cathedral].

PAGE 428

¹ Tam clare et articulate audies repetitum, ut perfectior sit echo quam ipse dixeris.
² Blowing of bellows, and knocking of hammers, if they apply their ear to the cliff.
³ Memb. 1, subs. 3, of this partition.   ⁴ Cap. 16 in 9 Rhasis.
⁵ Signa dæmonis nulla sunt nisi quod loquantur ea quæ ante nesciebant, ut Teutonicum aut aliud idioma, etc.
⁶ Cap. 12, tract. de mel.
⁷ Tract. 15, cap. 4.   ⁸ Cap. 9.
⁹ Mira vis concitat humores, ardorque vehemens mentem exagitat, quum, etc.

PAGE 429

¹ Præfat. Iamblichi mysteriis.
² Si melancholicis hæmorroides supervenerint, varices, vel ut quibusdam placet, aqua inter cutem, solvitur malum.
³ Cap. 10, de quartana.

PAGE 430

¹ Cum sanguis exit per superficiem et residet melancholia per scabiem, morpheam nigram, vel expurgatur per inferiores partes, vel urinam, etc., non erit, etc., splen magnificatur et varices apparent.
² Quia jam conversa in naturam.
³ In quocunque sit, a quacunque causa, hypocon. præsertim, semper est longa, morosa, nec facile curari potest.
⁴ Regina morborum et inexorabilis.
⁵ Omne delirium quod oritur a paucitate cerebri incurabile.—Hildesheim, Spicil. 2 de mania.
⁶ Si sola imaginatio lædatur, et non ratio.
⁷ Mala a sanguine fervente, deterior a bile assata, pessima ab atra bile putrefacta.
⁸ Difficilior cura ejus quæ fit vitio corporis totius et cerebri.
⁹ Difficilis curatu in viris, multo difficilior in feminis.
¹⁰ Ad interitum plerumque homines comitatur; licet medici levent plerumque, tamen non tollunt unquam, sed recidet acerbior quam antea minima occasione aut errore.
¹¹ Periculum est ne degeneret in epilepsiam, apoplexiam, convulsionem, cæcitatem.
¹² Montal. cap. 25; Laurentius; Nic. Piso.

PAGE 431

¹ Herc. de Saxonia, Aristotle, Capivaccius.
² Favent.   Humor frigidus sola delirii causa, furoris vero humor calidus.
³ Heurnius calls madness sobolem melancholiæ [the offspring of melancholy].   ⁴ Alexander, lib. 1, cap. 18.
⁵ Lib. 1, part. 2, cap. 11.
⁶ Montalt. cap. 15.   Raro mors aut nunquam, nisi sibi ipsis inferant.
⁷ Lib. de Insan. Fabio Calico interprete.
⁸ Nonnulli violentas manus sibi inferunt.
⁹ Lucret. lib. 3.

[10] Lib. 2 de intell. Sæpe mortem sibi consciscunt ob timorem et tristitiam, tædio vitæ affecti ob furorem et desperationem. Est enim infera, etc. Ergo sic perpetuo afflictati vitam oderunt, se præcipitant, his malis carituri, aut interficiunt se, aut tale quid committunt.

PAGE 432

[1] Psal. cvii, 10.   [2] Job, iii.   [3] Job vi, 8.
[4] Vi doloris et tristitiæ ad insaniam pene redactus.
[5] Seneca.
[6] In salutis suæ desperatione proponunt sibi mortis desiderium.—Oct. Horat. lib. 2, cap. 5.
[7] Lib. de insania. Sic, sic juvat ire per umbras.
[8] Cap. 3 de mentis alienat. Mœsti degunt, dum tandem mortem quam timent, suspendio aut submersione, aut aliqua alia vi, præcipitant, ut multa tristia exempla vidimus.
[9] Arculanus in 9 Rhasis, cap. 16. Cavendum ne ex alto se præcipitant aut alias lædent.

PAGE 433

[1] O omnium opinionibus incogitabile malum!—Lucian. Mortesque mille, mille dum vivit neces gerit, peritque.—Heinsius Austriaco.
[2] Regina morborum cui famulantur omnes et obediunt.—Cardan.
[3] Eheu, quis intus scorpio, etc.—Seneca, Herc. Œt. Act. 4.
[4] Silius Italicus.

PAGE 434

[1] Lib. 29.
[2] Hic omnis imbonitas et insuavitas consistit, ut Tertulliani verbis utar. Orat. ad Martyr.   [3] Plautus.
[4] Vit. Herculis.   [5] Persius. [Juv. 10, 188.]
[6] Quid est miserius in vita, quam velle mori?—Seneca.
[7] Tom. 2, Libello, an graviores passiones, etc.   [8] Ter.

PAGE 435

[1] Patet exitus; si pugnare non vultis, licet fugere; quis vos tenet invitos? —De provid. cap. 8
[2] Agamus Deo gratias, quod nemo invitus in vita teneri potest.
[3] Seneca, epist. 26, et de sacra. 2, cap. 15, et epist. 70, et 12.
[4] Lib. 2, cap. 83. Terra mater nostri miserta.
[5] Epist. 24, 71, 82.

PAGE 436

[1] 2 Macc. xiv, 42.   [2] Vindicatio Apoc. lib.

PAGE 437

[1] As amongst Turks and others.
[2] Bohemus, de moribus gent.
[3] Ælian, lib. 4, cap. 1. Omnes 70 annum egressos interficiunt.
[4] Lib. 2. Præsertim quum tormentum ei vita sit, bona spe fretus, acerba vita velut a carcere se eximat, vel ab aliis eximi sua voluntate patiatur.
[5] Nam quis amphoram exsiccans fæcem exsorberet? (Seneca, epist. 58). Quis in pœnas et risum viveret? Stulti est manere in vita cum sit miser.
[6] Expedit. ad Sinas, lib. 1, cap. 9. Vel bonorum desperatione vel malorum perpessione fracti et fatigati, vel manus violentas sibi inferunt vel ut inimicis suis ægre faciant, etc.

PAGE 438

[1] So did Anthony, Galba, Vitellius, Otho, Aristotle himself, etc.; Ajax in despair; Cleopatra to save her honour.

[2] Inertius deligitur diu vivere quam in timore tot morborum semel moriendo, nullum deinceps formidare.

[3] Curtius, lib. 8.

[4] Laqueus præcisus, contr. 1, lib. 5. Quidam naufragio facto, amissis tribus liberis et uxore, suspendit se; præcidit illi quidam ex prætereuntibus laqueum; a liberato reus fit maleficii.—Seneca.

[5] See Lipsius, Manuduc. ad Stoicam philosophiam, lib. 3, dissert. 22; Dr. King's 14th Lect. on Jonas; Dr. Abbot's 6th Lect. on the same prophet.

[6] Plautus.   [7] Martial.

PAGE 439

[1] As to be buried out of Christian burial with a stake. Idem Plato, 9 de legibus, vult separatim sepeliri, qui sibi ipsis mortem consciscunt, etc., lose their goods, etc.

[2] Navis destituta nauclero in terribilem aliquem scopulum impingit.

[3] Observat.

[4] Seneca, tract. 1, lib. 8, cap. 4. Lex, Homicida in se insepultus abjiciatur, contradicitur. Eo quod afferre sibi manus coactus sit assiduis malis; summam infelicitatem suam in hoc removit, quod existimabat licere misero mori.

[5] Buchanan, Eleg. lib.

THE SECOND PARTITION

THE SYNOPSIS OF THE SECOND PARTITION

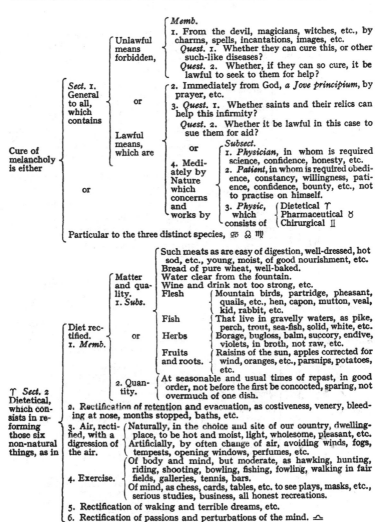

Cure of melancholy is either

Sect. 1. General to all, which contains

— Unlawful means forbidden,

Memb.
1. From the devil, magicians, witches, etc., by charms, spells, incantations, images, etc.
   Quest. 1. Whether they can cure this, or other such-like diseases?
   Quest. 2. Whether, if they can so cure, it be lawful to seek to them for help?

or

Lawful means, which are

2. Immediately from God, *a Jove principium*, by prayer, etc.
3. *Quest. 1.* Whether saints and their relics can help this infirmity?
   Quest. 2. Whether it be lawful in this case to sue them for aid?

or

4. Mediately by Nature which concerns and works by

Subsect.
1. *Physician*, in whom is required science, confidence, honesty, etc.
2. *Patient*, in whom is required obedience, constancy, willingness, patience, confidence, bounty, etc., not to practise on himself.
3. *Physic*, which consists of — Dietetical ♈ / Pharmaceutical ♉ / Chirurgical ♊

or

Particular to the three distinct species, ♋ ♌ ♍

♈ *Sect. 2* Dietetical, which consists in reforming those six non-natural things, as in

Diet rectified. 1. *Memb.*

Matter and quality. 1. *Subs.*

Such meats as are easy of digestion, well-dressed, hot sod, etc., young, moist, of good nourishment, etc.
Bread of pure wheat, well-baked.
Water clear from the fountain.
Wine and drink not too strong, etc.
Flesh — Mountain birds, partridge, pheasant, quails, etc., hen, capon, mutton, veal, kid, rabbit, etc.
Fish — That live in gravelly waters, as pike, perch, trout, sea-fish, solid, white, etc.
Herbs — Borage, bugloss, balm, succory, endive, violets, in broth, not raw, etc.
Fruits and roots. — Raisins of the sun, apples corrected for wind, oranges, etc., parsnips, potatoes, etc.

or

2. Quantity.

At seasonable and usual times of repast, in good order, not before the first be concocted, sparing, not overmuch of one dish.

2. Rectification of retention and evacuation, as costiveness, venery, bleeding at nose, months stopped, baths, etc.

3. Air, rectified, with a digression of the air.

Naturally, in the choice and site of our country, dwelling-place, to be hot and moist, light, wholesome, pleasant, etc.
Artificially, by often change of air, avoiding winds, fogs, tempests, opening windows, perfumes, etc.

4. Exercise.

Of body and mind, but moderate, as hawking, hunting, riding, shooting, bowling, fishing, fowling, walking in fair fields, galleries, tennis, bars.
Of mind, as chess, cards, tables, etc. to see plays, masks, etc., serious studies, business, all honest recreations.

5. Rectification of waking and terrible dreams, etc.

6. Rectification of passions and perturbations of the mind. ♎

I

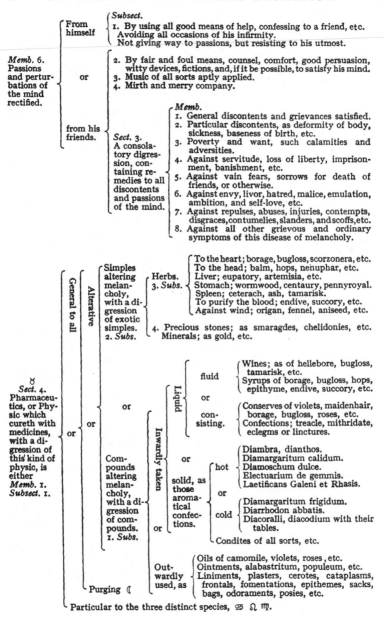

Memb. 6. Passions and perturbations of the mind rectified.

From himself
Subsect.
1. By using all good means of help, confessing to a friend, etc. Avoiding all occasions of his infirmity. Not giving way to passions, but resisting to his utmost.

or

from his friends.

2. By fair and foul means, counsel, comfort, good persuasion, witty devices, fictions, and, if it be possible, to satisfy his mind.
3. Music of all sorts aptly applied.
4. Mirth and merry company.

Sect. 3. A consolatory digression, containing remedies to all discontents and passions of the mind.

Memb.
1. General discontents and grievances satisfied.
2. Particular discontents, as deformity of body, sickness, baseness of birth, etc.
3. Poverty and want, such calamities and adversities.
4. Against servitude, loss of liberty, imprisonment, banishment, etc.
5. Against vain fears, sorrows for death of friends, or otherwise.
6. Against envy, livor, hatred, malice, emulation, ambition, and self-love, etc.
7. Against repulses, abuses, injuries, contempts, disgraces, contumelies, slanders, and scoffs, etc.
8. Against all other grievous and ordinary symptoms of this disease of melancholy.

♉ *Sect. 4.* Pharmaceutics, or Physic which cureth with medicines, with a digression of this kind of physic, is either *Memb. 1. Subsect. 1.*

General to all

Alterative

or

Simples altering melancholy, with a digression of exotic simples. 2. *Subs.*

Herbs. 3. *Subs.*
To the heart; borage, bugloss, scorzonera, etc.
To the head; balm, hops, nenuphar, etc.
Liver; eupatory, artemisia, etc.
Stomach; wormwood, centaury, pennyroyal.
Spleen; ceterach, ash, tamarisk.
To purify the blood; endive, succory, etc.
Against wind; origan, fennel, aniseed, etc.

4. Precious stones; as smaragdes, chelidonies, etc. Minerals; as gold, etc.

or

Compounds altering melancholy, with a digression of compounds. 1. *Subs.*

Inwardly taken

Liquid

fluid
Wines; as of hellebore, bugloss, tamarisk, etc.
Syrups of borage, bugloss, hops, epithyme, endive, succory, etc.

or

consisting.
Conserves of violets, maidenhair, borage, bugloss, roses, etc.
Confections; treacle, mithridate, eclegms or linctures.

or

solid, as those aromatical confections.

hot
Diambra, dianthos.
Diamargaritum calidum.
Diamoschum dulce.
Electuarium de gemmis.
Laetificans Galeni et Rhasis.

or

cold
Diamargaritum frigidum.
Diarrhodon abbatis.
Diacoralli, diacodium with their tables.

or

Condites of all sorts, etc.

Outwardly used, as
Oils of camomile, violets, roses, etc.
Ointments, alabastritum, populeum, etc.
Liniments, plasters, cerotes, cataplasms, frontals, fomentations, epithemes, sacks, bags, odoraments, posies, etc.

Purging ☾

Particular to the three distinct species, ♋ ♌ ♍.

Medicines purging melancholy, are either *Memb. 2.*

> **Simples purging melancholy.**
>> 1. *Subs.* Upward, as vomits. { Asarabacca, laurel, white hellebore, scilla, or sea-onion, antimony, tobacco.
>> Downward. 2. *Subs.*
>>> or { More gentle; as senna, epithyme, polypody, myrobalanes, fumitory, etc.
>>> { Stronger; aloes, lapis Armenus, lapis lazuli, black hellebore.

> or
> **3. *Subs.* Compounds purging melancholy.**
>> Superior parts.
>>> Mouth
>>>> swallowed, or
>>>>> { Liquid, as potions, juleps, syrups, wine of hellebore, bugloss, etc.
>>>>> Solid, as lapis Armenus and lazuli, pills of Indy, pills of fumitory, etc.
>>>>> Electuaries, diasenna, confection of hamech, hierologadium, etc.
>>>> Not swallowed, as gargarisms, masticatories, etc.
>>> or
>>> Nostrils, sneezing powders, odoraments, perfumes, etc.
>> Inferior parts, as clysters strong and weak, and suppositories of Castilian soap, honey boiled, etc.

II   Chirurgical physic, which consists of *Memb. 3.*
> Phlebotomy, to all parts almost, and all the distinct species.
> With knife, horseleeches.
> Cupping-glasses.
> Cauteries, and searing with hot irons, boring.
> Dropax and sinapismus.
> Issues to several parts, and upon several occasions.

℥ *Sect. 5.* Cure of head-melancholy. *Memb. 1.*

> 1. *Subsect.*
> Moderate diet, meat of good juice, moistening, easy of digestion.
> Good air.
> Sleep more than ordinary.
> Excrements daily to be voided by art or nature.
> Exercise of body and mind not too violent, or too remiss, passions of the mind, and perturbations to be avoided.

> 2. Blood-letting, if there be need, or that the blood be corrupt, in the arm, forehead, etc., or with cupping-glasses.

> 3. Preparatives and purgers.
>> Preparatives; as syrup of borage, bugloss, epithyme, hops, with their distilled waters, etc.
>> Purgers; as Montanus' and Matthiolus' helleborismus, Quercetanus' syrup of hellebore, extract of hellebore, pulvis Hali, antimony prepared, *Rulandi aqua mirabilis*; which are used, if gentler medicines will not take place, with Arnoldus' *vinum buglossatum*, senna, cassia, myrobalanes, *aurum potabile*, or before Hamech, pil. Indæ, hiera, pil. de lap. Armeno, lazuli.

> 4. Averters.
>> Cardan's nettles, frictions, clysters, suppositories, sneezings, masticatories, nasals, cupping-glasses.
>> To open the hemrods with horseleeches, to apply horseleeches to the forehead without scarification, to the shoulders, thighs.
>> Issues, boring, cauteries, hot irons in the suture of the crown.

> 5. Cordials, resolvers, hinderers.
>> A cup of wine or strong drink.
>> Bezoar's stone, amber, spice.
>> Conserves of borage, bugloss, roses, fumitory.
>> Confection of alkermes.
>> *Electuarium lætificans Galeni et Rhasis*, etc.
>> *Diamargaritum frigidum, diaboraginatum*, etc.

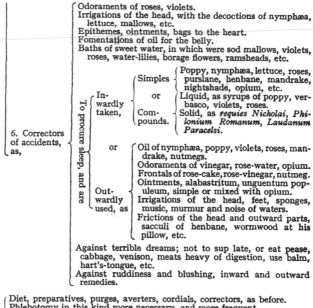

Odoraments of roses, violets.
Irrigations of the head, with the decoctions of nymphæa, lettuce, mallows, etc.
Epithemes, ointments, bags to the heart.
Fomentations of oil for the belly.
Baths of sweet water, in which were sod mallows, violets, roses, water-lilies, borage flowers, ramsheads, etc.

6. Correctors of accidents, as,

To procure sleep, and are

Inwardly taken, or Compounds.

Simples — Poppy, nymphæa, lettuce, roses, purslane, henbane, mandrake, nightshade, opium, etc.
or Liquid, as syrups of poppy, verbasco, violets, roses.
Solid, as *requies Nicholai, Philonium Romanum, Laudanum Paracelsi.*

or Outwardly used, as

Oil of nymphæa, poppy, violets, roses, mandrake, nutmegs.
Odoraments of vinegar, rose-water, opium.
Frontals of rose-cake, rose-vinegar, nutmeg.
Ointments, alabastritum, unguentum populeum, simple or mixed with opium.
Irrigations of the head, feet, sponges, music, murmur and noise of waters.
Frictions of the head and outward parts, sacculi of henbane, wormwood at his pillow, etc.

Against terrible dreams; not to sup late, or eat pease, cabbage, venison, meats heavy of digestion, use balm, hart's-tongue, etc.
Against ruddiness and blushing, inward and outward remedies.

Ω 2. *Memb.* Cure of melancholy over the body.

Diet, preparatives, purges, averters, cordials, correctors, as before.
Phlebotomy in this kind more necessary, and more frequent.
To correct and cleanse the blood with fumitory, senna, succory, dandelion, endive, etc.

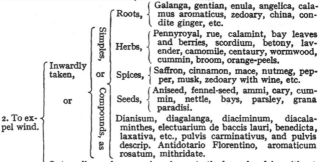

Subsect. 1.

Phlebotomy, if need require.
Diet, preparatives, averters, cordials, purgers, as before, saving that they must not be so vehement.
Use of pennyroyal, wormwood, centaury sod, which alone hath cured many.
To provoke urine with aniseed, daucus, asarum, etc., and stools, if need be, by clysters and suppositories.
To respect the spleen, stomach, liver, hypochondries.
To use treacle now and then in winter.
To vomit after meals sometimes, if it be inveterate.

℞ Cure of hypochondriacal or windy melancholy, 3. *Memb.*

2. To expel wind.

Inwardly taken, or

Simples, or Compounds, as

Roots, — Galanga, gentian, enula, angelica, calamus aromaticus, zedoary, china, condite ginger, etc.

Herbs, — Pennyroyal, rue, calamint, bay leaves and berries, scordium, betony, lavender, camomile, centaury, wormwood, cummin, broom, orange-peels.

Spices, — Saffron, cinnamon, mace, nutmeg, pepper, musk, zedoary with wine, etc.

Seeds, — Aniseed, fennel-seed, ammi, cary, cummin, nettle, bays, parsley, grana paradisi.

Dianisum, diagalanga, diaciminum, diacalaminthes, electuarium de baccis lauri, benedicta, laxativa, etc., pulvis carminativus, and pulvis descrip. Antidotario Florentino, aromaticum rosatum, mithridate.

Outwardly used, as cupping-glasses to the hypochondries without scarification, oil of camomile, rue, aniseed, their decoctions, etc.

THE SECOND PARTITION

THE CURE OF MELANCHOLY

THE FIRST SECTION, MEMBER, SUBSECTION

Unlawful Cures rejected

INVETERATE Melancholy, howsoever it may seem to be a continuate, inexorable disease, hard to be cured, accompanying them to their graves, most part, as Montanus observes,[1] yet many times it may be helped, even that which is most violent, or at least, according to the same author,[2] "it may be mitigated and much eased." *Nil desperandum* [never despair]. It may be hard to cure, but not impossible for him that is most grievously affected, if he be but willing to be helped.

Upon this good hope I will proceed, using the same method in the cure, which I have formerly used in the rehearsing of the causes; first general, then particular; and those according to their several species. Of these cures some be lawful, some again unlawful, which though frequent, familiar, and often used, yet justly censured, and to be controverted. As first, whether by these diabolical means which are commonly practised by the devil and his ministers, sorcerers, witches, magicians, etc., by spells, cabalistical words, charms, characters, images, amulets, ligatures, philters, incantations, etc., this disease and the like may be cured? and if they may, whether it be lawful to make use of them, those magnetical cures, or for our good to seek after such means in any case? The first, whether they can do any such cures, is questioned amongst many writers, some affirming, some denying. Valesius, *Cont. med. lib.* 5, *cap.* 6; *Malleus Maleficarum*; Heurnius, *lib.* 3 *pract. med. cap.* 28; Cælius, *lib.* 16, *cap.* 16; Delrio, *tom.* 3; Wierus, *lib.* 2 *de præstig. dæm.*; Libanius; Lavater, *de spect. part.* 2, *cap.* 7; Holbrenner the Lutheran, *in Pistorium*; Polydore Virg., *lib.* 1 *de prodig.*; Tandlerus; Lemnius (Hippocrates and Avicenna amongst the rest), deny that spirits or devils have any power over us, and refer all with Pomponatius of Padua to natural causes and humours. Of the other opinion are Bodinus, *Dæmonomantiæ lib.* 3, *cap.* 2;

Arnoldus; Marcellus Empiricus; J. Pistorius; Paracelsus, *Apodeix. Magic.*; Agrippa, *lib. 2 de occult. Philos. cap.* 36, 69, 71, 72, *et lib. 3, cap. 23 et* 10; Marsilius Ficinus, *de vit. cœlit. compar. cap.* 13, 15, 18, 21, etc.; Galeottus, *de promiscua doct. cap.* 24; Jovianus Pontanus, *tom.* 2; Plin., *lib.* 28, *cap.* 2; Strabo, *lib.* 15 *Geog.*; Leo Suavius; Goclenius, *de ung. armar.*; Oswaldus Crollius; Ernestus Burgravius; Dr. Flud, etc. Cardan, *de subt.*, brings many proofs out of *Ars Notoria* and Solomon's decayed works, old Hermes, Artesius, Costaben Luca, Picatrix, etc., that such cures may be done. They can make fire it shall not burn, fetch back thieves or stolen goods, show their absent faces in a glass, make serpents lie still, stanch blood, salve gouts, epilepsies, biting of mad dogs, toothache, melancholy, *et omnia mundi mala* [and all the ills of the world], make men immortal, young again as the Spanish marquess is said to have done by one of his slaves,[1] and some, which jugglers in China maintain still (as Tragaltius writes [2]) that they can do by their extraordinary skill in physic, and some of our modern chemists by their strange limbecks, by their spells, philosopher's stones and charms. "Many doubt," saith Nicholas Taurellus, "whether the devil can cure such diseases he hath not made, and some flatly deny it; howsoever, common experience confirms to our astonishment that magicians can work such feats, and that the devil without impediment can penetrate through all the parts of our bodies, and cure such maladies by means to us unknown." [3] Danæus, in his tract *de sortiariis*, subscribes to this of Taurellus; Erastus, *de lamiis*, maintaineth as much, and so do most divines, that out of their excellent knowledge and long experience they can commit *agentes cum patientibus*,[4] *colligere semina rerum, eaque materiæ applicare* [agents with patients, collect the seeds of things, and apply them to matter], as Austin infers, *de Civ. Dei, et de Trinit. lib. 3, cap. 7 et* 8; they can work stupend and admirable conclusions; we see the effects only, but not the causes of them. Nothing so familiar as to hear of such cures. Sorcerers are too common; cunning men, wizards, and white witches, as they call them, in every village, which, if they be sought unto, will help almost all infirmities of body and mind, *servatores* in Latin, and they have commonly St. Catherine's wheel printed in the roof of their mouth, or in some other part about them; *resistunt incantatorum præstigiis* (Boissardus writes [5]), *morbos a sagis motos propulsant* [they resist the tricks of enchanters, they repel the diseases brought by wizards], etc., that to doubt of it any longer, "or not to believe, were to

run into that other sceptical extreme of incredulity," [1] saith
Taurellus. Leo Suavius, in his Comment upon Paracelsus,
seems to make it an art, which ought to be approved; Pistorius
and others stiffly maintain the use of charms, words, characters,
etc. *Ars vera est, sed pauci artifices reperiuntur;* the art is true,
but there be but a few that have skill in it. Marcellus Donatus,
lib. 2 de hist. mir. cap. 1, proves out of Josephus' eighth book
of Antiquities, that "Solomon so cured all the diseases of the
mind by spells, charms, and drove away devils, and that Eleazar
did as much before Vespasian." [2]   Langius, in his *Med. epist.*,
holds Jupiter Menecrates, that did so many stupend cures
in his time, to have used this art, and that he was no other than
a magician. Many famous cures are daily done in this kind,
the devil is an expert physician, as Godelman calls him, *lib.* 1,
cap. 18, and God permits oftentimes these witches and magicians
to produce such effects, as Lavater, *cap.* 3, *lib.* 8, *part.* 3, *cap.* 1,
Polyd. Virg., *lib.* 1 *de prodigiis*, Delrio, and others admit.
Such cures may be done, and as Paracelsus, *tom.* 4, *de morb.
ament.*, stiffly maintains, "they cannot otherwise be cured but
by spells, seals, and spiritual physic." [3]   Arnoldus, *lib. de sigillis*,
sets down the making of them,[4] so doth Rulandus and many
others.

Hoc posito [this being granted, that] they can effect such cures,
the main question is whether it be lawful in a desperate case
to crave their help, or ask a wizard's advice. 'Tis a common
practice of some men to go first to a witch, and then to a
physician, if one cannot the other shall, *Flectere si nequeant
superos, Acheronta movebunt* [if they cannot move the gods
above, they will stir up those below]. "It matters not," saith
Paracelsus,[5] "whether it be God or the devil, angels or unclean
spirits cure him, so that he be eased." If a man fall into a
ditch, as he prosecutes it, what matter is it whether a friend
or an enemy help him out? and if I be troubled with such a
malady, what care I whether the devil himself, or any of his
ministers by God's permission, redeem me? He calls a magician
God's minister and His vicar,[6] applying that of *Vos estis dii* [7]
[ye are gods] profanely to them, for which he is lashed by
T. Erastus, *part.* 1, *fol.* 45. And elsewhere he encourageth his
patients to have a good faith, "a strong imagination, and they
shall find the effects: let divines say to the contrary what they
will." [8]   He proves and contends that many diseases cannot
otherwise be cured. *Incantatione orti, incantatione curari debent:*
if they be caused by incantation, they must be cured by

incantation.[1] Constantinus, *lib.* 4, approves of such remedies:
Bartolus the lawyer, Peter Ærodius, *rerum Judic. lib.* 3, *tit.* 7,
Salicetus, Godefridus, with others of that sect, allow of them,
modo sint ad sanitatem, quæ a magis fiunt, secus non, so they be
for the parties' good, or not at all.   But these men are confuted
by Remigius, Bodinus, *Dæm. lib.* 3, *cap.* 2; Godelmannus, *lib.* 1,
cap. 8; Wierus; Delrio, *lib.* 6, *quæst.* 2, *tom.* 3, *Mag. inquis.*;
Erastus, *de lamiis*; all our divines,[2] schoolmen, and such as write
cases of conscience are against it, the Scripture itself absolutely
forbids it as a mortal sin (Levit. xviii, xix, xx; Deut. xviii, etc.);
Rom. vii 19: "Evil is not to be done, that good may come
of it."   Much better it were for such patients that are so troubled,
to endure a little misery in this life, than to hazard their souls'
health for ever, and as Delrio counselleth, "much better die,
than be so cured."[3]   Some take upon them to expel devils by
natural remedies, and magical exorcisms, which they seem to
approve out of the practice of the primitive Church, as that
above cited of Josephus, Eleazar, Irenæus, Tertullian, Austin.
Eusebius makes mention of such, and magic itself hath been
publicly professed in some universities, as of old in Salamanca
in Spain, and Cracovia in Poland: but condemned, *anno* 1318,
by the chancellor and university of Paris.[4] Our pontificial
writers retain many of these adjurations and forms of exorcisms
still in the Church; besides those in baptism used, they exorcise
meats, and such as are possessed, as they hold, in Christ's name.
Read Hieron. Mengus, *cap.* 3, Pet. Thyræus, *part.* 3, *cap.* 8,
what exorcisms they prescribe, besides those ordinary means of
"fire, suffumigations, lights, cutting the air with swords,"[5]
cap. 57, herbs, odours: of which Tostatus treats, 2 *Reg. cap.* 16,
quæst. 43.   You shall find many vain and frivolous superstitious
forms of exorcisms among them, not to be tolerated or endured.

MEMB. II.

Lawful Cures, first from God

BEING so clearly evinced, as it is, all unlawful cures are to be
refused, it remains to treat of such as are to be admitted, and
those are commonly such which God hath appointed, by virtue
of stones, herbs, plants, meats, etc., and the like,[6] which are
prepared and applied to our use by art and industry of physicians,

who are the dispensers of such treasures for our good, and to be "honoured for necessity's sake," [1] God's intermediate ministers, to whom in our infirmities we are to seek for help. Yet not so that we rely too much, or wholly upon them: *a Jove principium*, we must first begin with prayer,[2] and then use physic; not one without the other, but both together. To pray alone, and reject ordinary means, is to do like him in Æsop, that when his cart was stalled, lay flat on his back, and cried aloud, "Help, Hercules!" but that was to little purpose, except (as his friend advised him, *Rotis tute ipse annitaris* [put your shoulder to the wheel yourself]) he whipped his horses withal, and put his shoulder to the wheel. God works by means, as Christ cured the blind man with clay and spittle: *Orandum est ut sit mens sana in corpore sano*. As we must pray for health of body and mind, so we must use our utmost endeavours to preserve and continue it. Some kind of devils are not cast out but by fasting and prayer, and both necessarily required, not one without the other. For all the physic we can use, art, excellent industry, is to no purpose without calling upon God, *nil juvat immensos Cratero promittere montes* [it avails not to promise Craterus a gold mine]: it is in vain to seek for help, run, ride, except God bless us.

> *Non Siculæ dapes*
> *Dulcem elaborabunt saporem,*
> *Non animum cithareæve cantus.*[3]

[No dainty meal, no song of bird or lyre shall coax him to sweet slumber.]

> *Non domus et fundus, non æris acervus et auri*
> *Ægroto possunt domino deducere febres.*[4]

With house, with land, with money, and with gold,
The master's fever will not be controll'd.[5]

We must use our prayer and physic both together: and so no doubt but our prayers will be available, and our physic take effect. 'Tis that Hezekiah practised (2 Kings, xx), Luke the Evangelist; and which we are enjoined (Coloss. iv), not the patient only, but the physician himself. Hippocrates, an heathen, required this in a good practitioner, and so did Galen, *lib. de Plat. et Hipp. dog. lib.* 9, *cap.* 15, and in that tract of his, *an mores sequantur temp. cor. cap.* 11; 'tis a rule which he doth inculcate, and many others.[6] Hyperius in his first book *de sacr. script. lect.*, speaking of that happiness and good success which all physicians desire and hope for in their cures, tells

them that "it is not to be expected, except with a true faith
they call upon God, and teach their patients to do the like."[1]
The Council of Lateran, Canon 22, decreed they should do so;
the Fathers of the Church have still advised as much. "Whatsoever thou takest in hand" (saith Gregory[2]) "let God be of
thy counsel, consult with Him, that healeth those that are
broken in heart (Ps. cxlvii, 3), and bindeth up their sores."
Otherwise, as the prophet Jeremiah, chap. xlvi, 11, denounced
to Egypt, "In vain shalt thou use many medicines, for thou
shalt have no health." It is the same counsel which Comineus,[3]
that politic historiographer, gives to all Christian princes, upon
occasion of that unhappy overthrow of Charles, Duke of Burgundy, by means of which he was extremely melancholy, and
sick to death, insomuch that neither physic nor persuasion
could do him any good, perceiving his preposterous error belike,
adviseth all great men in such cases, "to pray first to God with
all submission and penitency, to confess their sins, and then
to use physic."[4] The very same fault it was which the prophet
reprehends in Asa, King of Judah, that he relied more on physic
than on God, and by all means would have him to amend it.
And 'tis a fit caution to be observed of all other sorts of men.
The prophet David was so observant of this precept, that in his
greatest misery and vexation of mind he put this rule first in
practice: Ps. lxxvii, 3, "When I am in heaviness, I will think
on God"; Ps. lxxxvi, 4, "Comfort the soul of thy servant, for
unto thee I lift up my soul," and verse 7, "In the day of trouble
will I call upon thee, for thou hearest me"; Ps. liv, 1, "Save
me, O God, by thy name," etc.; Ps. lxxxii, Ps. xx. And 'tis
the common practice of all good men: Ps. cvii, 13, "When their
heart was humbled with heaviness, they cried to the Lord in
their trouble, and he delivered them from their distress."
And they have found good success in so doing, as David confesseth (Ps. xxx, 12), "Thou hast turned my mourning into joy,
thou hast loosed my sackcloth, and girded me with gladness."
Therefore he adviseth all others to do the like (Ps. xxxi, 24),
"All ye that trust in the Lord, be strong, and he shall establish
your heart." It is reported by Suidas,[5] speaking of Hezekiah,
that there was a great book of old, of King Solomon's writing,
which contained medicines for all manner of diseases, and lay
open still as they came into the temple: but Hezekiah, King of
Jerusalem, caused it to be taken away, because it made the
people secure, to neglect their duty in calling and relying upon
God, out of a confidence on those remedies. Minucius,[6] that

worthy consul of Rome, in an oration he made to his soldiers, was much offended with them, and taxed their ignorance, that in their misery called more on him than upon God. A general fault it is all over the world, and Minucius his speech concerns us all, we rely more on physic, and seek oftener to physicians, than to God himself. As much faulty are they that prescribe as they that ask, respecting wholly their gain, and trusting more to their ordinary receipts and medicines many times than to him that made them. I would wish all patients in this behalf, in the midst of their melancholy, to remember that of Siracides (Ecclus. i, 11 and 12), "The fear of the Lord is glory, and gladness, and rejoicing. The fear of the Lord maketh a merry heart, and giveth gladness, and joy, and long life": and all such as prescribe physic, to begin *in nomine Dei* [in the name of God], as Mesue did,[1] to imitate Lælius à Fonte Eugubinus, that in all his Consultations still concludes with a prayer for the good success of his business; and to remember that of Crato, one of their predecessors, *fuge avaritiam, et sine oratione et invocatione Dei nihil facias*, avoid covetousness, and do nothing without invocation upon God.

MEMB. III.

Whether it be lawful to seek to Saints for Aid in this Disease

THAT we must pray to God, no man doubts; but whether we should pray to saints in such cases, or whether they can do us any good, it may be lawfully controverted. Whether their images, shrines, relics, consecrated things, holy water, medals, benedictions, those divine amulets, holy exorcisms, and the sign of the cross, be available in this disease? The papists on the one side stiffly maintain how many melancholy, mad, demoniacal persons are daily cured at St. Anthony's Church in Padua, at St. Vitus' in Germany, by our Lady of Loretto in Italy, our Lady of Sichem in the Low Countries, *quæ et cæcis lumen, ægris salutem, mortuis vitam, claudis gressum reddit, omnes morbos corporis, animi, curat, et in ipsos dæmones imperium exercet:* [2] she cures halt, lame, blind, all diseases of body and mind, and commands the devil himself, saith Lipsius; "twenty-five thousand in a day come thither," *quis nisi numen in illum locum sic induxit?* [3] who brought them? *in auribus, in oculis*

omnium gesta, nova novitia: new news lately done, our eyes and
ears are full of her cures, and who can relate them all? They
have a proper saint almost for every peculiar infirmity: for
poison, gouts, agues, Petronella; St. Romanus for such as are
possessed; Valentine for the falling sickness; St. Vitus for madmen, etc.; and as of old Pliny reckons up gods for all diseases [1]
(*Febri fanum dicatum est* [a temple was dedicated to Fever];
Lilius Giraldus repeats many of her ceremonies), all affections
of the mind were heretofore accounted gods,[2] Love, and Sorrow,
Virtue, Honour, Liberty, Contumely, Impudency, had their
temples, tempests, seasons, *Crepitus Ventris, dea Vacuna, dea
Cloacina,* there was a goddess of idleness, a goddess of the
draught or jakes, Prema, Premunda, Priapus, bawdy gods, and
gods for all offices.[3] Varro reckons up 30,000 gods: Lucian
makes Podagra (the gout) a goddess, and assigns her priests
and ministers: and Melancholy comes not behind; for as Austin
mentioneth, *lib. 4 de Civit. Dei, cap.* 9, there was of old *Angerona
dea,* and she had her chapel and feasts, to whom (saith Macrobius [4]) they did offer sacrifice yearly, that she might be pacified
as well as the rest. 'Tis no new thing, you see this of papists;
and in my judgment, that old doting Lipsius might have fitter
dedicated his pen, after all his labours, to this our goddess of
melancholy, than to his *Virgo Hallensis,*[5] and been her chaplain,
it would have become him better: but he, poor man, thought
no harm in that which he did, and will not be persuaded but that
he doth well; he hath so many patrons, and honourable precedents in the like kind, that justify as much, as eagerly, and more
than he there saith of his lady and mistress: read but superstitious Coster and Gretser's tract *de Cruce Laur.*; Arcturus
Fanteus, *de Invoc. Sanct.*; Bellarmine; Delrio, *Dis. mag. tom.* 3,
lib. 6, *quæst.* 2, *sect.* 3; Greg. Tholosanus, *tom.* 2, *lib.* 8, *cap.* 24,
Syntax.; Strozzius Cicogna, *lib.* 4, *cap.* 9; Tyreus; Hieronymus
Mengus, and you shall find infinite examples of cures done in
this kind, by holy waters, relics, crosses, exorcisms, amulets,
images, consecrated beads, etc. Barradius the Jesuit boldly
gives it out, that Christ's countenance, and the Virgin Mary's,
would cure melancholy, if one had looked steadfastly on them.
P. Morales the Spaniard, in his book *de pulch, Jes. et Mar.*,
confirms the same out of Carthusianus and I know not whom,
that it was a common proverb in those days for such as were
troubled in mind to say, *Eamus ad videndum filium Mariæ,* let
us see the son of Mary, as they now do post to St. Anthony's
in Padua, or to St. Hilary's at Poictiers in France. In a closet

of that church, there is at this day St. Hilary's bed to be seen,
"to which they bring all the madmen in the country, and after
some prayers and other ceremonies, they lay them down there
to sleep, and so they recover." [1] It is an ordinary thing in
those parts to send all their madmen to St. Hilary's cradle.
They say the like of St. Tubery in another place.[2] Giraldus
Cambrensis, *Itin. Camb. cap.* 1, tells strange stories of St.
Ciricius' staff, that would cure this and all other diseases.
Others say as much (as Hospinian observes [3]) of the three kings
of Cologne; their names written in parchment, and hung about
a patient's neck, with the sign of the cross, will produce
like effects. Read Lipomannus, or that Golden Legend of
Jacobus de Voragine, you shall have infinite stories, or those
new relations of our Jesuits in Japan and China,[4] of Mat.
Riccius, Acosta, Loyola, Xaverius' life, etc. Jasper Belga,
a Jesuit, cured a mad woman by hanging St. John's Gospel
about her neck, and many such. Holy water did as much in
Japan, etc. Nothing so familiar in their works, as such
examples.

But we on the other side seek to God alone. We say with
David (Ps. xlvi, 1) "God is our hope and strength, and help in
trouble, ready to be found." For their catalogue of examples,
we make no other answer but that they are false fictions, or
diabolical illusions, counterfeit miracles. We cannot deny but
that it is an ordinary thing on St. Anthony's Day in Padua, to
bring divers madmen and demoniacal persons to be cured: yet
we make a doubt whether such parties be so affected indeed, but
prepared by their priests, by certain ointments and drams, to
cozen the commonalty, as Hildesheim well saith; [5] the like is
commonly practised in Bohemia, as Matthiolus gives us to understand in his preface to his Comment upon Dioscorides. But we
need not run so far for examples in this kind, we have a just
volume published at home to this purpose: "A Declaration of
egregious Popish Impostures, to withdraw the hearts of religious
men under pretence of casting out of devils, practised by
Father Edmunds, alias Weston, a Jesuit, and divers Romish
priests, his wicked associates, with the several parties' names,
confessions, examinations, etc., which were pretended to be
possessed." [6] But these are ordinary tricks only to get opinion
and money, mere impostures. Æsculapius of old, that counterfeit god, did as many famous cures; his temple (as Strabo
relates [7]) was daily full of patients, and as many several tables,
inscriptions, pendants, donaries, etc., to be seen in his church,

as at this day our Lady of Loretto's in Italy. It was a custom long since,

suspendisse potenti
Vestimenta maris deo.[1]

[For those who escaped shipwreck to hang up their
dripping garments in the temple of Neptune.]

To do the like, in former times they were seduced and deluded as they are now. 'Tis the same devil still, called heretofore Apollo, Mars, Neptune, Venus, Æsculapius, etc., as Lactantius, *lib. 2 de orig. erroris, cap.* 17, observes.[2] The same Jupiter and those bad angels are now worshipped and adored by the name of St. Sebastian, Barbara, etc.; Christopher and George are come in their places. Our Lady succeeds Venus (as they use her in many offices), the rest are otherwise supplied, as Lavater writes,[3] and so they are deluded. "And God often winks at these impostures, because they forsake His word, and betake themselves to the devil, as they do that seek after holy water, crosses," etc.[4] (Wierus, *lib.* 4, *cap.* 3). What can these men plead for themselves more than those heathen gods, the same cures done by both, the same spirit that seduceth; but read more of the pagan gods' effects in Austin, *de Civitate Dei, lib.* 10, *cap.* 6, and of Æsculapius especially in Cicogna, *lib.* 3, *cap.* 8; or put case they could help, why should we rather seek to them, than to Christ himself, since that he so kindly invites us unto him, "Come unto me all ye that are heavy laden, and I will ease you" (Matt. xi), and we know that there is one God, "one Mediator between God and man, Jesus Christ (1 Tim. ii, 5), who gave himself a ransom for all men." We know that "we have an Advocate with the Father, Jesus Christ" [5] (1 John, ii, 1), that "there is no other name under heaven, by which we can be saved, but by his," who is always ready to hear us, and sits at the right hand of God, and from whom we can have no repulse, *solus vult, solus potest, curat universos tanquam singulos,*[6] *et unumquemque nostrum ut solum;* [7] we are all as one to Him, He cares for us all as one, and why should we then seek to any other but to Him.

MEMB. IV.

Subsect. I.—*Physician, Patient, Physic*

Of those diverse gifts which our apostle Paul saith God hath
bestowed on man, this of physic is not the least, but most
necessary, and especially conducing to the good of mankind.
Next therefore to God in all our extremities ("for of the most
high cometh healing," Ecclus. xxxviii, 2) we must seek to, and
rely upon the physician, who is *manus Dei* [the hand of God],
saith Hierophilus, and to whom He hath given knowledge, that
He might be glorified in His wondrous works.[1] "With such
doth he heal men, and take away their pains" (Ecclus. xxxviii, 7);
"When thou hast need of him, let him not go from thee"
(verse 12); "The hour may come that their enterprises may have
good success" (verse 13). It is not therefore to be doubted,
that if we seek a physician as we ought, we may be eased of our
infirmities, such a one I mean as is sufficient, and worthily so
called; for there be many mountebanks, quacksalvers, empirics,
in every street almost, and in every village, that take upon
them this name, make this noble and profitable art to be evil
spoken of and contemned, by reason of these base and illiterate
artificers: but such a physician I speak of, as is approved,
learned, skilful, honest, etc., of whose duty Wecker, *Antid.
cap. 2, et Syntax. med.*, Crato, Julius Alexandrinus, *Medic.*,
Heurnius, *Prax. med. lib. 3, cap. 1*, etc., treat at large. For this
particular disease, him that shall take upon him to cure it,
Paracelsus will have to be a magician, a chemist, a philosopher,
an astrologer;[2] Thurnesserus, Severinus the Dane, and some
other of his followers, require as much: "many of them cannot
be cured but by magic." Paracelsus[3] is so stiff for those
chemical medicines that in his cures he will admit almost of no
other physic, deriding in the meantime Hippocrates, Galen,
and all their followers: but magic, and all such remedies, I have
already censured, and shall speak of chemistry elsewhere.[4]
Astrology is required by many famous physicians, by Ficinus,
Crato, Fernelius; doubted of, and exploded by others.[5] I will
not take upon me to decide the controversy myself; Johannes
Hossurtus, Thomas Boderius, and Maginus in the preface to
his Mathematical Physic, shall determine for me. "Many
physicians explode astrology in physic" (saith he), "there is no
use of it, *unam artem ac quasi temerarium insectantur, ac gloriam
sibi ab ejus imperitia aucupari* [they inveigh against it as mere

trickery, and take credit to themselves for being ignorant of it]: but I will reprove physicians by physicians, that defend and profess it, Hippocrates, Galen, Avicenna, etc., that count them butchers without it," *homicidas medicos astrologiæ ignaros*, etc. Paracelsus goes farther, and will have his physician predestinated to this man's cure,[1] this malady, and time of cure, the scheme of each geniture inspected, gathering of herbs, of administering, astrologically observed; in which Thurnesserus and some iatromathematical professors are too superstitious in my judgment. "Hellebore will help, but not alway, not given by every physician," etc.,[2] but these men are too peremptory and self-conceited, as I think. But what do I do, interposing in that which is beyond my reach? A blind man cannot judge of colours, nor I peradventure of these things. Only thus much I would require, honesty in every physician, that he be not over-careless or covetous, harpy-like to make a prey of his patient; *carnificis namque est* (as Wecker notes[3]) *inter ipsos cruciatus ingens pretium exposcere* [to demand a large fee from a patient in the midst of his agony is more worthy of a butcher than a physician], as a hungry chirurgeon often produces and wire-draws his cure, so long as there is any hope of pay, *Non missura cutem nisi plena cruoris hirudo* [like a leech that lets not go till it has sucked its fill]. Many of them, to get a fee, will give physic to every one that comes, when there is no cause, and they do so *irritare silentem morbum*, as Heurnius complains,[4] stir up a silent disease, as it often falleth out, which by good counsel, good advice alone, might have been happily composed, or by rectification of those six non-natural things otherwise cured. This is *naturæ bellum inferre*, to oppugn nature, and to make a strong body weak. Arnoldus in his eighth and eleventh Aphorisms gives cautions against, and expressly forbiddeth it. "A wise physician will not give physic, but upon necessity, and first try medicinal diet, before he proceed to medicinal cure."[5] In another place[6] he laughs those men to scorn, that think *longis syrupis expugnare dæmones et animi phantasmata*, they can purge fantastical imaginations and the devil by physic. Another caution is, that they proceed upon good grounds, if so be there be need of physic, and not mistake the disease; they are often deceived by the similitude of symptoms, saith Heurnius,[7] and I could give instance in many consultations, wherein they have prescribed opposite physic. Sometimes they go too perfunctorily to work, in not prescribing a just course of physic.[8] To stir up the humour, and not to purge it, doth often more harm than good. Montanus, *consil.* 30, inveighs against such perturbations, "that purge to the halves, tire nature, and molest the body to no purpose." 'Tis a crabbed humour to purge, and, as Laurentius calls this disease, the reproach of physicians; Bessardus, *flagellum medicorum*, their lash; and for that cause more carefully to be respected. Though the patient be averse, saith Laurentius, desire help, and refuse it again, though he neglect his own health, it behoves a good physician not to leave him helpless. But most part they offend in that other extreme, they prescribe too much physic, and tire out their bodies with continual potions, to no purpose. Aetius, *Tetrabib.* 2, 2 *ser. cap.* 90, will have them by all means therefore "to give some respite to nature," [1] to leave off now and then; and Lælius à Fonte Eugubinus, in his Consultations, found it (as he there witnesseth) often verified by experience, "that after a deal of physic to no purpose, left to themselves, they have recovered." [2] 'Tis that which Nic. Piso, Donatus Altomarus, still inculcate, *dare requiem naturæ*, to give nature rest.

SUBSECT. II.—*Concerning the Patient*

When these precedent cautions are accurately kept, and that we have now got a skilful, an honest physician to our mind, if his patient will not be conformable, and content to be ruled by him, all his endeavours will come to no good end. Many things are necessarily to be observed and continued on the patient's behalf. First that he be not too niggardly miserable of his purse, or think it too much he bestows upon himself, and to save charges endanger his health. The Abderites, when they sent for Hippocrates,[3] promised him what reward he would, "all the gold they had; if all the city were gold he should have it." [4] Naaman the Syrian, when he went into Israel to Elisha to be cured of his leprosy, took with him ten talents of silver, six thousand pieces of gold, and ten change of raiments (2 Kings v, 5). Another thing is, that out of bashfulness he do not conceal his grief; if aught trouble his mind, let him freely disclose it. *Stultorum incurata pudor malus ulcera celat* [the false shame of fools hides their festering wounds]. By that means he procures to himself much mischief, and runs into a greater inconvenience: he must be willing to be cured, and earnestly desire it. *Pars sanitatis velle sanari fuit* (Seneca). 'Tis a part of his cure to wish his own health; and not to defer it too long.

Qui blandiendo dulce nutrivit malum,
Sero recusat ferre quod subiit jugum.[1]

He that by cherishing a mischief doth provoke,
Too late at last refuseth to cast off his yoke.

Helleborum frustra cum jam cutis ægra tumebit,
Poscentes videas; venienti occurrite morbo.[2]

When the skin swells, to seek it to appease
With hellebore is vain; meet your disease.

By this means many times, or through their ignorance in not taking notice of their grievance and danger of it, contempt, supine negligence, extenuation, wretchedness, and peevishness; they undo themselves. The citizens, I know not of what city now, when rumour was brought their enemies were coming, could not abide to hear it; and when the plague begins in many places and they certainly know it, they command silence and hush it up; but after they see their foes now marching to their gates, and ready to surprise them, they begin to fortify and resist when 'tis too late; when the sickness breaks out and can be no longer concealed, then they lament their supine negligence: 'tis no otherwise with these men. And often out of prejudice, a loathing, and distaste of physic, they had rather die, or do worse, than take any of it. "Barbarous immanity" (Melancthon terms it [3]) "and folly to be deplored, so to contemn the precepts of health, good remedies, and voluntarily to pull death, and many maladies, upon their own heads." Though many again are in that other extreme too profuse, suspicious, and jealous of their health, too apt to take physic on every small occasion, to aggravate every slender passion, imperfection, impediment: if their finger do but ache, run, ride, send for a physician, as many gentlewomen do, that are sick, without a cause, even when they will themselves, upon every toy or small discontent, and when he comes, they make it worse than it is, by amplifying that which is not. Hier. Capivaccius [4] sets it down as a common fault of all "melancholy persons to say their symptoms are greater than they are, to help themselves"; and, which Mercurialis notes, *consil.* 53, "to be more troublesome to their physicians than other ordinary patients, that they may have change of physic." [5]

A third thing to be required in a patient is confidence, to be of good cheer, and have sure hope that his physician can help him. Damascen the Arabian requires likewise in the physician himself, that he be confident he can cure him, otherwise his

physic will not be effectual, and promise withal that he will
certainly help him, make him believe so at least.[1] Galeottus
gives this reason, because the form of health is contained in
the physician's mind,[2] and, as Galen holds "confidence and
hope do more good than physic," [3] he cures most in whom most
are confident. Axiochus, sick almost to death, at the very sight
of Socrates recovered his former health. Paracelsus assigns it
for an only cause why Hippocrates was so fortunate in his
cures, not for any extraordinary skill he had, but "because the
common people had a most strong conceit of his worth." [4] To
this of confidence we may add perseverance, obedience, and
constancy, not to change his physician, or dislike him upon
every toy; for he that so doth (saith Janus Damascen [5]) "or
consults with many, falls into many errors; or that useth many
medicines." It was a chief caveat of Seneca to his friend
Lucilius, that he should not alter his physician, or prescribed
physic: "Nothing hinders health more; a wound can never be
cured, that hath several plasters." [6] Crato, *consil.* 186, taxeth
all melancholy persons of this fault: "'Tis proper to them, if
things fall not out to their mind, and that they have not present
ease, to seek another and another" (as they do commonly that
have sore eyes), "twenty one after another, and they still promise
all to cure them, try a thousand remedies; and by this means
they increase their malady, make it most dangerous and difficult to be cured." [7] "They try many" (saith Montanus [8]) "and
profit by none": and for this cause, *consil.* 24, he enjoins his
patient, before he take him in hand, "perseverance and sufferance, for in such a small time no great matter can be effected,
and upon that condition he will administer physic, otherwise
all his endeavour and counsel would be to small purpose." [9]
And in his 31st counsel for a notable matron, he tells her, "if
she will be cured, she must be of a most abiding patience,
faithful obedience, and singular perseverance; if she remit, or
despair, she can expect or hope for no good success."[10] *Consil.* 230,
for an Italian abbot, he makes it one of the greatest reasons why
this disease is so incurable, "because the parties are so restless,
and impatient," [11] and will therefore have him that intends to
be eased, "to take physic, not for a month, a year, but to apply
himself to their prescriptions all the days of his life." [12] Last
of all, it is required that the patient be not too bold to practise
upon himself without an approved physician's consent, or to
try conclusions if he read a receipt in a book; for so many
grossly mistake, and do themselves more harm than good. That

which is conducing to one man, in one case, the same time is opposite to another. An ass and a mule went laden over a brook, the one with salt, the other with wool: the mule's pack was wet by chance, the salt melted, his burden the lighter, and he thereby much eased: he told the ass, who, thinking to speed as well, wet his pack likewise at the next water, but it was much the heavier, he quite tired.[1] So one thing may be good and bad to several parties, upon diverse occasions. "Many things" (saith Penottus[2]) "are written in our books, which seem to the reader to be excellent remedies, but they that make use of them are often deceived, and take for physic poison." I remember in Valleriola's Observations, a story of one John Baptist a Neapolitan, that finding by chance a pamphlet in Italian, written in praise of hellebore, would needs adventure on himself, and took one dram for one scruple, and had not he been sent for, the poor fellow had poisoned himself. From whence he concludes out of Damascenus, 2 *et* 3 *Aphoris.*, "that, without exquisite knowledge, to work out of books is most dangerous: how unsavoury a thing it is to believe writers, and take upon trust, as this patient perceived by his own peril." [3] I could recite such another example of mine own knowledge, of a friend of mine, that finding a receipt in Brassavola, would needs take hellebore in substance, and try it on his own person; but had not some of his familiars come to visit him by chance, he had by his indiscretion hazarded himself; many such I have observed. These are those ordinary cautions, which I should think fit to be noted, and he that shall keep them, as Montanus saith,[4] shall surely be much eased, if not thoroughly cured.

Subsect. III.—*Concerning Physic*

Physic itself in the last place is to be considered; "for the Lord hath created medicines of the earth, and he that is wise will not abhor them" (Ecclus. xxxviii, 4), and "of such doth the apothecary make a confection," etc. (verse 8). Of these medicines there be divers and infinite kinds, plants, metals, animals, etc., and those of several natures: some good for one, hurtful to another, some noxious in themselves, corrected by art, very wholesome and good, simples, mixed, etc., and therefore left to be managed by discreet and skilful physicians, and thence applied to man's use. To this purpose they have invented method, and several rules of art, to put these remedies in order for their particular ends. Physic (as Hippocrates defines it) is naught else but addition and subtraction;[1] and as it is required in all other diseases, so in this of melancholy it ought to be most accurate, it being (as Mercurialis acknowledgeth[2]) so common an affection in these our times, and therefore fit to be understood. Several prescripts and methods I find in several men, some take upon them to cure all maladies with one medicine, severally applied, as that panacea *aurum potabile* [liquid gold], so much controverted in these days, *herba solis*, etc. Paracelsus reduceth all diseases to four principal heads, to whom Severinus, Ravelascus, Leo Suavius, and others adhere and imitate: those are leprosy, gout, dropsy, falling sickness: to which they reduce the rest; as to leprosy, ulcers, itches, furfurs, scabs, etc.; to gout, stone, cholic, toothache, headache, etc.; to dropsy, agues, jaundice, cachexia, etc. To the falling sickness belong palsy, vertigo, cramps, convulsions, incubus, apoplexy, etc. "If any of these four principal be cured" (saith Ravelascus) "all the inferior are cured,"[3] and the same remedies commonly serve: but this is too general, and by some contradicted: for this peculiar disease of melancholy, of which I am now to speak, I find several cures, several methods and prescripts. They that intend the practic cure of melancholy, saith Duretus in his notes to Hollerius, set down nine peculiar scopes or ends; Savonarola prescribed seven especial canons. Ælianus Montaltus, *cap.* 26, Faventinus in his Empirics, Hercules de Saxonia, etc., have their several injunctions and rules, all tending to one end. The ordinary is threefold, which I mean to follow: Διαιτητική, *Pharmaceutica*, and *Chirurgica*, diet, or living, apothecary, chirurgery, which Wecker, Crato, Guianerius, etc., and most, prescribe; of which I will insist, and speak in their order.

SECT. II. MEMB. I.

Subsect. I.—*Diet rectified in substance*

DIET, διαιτητική, *victus*, or living, according to Fuchsius[4] and others, comprehend those six non-natural things, which I have before specified, are especial causes, and, being rectified, a sole or chief part of the cure. Johannes Arculanus, *cap.* 16, *in* 9 *Rhasis*, accounts the rectifying of these six a sufficient cure.[5] Guianerius, *tract.* 15, *cap.* 9, calls them *propriam et primam curam*, the principal cure; so doth Montanus, Crato, Mercurialis, Altomarus, etc., first to be tried; Lemnius, *Instit. cap.* 22, names them the hinges of our health, no hope of recovery without them.[1]   Reinerus Solenander, in his seventh consultation for a Spanish young gentlewoman, that was so melancholy she abhorred all company and would not sit at table with her familiar friends, prescribes this physic above the rest, no good to be done without it.[2]   Aretæus, *lib.* 1, *cap.* 7, an old physician, is of opinion that this is enough of itself, if the party be not too far gone in sickness.[3]   Crato, in a consultation of his for a noble patient,[4] tells him plainly, that if his highness will keep but a good diet, he will warrant him his former health.   Montanus, *consil.* 27, for a nobleman of France, admonisheth his lordship to be most circumspect in his diet, or else all his other physic will be to small purpose.[5]   The same injunction [6] I find verbatim in J. Cæsar Claudinus, *respon.* 34, *Scoltzii consil.* 183, Trallianus, *cap.* 16, *lib.* 1.   Lælius à Fonte Eugubinus often brags that he hath done more cures in this kind by rectification of diet than all other physic besides. So that in a word I may say to most melancholy men, as the fox said to the weasel that could not get out of the garner, *Macra cavum repetes, quem macra subisti* [lean went you in the hole, lean you 'll get out], the six non-natural things caused it, and they must cure it.   Which howsoever I treat of as proper to the meridian of melancholy, yet nevertheless, that which is here said, with him in Tully,[7] though writ especially for the good of his friends at Tarentum and Sicily, yet it will generally serve most other diseases,[8] and help them likewise, if it be observed.

Of these six non-natural things the first is diet, properly so called, which consists in meat and drink, in which we must consider substance, quantity, quality, and that opposite to the precedent.   In substance, such meats are generally commended which are moist, easy of digestion, and not apt to engender wind, not fried, nor roasted,[9] but sod (saith Valescus, Altomarus, Piso, etc.), hot and moist, and of good nourishment; Crato, *consil.* 21, *lib.* 2, admits roast meat, if the burned and scorched superficies, the brown we call it, be pared off.[10]   Salvianus, *lib.* 2, *cap.* 1, cries out on cold and dry meats; young flesh and tender is approved,[11] as of kid, rabbits, chickens, veal, mutton, capons, hens, partridge, pheasant, quails, and all mountain birds, which are so familiar in some parts of Africa, and in Italy, and as Dublinius reports,[12] the common food of

boors and clowns in Palestine. Galen takes exception at
mutton, but without question he means that rammy mutton
which is in Turkey and Asia Minor, which have those great
fleshy tails of forty-eight pound weight, as Vertomannus witnesseth, *Navig. lib. 2, cap.* 5.   The lean of fat meat is best, and
all manner of broths, and pottage, with borage, lettuce, and such
wholesome herbs are excellent good, especially of a cock boiled;
all spoon meat.   Arabians commend brains, but Laurentius,
cap. 8, excepts against them,[1] and so do many others.   Eggs
are justified as a nutritive wholesome meat,[2] butter and oil
may pass, but with some limitation; so Crato confines it,[3] and
"to some men sparingly at set times, or in sauce," and so sugar
and honey are approved.   All sharp and sour sauces must be
avoided,[4] and spices, or at least seldom used: and so saffron
sometimes in broth may be tolerated; but these things may be
more freely used, as the temperature of the party is hot or cold,
or as he shall find inconvenience by them.   The thinnest,
whitest, smallest wine is best, not thick, nor strong; and so of
beer, the middling is fittest.   Bread of good wheat, pure, well
purged from the bran, is preferred; Laurentius, *cap.* 8, would
have it kneaded with rain water if it may be gotten.

Pure, thin, light water by all means use, of good smell and
taste, like to the air in sight, such as is soon hot, soon cold,
and which Hippocrates so much approves, if at least it may
be had.   Rain water is purest, so that it fall not down in great
drops, and be used forthwith, for it quickly putrefies.   Next
to it fountain water that riseth in the east, and runneth eastward, from a quick running spring, from flinty, chalky, gravelly
grounds: and the longer a river runneth, it is commonly the
purest, though many springs do yield the best water at their
fountains.   The waters in hotter countries, as in Turkey, Persia,
India, within the tropics, are frequently purer than ours in the
north, more subtile, thin, and lighter, as our merchants observe,
by four ounces in a pound, pleasanter to drink, as good as our
beer, and some of them, as Choaspes in Persia, preferred by the
Persian kings before wine itself.

> *Clitorio quicunque sitim de fonte levarit*
> *Vina fugit gaudetque meris abstemius undis.*[5]

> [Who once hath tasted the Clitorian rill.
> Spurns wine, and of pure water drinks his fill.]

Many rivers, I deny not, are muddy still, white, thick, like those
in China, Nile in Egypt, Tiber at Rome, but after they be

settled two or three days, defecate and clear, very commodious,
useful and good.   Many make use of deep wells, as of old in the
Holy Land, lakes, cisterns, when they cannot be better provided; to fetch it in carts, or gondolas, as in Venice, or camels'
backs, as at Cairo in Egypt, Radzivilius [1] observed 8,000 camels
daily there, employed about that business; some keep it in tanks,
as in the East Indies, made four-square with descending steps,
and 'tis not amiss: for I would not have any one so nice as that
Grecian Calis, sister to Nicephorus, Emperor of Constantinople,
and married to Dominicus Silvius,[2] Duke of Venice, that, out of
incredible wantonness, *communi aqua uti nolebat*, would use no
vulgar water; but she died *tanta* (saith mine author) *fœtidissimi
puris copia*, of so fulsome a disease, that no water could wash
her clean.   Plato [3] would not have a traveller lodge in a city
that is not governed by laws, or hath not a quick stream running
by it; *illud enim animum, hoc corrumpit valetudinem*, one corrupts
the body, the other the mind.   But this is more than needs,
too much curiosity is naught, in time of necessity any water is
allowed.   Howsoever, pure water is best, and which (as Pindarus holds) is better than gold; an especial ornament it is, and
"very commodious to a city" (according to Vegetius [4]) "when
fresh springs are included within the walls," as at Corinth, in
the midst of the town almost, there was *arx altissima scatens
fontibus*, a goodly mount full of fresh-water springs: "if nature
afford them not they must be had by art."   It is a wonder to
read of those stupend aqueducts,[5] and infinite cost hath been
bestowed in Rome of old, Constantinople, Carthage, Alexandria,
and such populous cities, to convey good and wholesome waters:
read Frontinus,[6] Lipsius *de admir.*, Plinius,[7] *lib. 3, cap.* 11,
Strabo in his Geography.   That aqueduct of Claudius was most
eminent, fetched upon arches fifteen miles, every arch 109 feet
high: they had fourteen such other aqueducts, besides lakes
and cisterns, 700 as I take it; every house had private pipes
and channels to serve them for their use.[8]   Peter Gillius, in his
accurate description of Constantinople, speaks of an old cistern
which he went down to see, 336 foot long, 180 foot broad, built
of marble, covered over with arch-work and sustained by 336
pillars, 12 foot asunder, and in eleven rows, to contain sweet
water.   Infinite cost in channels and cisterns, from Nilus to
Alexandria, hath been formerly bestowed, to the admiration of
these times; their cisterns so curiously cemented and composed
that a beholder would take them to be all of one stone: when
the foundation is laid, and cistern made, their house is half

built.[1] That Segovian aqueduct in Spain is much wondered at in these days, upon three rows of pillars, one above another, conveying sweet water to every house:[2] but each city almost is full of such aqueducts. Amongst the rest he[3] is eternally to be commended that brought that new stream to the north side of London at his own charge; and Mr. Otho Nicholson, founder of our water-works and elegant conduit in Oxford. So much have all times attributed to this element, to be conveniently provided of it: although Galen hath taken exceptions at such waters which run through leaden pipes, *ob cerussam quæ in iis generatur*, for that unctuous ceruse, which causeth dysenteries and fluxes; yet, as Alsarius Crucius of Genoa well answers,[4] it is opposite to common experience. If that were true, most of our Italian cities, Montpelier in France, with infinite others, would find this inconvenience, but there is no such matter. For private families, in what sort they should furnish themselves, let them consult with P. Crescentius, *de Agric. lib.* 1, *cap.* 4, Pamphilus Hirelacus, and the rest.

Amongst fishes, those are most allowed of, that live in gravelly or sandy waters, pikes, perch, trout, gudgeon, smelts, flounders, etc. Hippolytus Salvianus takes exception at carp; but I dare boldy say with Dubravius,[5] it is an excellent meat, if it come not from muddy pools, that it retain not an unsavoury taste.[6] *Erinaceus marinus* [the sea-urchin] is much commended by Oribasius, Aetius, and most of our late writers.

Crato, *consil.* 21, *lib.* 2, censures all manner of fruits as subject to putrefaction, yet tolerable at some times; after meals, at second course, they keep down vapours, and have their use.[7] Sweet fruits are best, as sweet cherries, plums, sweet apples, pearmains, and pippins, which Laurentius extols as having a peculiar property against this disease, and Plater magnifies, *Omnibus modis appropriata conveniunt* [they are good in whatever way served], but they must be corrected for their windiness; ripe grapes are good, and raisins of the sun, musk-melons well corrected and sparingly used. Figs are allowed, and almonds blanched. Trallianus discommends figs, Salvianus[8] olives and capers, which others[9] especially like of, and so of pistick nuts. Montanus and Mercurialis, out of Avenzoar, admit peaches, pears, and apples baked, after meals, only corrected with sugar and aniseed or fennel-seed, and so they may be profitably taken, because they strengthen the stomach, and keep down vapours.[10] The like may be said of preserved cherries, plums, marmalade of plums, quinces, etc., but not to drink after them.   Pomegranates,[1] lemons, oranges are tolerated, if they be not too sharp.

Crato will admit of no herbs, but borage, bugloss, endive, fennel, aniseed, balm;[2] Calenus and Arnoldus tolerate lettuce, spinach, beets, etc.   The same Crato will allow no roots at all to be eaten.   Some approve of potatoes, parsnips, but all corrected for wind.   No raw sallets; but, as Laurentius prescribes, in broths; and so Crato commends many of them: or to use borage, hops, balm, steeped in their ordinary drink. Avenzoar[3] magnifies the juice of a pomegranate, if it be sweet, and especially rose-water, which he would have to be used in every dish, which they put in practice in those hot countries about Damascus, where (if we may believe the relations of Vertomannus) many hogsheads of rose-water are to be sold in the market at once, it is in so great request with them.

SUBSECT. II.—*Diet rectified in Quantity*

Man alone, saith Cardan,[4] eats and drinks without appetite, and useth all his pleasure without necessity, *animæ vitio* [through the corruption of his soul], and thence come many inconveniences unto him.   For there is no meat whatsoever, though otherwise wholesome and good, but if unseasonably taken, or immoderately used, more than the stomach can well bear, it will engender crudity and do much harm.   Therefore Crato [5] adviseth his patient to eat but twice a day, and that at his set meals, by no means to eat without an appetite or upon a full stomach, and to put seven hours' difference between dinner and supper.   Which rule if we did observe in our colleges, it would be much better for our healths: but custom, that tyrant, so prevails that, contrary to all good order and rules of physic, we scarce admit of five.   If after seven hours' tarrying he shall have no stomach, let him defer his meal, or eat very little at his ordinary time of repast.   This very counsel was given by Prosper Calenus to Cardinal Cæsius, labouring of this disease; and Platerus [6] prescribes it to a patient of his, to be most severely kept.   Guianerius admits of three meals a day, but Montanus, *consil. 23, pro Ab. Italo*, ties him precisely to two. And as he must not eat overmuch, so he may not absolutely fast; for as Celsus contends, *lib.* 1, Jacchinus, 15, *in* 9 *Rhasis*, repletion and inanition may both do harm in two contrary extremes.[7]   Moreover, that which he doth eat, must be well chewed, and not hastily gobbled, for that causeth crudity and wind;[1] and by all means to eat no more than he can well digest. "Some think (saith Trincavellius, *lib.* 11, *cap.* 29, *de curand. part. hum.*) "the more they eat the more they nourish themselves": eat and live, as the proverb is; "not knowing that only repairs man which is well concocted, not that which is devoured."[2]   Melancholy men most part have good appetites, but ill digestion,[3] and for that cause they must be sure to rise with an appetite: and, that which Socrates and Disarius the physicians in Macrobius[4] so much require, St. Hierome enjoins Rusticus to eat and drink no more than will satisfy hunger and thirst.[5] Lessius the Jesuit[6] holds twelve, thirteen, or fourteen ounces, or in our northern countries sixteen at most (for all students, weaklings, and such as lead an idle sedentary life), of meat, bread, etc., a fit proportion for a whole day, and as much or little more of drink. Nothing pesters the body and mind sooner than to be still fed, to eat and ingurgitate beyond all measure, as many do. "By overmuch eating and continual feasts they stifle nature, and choke up themselves; which, had they lived coarsely, or like galley-slaves been tied to an oar, might have happily prolonged many fair years."[7]

A great inconvenience comes by variety of dishes, which causeth the precedent distemperature, "than which" (saith Avicenna) "nothing is worse; to feed on diversity of meats, or overmuch,"[8] Sertorius-like, *in lucem cœnare* [to prolong supper till daylight], and, as commonly they do in Muscovy and Iceland, to prolong their meals all day long, or all night. Our northern countries offend especially in this, and we in this island (*ampliter viventes in prandiis et cœnis* [keeping a most liberal table], as Polydore notes[9]) are most liberal feeders, but to our own hurt. *Persicos odi, puer, apparatus*[10] [no Eastern luxury for me]. "Excess of meat breedeth sickness, and gluttony causeth choleric diseases: by surfeiting many perish, but he that dieteth himself prolongeth his life" (Ecclus. xxxvii, 29, 30). We account it a great glory for a man to have his table daily furnished with variety of meats; but hear the physician, he pulls thee by the ear as thou sittest, and telleth thee that nothing can be more noxious to thy health than such variety and plenty.[11] Temperance is a bridle of gold, and he that can use it aright, *ego non summis viris comparo, sed simillimum Deo judico*,[12] is liker a god than a man: for as it will transform a beast to a man again, so will it make a man a god. To preserve thine honour, health, and to avoid therefore all those

inflations, torments, obstructions, crudities, and diseases that
come by a full diet, the best way is to feed sparingly of one or
two dishes at most,[1] to have *ventrem bene moratum* [a stomach
in good order], as Seneca calls it, "to choose one of many, and
to feed on that alone," [2] as Crato adviseth his patient. The
same counsel Prosper Calenus gives to Cardinal Cæsius,[3] to use
a moderate and simple diet: and though his table be jovially
furnished by reason of his state and guests, yet for his own
part to single out some one savoury dish and feed on it. The
same is inculcated by Crato, *consil. 9. lib. 2*, to a noble personage
affected with this grievance; he would have his highness to dine
or sup alone, without all his honourable attendance and courtly
company, with a private friend or so, a dish or two, a cup of
Rhenish wine, etc.[4]   Montanus, *consil. 24*, for a noble matron,
enjoins her one dish,[5] and by no means to drink between meals.
The like, *consil. 229*, or not to eat till he be an-hungry, which
rule Berengarius did most strictly observe, as Hilbertus, *Ceno-
manensis Episcopus* [Bishop of Le Mans], writes in his life:

> *cui non fuit unquam*
> *Ante sitim potus, nec cibus ante famem*;

> [Who never drank before he was thirsty nor ate before
> he was hungry;]

and which all temperate men do constantly keep. It is a
frequent solemnity still used with us, when friends meet, to go
to the alehouse or tavern, they are not sociable otherwise: and
if they visit one another's houses, they must both eat and drink.
I reprehend it not moderately used; but to some men nothing
can be more offensive; they had better, I speak it with Saint
Ambrose,[6] pour so much water in their shoes.

It much avails likewise to keep order in our diet, "to eat
liquid things first, broths, fish, and such meats as are sooner
corrupted in the stomach; harder meats of digestion must come
last." [7]   Crato would have the supper less than the dinner,[8]
which Cardan, *Contradict. lib. 1, tract. 5, contradict. 18*, disallows, and that by the authority of Galen, *7 Art. curat. cap. 6*,
and for four reasons he will have the supper biggest. I have
read many treatises to this purpose, I know not how it may
concern some few sick men, but for my part, generally for all,
I should subscribe to that custom of the Romans, to make a
sparing dinner, and a liberal supper; all their preparation and
invitation was still at supper, no mention of dinner. Many
reasons I could give, but when all is said pro and con, Cardan's

rule [1] is best, to keep that we are accustomed unto, though it
be naught; and to follow our disposition and appetite in some
things is not amiss; to eat sometimes of a dish which is hurtful,
if we have an extraordinary liking to it.   Alexander Severus
loved hares and apples above all other meats, as Lampridius
relates in his life: [2] one pope pork, another peacock, etc.; what
harm came of it?   I conclude, our own experience is the best
physician; that diet which is most propitious to one is often
pernicious to another; such is the variety of palates, humours,
and temperatures, let every man observe, and be a law unto
himself.   Tiberius, in Tacitus,[3] did laugh at all such, that after
thirty years of age would ask counsel of others concerning
matters of diet; I say the same.

These few rules of diet he that keeps shall surely find great
ease and speedy remedy by it.   It is a wonder to relate that
prodigious temperance of some hermits, anchorites, and Fathers
of the Church: he that shall but read their lives, written by
Hierome, Athanasius, etc., how abstemious heathens have been
in this kind, those Curii and Fabricii, those old philosophers (as
Pliny records, *lib.* 11, Xenophon, *lib.* 1 *de vit. Socrat.*), emperors
and kings (as Nicephorus relates, *Eccles Hist. lib.* 18, *cap.* 8, of
Mauricius, Ludovicus Pius, etc.), and that admirable example
of Ludovicus Cornarus,[4] a patrician of Venice, cannot but
admire them   This have they done voluntarily and in health;
what shall these private men do that are visited with sickness,
and necessarily enjoined to recover, and continue their health? [5]
It is a hard thing to observe a strict diet, *et qui medice vivit, misere
vivit* [he who lives by the doctor's orders lives wretchedly], as
the saying is, *Quale hoc ipsum erit vivere, his si privatus fueris?*
as good be buried, as so much debarred of his appetite; *excessit
medicina malum,* the physic is more troublesome than the
disease, so he complained in the poet, so thou thinkest: yet he
that loves himself will easily endure this little misery to avoid
a greater inconvenience; *e malis minimum* [of evils choose the
least], better do this than do worse.   And, as Tully holds,[6]
"better be a temperate old man than a lascivious youth."
'Tis the only sweet thing (which he adviseth), so to moderate
ourselves, that we may have *senectutem in juventute, et in
juventute senectutem,* be youthful in our old age, staid in our
youth, discreet and temperate in both.

MEMB. II.

Retention and Evacuation rectified

I HAVE declared in the causes what harm costiveness hath done
in procuring this disease; if it be so noxious, the opposite must
needs be good, or mean at least, as indeed it is, and to this cure
necessarily required; *maxime conducit*, saith Montaltus, *cap*. 27,
it very much avails. Altomarus, *cap*. 7, commends walking in
a morning into some fair green pleasant fields, but by all means
first, by art or nature, he will have these ordinary excrements
evacuated.[1] Piso calls it *beneficium ventris*, the benefit, help,
or pleasure of the belly, for it doth much ease it. Laurentius,
cap. 8, Crato, *consil*. 21, *lib*. 2, prescribes it once a day at least:
where nature is defective, art must supply, by those lenitive
electuaries, suppositories, condite prunes, turpentine, clysters,
as shall be shown. Prosper Calenus, *lib. de atra bile*, commends
clysters in hypochondriacal melancholy, still to be used as
occasion serves; Peter Cnemander, in a consultation of his *pro
hypocondriaco*,[2] will have his patient continually loose, and to
that end sets down there many forms of potions and clysters.
Mercurialis, *consil*. 88, if this benefit come not of its own accord,
prescribes clysters in the first place:[3] so doth Montanus, *consil*. 24;
consil. 31 *et* 229, he commends turpentine to that purpose: the
same he ingeminates, *consil*. 230, for an Italian abbot. 'Tis
very good to wash his hands and face often, to shift his clothes,
to have fair linen about him, to be decently and comely attired,
for *sordes vitiant*, nastiness defiles and dejects any man that is
so voluntarily, or compelled by want, it dulleth the spirits.

Baths are either artificial or natural, both have their special
uses in this malady, and as Alexander supposeth, *lib*. 1, *cap*. 16,
yield as speedy a remedy as any other physic whatsoever.[4]
Aetius would have them daily used, *assidua balnea*, *Tetra*. 2,
sect. 2, *cap*. 9. Galen cracks how many several cures he hath
performed in this kind by use of baths alone, and Ruffus pills,
moistening them which are otherwise dry. Rhasis makes it a
principal cure, *tota cura sit in humectando*, to bathe and afterwards anoint with oil. Jason Pratensis, Laurentius, *cap*. 8,
and Montanus set down their peculiar forms of artificial baths.
Crato, *consil*. 17, *lib*. 2, commends mallows, camomile, violets,
borage to be boiled in it, and sometimes fair water alone, as in
his following counsel, *Balneum aquæ dulcis solum sæpissime*

profuisse compertum habemus [we have very frequently found a bath of sweet water to be beneficial]. So doth Fuchsius, *lib.* 1, *cap.* 33, Frisimelica, 2, *consil.* 42, in Trincavellius. Some beside herbs prescribe a ram's head and other things to be boiled. Fernelius, *consil.* 44, will have them used ten or twelve days together; to which he must enter fasting, and so continue in a temperate heat, and after that frictions all over the body.[1] Lælius Eugubinus, *consil.* 142, and Christoph. Ayrerus, in a consultation of his, hold once or twice a week sufficient to bathe, the "water to be warm, not hot, for fear of sweating." [2] Felix Plater, *Observ. lib.* 1, for a melancholy lawyer, will have lotions of the head still joined to these baths, with a lee wherein capital herbs have been boiled.[3] Laurentius speaks of baths of milk,[4] which I find approved by many others. And still, after bath, the body to be anointed with oil of bitter almonds, of violets, new or fresh butter, capon's grease,[5] especially the backbone, and then lotions of the head, embrocations, etc. These kinds of baths have been in former times much frequented, and diversely varied, and are still in general use in those eastern countries. The Romans had their public baths very sumptuous and stupend, as those of Antoninus and Dioclesian. Pliny, *lib.* 36, saith there were an infinite number of them in Rome, and mightily frequented: some bathed seven times a day, as Commodus the emperor is reported to have done: usually twice a day, and they were after anointed with most costly ointments: rich women bathed themselves in milk, some in the milk of five hundred she-asses at once. We have many ruins of such baths found in this island, amongst those parietines and rubbish of old Roman towns. Lipsius, *de mag. urb. Rom. lib.* 3, *cap.* 8, Rosinus, Scot of Antwerp, and other antiquaries, tell strange stories of their baths. Gillius, *lib.* 4, *cap. ult. Topogr. Constant.*, reckons up 155 public baths [6] in Constantinople, of fair building; they are still frequented in that city by the Turks of all sorts, men and women,[7] and all over Greece and those hot countries; to absterge belike that fulsomeness of sweat to which they are there subject. Busbequius, in his Epistles,[8] is very copious in describing the manner of them, how their women go covered, a maid following with a box of ointment to rub them. The richer sort have private baths in their houses; the poorer go to the common, and are generally so curious in this behalf, that they will not eat nor drink until they have bathed, before and after meals some, "and will not make water but they will wash their hands, or go to stool." [9]

Leo Afer, *lib*. 3, makes mention of an hundred several baths
at Fez in Africa, most sumptuous, and such as have great
revenues belonging to them.   Buxtorf., *cap*. 14 *Synagog. Jud.*,
speaks of many ceremonies amongst the Jews in this kind; they
are very superstitious in their baths, especially women.

Natural baths are praised by some, discommended by others;
but it is in a diverse respect.   Marcus de Oddis, *in Hyp. affect.*,
consulted about baths, condemns them for the heat of the
liver, because they dry too fast;[1] and yet by and by, in another
counsel for the same disease,[2] he approves them because they
cleanse by reason of the sulphur, and would have their water
to be drunk.   Aretæus, *cap*. 7, commends alum baths above the
rest; and Mercurialis, *consil*. 88, those of Lucca in that hypochondriacal passion.   "He would have his patient tarry there
fifteen days together, and drink the water of them, and to be
bucketed, or have the water poured on his head."[3]   John
Baptista Sylvaticus, *cont*. 64, commends all the paths in Italy,
and drinking of their water, whether they be iron, alum, sulphur;
so doth Hercules de Saxonia.[4]   But, in that they cause sweat,
and dry so much, he confines himself to hypochondriacal
melancholy alone, excepting that of the head and the other.
Trincavellius, *consil*. 14, *lib*. 1, prefers those Porrectan baths[5]
before the rest, because of the mixture of brass, iron, alum;
and, *consil*. 35, *lib*. 3, for a melancholy lawyer; and, *consil*. 36,
in that hypochondriacal passion, the baths of Aquaria;[6] and,
consil. 36, the drinking of them.   Frisimelica, consulted amongst
the rest in Trincavellius, *consil*. 42, *lib*. 2, prefers the waters of
Apona before all artificial baths whatsoever in this disease,
and would have one nine years affected with hypochondriacal
passions fly to them as to a holy anchor.[7][8]   Of the same mind is
Trincavellius himself there, and yet both put a hot liver in the
same party for a cause, and send him to the waters of St. Helen,
which are much hotter.   Montanus, *consil*. 230, magnifies the
Chalderinian baths,[9] and, *consil*. 237 *et* 239, he exhorteth to the
same, but with this caution, "that the liver be outwardly
anointed with some coolers that it be not overheated."[10]   But
these baths must be warily frequented by melancholy persons,
or if used, to such as are very cold of themselves, for as Gabelius
concludes of all Dutch baths, and especially of those of Baden,
"they are good for all cold diseases, naught for, choleric, hot and
dry, and all infirmities proceeding of choler, inflammations of
the spleen and liver."[11]   Our English baths, as they are hot,
must needs incur the same censure: but Dr. Turner of old, and

Dr. Jones, have written at large of them.   Of cold baths I find
little or no mention in any physician; some speak against them.
Cardan alone, out of Agathinus, commends "bathing in fresh
rivers, and cold waters, and adviseth all such as mean to live
long to use it, for it agrees with all ages and complexions, and is
most profitable for hot temperatures." [1]   As for sweating,
urine, blood-letting by hemrods, or otherwise, I shall elsewhere
more opportunely speak of them.

Immoderate Venus in excess, as it is a cause, or in defect;
so, moderately used, to some parties an only help, a present
remedy.   Peter Forestus calls it *aptissimum remedium*, a most
apposite remedy, "remitting anger, and reason, that was otherwise bound." [2]   Avicenna, *fen.* 3, 20, Oribasius, *Med. collect.
lib.* 6, *cap.* 37, contend out of Ruffus and others, "that many
madmen, melancholy, and labouring of the falling sickness,
have been cured by this alone.[3]   Montaltus, *cap.* 27 *de melan.*,
will have it drive away sorrow, and all illusions of the brain,
to purge the heart and brain from ill smokes and vapours that
offend them: "and if it be omitted," as Valescus supposeth,
"it makes the mind sad, the body dull and heavy." [4]   Many
other inconveniences are reckoned up by Mercatus, and by
Rodericus à Castro, in their tracts *de melancholia virginum et
monialium; ob seminis retentionem sæviunt sæpe moniales et
virgines,* but, as Platerus adds, *si nubant sanantur,* they rave
single, and pine away, much discontent, but marriage mends
all.   Marcellus Donatus, *lib.* 2 *Med. hist. cap.* 1, tells a story to
confirm this out of Alexander Benedictus, of a maid that was
mad, *ob menses inhibitos; cum in officinam meritoriam incidisset,
a quindecem viris eadem nocte compressa, mensium largo profluvio,
quod pluribus annis ante constiterat, non sine magno pudore menti
restituta discessit.*   But this must be warily understood, for, as
Arnoldus objects, *lib.* 1 *Breviar. cap.* 18, *Quid ccitus ad melancholicum succum?*   What affinity have these two? "except it
be manifest that superabundance of seed or fullness of blood be
a cause, or that love, or an extraordinary desire of Venus, have
gone before," [5] or that, as Lod. Mercatus excepts, they be very
flatuous, and have been otherwise accustomed unto it.   Montaltus, *cap.* 27, will not allow of moderate Venus to such as have
the gout, palsy, epilepsy, melancholy, except they be very lusty,
and full of blood.   Ludovicus Antonius, *lib. med. miscel.,* in his
chapter of Venus, forbids it utterly to all wrestlers, ditchers,
labouring men, etc.[6]   Ficinus and [7] Marsilius Cognatus [8] put
Venus one of the five mortal enemies of a student: "It

consumes the spirits, and weakeneth the brain." Halyabbas the Arabian, 5 *Theor. cap.* 36, and Jason Pratensis make it the fountain of most diseases, "but most pernicious to them who are cold and dry"; [1] a melancholy man must not meddle with it but in some cases. Plutarch in his book *de san. tuend.* accounts of it as one of the three principal signs and preservers of health, temperance in this kind: "to rise with an appetite, to be ready to work, and abstain from venery," [2] *tria saluberrima,* are three most healthful things. We see their opposites how pernicious they are to mankind, as to all other creatures they bring death, and many feral diseases: *Immodocis brevis est ætas et rara senectus* [fast livers are mostly short-lived, and rarely reach old age]. Aristotle gives instance in sparrows, which are *parum vivaces ob salacitatem,* short-lived because of their salacity, [3] which is very frequent, as Scioppius *in Priapeiis* will better inform you. The extremes being both bad, the medium is to be kept, which cannot easily be determined. [4] Some are better able to sustain, such as are hot and moist, phlegmatic, as Hippocrates insinuateth, some strong and lusty, well fed like Hercules, [5] Proculus the emperor, [6] lusty Laurence, *prostibulum feminæ* [that whore of a woman], Messalina the empress, [7] that by philters, and such kind of lascivious meats, use all means to enable themselves, [8] and brag of it in the end, *Confodi multas enim, occidi vero paucas per ventrem vidisti,* as that Spanish Celestina merrily said: [9] others impotent, of a cold and dry constitution, cannot sustain those gymnics without great hurt done to their own bodies, of which number (though they be very prone to it) are melancholy men for the most part.

MEMB. III.

Air rectified. With a digression of the Air

As a long-winged hawk, when he is first whistled off the fist, mounts aloft, and for his pleasure fetcheth many a circuit in the air, still soaring higher and higher till he be come to his full pitch, and in the end when the game is sprung, comes down amain, and stoops upon a sudden: so will I, having now come at last into these ample fields of air, wherein I may freely expatiate and exercise myself for my recreation, awhile rove, wander round about the world, mount aloft to those ethereal

orbs and celestial spheres, and so descend to my former elements
again. In which progress I will first see whether that relation
of the friar of Oxford [1] be true, concerning those northern parts
under the Pole (if I meet *obiter* [on the way] with the Wandering
Jew, Elias Artifex, or Lucian's Icaromenippus, they shall be
my guides) whether there be such four euripes, and a great rock
of loadstones, which may cause the needle in the compass still
to bend that way, and what should be the true cause of the
variation of the compass; is it a magnetical rock,[2] or the pole-
star, as Cardan will; or some other star in the Bear, as Marsilius
Ficinus; or a magnetical meridian, as Maurolicus; *vel situs in
vena terræ* [or a position in the interior of the earth], as Agricola;
or the nearness of the next continent, as Cabeus will; or some
other cause, as Scaliger, Cortesius, *Conimbricenses* [the philosophers of Coimbra], Peregrinus contend? why at the Azores
it looks directly north, otherwise not. In the Mediterranean or
Levant (as some observe) it varies 7 *grad.*, by and by 12, and
then 22. In the Baltic Seas, near Rasceburg in Finland, the
needle runs round if any ships come that way, though Martin
Ridley write otherwise,[3] that the needle near the Pole will
hardly be forced from his direction. 'Tis fit to be inquired
whether certain rules may be made of it, as 11 *grad. Lond.
variat. alibi* 36, etc., and, that which is more prodigious, the
variation varies in the same place; now taken accurately, 'tis
so much after a few years quite altered from that it was: till we
have better intelligence, let our Dr. Gilbert, and Nicholas
Cabeus the Jesuit,[4] that have both written great volumes of
this subject, satisfy these inquisitors. Whether the sea be open
and navigable by the Pole Arctic, and which is the likeliest way,
that of Bartison the Hollander, under the Pole itself, which for
some reasons I hold best: or by *Fretum Davis* [Davis Strait], or
Nova Zembla. Whether Hudson's discovery [5] be true of a new-
found ocean, any likelihood of Button's Bay in 50 degrees,
Hubberd's Hope in 60, that of *ut ultra* near Sir Thomas Roc's
Welcome in North-west Fox, being that the sea ebbs and flows
constantly there 15 foot in 12 hours, as our new cards [6] inform
us that California is not a cape, but an island, and the west
winds make the neap tides equal to the spring, or that there be
any probability to pass by the Straits of Anian to China, by
the promontory of Tabin. If there be, I shall soon perceive
whether Marcus Polus the Venetian's narration [7] be true or
false, of that great city of Quinsay and Cambalu; whether there
be any such places, or that, as Matth. Riccius the Jesuit hath

written,[1] China and Cataia be all one, the great Cham of Tartary and the King of China be the same, Xuntain and Quinsay, and the city of Cambalu be that new Peking, or such a wall 400 leagues long to part China from Tartary: whether Presbyter John be in Asia or Africa;[2] M. Polus Venetus puts him in Asia; the most received opinion[3] is, that he is emperor of the Abyssines, which of old was Ethiopia, now Nubia, under the Equator in Africa. Whether Guinea[4] be an island or part of the continent, or that hungry Spaniard's[5] discovery of *Terra Australis Incognita*, [the Unknown Land in the South] or *Magellanica*, be as true as that of Mercurius Britannicus, or his of Utopia, or his of Lucinia. And yet in likelihood it may be so, for without all question it being extended from the Tropic of Capricorn to the Circle Antarctic, and lying as it doth in the temperate zone, cannot choose but yield in time some flourishing kingdoms to succeeding ages, as America did unto the Spaniards. Schouten and Le Meir have done well in the discovery of the Straits of Magellan, in finding a more convenient passage to *Mare Pacificum* [the Pacific Ocean]: methinks some of our modern Argonauts should prosecute the rest. As I go by Madagascar, I would see that great bird ruck,[6] that can carry a man and horse or an elephant, with that Arabian phœnix described by Adricomius;[7] see the pelicans of Egypt, those Scythian gryphes in Asia; and afterwards in Africa examine the fountains of Nilus, whether Herodotus, Seneca,[8] Pliny, *lib.* 5, *cap.* 9. Strabo, *lib.* 5, give a true cause of his annual flowing, Pagaphetta[9] discourse rightly of it, or of Niger and Senegal; examine Cardan, Scaliger's reasons,[10] and the rest. Is it from those etesian winds, or melting of snow in the mountains under the Equator (for Jordan yearly overflows when the snow melts in Mount Libanus), or from those great dropping perpetual showers, which are so frequent to the inhabitants within the tropics, when the sun is vertical, and cause such vast inundations in Senegal, Maragnan, Orinoco and the rest of those great rivers in *Zona Torrida*, which have all commonly the same passions at set times: and by good husbandry and policy hereafter no doubt may come to be as populous, as well tilled, as fruitful, as Egypt itself or Cochin-China? I would observe all those motions of the sea, and from what cause they proceed, from the moon (as the vulgar hold) or earth's motion, which Galileus, in the fourth dialogue of his System of the World, so eagerly proves and firmly demonstrates; or winds, as some will.[11] Why in that quiet Ocean of Zur, *in Mari Pacifico* [in

the Pacific Ocean], it is scarce perceived, in our British seas
most violent, in the Mediterranean and Red Sea so vehement,
irregular, and diverse?   Why the current in that Atlantic Ocean
should still be in some places from, in some again towards the
north, and why they come sooner than go? and so from Moabar
to Madagascar in that Indian Ocean, the merchants come in
three weeks, as Scaliger discusseth,[1] they return scarce in three
months, with the same or like winds: the continual current is
from east to west.   Whether Mount Athos, Pelion, Olympus,
Ossa, Caucasus, Atlas, be so high as Pliny, Solinus, Mela relate,
above clouds, meteors, *ubi nec auræ nec venti spirant* [where
there are no winds or breezes] (insomuch that they that ascend
die suddenly very often, the air is so subtile), 1,250 paces high,
according to that measure of Dicæarchus, or 78 miles perpendicularly high, as Jacobus Mazonius, *sec.* 3 *et* 4, expounding
that place of Aristotle about Caucasus,[2] and as Blancanus the
Jesuit [3] contends out of Clavius' and Nonius' demonstrations
de crepusculis [on twilights]; or rather 32 stadiums, as the most
received opinion is; or 4 miles, which the height of no mountain
doth perpendicularly exceed, and is equal to the greatest depths
of the sea, which is, as Scaliger holds, 1,580 paces (*Exer.* 38),
others 100 paces.   I would see those inner parts of America,
whether there be any such great city of Manoa or Eldorado in
that golden empire, where the highways are as much beaten
(one reports) as between Madrid and Valladolid in Spain; or
any such Amazons as he relates, or gigantic Patagones in Chica;
with that miraculous mountain Ybouyapab in the Northern
Brazil, *cujus jugum sternitur in amœnissimam planitiem* [4] [the
top of which spreads out into a most pleasant tableland], etc.
or that of Pariacacca, so high elevated in Peru.   The pike of
Teneriffe [5] how high it is?   70 miles? or 50, as Patricius holds?
or 9, as Snellius demonstrates in his *Eratosthenes?*   See that
strange Cirknickzerkscy lake in Carniola, whose waters gush so
fast out of the ground that they will overtake a swift horseman,
and by and by with as incredible celerity are supped up: [6]
which Lazius and Wernerus make an argument of the Argonauts
sailing under ground.   And that vast den or hole called Esmellen
in Muscovia, *quæ visitur horrendo hiatu,* [which presents a fright-
ful chasm], etc. which if anything casually fall in, makes such
a roaring noise, that no thunder or ordnance or warlike engine
can make the like; [7] such another is Gilber's Cave in Lapland,
with many the like.   I would examine the Caspian Sea, and
see where and how it exonerates itself, after it hath taken in

Volga, Iaxartes, Oxus, and those great rivers; at the mouth of
Obi, or where? What vent the Mexican lake hath, the Titicacan
in Peru, or that circular pool in the vale of Terapeia, of which
Acosta, *lib.* 3, *cap.* 16, hot in a cold country, the spring of
which boils up in the middle twenty foot square, and hath no
vent but exhalation: and that of *Mare mortuum* [the Dead Sea]
in Palestine, of Thrasymene, at Perusium in Italy: the Mediterranean itself. For from the ocean, at the Straits of Gibraltar,
there is a perpetual current into the Levant, and so likewise by
the Thracian Bosphorus out of the Euxine or Black Sea, besides
all those great rivers of Nile, Padus, Rhodanus, etc., how is this
water consumed? by the sun or otherwise? I would find out
with Trajan the fountains of Danubius, of Ganges, Oxus, see
those Egyptian pyramids, Trajan's bridge, *Grotta de Sibylla*,
Lucullus' fish-ponds, the temple of Nidrose, etc., and, if I could,
observe what becomes of swallows, storks, cranes, cuckoos,
nightingales, redstarts, and many other kind of singing-birds,
water-fowls, hawks, etc.; some of them are only seen in summer,
some in winter; some are observed in the snow and at no other
times,[1] each have their seasons. In winter not a bird is in
Muscovy to be found, but at the spring in an instant the woods
and hedges are full of them, saith Herbastein:[2] how comes it
to pass? Do they sleep in winter, like Gesner's Alpine mice;
or do they lie hid (as Olaus affirms[3]) "in the bottom of lakes
and rivers, *spiritum continentes* [keeping in their breath]? often
so found by fishermen in Poland and Scandia, two together,
mouth to mouth, wing to wing; and when the spring comes
they revive again, or if they be brought into a stove, or to the
fire-side." Or do they follow the sun, as Peter Martyr, *Legat.
Babylonica, lib.* 2, manifestly convicts, out of his own knowledge; for when he was ambassador in Egypt, he saw swallows,
Spanish kites, and many such other European birds,[4] in December
and January very familiarly flying, and in great abundance,
about Alexandria, *ubi floridæ tunc arbores ac viridaria* [where
trees and gardens are then in bloom]. Or lie they hid in caves,
rocks, and hollow trees, as most think, in deep tin-mines or sea-
cliffs, as Mr. Carew gives out?[5] I conclude of them all, for my
part, as Munster doth of cranes and storks; whence they come,
whither they go, *incompertum adhuc*, as yet we know not. We
see them here, some in summer, some in winter; "their coming
and going is sure in the night: in the plains of Asia" (saith he)
"the storks meet on such a set day, he that comes last is torn
in pieces, and so they get them gone."[6] Many strange places,

isthmi, euripi, Chersonesi [isthmuses, narrow channels, penin-
sulas], creeks, havens, promontories, straits, lakes, baths, rocks,
mountains; places and fields where cities have been ruined or
swallowed, battles fought; creatures, sea-monsters, remora, etc.,
minerals, vegetals. Zoophytes were fit to be considered in
such an expedition, and amongst the rest that of Herbastein
his Tartar lamb,[1] Hector Boethius' goose-bearing tree in the
Orcades,[2] to which Cardan, *lib. 7, cap. 36, de rerum varietate*,
subscribes: Vertomannus' wonderful palm;[3] that fly in His-
paniola, that shines like a torch in the night, that one may well
see to write;[4] those spherical stones in Cuba which nature hath
so made, and those like birds, beasts, fishes, crowns, swords,
saws, pots, etc., usually found in the metal mines in Saxony
about Mansfield, and in Poland near Nokow and Pallukie, as
Munster[5] and others relate. Many rare creatures and novelties
each part of the world affords: amongst the rest, I would know
for a certain whether there be any such men, as Leo Suavius,
in his Comment on Paracelsus *de sanit. tuend.*, and Gaguinus
records in his description of Muscovy, "that in Lucomoria, a
province in Russia, lie fast asleep as dead all winter, from the
27th of November, like frogs and swallows, benumbed with
cold, but about the 24th of April in the spring they revive
again, and go about their business."[6] I would examine that
demonstration of Alexander Piccolomineus, whether the earth's
superficies be bigger than the sea's: or that of Archimedes be
true, the superficies of all water is even? Search the depth,
and see that variety of sea-monsters and fishes, mermaids, seamen, horses, etc., which it affords. Or whether that be true
which Jordanus Brunus scoffs at, that if God did not detain it,
the sea would overflow the earth by reason of his higher site,
and which Josephus Blancanus the Jesuit, in his interpretation
on those mathematical places of Aristotle, foolishly fears, and in
a just tract proves by many circumstances that in time the sea
will waste away the land, and all the globe of the earth shall
be covered with waters; *risum teneatis, amici?* [can you contain
your laughter, friends?] what the sea takes away in one place
it adds in another. Methinks he might rather suspect the sea
should in time be filled by land, trees grow up, carcasses, etc.,
that all-devouring fire, *omnia devorans et consumens*, will sooner
cover and dry up the vast ocean with sand and ashes. I would
examine the true seat of that terrestrial paradise,[7] and where
Ophir was, whence Solomon did fetch his gold: from Peruana,
which some suppose, or that Aurea Chersonesus, as Dominicus

Niger, Arias Montanus, Goropius, and others will. I would
censure all Pliny's, Solinus', Strabo's, Sir John Mandeville's,
Olaus Magnus', Marcus Polus' lies, correct those errors in navigation, reform cosmographical charts, and rectify longitudes, if
it were possible; not by the compass, as some dream, with Mark
Ridley in his Treatise of Magnetical Bodies, *cap.* 43, for as
Cabeus, *Magnet. philos. lib.* 3, *cap.* 4, fully resolves, there is no
hope thence; yet I would observe some better means to find
them out.

I would have a convenient place to go down with Orpheus,
Ulysses, Hercules, Lucian's Menippus,[1] at St. Patrick's Purgatory, at Trophonius' den,[2] Hecla in Iceland, Ætna in Sicily, to
descend and see what is done in the bowels of the earth; do
stones and metals grow there still? how come fir-trees to be
digged out from the tops of hills,[3] as in our mosses and marshes
all over Europe? How come they to dig up fish-bones, shells,
beams, iron-works, many fathoms underground, and anchors in
mountains far remote from all seas? *Anno* 1460, at Berne
in Switzerland, 50 fathom deep, a ship was digged out of a
mountain where they got metal ore, in which were 48 carcasses
of men, with other merchandise.[4] That such things are ordinarily found in tops of hills, Aristotle insinuates in his Meteors,
Pomponius Mela in his first book, *cap. de Numidia,*[5] and familiarly
in the Alps, saith Blancanus the Jesuit,[6] the like is to be seen.
Came this from earthquakes, or from Noah's flood, as Christians
suppose? or is there a vicissitude of sea and land, as Anaximenes
held of old the mountains of Thessaly would become seas, and
seas again mountains? The whole world belike should be new-
moulded, when it seemed good to those all-commanding powers,
and turned inside out, as we do hay-cocks in harvest, top to
bottom, or bottom to top: or as we turn apples to the fire, move
the world upon his centre; that which is under the poles now,
should be translated to the equinoctial, and that which is under
the torrid zone to the Circle Arctic and Antarctic another while,
and so be reciprocally warmed by the sun: or if the worlds be
infinite, and every fixed star a sun, with his compassing planets
(as Brunus and Campanella conclude), cast three or four worlds
into one; or else of one world make three or four new, as it shall
seem to them best. To proceed, if the earth be 21,500 miles
in compass,[7] its diameter is 7,000 from us to our antipodes,
and what shall be comprehended in all that space? What is
the centre of the earth? is it pure element only, as Aristotle
decrees, inhabited (as Paracelsus thinks [8]) with creatures whose

chaos is the earth: or with fairies, as the woods and waters (according to him) are with nymphs, or as the air with spirits? Dionysiodorus, a mathematician in Pliny,[1] that sent a letter *ad superos* [to the upper world] after he was dead, from the centre of the earth, to signify what distance the same centre was from the superficies of the same, viz. 42,000 stadiums, might have done well to have satisfied all these doubts. Or is it the place of hell, as Virgil in his Æneid, Plato, Lucian, Dante, and others poetically describe it, and as many of our divines think? In good earnest, Anthony Rusca, one of the society of that Ambrosian College, in Milan, in his great volume *de Inferno, lib. 1, cap.* 47, is stiff in this tenent, 'tis a corporeal fire tow, *cap. 5, lib.* 2, as he there disputes. "Whatsoever philosophers write" (saith Surius [2]), "there be certain mouths of hell, and places appointed for the punishment of men's souls, as at Hecla in Iceland, where the ghosts of dead men are familiarly seen, and sometimes talk with the living: God would have such visible places, that mortal men might be certainly informed that there be such punishments after death, and learn hence to fear God." Cranzius, *Dan. hist. lib.* 2, *cap.* 24, subscribes to this opinion of Surius, so doth Colerus, *cap.* 12, *lib. de immortal. animæ* (out of the authority belike of St. Gregory, Durand, and the rest of the Schoolmen, who derive as much from Ætna in Sicily, Lipari, Hiera, and those sulphureous vulcanian islands), making Terra del Fuego and those frequent volcanoes in America (of which Acosta, *lib.* 3, *cap.* 24), that fearful mount Hecklebirg in Norway, an especial argument to prove it, "where lamentable screeches and howlings are continually heard, which strike a terror to the auditors; fiery chariots are commonly seen to bring in the souls of men in the likeness of crows, and devils ordinarily go in and out." [3] Such another proof is that place near the Pyramids in Egypt, by Cairo, as well to confirm this as the resurrection, mentioned by Kornmannus, *Mirac. mort. lib. 1, cap.* 38, Camerarius, *Oper. subcis. cap.* 37, Bredenbachius, *Pereg. Ter. Sanct.*, and some others, "where once a year dead bodies arise about March, and walk, after awhile hide themselves again: thousands of people come yearly to see them." [4] But these and such like testimonies others reject, as fables, illusions of spirits, and they will have no such local known place, more than Styx or Phlegethon, Pluto's court, or that poetical *Infernus,* where Homer's soul was seen hanging on a tree, etc., to which they ferried over in Charon's boat, or went down at Hermione in Greece, *compendiaria ad inferos via,*

II—D 887

which is the shortest cut, *quia nullum a mortuis naulum eo loci
exposcunt* (saith Gerbelius [1]), and besides there were no fees to
be paid. Well then, is it hell, or purgatory, as Bellarmine, or
Limbus patrum [limbo], as Gallucius will, and as Rusca will
(for they have made maps of it), or Ignatius' parlour? [2] Virgil,
sometime Bishop of Salzburg (as Aventinus, *anno* 745, relates),
by Bonifacius, Bishop of Mentz, was therefore called in question,
because he held antipodes (which they made a doubt whether
Christ died for) and so by that means took away the seat of
hell, or so contracted it that it could bear no proportion to
heaven, and contradicted that opinion of Austin, Basil, Lactantius, that held the earth round as a trencher (whom Acosta
and common experience more largely confute) but not as a ball;
and Jerusalem, where Christ died, the middle of it; or Delos,
as the fabulous Greeks feigned: because when Jupiter let two
eagles loose, to fly from the world's ends east and west, they
met at Delos. But that scruple of Bonifacius is now quite
taken away by our latter divines: Franciscus Ribera, *in cap.* 14
Apocalyps., will have hell a material and local fire in the centre
of the earth, 200 Italian miles in diameter, as he defines it out
of those words, *Exivit sanguis de terra . . . per stadia mille
sexcenta* [blood came out of the earth for 1,600 furlongs], etc.
But Lessius, *lib.* 13 *de moribus divinis, cap.* 24, will have this
local hell far less, one Dutch mile in diameter, all filled with
fire and brimstone; because, as he there demonstrates, that
space, cubically multiplied, will make a sphere able to hold
800,000 millions of damned bodies (allowing each body six
foot square), which will abundantly suffice; *cum certum sit,
inquit, facta subductione, non futuros centies mille milliones
damnandorum* [since it is beyond question that, after proper
subtraction is made, there will not be 100,000 millions
damned]. But if it be no material fire (as Scotus, Thomas,
Bonaventure, Soncinas, Vossius, and others argue), it may be
there or elsewhere, as Keckerman disputes, *System. Theol.*, for
sure somewhere it is, *certum est alicubi, etsi definitus circulus non
assignetur* [it is certainly somewhere, although a definite zone
cannot be assigned to it]. I will end the controversy in Austin's
words, " Better doubt of things concealed, than to contend about
uncertainties, where Abraham's bosom is, and hell-fire "; [3] *vix a
mansuetis, a contentiosis nunquam invenitur:* [4] scarce the meek,
the contentious shall never find. If it be solid earth, 'tis the
fountain of metals, waters, which by his innate temper turns
air into water, which springs up in several chinks to moisten

the earth's superficies, and that in a tenfold proportion (as Aristotle holds); or else these fountains come directly from the sea by secret passages,[1] and so made fresh again by running through the bowels of the earth; and are either thick, thin, hot, cold, as the matter or minerals are by which they pass; or, as Peter Martyr, *Ocean. decad. lib.* 9, and some others hold, from abundance of rain that falls,[2] or from that ambient heat and cold, which alters that inward heat, and so *per consequens* the generation of waters. Or else it may be full of wind, or a sulphureous innate fire, as our meteorologists inform us, which sometimes breaking out, causeth those horrible earthquakes which are so frequent in these days in Japan, China, and oftentimes swallow up whole cities. Let Lucian's Menippus consult with or ask of Tiresias, if you will not believe philosophers; he shall clear all your doubts when he makes a second voyage.

In the meantime let us consider of that which is *sub dio* [in the open], and find out a true cause, if it be possible, of such accidents, meteors, alterations, as happen above ground. Whence proceed that variety of manners, and a distinct character (as it were) to several nations? Some are wise, subtile, witty; others dull, sad, and heavy; some big, some little, as Tully *de Fato*, Plato *in Timæo*, Vegetius, and Bodine proves at large, *Method cap.* 5; some soft, and some hardy, barbarous, civil, black, dun, white; is it from the air, from the soil, influence of stars, or some other secret cause? Why doth Africa breed so many venomous beasts, Ireland none? Athens owls, Crete none? Why hath Daulis and Thebes no swallows (so Pausanias informeth us[3]) as well as the rest of Greece, Ithaca no hares,[4] Pontus asses, Scythia swine? Whence comes this variety of complexions, colours, plants, birds, beasts, metals,[5] peculiar almost to every place? Why so many thousand strange birds and beasts proper to America alone, as Acosta demands, *lib.* 4, *cap.* 36? Were they created in the six days, or ever in Noah's ark? if there, why are they not dispersed and found in other countries? It is a thing (saith he) hath long held me in suspense; no Greek, Latin, Hebrew ever heard of them before, and yet as differing from our European animals as an egg and a chestnut: and, which is more, kine, horses, sheep, etc., till the Spaniards brought them, were never heard of in those parts. How comes it to pass, that in the same site, in one latitude, to such as are *periœci* [neighbours], there should be such difference of soil, complexion, colour, metal, air, etc. The

Spaniards are white, and so are Italians, whenas the inhabitants about *Caput Bonæ Spei* [1] [the Cape of Good Hope] are blacka-moors, and yet both alike distant from the Equator: nay, they that dwell in the same parallel line with these negroes, as those the Straits of Magellan, are white-coloured, and yet some in Presbyter John's country in Æthiopia are dun; they in Zeilan and Malabar parallel with them again black: Monomotapa in Africa and St. Thomas' Isle are extreme hot, both under the line, coal-black their inhabitants, whereas in Peru they are quite opposite in colour, very temperate, or rather cold, and yet both alike elevated. Moscow in 53 degrees of latitude extreme cold, as those northern countries usually are, having one per-petual hard frost all winter long; and in 52 deg. lat. sometimes hard frost and snow all summer, as in Button's Bay, etc., or by fits; and yet England, near the same latitude, and Ireland, very moist, warm, and more temperate in winter than Spain, Italy, or France.[2] Is it the sea that causeth this difference, and the air that comes from it? Why then is Ister[3] so cold near the Euxine, Pontus, Bithynia, and all Thrace? *frigidas regiones* [chilly regions] Maginus calls them, and yet their latitude is but 42, which should be hot: Quevira,[4] or Nova Albion in America, bordering on the sea, was so cold in July that our Englishmen could hardly endure it.[5] At Norembega, in 45 lat., all the sea is frozen ice, and yet in a more southern latitude than ours. New England, and the island of Cambriol Colchis,[6] which that noble gentleman Mr. Vaughan, or Orpheus Junior, describes in his Golden Fleece, is in the same latitude with Little Britain in France, and yet their winter begins not till January, their spring till May; which search he accounts worthy of an astrologer: is this from the easterly winds, or melting of ice and snow dissolved within the Circle Arctic; or that the air being thick, is longer before it be warm by the sunbeams, and once heated like an oven will keep itself from cold? Our climes breed lice, Hungary[7] and Ireland *male audiunt* [have a bad name] in this kind; come to the Azores, by a secret virtue of that air they are instantly consumed, and all our European vermin almost, saith Ortelius. Egypt is watered with Nilus not far from the sea, and yet there it seldom or never rains: Rhodes, an island of the same nature, yields not a cloud, and yet our islands ever dropping and inclining to rain. The Atlantic Ocean is still subject to storms, but in Del Zur, or *Mari Pacifico* [the Pacific Ocean], seldom or never any. Is it from topic stars, *apertio portarum* [the opening of the gates], in the dode-

catemories or constellations, the moon's mansions, such aspects
of planets, such winds, or dissolving air, or thick air, which
causeth this and the like differences of heat and cold? Bodine
relates of a Portugal ambassador, that coming from Lisbon [1]
to Dantzic [2] in Spruce, found greater heat there than at any time
at home. Don Garcia de Silva, legate to Philip III, King of
Spain, residing at Ispahan in Persia, 1619, in his letter to the
Marquess of Bedmar, makes mention of greater cold in Ispahan,
whose lat. is 31 gr., than ever he felt in Spain, or any part of
Europe. The torrid zone was by our predecessors held to be
uninhabitable, but by our modern travellers found to be most
temperate, bedewed with frequent rains and moistening showers,
the brise and cooling blasts in some parts, as Acosta describes,[3]
most pleasant and fertile (Arica in Chili is by report one of the
sweetest places that ever the sun shined on, *Olympus terræ*, a
heaven on earth: how incomparably do some extol Mexico in
Nova Hispania, Peru, Brazil, etc.!); in some again hard, dry,
sandy, barren, a very desert, and still in the same latitude.
Many times we find great diversity of air in the same country,[4]
by reason of the site to seas, hills, or dales, want of water, nature
of soil, and the like: as in Spain Aragon is *aspera et sicca*, harsh
and evil inhabited; Estremadura is dry, sandy, barren most
part, extreme hot by reason of his plains; Andalusia another
paradise; Valencia a most pleasant air, and continually green;
so is it about Granada,[5] on the one side fertile plains, on the
other continual snow to be seen all summer long on the hill-
tops. That their houses in the Alps are three-quarters of the
year covered with snow, who knows not? That Teneriffe is so
cold at the top, extreme hot at the bottom; Mons Atlas in
Africa, Libanus in Palestine, with many such, *tantos inter ardores
fidos nivibus* [invariably snow-clad even in that hot climate],
Tacitus calls them,[6] and Radzivilius, *Epist. 2, fol.* 27, yields it
to be far hotter there than in any part of Italy: 'tis true; but
they are highly elevated, near the middle region, and therefore
cold, *ob paucam solarium radiorum refractionem* [on account of
the slight refraction of the sun's rays], as Serrarius answers,
Com. in 3 *cap. Josua, quæst.* 5, Abulensis, *quæst.* 37. In the
heat of summer, in the king's palace in Escurial, the air is most
temperate, by reason of a cold blast which comes from the
snowy mountains of Sierra de Guadarama hard by, whenas in
Toledo it is very hot: so in all other countries. The causes of
these alterations are commonly by reason of their nearness
(I say) to the middle region: but this diversity of air, in places

equally site, elevated, and distant from the Pole, can hardly
be satisfied with that diversity of plants, birds, beasts which is
so familiar with us: with Indians, everywhere, the sun is equally
distant, the same vertical stars, the same irradiations of planets,
aspects like, the same nearness of seas, the same superficies,
the same soil, or not much different. Under the Equator itself,
amongst the sierras, Andes, llanos, as Herrera, Laet, and
Acosta [1] contend, there is *tam mirabilis et inopinata varietas*,
such variety of weather, *ut merito exerceat ingenia*, that no
philosophy can yet find out the true cause of it. When I consider how temperate it is in one place, saith Acosta,[2] within the
Tropic of Capricorn, as about La Plata, and yet hard by at
Potosi, in that same altitude, mountainous alike, extreme cold;
extreme hot in Brazil, etc.; *hic ego*, saith Acosta, *philosophiam
Aristotelis meteorologicam vehementer irrisi, cum* [I had to laugh
at Aristotle's meteorology, since], etc.; when the sun comes
nearest to them, they have great tempests, storms, thunder
and lightning, great store of rain, snow, and the foulest
weather: when the sun is vertical, their rivers overflow, the
morning fair and hot, noon-day cold and moist: all which is
opposite to us. How comes it to pass? Scaliger, *Poetices
lib.* 3, *cap.* 16, discourseth thus of this subject. How
comes, or wherefore is, this *temeraria siderum dispositio*,
this rash placing of stars, or, as Epicurus will, *fortuita*, or
accidental? Why are some big, some little? Why are they
so confusedly, unequally site in the heavens, and set so
much out of order? In all other things nature is equal, pro-
portionable, and constant; there be *justæ dimensiones, et prudens
partium dispositio* [just dimensions, and a wise arrangement
of parts]; as in the fabric of man, his eyes, ears, nose, face,
members are correspondent, *cur non idem cœlo opere omnium
pulcherrimo?* [why is it not so in the sky, the fairest part of
creation?] Why are the heavens so irregular, *neque paribus
molibus, neque paribus intervallis* [as regards both mass and
interstices]? whence is this difference? *Diversos* (he concludes)
efficere locorum genios, to make diversity of countries, soils,
manners, customs, characters, and constitutions among us, *ut
quantum vicinia ad caritatem addat, sidera distrahant ad perniciem*
[in order that the stars may sunder those whom proximity
would naturally make friends], and so by this means *fluvio vel
monte distincti sunt dissimiles* [people separated only be a river
or a mountain are dissimilar], the same places almost shall be
distinguished in manners. But this reason is weak and most

insufficient. The fixed stars are removed since Ptolemy's time
26 gr. from the first of Aries, and if the earth be immovable,
as their site varies, so should countries vary, and divers alterations would follow. But this we perceive not; as in Tully's
time with us in Britain, *cœlum visu fœdum, et in quo facile
generantur nubes* [their sky is gloomy and quickly becomes
overcast], etc., 'tis so still. Wherefore Bodine, *Theat. nat.
lib.* 2, and some others, will have all these alterations and
effects immediately to proceed from those genii, spirits, angels,
which rule and domineer in several places; they cause storms,
thunder, lightning, earthquakes, ruins, tempests, great winds,
floods, etc. The philosophers of Coimbra will refer this diversity
to the influence of that empyrean heaven: for some say the
eccentricity of the sun is come nearer to the earth than in
Ptolemy's time, the virtue therefore of all the vegetals is
decayed, men grow less, etc.[1] There are that observe new
motions of the heavens, new stars, *palantia sidera* [wandering
stars], comets, clouds, call them what you will, like those
Medicean, Bourbonian, Austrian planets lately detected, which
do not decay, but come and go, rise higher and lower, hide and
show themselves amongst the fixed stars, amongst the planets,
above and beneath the moon, at set times, now nearer, now
farther off, together, asunder; as he that plays upon a sackbut
by pulling it up and down alters his tones and tunes, do they
their stations and places, though to us undiscerned; and from
those motions proceed (as they conceive) divers alterations.
Clavius conjectures otherwise, but they be but conjectures.
About Damascus in Cœle-Syria is a paradise,[2] by reason of the
plenty of waters, *in promptu causa est* [the cause is obvious],
and the deserts of Arabia barren, because of rocks, rolling seas
of sands, and dry mountains, *quod inaquosa* (saith Adricomius)
*montes habens asperos, saxosos, præcipites, horroris et mortis
speciem præ se ferentes,* uninhabitable therefore of men, birds,
beasts, void of all green trees, plants, and fruits, a vast rocky
horrid wilderness, which by no art can be manured, 'tis evident.
Bohemia is cold, for that it lies all along to the north. But
why should it be so hot in Egypt, or there never rain? Why
should those etesian and north-eastern winds blow continually
and constantly so long together, in some places, at set times,
one way still, in the dog-days only:[3] here perpetual drought,
there dropping showers; here foggy mists, there a pleasant
air;[4] here terrible thunder and lightning at such set seasons,
here frozen seas all the year, there open in the same latitude,

to the rest no such thing, nay, quite opposite is to be found?
Sometimes (as in Peru[1]) on the one side of the mountains it is
hot, on the other cold, here snow, there wind, with infinite
such.   Fromundus, in his Meteors, will excuse or solve all this
by the sun's motion, but when there is such diversity to such as
[are] *periœci* [neighbours], or very near site, how can that
position hold?

Who can give a reason of this diversity of meteors, that it
should rain stones,[2] frogs, mice, etc., rats, which they call
lemmer in Norway, and are manifestly observed (as Munster
writes[3]) by the inhabitants to descend and fall with some
feculent showers, and like so many locusts, consume all that
is green.   Leo Afer speaks as much of locusts, about Fez in
Barbary there be infinite swarms in their fields upon a sudden:
so at Arles in France, 1553, the like happened by the same mischief, all their grass and fruits were devoured, *magna incolarum
admiratione et consternatione* (as Valleriola, *Obser. med. lib.* 1,
obser. 1, relates) *cœlum subito obumbrabant* [to the amazement
and consternation of the inhabitants, they suddenly darkened
the heavens], etc.; he concludes it could not be from natural
causes, they cannot imagine whence they come, but from
heaven.[4]   Are these and such creatures, corn, wood, stones,
worms, wool, blood, etc., lifted up into the middle region by
the sunbeams, as Baracellus the physician disputes,[5] and thence
let fall with showers, or there engendered?   Cornelius Gemma [6]
is of that opinion, they are there conceived by celestial influences:
others suppose they are immediately from God, or prodigies
raised by art and illusions of spirits, which are princes of the
air; to whom Bodine, *lib.* 2 *Theat. Nat.*, subscribes.   In fine,
of meteors in general, Aristotle's reasons are exploded by
Bernardinus Telesius, by Paracelsus his principles confuted, and
other causes assigned, *sal* [salt], sulphur, mercury, in which
his disciples are so expert, that they can alter elements, and
separate at their pleasure, make perpetual motions, not as
Cardan, Taisnier, Peregrinus, by some magnetical virtue, but
by mixture of elements; imitate thunder, like Salmoneus, snow,
hail, the sea's ebbing and flowing, give life to creatures (as they
say) without generation, and what not?   P. Nonius Saluciensis
and Kepler take upon them to demonstrate that no meteors,
clouds, fogs, vapours,[7] arise higher than fifty or eighty miles,
and all the rest to be purer air or element of fire: which Cardan,[8]
Tycho,[9] and John Pena [10] manifestly confute by refractions, and
many other arguments, there is no such element of fire at all.

If, as Tycho proves, the moon be distant from us fifty and sixty semi-diameters of the earth, and, as Peter Nonius will have it, the air be so angust, what proportion is there betwixt the other three elements and it? To what use serves it? Is it full of spirits which inhabit it, as the Paracelsians and Platonists hold, the higher the more noble, full of birds,[1] or a mere vacuum to no purpose? It is much controverted between Tycho Brahe and Christopher Rotman, the Landgrave of Hesse's mathematician, in their Astronomical Epistles, whether it be the same *diaphanum*, clearness, matter of air and heavens, or two distinct essences? Christopher Rotman, John Pena, Jordanus Brunus, with many other late mathematicians, contend it is the same and one matter throughout, saving that the higher still the purer it is, and more subtile; as they find by experience in the top of some hills in America;[2] if a man ascend, he faints instantly for want of thicker air to refrigerate the heart. Acosta, *lib. 3, cap.* 9, calls this mountain Periacacca in Peru; it makes men cast and vomit, he saith, that climb it, as some other of those Andes do in the deserts of Chile for five hundred miles together, and for extremity of cold to lose their fingers and toes. Tycho will have two distinct matters of heaven and air; but to say truth, with some small qualification, they have one and the self-same opinion about the essence and matter of heavens; that it is not hard and impenetrable, as Peripatetics hold, transparent, of a *quinta essentia* [fifth essence], "but that it is penetrable and soft as the air itself is, and that the planets move in it, as birds in the air, fishes in the sea."[3] This they prove by motion of comets, and otherwise (though Claremontius in his *Antitycho* stiffly oppose), which are not generated, as Aristotle teacheth, in the aerial region, of a hot and dry exhalation, and so consumed: but, as Anaxagoras and Democritus held of old, of a celestial matter: and as Tycho,[4] Helisæus,[5] Rœslin, Thaddæus Haggesius, Pena, Rotman, Fracastorius, demonstrate by their progress, parallaxes, refractions, motions of the planets, which interfere and cut one another's orbs, now higher, and then lower, as ♂ amongst the rest, which sometimes, as Kepler[6] confirms by his own and Tycho's accurate observations, comes nearer the earth than the ☉, and is again eftsoons aloft in Jupiter's orb; and other sufficient reasons, far above the moon:[7] exploding in the meantime that element of fire, those fictitious first watery movers, those heavens, I mean, above the firmament, which Delrio, Lodovicus Imola, Patricius, and many of the Fathers affirm; those monstrous orbs of

eccentrics, and *eccentre epicycles deserentes* [epicycles leaving
the eccentric], which, howsoever Ptolemy, Alhazen, Vitellio,
Purbachius, Maginus, Clavius, and many of their associates,
stiffly maintain to be real orbs, eccentric, concentric, circles
equant, etc., are absurd and ridiculous. For who is so mad
to think that there should be so many circles, like subordinate
wheels in a clock, all impenetrable and hard, as they feign, add
and subtract at their pleasure. Maginus makes eleven heavens,[1]
subdivided into their orbs and circles, and all too little to serve
those particular appearances: Fracastorius, seventy-two homocentrics; Tycho Brahe, Nicholas Ramerus, Helisæus Rœslin,
have peculiar hypotheses of their own inventions; and they
be but inventions, as most of them acknowledge, as we admit
of equators, tropics, colures, circles arctic and antarctic, for
doctrine's sake (though Ramus thinks them all unnecessary),
they will have them supposed only for method and order. Tycho
hath feigned I know not how many subdivisions of epicycles in
epicycles, etc., to calculate and express the moon's motion:
but when all is done, as a supposition, and no otherwise; not
(as he holds) hard, impenetrable, subtile, transparent, etc., or
making music, as Pythagoras maintained of old, and Robert
Constantine of late, but still quiet, liquid, open, etc.

If the heavens then be penetrable, as these men deliver, and
no lets, it were not amiss in this aerial progress to make wings
and fly up, which that Turk in Busbequius made his fellow-
citizens in Constantinople believe he would perform: and some
newfangled wits, methinks, should some time or other find out:
or if that may not be, yet with a Galileo's glass, or Icaromenippus'
wings in Lucian, command the spheres and heavens, and see
what is done amongst them. Whether there be generation and
corruption, as some think, by reason of ethereal comets, that
in Cassiopea, 1572, that in Cygnus, 1600, that in Sagittarius,
1604, and many like, which by no means Julius Cæsar la Galla,
that Italian philosopher, in his physical disputation with
Galileus *de phenomenis in orbe lunæ* [concerning the phenomena
in the orb of the moon], *cap.* 9, will admit: or that they were
created *ab initio* [from the beginning], and show themselves at
set times: and as Helisæus Rœslin contends,[2] have poles, axle-
trees, circles of their own, and regular motions. For, *non
pereunt, sed minuuntur et disparent* [they do not dissolve, but
diminish and finally disappear], Blancanus holds,[3] they come
and go by fits, casting their tails still from the sun, some of
them, as a burning-glass projects the sunbeams from it; though

not always neither: for sometimes a comet casts his tail from
Venus, as Tycho observes; and, as Helisæus Rœslin of some
others,[1] from the moon, with little stars about them *ad stuporem*
astronomorum; *cum multis aliis in cœlo miraculis* [to the amazement of astronomers; with many other wonders in the heavens],
all which argue, with those Medicean, Austrian, and Bourbonian
stars, that the heaven of the planets is indistinct, pure, and
open, in which the planets move *certis legibus ac metis* [regularly
and in fixed orbits].   Examine likewise *An cœlum sit coloratum*
[whether the sky is coloured]?   Whether the stars be of that
bigness, distance, as astronomers relate, so many in number,[2]
1026, or 1725, as J. Bayerus; or as some rabbins, 29,000 myriads;
or as Galileo discovers by his glasses, infinite, and that *via*
lactea [Milky Way] a confused light of small stars, like so many
nails in a door: or all in a row, like those 12,000 isles of the
Maldives in the Indian Ocean?   Whether the least visible star
in the eighth sphere be eighteen times bigger than the earth,
and, as Tycho calculates, 14,000 semidiameters distant from it?
Whether they be thicker parts of the orbs, as Aristotle delivers:
or so many habitable worlds, as Democritus?   Whether they
have light of their own, or from the sun, or give light round, as
Patricius discourseth?   *An æque distent a centro mundi* [whether
they are equally distant from the centre of the world]?   Whether
light be of their essence; and that light be a substance or an
accident?   Whether they be hot by themselves, or by accident
cause heat?   Whether there be such a precession of the equi-
noxes as Copernicus holds, or that the eighth sphere move?
An bene philosophentur R. Bacon and J. Dee, *aphorism. de*
multiplicatione specierum [whether Roger Bacon and John Dee
reason well in their aphorisms on the multiplication of images]?
Whether there be any such images ascending with each degree
of the zodiac in the east, as Aliacensis feigns?   *An aqua super*
cœlum [whether there is water above the sky]? as Patricius and
the schoolmen will, a crystalline watery heaven,[3] which is certainly to be understood of that in the middle region;[4] for
otherwise, if at Noah's flood the water came from thence, it
must be above an hundred years falling down to us, as some
calculate.[5]   Besides, *an terra sit animata* [whether the earth is
animate]? which some so confidently believe, with Orpheus,
Hermes, Averroes, from which all other souls of men, beasts,
devils, plants, fishes, etc. are derived, and into which again,
after some revolutions, as Plato in his *Timæus*, Plotinus in his
Enneades, more largely discuss, they return (see Chalcidius and

Bennius, Plato's commentators), as all philosophical matter, *in materiam primam* [to their original material]. Keplerus, Patricius, and some other neoterics have in part revived this opinion; and that every star in heaven hath a soul, angel, or intelligence to animate or move it, etc. Or, to omit all smaller controversies, as matters of less moment, and examine that main paradox of the earth's motion, now so much in question: Aristarchus Samius, Pythagoras, maintained it of old, Democritus, and many of their scholars. Didacus Astunica, Anthony Fascarinus, a Carmelite, and some other commentators, will have Job to insinuate as much, *cap.* 9, *ver.* 6, *Qui commovet terram de loco suo* [which shaketh the earth out of her place], etc., and that this one place of Scripture makes more for the earth's motion than all the other prove against it; whom Pineda confutes, most contradict. Howsoever, it is revived since by Copernicus, not as a truth, but a supposition, as he himself confesseth in the Preface to Pope Nicholas, but now maintained in good earnest by Calcagninus,[1] Telesius, Kepler, Rotman, Gilbert, Digges, Galileo, Campanella, and especially by Lansbergius,[2] *naturæ, rationi, et veritati consentaneum* [as agreeing with nature, reason, and truth], by Origanus, and some others of his followers.[3] For if the earth be the centre of the world, stand still, and the heavens move, as the most received opinion is,[4] which they call *inordinatam cœli dispositionem* [an ill-regulated disposition of the sky], though stiffly maintained by Tycho, Ptolemæus, and their adherents, *quis ille furor?* etc., what fury is that, saith Dr. Gilbert,[5] *satis animose* [with a good deal of temper], as Cabeus notes, that shall drive the heavens about with such incomprehensible celerity in twenty-four hours? whenas every point of the firmament, and in the Equator, must needs move (so Clavius calculates[6]) 176,660 in one 246th part of an hour: and an arrow out of a bow must go seven times about the earth, whilst a man can say an Ave Maria, if it keep the same space, or compass the earth 1,884 times in an hour, which is *supra humanam cogitationem*, beyond human conceit: *Ocior et jaculo, et ventos æquante sagitta* [swifter than a dart, or arrow swift as wind]. A man could not ride so much ground, going 40 miles a day, in 2,904 years as the firmament goes in 24 hours, or so much in 2·3 years as the firmament in one minute: *quod incredibile videtur* [which seems incredible]: and the pole-star,[7] which to our thinking scarce moveth out of his place, goeth a bigger circuit than the sun, whose diameter is much larger than the diameter of the heaven of the sun, and

20,000 semi-diameters of the earth from us, with the rest of
the fixed stars, as Tycho proves. To avoid therefore these
impossibilities, they ascribe a triple motion to the earth, the
sun immovable in the centre of the whole world, the earth centre
of the moon alone, above ♀ and ☿, beneath ♄, ♃, ♂ (or, as
Origanus [1] and others will, one single motion to the earth, still
placed in the centre of the world, which is more probable); a
single motion to the firmament, which moves in 30 or 26 thousand
years; and so the planets, Saturn in thirty years absolves
his sole and proper motion, Jupiter in 12, Mars in 3, etc., and
so solve all appearances better than any way whatsoever: calculate all motions, be they in *longum* [lengthwise] or *latum* [breadth-
wise], direct, stationary, retrograde, ascent or descent, without
epicycles, intricate eccentrics, etc., *rectius commodiusque per
unicum mótum terræ* [more accurately and more simply by the
single motion of the earth], saith Lansbergius, much more
certain than by those Alphonsine, or any such tables, which
are grounded from those other suppositions. And 'tis true
they say, according to optic principles, the visible appearances
of the planets do so indeed answer to their magnitudes and
orbs, and come nearest to mathematical observations and precedent calculations; there is no repugnancy to physical axioms,
because no penetration of orbs; but then, between the sphere
of Saturn and the firmament, there is such an incredible and
vast space [2] or distance (7,000,000 semi-diameters of the earth,
as Tycho calculates) void of stars: and besides, they do so
enhance the bigness of the stars, enlarge their circuit, to solve
those ordinary objections of parallaxes and retrogradations of
the fixed stars, that alteration of the poles, elevation in several
places or latitude of cities here on earth (for, say they, if a man's
eye were in the firmament, he should not at all discern that
great annual motion of the earth, but it would still appear
punctum indivisibile [an indivisible point], and seem to be fixed
in one place, of the same bigness), that it is quite opposite to
reason, to natural philosophy, and all out as absurd as dis-
proportional (so some will), as prodigious, as that of the sun's
swift motion of heavens. But *hoc posito*, to grant this their
tenent of the earth's motion: if the earth move, it is a planet,
and shines to them in the moon, and to the other planetary
inhabitants, as the moon and they do to us upon the earth:
but shine she doth, as Galileo, Kepler,[3] and others prove, and
then, *per consequens*, the rest of the planets are inhabited, as
well as the moon, which he grants in his dissertation with

Galileo's *nuncius sidereus* [messenger from the stars], "that
there be Jovial and Saturnine inhabitants,"[1] etc., and those
several planets have their several moons about them, as the
earth hath hers, as Galileo hath already evinced by his glasses:
four about Jupiter,[2] two about Saturn (though Sitius the
Florentine, Fortunius Licetus, and Jul. Cæsar la Galla cavil at
it, yet Kepler, the emperor's mathematician, confirms out of
his experience that he saw as much by the same help), and
more about Mars, Venus; and the rest they hope to find out,
peradventure even amongst the fixed stars, which Brunus and
Brutius have already averred. Then (I say) the earth and
they be planets alike, inhabited alike, moved about the sun,
the common centre of the world alike, and it may be those two
green children which Nubrigensis speaks of[3] in his time, that
fell from heaven, came from thence; and that famous stone
that fell from heaven in Aristotle's time, Olymp. 84, *anno
tertio, ad Capuæ fluenta* [in the third year, near the streams of
Capua], recorded by Laertius and others, or *ancile* or buckler in
Numa's time, recorded by Festus. We may likewise insert with
Campanella and Brunus that which Pythagoras, Aristarchus
Samius, Heraclitus, Epicurus, Melissus, Democritus, Leucippus
maintained in their ages: there be infinite worlds,[4] and infinite
earths or systems, *in infinito æthere* [in the infinite ether], which
Eusebius collects out of their tenents,[5] because infinite stars
and planets like unto this of ours, which some stick not still
to maintain and publicly defend, *sperabundus exspecto innumera-
bilium mundorum in æternitate perambulationem* [I confidently
count upon the eternal movement of innumerable worlds], etc.
(Nic. Hill, Londinensis, *Philos. Epicur.*). For if the firmament
be of such an incomparable bigness as these Copernical giants
will have it, *infinitum, aut infinito proximum* [infinite, or very
nearly infinite], so vast and full of innumerable stars, as being
infinite in extent, one above another, some higher, some lower,
some nearer, some farther off, and so far asunder, and those
so huge and great, insomuch that if the whole sphere of Saturn,
and all that is included in it, *totum aggregatum* (as Fromundus
of Louvain in his tract *de immobilitate terræ* argues) *evehatur
inter stellas, videri a nobis non poterat, tam immanis est distantia
inter tellurem et fixas, sed instar puncti, etc.* [if the whole aggre-
gate were carried away to the stars, it would not be visible to
us, so immense is the distance between the earth and the fixed
stars, but like a point, etc.]. If our world be small in respect,
why may we not suppose a plurality of worlds, those infinite

stars visible in the firmament to be so many suns, with particular fixed centres; to have likewise their subordinate planets,
as the sun hath his dancing still round him? which Cardinal
Cusanus, Walkarinus, Brunus, and some others have held, and
some still maintain. *Animæ Aristotelismo innutritæ, et minutis
speculationibus assuetæ, secus forsan* [minds brought up on
Aristotelianism and accustomed to minute speculations might
think differently], etc. Though they seem close to us, they are
infinitely distant, and so, *per consequens*, there are infinite
habitable worlds: what hinders? Why should not an infinite
cause (as God is) produce infinite effects? as Nic. Hill, *Democrit.
philos.*, disputes. Kepler (I confess) will by no means admit
of Brunus' infinite worlds, or that the fixed stars should be so
many suns, with their compassing planets, yet the said Kepler [1]
betwixt jest and earnest in his Perspectives, Lunar Geography,
et Somnio suo,[2] *Dissertat. cum nunc. sider.*; seems in part to
agree with this, and partly to contradict; for the planets, he
yields them to be inhabited, he doubts of the stars; and so
doth Tycho in his Astronomical Epistles, out of a consideration
of their vastity and greatness, break out into some such-like
speeches, that he will never believe those great and huge bodies
were made to no other use than this that we perceive, to illuminate the earth, a point insensible in respect of the whole.
But who shall dwell in these vast bodies, earths, worlds, "if
they be inhabited? rational creatures?" as Kepler demands,
"or have they souls to be saved? or do they inhabit a better
part of the world than we do? Are we or they lords of the
world? And how are all things made for man?"[3] *Difficile
est nodum hunc expedire, eo quod nondum omnia quæ huc pertinent explorata habemus* [it is hard to resolve this difficulty,
because we do not yet possess all the requisite data]: 'tis hard
to determine; this only he proves, that we are in *præcipuo
mundi sinu,* in the best place, best world, nearest the heart of
the sun. Thomas Campanella, a Calabrian monk, in his second
book *de sensu rerum,*[4] *cap.* 4, subscribes to this of Kepler; that
they are inhabited he certainly supposeth, but with what kind
of creatures he cannot say; he labours to prove it by all means,
and that there are infinite worlds, having made an apology
for Galileo, and dedicates this tenent of his to Cardinal Cajetanus. Others freely speak, mutter, and would persuade the
world (as Marinus Marcennus complains[5]) that our modern
divines are too severe and rigid against mathematicians, ignorant
and peevish in not admitting their true demonstrations and

certain observations, that they tyrannize over art, science, and
all philosophy, in suppressing their labours (saith Pomponatius),
forbidding them to write, to speak a truth, all to maintain their
superstition, and for their profit's sake. As for those places of
Scripture which oppugn it, they will have spoken *ad captum
vulgi* [for the popular intelligence], and if rightly understood,
and favourably interpreted, not at all against it: and as Otho
Casman, *Astrol. cap.* 1, *part.* 1, notes, many great divines,
besides Porphyrius, Proclus, Simplicius, and those heathen
philosophers, *doctrina et ætate venerandi, Mosis Genesin mun-
danam popularis nescio cujus ruditatis, quæ longa absit a vera
philosophorum eruditione, insimulant* [venerable for age and
learning, accuse the Mosaic cosmology of being a crude popular
account, far removed from true philosophical learning]. For
Moses makes mention but of two planets, ⊙ and ☾, no four
elements, etc. Read more on him, in Grossius [1] and Junius.
But to proceed, these and such-like insolent and bold attempts,
prodigious paradoxes, inferences, must needs follow, if it once
be granted, which Rotman, Kepler, Gilbert, Diggeus, Origanus,
Galileo, and others maintain of the earth's motion, that 'tis a
planet, and shines as the moon doth, which contains in it "both
land and sea as the moon doth"; for so they find by their glasses
that *maculæ in facie lunæ* [the spots on the face of the moon],
"the brighter parts are earth, the dusky sea," [2] which Thales,
Plutarch, and Pythagoras formerly taught; and manifestly
discern hills and dales, and such-like concavities, if we may
subscribe to and believe Galileo's observations. But to avoid
these paradoxes of the earth's motion (which the Church of
Rome hath lately condemned as heretical,[3] as appears by
Blancanus' and Fromundus' writings) our latter mathematicians
have rolled all the stones that may be stirred: and, to solve all
appearances and objections, have invented new hypotheses,
and fabricated new systems of the world, out of their own
Dædalian heads. Fracastorius will have the earth stand still,
as before; and to avoid that supposition of eccentrics and epicycles, he hath coined seventy-two homocentrics, to solve all
appearances. Nicholas Ramerus will have the earth the centre
of the world, but movable, and the eighth sphere immovable,
the five upper planets to move about the sun, the sun and moon
about the earth. Of which orbs Tycho Brahe puts the earth
the centre immovable, the stars immovable, the rest with
Ramerus, the planets without orbs to wander in the air, keep
time and distance, true motion, according to that virtue which

God hath given them.   Helisæus Rœslin censureth both,[1] with Copernicus (whose hypothesis *de terræ motu* [about the motion of the earth] Philippus Lansbergius hath lately vindicated, and demonstrated with solid arguments in a just volume, Jansonius Cæsius hath illustrated in a sphere.)   The said Johannes Lansbergius, 1633,[2] hath since defended his assertion against all the cavils and calumnies of Fromundus his *Anti-Aristarchus*, Baptista Morinus, and Petrus Bartholinus; Fromundus, 1634, hath written against him again, J. Rosseus of Aberdeen, etc. (sound drums and trumpets), whilst Rœslin (I say) censures all, and Ptolemæus himself as insufficient: one offends against natural philosophy, another against optic principles, a third against mathematical, as not answering to astronomical observations; one puts a great space between Saturn's orb and the eighth sphere, another too narrow.   In his own hypothesis he makes the earth as before the universal centre, the sun to the five upper planets, to the eighth sphere he ascribes diurnal motion, eccentrics and epicycles to the seven planets, which hath been formerly exploded; and so, *Dum vitant stulti vitia in contraria currunt* [while they run away from one vice, they foolishly fall into the opposite one], as a tinker stops one hole and makes two, he corrects them and doth worse himself, reforms some and mars all.   In the meantime, the world is tossed in a blanket amongst them, they hoist the earth up and down like a ball, make it stand and go at their pleasures: one saith the sun stands, another he moves; a third comes in, taking them all at rebound, and, lest there should any paradox be wanting, he finds certain spots and clouds in the sun,[3] by the help of glasses, which multiply (saith Keplerus) a thing seen a thousand times bigger *in plano* [in clear air], and makes it come thirty-two times nearer to the eye of the beholder: but see the demonstration of this glass in Tarde,[4] by means of which the sun must turn round upon his own centre, or they about the sun.   Fabricius puts only three, and those in the sun: Apelles fifteen, and those without the sun, floating like the Cyanean Isles in the Euxine Sea.   Tarde, the Frenchman,[5] hath observed thirty-three, and those neither spots nor clouds, as Galileo, *Epist. ad Velserum*, supposeth, but planets concentric with the sun, and not far from him with regular motions.   Christopher Scheiner, a German Suisser Jesuit, *Ursica Rosa*,[6] divides them *in maculas et faculas* [into spots and faculæ], and will have them to be fixed *in solis superficie* [on the surface of the sun], and to absolve their periodical and regular motion in twenty-seven or twenty

eight days, holding withal the rotation of the sun upon his
centre; and all are so confident that they have made schemes
and tables of their motions. The Hollander, in his *disserta-
tiuncula cum Apelle*,[1] censures all; and thus they disagree
amongst themselves, old and new, irreconcilable in their
opinions; thus Aristarchus, thus Hipparchus, thus Ptolemæus,
thus Albateginus, thus Alfraganus, thus Tycho, thus Ramerus,
thus Rœslinus, thus Fracastorius, thus Copernicus and his
adherents, thus Clavius and Maginus, etc., with their followers,
vary and determine of these celestial orbs and bodies: and so,
whilst these men contend about the sun and moon, like the
philosophers in Lucian, it is to be feared the sun and moon will
hide themselves, and be as much offended as she was with
those,[2] and send another message to Jupiter, by some new-
fangled Icaromenippus, to make an end of all those curious
controversies, and scatter them abroad.

But why should the sun and moon be angry, or take exceptions at mathematicians and philosophers, whenas the like
measure is offered unto God Himself, by a company of theologasters? They are not contented to see the sun and moon,
measure their site and biggest distance in a glass, calculate their
motions, or visit the moon in a poetical fiction, or a dream, as
he saith, *Audax facinus et memorabile nunc incipiam, neque hoc
sæculo usurpatum prius, quid in lunæ regno hac nocte gestum sit
exponam, et quo nemo unquam nisi somniando pervenit* [I will
now adventure a daring and memorable exploit, never before
attempted in this age—to set forth what has taken place this
night in the kingdom of the moon, in regions to which no one
has ever penetrated, save in a dream], but he and Menippus:[3]
or as Peter Cuneus,[4] *Bona fide agam, nihil eorum quæ scripturus
sum, verum esse scitote, etc.; quæ nec facta, nec futura sunt, dicam,
stili tantum et ingenii causa* [5] [I will be honest, and admit that
nothing of what I am about to relate is true; I shall relate
things which never have happened and never will happen,
merely to show my literary skill], not in jest, but in good earnest
these gigantical Cyclopes will transcend spheres, heaven, stars,
into that empyrean heaven; soar higher yet, and see what
God Himself doth. The Jewish Talmudists take upon them to
determine how God spends His whole time, sometimes playing
with Leviathan, sometimes overseeing the world, etc., like
Lucian's Jupiter, that spent much of the year in painting butterflies' wings, and seeing who offered sacrifice; telling the hours
when it should rain, how much snow should fall in such a place,

which way the wind should stand in Greece, which way in
Africa. In the Turks' Alcoran, Mahomet is taken up to heaven
upon a Pegasus sent on purpose for him, as he lay in bed with
his wife, and after some conference with God is set on ground
again. The pagans paint Him and mangle Him after a thousand
fashions; our heretics, schismatics, and some schoolmen, come
not far behind: some paint Him in the habit of an old man,
and make maps of heaven, number the angels, tell their several
names, offices:[1] some deny God and His providence, some take
His office out of His hand, will bind and loose in heaven,[2] release,
pardon, forgive, and be quartermaster with Him; some call
His Godhead in question, His power and attributes, His mercy,
justice, providence: they will know with Cæcilius,[3] why good and
bad are punished together, war, fires, plagues infest all alike,
why wicked men flourish, good are poor, in prison, sick, and
ill at ease. Why doth He suffer so much mischief and evil to
be done, if He be able to help?[4] why doth He not assist good,
or resist bad, reform our wills, if He be not the author of sin,
and let such enormities be committed, unworthy of His knowledge, wisdom, government, mercy, and providence? why lets
He all things be done by fortune and chance? Others as prodigiously inquire after His omnipotency, *an possit plures similes
creare deos? an ex scarabæo deum? etc.; et quo demum ruetis,
sacrificuli?* [Can he create many similar gods? A god from a
scarab? Whither then will you priests rush to sacrifice?]
Some, by visions and revelations, take upon them to be familiar
with God, and to be of privy council with Him; they will tell
how many, and who, shall be saved, when the world shall come
to an end, what year, what month, and whatsoever else God
hath reserved unto Himself, and to His angels. Some again,
curious phantastics, will know more than this, and inquire with
Epicurus, what God did before the world was made? was He
idle?[5] Where did He bide? What did He make the world
of? Why did He then make it, and not before? If He made it
new, or to have an end, how is He unchangeable, infinite, etc.
Some will dispute, cavil, and object, as Julian did of old, whom
Cyril confutes, as Simon Magus is feigned to do in that dialogue
betwixt him and Peter,[6] and Ammonius the philosopher in
that dialogical disputation with Zacharias the Christian. If
God be infinitely and only good, why should He alter or destroy
the world? if He confound that which is good, how shall Himself
continue good? If He pull it down because evil, how shall He
be free from the evil that made it evil? etc., with many such

absurd and brain-sick questions, intricacies, froth of human wit,
and excrements of curiosity, etc., which, as our Saviour told
His inquisitive disciples, are not fit for them to know. But hoo!
I am now gone quite out of sight, I am almost giddy with
roving about: I could have ranged farther yet, but I am an
infant, and not able to dive into these profundities or sound these
depths,[1] not able to understand, much less to discuss. I leave
the contemplation of these things to stronger wits, that have
better ability and happier leisure to wade into such philosophical
mysteries; for put case I were as able as willing, yet what can
one man do? I will conclude with Scaliger,[2] *Nequaquam nos
homines sumus, sed partes hominis; ex omnibus aliquid fieri
potest, idque non magnum; ex singulis fere nihil* [we are not
whole men but parts of men; from all of us together something
might be made and that not much; from each of us individually
nothing]. Besides (as Nazianzen hath it) *Deus latere nos multa
voluit* [God willed that much should remain hidden from us]:
and with Seneca, *cap.* 35 *de Cometis, Quid miramur tam rara
mundi spectacula non teneri certis legibus, nondum intelligi?
Multæ sunt gentes quæ tantum de facie sciunt cælum; veniet
tempus fortasse, quo ista quæ nunc latent in lucem diei extrahat
longioris ævi diligentia; una ætas non sufficit, posteri, etc.*
[Why are we surprised that such unusual phenomena do not
obey fixed laws, so far as we understand? There are many
peoples who know nothing more of the sky than its appearance.
A day will perhaps come when the labours of succeeding ages
will reveal things at present obscure; one age is not sufficient,
our descendants, etc.]; when God sees His time, He will reveal
these mysteries to mortal men, and show that to some few at
last, which He hath concealed so long. For I am of his mind,[3]
that Columbus did not find out America by chance, but God
directed him at that time to discover it: it was contingent to
him, but necessary to God; He reveals and conceals to whom
and when He will. And which one said [4] of history and records
of former times, "God in His providence, to check our presumptuous inquisition, wraps up all things in uncertainty, bars
us from long antiquity, and bounds our search within the compass of some few ages": many good things are lost which our
predecessors made use of, as Pancirolli will better inform you;
many new things are daily invented, to the public good; so
kingdoms, men, and knowledge ebb and flow, are hid and
revealed, and when you have all done, as the Preacher concluded, *Nihil est sub sole novum* [there is nothing new under

the sun]. But my melancholy spaniel's quest, my game, is sprung, and I must suddenly come down and follow.

Jason Pratensis, in his book *de morbis capitis*, and chapter of melancholy, hath these words out of Galen, "Let them come to me to know what meat and drink they shall use, and besides that, I will teach them what temper of ambient air they shall make choice of, what wind, what countries they shall choose, and what avoid." [1] Out of which lines of his thus much we may gather, that to this cure of melancholy, amongst other things, the rectification of air is necessarily required. This is performed either in reforming natural or artificial air. Natural is that which is in our election to choose or avoid: and 'tis either general, to countries, provinces; [or] particular, to cities, towns, villages, or private houses. What harm those extremities of heat or cold do in this malady, I have formerly showed: the medium must needs be good, where the air is temperate, serene, quiet, free from bogs, fens, mists, all manner of putrefaction, contagious and filthy noisome smells. The Egyptians by all geographers [2] are commended to be *hilares*, a conceited and merry nation: which I can ascribe to no other cause than the serenity of their air. They that live in the Orcades are registered by Hector Boethius [3] and Cardan [4] to be fair of complexion, long-lived, most healthful, free from all manner of infirmities of body and mind, by reason of a sharp purifying air, which comes from the sea. The Bœotians in Greece were dull and heavy, *crassi Bœoti*, by reason of a foggy air in which they lived (*Bœotum in crasso jurares aere natum* [5] [you would swear he had been born in the thick air of Boeotia]); Attica most acute, pleasant, and refined. The clime changes not so much customs, manners, wits (as Aristotle, *Polit. lib.* 6, *cap.* 4, Vegetius, Plato, Bodine, *Method. hist. cap.* 5, hath proved at large) as constitutions of their bodies, and temperature itself. In all particular provinces we see it confirmed by experience; as the air is, so are the inhabitants, dull, heavy, witty, subtle, neat, cleanly, clownish, sick, and sound. In Périgord [6] in France the air is subtile, healthful, seldom any plague or contagious disease, but hilly and barren: the men sound, nimble, and lusty; but in some parts of Guienne, full of moors and marshes, the people dull, heavy, and subject to many infirmities. Who sees not a great difference between Surrey, Sussex, and Romney Marsh, the wolds in Lincolnshire and the fens? He therefore that loves his health, if his ability will give him leave, must often shift places, and make choice of such as are wholesome, pleasant, and convenient: there is nothing better than change of air in this malady, and generally for health to wander up and down, as those *Tartari Zamolhenses*,[1] that live in hordes, and take opportunity of times, places, seasons.   The kings of Persia had their summer and winter houses; in winter at Sardis, in summer at Susa; now at Persepolis, then at Pasargada.   Cyrus lived seven cold months at Babylon, three at Susa, two at Ecbatana, saith Xenophon,[2] and had by that means a perpetual spring. The Great Turk sojourns sometimes at Constantinople, sometimes at Adrianople, etc.   The kings of Spain have their Escurial in heat of summer, Madrid for a wholesome seat,[3] Valladolid a pleasant site, etc., variety of *secessus* [retreats] as all princes and great men have, and their several progresses to this purpose.   Lucullus the Roman had his house at Rome, at Baiæ, etc.   When Cn. Pompeius, Marcus Cicero (saith Plutarch),[4] and many noblemen in the summer came to see him, at supper Pompeius jested with him, that it was an elegant and pleasant village, full of windows, galleries, and all offices fit for a summer house, but in his judgment very unfit for winter: Lucullus made answer that the lord of the house had wit like a crane, that changeth her country with the season; he had other houses furnished and built for that purpose, all out as commodious as this.   So Tully had his Tusculan, Plinius his Lauretan [Larian] village, and every gentleman of any fashion in our times hath the like.   The Bishop of Exeter had fourteen several houses all furnished, in times past.[5]   In Italy, though they bide in cities in winter, which is more gentlemanlike, all the summer they come abroad to their country-houses, to recreate themselves.   Our gentry in England live most part in the country (except it be some few castles), building still in bottoms (saith Jovius[6]) or near woods, *corona arborum virentium* [with a ring of lofty trees]; you shall know a village by a tuft of trees at or about it, to avoid those strong winds wherewith the island is infested, and cold winter blasts.   Some discommend moated houses, as unwholesome (so Camden saith of Ewelme[7] that it was therefore unfrequented *ob stagni vicini halitus* [on account of the vapours from the neighbouring pond]), and all such places as be near lakes or rivers.   But I am of opinion that these inconveniences will be mitigated, or easily corrected, by good fires, as one[8] reports of Venice, that *graveolentia* [fetidness] and fog of the moors is sufficiently qualified by those innumerable smokes.   Nay more, Thomas Philol. Ravennas,[9] a great physician, contends that the Venetians are generally longer-lived than any city in Europe, and live many of them 120 years. But it is not water simply that so much offends as the slime and noisome smells that accompany such overflowed places, which is but at some few seasons after a flood, and is sufficiently recompensed with sweet smells and aspects in summer—*Ver pinget vario gemmantia prata colore* [Spring paints with varied hues the sparkling mead] and many other commodities of pleasure and profit; or else may be corrected by the site, if it be somewhat remote from the water, as Lindley, Orton *super montem*,[1] Drayton,[2] or a little more elevated, though nearer, as Caucut,[3] Amington,[4] Polesworth,[5] Weddington [6] (to insist in such places best to me known), upon the river of Anker in Warwickshire, Swarston,[7] and Drakesly [8] upon Trent. Or howsoever they be unseasonable in winter, or at some times, they have their good use in summer. If so be that their means be so slender as they may not admit of any such variety, but must determine once for all, and make one house serve each season, I know no men that have given better rules in this behalf than our husbandry writers. Cato [9] and Columella prescribe a good house to stand by a navigable river, good highways, near some city, and in a good soil, but that is more for commodity than health.

The best soil commonly yields the worst air, a dry sandy plat is fittest to build upon, and such as is rather hilly than plain, full of downs, a Cotswold country, as being most commodious for hawking, hunting, wood, waters, and all manner of pleasures. Périgord in France is barren, yet by reason of the excellency of the air, and such pleasures that it affords, much inhabited by the nobility; as Nuremberg in Germany, Toledo in Spain. Our countryman Tusser will tell us so much, that the fieldone is for profit, the woodland for pleasure and health; the one commonly a deep clay, therefore noisome in winter, and subject to bad highways: the other a dry sand. Provision may be had elsewhere, and our towns are generally bigger in the woodland than the fieldone, more frequent and populous, and gentlemen more delight to dwell in such places. Sutton Coldfield in Warwickshire (where I was once a grammar scholar) may be a sufficient witness, which stands, as Camden notes, *loco ingrato et sterili* [in a cheerless and barren spot], but in an excellent air, and full of all manner of pleasures. Wadley [10] in Berkshire is situate in a vale, though not so fertile a soil as some vales afford, yet a most commodious site, wholesome, in a delicious air, a rich and pleasant seat. So Segrave in Leicestershire (which town I am now bound to remember [1]) is sited in a champaign at the edge of the wolds, and more barren than the villages about it, yet no place likely yields a better air. And he that built that fair house, Wollerton in Nottinghamshire,[2] is much to be commended (though the tract be sandy and barren about it) for making choice of such a place. Constantine, *lib.* 2, *cap. de agricult.*, praiseth mountains, hilly, steep places, above the rest by the seaside, and such as look toward the north [3] upon some great river, as Farmack in Derbyshire,[4] on the Trent, environed with hills, open only to the north, like Mount Edgemond [5] in Cornwall, which Mr. Carew so much admires for an excellent seat: [6] such is the general site of Bohemia: *serenat Boreas*, the north wind clarifies, but near lakes or marshes, in holes, obscure places, or to the south and west, he utterly disproves; those winds are unwholesome, putrefying, and make men subject to diseases.[7] The best building for health, according to him, is "in high places, and in an excellent prospect," [8] like that of Cuddesdon in Oxfordshire (which place I must *honoris ergo* [out of respect] mention), is lately and fairly built [9] in a good air, good prospect, good soil, both for profit and pleasure, not so easily to be matched. P. Crescentius, in his *lib.* 1 *de agric. cap.* 5, is very copious in this subject, how a house should be wholesomely sited, in a good coast, good air, wind, etc. Varro, *de re rust. lib.* 1, *cap.* 12, forbids lakes and rivers, marish and manured grounds; they cause a bad air, gross diseases, hard to be cured: [10] "if it be so that he cannot help it, better" (as he adviseth) "sell thy house and land than lose thine health." [11] He that respects not this in choosing of his seat or building his house, is *mente captus*, mad, Cato saith "and his dwelling next to hell itself," according to Columella: [12] he commends, in conclusion, the middle of a hill, upon a descent. Baptista Porta, *Villæ*, *lib.* 1, *cap.* 22, censures Varro, Cato, Columella, and those ancient rustics, approving many things, disallowing some, and will by all means have the front of a house stand to the south, which how it may be good in Italy and hotter climes, I know not, in our northern countries I am sure it is best: Stephanus, a Frenchman, *Prædio rustic. lib.* 1, *cap.* 4, subscribes to this, approving especially the descent of an hill south or south-east, with trees to the north, so that it be well watered; a condition in all sites which must not be omitted, as Herbastein inculcates, *lib.* 1. Julius Cæsar Claudinus, a physician, *consult.* 24, for a nobleman in Poland, melancholy given, adviseth him to dwell in a house inclining to the east,[13]

and by all means to provide the air be clear and sweet;[1] which,
Montanus, *consil.* 229, counselleth the Earl of Montfort, his
patient, to inhabit a pleasant house, and in a good air.　If it
be so the natural site may not be altered of our city, town,
village, yet by artificial means it may be helped.　In hot
countries, therefore, they make the streets of their cities very
narrow, all over Spain, Africa, Italy, Greece, and many cities
of France, in Languedoc especially, and Provence, those southern
parts: Montpelier, the habitation and university of physicians,
is so built, with high houses, narrow streets, to divert the sun's
scalding rays, which Tacitus commends, *lib.* 15 *Annal.*, as most
agreeing to their health, "because the height of buildings, and
narrowness of streets, keep away the sunbeams." [2]　Some cities
use galleries, or arched cloisters towards the street, as Damascus,
Bologna, Padua, Berne in Switzerland, Westchester [3] with us,
as well to avoid tempests as the sun's scorching heat.　They
build on high hills in hot countries for more air; or to the seaside, as Baiæ, Naples, etc.　In our northern coasts we are
opposite; we commend straight, broad, open, fair streets, as
most befitting and agreeing to our clime.　We build in bottoms
for warmth; and that site of Mitylene in the island of Lesbos,
in the Ægean Sea (which Vitruvius so much discommends,
magnificently built with fair houses, *sed imprudenter positam,*
[but] unadvisedly sited, because it lay along to the south, and
when the south wind blew, the people were all sick), would
make an excellent site in our northern climes.

Of that artificial site of houses I have sufficiently discoursed:
if the seat of the dwelling may not be altered, yet there is
much in choice of such a chamber or room, in opportune opening
and shutting of windows, excluding foreign air and winds, and
walking abroad at convenient times.　Crato, a German,[4] commends east and south site (disallowing cold air and northern
winds in this case, rainy weather and misty days), free from
putrefaction, fens, bogs, and muck-hills.　If the air be such,
open no windows, come not abroad.　Montanus will have his
patient not to stir at all, if the wind be big or tempestuous,[5]
as most part in March it is with us; or in cloudy, lowering, dark
days, as in November, which we commonly call the black
month; or stormy, let the wind stand how it will (*consil.* 27),
and (30) he must not "open a casement in bad weather," [6] or in
a boisterous season; *consil.* 299, he especially forbids us to open
windows to a south wind.　The best sites for chamber windows,
in my judgment, are north, east, south, and, which is the worst,

west. Levinus Lemnius, *lib. 3, cap. 3, de occult. nat. mir.*, attributes so much to air, and rectifying of wind and windows, that he holds it alone sufficient to make a man sick or well, to alter body and mind. "A clear air cheers up the spirits, exhilarates the mind; a thick, black, misty, tempestuous, contracts, overthrows." [1] Great heed is therefore to be taken at what times we walk, how we place our windows, lights, and houses, how we let in or exclude this ambient air. The Egyptians, to avoid immoderate heat, make their windows on the top of the house like chimneys, with two tunnels to draw a through air. In Spain they commonly make great opposite windows without glass, still shutting those which are next to the sun: so likewise in Turkey and Italy (Venice excepted, which brags of her stately glazed palaces) they use paper windows to like purpose; and lie *sub dio* [under the open sky], in the top of their flat-roofed houses, so sleeping under the canopy of heaven. In some parts of Italy they have windmills, to draw a cooling air out of hollow caves, and disperse the same through all the chambers of their palaces, to refresh them; [2] as at Custozza, the house of Cesareo Trento, a gentleman of Vicenza, and elsewhere. Many excellent means are invented to correct nature by art. If none of these courses help, the best way is to make artificial air, which howsoever is profitable and good, still to be made hot and moist, and to be seasoned with sweet perfumes, pleasant and lightsome as it may be; [3] to have roses, violets, and sweet-smelling flowers ever in their windows, posies in their hand. Laurentius commends water-lilies, a vessel of warm water to evaporate in the room, which will make a more delightsome perfume, if there be added orange-flowers, peels of citrons, rosemary, cloves, bays, rosewater, rose-vinegar, benzoin, ladanum, styrax, and such-like gums, which make a pleasant and acceptable perfume. Bessardus Bisantinus [4] prefers the smoke of juniper to melancholy persons, which is in great request with us at Oxford, to sweeten our chambers. Guianerius [5] prescribes the air to be moistened with water, and sweet herbs boiled in it, vine, and sallow leaves, etc., to besprinkle the ground and posts with rose-water, rose-vinegar, [6] which Avicenna much approves. Of colours it is good to behold green, red, yellow, and white, and by all means to have light enough, with windows in the day, wax candles in the night, neat chambers, good fires in winter, merry companions; for though melancholy persons love to be dark and alone, yet darkness is a great increaser of the humour.

Although our ordinary air be good by nature or art, yet it is not amiss, as I have said, still to alter it; no better physic for a melancholy man than change of air and variety of places, to travel abroad and see fashions. Leo Afer speaks of many of his countrymen so cured, without all other physic: amongst the negroes, "there is such an excellent air, that if any of them be sick elsewhere and brought thither, he is instantly recovered, of which he was often an eye-witness." [1] Lipsius,[2] Zuinger, and some others, add as much of ordinary travel. "No man," saith Lipsius, in an epistle to Phil. Lanoius, a noble friend of his, now ready to make a voyage, "can be such a stock or stone, whom that pleasant speculation of countries, cities, towns, rivers, will not affect." [3] Seneca the philosopher [4] was infinitely taken with the sight of Scipio Africanus' house near Linternum, to view those old buildings, cisterns, baths, tombs, etc. And how was Tully [5] pleased with the sight of Athens, to behold those ancient and fair buildings, with a remembrance of their worthy inhabitants! Paulus Æmilius, that renowned Roman captain, after he had conquered Perseus, the last king of Macedonia, and now made an end of his tedious wars, though he had been long absent from Rome, and much there desired, about the beginning of autumn (as Livy describes it [6]) made a pleasant peregrination all over Greece, accompanied with his son Scipio and Athenæus the brother of King Eumenes, leaving the charge of his army with Sulpicius Gallus. By Thessaly he went to Delphi, thence to Megaris, Aulis, Athens, Argos, Lacedæmon, Megalopolis, etc. He took great content, exceeding delight in that his voyage, as who doth not that shall attempt the like, though his travel be *ad jactationem magis quam ad usum reipub.* (as one [7] well observes), to crack, gaze, see fine sights and fashions, spend time, rather than for his own or public good (as it is to many gallants that travel out their best days, together with their means, manners, honesty, religion)? yet it availeth howsoever. For peregrination charms our senses with such unspeakable and sweet variety that some count him unhappy that never travelled,[8] and pity his case that from his cradle to his old age beholds the same still; still, still the same, the same. Insomuch that Rhasis, *Cont. lib.* 1, *tract.* 2, doth not only commend, but enjoin travel, and such variety of objects to a melancholy man, "and to lie in diverse inns, to be drawn into several companies": [9] Montaltus, *cap.* 36, and many neoterics are of the same mind: Celsus adviseth him therefore that will continue his health to have *varium vitæ genus*, diversity of callings, occupations, to be busied about, "sometimes to live in the city, sometimes in the country; now to study or work, to be intent, then again to hawk or hunt, swim, run, ride, or exercise himself."[1] A good prospect alone will ease melancholy, as Gomesius contends, *lib. 2, cap. 7, de sale.* The citizens of Barcino,[2] saith he, otherwise penned in, melancholy, and stirring little abroad, are much delighted with that pleasant prospect their city hath into the sea, which, like that of old Athens, besides Ægina, Salamis, and many pleasant islands, had all the variety of delicious objects; so are those Neapolitans, and inhabitants of Genoa, to see the ships, boats, and passengers go by, out of their windows, their whole cities being sited on the side of a hill, like Pera by Constantinople, so that each house almost hath a free prospect to the sea, as some part of London to the Thames: or to have a free prospect all over the city at once, as at Granada in Spain and Fez in Africa, the river running betwixt two declining hills, the steepness causeth each house, almost, as well to oversee as to be overseen of the rest. Every country is full of such delightsome prospects,[3] as well within land as by sea, as Hermon and Ramah[4] in Palestine, Collalto in Italy, the top of Taygetus or Acrocorinthus, that old decayed castle in Corinth, from which Peloponnesus, Greece, the Ionian and Ægean Seas were *semel et simul* at one view to be taken. In Egypt the square top of the Great Pyramid, three hundred yards in height, and so the Sultan's palace in Grand Cairo, the country being plain, hath a marvellous fair prospect as well over Nilus as that great city, five Italian miles long, and two broad, by the river-side: from Mount Sion in Jerusalem, the Holy Land is of all sides to be seen: such high places are infinite: with us those of the best note are Glastonbury tower, Box Hill in Surrey, Bever Castle, Rodway Grange, Walsby in Lincolnshire, where I lately received a real kindness by the munificence of the right honourable my noble lady and patroness, the Lady Frances, Countess Dowager of Exeter;[5] and two amongst the rest, which I may not omit for vicinity's sake: Oldbury in the confines of Warwickshire, where I have often looked about me with great delight, at the foot of which hill I was born;[6] and Hanbury in Staffordshire, contiguous to which is Falde, a pleasant village, and an ancient patrimony belonging to our family, now in the possession of mine elder brother, William Burton, Esquire. Barclay the Scot[7] commends that of Greenwich tower for one of the best prospects in Europe, to see London on the one side, the Thames, ships, and pleasant

meadows on the other.   There be those that say as much and
more of St. Mark's steeple in Venice.   Yet these are at too great
a distance; some are especially affected with such objects as
be near, to see passengers go by in some great roadway, or boats
in a river, *in subjectum forum despicere*, to oversee a fair, a
market-place, or, out of a pleasant window into some thorough-
fare street, to behold a continual concourse, a promiscuous
rout, coming and going, or a multitude of spectators at a
theatre, a mask, or some such-like show.   But I rove: the sum
is this, that variety of actions, objects, air, places, are excellent
good in this infirmity and all others, good for man, good for
beast.   Constantine the emperor, *lib.* 18, *cap.* 13, *ex Leontio,*
holds it an only cure for rotten sheep, and any manner of sick
cattle.[1]   Lælius à Fonte Eugubinus, that great doctor, at the
latter end of many of his consultations (as commonly he doth
set down what success his physic had), in melancholy most
especially approves of this above all other remedies whatsoever, as appears *consult.* 69, *consult.* 229, etc.: "Many other things
helped, but change of air was that which wrought the cure,
and did most good." [2]

MEMB. IV.

Exercise rectified of Body and Mind

To that great inconvenience which comes on the one side
by immoderate and unseasonable exercise, too much solitariness
and idleness on the other, must be opposed as an antidote, a
moderate and seasonable use of it, and that both of body and
mind, as a most material circumstance, much conducing to this
cure and to the general preservation of our health.   The heavens
themselves run continually round, the sun riseth and sets, the
moon increaseth and decreaseth, stars and planets keep their
constant motions, the air is still tossed by the winds, the waters
ebb and flow, to their conservation no doubt, to teach us that
we should ever be in action.   For which cause Hierome prescribes Rusticus the monk, that he be always occupied about
some business or other, "that the devil do not find him idle." [3]
Seneca would have a man do something, though it be to no
purpose.[4]   Xenophon wisheth one rather to play at tables,
dice, or make a jester of himself (though he might be far better

employed) than do nothing.[1] The Egyptians of old,[2] and many flourishing commonwealths since, have enjoined labour and exercise to all sorts of men, to be of some vocation and calling, and to give an account of their time, to prevent those grievous mischiefs that come by idleness; "for as fodder, whip, and burthen belong to the ass, so meat, correction, and work unto the servant" (Ecclus. xxx, 24). The Turks enjoin all men whatsoever, of what degree, to be of some trade or other, the Grand Seignior himself is not excused. "In our memory" (saith Sabellicus) "Mahomet the Turk, he that conquered Greece, at that very time when he heard ambassadors of other princes, did either carve or cut wooden spoons, or frame something upon a table." [3] This present Sultan makes notches for bows.[4] The Jews are most severe in this examination of time. All well-governed places, towns, families, and every discreet person will be a law unto himself. But amongst us the badge of gentry is idleness: to be of no calling, not to labour, for that's derogatory to their birth, to be a mere spectator, a drone, *fruges consumere natus* [born only to consume his food], to have no necessary employment to busy himself about in church and commonwealth (some few governors exempted), "but to rise to eat," etc., to spend his days in hawking, hunting, etc., and such-like disports and recreations (which our casuists tax[5]), are the sole exercise almost, and ordinary actions of our nobility, and in which they are too immoderate. And thence it comes to pass, that in city and country so many grievances of body and mind, and this feral disease of melancholy so frequently rageth, and now domineers almost all over Europe amongst our great ones. They know not how to spend their time (disports excepted, which are all their business), what to do, or otherwise how to bestow themselves: like our modern Frenchmen, that had rather lose a pound of blood in a single combat than a drop of sweat in any honest labour. Every man almost hath something or other to employ himself about, some vocation, some trade, but they do all by ministers and servants, *ad otia duntaxat se natos existimant, immo ad sui ipsius plerumque et aliorum perniciem* [they think themselves born only for idleness—nay, for their own and other people's ruin], as one [6] freely taxeth such kind of men; they are all for pastimes, 'tis all their study; all their invention tends to this alone, to drive away time, as if they were born some of them to no other ends. Therefore to correct and avoid these errors and inconveniences, our divines, physicians, and politicians so much labour, and so

seriously exhort; and for this disease in particular, "there can
be no better cure than continual business," as Rhasis holds,
"to have some employment or other, which may set their mind
awork and distract their cogitations." [1] Riches may not easily
be had without labour and industry, nor learning without study,
neither can our health be preserved without bodily exercise.
If it be of the body, Guianerius allows that exercise which is
gentle, "and still after those ordinary frications," [2] which must
be used every morning.   Montaltus, *cap.* 26, and Jason Pratensis
use almost the same words, highly commending exercise if it
be moderate; "a wonderful help so used," Crato calls it, "and
a great means to preserve our health, as adding strength to the
whole body, increasing natural heat, by means of which the
nutriment is well concocted in the stomach, liver, and veins, few
or no crudities left, is happily distributed over all the body."
Besides, it expels excrements by sweat and other insensible
vapours; insomuch that Galen [3] prefers exercise before all
physic, rectification of diet, or any regiment in what kind
soever; 'tis nature's physician.   Fulgentius, out of Gordonius,
de conserv. vit. hom. lib. 1, *cap.* 7, terms exercise "a spur of a
dull, sleepy nature, the comforter of the members, cure of
infirmity, death of diseases, destruction of all mischiefs and
vices." [4]   The fittest time for exercise is a little before dinner,
a little before supper, or at any time when the body is empty.[5]
Montanus, *consil.* 31, prescribes it every morning to his patient,
and that, as Calenus adds, "after he hath done his ordinary
needs, rubbed his body, washed his hands and face, combed his
head and gargarized." [6]   What kind of exercise he should use,
Galen tells us, *lib.* 2 *et* 3 *de sanit. tuend.*, and in what measure,
"till the body be ready to sweat," [7] and roused up; *ad ruborem*
[till they become flushed], some say, *non ad sudorem* [not till
they sweat], lest it should dry the body too much; others enjoin
those wholesome businesses, as to dig so long in his garden, to
hold the plough, and the like. Some prescribe frequent and
violent labour and exercises, as sawing every day so long together
(*Epid.* 6, Hippocrates confounds them), but that is in some
cases, to some peculiar men; the most forbid,[8] and by no
means will have it go farther than a beginning sweat, as being
perilous if it exceed.[9]

Of these labours, exercises, and recreations, which are likewise included, some properly belong to the body, some to the
mind, some more easy, some hard, some with delight, some
without, some within doors, some natural, some are artificial.

Amongst bodily exercises, Galen commends *ludum parvæ pilæ*,
to play at ball, be it with the hand or racket, in tennis-courts
or otherwise; it exerciseth each part of the body, and doth
much good, so that they sweat not too much. It was in great
request of old amongst the Greeks, Romans, Barbarians, mentioned by Homer, Herodotus, and Plinius. Some write that
Aganella, a fair maid of Corcyra, was the inventor of it, for
she presented the first ball that ever was made to Nausicaa, the
daughter of King Alcinous, and taught her how to use it.

The ordinary sports which are used abroad are hawking,
hunting, *hilares venandi labores* [the cheerful toils of the chase],
one calls them,[1] because they recreate body and mind; another,[2]
"the best exercise that is,[3] by which alone many have been
freed from all feral diseases."[4]   Hegesippus, *lib.* 1, *cap.* 37,
relates of Herod, that he was eased of a grievous melancholy
by that means. Plato, 7 *de leg.*, highly magnifies it, dividing
it into three parts, "by land, water, air." Xenophon, in
Cyropæd., graces it with a great name, *deorum munus*, the gift
of the gods, a princely sport, which they have ever used, saith
Langius, *epist.* 59, *lib.* 2, as well for health as pleasure, and do
at this day, it being the sole almost and ordinary sport of our
noblemen in Europe, and elsewhere all over the world. Bohemus,
de mor. gent. lib. 3, *cap.* 12, styles it therefore *studium nobilium;
communiter venantur, quod sibi solis licere contendunt* [the occupation of nobles; they are commonly a-hunting, and maintain
that they alone have liberty to do this], 'tis all their study, their
exercise, ordinary business, all their talk: and indeed some dote
too much after it, they can do nothing else, discourse of naught
else. Paulus Jovius, *Descr. Brit.*, doth in some sort tax our
English nobility for it, for living in the country so much, and
too frequent use of it, as if they had no other means but hawking
and hunting to approve themselves gentlemen with.[5]

Hawking comes near to hunting, the one in the air, as the
other on the earth, a sport as much affected as the other, by some
preferred. It was never heard of amongst the Romans, invented
some twelve hundred years since, and first mentioned by Firmi-
cus, *lib.* 5, *cap.* 8.[6] The Greek emperors began it, and now
nothing so frequent: he is nobody that in the season hath not
a hawk on his fist. A great art, and many books written of it.[7]
It is a wonder to hear what is related of the Turks' officers in
this behalf,[8] how many thousand men are employed about it,
how many hawks of all sorts, how much revenues consumed on
that only disport, how much time is spent at Adrianople alone

every year to that purpose. The Persian kings hawk after butterflies with sparrows made to that use, and stares: lesser hawks for lesser games they have, and bigger for the rest, that they may produce their sport to all seasons.[1] The Muscovian emperors reclaim eagles to fly at hinds, foxes, etc., and such a one was sent for a present to Queen Elizabeth:[2] some reclaim ravens, castrils, pies, etc., and man them for their pleasures.

Fowling is more troublesome, but all out as delightsome to some sorts of men, be it with guns, lime, nets, glades, gins, strings, baits, pitfalls, pipes, calls, stalking-horses, setting-dogs, decoy-ducks, etc., or otherwise. Some much delight to take larks with day-nets, small birds with chaff-nets, plovers, partridge, herons, snite, etc. Henry the Third, King of Castile (as Mariana the Jesuit reports of him, *lib.* 3, *cap.* 7), was much affected "with catching of quails,"[3] and many gentlemen take a singular pleasure at morning and evening to go abroad with their quail-pipes, and will take any pains to satisfy their delight in that kind. The Italians have gardens fitted to such use, with nets, bushes, glades, sparing no cost or industry, and are very much affected with the sport.[4] Tycho Brahe, that great astronomer, in the Chorography of his Isle of Huena and Castle of Uraniburg, puts down his nets, and manner of catching small birds, as an ornament and a recreation, wherein he himself was sometimes employed.

Fishing is a kind of hunting by water, be it with nets, weels, baits, angling, or otherwise, and yields all out as much pleasure to some men as dogs or hawks, "when they draw their fish upon the bank,"[5] saith Nic. Henselius, *Silesiographiæ, cap.* 3, speaking of that extraordinary delight his countrymen took in fishing and in making of pools. James Dubravius, that Moravian, in his book *de pisc.*, telleth how, travelling by the highway side in Silesia, he found a nobleman, "booted up to the groins,"[6] wading himself, pulling the nets, and labouring as much as any fisherman of them all: and when some belike objected to him the baseness of his office, he excused himself, "that if other men might hunt hares, why should not he hunt carps?"[7] Many gentlemen in like sort with us will wade up to the arm-holes upon such occasions, and voluntarily undertake that, to satisfy their pleasure, which a poor man for a good stipend would scarce be hired to undergo. Plutarch, in his book *de soler. animal.*, speaks against all fishing, "as a filthy, base, illiberal employment, having neither wit nor perspicacity in it, nor worth the

labour." [1]   But he that shall consider the variety of baits for
all seasons, and pretty devices which our anglers have invented,
peculiar lines, false flies, several sleights, etc., will say that it
deserves like commendation, requires as much study and perspicacity as the rest, and is to be preferred before many of
them.   Because hawking and hunting are very laborious, much
riding, and many dangers accompany them; but this is still
and quiet: and if so be the angler catch no fish, yet he hath a
wholesome walk to the brookside, pleasant shade by the sweet
silver streams; he hath good air, and sweet smells of fine fresh
meadow flowers, he hears the melodious harmony of birds, he
sees the swans, herons, ducks, water-hens, coots, etc., and many
other fowl, with their brood, which he thinketh better than
the noise of hounds, or blast of horns, and all the sport that
they can make.

Many other sports and recreations there be, much in use, as
ringing, bowling, shooting, which Ascham commends in a just
volume, and hath in former times been enjoined by statute as
a defensive exercise and an honour to our land,[2] as well may
witness our victories in France; keelpins, trunks, quoits, pitching
bars, hurling, wrestling, leaping, running, fencing, mustering,
swimming, wasters, foils, football, balloon, quintain, etc., and
many such, which are the common recreations of the country
folks; riding of great horses, running at rings, tilts and tournaments, horse-races, wild-goose chases, which are the disports
of greater men, and good in themselves, though many gentlemen
by that means gallop quite out of their fortunes.

But the most pleasant of all outward pastimes is that of
Aretæus,[3] *deambulatio per amœna loca* [strolling through pleasant
scenery], to make a petty progress, a merry journey now and
then with some good companions, to visit friends, see cities
castles, towns,

> *Visere sæpe amnes nitidos, peramœnaque Tempe,*
> *Et placidas summis sectari in montibus auras:*[4]

To see the pleasant fields, the crystal fountains,
And take the gentle air amongst the mountains:

to walk amongst orchards, gardens, bowers, mounts, and
arbours,[5] artificial wildernesses, green thickets, arches, groves,
lawns, rivulets, fountains, and such-like pleasant places, like
that Antiochian Daphne, brooks, pools, fishponds, between wood
and water, in a fair meadow, by a river-side, *ubi variæ avium*

cantationes, florum colores, pratorum frutices [1] [to enjoy the songs of the birds, the colours of the flowers, the verdure of the meadows], etc., to disport in some pleasant plain, park, run up a steep hill sometimes, or sit in a shady seat, must needs be a delectable recreation. *Hortus principis et domus ad delectationem facta, cum sylva, monte et piscina, vulgo La Montagna:* the prince's garden at Ferrara Schottus [2] highly magnifies, with the groves, mountains, ponds, for a delectable prospect, he was much affected with it; a Persian paradise, or pleasant park, could not be more delectable in his sight. St. Bernard, in the description of his monastery, is almost ravished with the pleasures of it. "A sick man" (saith he) "sits upon a green bank, and when the dog-star parcheth the plains and dries up rivers, he lies in a shady bower," *Fronde sub arborea ferventia temperat astra,* "and feeds his eyes with variety of objects, herbs, trees, to comfort his misery, he receives many delightsome smells, and fills his ears with that sweet and various harmony of birds. Good God" (saith he), "what a company of pleasures hast Thou made for man!" [3] He that should be admitted on a sudden to the sight of such a palace as that of Escurial in Spain, or to that which the Moors built at Granada, Fontainebleau in France, the Turk's gardens in his seraglio, wherein all manner of birds and beasts are kept for pleasure, wolves, bears, lynxes, tigers, lions, elephants, etc., or upon the banks of that Thracian Bosphorus: the Pope's Belvedere in Rome, as pleasing as those *horti pensiles* [hanging gardens] in Babylon,[4] or that Indian king's delightsome garden in Ælian; [5] or those famous gardens of the Lord Cantelow in France, could not choose, though he were never so ill paid, but be much recreated for the time; [6] or many of our nobleman's gardens at home. To take a boat in a pleasant evening, and with music to row upon the waters,[7] which Plutarch so much applauds, Ælian admires, upon the river Peneus, in those Thessalian fields, beset with green bays, where birds so sweetly sing that passengers, enchanted as it were with their heavenly music, *omnium laborum et curarum obliviscantur,* forget forthwith all labours, care, and grief; or in a gondola through the Grand Canal in Venice, to see those goodly palaces, must needs refresh and give content to a melancholy dull spirit. Or to see the inner rooms of a fair-built and sumptuous edifice, as that of the Persian kings so much renowned by Diodorus and Curtius, in which all was almost beaten gold,[8] chairs, stools, thrones, tabernacles, and pillars of gold, plane-trees and vines of gold, grapes of precious stones, all the other ornaments of pure gold,

> *Fulget gemma toris, et jaspide fulva supellex,*
> *Strata micant Tyrio,*[3]

> [The couches flash with jewels, the furniture is ablaze
> with jasper, the coverlets are of gleaming purple,]

with sweet odours and perfumes, generous wines, opiparous fare, etc., besides the gallantest young men, the fairest virgins,[2] *puellæ scitulæ ministrantes*, the rarest beauties the world could afford, and those set out with costly and curious attires, *ad stuporem usque spectantium* [throwing the spectators into amazement], with exquisite music, as in Trimalchio's house,[3] in every chamber sweet voices ever sounding day and night, *incomparabilis luxus* [unheard-of luxury], all delights and pleasures in each kind which to please the senses could possibly be devised or had, *convivæ coronati, deliciis ebrii* [guests wearing garlands and running riot], etc. Telemachus, in Homer, is brought in as one ravished almost at the sight of that magnificent palace and rich furniture of Menelaus, when he beheld

> *Æris fulgorem et resonantia tecta corusco*
> *Auro, atque electro nitido, sectoque elephanto,*
> *Argentoque simul. Talis Jovis ardua sedes,*
> *Aulaque cælicolum stellans splendescit Olympo.*[4]

> Such glittering of gold and brightest brass to shine,
> Clear amber, silver pure, and ivory so fine:
> Jupiter's lofty palace, where the gods do dwell,
> Was even such a one, and did it not excel.

It will *laxare animos*, refresh the soul of man, to see fair-built cities, streets, theatres, temples, obelisks, etc. The temple of Jerusalem was so fairly built of white marble, with so many pyramids covered with gold; *tectumque templi, fulvo coruscans auro, nimio suo fulgore obcæcabat oculos itinerantium*, [and the roof of the temple] was so glorious, and so glistered afar off, that the spectators might not well abide the sight of it. But the inner parts were all so curiously set out with cedar, gold, jewels, etc., as he said of Cleopatra's palace in Egypt, *Crassumque trabes absconderat aurum*[5] [and solid gold hid the beams], that the beholders were amazed. What so pleasant as to see some pageant or sight go by, as at coronations, weddings, and suchlike solemnities, to see an ambassador or a prince met, received, entertained with masks, shows, fireworks, etc. To see two kings fight in single combat, as Porus and Alexander; Canutus and Edmund Ironside; Scanderbeg and Ferat Bassa the Turk; when not honour alone but life itself is at stake, as the poet [1] of Hector,

> *Nec enim pro tergore tauri,*
> *Pro bove nec certamen erat, quæ præmia cursus*
> *Esse solent, sed pro magni vitaque animaque*
> *Hectoris.*

[For not for any common prize,
For hide of ox or sacrificial steer
The race was run, but for great Hector's life.]

To behold a battle fought, like that of Cressy, or Agincourt, or Poictiers, *qua nescio* (saith Froissart) *an vetustas ullam proferre possit clariorem* [than which I doubt if antiquity can show any more glorious]. To see one of Cæsar's triumphs in old Rome revived, or the like. To be present at an interview,[2] as that famous of Henry the Eighth and Francis the First, so much renowned all over Europe; *ubi tanto apparatu* (saith Hubertus Vellius) *tamque triumphali pompa ambo reges cum eorum conjugibus coiere* [where the two kings, with their wives, met with such state and pomp], *ut nulla unquam ætas tam celebria festa viderit aut audierit,* [that] no age ever saw the like. So infinitely pleasant are such shows, to the sight of which oftentimes they will come hundreds of miles, give any money for a place, and remember many years after with singular delight. Bodine, when he was ambassador in England, said he saw the noblemen go in their robes to the parliament-house, *summa cum jucunditate vidimus,* he was much affected with the sight of it. Pomponius Columna, saith Jovius in his Life, saw thirteen Frenchmen and so many Italians once fight for a whole army: *quod jucundissimum spectaculum in vita dicit sua,* the pleasantest sight that ever he saw in his life. Who would not have been affected with such a spectacle? Or that single combat of Breauté the Frenchman, and Anthony Schets a Dutchman, before the walls of Sylvaducis [3] in Brabant, *anno* 1600.[4] They were twenty-two horse on the one side, as many on the other, which like Livy's Horatii, Torquati, and Corvini fought for their own glory and country's honour, in the sight and view of their whole city and army. When Julius Cæsar warred about the banks of Rhone,[5] there came a barbarian prince to see him and the Roman army, and when he had beheld Cæsar a good while, "I see the gods now" (saith he) "which before I heard of,[6] *nec feliciorem ullam vitæ meæ aut optavi, aut sensi diem*": it was the happiest day that ever he had in his life. Such a sight alone were able of itself to drive away melancholy; if not for ever, yet it must needs expel it for a time. Radzivilius was much taken with the bassa's palace in Cairo, and, amongst many other objects which that place afforded, with that solemnity of cutting the banks of Nilus by Imbram Bassa, when it overflowed; besides two or three hundred gilded galleys on the water, he saw two millions of men gathered together on the land, with turbans as white as snow, and 'twas a goodly sight. The very reading of feasts, triumphs, interviews, nuptials, tilts, tournaments, combats, and monomachies is most acceptable and pleasant. Franciscus Modius hath made a large collection of such solemnities in two great tomes,[1] which whoso will may peruse. The inspection alone of those curious iconographies of temples and palaces, as that of the Lateran Church in Albertus Durer, that of the temple of Jerusalem in Josephus,[2] Adricomius, and Villalpandus; that of the Escurial in Guadas, of Diana at Ephesus in Pliny, Nero's golden palace in Rome, Justinian's in Constantinople,[3] that Peruvian Inca's in Cusco, *ut non ab hominibus, sed a dæmoniis constructum videatur* [4] [which seemed to have been constructed not by men but by demons]; St. Mark's in Venice, by Ignatius, with many such; *priscorum artificum opera* (saith that interpreter of Pausanias [5]), the rare workmanship of those ancient Greeks, in theatres, obelisks, temples, statues, gold, silver, ivory, marble images, *non minore ferme quum leguntur, quam quum cernuntur, animum delectatione complent*, affect one as much by reading almost as by sight.

The country hath his recreations, the city his several gymnics and exercises, May-games, feasts, wakes, and merry meetings, to solace themselves; the very being in the country, that life itself is a sufficient recreation to some men, to enjoy such pleasures as those old patriarchs did. Diocletian, the emperor, was so much affected with it that he gave over his sceptre and turned gardener. Constantine wrote twenty books of husbandry. Lysander, when ambassadors came to see him, bragged of nothing more than of his orchard: *Hi sunt ordines mei* [these are my ranks]. What shall I say of Cincinnatus, Cato, Tully, and many such? how they have been pleased with it, to prune, plant, inoculate, and graft, to show so many several kinds of pears, apples, plums, peaches, etc.:

> *Nunc captare feras laqueo, nunc fallere visco,*
> *Atque etiam magnos canibus circundare saltus,*
> *Insidias avibus moliri, incendere vepres.*[6]

Sometimes with traps deceive, with line and string
To catch wild birds and beasts, encompassing
The grove with dogs, and out of bushes firing.

Et nidos avium scrutari, etc.

[And to go birds'-nesting, etc.]

Jucundus, in his preface to Cato, Varro, Columella, etc., put out
by him, confesseth of himself, that he was mightily delighted
with these husbandry studies, and took extraordinary pleasure
in them: if the theoric or speculation can so much affect, what
shall the place and exercise itself, the practic part, do? The
same confession I find in Herbastein, Porta, Camerarius, and
many others which have written of that subject. If my testimony were aught worth, I could say as much of myself; I am
vere Saturnius [a true lover of the country]; no man ever took
more delight in springs, woods, groves, gardens, walks, fish-
ponds, rivers, etc. But

*Tantalus a labris sitiens fugientia captat
Flumina;*

[Tantalus is fain to slake his thirsty need
In streams that ever from his lips recede;]

and so do I; *velle licet, potiri non licet* [I may desire, I may
not have].

Every palace, every city almost, hath his peculiar walks,
cloisters, terraces, groves, theatres, pageants, games, and
several recreations; every country some professed gymnics to
exhilarate their minds, and exercise their bodies. The Greeks
had their Olympian, Pythian, Isthmian, Nemean games, in
honour of Neptune, Jupiter, Apollo;[1] Athens hers: some for
honour, garlands, crowns; for beauty, dancing, running, leaping,[2]
like our silver games. The Romans had their feasts,[3] as the
Athenians, and Lacedæmonians held their public banquets, *in
Prytaneo, Panathenæis, Thesmophoriis, Phiditiis,* plays, nau-
machies, places for sea-fights, theatres, amphitheatres able to
contain 70,000 men, wherein they had several delightsome
shows to exhilarate the people;[4] gladiators, combats of men
with themselves, with wild beasts, and wild beasts one with
another,[5] like our bull-baitings or bear-baitings (in which many
countrymen and citizens amongst us so much delight and so
frequently use), dancers on ropes, jugglers, wrestlers, comedies,
tragedies, publicly exhibited at the emperor's and city's charge,
and that with incredible cost and magnificence. In the Low

Countries (as Meteran relates [1]) before these wars, they had
many solemn feasts, plays, challenges, artillery gardens, colleges
of rhymers, rhetoricians, poets: and to this day such places are
curiously maintained in Amsterdam, as appears by that description of Isaacus Pontanus, *Rerum Amstelrod. lib. 2, cap. 25.* So
likewise not long since at Freiburg in Germany, as is evident
by that relation of Neander,[2] they had *ludos septennales,* solemn
plays every seven years, which Bocerus, one of their own
poets, hath elegantly described:

> *At nunc magnifico spectacula structa paratu*
> *Quid memorem, vereti non concessura Quirino,*
> *Ludorum pompa,* etc.

> [What shall I say of the magnificence of their shows, not
> inferior to the games of ancient Rome?]

In Italy thay have solemn declarations of certain select young
gentlemen in Florence (like those reciters in old Rome), and
public theatres in most of their cities, for stage-players and
others, to exercise and recreate themselves. All seasons almost,
all places have their several pastimes; some in summer, some in
winter; some abroad, some within; some of the body, some of
the mind: and diverse men have diverse recreations and exercises. Domitian, the emperor, was much delighted with
catching flies, Augustus to play with nuts amongst children;
Alexander Severus was often pleased to play with whelps and
young pigs;[3] Hadrian was so wholly enamoured with dogs and
horses that he bestowed monuments and tombs on them, and
buried them in graves.[4] In foul weather, or when they can
use no other convenient sports by reason of the time, as we
do cock-fighting, to avoid idleness, I think (though some be
more seriously taken with it, spend much time, cost and charges,
and are too solicitous about it), Severus used partridges and
quails,[5] as many Frenchmen do still, and to keep birds in
cages, with which he was much pleased when at any time he
had leisure from public cares and businesses. He had (saith
Lampridius) tame pheasants, ducks, partridges, peacocks, and
some 20,000 ring-doves and pigeons. Busbequius, the emperor's
orator, when he lay in Constantinople and could not stir much
abroad, kept for his recreation, busying himself to see them
fed, almost all manner of strange birds and beasts; this was
something, though not to exercise his body, yet to refresh his
mind. Conradus Gesner, at Zurich in Switzerland, kept so
likewise for his pleasure a great company of wild beasts; and

(as he saith) took great delight to see them eat their meat. Turkey gentlewomen, that are perpetual prisoners, still mewed up according to the custom of the place, have little else besides their household business, or to play with their children to drive away time, but to dally with their cats, which they have *in deliciis* [as pets], as many of our ladies and gentlewomen use monkeys and little dogs. The ordinary recreations which we have in winter, and in most solitary times busy our minds with, are cards, tables and dice, shovelboard, chess-play, the philosopher's game, small trunks, shuttlecock, billiards, music, masks, singing, dancing, Yule-games, frolics, jests, riddles, catches, purposes, questions and commands, merry tales [1] of errant knights, queens, lovers, lords, ladies, giants, dwarfs, thieves, cheaters, witches, fairies, goblins, friars, etc., such as the old woman told [of] Psyche in Apuleius,[2] Boccace novels, and the rest, *quarum auditione pueri delectantur, senes narratione*, which some delight to hear, some to tell, all are well pleased with. Amaranthus, the philosopher, met Hermocles, Diophantus, and Philolaus, his companions, one day busily discoursing about Epicurus' and Democritus' tenents, very solicitous which was most probable and came nearest to truth: to put them out of that surly controversy, and to refresh their spirits, he told them a pleasant tale of Stratocles the physician's wedding, and of all the particulars, the company, the cheer, the music, etc., for he was new come from it; with which relation they were so much delighted, that Philolaus wished a blessing to his heart, and many a good wedding, many such merry meetings might he be at "to please himself with the sight, and others with the narration of it." [3] News are generally welcome to all our ears, *avide audimus, aures enim hominum novitate lætantur* [we listen greedily, for men's ears are charmed with novelty] (as Pliny observes[4]), we long after rumour to hear and listen to it, *densum humeris bibit aure vulgus* [5] [close packed the crowd drinks in the news]. We are most part too inquisitive and apt to hearken after news, which Cæsar in his Commentaries [6] observes of the old Gauls; they would be inquiring of every carrier and passenger what they had heard or seen, what news abroad?

> *Quid toto fiat in orbe,*
> *Quid Seres, quid Thraces agant, secreta novercæ*
> *Et pueri, quis amet,* etc.,

> [What news in all the world;
> What China does, what Thrace, the love affair
> Of son and stepmother, the latest scandal,]

as at an ordinary with us, bakehouse, or barber's shop.   When
that great Gonsalvo was upon some displeasure confined by
King Ferdinand to the city of Loxa in Andalusia, the only
comfort (saith Jovius [1]) he had to ease his melancholy thoughts,
was to hear news, and to listen after those ordinary occurrents,
which were brought him *cum primis* [among the very first], by
letters or otherwise, out of the remotest parts of Europe.   Some
men's whole delight is to take tobacco, and drink all day long
in a tavern or alehouse, to discourse, sing, jest, roar, talk of
a cock and bull over a pot, etc.   Or when three or four good
companions meet, tell old stories by the fireside or in the sun,
as old folks usually do, *quæ aprici meminere senes*, remembering
afresh and with pleasure ancient matters, and such-like accidents, which happened in their younger years.   Others' best
pastime is to game, nothing to them so pleasant.   *Hic Veneri
indulget, hunc decoquit alea* [2] [one spends on women, another
ruins himself with gaming].   Many too nicely take exceptions
at cards, tables, and dice, and such mixed lusorious lots,[3] whom
Gataker well confutes; which, though they be honest recreations
in themselves, yet may justly be otherwise excepted at, as they
are often abused, and forbidden as things most pernicious;
insanam rem et damnosam [a mad and ruinous proceeding],
Lemnius calls it.[4]   "For most part in these kind of disports
'tis not art or skill, but subtlety, cony-catching, knavery,
chance and fortune carries all away:" 'tis *ambulatoria pecunia*
[money on the move],

*Puncto mobilis horæ
Permutat dominos, et cedit in altera jura.*

[In one brief hour it changes owners, gets a new master.]

They labour most part not to pass their time in honest disport,
but for filthy lucre and covetousness of money.   *In fœdissimum
lucrum et avaritiam hominum convertitur*, as Danæus observes.
Fons fraudum et maleficiorum, 'tis the fountain of cozenage and
villainy, "a thing so common all over Europe at this day, and
so generally abused, that many men are utterly undone by
it, their means spent, patrimonies consumed, they and their
posterity beggared"; [5] besides swearing, wrangling, drinking,
loss of time, and such inconveniences, which are ordinary concomitants; "for when once they have got a haunt of such
companies, and habit of gaming, they can hardly be drawn
from it, but as an itch it will tickle them, and as it is with
whoremasters, once entered, they cannot easily leave it off": [6]

vexat mentes insana cupido, they are mad upon their sport. And in conclusion (which Charles the Seventh, that good French king, published in an edict against gamesters), *unde piæ et hilaris vitæ suffugium sibi suisque liberis, totique familiæ,* etc., "that which was once their livelihood, should have maintained wife, children, family, is now spent and gone"; *mæror et egestas,* etc., sorrow and beggary succeeds. So good things may be abused, and that which was first invented to refresh men's weary spirits, when they come from other labours and studies, to exhilarate the mind,[1] to entertain time and company, tedious otherwise in those long solitary winter nights, and keep them from worse matters, an honest exercise, is contrarily perverted.

Chess-play is a good and witty exercise of the mind for some kind of men, and fit for such melancholy, Rhasis holds, as are idle, and have extravagant impertinent thoughts, or troubled with cares, nothing better to distract their mind and alter their meditations; invented (some say) by the general of an army in a famine, to keep soldiers from mutiny;[2] but if it proceed from overmuch study, in such a case it may do more harm than good; it is a game too troublesome for some men's brains, too full of anxiety, all out as bad as study; besides it is a testy, choleric game, and very offensive to him that loseth the mate. William the Conqueror,[3] in his younger years, playing at chess with the Prince of France (Dauphiné was not annexed to that crown in those days), losing a mate, knocked the chess-board about his pate, which was a cause afterward of much enmity between them. For some such reason it is, belike, that Patricius, in his third book, *tit.* 12, *de reg. instit.,* forbids his prince to play at chess; hawking and hunting, riding, etc., he will allow, and this to other men, but by no means to him. In Muscovy, where they live in stoves and hot-houses all winter long, come seldom or little abroad, it is again very necessary, and therefore in those parts (saith Herbastein[4]), much used. At Fez in Africa, where the like inconvenience of keeping within doors is through heat, it is very laudable, and (as Leo Afer relates[5]) as much frequented. A sport fit for idle gentlewomen, soldiers in garrison, and courtiers that have naught but love-matters to busy themselves about, but not altogether so convenient for such as are students. The like I may say of Cl. Bruxer's philosophy game, Dr. Fulke's *Metromachia* and his *Ouranomachia,* with the rest of those intricate astrological and geometrical fictions, for such especially as are mathematically given; and the rest of those curious games.

Dancing, singing, masking, mumming, stage-plays, howso-ever they be heavily censured by some severe Catos, yet, if opportunely and soberly used, may justly be approved. *Melius est fodere quam saltare* [it is better to dig than to dance], saith Austin; but what is that if they delight in it? *Nemo saltat sobrius* [1] [no sensible man dances]. But in what kind of dance? I know these sports have many oppugners, whole volumes writ against them; when as all they say (if duly considered) is but *ignoratio elenchi*; and some again, because they are now cold and wayward, past themselves, cavil at all such youthful sports in others, as he did in the comedy; they think them *illico nasci senes* [that they are born old], etc. Some out of preposterous zeal object many times trivial arguments, and because of some abuse will quite take away the good use, as if they should forbid wine because it makes men drunk; but in my judgment they are too stern: "there is a time for all things, a time to mourn, a time to dance" (Eccles. iii, 4), "a time to embrace, a time not to embrace" (verse 5), and "nothing better than that a man should rejoice in his own works" (verse 22); for my part, I will subscribe to the king's declaration,[2] and was ever of that mind, those May-games, wakes, and Whitsun ales, etc., if they be not at unseasonable hours, may justly be permitted. Let them freely feast, sing and dance, have their poppet-plays, hobby-horses, tabors, crowds, bagpipes, etc., play at ball, and barley-breaks, and what sports and recreations they like best. In Franconia, a province of Germany (saith Aubanus Bohemus [3]), the old folks, after evening prayer, went to the alehouse, the younger sort to dance: and to say truth with Sarisburiensis,[4] *satius fuerat sic otiari quam turpius occupari*, better do so than worse, as without question otherwise (such is the corruption of man's nature) many of them will do. For that cause, plays, masks, jesters, gladiators, tumblers, jugglers, etc., and all that crew is admitted and winked at: *Tota jocularium scena procedit, et ideo spectacula admissa sunt, et infinita tirocinia vanitatum, ut his occupentur, qui perniciosius otiari solent:* [5] that they might be busied about such toys, that would otherwise more perniciously be idle. So that as Tacitus said of the astrologers in Rome,[6] we may say of them, *genus hominum est quod in civitate nostra et vitabitur semper et retinebitur*, they are a deboshed company most part, still spoken against, as well they deserve some of them (for I so relish and distinguish them as fiddlers, and musicians), and yet ever retained. "Evil is not to be done" (I confess) "that good may come of it": but this is evil

per accidens, and in a qualified sense, to avoid a greater inconvenience, may justly be tolerated. Sir Thomas More, in his
Utopian commonwealth, as he will have none idle, so will he
have no man labour over-hard, to be toiled out like a horse;
'tis more than slavish infelicity, the life of most of our hired
servants and tradesmen elsewhere (excepting his Utopians);
but half the day allotted for work, and half for honest recreation
or whatsoever employment they shall think fit themselves.[1] If
one half-day in a week were allowed to our household servants
for their merry-meetings by their hard masters, or in a year
some feasts, like those Roman Saturnals, I think they would
labour harder all the rest of their time, and both parties be
better pleased: but this needs not (you will say), for some of
them do naught but loiter all the week long.

This which I aim at, is for such as are *fracti animis*, troubled
in mind, to ease them: over-toiled on the one part, to refresh;
over-idle on the other, to keep themselves busied. And to this
purpose, as any labour or employment will serve to the one,
any honest recreation will conduce to the other, so that it be
moderate and sparing, as the use of meat and drink; not to
spend all their life in gaming, playing, and pastimes, as too
many gentlemen do; but to revive our bodies and recreate our
souls with honest sports: of which as there be divers sorts, and
peculiar to several callings, ages, sexes, conditions, so there be
proper for several seasons, and those of distinct natures, to fit
that variety of humours which is amongst them, that if one will
not, another may: some in summer, some in winter, some gentle,
some more violent, some for the mind alone, some for the body
and mind (as to some it is both business and a pleasant recreation
to oversee workmen of all sorts, husbandry, cattle, horse, etc.,
to build, plot, project, to make models, cast up accounts, etc.);
some without, some within doors; new, old, etc., as the season
serveth, and as men are inclined. It is reported of Philippus
Bonus, that good Duke of Burgundy (by Lodovicus Vives *in
Epist.* and Pont. Heuter in his History[2]), that the said duke, at
the marriage of Eleonora, sister to the King of Portugal, at
Bruges in Flanders, which was solemnized in the deep of winter,
whenas by reason of unseasonable weather he could neither
hawk nor hunt, and was now tired with cards, dice, etc., and
such other domestical sports, or to see ladies dance, with some
of his courtiers he would in the evening walk disguised all about
the town. It so fortuned, as he was walking late one night, he
found a country fellow dead-drunk, snorting on a bulk; he

caused his followers to bring him to his palace, and there stripping him of his old clothes, and attiring him after the court fashion, when he waked, he and they were all ready to attend upon his excellency, persuading him he was some great duke.[1] The poor fellow, admiring how he came there, was served in state all the day long; after supper he saw them dance, heard music, and the rest of those court-like pleasures: but late at night, when he was well tippled, and again fast asleep, they put on his old robes, and so conveyed him to the place where they first found him. Now the fellow had not made them so good sdort the day before as he did when he returned to himself; all the jest was to see how he looked upon it.[2] In conclusion, after some little admiration, the poor man told his friends he had seen a vision, constantly believed it, would not otherwise be persuaded, and so the jest ended. Antiochus Epiphanes would often disguise himself, steal from his court, and go into merchants', goldsmiths', and other tradesmen's shops, sit and talk with them, and sometimes ride or walk alone, and fall aboard with any tinker, clown, serving man, carrier, or whomsoever he met first.[3] Sometimes he did *ex insperato* [unexpectedly] give a poor fellow money, to see how he would look, or on set purpose lose his purse as he went, to watch who found it, and withal how he would be affected, and with such objects he was much delighted. Many such tricks are ordinarily put in practice by great men, to exhilarate themselves and others, all which are harmless jests, and have their good uses.

But amongst those exercises or recreations of the mind within doors, there is none so general, so aptly to be applied to all sorts of men, so fit and proper to expel idleness and melancholy, as that of study. *Studia senectutem oblectant, adolescentiam alunt, secundas res ornant, adversis perfugium et solatium præbent, domi delectant* [study is the delight of old age, the training of youth, the ornament of prosperity, the refuge and solace of adversity; it entertains us at home], etc., find the rest in Tully, *pro Archia Poeta.* What so full of content, as to read, walk, and see maps, pictures, statues, jewels, marbles, which some so much magnify, as those that Phidias made of old so exquisite and pleasing to be beheld, that, as Chrysostom thinketh, "if any man be sickly, troubled in mind, or that cannot sleep for grief, and shall but stand over against one of Phidias' images, he will forget all care, or whatsoever else may molest him, in an instant"?[4] There be those so much taken with Michael Angelo's, Raphael de Urbino's, Francesco Francia's pieces, and many of those Italian and Dutch painters, which were excellent in their ages; and esteem of it as a most pleasing sight to view those neat architectures, devices, escutcheons, coats of arms, read such books, to peruse old coins of several sorts in a fair gallery; artificial works, perspective glasses, old relics, Roman antiquities, variety of colours. A good picture is *falsa veritas et muta poesis* [a counterfeit reality, a poem without words]; and though (as Vives saith[1]) *artificialia delectant, sed mox fastidimus*, artificial toys please but for a time, yet who is he that will not be moved with them for the present? When Achilles was tormented and sad for the loss of his dear friend Patroclus, his mother Thetis brought him a most elaborate and curious buckler made by Vulcan, in which were engraven sun, moon, stars, planets, sea, land, men fighting, running, riding, women scolding, hills, dales, towns, castles, brooks, rivers, trees, etc., with many pretty landskips and perspective pieces: with sight of which he was infinitely delighted, and much eased of his grief.

> *Continuo eo spectaculo captus delenito mœrore*
> *Oblectabatur in manibus tenens dei splendida dona.*[2]

Who will not be affected so in like case, or to see those well-furnished cloisters and galleries of the Roman cardinals, so richly stored with all modern pictures, old statues and antiquities? *Cum se Spectando recreet simul atque legendo,* to see their pictures alone and read the description, as Boissardus well adds,[3] whom will it not affect? which Bozius, Pomponius Lætus, Marlianus, Schottus, Cavelerius, Ligorius, etc., and he himself hath well performed of late. Or in some prince's cabinets, like that of the great duke's in Florence, of Felix Platerus in Basil, or noblemen's houses, to see such variety of attires, faces, so many, so rare, and such exquisite pieces, of men, birds, beasts, etc., to see those excellent landskips, Dutch works, and curious cuts of Sadeler of Prague, Albertus Durer, Goltzius, Vrintes, etc., such pleasant pieces of perspective, Indian pictures made of feathers, China works, frames, thaumaturgical motions, exotic toys, etc. Who is he that is now wholly overcome with idleness, or otherwise involved in a labyrinth of worldly cares, troubles, and discontents, that will not be much lightened in his mind by reading of some enticing story, true or feigned, where as in a glass he shall observe what our forefathers have done, the beginnings, ruins, falls, periods of commonwealths, private men's actions displayed to the life, etc. Plutarch therefore calls them

secundas mensas et bellaria, the second course and junkets,
because they were usually read at noblemen's feasts.[1] Who is
not earnestly affected with a passionate speech, well penned,
an elegant poem, or some pleasant bewitching discourse, like
that of Heliodorus, *ubi oblectatio quædam placide fluit, cum
hilaritate conjuncta?*[2]   Julian the Apostate was so taken with
an oration of Libanius the Sophister, that, as he confesseth, he
could not be quiet till he had read it all out. *Legi orationem
tuam magna ex parte hesterna die ante prandium, pransus vero
sine ulla intermissione totam absolvi. O argumenta! O composi-
tionem!* [I read a great part of your speech yesterday before
dinner, and after dinner I finished it without a stop. What arguments! What style!] I may say the same of this or that pleasing
tract, which will draw his attention along with it. To most kind
of men it is an extraordinary delight to study. For what a world
of books offers itself, in all subjects, arts, and sciences, to the
sweet content and capacity of the reader! In arithmetic,
geometry, perspective, optics, astronomy, architecture, *sculp-
tura, pictura* [sculpture, painting], of which so many and such
elaborate treatises are of late written; in mechanics and their
mysteries, military matters, navigation, riding of horses,[3]
fencing,[4] swimming, gardening, planting, great tomes of husbandry, cookery, falconry, hunting, fishing, fowling, etc., with
exquisite pictures of all sports, games, and what not? In
music, metaphysics, natural and moral philosophy, philology,
in policy, heraldry, genealogy, chronology, etc., they afford
great tomes; or those studies of antiquity,[5] etc.; *et quid subtilius
arithmeticis inventionibus, quid jucundius musicis rationibus,
quid divinius astronomicis, quid rectius geometricis demonstra-
tionibus?*[6] [and what could be more ingenious than the devices
of arithmetic, more pleasing than the theories of music, more
elevating than the discoveries of astronomy, more convincing
than the proofs of geometry?] What so sure, what so pleasant?
He that shall but see that geometrical tower of Garisenda at
Bologna in Italy, the steeple and clock at Strasburg, will admire
the effects of art, or that engine of Archimedes, to remove the
earth itself, if he had but a place to fasten his instrument,
Archimedes' *cochlea* [water-screw], and rare devices to corrivate
waters, music instruments, and trisyllable echoes again, again,
and again repeated, with myriads of such. What vast tomes
are extant in law, physic, and divinity, for profit, pleasure,
practice, speculation, in verse or prose, etc.! Their names alone
are the subject of whole volumes, we have thousands of authors

of all sorts, many great libraries full well furnished, like so many
dishes of meat served out for several palates; and he is a very
block that is affected with none of them. Some take an infinite
delight to study the very languages wherein these books are
written, Hebrew, Greek, Syriac, Chaldee, Arabic, etc. Methinks
it would please any man to look upon a geographical map,
*suavi animum delectatione allicere, ob incredibilem rerum varieta-
tem et jucunditatem, et ad pleniorem sui cognitionem excitare* [1]
[which insensibly charms the mind with the great and pleasing
variety of objects that it offers, and incites it to further study],
chorographical, topographical delineations, to behold, as it were,
all the remote provinces, towns, cities of the world, and never
to go forth of the limits of his study, to measure by the scale
and compass their extent, distance, examine their site. Charles
the Great, as Platina writes, had three fair silver tables, in one
of which superficies was a large map of Constantinople, in the
second Rome neatly engraved, in the third an exquisite description of the whole world, and much delight he took in them.
What greater pleasure can there now be, than to view those
elaborate maps of Ortelius, Mercator,[2] Hondius, etc.? To
peruse those books of cities, put out by Braunus and Hogen-
bergius? To read those exquisite descriptions of Maginus,
Munster, Herrera, Laet, Merula, Boterus, Leander, Albertus,
Camden, Leo Afer, Adricomius, Nic. Gerbelius, etc.? Those
famous expeditions of Christoph. Columbus, Amoricus Vespuccius, Marcus Polus the Venetian, Lod. Vertomannus, Aloysius
Cadamustus, etc.? Those accurate diaries of Portugals, Hollanders, of Bartison, Oliver à Nort, etc., Hakluyt's Voyages,
Pet. Martyr's Decades, Benzo, Lerius, Linschoten's Relations,
those Hodœporicons of Joh. à Meggen, Brocard the monk,
Bredenbachius, Jo. Dublinius, Sandys, etc., to Jerusalem,
Egypt, and other remote places of the world? those pleasant
itineraries of Paulus Hentznerus, Jodocus Sincerus, Dux
Polonus,[3] etc., to read Bellonius' Observations, P. Gillius his
Surveys; those parts of America, set out, and curiously cut in
pictures, by Fratres à Bry. To see a well-cut herbal, herbs,
trees, flowers, plants, all vegetals expressed in their proper
colours to the life, as that of Matthiolus upon Dioscorides, Delacampius, Lobel, Bauhinus, and that last voluminous and mighty
herbal of Besler of Nuremburg, wherein almost every plant is
to his own bigness. To see birds, beasts, and fishes of the sea,
spiders, gnats, serpents, flies, etc., all creatures set out by the
same art, and truly expressed in lively colours, with an exact

description of their natures, virtues, qualities, etc., as hath
been accurately performed by Ælian, Gesner, Ulysses Aldrovandus, Bellonius, Rondeletius, Hippolytus Salvianus, etc.
*Arcana cœli, naturæ secreta, ordinem universi scire, majoris
felicitatis et dulcedinis est, quam cogitatione quis assequi possit,
aut mortalis sperare* [1] [to discover the mysteries of the heavens,
the secrets of nature, and the order of the universe, would
confer greater happiness and pleasure than can be imagined,
or than any mortal could hope to attain]. What more pleasing
studies can there be than the mathematics, theoric or practic
parts? as to survey land, make maps, models, dials, etc., with
which I was ever much delighted myself. *Talis est mathematum
pulchritudo* (saith Plutarch [2]), *ut his indignum sit divitiarum
phaleras istas et bullas et puellaria spectacula comparari;* such
is the excellency of these studies, that all those ornaments and
childish bubbles of wealth are not worthy to be compared to
them; *Crede mihi* (saith one [3]), *extingui dulce erit mathematicarum
artium studio,* I could even live and die with such meditations,
and take more delight, true content of mind in them, than thou
hast in all thy wealth and sport, how rich soever thou art. [4]
And as Cardan well seconds me, [5] *Honorificum magis est et
gloriosum hæc intelligere, quam provinciis præesse, formosum aut
ditem juvenem esse* [it is more honourable and glorious to understand these things than to rule over provinces or be young,
handsome, and rich]. The like pleasure there is in all other
studies, to such as are truly addicted to them. *Ea suavitas*
(one holds [6]) *ut cum quis ea degustaverit, quasi poculis Circeis
captus, non possit unquam ab illis divelli:* the like sweetness,
which as Circe's cup bewitcheth a student, he cannot leave off,
as well may witness those many laborious hours, days, and
nights, spent in the voluminous treatises written by them; the
same content. Julius Scaliger [7] was so much affected with
poetry that he brake out into a pathetical protestation, he had
rather be the author of twelve verses in Lucan, or such an ode
in Horace, [8] than emperor of Germany. Nicholas Gerbelius, [9]
that good old man, was so much ravished with a few Greek
authors restored to light, with hope and desire of enjoying the
rest, that he exclaims forthwith, *Arabibus atque Indis omnibus
erimus ditiores,* we shall be richer than all the Arabic or Indian
princes; of such esteem they were with him, incomparable worth
and value. [10] Seneca prefers Zeno and Chrysippus, two doting
Stoics (he was so much enamoured of their works), before any
prince or general of an army; and Orontius the mathematician

so far admires Archimedes, that he calls him *divinum et homine majorem*, a petty god, more than a man; and well he might, for aught I see, if you respect fame or worth. Pindarus of Thebes is as much renowned for his poems as Epaminondas, Pelopidas, Hercules, or Bacchus, his fellow-citizens, for their warlike actions; *et si famam respicias, non pauciores Aristotelis quam Alexandri meminerunt* (as Cardan notes), Aristotle is more known than Alexander; for we have a bare relation of Alexander's deeds, but Aristotle *totus vivit in monumentis*, is whole in his works: yet I stand not upon this; the delight is it which I aim at; so great pleasure, such sweet content there is in study. King James, 1605,[1] when he came to see our University of Oxford, and amongst other edifices now went to view that famous library, renewed by Sir Thomas Bodley, in imitation of Alexander, at his departure brake out into that noble speech: "If I were not a king, I would be a university man: and if it were so that I must be a prisoner, if I might have my wish, I would desire to have no other prison than that library, and to be chained together with so many good authors *et mortuis magistris* [deceased teachers]."[2]　So sweet is the delight of study, the more learning they have (as he that hath a dropsy, the more he drinks the thirstier he is), the more they covet to learn, and the last day is *prioris discipulus* [the disciple of the preceding]; harsh at first learning is, *radices amaræ* [the roots are bitter], but *fructus dulces* [the fruit is sweet], according to that of Isocrates, pleasant at last; the longer they live, the more they are enamoured with the Muses. Heinsius, the keeper of the library at Leyden in Holland, was mewed up in it all the year long; and that which to thy thinking should have bred a loathing, caused in him a greater liking. "I no sooner" (saith he) "come into the library, but I bolt the door to me, excluding lust, ambition, avarice, and all such vices, whose nurse is idleness, the mother of ignorance, and melancholy herself, and in the very lap of eternity, amongst so many divine souls, I take my seat, with so lofty a spirit and sweet content that I pity all our great ones and rich men that know not this happiness."[3]　I am not ignorant in the meantime (notwithstanding this which I have said) how barbarously and basely, for the most part, our ruder gentry esteem of libraries and books, how they neglect and contemn so great a treasure, so inestimable a benefit, as Æsop's cock did the jewel he found in the dunghill; and all through error, ignorance, and want of education. And 'tis a wonder withal to observe how much they will vainly cast away in unnecessary expenses, *quot modis pereant* (saith Erasmus [1]) *magnatibus pecuniæ, quantum absumant alea, scorta, compotationes, profectiones non necessariæ, pompæ, bella quæsita, ambitio, colax, morio, ludio,* etc., what in hawks, hounds, lawsuits, vain building, gormandizing, drinking, sports, plays, pastimes, etc. If a well-minded man to the Muses would sue to some of them for an exhibition, to the farther mainte-nance or enlargement of such a work, be it college, lecture, library, or whatsoever else may tend to the advancement of learning, they are so unwilling, so averse, they had rather see these which are already with such cost and care erected, utterly ruined, demolished, or otherwise employed; for they repine many and grudge at such gifts and revenues so bestowed: and therefore it were in vain, as Erasmus well notes, *vel ab his, vel a negotiatoribus qui se Mammonæ dediderunt, improbum fortasse tale officium exigere,* to solicit or ask anything of such men that are likely damned to riches, to this purpose. For my part I pity these men, *stultos jubeo esse libenter,* let them go as they are, in the catalogue of ignoramus[es]. How much, on the other side, are all we bound that are scholars, to those munificent Ptolemies, bountiful Mæcenases, heroical patrons, divine spirits, *qui nobis hæc otia fecerunt* [who gave us all this comfort],

Namque erit ille mihi semper deus, [2]
[For never can I deem him less than god,]

that have provided for us so many well-furnished libraries, as well in our public academies in most cities, as in our private colleges! How shall I remember Sir Thomas Bodley,[3] amongst the rest, Otho Nicholson,[4] and the Right Reverend John Williams, Lord Bishop of Lincoln (with many other pious acts), who besides that at St. John's College in Cambridge, that in Westminster, is now likewise *in fieri* [proceeding] with a library at Lincoln (a noble precedent for all corporate towns and cities to imitate), *O quam te memorem (vir illustrissime), quibus elogiis?* [How shall I speak of thee, most illustrious man, how praise thee worthily?] But to my task again.

Whosoever he is, therefore, that is overrun with solitariness, or carried away with pleasing melancholy and vain conceits, and for want of employment knows not how to spend his time, or crucified with worldly care, I can prescribe him no better remedy than this of study, to compose himself to the learning of some art or science. Provided always that his malady pro-ceed not from overmuch study; for in such case he adds fuel

to the fire, and nothing can be more pernicious; let him take
heed he do not overstretch his wits, and make a skeleton of
himself; or such inamoratoes as read nothing but play-books,
idle poems, jests, Amadis de Gaul, the Knight of the Sun, the
Seven Champions, Palmerin de Oliva, Huon of Bordeaux, etc.
Such many times prove in the end as mad as Don Quixote.
Study is only prescribed to those that are otherwise idle,
troubled in mind, or carried headlong with vain thoughts and
imaginations, to distract their cogitations (although variety of
study, or some serious subject, would do the former no harm),
and divert their continual meditations another way. Nothing
in this case better than study; *semper aliquid memoriter ediscant,*
saith Piso, let them learn something without book, transcribe,
translate, etc., read the Scriptures, which Hyperius, *lib.* 1 *de
quotid. script. lec. fol.* 77, holds available of itself; "the mind is
erected thereby from all worldly cares, and hath much quiet
and tranquillity." [1] For, as Austin [2] well hath it, 'tis *scientia
scientiarum, omni melle dulcior, omni pane suavior, omni vino
hilarior* [the all-embracing knowledge, sweeter than honey, more
gladdening than wine]; 'tis the best nepenthes, surest cordial,
sweetest alterative, presentest diverter: for neither, as Chrysostom well adds,[3] "those boughs and leaves of trees which are
plashed for cattle to stand under, in the heat of the day, in
summer, so much refresh them with their acceptable shade, as
the reading of the Scripture doth recreate and comfort a· distressed soul, in sorrow and affliction." Paul bids "pray continually"; *quod cibus corpori, lectio animæ facit,* saith Seneca,
as meat is to the body, such is reading to the soul. "To be at
leisure without books is another hell, and to be buried alive." [4]
Cardan [5] calls a library the physic of the soul; "divine authors
fortify the mind, make men bold and constant; and" (as
Hyperius adds) "godly conference will not permit the mind
to be tortured with absurd cogitations." [6] Rhasis enjoins continual conference to such melancholy men, perpetual discourse
of some history, tale, poem, news, etc., *alternos sermones edere
ac bibere, æque jucundum quam cibus, sive potus,* which feeds
the mind as meat and drink doth the body, and pleaseth as
much: and therefore the said Rhasis, not without good cause,
would have somebody still talk seriously, or dispute with them,
and sometimes "to cavil and wrangle" (so that it break not out
to a violent perturbation), "for such altercation is like stirring
of a dead fire to make it burn afresh," it whets a dull spirit,
"and will not suffer the mind to be drowned in those profound

cogitations which melancholy men are commonly troubled
with." [1]   Ferdinand and Alphonsus, kings of Aragon and
Sicily, were both cured by reading the history, one of Curtius,
the other of Livy, when no prescribed physic would take place.[2]
Camerarius [3] relates as much of Laurence Medices.[4] Heathen
philosophers are so full of divine precepts in this kind, that, as
some think, they alone are able to settle a distressed mind—
Sunt verba et voces, quibus hunc lenire dolorem [5] [words there are,
and discourse, with which to assuage this grief], etc.—Epictetus,
Plutarch, and Seneca. *Qualis ille, quæ tela*, saith Lipsius,
*adversus omnes animi casus administrat, et ipsam mortem,
quomodo vitia eripit, infert virtutes !* [What a man was he! What
weapons doth he furnish against all sufferings of the mind,
against the fear of death itself! How he eradicates vice and
implants virtue!] When I read Seneca, "methinks I am beyond
all human fortunes, on the top of a hill above mortality." [6]
Plutarch saith as much of Homer, for which cause belike Nicera-
tus, in Xenophon, was made by his parents to con Homer's
Iliads and Odysseys without book, *ut in virum bonum evaderet*,
as well to make him a good and honest man as to avoid idleness.
If this comfort may be got from philosophy, what shall be had
from divinity?   What shall Austin, Cyprian, Gregory, Bernard's
divine meditations afford us?

> *Qui quid sit pulchrum, quid turpe, quid utile, quid non,*
> *Plenius et melius Chrysippo et Crantore dicunt.*
>
> [Who can indicate
> What we should praise or blame, choose or reject,
> More fully and with judgment more correct
> Than Crantor and Chrysippus.]

Nay, what shall the Scripture itself?—which is like an apothecary's shop, wherein are all remedies for all infirmities of mind,
purgatives, cordials, alteratives, corroboratives, lenitives, etc.
"Every disease of the soul," saith Austin,[7] "hath a peculiar
medicine in the Scripture; this only is required, that the sick
man take the potion which God hath already tempered."
Gregory [8] calls it "a glass wherein we may see all our infirmities,"
ignitum colloquium [a fiery discourse] (Ps. cxix, 140); Origen,[9] a
charm.   And therefore Hierome prescribes Rusticus the monk,
"continually to read the Scripture, and to meditate on that
which he hath read; for as mastication is to meat, so is meditation on that which we read." [10]   I would for these causes wish
him that is melancholy to use both human and divine authors,

voluntarily to impose some task upon himself, to divert his melancholy thoughts: to study the art of memory, Cosmus Rosselius, Pet. Ravennas, *Scenkelius detectus*, or practise brachygraphy, etc., that will ask a great deal of attention: or let him demonstrate a proposition in Euclid, in his five last books, extract a square root, or study algebra: than which, as Clavius [1] holds, "in all human disciplines nothing can be more excellent and pleasant, so abstruse and recondite, so bewitching, so miraculous, so ravishing, so easy withal and full of delight," *omnem humanum captum superare videtur.* By this means you may define *ex ungue leonem*, as the diverb is, by his thumb alone the bigness of Hercules, or the true dimensions of the great Colossus,[2] Solomon's temple, and Domitian's amphitheatre out of a little part. By this art you may contemplate the variation of the twenty-three letters, which may be so infinitely varied, that the words complicated and deduced thence will not be contained within the compass of the firmament; ten words may be varied 40,320 several ways: by this art you may examine how many men may stand one by another in the whole superficies of the earth, some say 148,456,800,000,000, *assignando singulis passum quadratum* [assigning a square foot to each]; how many men, supposing all the world as habitable as France, as fruitful and so long-lived, may be born in 60,000 years; and so may you demonstrate with Archimedes [3] how many sands the mass of the whole world might contain if all sandy, if you did but first know how much a small cube as big as a mustard-seed might hold; with infinite such. But in all nature what is there so stupend as to examine and calculate the motion of the planets, their magnitudes, apogeums, perigeums, eccentricities, how far distant from the earth, the bigness, thickness, compass of the firmament, each star, with their diameters and circumference, apparent area, superficies, by those curious helps of glasses, astrolabes, sextants, quadrants, of which Tycho Brahe in his Mechanics, optics (divine optics [4]), arithmetic, geometry, and such-like arts and instruments? What so intricate and pleasing withal, as to peruse and practise Hero Alexandrinus' works, *de spiritalibus, de machinis bellicis, de machina se movente* [about pneumatic machines, about military engines, about a self-moving machine], *Jordani Nemorarii de ponderibus proposit.* 13, that pleasant tract of Machometes Bragdedinus *de superficierum divisionibus* [of the divisions of plane surfaces], Apollonius' Conics, or Commandinus' labours in that kind, *de centro gravitatis*, with many such

geometrical theorems and problems? Those rare instruments
and mechanical inventions of Jac. Bessonus and Cardan to this
purpose, with many such experiments intimated long since by
Roger Bacon, in his tract *de secretis artis et naturæ* [1] [of the
secrets of nature and art], as to make a chariot to move *sine
animali* [without animal traction], diving-boats, to walk on the
water by art and to fly in the air, to make several cranes and
pulleys, *quibus homo trahat ad se mille homines* [by which one
man can draw to himself a thousand], lift up and remove great
weights, mills to move themselves, Archytas' dove, Albertus'
brazen head, and such thaumaturgical works. But especially
to do strange miracles by glasses, of which Proclus and Bacon
writ of old, burning-glasses, multiplying glasses, perspectives,
ut unus homo appareat exercitus [which make one man look like
an army], to see afar off, to represent solid bodies by cylinders
and concaves, to walk in the air, *ut veraciter videant* (saith
Bacon) *aurum et argentum et quicquid aliud volunt, et quum
veniant ad locum visionis, nihil inveniant* [so that they are positive
they see gold and silver and whatever else they want, yet when
they come to the spot they see nothing], which glasses are much
perfected of late by Baptista Porta and Galileo, and much more
is promised by Maginus and Midorgius, to be performed in this
kind. Otacousticons some speak of, to intend hearing, as the
other do sight; Marcellus Vrencken, an Hollander, in his epistle
to Burgravius, makes mention of a friend of his that is about an
instrument, *quo videbit quæ in altero horizonte sint* [by which he
will see things beyond the horizon]. But our alchemists,
methinks, and Rosy-cross men,[2] afford most rarities, and are
fuller of experiments: they can make gold, separate and alter
metals, extract oils, salts, lees, and do more strange works than
Geber, Lullius, Bacon, or any of those ancients. Crollius hath
made, after his master Paracelsus, *aurum fulminans*, or *aurum
volatile* [explosive or volatile gold], which shall imitate thunder
and lightning, and crack louder than any gunpowder; Cornelius
Drible a perpetual motion, inextinguible lights, *linum non
ardens* [non-inflammable flax], with many such feats (see his
book *de natura elementorum*), besides hail, wind, snow, thunder,
lightning, etc., those strange fireworks, devilish petards, and
such-like warlike machinations derived hence, of which read
Tartalea and others. Ernestus Burgravius, a disciple of Paracelsus, hath published a discourse, in which he specifies a lamp
to be made of man's blood, *lucerna vitæ et mortis index* [a lamp
which shall be an index of life and death], so he terms it, which

chemically prepared forty days, and afterwards kept in a glass, shall show all the accidents of this life; *si lampas hic clarus, tunc homo hilaris et sanus corpore et animo; si nebulosus et depressus, male afficitur, et sic pro statu hominis variatur, unde sumptus sanguis* [if the lamp burns clearly, then the man is cheerful and healthy in mind and body; if dim and cloudy, he is in low spirits; and so it varies with the condition of the man whose blood has been taken]; and, which is most wonderful, it dies with the party, *cum homine perit, et evanescit,* the lamp and the man whence the blood was taken are extinguished together. The same author hath another tract of *Mummia* (all out as vain and prodigious as the first), by which he will cure most diseases, and transfer them from a man to a beast, by drawing blood from one and applying it to the other, *vel in plantam derivare* [or even divert it to a plant], and an *alexipharmacum,* of which Roger Bacon of old in his *tract. de retardanda senectuie,* to make a man young again, live three or four hundred years; besides panaceas, martial amulets, *unguentum armarium* [the weapon-salve], balsams, strange extracts, elixirs, and such-like magico-magnetical cures. Now what so pleasing can there be as the speculation of these things, to read and examine such experiments, or, if a man be more mathematically given, to calculate, or peruse Napier's Logarithms, or those tables of artificial sines and tangents,[1] not long since set out by mine old collegiate, good friend, and late fellow-student of Christ Church in Oxford, Mr. Edmund Gunter,[2] which will perform that by addition and subtraction only, which heretofore Regiomontanus' tables did by multiplication and division, or those elaborate conclusions of his Sector, Quadrant, and Crossstaff.[3] Or let him that is melancholy calculate spherical triangles, square a circle, cast a nativity, which, howsoever some tax, I say with Garcæus,[4] *dabimus hoc petulantibus ingeniis* [we will concede to wayward minds], we will in some cases allow: or let him make an ephemerides, read Suisset the calculator's works, Scaliger *de emendatione temporum,* and Petavius his adversary, till he understand them, peruse subtle Scotus' and Suarez' metaphysics, or school divinity, Occam, Thomas, Entisberus, Durand, etc. If those other do not affect him, and his means be great, to employ his purse and fill his head, he may go find the philosopher's stone; he may apply his mind, I say, to heraldry, antiquity, invent impresses, emblems; make epithalamiums, epitaphs, elegies, epigrams, *palindroma epigrammata,*[5] anagrams, chronograms, acrostics upon his friends' names; or write a comment on Martianus Capella, Tertullian *de pallio*, the Nubian geography, or upon *Ælia Lælia Crispis*,[1] as many idle fellows have essayed; and rather than do nothing, vary a verse a thousand ways with Putean,[2] so torturing his wits, or as Rainnerus of Luneberg, 2,150 times in his *Proteus Poeticus*,[3] or Scaliger, Chrysolithus, Cleppisius, and others, have in like sort done. If such voluntary tasks, pleasure and delight, or crabbedness of these studies, will not yet divert their idle thoughts and alienate their imaginations, they must be compelled, saith Christophorus à Vega, *cogi debent (lib. 5, cap.* 14), upon some mulct if they perform it not, *quod ex officio incumbat* [which is incumbent on them in virtue of their office], loss of credit or disgrace, such as our public university exercises. For, as he that plays for nothing will not heed his game, no more will voluntary employment so throughly affect a student, except he be very intent of himself, and take an extraordinary delight in the study about which he is conversant. It should be of that nature his business, which *volens nolens* he must necessarily undergo, and without great loss, mulct, shame, or hindrance, he may not omit.

Now for women, instead of laborious studies, they have curious needleworks, cut-works, spinning, bone-lace, and many pretty devices of their own making, to adorn their houses, cushions, carpets, chairs, stools ("for she eats not the bread of idleness," Prov. xxxi, 27, *quæsivit lanam et linum* [she hath sought out wool and flax]) confections, conserves, distillations, etc., which they show to strangers.

> *Ipsa comes præsesque operis venientibus ultro*
> *Hospitibus monstrare solet, non segniter horas*
> *Contestata suas, sed nec sibi deperiisse.*[4]

> Which to her guests she shows, with all her pelf,
> Thus far my maids, but this I did myself.

This they have to busy themselves about, household offices, etc., neat gardens,[5] full of exotic, versicolour, diversely varied, sweet-smelling flowers, and plants in all kinds, which they are most ambitious to get, curious to preserve and keep, proud to possess, and much many times brag of. Their merry meetings and frequent visitations, mutual invitations in good towns, I voluntarily omit, which are so much in use, gossiping among the meaner sort, etc. Old folks have their beads: an excellent invention to keep them from idleness that are by nature melancholy and past all affairs, to say so many paternosters, Ave

Maries, creeds, if it were not profane and superstitious. In a word, body and mind must be exercised, not one, but both, and that in a mediocrity; otherwise it will cause a great inconvenience. If the body be overtired, it tires the mind. The mind oppresseth the body, as with students it oftentimes falls out, who (as Plutarch observes [1]) have no care of the body, "but compel that which is mortal to do as much as that which is immortal: that which is earthly, as that which is ethereal. But as the ox, tired, told the camel (both serving one master) that refused to carry some part of his burden, before it were long he should be compelled to carry all his pack, and skin to boot (which by and by, the ox being dead, fell out), the body may say to the soul that will give him no respite or remission: a little after, an ague, vertigo, consumption, seizeth on them both, all his study is omitted, and they must be compelled to be sick together." He that tenders his own good estate and health must let them draw with equal yoke, both alike, "that so they may happily enjoy their wished health." [2]

MEMB. V.

Waking and terrible Dreams rectified

As waking, that hurts, by all means must be avoided, so sleep, which so much helps, by like ways "must be procured, by nature or art, inward or outward medicines, and be protracted longer than ordinary, if it may be, as being an especial help." [3] It moistens and fattens the body, concocts, and helps digestion, as we see in dormice, and those Alpine mice that sleep all winter, which Gesner speaks of, when they are so found sleeping under the snow in the dead of winter, as fat as butter. It expels cares, pacifies the mind, refresheth the weary limbs after long work:

> Somne quies rerum, placidissime somne deorum,
> Pax animi, quem cura fugit, qui corpora duris
> Fessa ministeriis mulces reparasque labori. [4]

> Sleep, rest of things, O pleasing deity,
> Peace of the soul, which cares dost crucify,
> Weary bodies refresh and mollify.

The chiefest thing in all physic, Paracelsus [5] calls it, *omnia arcana gemmarum superans et metallorum* [better than all the

secret powers of precious stones and metals]. The fittest time
is "two or three hours after supper, whenas the meat is now
settled at the bottom of the stomach, and 'tis good to lie on
the right side first, because at that site the liver doth rest under
the stomach, not molesting any way, but heating him as a fire
doth a kettle that is put to it. After the first sleep 'tis not
amiss to lie on the left side, that the meat may the better
descend"; [1] and sometimes again on the belly, but never on the
back. Seven or eight hours is a competent time for a melancholy man to rest, as Crato thinks; but as some do, to lie in bed
and not sleep, a day, or half a day together, to give assent to
pleasing conceits and vain imagination, is many ways pernicious.
To procure this sweet moistening sleep, it's best to take away
the occasions (if it be possible) that hinder it, and then to use
such inward or outward remedies which may cause it. *Constat
hodie* (saith Boissardus in his tract *de magia, cap.* 4) *multos ita
fascinari ut noctes integras exigant insomnes, summa inquietudine
animorum et corporum;* many cannot sleep for witches and
fascinations, which are too familiar in some places; they call it,
dare alicui malam noctem [giving a person a bad night]. But
the ordinary causes are heat and dryness, which must first be
removed; a hot and dry brain never sleeps well; [2] grief, fears,
cares, expectations, anxieties, great businesses, *in aurem utramque otiose ut dormias* [3] [that you may slumber peacefully on
either ear], and all violent perturbations of the mind, must in
some sort be qualified, before we can hope for any good repose.
He that sleeps in the day-time, or is in suspense, fear, anyway
troubled in mind, or goes to bed upon a full stomach,[4] may
never hope for quiet rest in the night; *nec enim meritoria somnos
admittunt,* as the poet saith; [5] inns and such-like troublesome
places are not for sleep; one calls "Ostler!" another, "Tapster!"
one cries and shouts, another sings, whoops, halloos:

> *Absentem cantat amicam,*
> *Multa prolutus vappa nauta atque viator.* [6]

[Well moistened with cheap wine, the sailor and the
wayfarer sing of their absent sweethearts.]

Who not accustomed to such noises can sleep amongst them?
He that will intend to take his rest must go to bed *animo securo,
quieto et libero,* with a secure and composed mind,[7] in a quiet
place: *omnia noctis erunt placida composta quiete* [at night all
will be hushed in calm tranquillity]: and if that will not serve,
or may not be obtained, to seek then such means as are requisite.

To lie in clean linen and sweet; before he goes to bed, or in bed, to hear "sweet music," [1] which Ficinus commends, *lib. 1, cap. 24,* or, as Jobertus, *Med. pract. lib. 3, cap.* 10, "to read some pleasant author till he be asleep, to have a basin of water still dropping by his bedside," [2] or to lie near that pleasant murmur, *lene sonantis aquæ* [3] [of gently trickling water], some flood-gates, arches, falls of water, like London Bridge, or some continuate noise which may benumb the senses; *lenis motus, silentium et tenebra, tum et ipsa voluntas somnos faciunt:* as a gentle noise to some procures sleep, so, which Bernardinus Tilesius, *lib. de somno,* well observes, silence, in a dark room, and the will itself, is most available to others.   Piso commends frications, Andrew Borde a good draught of strong drink before one goes to bed; I say, a nutmeg and ale, or a good draught of muscadine, with a toast and nutmeg, or a posset of the same, which many use in a morning, but, methinks, for such as have dry brains, are much more proper at night: some prescribe a sup of vinegar [4] as they go to bed, a spoonful, saith Aetius, *Tetrabib. lib. 2, ser. 2, cap.* 10, *lib.* 6, *cap.* 10. Ægineta, *lib. 3, cap.* 14; Piso, "a little after meat, because it rarefies melancholy, and procures an appetite to sleep." [5]   Donat. ab Altomar., *cap.* 7, and Mercurialis approve of it, if the malady proceed from the spleen. [6]   Sallust. Salvian., *lib. 2, cap. 1, de remed.,* Hercules de Saxonia, *in Pan.,* Ælianus Montaltus, *de morb. capitis, cap.* 28 *de melan.,* are altogether against it.   Lod. Mercatus, *de inter. morb. cau. lib.* 1, *cap.* 17, in some cases doth allow it.   Rhasis [7] seems to deliberate of it; though Simeon commend it (in sauce peradventure), he makes a question of it.   As for baths, fomentations, oils, potions, simples or compounds, inwardly taken to this purpose, I shall speak of them elsewhere. [8]   If in the midst of the night when they lie awake, which is usual to toss and tumble, and not sleep, Ranzovius [9] would have them, if it be in warm weather, to rise and walk three or four turns (till they be cold) about the chamber, and then go to bed again.

Against fearful and troublesome dreams, *incubus* [nightmare], and such inconveniences, wherewith melancholy men are molested, the best remedy is to eat a light supper, and of such meats as are easy of digestion, no hare, venison, beef, etc., not to lie on his back, not to meditate or think in the day-time of any terrible objects, or especially talk of them before he goes to bed.   For, as he said in Lucian after such conference, *Hecates somniare mihi videor,* I can think of nothing but hobgoblins: and, as Tully notes, [10] "for the most part our speeches in the

day-time cause our phantasy to work upon the like in our
sleep," which Ennius writes of Homer: *Et canis in somnis
leporis vestigia latrat:* as a dog dreams of a hare, so do men on
such subjects they thought on last.

> *Somnia quæ mentes ludunt volitantibus umbris,*
> *Nec delubra deum, nec ab æthere numina mittunt,*
> *Sed sibi quisque facit,* etc.[1]

> [The dreams which mock us with fleeting shadows are sent
> neither from the shrines of the gods nor by the gods
> themselves, but each of us makes his own.]

For that cause when Ptolemy, King of Egypt, had posed the
seventy interpreters in order, and asked the nineteenth man
what would make one sleep quietly in the night, he told him,
"the best way was to have divine and celestial meditations,
and to use honest actions in the day-time." [2] Lod. Vives [3]
"wonders how schoolmen could sleep quietly, and were not
terrified in the night, or walk in the dark, they had such monstrous questions, and thought of such terrible matters all day
long." They had need, amongst the rest, to sacrifice to God
Morpheus, whom Philostratus [4] paints in a white and black
coat, with a horn and ivory box full of dreams, of the same
colours, to signify good and bad. If you will know how to
interpret them, read Artemidorus, Sambucus, and Cardan; but
how to help them, I must refer you to a more convenient place.[5]

MEMB. VI.

SUBSECT. I.—*Perturbations of the Mind rectified. From himself,
by resisting to the utmost, confessing his grief to a friend, etc.*

WHOSOEVER he is that shall hope to cure this malady in himself.
or any other, must first rectify these passions and perturbations
of the mind; the chiefest cure consists in them. A quiet mind is
that *voluptas* [pleasure], or *summum bonum*, of Epicurus, *non
dolere, curis vacare, animo tranquillo esse*, not to grieve, but to
want cares and have a quiet soul, is the only pleasure of the
world, as Seneca truly recites his opinion, not that of eating
and drinking, which injurious Aristotle maliciously puts upon
him, and for which he is still mistaken, *male audit et vapulat*,
slandered without a cause, and lashed by all posterity. "Fear
and sorrow, therefore, are especially to be avoided, and the

mind to be mitigated with mirth, constancy, good hope; vain
terror, bad objects, are to be removed, and all such persons in
whose companies they be not well pleased." [1]　Gualter Bruel,
Fernelius, *consil.* 43, Mercurialis, *consil.* 6, Piso, Jacchinus,
cap. 15, *in* 9 *Rhasis*, Capivaccius, Hildesheim, etc., all inculcate this as an especial means of their cure, that their "minds
be quietly pacified, vain conceits diverted, if it be possible,
with terrors, cares,[2] fixed studies, cogitations, and whatsoever
it is that shall any way molest or trouble the soul," [3] because
that otherwise there is no good to be done.　"The body's mischiefs," as Plato proves, "proceed from the soul: and if the
mind be not first satisfied, the body can never be cured." [4]
Alcibiades raves (saith Maximus Tyrius [5]) and is sick, his furious
desires carry him from Lyceum to the pleading-place, thence
to the sea, so into Sicily, thence to Lacedæmon, thence to Persia,
thence to Samos, then again to Athens; Critias tyrannizeth
over all the city; Sardanapalus is love-sick; these men are
ill-affected all, and can never be cured till their minds be
otherwise qualified.　Crato, therefore, in that often-cited counsel
of his for a nobleman his patient, when he had sufficiently
informed him in diet, air, exercise, Venus, sleep, concludes with
these as matters of greatest moment, *Quod reliquum est, animæ
accidentia corrigantur* [it remains to correct the maladies of the
mind], from which alone proceeds melancholy; they are the
fountain, the subject, the hinges whereon it turns, and must
necessarily be reformed.　"For anger stirs choler, heats the
blood and vital spirits; sorrow on the other side refrigerates
the body, and extinguisheth natural heat, overthrows appetite,
hinders concoction, dries up the temperature, and perverts the
understanding";[6] fear dissolves the spirits, infects the heart,
attenuates the soul; and for these causes all passions and
perturbations must, to the uttermost of our power and most
seriously, be removed.　Ælianus Montaltus attributes so much
to them that he holds the rectification of them alone to be
sufficient to the cure of melancholy in most patients.[7]　Many
are fully cured when they have seen or heard, etc., enjoy their
desires, or be secured and satisfied in their minds; Galen, the
common master of them all, from whose fountain they fetch
water, brags, *lib.* 1 *de san. tuend.*, that he for his part hath
cured divers of this infirmity, *solum animis ad rectum institutis,*
by right settling alone of their minds.

　　Yea, but you will here infer that this is excellent good indeed
if it could be done; but how shall it be effected, by whom, what

art, what means? *hic labor, hoc opus est* [this is the task, this
the labour]. 'Tis a natural infirmity, a most powerful adversary; all men are subject to passions, and melancholy above all
others, as being distempered by their innate humours, abundance
of choler adust, weakness of parts, outward occurrences; and
how shall they be avoided? The wisest men, greatest philosophers, of most excellent wit, reason, judgment, divine spirits,
cannot moderate themselves in this behalf; such as are sound
in body and mind, Stoics, heroes, Homer's gods, all are passionate, and furiously carried sometimes; and how shall we that
are already crazed, *fracti animis*, sick in body, sick in mind,
resist? We cannot perform it. You may advise and give
good precepts, as who cannot? But how shall they be put in
practice? I may not deny but our passions are violent, and
tyrannize of us, yet there be means to curb them; though they
be headstrong, they may be tamed, they may be qualified, if
he himself or his friends will but use their honest endeavours, or
make use of such ordinary helps as are commonly prescribed.

"He himself," I say; from the patient himself the first and
chiefest remedy must be had; for if he be averse, peevish,
waspish, give way wholly to his passions, will not seek to be
helped or be ruled by his friends, how is it possible he should
be cured? But if he be willing at least, gentle, tractable, and
desire his own good, no doubt but he may *magnam morbi
deponere partem*, be eased at least, if not cured. He himself
must do his utmost endeavour to resist and withstand the
beginnings. *Principiis obsta.* "Give not water passage, no
not a little" (Ecclus. xxv, 25). If they open a little, they will
make a greater breach at length. Whatsoever it is that runneth
in his mind, vain conceit, be it pleasing or displeasing, which
so much affects or troubleth him, "by all possible means he
must withstand it, expel those vain, false, frivolous imaginations,
absurd conceits, feigned fears and sorrows; from which," saith
Piso, "this disease primarily proceeds, and takes his first
occasion or beginning, by doing something or other that shall
be opposite unto them, thinking of something else, persuading
by reason, or howsoever, to make a sudden alteration of them." [1]
Though he have hitherto run in a full career, and precipitated
himself, following his passions, giving reins to his appetite, let
him now stop upon a sudden, curb himself in; and, as Lemnius
adviseth,[2] "strive against with all his power, to the utmost
of his endeavour, and not cherish those fond imaginations which
so covertly creep into his mind, most pleasing and amiable at

first, but bitter as gall at last, and so headstrong that by no reason, art, counsel, or persuasion they may be shaken off." Though he be far gone, and habituated unto such phantastical imaginations, yet, as Tully and Plutarch advise,[1] let him oppose, fortify, or prepare himself against them, by premeditation, reason, or, as we do by a crooked staff, bend himself another way.

> *Tu tamen interea effugito quæ tristia mentem*
> *Sollicitant, procul esse jube curasque metumque*
> *Pallentem, ultrices iras; sint omnia læta.*[2]

> In the meantime expel them from thy mind,
> Pale fears, sad cares, and griefs which do it grind,
> Revengeful anger, pain and discontent;
> Let all thy soul be set on merriment.

Curas tolle graves, irasci crede profanum [dismiss all serious cares, count it sin to be angry]. If it be idleness hath caused this infirmity, or that he perceive himself given to solitariness, to walk alone, and please his mind with fond imaginations, let him by all means avoid it; 'tis a bosom enemy, 'tis delightsome melancholy, a friend in show, but a secret devil, a sweet poison, it will in the end be his undoing; let him go presently, task or set himself a work, get some good company. If he proceed, as a gnat flies about a candle, so long till at length he burn his body, so in the end he will undo himself; if it be any harsh object, ill company, let him presently go from it. If by his own default, through ill diet, bad air, want of exercise, etc., let him now begin to reform himself. "It would be a perfect remedy against all corruption, if," as Roger Bacon hath it,[3] "we could but moderate ourselves in those six non-natural things." "If it be any disgrace, abuse, temporal loss, calumny, death of friends, imprisonment, banishment, be not troubled with it, do not fear, be not angry, grieve not at it, but with all courage sustain it"[4] (Gordonius, *lib.* 1, *cap.* 15, *de conser. vit.*). *Tu contra audentior ito* [advance boldly to meet it]. If it be sickness, ill success, or any adversity that hath caused it, oppose an invincible courage, "fortify thyself by God's word, or otherwise,"[5] *mala bonis persuadenda*, set prosperity against adversity, as we refresh our eyes by seeing some pleasant meadow, fountain, picture, or the like; recreate thy mind by some contrary object, with some more pleasing meditation divert thy thoughts.

Yea, but you infer again, *facile consilium damus aliis*, we can easily give counsel to others; every man, as the saying is,

II—H 887

can tame a shrew but he that hath her; *si hic esses, aliter sentires*, if you were in our misery, you would find it otherwise, 'tis not so easily performed. We know this to be true; we should moderate ourselves, but we are furiously carried, we cannot make use of such precepts, we are overcome, sick, *male sani*, distempered and habituated to these courses, we can make no resistance; you may as well bid him that is diseased not to feel pain, as a melancholy man not to fear, not to be sad: 'tis within his blood, his brains, his whole temperature, it cannot be removed. But he may choose whether he will give way too far unto it, he may in some sort correct himself. A philosopher was bitten with a mad dog, and as the nature of that disease is to abhor all waters and liquid things, and to think still they see the picture of a dog before them, he went for all this, *reluctante se* [forcing himself], to the bath, and seeing there (as he thought) in the water the picture of a dog, with reason overcame this conceit; *Quid cani cum balneo?* what should a dog do in a bath? a mere conceit. Thou thinkest thou hearest and seest devils, black men, etc., 'tis not so, 'tis thy corrupt phantasy; settle thine imagination, thou art well. Thou thinkest thou hast a great nose, thou art sick, every man observes thee, laughs thee to scorn; persuade thyself 'tis no such matter: this is fear only, and vain suspicion. Thou art discontent, thou art sad and heavy; but why? upon what ground? consider of it: thou art jealous, timorous, suspicious; for what cause? examine it thoroughly, thou shalt find none at all, or such as is to be contemned, such as thou wilt surely deride, and contemn in thyself, when it is past. Rule thyself then with reason, satisfy thyself, accustom thyself, wean thyself from such fond conceits, vain fears, strong imaginations, restless thoughts. Thou mayest do it; *Est in nobis assuescere* (as Plutarch saith), we may frame ourselves as we will. As he that useth an upright shoe may correct the obliquity or crookedness by wearing it on the other side, we may overcome passions if we will. *Quicquid sibi imperavit animus obtinuit* (as Seneca saith[1]): *nulli tam feri affectus, ut non disciplina perdomentur:* whatsoever the will desires, she may command: no such cruel affections, but by discipline they may be tamed; voluntarily thou wilt not do this or that, which thou oughtest to do, or refrain, etc., but when thou art lashed like a dull jade, thou wilt reform it; fear of a whip will make thee do, or not do. Do that voluntarily then which thou canst do, and must do by compulsion: thou mayst refrain if thou wilt, and master thine affections. "As in a

city" (saith Melancthon) "they do by stubborn rebellious rogues
that will not submit themselves to political judgment, compel
them by force; so must we do by our affections. If the heart
will not lay aside those vicious motions, and the phantasy those
fond imaginations, we have another form of government to
enforce and refrain our outward members, that they be not led
by our passions." [1] If appetite will not obey, let the moving
faculty overrule her, let her resist and compel her to do otherwise. In an ague the appetite would drink; sore eyes that itch
would be rubbed; but reason saith no, and therefore the moving
faculty will not do it. Our phantasy would intrude a thousand
fears, suspicions, chimeras upon us, but we have reason to
resist, yet we let it be overborne by our appetite; "Imagination
enforceth spirits, which, by an admirable league of nature,
compel the nerves to obey, and they our several limbs": [2] we
give too much way to our passions. And as to him that is
sick of an ague all things are distasteful and unpleasant, *non
ex cibi vitio,* saith Plutarch, not in the meat, but in our taste,
so many things are offensive to us, not of themselves, but out of
our corrupt judgment, jealousy, suspicion, and the like; we pull
these mischiefs upon our own heads.

If then our judgment be so depraved, our reason overruled,
will precipitated, that we cannot seek our own good, or moderate
ourselves, as in this disease commonly it is, the best way for
ease is to impart our misery to some friend, not to smother it
up in our own breast; *alitur vitium crescitque tegendo* [a fault
grows and becomes stronger by being covered up], etc., and
that which was most offensive to us, a cause of fear and grief,
quod nunc te coquit, another hell; for *strangulat inclusus dolor
atque excestuat intus,*[3] grief concealed strangles the soul; but
whenas we shall but import it to some discreet, trusty, loving
friend, it is instantly removed,[4] by his counsel haply, wisdom,
persuasion, advice, his good means, which we could not otherwise apply unto ourselves. A friend's counsel is a charm, like
mandrake wine, *curas sopit* [it assuages our care]; and as a bull
that is tied to a fig-tree becomes gentle on a sudden [5] (which
some, saith Plutarch,[6] interpret of good words), so is a savage,
obdurate heart mollified by fair speeches. "All adversity finds
ease in complaining" (as Isidore holds [7]), "and 'tis a solace to
relate it," ἀγαθὴ δὲ παραίφασίς ἐστιν ἐταίρου [8] [sweet is the com-
forting of a comrade]. Friends' confabulations are comfortable
at all times, as fire in winter, shade in summer, *quale sopor
fessis in gramine* [like sleep on the grass to the weary], meat

and drink to him that is hungry or athirst; Democritus' colly-
rium is not so sovereign to the eyes as this is to the heart; good
words are cheerful and powerful of themselves, but much more
from friends, as so many props, mutually sustaining each other
like ivy and a wall, which Camerarius hath well illustrated in
an emblem.[1] *Lenit animum simplex vel sæpe narratio*, the
simple narration many times easeth our distressed mind, and
in the midst of greatest extremities; so divers have been relieved,
by exonerating themselves to a faithful friend:[2] he sees that
which we cannot see for passion and discontent, he pacifies our minds, he will ease our pain, assuage our anger;
Quanta inde voluptas! quanta securitas! Chrysostom adds, what
pleasure, what security by that means! "Nothing so available,
or that so much refresheth the soul of man."[3] Tully, as I
remember, in an epistle to his dear friend Atticus, much condoles the defect of such a friend. "I live here" (saith he) "in
a great city, where I have a multitude of acquaintance, but not
a man of all that company with whom I dare familiarly breathe,
or freely jest. Wherefore I expect thee, I desire thee, I send
for thee; for there be many things which trouble and molest
me, which, had I but thee in presence, I could quickly disburden myself of in a walking discourse."[4] The like, peradventure, may he and he say with that old man in the comedy,

Nemo est meorum amicorum hodie,
Apud quem expromere occulta mea audeam,

[I have not one friend to-day to whom I can open my heart,]

and much inconvenience may both he and he suffer in the
meantime by it. He or he, or whosoever then labours of this
malady, by all means let him get some trusty friend, *Semper
habens Pyladémque aliquem qui curet Orestem,*[5] a Pylades, to
whom freely and securely he may open himself. For as in all
other occurrences, so it is in this, *Si quis in cœlum ascendisset,*
etc., as he said in Tully,[6] if a man had gone to heaven, "seen
the beauty of the skies," stars errant, fixed, etc., *insuavis erit
admiratio*, it will do him no pleasure, except he have somebody
to impart what he hath seen. It is the best thing in the world,
as Seneca therefore adviseth in such a case,[7] "to get a trusty
friend, to whom we may freely and sincerely pour out our
secrets; nothing so delighteth and easeth the mind, as when
we have a prepared bosom, to which our secrets may descend,
of whose conscience we are assured as our own, whose speech
may ease our succourless estate, counsel relieve, mirth expel

our mourning, and whose very sight may be acceptable unto us." It was the counsel which that politic Comineus [1] gave to all princes, and others distressed in mind, by occasion of Charles, Duke of Burgundy, that was much perplexed, "first to pray to God, and lay himself open to Him, and then to some special friend, whom we hold most dear, to tell all our grievances to him; nothing so forcible to strengthen, recreate, and heal the wounded soul of a miserable man."

SUBSECT. II.—*Help from friends by counsel, comfort, fair and foul means, witty devices, satisfaction, alteration of his course of life, removing objects, etc.*

When the patient of himself is not able to resist or overcome these heart-eating passions, his friends or physician must be ready to supply that which is wanting. *Suæ erit humanitatis et sapientiæ* (which Tully [2] enjoineth in like case) *siquid erratum, curare, aut improvisum, sua diligentia corrigere* [he must exercise his own friendship and wisdom to set right any mistake or remedy any unforeseen ill]. They must all join; *nec satis medico*, saith Hippocrates,[3] *suum fecisse officium, nisi suum quoque ægrotus, suum astantes* [it is not enough for the physician to do his duty, the patient and his friends must also do theirs], etc. First, they must especially beware, a melancholy discontented person (be it in what kind of melancholy soever) never be left alone or idle; but as physicians prescribe physic, *cum custodia*, let them not be left unto themselves, but with some company or other, lest by that means they aggravate and increase their disease; *non oportet ægros hujusmodi esse solos vel inter ignotos, vel inter eos quos non amant aut negligunt* [such sick persons should not be left by themselves or among strangers, or with persons whom they do not care for], as Rod. à Fonseca, *tom.* 1, *consult.* 35, prescribes. *Lugentes custodire solemus* (saith Seneca[4]) *ne solitudine male utantur*: we watch a sorrowful person, lest he abuse his solitariness, and so should we do a melancholy man; set him about some business, exercise or recreation, which may divert his thoughts, and still keep him otherwise intent; for his phantasy is so restless, operative and quick, that if it be not in perpetual action, ever employed, it will work upon itself, melancholize, and be carried away instantly, with some fear, jealousy, discontent, suspicion, some vain conceit or other.

If his weakness be such that he cannot discern what is amiss, correct, or satisfy, it behoves them by counsel, comfort, or persuasion, by fair or foul means, to alienate his mind, by some artificial invention, or some contrary persuasion, to remove all objects, causes, companies, occasions, as may anyways molest him, to humour him, please him, divert him, and, if it be possible, by altering his course of life, to give him security and satisfaction. If he conceal his grievances, and will not be known of them, "they must observe by his looks, gestures, motions, phantasy, what it is that offends," [1] and then to apply remedies unto him. Many are instantly cured, when their minds are satisfied. Alexander makes mention of a woman, "that, by reason of her husband's long absence in travel, was exceeding peevish and melancholy, but when she heard her husband was returned, beyond all expectation, at the first sight of him, she was freed from all fear, without help of any other physic restored to her former health." [2]   Trincavellius, *consil.* 12, *lib.* 1, hath such a story of a Venetian that, being much troubled with melancholy, "and ready to die for grief, when he heard his wife was brought to bed of a son, instantly recovered." [3]   As Alexander concludes, "If our imaginations be not inveterate, by this art they may be cured, especially if they proceed from such a cause." [4]   No better way to satisfy than to remove the object, cause, occasion, if by any art or means possible we may find it out.   If he grieve, stand in fear, be in suspicion, suspense, or anyway molested, secure him, *solvitur malum*, give him satisfaction, the cure is ended; alter his course of life, there needs no other physic.   If the party be sad, or otherwise affected, "consider" (saith Trallianus [5]) "the manner of it, all circumstances, and forthwith make a sudden alteration," by removing the occasions; avoid all terrible objects, heard or seen, "monstrous and prodigious aspects," [6] tales of devils, spirits, ghosts, tragical stories; to such as are in fear they strike a great impression, renew many times, and recall such chimeras and terrible fictions into their minds.   "Make not so much as mention of them in private talk, or a dumb show tending to that purpose: such things" (saith Galatæus) "are offensive to their imaginations." [7]   And to those that are now in sorrow, Seneca [8] forbids "all sad companions, and such as lament; a groaning companion is an enemy to quietness."   "Or if there be any such party, at whose presence the patient is not well pleased, he must be removed: gentle speeches and fair means must first be tried; no harsh language used, or uncomfortable words; and

not expel, as some do, one madness with another; he that so
doth is madder than the patient himself": [1] all things must be
quietly composed; *eversa non evertenda, sed erigenda*, things
down must not be dejected, but reared, as Crato counselleth;
"he must be quietly and gently used," [2] and we should not do
anything against his mind, but by little and little effect it.
As a horse that starts at a drum or trumpet, and will not endure
the shooting of a piece, may be so manned by art, and animated,
that he cannot only endure, but is much more generous at the
hearing of such things, much more courageous than before, and
much delighteth in it: they must not be reformed *ex abrupto*
[abruptly], but by all art and insinuation, made to such companies, aspects, objects they could not formerly away with.
Many at first cannot endure the sight of a green wound, a sick
man, which afterward become good chirurgeons, bold empirics:
a horse starts at a rotten post afar off, which coming near he
quietly passeth.   'Tis much in the manner of making such kind
of persons; be they never so averse from company, bashful,
solitary, timorous, they may be made at last, with those Roman
matrons, to desire nothing more than, in a public show, to see
a full company of gladiators breathe out their last.

If they may not otherwise be accustomed to brook such distasteful and displeasing objects, the best way then is generally
to avoid them.   Montanus, *consil. 229*, to the Earl of Montfort,
a courtier, and his melancholy patient, adviseth him to leave
the court, by reason of those continual discontents, crosses,
abuses, "cares, suspicions, emulations, ambition, anger, jealousy,
which that place afforded, and which surely caused him to be
so melancholy at the first." [3]   *Maxima quæque domus servis
est plena superbis* [every great house is full of haughty slaves];
a company of scoffers and proud Jacks are commonly conversant and attendant in such places, and able to make any
man that is of a soft, quiet disposition (as many times they do)
ex stulto insanum, if once they humour him, a very idiot, or
stark mad.   A thing too much practised in all common societies;
and they have no better sport than to make themselves merry
by abusing some silly fellow, or to take advantage of another
man's weakness.   In such cases, as in a plague, the best remedy
is *cito, longe, tarde* (for to such a party, especially if he be
apprehensive, there can be no greater misery), to get him quickly
gone, far enough off, and not to be overhasty in his return.   If
he be so stupid that he do not apprehend it, his friends should
take some order, and by their discretion supply that which is

wanting in him, as in all other cases they ought to do. If
they see a man melancholy given, solitary, averse from company, please himself with such private and vain meditations,
though he delight in it, they ought by all means seek to divert
him, to dehort him, to tell him of the event and danger that may
come of it. If they see a man idle, that by reason of his means
otherwise will betake himself to no course of life, they ought
seriously to admonish him he makes a noose to entangle
himself, his want of employment will be his undoing. If he have
sustained any great loss, suffered a repulse, disgrace, etc., if
it be possible, relieve him. If he desire aught, let him be
satisfied; if in suspense, fear, suspicion, let him be secured: and
if it may conveniently be, give him his heart's content; for the
body cannot be cured till the mind be satisfied. Socrates, in
Plato, would prescribe no physic for Charmides' headache, "till
first he had eased his troublesome mind; body and soul must
be cured together, as head and eyes." [1]

> *Oculum non curabis sine toto capite,*
> *Nec caput sine toto corpore,*
> *Nec totum corpus sine anima.* [2]

[The eye cannot be cured without the whole head,
   nor the head without the whole body, nor the
   body without the mind.]

If that may not be hoped or expected, yet ease him with comfort, cheerful speeches, fair promises, and good words; persuade
him, advise him. "Many," saith Galen, "have been cured by
good counsel and persuasion alone." [3] "Heaviness of the heart
of man doth bring it down, but a good word rejoiceth it"
(Prov. xii, 25). "And there is he that speaketh words like
the pricking of a sword, but the tongue of a wise man is health"
(ver. 18). *Oratio namque saucii animi est remedium,* a gentle
speech is the true cure of a wounded soul, as Plutarch [4] contends out of Æschylus and Euripides; "if it be wisely administered it easeth grief and pain, as divers remedies do many
other diseases." 'Tis *incantationis instar,* a charm, *æstuantis
animi refrigerium* [to calm a storm-tossed mind], that true
nepenthe of Homer, which was no Indian plant, or feigned
medicine, which Epidamna, Thon's wife, sent Helena for a
token, as Macrobius, 7 *Saturnal.,* Goropius, *Hermath., lib.* 9,
Greg. Nazianzen, and others suppose, but opportunity of
speech: for Helena's bowl, Medea's unction, Venus' girdle,
Circe's cup, cannot so enchant, so forcibly move or alter as it

doth. A letter sent or read will do as much; *Multum allevor
quum tuas literas lego,* "I am much eased," as Tully writ to
Pomponius Atticus,[1] "when I read thy letters"; and as Julianus
the Apostate once signified to Maximus the philosopher, "As
Alexander slept with Homer's works, so do I with thine epistles,
*tanquam Pæoniis medicamentis, easque assidue tanquam recentes
et novas iteramus; scribe ergo, et assidue scribe* [as though they
were the finest medicine. I peruse them again greedily as
though they were fresh; write, therefore, and write diligently],
or else come thyself; *amicus ad amicum venies* [come to your
old friend]." Assuredly a wise and well-spoken man may do
what he will in such a case; a good orator alone, as Tully holds,[2]
can alter affections by power of his eloquence, "comfort such
as are afflicted, erect such as are depressed, expel and mitigate
fear, lust, anger," etc. And how powerful is the charm of a
discreet and dear friend! *Ille regit dictis animos et temperat
iras* [he soothes their angry passions with his words]. What
may not he effect? As Chremes told Menedemus,[3] "Fear not,
conceal it not, O friend! but tell me what it is that troubles thee,
and I shall surely help thee by comfort, counsel, or in the matter
itself." Arnoldus, *lib.* 1 *Breviar. cap.* 18, speaks of a usurer
in his time, that upon a loss, much melancholy and discontent,
was so cured.[4] As imagination, fear, grief, cause such passions,
so conceits alone, rectified by good hope, counsel, etc., are able
again to help; and 'tis incredible how much they can do in
such a case, as Trincavellius [5] illustrates by an example of a
patient of his. Porphyrius, the philosopher, in Plotinus' life
(written by him), relates that, being in a discontented humour
through unsufferable anguish of mind, he was going to make
away himself; but meeting by chance his master Plotinus, who,
perceiving by his distracted looks all was not well, urged him
to confess his grief; which when he had heard, he used such
comfortable speeches, that he redeemed him *e faucibus Erebi*
[from the jaws of Hades], pacified his unquiet mind, insomuch
that he was easily reconciled to himself, and much abashed to
think afterwards that he should ever entertain so vile a motion.
By all means, therefore, fair promises, good words, gentle persuasions are to be used, not to be too rigorous at first, "or to
insult over them, not to deride, neglect, or contemn, but rather,"
as Lemnius exhorteth, "to pity, and by all plausible means to
seek to reduce them"; [6] but if satisfaction may not be had,
mild courses, promises, comfortable speeches, and good counsel
will not take place; then, as Christopherus à Vega determines,

lib. 3, *cap.* 14, *de mel.* to handle them more roughly, to threaten
and chide, saith Altomarus,[1] terrify sometimes, or, as Salvianus
will have them, to be lashed and whipped, as we do by a starting
horse that is affrighted without a cause,[2] or, as Rhasis adviseth,
"one while to speak fair and flatter, another while to terrify
and chide,[3] as they shall see cause."

When none of these precedent remedies will avail, it will not
be amiss, which Savonarola and Ælian Montaltus so much
commend, *clavum clavo pellere* [to drive out a nail with a nail],
"to drive out one passion with another, or by some contrary
passion,"[4] as they do bleeding at nose by letting blood in the
arm, to expel one fear with another, one grief with another.
Christopherus à Vega [5] accounts it rational physic, *non alienum
a ratione*; and Lemnius much approves it, "to use an hard
wedge to an hard knot," to drive out one disease with another,
to pull out a tooth, or wound him, to geld him, saith Platerus,[6]
as they did epileptical patients of old, because it quite alters the
temperature, that the pain of the one may mitigate the grief
of the other; "and I knew one that was so cured of a quartan
ague, by the sudden coming of his enemies upon him."[7] If
we may believe Pliny,[8] whom Scaliger calls *mendaciorum patrem*,
the father of lies, Q. Fabius Maximus, that renowned consul of
Rome, in a battle fought with the king of the Allobroges at the
river Isaurus, was so rid of a quartan ague. Valesius, in his
Controversies, holds this an excellent remedy, and, if it be
discreetly used in this malady, better than any physic.

Sometimes again by some feigned lie, strange news, witty
device, artificial invention, it is not amiss to deceive them.[9]
"As they hate those," saith Alexander,[10] "that neglect or deride,
so they will give ear to such as will soothe them up. If they
say they have swallowed frogs or a snake, by all means grant
it, and tell them you can easily cure it"; 'tis an ordinary thing.
Philodotus the physician cured a melancholy king that thought
his head was off, by putting a leaden cap thereon; the weight
made him perceive it, and freed him of his fond imagination.
A woman, in the said Alexander, swallowed a serpent as she
thought; he gave her a vomit, and conveyed a serpent, such
as she conceived, into the basin; upon the sight of it she was
amended. The pleasantest dotage that ever I read, saith
Laurentius,[11] was of a gentleman at Senes in Italy, who was
afraid to piss, lest all the town should be drowned; the physicians
caused the bells to be rung backward, and told him the town
was on fire, whereupon he made water, and was immediately

cured. Another supposed his nose so big that he should dash
it against the wall if he stirred; his physician took a great piece
of flesh, and holding it in his hand .pinched him by the nose,
making him believe that flesh was cut from it. Forestus, *Obs.
lib.* 1, had a melancholy patient who thought he was dead;
"he put a fellow in a chest, like a dead man, by his bed's side,
and made him rear himself a little, and eat: the melancholy
man asked the counterfeit whether dead men use to eat meat?
he told him yea; whereupon he did eat likewise and was cured."[1]
Lemnius, *lib. 2, cap. 6, de 4 complex.*, hath many such instances,
and Jovianus Pontanus, *lib. 4, cap. 2*, of Wisdom, of the like:
but amongst the rest I find one most memorable, registered in
the French chronicles,[2] of an advocate of Paris before mentioned,
who believed verily he was dead, etc. I read a multitude of
examples of melancholy men cured by such artificial inventions.

SUBSECT. III.—*Music a Remedy*

Many and sundry are the means which philosophers and
physicians have prescribed to exhilarate a sorrowful heart, to
divert those fixed and intent cares and meditations, which in
this malady so much offend; but in my judgment none so
present, none so powerful, none so apposite as a cup of strong
drink, mirth, music, and merry company. Ecclus. xl, 20,
"Wine and music rejoice the heart." Rhasis, *Cont. 9, tract. 15,*
Altomarus, *cap. 7,* Ælianus Montaltus, *cap. 26,* Ficinus, Bened.
Victor. Faventinus, are almost immoderate in the commendation of it; a most forcible medicine Jacchinus [3] calls it; Jason
Pratensis,[4] "a most admirable thing, and worthy of consideration, that can so mollify the mind, and stay those tempestuous
affections of it." *Musica est mentis medicina mœstæ,* [music is] a
roaring-meg against melancholy, to rear and revive the languishing soul; "affecting not only the ears, but the very arteries,
the vital and animal spirits, it erects the mind, and makes it
nimble" [5] (Lemnius, *Instit. cap.* 44). This it will effect in the
most dull, severe, and sorrowful souls, "expel grief with mirth,
and if there be any clouds, dust, or dregs of cares yet lurking
in our thoughts, most powerfully it wipes them all away" [6]
(Sarisbur. *Polycrat. lib. 1, cap.* 6), and that which is more, it
will perform all this in an instant: "cheer up the countenance,
expel austerity, bring in hilarity" (Girald. Camb. *cap. 12 Topog.
Hiber.*), "inform our manners, mitigate anger." [7] Athenæus
(*Deipnosophist. lib. 14, cap.* 10) calleth it an infinite treasure to

such as are endowed with it. *Dulcisonum reficit tristia corda
melos* [a sweet melody restoreth a sad heart] (Eobanus Hessus).
Many other properties Cassiodorus, *epist.* 4, reckons up of this
our divine music, not only to expel the greatest griefs, but
"it doth extenuate fears and furies, appeaseth cruelty, abateth
heaviness, and to such as are watchful it causeth quiet rest;
it takes away spleen and hatred,"[1] be it instrumental, vocal,
with strings, wind, *quæ a spiritu, sine manuum dexteritate
gubernetur*[2] [such as are played with the breath, without any
action of the hands], etc.; it cures all irksomeness and heaviness
of the soul. Labouring men that sing to their work can tell
as much,[3] and so can soldiers when they go to fight, whom
terror of death cannot so much affright as the sound of trumpet,
drum, fife, and such-like music animates; *metus enim mortis*,
as Censorinus informeth us,[4] *musica depellitur* [for the fear of
death can be banished by music]. "It makes a child quiet,"
the nurse's song; and many times the sound of a trumpet on a
sudden, bells ringing, a carman's whistle, a boy singing some
ballad tune early in the street, alters, revives, recreates a
restless patient that cannot sleep in the night, etc. In a word,
it is so powerful a thing that it ravisheth the soul, *regina sensuum*,
the queen of the senses, by sweet pleasure (which is a happy
cure), and corporal tunes pacify our incorporeal soul; *sine ore
loquens, dominatum in animam exercet* [speaking without a
mouth, it exercises domination over the soul], and carries it
beyond itself, helps, elevates, extends it. Scaliger, *exercit.* 302,
gives a reason of these effects, "because the spirits about the
heart take in that trembling and dancing air into the body,
are moved together, and stirred up with it,"[5] or else the mind,
as some suppose, harmonically composed, is roused up at the
tunes of music. And 'tis not only men that are so affected,
but almost all other creatures. You know the tale of Hercules
Gallus, Orpheus, and Amphion, *felices animas* [blessed souls]
Ovid calls them, that could *saxa movere sono testudinis*, etc.
make stocks and stones, as well as beasts and other animals,
dance after their pipes: the dog and hare, wolf and lamb;
vicinumque lupo præbuit agna latus [the lamb lay down by the
side of the wolf]; *clamosus graculus, stridula cornix, et Jovis
aquila* [the chattering daw, the croaking rook, the eagle of Jove],
as Philostratus describes it in his Images, stood all gaping upon
Orpheus; and trees pulled up by the roots came to hear him,[6]
Et comitem quercum pinus amica trahit [the pine brought the oak
in company].

Arion made fishes follow him, which, as common experience
evinceth, are much affected with music.[1] All singing-birds are
much pleased with it, especially nightingales, if we may believe
Calcagninus; and bees amongst the rest, though they be flying
away, when they hear any tingling sound, will tarry behind.
"Harts, hinds, horses, dogs, bears, are exceedingly delighted
with it" (Scal. *exerc.* 302);[2] elephants, Agrippa adds, *lib. 2,
cap.* 24; and in Lydia in the midst of a lake there be certain
floating islands (if ye will believe it), that after music will dance.

But to leave all declamatory speeches in praise of divine
music,[3] I will confine myself to my proper subject: besides that
excellent power it hath to expel many other diseases, it is a
sovereign remedy against despair and melancholy,[4] and will
drive away the devil himself. Canus, a Rhodian fiddler in
Philostratus,[5] when Apollonius was inquisitive to know what
he could do with his pipe, told him, "that he would make a
melancholy man merry, and him that was merry much merrier
than before, a lover more enamoured, a religious man more
devout." Ismenias the Theban, Chiron the centaur,[6] is said
to have cured this and many other diseases by music alone: as
now they do those, saith Bodine,[7] that are troubled with St.
Vitus' Bedlam dance. Timotheus, the musician, compelled
Alexander to skip up and down, and leave his dinner [9] (like the
tale of the Friar and the Boy), whom Austin, *de Civ. Dei, lib.* 17,
cap. 14, so much commends for it. Who hath not heard how
David's harmony drove away the evil spirits from King Saul
(1 Sam. xvi); and Elisha, when he was much troubled by
importunate kings, called for a minstrel, "and when he played,
the hand of the Lord came upon him" (2 Kings iii). Censorinus,
de natali, cap. 12, reports how Asclepiades the physician helped
many frantic persons by this means, *phreneticorum mentes morbo
turbatas.* Jason Pratensis, *cap. de mania,* hath many examples,
how Clinias and Empedocles cured some desperately melancholy,
and some mad, by this our music. Which because it hath such
excellent virtues, belike Homer [9] brings in Phemius playing,
and the Muses singing, at the banquet of the gods. Aristotle,
Polit. lib. 8, *cap.* 5, Plato, 2 *de legibus,* highly approve it, and so
do all politicians. The Greeks, Romans, have graced music,
and made it one of the liberal sciences, though it be now become
mercenary. All civil commonwealths allow it: Cneius Manlius
(as Livius relates [10]), *anno ab urb. cond.* 567, brought first out of
Asia to Rome singing-wenches, players, jesters, and all kind of
music to their feasts. Your princes, emperors, and persons of

any quality, maintain it in their courts; no mirth without music. Sir Thomas More, in his absolute Utopian common-wealth, allows music as an appendix to every meal, and that throughout, to all sorts. Epictetus calls *mensam mutam præsepe*, a table without music a manger; for "the concent of musicians at a banquet is a carbuncle set in gold; and as the signet of an emerald well trimmed with gold, so is the melody of music in a pleasant banquet" (Ecclus. xxxii, 5, 6). Louis the Eleventh,[1] when he invited Edward the Fourth to come to Paris, told him that, as a principal part of his entertainment, he should hear sweet voices of children, Ionic and Lydian tunes, exquisite music, he should have a ——, and the Cardinal of Bourbon to be his confessor, which he used as a most plausible argument; as to a sensual man indeed it is. Lucian, in his book *de saltatione*, is not ashamed to confess that he took infinite delight in singing, dancing, music, women's company, and such-like pleasures: "and if thou" (saith he) "didst but hear them play and dance, I know thou wouldst be so well pleased with the object that thou wouldst dance for company thyself, without doubt thou wilt be taken with it."[2] So Scaliger ingenuously confesseth, *exercit.* 274, "I am beyond all measure affected with music, I do most willingly behold them dance, I am mightily detained and allured with that grace and comeliness of fair women, I am well pleased to be idle amongst them."[3] And what young man is not? As it is acceptable and conducing to most, so especially to a melancholy man; provided always, his disease proceed not originally from it, that he be not some light *inamorato*, some idle phantastic, who capers in conceit all the day long, and thinks of nothing else but how to make jigs, sonnets, madrigals, in commendation of his mistress. In such cases music is most pernicious, as a spur to a free horse will make him run himself blind, or break his wind; *incitamentum enim amoris musica* [for music is a stimulus to love], for music enchants, as Menander holds, it will make such melancholy persons mad, and the sound of those jigs and hornpipes will not be removed out of the ears a week after. Plato[4] for this reason forbids music and wine to all young men, because they are most part amorous, *ne ignis addatur igni*, lest one fire increase another. Many men are melancholy by hearing music, but it is a pleasing melancholy that it causeth; and therefore to such as are discontent, in woe, fear, sorrow, or dejected, it is a most present remedy: it expels cares, alters their grieved minds, and easeth in an instant. Otherwise, saith

Plutarch,[1] *musica magis dementat quam vinum* [music maddens
more than wine]; music makes some men mad as a tiger; like
Astolpho's horn in Ariosto, or Mercury's golden wand in Homer,
that made some wake, others sleep, it hath divers effects; and
Theophrastus right well prophesied that diseases were either
procured by music or mitigated.[2]

SUBSECT. IV.—*Mirth and merry company, fair objects, Remedies*

   Mirth and merry company may not be separated from music,
both concerning and necessarily required in this business.
"Mirth" (saith Vives[3]) "purgeth the blood, confirms health,
causeth a fresh, pleasing, and fine colour," prorogues life, whets
the wit, makes the body young, lively, and fit for any manner
of employment. The merrier the heart the longer the life;
"A merry heart is the life of the flesh" (Prov. xiv, 30); "Gladness prolongs his days" (Ecclus. xxx, 22); and this is one of the
three Salernitan doctors, Dr. Merryman, Dr. Diet, Dr. Quiet,
which cures all diseases[4]—*Mens hilaris, requies, moderata diæta*
[cheerfulness, rest, temperate diet]. Gomesius, *præfat. lib. 3
de sal. gen.*, is a great magnifier of honest mirth, by which (saith
he) "we cure many passions of the mind in ourselves, and in
our friends";[5] which Galatæus[6] assigns for a cause why we love
merry companions: and well they deserve it, being that, as
Magninus holds,[7] a merry companion is better than any music,
and, as the saying is, *comes jucundus in via pro vehiculo*, as a
wagon to him that is wearied on the way. *Jucunda confabu-
latio, sales, joci*, pleasant discourse, jests, conceits, merry tales,
melliti verborum globuli ["dainty-fine honey-pellets of words"],
as Petronius, Pliny,[8] Spondanus,[9] Cælius,[10] and many good
authors plead, arc that sole nepenthes of Homer, Helena's
bowl, Venus' girdle, so renowned of old to expel grief and care,
to cause mirth and gladness of heart,[11] if they be rightly understood, or seasonably applied. In a word,

> *Amor, voluptas, Venus, gaudium,*
> *Jocus, ludus, sermo suavis, suaviatio,*[12]

   [Love, pleasure, Venus, joy, merriment, pleasant
   conversation, kissing,]

are the true nepenthes. For these causes our physicians
generally prescribe this as a principal engine to batter the
walls of melancholy, a chief antidote, and a sufficient cure of

itself. "By all means" (saith Mesue[1]) "procure mirth to these
men in such things as are heard, seen, tasted, or smelled, or
anyway perceived, and let them have all enticements and fair
promises, the sight of excellent beauties, attires, ornaments,
delightsome passages, to distract their minds from fear and
sorrow, and such things on which they are so fixed and intent."
"Let them use hunting, sports, plays, jests, merry company,"
as Rhasis prescribes, "which will not let the mind be molested,
a cup of good drink now and then, hear music, and have such
companions with whom they are especially delighted"; [2] "merry
tales or toys, drinking, singing, dancing, and whatsoever else
may procure mirth"; [3] and by no means, saith Guianerius,
suffer them to be alone. Benedictus Victorius Faventinus, in
his Empirics, accounts it an especial remedy against melancholy, "to hear and see singing, dancing, maskers, mummers,
to converse with such merry fellows and fair maids."[4] For
"the beauty of a woman cheereth the countenance" (Ecclus.
xxxvi, 22). Beauty alone is a sovereign remedy against fear,
grief, and all melancholy fits; a charm, as Peter de la Seine [5]
and many other writers affirm, a banquet itself; he gives instance
in discontented Menelaus, that was so often freed by Helena's
fair face: and Tully, 3 *Tusc.*, cites Epicurus as a chief patron of
this tenent.[6] To expel grief, and procure pleasance, sweet smells,
good diet, touch, taste, embracing, singing, dancing, sports,
plays, and, above the rest, exquisite beauties, *quibus oculi
jucunde moventur et animi* [which take the eye and charm the
mind], are most powerful means, *obvia forma*, to meet or see a
fair maid pass by, or to be in company with her. He found it
by experience, and made good use of it in his own person, if
Plutarch belie him not; for he reckons up the names of some
more elegant pieces, Leontium, Boedina, Hedeia, Nicidium, that
were frequently seen in Epicurus' garden,[7] and very familiar
in his house. Neither did he try it himself alone, but if we may
give credit to Athenæus,[8] he practised it upon others. For when
a sad and sick patient was brought unto him to be cured, "he
laid him on a down bed, crowned him with a garland of sweet-
smelling flowers, in a fair perfumed closet delicately set out, and,
after a potion or two of good drink which he administered, he
brought in a beautiful young wench [9] that could play upon a
lute, sing and dance," etc. Tully, 3 *Tusc.*, scoffs at Epicurus
for this his profane physic (as well he deserved), and yet
Favorinus and Stobæus highly approve of it. Most of our
looser physicians in some cases, to such parties especially, allow

of this; and all of them will have a melancholy, sad, and discontented person make frequent use of honest sports, companies, and recreations, *et incitandos ad Venerem*, as Rodericus à Fonseca will,[1] *aspectu et contactu pulcherrimarum feminarum* [and] to be drawn to such consorts [with beautiful women], whether they will or no. Not to be an auditor only, or a spectator, but sometimes an actor himself. *Dulce est desipere in loco*, to play the fool now and then is not amiss, there is a time for all things. Grave Socrates would be merry by fits, sing, dance, and take his liquor too, or else Theodoret belies him; so would old Cato, Tully by his own confession,[2] and the rest. Xenophon, in his *Sympos.*, brings in Socrates as a principal actor, no man merrier than himself, and sometimes he would "ride a cock-horse with his children,"[3] *equitare in arundine longa* (though Alcibiades scoffed at him for it), and well he might; for now and then (saith Plutarch) the most virtuous, honest, and gravest men will use feasts, jests, and toys, as we do sauce to our meats. So did Scipio and Lælius:

> *Quin ubi se a vulgo et scena in secreta remorant,*
> *Virtus Scipiadæ et mitis sapientia Læli,*
> *Nugari cum illo, et discincti ludere, donec*
> *Decoqueretur olus, soliti.*[4]

> Valorous Scipio and gentle Lælius,
> Removed from the scene and rout so clamorous,
> Were wont to recreate themselves, their robes laid by,
> Whilst supper by the cook was making ready.

Machiavel, in the eighth book of his Florentine History, gives this note of Cosmus Medices,[5] the wisest and gravest man of his time in Italy, that he would "now and then play the most egregious fool in his carriage, and was so much given to jesters, players and childish sports, to make himself merry, that he that should but consider his gravity on the one part, his folly and lightness on the other, would surely say, there were two distinct persons in him."[6] Now methinks he did well in it, though Sarisburiensis[7] be of opinion that magistrates, senators, and grave men should not descend to lighter sports, *ne respublica ludere videatur* [lest the State should seem to trifle], but, as Themistocles, still keep a stern and constant carriage. I commend Cosmus Medices, and Castruccius Castrucanus, than whom Italy never knew a worthier captain, another Alexander, if Machiavel do not deceive us in his life: "When a friend of his reprehended him for dancing beside his dignity" (belike at some cushion dance), he told him again, *qui sapit interdiu vix unquam noctu desipit*, he that is wise in the day may dote a little in the night.[1] Paulus Jovius relates as much of Pope Leo Decimus, that he was a grave, discreet, staid man, yet sometimes most free, and too open in his sports. And 'tis not altogether unfit or misbeseeming the gravity of such a man, if that decorum of time, place, and such circumstances be observed.[2] *Misce stultitiam consiliis brevem* [3] [mix a little folly with serious business]; and, as he said [4] in an epigram to his wife, I would have every man say to himself, or to his friend:

> Moll, once in pleasant company by chance,
> I wished that you for company would dance:
> Which you refused, and said, your years require,
> Now, matron-like, both manners and attire.
> Well, Moll, if needs you will be matron-like,
> Then trust to this, I will thee matron like:
> Yet so to you my love may never lessen,
> As you for church, house, bed, observe this lesson:
> Sit in the church as solemn as a saint,
> No deed, word, thought, your due devotion taint:
> Veil, if you will, your head, your soul reveal
> To him that only wounded souls can heal:
> Be in my house as busy as a bee,
> Having a sting for every one but me;
> Buzzing in every corner, gath'ring honey:
> Let nothing waste, that costs or yieldeth money.
> And when thou seest my heart to mirth incline,
> Thy tongue, wit, blood, warm with good cheer and wine:
> > Then of sweet sports let no occasion scape,
> > But be as wanton, toying, as an ape.[5]

Those old Greeks had their *Lubentiam deam*, goddess of pleasance,[6] and the Lacedemonians, instructed from Lycurgus, did *deo Risui sacrificare* [sacrifice to the god Laughter] after their wars especially, and in times of peace, which was used in Thessaly, as it appears by that of Apuleius,[7] who was made an instrument of their laughter himself, "because laughter and merriment was to season their labours and modester life." [8] *Risus enim divum atque hominum est æterna voluptas* [9] [for laughter is for ever the pleasure of men and gods]. Princes use jesters, players, and have those masters of revels in their courts. The Romans at every supper (for they had no solemn dinner) used music, gladiators, jesters, etc., as Suetonius relates of Tiberius,[10] Dion of Commodus, and so did the Greeks. Besides music, in Xenophon's *Sympos.*, *Philippus, ridendi artifex*, Philip, a jester, was brought to make sport. Paulus Jovius, in the eleventh book of his History, hath a pretty digression of

our English customs, which howsoever some may misconster,
I, for my part, will interpret to the best. "The whole nation
beyond all other mortal men is most given to banqueting and
feasts; for they prolong them many hours together, with dainty
cheer, exquisite music, and facete jesters, and afterwards they
fall a-dancing and courting their mistresses, till it be late in
the night." [1] Volaterran gives the same testimony of this
island, commending our jovial manner of entertainment and
good mirth, and methinks he saith well, there is no harm in it;
long may they use it, and all such modest sports. Ctesias reports
of a Persian king, that had 150 maids attending at his table,
to play, sing, and dance by turns; and Lil. Giraldus [2] of an
Egyptian prince, that kept nine virgins still to wait upon him,
and those of most excellent feature and sweet voices, which
afterwards gave occasion to the Greeks of that fiction of the
nine Muses. The king of Ethiopia in Africa, most of our Asiatic
princes have done so and do; those Sophies, Mogors, Turks, etc.,
solace themselves after supper amongst their queens and concubines, *quæ jucundioris oblectamenti causa* (saith mine author [3])
coram rege psallere et saltare consueverant, taking great pleasure
to see and hear them sing and dance. This and many such
means to exhilarate the heart of men have been still practised
in all ages, as knowing there is no better thing to the preservation of man's life. What shall I say then, but to every
melancholy man,

> *Utere convivis, non tristibus utere amicis,*
> *Quos nugæ et risus, et joca salsa juvant.* [4]

> Feast often, and use friends not still so sad,
> Whose jests and merriments may make thee glad.

Use honest and chaste sports, scenical shows, plays, games:
Accedant juvenumque chori, mistæque puellæ [5] [bring choruses
of youths and maidens together]. And, as Marsilius Ficinus
concludes an epistle to Bernard Canisianus and some other of
his friends, will I this tract to all good students: "Live merrily,
O my friends, free from cares, perplexity, anguish, grief of
mind, live merrily, [6] *lætitiæ cælum vos creavit* [Heaven created
you for mirth]. Again and again I request you to be merry,
if anything trouble your hearts, or vex your souls, neglect and
contemn it, [7] let it pass. [8] And this I enjoin you, not as a divine
alone, but as a physician; for without this mirth, which is the
life and quintessence of physic, medicines, and whatsoever is
used and applied to prolong the life of man, is dull, dead, and

of no force." [1]   *Dum fata sinunt, vivite læti* [while the fates
permit, live joyfully] (Seneca).   I say, be merry.

> *Nec lusibus virentem*
> *Viduemus hanc juventam.* [2]

> [Youth, whose month is May,
> From its merry play
> 'Twere not well to stay.]

It was Tiresias the prophet's counsel to Menippus, [3] that travelled
all the world over, even down to hell itself, to seek content, and
his last farewell to Menippus, to be merry.   "Contemn the
world" (saith he) "and count that is in it vanity and toys;
this only covet all thy life long; be not curious or over-solicitous
in anything, but with a well-composed and contented estate to
enjoy thyself, and above all things to be merry." [4]

> *Si, Mimnermus uti conset, sine amore jocisque*
> *Nil est jucundum, vivas in amore jocisque.*

> [If, as Mimnermus thinks, there is no pleasure in
> life without mirth and love, then live for
> mirth and love.]

"Nothing better" (to conclude with Solomon, Eccles. iii, 22)
"than that a man should rejoice in his affairs."   'Tis the same
advice which every physician in this case rings to his patient,
as Capivaccius to his, "Avoid overmuch study and perturbations of the mind, and as much as in thee lies live at heart's
ease"; [5] Prosper Calenus to that melancholy Cardinal Cæsius,
"Amidst thy serious studies and business, use jests and conceits, plays and toys, and whatsoever else may recreate thy
mind." [6]   Nothing better than mirth and merry company in
this malady.   "It begins with sorrow" (saith Montanus), "it
must be expelled with hilarity." [7]

But see the mischief; many men, knowing that merry company is the only medicine against melancholy, will therefore
neglect their business, and, in another extreme, spend all their
days among good fellows in a tavern or an ale-house, and know
not otherwise how to bestow their time but in drinking; malt-
worms, men-fishes, or water-snakes, *qui bibunt solum ranarum
more, nihil comedentes,* [8] like so many frogs in a puddle.   'Tis
their sole exercise to eat, and drink; to sacrifice to Volupia,
Rumina, Edulica, Potina, Mellona, is all their religion.   They
wish for Philoxenus' neck, Jupiter's *trinoctium,* and that the
sun would stand still as in Joshua's time, to satisfy their lust,
that they might *dies noctesque pergræcari et bibere* [to revel and

carouse day and night]. Flourishing wits, and men of good
parts, good fashion, and good worth, basely prostitute themselves to every rogue's company, to take tobacco and drink,
to roar and sing scurrile songs in base places.

> *Invenies aliquem cum percussore jacentem,*
> *Permixtum nautis, aut furibus, aut fugitivis.*[1]

> [You will find him lying beside a cut-throat, amid
>   a crowd of sailors, or thieves, or runaway
>   slaves.]

Which Thomas Erastus objects to Paracelsus, that he would lie
drinking all day long with carmen and tapsters in a brothel-
house, is too frequent amongst us, with men of better note:
like Timocreon of Rhodes, *multa bibens et multa vorans*, etc.,
they drown their wits, seethe their brains in ale, consume their
fortunes, lose their time, weaken their temperatures, contract
filthy diseases, rheums, dropsies, calentures, tremor, get swollen
jugulars, pimpled red faces, sore eyes, etc., heat their livers,
alter their complexions, spoil their stomachs, overthrow their
bodies; for drink drowns more than the sea and all the rivers
that fall into it (mere funges and casks), confound their souls,
suppress reason, go from Scylla to Charybdis, and use that
which is a help to their undoing. *Quid refert morbo an ferro
pereamve ruina?*[2] [What matters whether illness or the sword or
a falling building causes my death?] When the Black Prince
went to set the exiled King of Castile into his kingdom, there
was a terrible battle fought between the English and the
Spanish: at last the Spanish fled, the English followed them to
the river-side, where some drowned themselves to avoid their
enemies, the rest were killed.[3] Now tell me what difference
is between drowning and killing? As good be melancholy still,
as drunken beasts and beggars. Company, a sole comfort, and
an only remedy to all kind of discontent, is their sole misery
and cause of perdition. As Hermione lamented in Euripides,
Malæ mulieres me fecerunt malam [bad women have corrupted
me], evil company marred her, may they justly complain, bad
companions have been their bane. For, *malus malum vult ut
sui similis*[4] [the bad man wants others to be like himself];
one drunkard in a company, one thief, one whoremaster, will
by his good will make all the rest as bad as himself;

> *Etsi*
> *Nocturnos jures te formidare vapores,*[5]

> [Even though you swear you dread the damp night air,]

be of what complexion you will, inclination, love or hate, be it
good or bad, if you come amongst them, you must do as they do;
yea, though it be to the prejudice of your health, you must
drink [1] *venenum pro vino* [poison for wine]. And so, like grasshoppers, whilst they sing over their cups all summer, they
starve in winter; and for a little vain merriment shall find a
sorrowful reckoning in the end.

SECT. III. MEMB. I.

SUBSECT. I.—*A Consolatory Digression, containing the Remedies
of all manner of Discontents*

BECAUSE in the precedent section I have made mention of good
counsel, comfortable speeches, persuasion, how necessarily they
are required to the cure of a discontented or troubled mind,
how present a remedy they yield, and many times a sole sufficient
cure of themselves; I have thought fit, in this following section,
a little to digress (if at least it be to digress in this subject),
to collect and glean a few remedies and comfortable speeches
out of our best orators, philosophers, divines, and Fathers of
the Church, tending to this purpose. I confess, many have
copiously written of this subject, Plato, Seneca, Plutarch,
Xenophon, Epictetus, Theophrastus, Xenocrates, Crantor,
Lucian, Boethius: and some of late, Sadoletus, Cardan, Budæus,
Stella, Petrarch, Erasmus, besides Austin, Cyprian, Bernard,
etc. And they so well, that as Hierome in like case said, *si
nostrum areret ingenium, de illorum posset fontibus irrigari*, if
our barren wits were dried up, they might be copiously irrigated
from those well-springs: and I shall but *actum agere* [go over
beaten ground], yet, because these tracts are not so obvious and
common, I will epitomize and briefly insert some of their divine
precepts, reducing their voluminous and vast treatises to my
small scale; for it were otherwise impossible to bring so great
vessels into so little a creek. And although (as Cardan said of
his book *de consol.*) "I know beforehand, this tract of mine
many will contemn and reject; they that are fortunate, happy,
and in flourishing estate have no need of such consolatory
speeches; they that are miserable and unhappy think them
unsufficient to ease their grieved minds and comfort their
misery"; [2] yet I will go on; for this must needs do some good

to such as are happy, to bring them to a moderation, and make them reflect and know themselves, by seeing the inconstancy of human felicity, others' misery; and to such as are distressed, if they will but attend and consider of this, it cannot choose but give some content and comfort. 'Tis true, "no medicine can cure all diseases, some affections of the mind are altogether incurable; yet these helps of art, physic, and philosophy must not be contemned."[1] Arrianus and Plotinus are stiff in the contrary opinion, that such precepts can do little good. Boethius himself cannot comfort in some cases, they will reject such speeches like bread of stones, *Insana stultæ mentis hæc solatia.*[2]

"Words add no courage" (which Catiline once said to his soldiers),[3] "a captain's oration doth not make a coward a valiant man": and, as Job feelingly said to his friends, "You are but miserable comforters all."[4] 'Tis to no purpose in that vulgar phrase to use a company of obsolete sentences and familiar sayings: as Plinius Secundus,[5] being now sorrowful and heavy for the departure of his dear friend Cornelius Rufus, a Roman senator, wrote to his fellow Tiro in like case, *Adhibe solatia, sed nova aliqua, sed fortia, quæ audierim nunquam, legerim nunquam; nam quæ audivi, quæ legi omnia, tanto dolore superantur* [suggest new and strong grounds of comfort such as I never heard or read before; for all that I have heard or read is inadequate for my great grief], either say something that I never read nor heard of before, or else hold thy peace. Most men will here except: Trivial consolations, ordinary speeches, and known persuasions in this behalf will be of small force; what can any man say that hath not been said? To what end are such parænetical discourses? You may as soon remove Mount Caucasus as alter some men's affections. Yet sure I think they cannot choose but do some good, and comfort and ease a little; though it be the same again, I will say it, and upon that hope I will adventure. *Non meus hic sermo,*[6] 'tis not my speech this, but of Seneca, Plutarch, Epictetus, Austin, Bernard, Christ and His Apostles. If I make nothing, as Montaigne said in like case,[7] I will mar nothing; 'tis not my doctrine but my study, I hope I shall do nobody wrong to speak what I think, and deserve not blame in imparting my mind. If it be not for thy ease, it may for mine own; so Tully, Cardan, and Boethius wrote *de consol.* as well to help themselves as others; be it as it may, I will essay.

Discontents and grievances are either general or particular; general are wars, plagues, dearths, famine, fires, inundations, unseasonable weather, epidemical diseases which afflict whole kingdoms, territories, cities: or peculiar to private men, as cares, crosses, losses, death of friends, poverty, want, sickness, orbities, injuries, abuses, etc.,[1] generally all discontent, *homines quatimur fortunæ salo* [2] [we mortals are tossed on the tide of fortune]. No condition free, *quisque suos patimur manes* [each of us suffers his own fate]. Even in the midst of our mirth and jollity, there is some grudging, some complaint; as he saith,[3] our whole life is a *glucupicron,* a bitter-sweet passion, honey and gall mixed together, we are all miserable and discontent, who can deny it? If all, and that it be a common calamity, an inevitable necessity, all distressed, then, as Cardan infers, "who art thou that hopest to go free? Why dost thou not grieve thou art a mortal man, and not governor of the world?" [4] *Ferre quam sortem patiuntur omnes, Nemo recuset.* "If it be common to all, why should one man be more disquieted than another?" [5] If thou alone wert distressed, it were indeed more irksome, and less to be endured; but when the calamity is common, comfort thyself with this, thou hast more fellows, *Solamen miseris socios habuisse doloris;* 'tis not thy sole case, and why shouldst thou be so impatient? "Ay, but, alas! we are more miserable than others; what shall we do? Besides private miseries, we live in perpetual fear and danger of common enemies: we have Bellona's whips, and pitiful outcries, for epithalamiums; for pleasant music, that fearful noise of ordnance, drums, and warlike trumpets still sounding in our ears; instead of nuptial torches, we have firing of towns and cities; for triumphs, lamentations; for joy, tears.[6] So it is, and so it was, and so it ever will be. He that refuseth to see and hear, to suffer this, is not fit to live in this world, and knows not the common condition of all men, to whom so long as they live, with a reciprocal course, joys and sorrows are annexed, and succeed one another." [7] It is inevitable, it may not be avoided, and why then shouldst thou be so much troubled? *Grave nihil est homini quod fert necessitas,* as Tully deems out of an old poet,[8] that which is necessary cannot be grievous. If it be so, then comfort thyself in this, "that, whether thou wilt or no, it must be endured": [9] make a virtue of necessity, and conform thyself to undergo it. *Si longa est, levis est; si gravis est, brevis est:* [10] if it be long, 'tis light; if grievous, it cannot last. It will away, *dies dolorem minuit,* and if naught else, time will wear it out; custom will ease it; oblivion is a common medicine for all losses, injuries, griefs, and detriments whatsoever,[11] "and when they are once past, this commodity comes of infelicity, it makes the rest of our life sweeter

unto us":[1] *atque hæc olim meminisse juvabit*[2] [some day we shall
take pleasure in these memories]; "the privation and want of a
thing many times makes it more pleasant and delightsome than
before it was." We must not think the happiest of us all to
escape here without some misfortunes:

> *Usque adeo nulla est sincera voluptas,*
> *Sollicitumque aliquid lætis intervenit.*[3]

> [Of a truth no pleasure is unmixed; in all joy there
> lurks some sorrow.]

Heaven and earth are much unlike; "Those heavenly bodies
indeed are freely carried in their orbs without any impediment
or interruption, to continue their course for innumerable ages,
and make their conversions: but men are urged with many
difficulties, and have divers hindrances, oppositions, still crossing, interrupting their endeavours and desires, and no mortal
man is free from this law of nature."[4] We must not therefore
hope to have all things answer our own expectation, to have a
continuance of good success and fortunes; *Fortuna nunquam
perpetuo est bona* [good fortune cannot last for ever]. And as
Minucius Felix, the Roman consul, told that insulting Coriolanus, drunk with his good fortunes, "Look not for that success
thou hast hitherto had; it never yet happened to any man since
the beginning of the world, nor ever will, to have all things
according to his desire, or to whom fortune was never opposite
and adverse."[5] Even so it fell out to him as he foretold. And
so to others, even to that happiness of Augustus; though he were
Jupiter's almoner, Pluto's treasurer, Neptune's admiral, it
could not secure him. Such was Alcibiades' fortune, Narses',
that great Gonsalvo's and most famous men's, that, as Jovius
concludes,[6] "it is almost fatal to great princes, through their
own default or otherwise circumvented with envy and malice,
to lose their honours, and die contumeliously." 'Tis so, still
hath been, and ever will be, *Nihil est ab omni parte beatum*
[no happiness is complete],

> There's no perfection is so absolute,
> That some impurity doth not pollute.

Whatsoever is under the moon is subject to corruption, alteration; and so long as thou livest upon earth look not for other.
"Thou shalt not here find peaceable and cheerful days, quiet
times, but rather clouds, storms, calumnies, such is our fate."[7]
And as those errant planets in their distinct orbs have their

several motions, sometimes direct, stationary, retrograde, in
apogee, perigee, oriental, occidental, combust, feral, free, and,
as our astrologers will, have their fortitudes and debilities, by
reason of those good and bad irradiations, conferred to each
other's site in the heavens, in their terms, houses, case, detriments, etc.; so we rise and fall in this world, ebb and flow, in
and out, reared and dejected, lead a troublesome life, subject
to many accidents and casualties of fortunes, variety of passions,
infirmities as well from ourselves as others.

Yea, but thou thinkest thou art more miserable than the rest,
other men are happy in respect of thee, their miseries are
but flea-bitings to thine, thou alone art unhappy, none so bad
as thyself. Yet "if," as Socrates said, "all men in the world
should come and bring their grievances together, of body,
mind, fortune, sores, ulcers, madness, epilepsies, agues, and all
those common calamities of beggary, want, servitude, imprisonment, and lay them on a heap to be equally divided, wouldst
thou share alike, and take thy portion? or be as thou art?
Without question thou wouldst be as thou art." [1] If some
Jupiter should say, to give us all content,

> *Jam faciam quod vultis; eris tu, qui modo miles,*
> *Mercator; tu consultus modo, rusticus; hinc vos,*
> *Vos hinc mutatis discodite partibus; eia !*
> *Quid statis? nolint.*[2]

> Well, be 't so then; you, master soldier,
> Shall be a merchant; you, sir lawyer,
> A country gentleman: go you to this,
> That side you; why stand ye? It 's well as 'tis.

"Every man knows his own, but not others' defects and miseries;
and 'tis the nature of all men still to reflect upon themselves,
their own misfortunes," [3] not to examine or consider other
men's, not to confer themselves with others: to recount their
miseries, but not their good gifts, fortunes, benefits, which they
have, to ruminate on their adversity, but not once to think on
their prosperity, not what they have, but what they want: to
look still on them that go before, but not on those infinite
numbers that come after. "Whereas many a man would think
himself in heaven, a petty prince, if he had but the least part
of that fortune which thou so much repinest at, abhorrest, and
accountest a most vile and wretched estate." [4] How many
thousands want that which thou hast! how many myriads of
poor slaves, captives, of such as work day and night in coal-pits,

tin-mines, with sore toil to maintain a poor living, of such as
labour in body and mind, live in extreme anguish and pain,
all which thou art free from! *O fortunatos nimium bona si sua
norint!* Thou art most happy if thou couldst be content, and
acknowledge thy happiness. *Rem carendo, non fruendo cog-
noscimus* [we know the value of a thing when we miss it, not
when we have it]; when thou shalt hereafter come to want that
which thou now loathest, abhorrest, and art weary of and tired
with, when 'tis past thou wilt say thou werest most happy:
and, after a little miss, wish with all thine heart thou hadst
the same content again, mightst lead but such a life, a world for
such a life: the remembrance of it is pleasant. Be silent then,
rest satisfied,[1] *desine, intuensque in aliorum infortunia solare
mentem,* comfort thyself with other men's misfortunes, and, as
the moldiwarp in Æsop told the fox, complaining for want of a
tail, and the rest of his companions, *Tacete, quando me oculis
captum videtis,* you complain of toys, but I am blind, be quiet;
I say to thee, be thou satisfied. It is recorded [2] of the hares,
that with a general consent they went to drown themselves,
out of a feeling of their misery; but when they saw a company
of frogs more fearful than they were, they began to take courage
and comfort again. Confer thine estate with others. *Similes
aliorum respice casus, mitius ista feres.* Be content and rest
satisfied, for thou art well in respect to others: be thankful
for that thou hast, that God hath done for thee, He hath not
made thee a monster, a beast, a base creature, as He might, but
a man, a Christian, such a man; consider aright of it, thou art
full well as thou art. *Quicquid vult habere nemo potest,*[3] no man
can have what he will, *illud potest nolle quod non habet,* he may
choose whether he will desire that which he hath not. Thy lot
is fallen, make the best of it. "If we should all sleep at all
times" (as Endymion is said to have done), "who then were
happier than his fellow?" [4] Our life is but short, a very dream,
and while we look about, *immortalitas adest,*[4] eternity is at hand:
"Our life is a pilgrimage on earth, which wise men pass with
great alacrity." [6] If thou be in woe, sorrow, want, distress, in
pain, or sickness, think of that of our apostle, "God chastiseth
them whom he loveth." "They that sow in tears, shall reap in
joy" (Ps. cxxvi, 6). "As the furnace proveth the potter's vessel,
so doth temptation try men's thoughts" (Ecclus. xxvii, 5);
'tis for thy good,[7] *periisses nisi periisses:* hadst thou not been so
visited, thou hadst been utterly undone; "as gold in the fire,"
so men are tried in adversity. *Tribulatio ditat* [tribulation

enriches]: and, which Camerarius hath well shadowed in an emblem of a thresher and corn:

> *Si tritura absit paleis sunt abdita grana,*
> *Nos crux mundanis separat a paleis.*

> As threshing separates from straw the corn,
> By crosses from the world's chaff are we born.

'Tis the very same which Chrysostom comments, *Hom.* 2, *in* 3 *Matt.*: "Corn is not separated but by threshing, nor men from worldly impediments but by tribulation." [1] 'Tis that which Cyprian ingeminates, *Ser. 4 de immort.*[2] 'Tis that which Hierome, which all the Fathers inculcate: "So we are catechized for eternity." [3] 'Tis that which the proverb insinuates: *Nocumentum documentum* [hurting is teaching]; 'tis that which all the world rings into our ears. *Deus unicum habet filium sine peccato, nullum sine flagello:* God, saith Austin,[4] hath one son without sin, none without correction. "An expert seaman is tried in a tempest, a runner in a race, a captain in a battle, a valiant man in adversity, a Christian in tentation and misery" [5] (Basil, *Hom.* 8). We are sent as so many soldiers into this world, to strive with it, the flesh, the devil; our life is a warfare, and who knows it not? *Non est ad astra mollis e terris via* [6] [not easy is the way from earth to heaven]; "and therefore peradventure this world here is made troublesome unto us, that," as Gregory notes, "we should not be delighted by the way, and forget whither we are going." [7]

> *Ite nunc fortes, ubi celsa magni*
> *Ducit exempli via; cur inertes*
> *Terga nudatis? superata tellus*
>   *Sidera domat.*[8]

> [Advance now, ye brave, follow the lofty path of a
>   great example. Why do you tamely show
>   your backs? By conquering the earth you
>   win the stars.]

Go on then merrily to heaven. If the way be troublesome, and you in misery, in many grievances, on the other side you have many pleasant sports, objects, sweet smells, delightsome tastes, music, meats, herbs, flowers, etc., to recreate your senses. Or put case thou art now forsaken of the world, dejected, contemned, yet comfort thyself; as it was said to Hagar in the wilderness, "God sees thee, he takes notice of thee": [9] there is a God above that can vindicate thy cause, that can relieve thee. And surely Seneca [10] thinks He takes delight in seeing thee: "The gods are well pleased when they see great men contending with adversity," as we are to see men fight, or a man with a beast. But these are toys in respect. "Behold," saith he, "a spectacle worthy of God; a good man contented with his estate."[1] A tyrant is the best sacrifice to Jupiter, as the ancients held, and his best object a contented mind. For thy part then rest satisfied, "cast all thy care on him, thy burden on him, rely on him, trust on him, and he shall nourish thee, care for thee, give thee thine heart's desire";[2] say with David, "God is our hope and strength, in troubles ready to be found" (Ps. xlvi, 1). "For they that trust in the Lord shall be as Mount Zion, which cannot be removed. As the mountains are about Jerusalem, so is the Lord about his people, from henceforth and for ever" (Ps. cxxv, 1, 2).

MEMB. II.

Deformity of Body, Sickness, Baseness of Birth, Peculiar Discontents

PARTICULAR discontents and grievances are either of body, mind, or fortune, which, as they wound the soul of man, produce this melancholy and many great inconveniences, by that anti-dote of good counsel and persuasion may be eased or expelled. Deformities and imperfections of our bodies, as lameness, crookedness, deafness, blindness, be they innate or accidental, torture many men; yet this may comfort them, that those imperfections of the body do not a whit blemish the soul, or hinder the operations of it, but rather help and much increase it. Thou art lame of body, deformed to the eye, yet this hinders not but that thou mayest be a good, a wise, upright, honest man. "Seldom," saith Plutarch, "honesty and beauty dwell together,"[3] and oftentimes under a threadbare coat lies an excellent under-standing, *sæpe sub attrita latitat sapientia veste.* Cornelius Mussus,[4] that famous preacher in Italy, when he came first into the pulpit in Venice, was so much contemned by reason of his outside, a little, lean, poor, dejected person, they were all ready to leave the church; but when they heard his voice they did admire him,[5] and happy was that senator could enjoy his company, or invite him first to his house. A silly fellow to look to may have more wit, learning, honesty than he that struts it out *ampullis jactans* [talking big], etc., *grandia gradiens* [strutting

about], and is admired in the world's opinion. *Vilis sæpe cadus
nobile nectar habet*, the best wine comes out of an old vessel.
How many deformed princes, kings, emperors, could I reckon
up, philosophers, orators! Hannibal had but one eye; Appius
Claudius, Timoleon blind, Muleasses,[1] King of Tunis, John,
King of Bohemia, and Tiresias the prophet. "The night hath
his pleasure";[2] and for the loss of that one sense such men are
commonly recompensed in the rest; they have excellent
memories, other good parts, music, and many recreations; much
happiness, great wisdom, as Tully well discourseth in his Tusculan Questions.[3] Homer was blind, yet who (saith he) made
more accurate, lively, or better descriptions, with both his
eyes? Democritus was blind, yet, as Laertius writes of him, he
saw more than all Greece besides; as Plato concludes,[4] *Tum
sane mentis oculus acute insipit cernere, quum primum corporis
oculus deflorescit*, when our bodily eyes are at worst, generally
the eyes of our soul see best. Some philosophers and divines
have evirated themselves, and put out their eyes voluntarily,
the better to contemplate. Angelus Politianus had a tetter in
his nose continually running, fulsome in company, yet no man
so eloquent and pleasing in his works. Æsop was crooked,
Socrates purblind, long-legged, hairy, Democritus withered,
Seneca lean and harsh, ugly to behold; yet show me so many
flourishing wits, such divine spirits: Horace a little blear-eyed
contemptible fellow, yet who so sententious and wise? Marsilius
Ficinus, Faber Stapulensis, a couple of dwarfs, Melancthon a
short hard-favoured man,[5] *parvus erat, sed magnus erat*, etc.,
yet of incomparable parts all three. Ignatius Loyola,[6] the
founder of the Jesuits, by reason of a hurt he received in his
leg at the siege of Pampeluna, the chief town of Navarre in
Spain, unfit for wars and less serviceable at court, upon that
accident betook himself to his beads, and by those means got
more honour than ever he should have done with the use of his
limbs and properness of person: *vulnus non penetrat animum*,[7]
a wound hurts not the soul. Galba the emperor was crook-
backed, Epictetus lame; that great Alexander a little man of
stature, Augustus Cæsar of the same pitch;[8] Agesilaus *despicabili
forma* [contemptible in appearance]; Boccharis a most deformed
prince as ever Egypt had, yet, as Diodorus Siculus records of
him,[9] in wisdom and knowledge far beyond his predecessors.
Anno Dom. 1306, Uladislaus Cubitalis, that pigmy King of
Poland, reigned and fought more victorious battles than any of
his long-shanked predecessors.[10] *Nullam virtus respuit staturam,*

virtue refuseth no stature, and commonly your great vast bodies and fine features are sottish, dull, and leaden spirits. What's in them? *Quid nisi pondus iners stolidæque ferocia mentis?*[1] [What but sheer bulk and stupid insolence?] What in Otus and Ephialtes (Neptune's sons in Homer), nine acres long?

> *Qui ut magnus Orion,*
> *Cum pedes incedit, medii per maxima Nerei*
> *Stagna, viam findens humero supereminet undas.*[2]

> [Like tall Orion stalking o'er the flood:
> When with his brawny breast he cuts the waves.
> His shoulder scarce the topmost billow laves.]

What in Maximinus, Ajax, Caligula, and the rest of those great Zamzummims,[3] or gigantical Anakims, heavy, vast, barbarous lubbers?

> *Si membra tibi dant grandia Parcæ,*
> *Mentis eges.*

> [If the Fates give thee huge limbs,
> thou art short of wit.]

Their body, saith Lemnius,[4] "is a burden to them, and their spirits not so lively, nor they so erect and merry." *Non est in magno corpore mica salis* [there is no spark of wit in a huge frame]: a little diamond is more worth than a rocky mountain: which made Alexander Aphrodisiæus positively conclude, "The lesser, the wiser, because the soul was more contracted in such a body."[5] Let Bodine in his *5th cap. Method. hist.* plead the rest: the lesser they are, as in Asia, Greece, they have generally the finest wits. And for bodily stature, which some so much admire, and goodly presence, 'tis true, to say the best of them, great men are proper, and tall, I grant, *caput inter nubila condunt* [hide their heads in the clouds]; but *belli pusilli*, little men are pretty: *Sed si bellus homo est Cotta, pusillus homo est* [if Cotta is a pretty man, he is also a little man]. Sickness, diseases, trouble many, but without a cause; "It may be 'tis for the good of their souls";[6] *pars fati fuit* ['twas part of their destiny], the flesh rebels against the spirit; that which hurts the one must needs help the other. Sickness is the mother of modesty, putteth us in mind of our mortality; and when we are in the full career of wordly pomp and jollity, she pulleth us by the ear, and maketh us know ourselves. Pliny[7] calls it the sum of philosophy, "if we could but perform that in our health, which we promise in our sickness." *Quum infirmi sumus, optimi sumus* [when we are sick we are most virtuous]; for "what sick man" (as

Secundus expostulates with Rufus [1]) "was ever lascivious,
covetous, or ambitious? he envies no man, admires no man,
flatters no man, despiseth no man, listens not after lies and
tales," etc.   And were it not for such gentle remembrances,
men would have no moderation of themselves, they would be
worse than tigers, wolves, and lions: who should keep them in
awe? "Princes, masters, parents, magistrates, judges, friends,
enemies, fair or foul means cannot contain us, but a little sickness" (as Chrysostom observes) "will correct and amend us." [2]
And therefore, with good discretion, Jovianus Pontanus caused
his short sentence to be engraven on his tomb in Naples:
"Labour, sorrow, grief, sickness, want and woe, to serve proud
masters, bear that superstitious yoke, and bury your dearest
friends, etc., are the sauces of our life." [3]   If thy disease be
continuate and painful to thee, it will not surely last; "and a
light affliction, which is but for a moment, causeth unto us a
far more excellent and eternal weight of glory" (2 Cor. iv, 17).
Bear it with patience; women endure much sorrow in childbed,
and yet they will not contain; and those that are barren wish
for this pain; "be courageous, there is as much valour to be
shown in thy bed as in an army or at a sea fight": [4] *aut vincetur,
aut vincet* [he will either be victor or vanquished], thou shalt
be rid at last.   In the meantime, let it take its course, thy mind
is not anyway disabled.   Bilibaldus Pirkimerus,[5] senator to
Charles the Fifth, ruled all Germany, lying most part of his
days sick of the gout upon his bed.   The more violent thy
torture is, the less it will continue: and though it be severe and
hideous for the time, comfort thyself as martyrs do, with honour
and immortality.   That famous philosopher Epicurus, being
in as miserable pain of stone and colic as a man might endure,
solaced himself with a conceit of immortality; "the joy of his
soul for his rare inventions repelled the pain of his bodily
torments." [6]

Baseness of birth is a great disparagement to some men,
especially if they be wealthy, bear office, and come to promotion
in a commonwealth; then (as he [7] observes) if their birth be not
answerable to their calling and to their fellows, they are much
abashed and ashamed of themselves.   Some scorn their own
father and mother, deny brothers and sisters, with the rest of
their kindred and friends, and will not suffer them to come near
them when they are in their pomp, accounting it a scandal to
their greatness to have such beggarly beginnings.   Simon in
Lucian, having now got a little wealth, changed his name from

Simon to Simonides, for that there were so many beggars of his
kin, and set the house on fire where he was born, because nobody
should point at it.   Others buy titles, coats of arms, and by all
means screw themselves into ancient families, falsifying pedigrees, usurping scutcheons, and all because they would not seem
to be base.   The reason is, for that this gentility is so much
admired by a company of outsides, and such honour attributed
unto it, as amongst Germans,[1] Frenchmen, and Venetians, the
gentry scorn the commonalty, and will not suffer them to match
with them; they depress, and make them as so many asses, to
carry burdens.   In our ordinary talk and fallings out, the most
opprobrious and scurrile name we can fasten upon a man, or
first give, is to call him base rogue, beggarly rascal, and the like:
whereas, in my judgment, this ought of all other grievances to
trouble men least.   Of all vanities and fopperies, to brag of
gentility is the greatest; for what is it they crack so much of,
and challenge such superiority, as if they were demi-gods?
Birth?   *Tantane vos generis tenuit fiducia vestri?* [Do ye presume
so much on your descent?]   It is *non ens*, a mere flash, a ceremony, a toy, a thing of naught.   Consider the beginning, present estate, progress, ending of gentry, and then tell me what it
is.   "Oppression, fraud, cozening, usury, knavery, bawdry,
murder, and tyranny, are the beginning of many ancient
families.[2]   One hath been a blood-sucker, a parricide, the death
of many a silly soul in some unjust quarrels, seditions, made
many an orphan and poor widow, and for that he is made
a lord or an earl, and his posterity gentlemen for ever after.[3]
Another hath been a bawd, a pander to some great men, a
parasite, a slave, prostituted himself, his wife, daughter,"[4]
to some lascivious prince, and for that he is exalted.   Tiberius
preferred many to honours in his time, because they were
famous whoremasters and sturdy drinkers; many come into this
parchment-row (so one calls it [5]) by flattery or cozening; search
your old families, and you shall scarce find of a multitude (as
Æneas Sylvius observes) *qui sceleratum non habent ortum*, that
have not a wicked beginning; *aut qui vi et dolo eo fastigii non
ascendunt* [or who did not reach their present position through
violence or deceit], as that plebeian in Machiavel in a set oration
proved to his fellows, that do not rise by knavery, force, foolery,
villainy, or such indirect means.   "They are commonly able
that are wealthy; virtue and riches seldom settle on one man:
who then sees not the base beginning of nobility? spoils enrich
one, usury another, treason a third, witchcraft a fourth, flattery a

II—K 887

fifth, lying, stealing, bearing false witness a sixth, adultery the seventh."[1] etc. One makes a fool of himself to make his lord merry, another dandles my young master, bestows a little nag on him, a third marries a cracked piece, etc. Now may it please your good worship, your lordship, who was the first founder of your family? The poet answers, *Aut pastor fuit, aut illud quod dicere nolo*[2] [he was either a shepherd or something which I prefer not to mention]. Are he or you the better gentleman? If he, then we have traced him to his form. If you, what is it of which thou boastest so much? That thou art his son. It may be his heir, his reputed son, and yet indeed a priest or a serving-man may be the true father of him; but we will not controvert that now; married women are all honest; thou art his son's son's son, begotten and born *intra quatuor maria* [within the four seas], etc. Thy great-great-great-grandfather was a rich citizen, and then in all likelihood a usurer, a lawyer, and then a ——, a courtier, and then a ——, a country gentleman, and then he scraped it out of sheep, etc. And you are the heir of all his virtues, fortunes, titles; so then, what is your gentry but, as Hierome saith, *opes antiquæ, inveteratæ divitiæ*, ancient wealth? that is the definition of gentility. The father goes often to the devil to make his son a gentleman. For the present, what is it? "It began" (saith Agrippa[3]) "with strong impiety, with tyranny, oppression," etc., and so it is maintained: wealth began it (no matter how got), wealth continueth and increaseth it. Those Roman knights were so called, if they could dispend *per annum* so much. In the kingdom of Naples and France, he that buys such lands buys the honour, title, barony together with it;[4] and they that can dispend so much amongst us must be called to bear office, to be knights, or fine for it; as one observes, *nobiliorum ex censu judicant*,[5] our nobles are measured by their means. And what now is the object of honour? What maintains our gentry but wealth? *Nobilitas sine re projecta vilior alga*,[6] without means gentry is naught worth; nothing so contemptible and base. *Disputare de nobilitate generis, sine divitiis, est disputare de nobilitate stercoris*, saith Nevisanus the lawyer,[7] to dispute of gentry without wealth is (saving your reverence) to discuss the original of a mard. So that it is wealth alone that denominates, money which maintains it, gives *esse* to it, for which every man may have it. And what is their ordinary exercise? "Sit to eat, drink, lie down to sleep, and rise to play."[8] Wherein lies their worth and sufficiency? In a few coats of arms, eagles, lions, serpents, bears, tigers, dogs, crosses, bends, fesses, etc., and such-like baubles, which they commonly set up in their galleries, porches, windows, on bowls, platters, coaches, in tombs, churches, men's sleeves, etc. "If he can hawk and hunt, ride a horse, play at cards and dice, swagger, drink, swear," [1] take tobacco with a grace, sing, dance, wear his clothes in fashion, court and please his mistress, talk big fustian, insult, scorn, strut, contemn others,[2] and use a little mimical and apish complement above the rest, he is a complete (*Egregiam vero laudem* [a truly noble compliment]), a well-qualified gentleman; these are most of their employments, this their greatest commendation. What is gentry, this parchment nobility then, but, as Agrippa defines it, "a sanctuary of knavery and naughtiness, a cloak for wickedness and execrable vices, of pride, fraud, contempt, boasting, oppression, dissimulation, lust, gluttony, malice, fornication, adultery, ignorance, impiety"? [3] A nobleman therefore, in some likelihood, as he concludes, is "an atheist, an oppressor, an epicure, a gull,[4] a dizzard, an illiterate idiot, an outside, a glow-worm, a proud fool, an arrant ass," *ventris et inguinis mancipium*, a slave to his lust and belly, *solaque libidine fortis*. And as Salvianus observed of his countrymen the Aquitanes in France; *Sicut titulis primi fuere, sic et vitiis* [as they were the first in rank, so also in rottenness]; and Cabinet du Roy, their own writer, distinctly of the rest: "the nobles of Berry are most part lechers. they of Touraine thieves, they of Narbonne covetous, they of Guienne coiners, they of Provence atheists, they of Rheims superstitious, they of Lyons treacherous, of Normandy proud, of Picardy insolent," etc.; we may generally conclude, the greater men, the more vicious. In fine, as Æneas Sylvius adds,[5] "they are most part miserable, sottish, and filthy fellows, like the walls of their houses, fair without, foul within." What dost thou vaunt of now? "What dost thou gape and wonder at? admire him for his brave apparel, horses, dogs, fine houses, manors, orchards, gardens, walks? Why, a fool may be possessor of this as well as he; and he that accounts him a better man, a nobleman for having of it, he is a fool himself." [6] Now go and brag of thy gentility. This is it belike which makes the Turks at this day scorn nobility,[7] and all those huffing bombast titles which so much elevate their poles; except it be such as have got it at first, maintain it by some supereminent quality or excellent worth. And for this cause, the Ragusian commonwealth, Switzers, and the United Provinces, in all their aristocracies, or democratical monarchies (if I may so

call them), exclude all these degrees of hereditary honours,
and will admit of none to bear office, but such as are learned,
like those Athenian Areopagites, wise, discreet, and well brought
up. The Chinenses [1] observe the same customs; no man
amongst them noble by birth; out of their philosophers and
doctors they choose magistrates: their politic nobles are taken
from such as be *moraliter nobiles*, virtuous noble; *nobilitas ut
olim ab officio, non a natura* [nobility, as of old, is derived from
office, not from birth], as in Israel of old, and their office was to
defend and govern their country in war and peace, not to hawk,
hunt, eat, drink, game alone, as too many do. Their *Loysii*,
Mandarini, literati, licentiati, and such as have raised themselves by their worth, are their noblemen only, thought fit to
govern a state; and why then should any that is otherwise of
worth be ashamed of his birth? why should not he be as much
respected that leaves a noble posterity, as he that hath had
noble ancestors? nay, why not more? for *plures solem orientem*,
we adore the sun rising most part; and how much better is it
to say, *Ego meis majoribus virtute præluxi* [I have outshone my
ancestors in virtue], to boast himself of his virtues, than of his
birth? Cathesbeius, Sultan of Egypt and Syria, was by his
condition a slave, but for worth, valour, and manhood second
to no king, and for that cause (as Jovius writes [2]) elected
Emperor of the Mamelukes. That poor Spanish Pizarro for
his valour made by Charles the Fifth Marquess of Anatillo; the
Turkey bassas are all such. Pertinax, Philippus Arabs, Maximinus, Probus, Aurelius, etc., from common soldiers, became
emperors; Cato, Cincinnatus, etc., consuls; Pius Secundus,
Sixtus Quintus, Johannes Secundus, Nicholas Quintus, etc.,
popes. Socrates, Virgil, Horace, *libertino patre natus* [the son
of a freedman]. The kings of Denmark fetch their pedigree,
as some say,[3] from one Ulfo, that was the son of a bear. *E tenui
casa sæpe vir magnus exit*,[4] many a worthy man comes out of
a poor cottage. Hercules, Romulus, Alexander (by Olympia's
confession), Themistocles, Jugurtha, King Arthur, William the
Conqueror, Homer, Demosthenes, P. Lombard, P. Comestor,
Bartholus, Adrian the Fourth, Pope, etc., bastards; and almost
in every kingdom the most ancient families have been at first
princes' bastards; their worthiest captains, best wits, greatest
scholars, bravest spirits in all our annals, have been base.
Cardan, in his Subtleties, gives a reason why they are most
part better able than others in body and mind, and so, *per
consequens*, more fortunate.[5] Castruccius Castrucanus, a poor

child, found in the field, exposed to misery, became Prince of
Lucca and Senes in Italy, a most complete soldier and worthy
captain; Machiavel compares him to Scipio or Alexander.
"And 'tis a wonderful thing" (saith he [1]) "to him that shall
consider of it, that all those, or the greatest part of them, that
have done the bravest exploits here upon earth, and excelled
the rest of the nobles of their time, have been still born in some
abject, obscure place, or of base and obscure abject parents."
A most memorable observation, Scaliger [2] accounts it, *et non
prætereundum, maximorum virorum plerosque patres ignoratos,
matres impudicas fuisse* [and not to be passed over, that for
the most part the fathers of the greatest men were unknown
and their mothers unchaste]. "I could recite a great catalogue
of them," every kingdom, every province will yield innumerable
examples; and why then should baseness of birth be objected
to any man?   Who thinks worse of Tully for being *Arpinas*
[from Arpinum], an upstart?   Or Agathocles, that Sicilian king,
for being a potter's son?   Iphicrates and Marius were meanly
born.   What wise man thinks better of any person for his
nobility? as he said in Machiavel,[3] *omnes eodem patre nati*
[all descended from one ancestor], Adam's sons, conceived all
and born in sin, etc.   "We are by nature all as one, all alike, if
you see us naked; let us wear theirs and they our clothes, and
what's the difference?"   To speak truth, as Bale did of P.
Schalichius,[4] "I more esteem thy worth, learning, honesty,
than thy nobility; honour thee more that thou art a writer, a
doctor of divinity, than Earl of the Huns, Baron of Skradine,
or hast title to such and such provinces," etc.   "Thou art more
fortunate and great" (so Jovius writes [5] to Cosmus Medices,
then Duke of Florence) "for thy virtues, than for thy lovely
wife and happy children, friends, fortunes, or great duchy
of Tuscany."   So I account thee; and who doth not so indeed?
Abdolonymus was a gardener, and yet by Alexander for his
virtues made King of Syria.[6]   How much better is it to be born
of mean parentage, and to excel in worth, to be morally noble,
which is preferred before that natural nobility, by divines,
philosophers, and politicians,[7] to be learned, honest, discreet,
well qualified, to be fit for any manner of employment, in
country and commonwealth, war and peace, than to be *degeneres
Neoptolemi* [degenerate Neoptolemuses], as many brave nobles
are, only wise because rich, otherwise idiots, illiterate, unfit for
any manner of service!   Udalricus, Earl of Cilia, upbraided
John Huniades with the baseness of his birth, but he replied,

*In te Ciliensis comitatus turpiter extinguitur, in me gloriose
Bistricensis exoritur,* thine earldom is consumed with riot, mine
begins with honour and renown.[1]   Thou hast had so many
noble ancestors; what is that to thee?   *Vix ea nostra voco* [I
scarce call that ours], when thou art a dizzard thyself: [2] *Quid
prodest, Pontice, longo stemmate censeri?* [What boots it, Ponticus,
to have an ancestry?], etc.   I conclude, hast thou a sound body,
and a good soul, good bringing up?   Art thou virtuous, honest,
learned, well-qualified, religious, are thy conditions good?
Thou art a true nobleman, perfectly noble, although born of
Thersites, *dummodo tu sis Æacidæ similis, non natus, sed factus*
[provided thou be like Achilles, not born so but made], noble
κατ' ἐξοχὴν [in the truest sense of the word], "for neither sword,
nor fire, nor water, nor sickness, nor outward violence, nor the
devil himself can take thy good parts from thee." [3]   Be not
ashamed of thy birth then, thou art a gentleman all the world
over, and shalt be honoured, whenas he, strip him of his fine
clothes, dispossess him of his wealth,[4] is a funge (which Polynices
in his banishment found true by experience, gentry was not
esteemed [5]), like a piece of coin in another country, that no man
will take, and shall be contemned.   Once more, though thou be
a barbarian, born at Tontonteac, a villain, a slave, a Saldanian
negro, or a rude Virginian in Dasamonquepeuc, he a French
monsieur, a Spanish don, a seignior of Italy, I care not how
descended, of what family, of what order, baron, count, prince,
if thou be well qualified, and he not, but a degenerate Neo-
ptolemus, I tell thee in a word, thou art a man, and he is a beast.

    Let no *terræ filius*, or upstart, insult at this which I have said,
no worthy gentleman take offence.   I speak it not to detract
from such as are well deserving, truly virtuous and noble: I do
much respect and honour true gentry and nobility; I was born
of worshipful parents myself, in an ancient family, but I am a
younger brother, it concerns me not: or had I been some great
heir, richly endowed, so minded as I am, I should not have been
elevated at all, but so esteemed of it as of all other human
happiness, honours, etc.; they have their period, are brittle and
unconstant.   As he said of that great river Danubius, it riseth
from a small fountain, a little brook at first, sometimes broad,
sometimes narrow, now slow, then swift, increased at last to
an incredible greatness by the confluence of sixty navigable
rivers; it vanisheth in conclusion, loseth his name, and is
suddenly swallowed up of the Euxine Sea: [6] I may say of our
greatest families, they were mean at first, augmented by rich

marriages, purchases, offices, they continue for some ages, with some little alteration of circumstances, fortunes, places, etc.; by some prodigal son, for some default, or for want of issue they are defaced in an instant, and their memory blotted out.

So much in the meantime I do attribute to gentility, that if he be well-descended, of worshipful or noble parentage, he will express it in his conditions:

> *Nec enim feroces*
> *Progenerant aquilæ columbas.*

[For fierce eagles beget not timid doves.]

And although the nobility of our times be much like our coins, more in number and value, but less in weight and goodness, with finer stamps, cuts, or outsides than of old, yet if he retain those ancient characters of true gentry, he will be more affable, courteous, gently disposed, of fairer carriage, better temper, or a more magnanimous, heroical, and generous spirit, than that *vulgus hominum,* those ordinary boors and peasants, *qui adeo improbi, agrestes, et inculti plerumque sunt, ne dicam malitiosi, ut nemini ullum humanitatis officium præstent, ne ipsi Deo si advenerit,* as one [1] observes of them, a rude, brutish, uncivil, wild, a currish generation, cruel and malicious, uncapable of discipline, and such as have scarce common sense. And it may be generally spoken of all, which Lemnius the physician said of his travel into England,[2] the common people were silly, sullen, dogged clowns, *sed mitior nobilitas, ad omne humanitatis officium paratissima,* the gentlemen were courteous and civil. If it so fall out (as often it doth) that such peasants are preferred by reason of their wealth, chance, error, etc., or otherwise, yet (as the cat in the fable, when she was turned to a fair maid, would play with mice) a cur will be a cur, a clown will be a clown, he will likely savour of the stock whence he came, and that innate rusticity can hardly be shaken off.

> *Licet superbus umbulot pecunia,*
> *Fortuna non mutat genus.*[3]

[Let him strut as proudly as he will, his fortune does
not change his birth.]

And though by their education such men may be better qualified and more refined, yet there be many symptoms by which they may likely be descried, an affected phantastical carriage, a tailor-like spruceness, a peculiar garb in all their proceedings; choicer than ordinary in his diet, and, as Hierome [4] well describes such a one to his Nepotian: "An upstart born in a base cottage, that scarce at first had coarse bread to fill his hungry guts, must now feed on kickshaws and made dishes, will have all variety of flesh and fish, the best oysters," etc. A beggar's brat will be commonly more scornful, imperious, insulting, insolent, than another man of his rank: "Nothing so intolerable as a fortunate fool,"[1] as Tully found long since out of his experience. *Asperius nihil est humili cum surgit in altum*, set a beggar on horseback, and he will ride a gallop, a gallop, etc.

> *Desævit in omnes*
> *Dum se posse putat, nec bellua sævior ulla est,*
> *Quam servi rabies in libera colla furentis;*[2]

[He rages against all as long as he thinks he has
power; no wild beast so savage as a slave
venting his fury on the free;]

he forgets what he was, domineers, etc., and many such other symptoms he hath, by which you may know him from a true gentleman. Many errors and obliquities are on both sides, noble, ignoble, *factis, natis* [made or born so]; yet still in all callings, as some degenerate, some are well deserving, and most worthy of their honours. And as Busbequius said of Solyman the Magnificent, he was *tanto dignus imperio*, worthy of that great empire. Many meanly descended are most worthy of their honour, *politice nobiles* [ennobled through their statesmanship], and well deserve it. Many of our nobility so born (which one said of Hephæstion, Ptolemæus, Seleucus, Antigonus, etc., and the rest of Alexander's followers, they were all worthy to be monarchs and generals of armies) deserve to be princes. And I am so far forth of Sesellius his mind,[3] that they ought to be preferred (if capable) before others, "as being nobly born, ingenuously brought up, and from their infancy trained to all manner of civility." For learning and virtue in a nobleman is more eminent, and, as a jewel set in gold is more precious, and much to be respected; such a man deserves better than others, and is as great an honour to his family as his noble family to him. In a word, many noblemen are an ornament to their order: many poor men's sons are singularly well endowed, most eminent, and well deserving for their worth, wisdom, learning, virtue, valour, integrity; excellent members and pillars of a commonwealth. And therefore, to conclude that which I first intended, to be base by birth, meanly born, is no such disparagement. *Et sic demonstratur, quod erat demonstrandum* and so what was to be proved has been proved].

MEMB. III.

Against Poverty and Want, with such other Adversities

ONE of the greatest miseries that can befall a man, in the world's esteem, is poverty or want, which makes men steal, bear false witness, swear, forswear, contend, murder and rebel, which breaketh sleep, and causeth death itself. οὐδὲν πενίας βαρύτερόν ἐστι φορτίον,[1] no burden (saith Menander) so intolerable as poverty: it makes men desperate, it erects and dejects, *census honores, census amicitias* [money procures honours, money procures friendships]; money makes, but poverty mars, etc., and all this in the world's esteem: yet, if considered aright, it is a great blessing in itself, a happy estate, and yields no cause of discontent, or that men should therefore account themselves vile, hated of God, forsaken, miserable, unfortunate. Christ Himself was poor, born in a manger, and had not a house to hide His head in all His life, "lest any man should make poverty a judgment of God, or an odious estate." [2]   And as He was himself, so He informed His apostles and disciples, they were all poor, prophets poor, apostles poor (Acts iii, "Silver and gold have I none"). "As sorrowing" (saith Paul) "and yet always rejoicing; as having nothing, and yet possessing all things" (1 Cor. vi, 10). Your great philosophers have been voluntarily poor, not only Christians, but many others. Crates Thebanus was adored for a god in Athens, "a nobleman by birth, many servants he had, an honourable attendance, much wealth, many manors, fine apparel; but when he saw this, that all the wealth of the world was but brittle, uncertain and no whit availing to live well, he flung his burden into the sea, and renounced his estate." [3]   Those Curii and Fabricii will be ever renowned for contempt of these fopperies, wherewith the world is so much affected. Amongst Christians I could reckon up many kings and queens that have forsaken their crowns and fortunes, and wilfully abdicated themselves from these so much esteemed toys; many that have refused honours, titles, and all this vain pomp and happiness, which others so ambitiously seek, and carefully study to compass and attain.[4] Riches, I deny not, are God's good gifts and blessings; and *honor est in honorante*, honours are from God; both rewards of virtue, and fit to be sought after, sued for, and may well be possessed: yet no such great happiness in having, or misery in wanting of them. *Dantur quidem bonis*, saith Austin, *ne quis mala æstimet:*

malis autem ne quis nimis bona, good men have wealth that we
should not think it evil, and bad men that they should not rely
on or hold it so good; as the rain falls on both sorts, so are
riches given to good and bad, *sed bonis in bonum,* but they are
good only to the godly. But confer both estates, for natural
parts they are not unlike;[1] and a beggar's child, as Cardan
well observes,[2] "is no whit inferior to a prince's, most part
better"; and for those accidents of fortune, it will easily appear
there is no such odds, no such extraordinary happiness in the
one, or misery in the other. He is rich, wealthy, fat; what
gets he by it? pride, insolency, lust, ambition, cares, fears,
suspicion, trouble, anger, emulation, and many filthy diseases
of body and mind. He hath indeed variety of dishes, better
fare, sweet wine, pleasant sauce, dainty music, gay clothes,
lords it bravely out, etc., and all that which Micyllus admired
in Lucian;[3] but with them he hath the gout, dropsies, apoplexies,
palsies, stone, pox, rheums, catarrhs, crudities, oppilations,
melancholy, etc.;[4] lust enters in, anger, ambition; according
to Chrysostom, "the sequel of riches is pride, riot, intemperance,
arrogancy, fury, and all irrational courses."[5]

> *Turpi fregerunt sæcula luxu*
> *Divitiæ molles.*[6]

[Effeminate riches have corrupted the age with base
luxury,]

with their variety of dishes, many such maladies of body and
mind get in, which the poor man knows not of. As Saturn,
in Lucian,[7] answered the discontented commonalty (which,
because of their neglected Saturnal feasts in Rome, made a
grievous complaint and exclamation against rich men) that they
were much mistaken in supposing such happiness in riches;
'You see the best" (said he) "but you know not their several
gripings and discontents":[8] they are like painted walls, fair
without, rotten within: diseased, filthy, crazy, full of intemperance's effects; "and who can reckon half? if you but knew
their fears, cares, anguish of mind, and vexation, to which they
are subject, you would hereafter renounce all riches."[9]

> *O si pateant pectora divitum*
> *Quantos intus sublimis agit*
> *Fortuna metus ! Bruttia Coro*
> *Pulsante fretum mitior unda est.*[10]

O that their breasts were but conspicuous,
How full of fear within, how furious!
The narrow seas are not so boisterous.

Yea, but he hath the world at will that is rich, the good things
of the earth: *suave est de magno tollere acervo* [it is sweet to draw
from a great heap], he is a happy man, adored like a god,[1] a
prince, every man seeks to him, applauds, honours, admires
him. He hath honours indeed, abundance of all things; but
(as I said) withal "pride, lust, anger, faction, emulation, fears,
cares, suspicion enter with his wealth"; [2] for his intemperance
he hath aches, crudities, gouts, and, as fruits of his idleness and
fullness, lust, surfeiting, and drunkenness, all manner of diseases:
pecuniis augetur improbitas, the wealthier, the more dishonest.
"He is exposed to hatred, envy, peril, and treason, fear of
death, degradation," [3] etc.; 'tis *lubrica statio et proxima præcipitio* [a slippery position, on the edge of a precipice], and the
higher he climbs, the greater is his fall.

> *Celsæ graviore casu*
> *Decidunt turres, feriuntque summos*
> *Fulgura montes,*[4]

the lightning commonly sets on fire the highest towers; in the
more eminent place he is, the more subject to fall.[5]

> *Rumpitur innumeris arbos uberrima pomis,*
> *Et subito nimiæ præcipitantur opes.*

As a tree that is heavy laden with fruit breaks her own boughs,
with their own greatness they ruin themselves; which Joachimus
Camerarius hath elegantly expressed in his 13th Emblem,
cent. 1. *Inopem se copia fecit* [plenty has led to want] Their
means is their misery, though they do apply themselves to the
times, to lie, dissemble, collogue and flatter their lieges, obey,
second his will and commands, as much as may be, yet too
frequently they miscarry, they fat themselves like so many
hogs, as Æneas Sylvius observes,[6] that when they are full fed,
they may be devoured by their princes, as Seneca by Nero was
served, Sejanus by Tiberius, and Haman by Ahasuerus. I
resolve with Gregory, *potestas culminis est tempestas mentis;
et quo dignitas altior, casus gravior*, honour is a tempest, the
higher they are elevated, the more grievously depressed. For
the rest of his prerogatives which wealth affords, as he hath
more, his expenses are the greater. "When goods increase,
they are increased that eat them; and what good cometh to the
owners, but the beholding thereof with the eyes?" (Eccles. v, 11).

> *Millia frumenti tua triverit area centum,*
> *Non tuus hinc capiet venter plus quam meus.*[7]

[Though endless corn come to your threshing floor,
You can, like me, but eat your fill, no more.]

"An evil sickness," Solomon calls it, "and reserved to them for an evil" (13th verse). "They that will be rich fall into many fears and temptations, into many foolish and noisome lusts, which drown men in perdition" (1 Tim. vi, 9). "Gold and silver hath destroyed many" (Ecclus. viii, 2). *Divitiæ sæculi sunt laquei diaboli:* so writes Bernard; worldly wealth is the devil's bait: and as the moon when she is fuller of light is still farthest from the sun, the more wealth they have, the farther they are commonly from God. (If I had said this of myself, rich men would have pulled me a-pieces; but hear who saith, and who seconds it, an Apostle.) Therefore St. James bids them "weep and howl for the miseries that shall come upon them; their gold shall rust and canker, and eat their flesh as fire" (James v, 1, 2, 3). I may then boldly conclude with Theodoret,[1] *Quotiescunque divitiis affluentem,* etc., "As often as you shall see a man abounding in wealth," *qui gemmis bibit et Sarrano dormit in ostro* [who drinks from jewelled cups and sleeps on purple], "and naught withal, I beseech you call him not happy, but esteem him unfortunate, because he hath many occasions offered to live unjustly; on the other side, a poor man is not miserable if he be good, but therefore happy that those evil occasions are taken from him."

> *Non possidentem multa vocaveris*
> *Recte beatum'; rectius occupat*
> *Nomen beati, qui deorum*
> *Muneribus sapienter uti,*
> *Duramque callet pauperiem pati,*
> *Pejusque leto flagitium timet.*[2]

He is not happy that is rich,
  And hath the world at will,
But he that wisely can God's gifts
  Possess and use them still:
That suffers and with patience
  Abides hard poverty,
And chooseth rather for to die;
  Than do such villainy.

Wherein now consists his happiness? What privileges hath he more than other men? Or rather what miseries, what cares and discontents hath he not more than other men?

> *Non enim gazæ, neque consularis*
> *Summovet lictor miseros tumultus*
> *Mentis, et curas laqueata circum*
> * Tecta volantes.*[3]

> Nor treasures, nor mayors' officers remove
> The miserable tumults of the mind:
> Or cares that lie about, or fly above
> Their high-roofed houses, with huge beams combin'd.

'Tis not his wealth can vindicate him, let him have Job's inventory, *sint Crœsi et Crassi licet, non hos Pactolus aureas undas agens, eripiat unquam e miseriis*, Crœsus or rich Crassus cannot now command health, or get himself a stomach. "His worship," as Apuleius describes him,[1] "in all his plenty and great provision, is forbidden to eat, or else hath no appetite" (sick in bed, can take no rest, sore grieved with some chronic disease, contracted with full diet and ease, or troubled in mind), "whenas, in the meantime, all his household are merry, and the poorest servant that he keeps doth continually feast." 'Tis *bracteata felicitas*, as Seneca terms it,[2] tinfoiled happiness, *infelix felicitas*, an unhappy kind of happiness, if it be happiness at all. His gold, guard, clattering of harness, and fortifications against outward enemies, cannot free him from inward fears and cares.

> *Reveraque metus hominum, curæque sequaces*
> *Nec metuunt fremitus armorum, aut ferrea tela,*
> *Audacterque inter reges regumque potentes*
> *Versantur, neque fulgorem reverentur ab auro.*

> Indeed men still attending fears and cares
> Nor armours clashing, nor fierce weapons fears:
> With kings converse they boldly, and kings' peers,
> Fearing no flashing that from gold appears.

Look how many servants he hath, and so many enemies he suspects; for liberty he entertains ambition; his pleasures are no pleasures; and that which is worst, he cannot be private or enjoy himself as other men do, his state is a servitude. A countryman may travel from kingdom to kingdom, province to province, city to city, and glut his eyes with delightful objects, hawk, hunt, and use those ordinary disports, without any notice taken, all which a prince or a great man cannot do.[3] He keeps in for state, *ne majestatis dignitas evilescat* [in order not to make his royal dignity cheap], as our China kings, of Borneo, and Tartarian Chams, those *aurea mancipia* [golden slaves], are said to do, seldom or never seen abroad, *ut major sit hominum erga se observantia* [to inspire greater respect in their subjects], which the Persian kings so precisely observed of old.[4] A poor man takes more delight in an ordinary meal's meat, which he hath but seldom, than they do with all their exotic dainties and continual viands; *Quippe voluptatem commendat rarior usus*, 'tis the rarity and necessity that makes a thing acceptable and pleasant. Darius, put to flight by Alexander, drank puddle water to quench his thirst, and it was pleasanter, he swore, than any wine or mead. All excess, as Epictetus argues,[1] will cause a dislike; sweet will be sour, which made that temperate Epicurus sometimes voluntarily fast. But they, being always accustomed to the same dishes (which are nastily dressed by slovenly cooks, that after their obscenities never wash their bawdy hands[2]), be they fish, flesh, compounded, made dishes, or whatsoever else, are therefore cloyed; nectar's self grows loathsome to them, they are weary of all their fine palaces, they are to them but as so many prisons. A poor man drinks in a wooden dish, and eats his meat in wooden spoons, wooden platters, earthen vessels, and such homely stuff: the other in gold, silver, and precious stones; but with what success? *In auro bibitur venenum*, fear of poison in the one, security in the other. A poor man is able to write, to speak his mind, to do his own business himself; *locuples mittit parasitum*, saith Philostratus,[3] a rich man employs a parasite, and, as the mayor of a city, speaks by the town clerk, or by Mr. Recorder, when he cannot express himself. Nonius the senator[4] hath a purple coat as stiff with jewels as his mind is full of vices; rings on his fingers worth 20,000 sesterces, and as Perozes the Persian king,[5] an union in his ear worth an hundred pounds' weight of gold: Cleopatra hath whole boars and sheep served up to her table at once, drinks jewels dissolved, 40,000 sesterces in value;[6] but to what end?

> *Num tibi cum fauces urit sitis, aurea quæris Pocula?*[7]

Doth a man that is adry desire to drink in gold? Doth not a cloth suit become him as well, and keep him as warm, as all their silks, satins, damasks, taffeties and tissues? Is not homespun cloth as great a preservative against cold as a coat of Tartar lamb's-wool, dyed in grain, or a gown of giants' beards? Nero, saith Suetonius,[8] never put on one garment twice, and thou hast scarce one to put on? what's the difference? one's sick, the other sound: such is the whole tenor of their lives, and that which is the consummation and upshot of all, death itself, makes the greatest difference. One like a hen feeds on the dunghill all his days, but is served up at last to his Lord's table; the other as a falcon is fed with partridge and pigeons, and carried on his master's fist, but when he dies is flung to the muckhill, and there lies. The rich man lives like Dives jovially here on earth, *temulentus divitiis* [drunk with riches], makes the best of it; and "boasts himself in the multitude of his riches" (Ps. xlix, 6); he thinks his house, "called after his own name," shall continue for ever (verse 11); "but he perisheth like a beast" (verse 20), "his way utters his folly" (verse 13); *male parta male dilabuntur* [ill-gotten gains are soon squandered]; "like sheep they lie in the grave" (verse 14). *Puncto descendunt ad infernum,* "they spend their days in wealth, and go suddenly down to hell" (Job xxi, 13). For all physicians and medicines enforcing nature, a swooning wife, families' complaints, friends' tears, dirges, masses, *nœnias* [wailing women], funerals, for all orations, counterfeit hired acclamations, elogiums, epitaphs, hearses, heralds, black mourners, solemnities, obelisks, and Mausolean tombs if he have them, at least, he, like a hog, goes to hell [1] with a guilty conscience (*propter hos dilatavit infernus os suum* [for these Hell opened wide her mouth]), and a poor man's curse: his memory stinks like the snuff of a candle when it is put out; scurrile libels and infamous obloquies accompany him; whenas poor Lazarus is *Dei sacrarium,* the temple of God, lives and dies in true devotion, hath no more attendants but his own innocency, the heaven a tomb, desires to be dissolved, buried in his mother's lap, and hath a company of angels ready to convey his soul into Abraham's bosom,[2] he leaves an everlasting and a sweet memory behind him. Crassus and Sylla are indeed still recorded, but not so much for their wealth as for their victories; Crœsus for his end, Solomon for his wisdom. In a word, "to get wealth is a great trouble, anxiety to keep, grief to lose it." [3]

> *Quid dignum stolidis mentibus imprecer?*
> *Opes, honores ambiant;*
> *Et cum falsa gravi mole paraverint,*
> *Tum vera cognoscant bona.*[4]

[For fools what fitting curse should I call down?
That they should wealth and honours court,
And with much toil make these false goods their own.
Then learn to know the better sort.]

But consider all those other unknown, concealed happinesses which a poor man hath (I call them unknown, because they be not acknowledged in the world's esteem, or so taken); *O fortunatos nimium bona si sua norint:* happy they are in the meantime if they would take notice of it, make use, or apply

it to themselves. "A poor man wise is better than a foolish
king" (Eccles. iv, 13). "Poverty is the way to heaven,"[1] the
mistress of philosophy,[2] the mother of religion, virtue, sobriety,
sister of innocency, and an upright mind.[3] How many such
encomiums might I add out of the Fathers, philosophers, orators!
It troubles many that are poor, they account of it as a great
plague, curse, a sign of God's hatred, *ipsum scelus*, damned
villainy itself, a disgrace, shame and reproach; but to whom,
or why? "If fortune hath envied me wealth, thieves have
robbed me, my father have not left me such revenues as
others have," that I am a younger brother, basely born,

> *Cui sine luce genus, surdumque parentum*
> *Nomen,*

of mean parentage, a dirt-dauber's son, "am I therefore to be
blamed? an eagle, a bull, a lion is not rejected for his poverty,
and why should a man?"[4] 'Tis *fortunæ telum, non culpæ,*[5]
fortune's fault, not mine. "Good sir, I am a servant" (to use
Seneca's words[6]), "howsoever your poor friend; a servant, and
yet your chamber-fellow, and, if you consider better of it, your
fellow-servant." I am thy drudge in the world's eyes, yet in
God's sight peradventure thy better, my soul is more precious,
and I dearer unto Him. *Etiam servi diis curæ sunt,* as Evangelus
at large proves in Macrobius, the meanest servant is most
precious in His sight. Thou art an Epicure, I am a good Christian;
thou art many parasangs before me in means, favour, wealth,
honour, Claudius his Narcissus, Nero's Massa, Domitian's Parthenius, a favourite, a golden slave; thou coverest thy floors
with marble, thy roofs with gold, thy walls with statues, fine
pictures, curious hangings, etc.; what of all this? *calcas opes*
[you tread on wealth], etc., what's all this to true happiness?
I live and breathe under that glorious heaven, that august
Capitol of nature, enjoy the brightness of stars, that clear light
of sun and moon, those infinite creatures, plants, birds, beasts,
fishes, herbs, all that sea and land afford, far surpassing all
that art and *opulentia* can give. I am free, and which Seneca
said of Rome,[7] *culmus liberos texit, sub marmore et auro postea
servitus habitavit* [when free they lived under thatch, their
slavery was housed in marble and gold]. Thou hast *Amaltheæ
cornu* [cornucopia], plenty, pleasure, the world at will, I am
despicable and poor; but a word overshot, a blow in choler, a
game at tables, a loss at sea, a sudden fire, the prince's dislike,
a little sickness, etc., may make us equal in an instant; how-

soever take thy time, triumph and insult awhile, *cinis æquat*, as Alphonsus said,[1] death will equalize us all at last. I live sparingly in the meantime, am clad homely, fare hardly; is this a reproach? am I the worse for it? am I contemptible for it? am I to be reprehended? A learned man in Nevisanus[2] was taken down for sitting amongst gentlemen, but he replied, "My nobility is about the head, yours declines to the tail," and they were silent. Let them mock, scoff, and revile, 'tis not thy scorn, but his that made thee so; "He that mocketh the poor, reproacheth him that made him" (Prov. xvii, 5), "and he that rejoiceth at affliction shall not be unpunished." For the rest, the poorer thou art, the happier thou art,[3] *ditior est, at non melior*, saith Epictetus, he is richer, not better than thou art, not so free from lust, envy, hatred, ambition.

> *Beatus ille qui procul negotiis*
> *Paterna rura bobus exercet suis.*

Happy he, in that he is freed from the tumults of the world, he seeks no honours, gapes after no preferment, flatters not, envies not, temporizeth not, but lives privately, and well contented with his estate;[4]

> *Nec spes corde avidas, nec curam pascit inanem,*
> *Securus quo fata cadant.*

> [He is not troubled with ambition nor vexed with care; indifferent to the fate of kingdoms.]

He is not troubled with state matters, whether kingdoms thrive better by succession or election; whether monarchies should be mixed, temperate, or absolute; the house of Ottomon's and Austria is all one to him; he inquires not after colonies or new discoveries; whether Peter were at Rome, or Constantine's donation be of force; what comets or new stars signify, whether the earth stand or move, there be a new world in the moon, or infinite worlds, etc. He is not touched with fear of invasions, factions, or emulations.

> *Felix ille animi, divisque simillimus ipsis,*
> *Quem non mordaci resplendens gloria fuco*
> *Sollicitat, non jastosi mala gaudia luxus,*
> *Sed tacitos sinit ire dies, et paupere cultu*
> *Exigit innocuæ tranquilla silentia vitæ.*[5][6]

> An happy soul, and like to God himself,
> Whom not vain glory macerates or strife,
> Or wicked joys of that proud swelling pelf,
> But leads a still, poor, and contented life.

A secure, quiet, blissful state he hath, if he could acknowledge it.[1] But here is the misery, that he will not take notice of it; he repines at rich men's wealth, brave hangings, dainty fare, as Simonides objecteth to Hiero, he hath all the pleasures of the world, *in lectis eburneis dormit, vinum phialis bibit, optimis unguentis delibuitur*, "he knows not the affliction of Joseph, stretching himself on ivory beds, and singing to the sound of the viol."[2] And it troubles him that he hath not the like: there is a difference (he grumbles) between laplolly and pheasants, to tumble i' th' straw and lie in a down bed, betwixt wine and water, a cottage and a palace. "He hates nature" (as Pliny characterizeth him[3]) "that she hath made him lower than a god, and is angry with the gods that any man goes before him"; and although he hath received much, yet (as Seneca follows it[4]) "he thinks it an injury that he hath no more, and is so far from giving thanks for his tribuneship, that he complains he is not prætor; neither doth that please him, except he may be consul." Why is he not a prince, why not a monarch, why not an emperor? Why should one man have so much more than his fellows, one have all, another nothing? Why should one man be a slave or drudge to another? one surfeit, another starve, one live at ease, another labour, without any hope of better fortune? Thus they grumble, mutter, and repine: not considering that inconstancy of human affairs, judicially conferring one condition with another, or well weighing their own present estate. What they are now, thou mayest shortly be; and what thou art, they shall likely be. Expect a little, confer future and times past with the present, see the event, and comfort thyself with it. It is as well to be discerned in commonwealths, cities, families, as in private men's estates. Italy was once lord of the world, Rome, the queen of cities, vaunted herself of two myriads of inhabitants;[5] now that all-commanding country is possessed by petty princes, Rome a small village in respect.[6] Greece of old the seat of civility, mother of sciences. and humanity; now forlorn, the nurse of barbarism, a den of thieves. Germany then, saith Tacitus, was incult and horrid, now full of magnificent cities: Athens, Corinth, Carthage, how flourishing cities! now buried in their own ruins: *corvorum, ferarum, aprorum, et bestiarum lustra*, like so many wildernesses, a receptacle of wild beasts. Venice, a poor fisher-town, Paris, London, small cottages in Cæsar's time, now most noble emporiums. Valois, Plantagenet, and Scaliger, how fortunate families! how likely to continue! now quite extinguished and rooted out. He stands aloft to-day, full of favour, wealth, honour, and prosperity, in the top of fortune's wheel: to-morrow in prison, worse than nothing, his son's a beggar. Thou art a poor servile drudge, *fæx populi* [the dregs of the people], a very slave; thy son may come to be a prince, with Maximinus, Agathocles, etc., a senator, a general of an army. Thou standest bare to him now, workest for him, drudgest for him and his, takest an alms of him; stay but a little, and his next heir peradventure shall consume all with riot, be degraded, thou exalted, and he shall beg of thee. Thou shalt be his most honourable patron, he thy devout servant, his posterity shall run, ride, and do as much for thine; as it was with Frescobald and Cromwell,[1] it may be for thee. Citizens devour country gentlemen, and settle in their seats; after two or three descents, they consume all in riot, it returns to the city again.

> *Novus incola venit;*
> *Nam propriæ telluris herum natura, neque illum,*
> *Nec me, nec quenquam statuit; nos expulit ille;*
> *Illum aut nequities, aut vafri inscitia furis.*[2]

> [Have we liv'd at a more frugal rate
> Since this new stranger seiz'd on our estate?
> Nature will no perpetual heir assign,
> Or make the farm his property or mine.
> He turn'd us out; but follies all his own,
> Or law-suits and their knaveries yet unknown,
> Or, all his follies and his law-suits past,   ·
> Some long-liv'd heir shall turn him out at last.]

A lawyer buys out his poor client, after a while his client's posterity buy out him and his; so things go round, ebb and flow.

> *Nunc ager Umbreni sub nomine, nuper Ofellæ*
> *Dictus erat, nulli proprius, sed cedit in usum*
> *Nunc mihi, nunc aliis.*

> [The farm, once mine, now bears Umbrenus' name;
> The use alone, not property, we claim.]

As he said then, *Ager cujus, quot habes dominos?* [Whose art thou, field? How many masters hast thou?] so say I of land, houses, movables and money, mine to-day, his anon, whose to-morrow? In fine (as Machiavel observes[3]), "virtue and prosperity beget rest; rest idleness; idleness riot; riot destruction: from which we come again to good laws; good laws engender virtuous actions; virtue, glory, and prosperity"; and "'tis no dishonour then" (as Guicciardine adds) "for a flourishing man, city, or state to come to ruin, nor infelicity to be subject to the law of nature."[1] *Ergo terrena calcanda, sitienda cœlestia*, therefore (I say) scorn this transitory state, look up to heaven, think not what others are, but what thou art, *qua parte locatus es in re*,[2] and what thou shalt be, what thou mayest be. Do (I say) as Christ Himself did, when He lived here on earth, imitate Him as much as in thee lies. How many great Cæsars, mighty monarchs, tetrarchs, dynasts, princes lived in His days, in what plenty, what delicacy, how bravely attended, what a deal of gold and silver, what treasure, how many sumptuous palaces had they, what provinces and cities, ample territories, fields, rivers, fountains, parks, forests, lawns, woods, cells, etc.! Yet Christ had none of all this, He would have none of this, He voluntarily rejected all this, He could not be ignorant, He could not err in His choice, He contemned all this, He chose that which was safer, better, and more certain, and less to be repented, a mean estate, even poverty itself; and why dost thou then doubt to follow Him, to imitate Him, and His apostles, to imitate all good men? So do thou tread in His divine steps, and thou shalt not err eternally, as too many worldlings do, that run on in their own dissolute courses, to their confusion and ruin, thou shalt not do amiss. Whatsoever thy fortune is, be contented with it, trust in Him, rely on Him, refer thyself wholly to Him. For know this, in conclusion, *non est volentis nec currentis, sed miserentis Dei*, 'tis not as men, but as God will. "The Lord maketh poor and maketh rich, bringeth low, and exalteth" (1 Sam. ii, ver. 7, 8), "he lifteth the poor from the dust, and raiseth the beggar from the dunghill, to set them amongst princes, and make them inherit the seat of glory"; 'tis all as He pleaseth, how, and when, and whom; He that appoints the end (though to us unknown) appoints the means likewise subordinate to the end.

Yea, but their present estate crucifies and torments most mortal men, they have no such forecast to see what may be, what shall likely be, but what is, though not wherefore, or from whom; *hoc angit*, their present misfortunes grind their souls, and an envious eye which they cast upon other men's prosperities; *Vicinumque pecus grandius uber habet* [your neighbour's cattle give more milk], how rich, how fortunate, how happy is he! But in the meantime he doth not consider the other miseries, his infirmities of body and mind, that accompany his estate, but still reflects upon his own false conceived woes and wants, whereas if the matter were duly examined, he is in no distress at all, he hath no cause to complain: [1]

> *Tolle querelas,*
> *Pauper enim non est cui rerum suppetit usus,* [2]

[Then cease complaining, friend, and learn to live.
He is not poor to whom kind fortune grants,
Even with a frugal hand, what nature wants,]

he is not poor, he is not in need. "Nature is content with bread and water; and he that can rest satisfied with that, may contend with Jupiter himself for happiness." [3] In that golden age, *somnos dedit umbra salubres, potum quoque lubricus amnis,* [4] the tree gave wholesome shade to sleep under, and the clear rivers drink. The Israelites drank water in the wilderness; Samson, David, Saul, Abraham's servant when he went for Isaac's wife, the Samaritan woman, and how many besides might I reckon up, Egypt, Palestine, whole countries in the Indies, [5] that drank water all their lives. The Persian kings themselves drank no other drink than the water of Choaspes, that runs by Susa, which was carried in bottles after them whithersoever they went. [6] Jacob desired no more of God, but bread to eat, and clothes to put on in his journey (Gen. xxviii, 20). *Bene est cui deus obtulit Parca quod satis est manu* [happy he to whom heaven hath given enough, yet sparingly]; bread is enough "to strengthen the heart." [7] And if you study philosophy aright, saith Madaurensis, "whatsoever is beyond this moderation, is not useful, but troublesome." [8] A. Gellius, [9] out of Euripides, accounts bread and water enough to satisfy nature, "of which there is no surfeit; the rest is not a feast, but a riot." St. Hierome esteems him rich "that hath bread to eat, and a potent man that is not compelled to be a slave: hunger is not ambitious, so that it have to eat, and thirst doth not prefer a cup of gold." [10] It was no Epicurean speech of an Epicure, "He that is not satisfied with a little will never have enough:" and very good counsel of him in the poet, [11] "O my son, mediocrity of means agrees best with men; too much is pernicious."

> *Divitiæ grandes homini sunt vivere parce,*
> *Æquo animo.*

[Great fortune 'tis, and riches of a kind,
To live on little with contented mind.]

And if thou canst be content, thou hast abundance, *nihil est, nihil deest,* thou hast little, thou wantest nothing. 'Tis all one to be hanged in a chain of gold, or in a rope; to be filled with dainties, or coarser meat.

> *Si ventri bene, si lateri, pedibusque tuis, nil*
> *Divitiæ poterunt regales addere majus.*[1]

> If belly, sides and feet be well at ease,
> A prince's treasure can thee no more please.

Socrates in a fair, seeing so many things bought and sold, such a multitude of people convented to that purpose, exclaimed forthwith, "O ye gods, what a sight of things do not I want! 'Tis thy want alone that keeps thee in health of body and mind, and that which thou persecutest and abhorrest as a feral plague is thy physician and chiefest friend,[2] which makes thee a good man, a healthful, a sound, a virtuous, an honest and happy man." For when Virtue came from heaven (as the poet feigns) rich men kicked her up, wicked men abhorred her, courtiers scoffed at her, citizens hated her, and that she was thrust out of doors in every place; she came at last to her sister Poverty, where she had found good entertainment.[3] Poverty and Virtue dwell together.

> *O vitæ tuta facultas*
> *Pauperis, angustique lares, o munera nondum*
> *Intellecta deum.*[4]

> [To need but little and to feel secure—
> The great though unmarked blessing of the poor.]

How happy art thou if thou couldst be content! "Godliness is great gain, if a man can be content with that which he hath" (1 Tim. vi, 6); and all true happiness is in a mean estate. I have a little wealth, as he said,[5] *sed quas animus magnas facit*, a kingdom in conceit:

> *Nil amplius opto,*
> *Maia nate, nisi ut propria hæc mihi munera faxis;* [6]

> [Naught more I desire, O son of Maia, than that thou
> shouldst make these gifts my own;]

I have enough and desire no more.

> *Di bene fecerunt inopis me quodque pusilli*
> *Fecerunt animi;* [7]

> [The gods did well when they made me lacking in
> ideas and in spirit;]

'tis very well, and to my content. *Vestem et fortunam concinnam potius quam laxam probo*,[8] let my fortune and my garments be both alike fit for me. And which Sebastian Foscarinus, sometime Duke of Venice, caused to be engraven on his tomb in St. Mark's Church, "Hear, O ye Venetians, and I will tell you which is the best thing in the world: to contemn it":[1] I will engrave it in my heart, it shall be my whole study to contemn it. Let them take wealth, *stercora stercus amet* [let dung delight in dung], so that I may have security; *bene qui latuit, bene vixit:* though I live obscure, yet I live clean and honest;[2] and whenas the lofty oak is blown down, the silly reed may stand. Let them take glory, for that's their misery; let them take honour, so that I may have heart's ease. *Duc me, O Jupiter, et tu fatum,* etc.[3] Lead me, O God, whither thou wilt, I am ready to follow; command, I will obey. I do not envy at their wealth, titles, offices;

> *Stet quicunque volet potens*
> *Aulæ culmine lubrico,*
> *Me dulcis saturet quies,*

[Let who will stand on the slippery slope of fame,
I want but sweet tranquillity,]

let me live quiet and at ease. *Erimus fortasse* (as he[4] comforted himself) *quando illi non erunt,* when they are dead and gone, and all their pomp vanished, our memory may flourish:

> *Dant perennes*
> *Stemmata non peritura Musæ.*[5]

[The immortal Muses confer a pedigree that shall not fade.]

Let him be my lord, patron, baron, earl, and possess so many goodly castles, 'tis well for me that I have a poor house, and a little wood, and a well by it, etc.[6]

> *His me consolor victurum suavius, ac si*
> *Quæstor avus pater atque meus, patruusque fuissent.*

[With which I feel myself more truly blest
Than if my sires the quæstor's power possess'd.]

I live, I thank God, as merrily as he, and triumph as much in this my mean estate, as if my father and uncle had been Lord Treasurer, or my Lord Mayor. He feeds of many dishes, I of one; *qui Christum curat, non multum curat quam de pretiosis cibis stercus conficiat:*[7] what care I of what stuff my excrements be made? "He that lives according to nature cannot be poor, and he that exceeds can never have enough,"[8] *totus non sufficit orbis,* the whole world cannot give him content. "A small thing that the righteous hath, is better than the riches

of the ungodly" (Ps. xxxvii, 19); "and better is a poor morsel
with quietness, than abundance with strife" (Prov. xvii, 7).

Be content then, enjoy thyself, and, as Chrysostom adviseth,[1]
"be not angry for what thou hast not, but give God hearty
thanks for what thou hast received."

> *Si dat oluscula*
> *Mensa minuscula*
> *Pace referta,*
> *Ne pete grandia,*
> *Lautaque prandia*
> *Lite repleta.*[2]

[If your humble table offer you but herbs along with
peace, seek not rich and elegant banquets full
of strife.]

But what wantest thou, to expostulate the matter? or what
hast thou not better than a rich man? "Health, competent
wealth, children, security, sleep, friends, liberty, diet, apparel,
and what not," [3] or at least mayest have (the means being so
obvious, easy, and well known); for as he inculcated to himself,

> *Vitam quæ faciunt beatiorem,*
> *Jucundissime Martialis, hæc sunt;*
> *Res non parta labore, sed relicta,*
> *Lis nunquam, etc.,*[4]

[The things which make life happy, my sweet Martial,
are these: a fortune gained not by work but by
inheritance, freedom from law-suits, etc.,]

I say again thou hast, or at least mayst have it, if thou wilt
thyself, and that which I am sure he wants, a merry heart.
"Passing by a village in the territory of Milan," saith St. Austin,[5]
"I saw a poor beggar that had got belike his bellyful of meat,
jesting and merry; I sighed, and said to some of my friends
that were then with me, What a deal of trouble, madness,
pain and grief do we sustain and exaggerate unto ourselves, to
get that secure happiness which this poor beggar hath prevented
us of, and which we peradventure shall never have! For that
which he hath now attained with the begging of some small
pieces of silver, a temporal happiness, and present heart's ease,
I cannot compass with all my careful windings, and running in
and out. And surely [6] the beggar was very merry, but I was
heavy; he was secure, but I timorous. And if any man should
ask me now, whether I had rather be merry, or still so solicitous
and sad, I should say, merry. If he should ask me again,
whether I had rather be as I am, or as this beggar was, I should

sure choose to be as I am, tortured still with cares and fears;
but out of peevishness, and not out of truth." That which
St. Austin said of himself here in this place, I may truly say to
thee, thou discontented wretch, thou covetous niggard, thou
churl, thou ambitious and swelling toad, 'tis not want but
peevishness which is the cause of thy woes; settle thine affection,
thou hast enough.

> Denique sit finis quærendi, quoque habeas plus,
> Pauperiem metuas minus, et finire laborem
> Incipias; parto, quod avebas, utere.[1]

> [Make an end of acquiring, with so much in hand
> cease to fear poverty, and begin to wind up your
> labours; having got what you desired, use it.]

Make an end of scraping, purchasing this manor, this field, that
house, for this and that child; thou hast enough for thyself
and them:

> Quod petis hic est,
> Est Ulubris, animus si te non deficit æquus,[2]

> [What you are looking for is here, in this village, if
> you keep a cheerful mind,]

'tis at hand, at home already, which thou so earnestly seekest.
But

> O si angulus ille
> Proximus accedat, qui nunc denormat agellum!

> [If I but had that next corner to round off my estate!]

O that I had but that one nook of ground, that field there,
that pasture! *O si urnam argenti fors quis mihi monstret!* O
that I could but find a pot of money now, to purchase, etc.,
to build me a new house, to marry my daughter, place my
son, etc. "O if I might but live a while longer to see all things
settled, some two or three years, I would pay my debts," make
all my reckonings even: but they are come and past, and thou
hast more business than before. "O madness, to think to settle
that in thine old age when thou hast more, which in thy youth
thou canst not now compose, having but a little." [3] Pyrrhus
would first conquer Africa, and then Asia, *et tum suaviter agere,*
and then live merrily and take his ease: but when Cineas the
orator told him he might do that already, *id jam posse fieri,*
he rested satisfied, condemning his own folly.[4] *Si parva licet
componere magnis* [to compare small things with great], thou
mayst do the like, and therefore be composed in thy fortune.
Thou hast enough: he that is wet in a bath, can be no more wet

if he be flung into Tiber, or into the ocean itself; and if thou
hadst all the world, or a solid mass of gold as big as the world,
thou canst not have more than enough; enjoy thyself at length,
and that which thou hast; the mind is all; be content, thou art
not poor, but rich, and so much the richer, as Censorinus [1]
well writ to Cerellius, *quanto pauciora optas, non quo plura
possides*, in wishing less, not having more. I say then, *Non
adjice opes, sed minue cupiditates* ('tis Epicurus' advice [2]), add
no more wealth, but diminish thy desires; and as Chrysostom [3]
well seconds him, *Si vis ditari, contemne divitias* [if thou wilt be
rich despise riches]; that's true plenty, not to have, but not to
want riches, *non habere, sed non indigere, vera abundantia*; 'tis
more glory to contemn than to possess; *et nihil egere est deorum*
[and to want nothing is divine]. How many deaf, dumb, halt,
lame, blind, miserable persons could I reckon up that are poor,
and withal distressed, in imprisonment, banishment, galley-slaves,
condemned to the mines, quarries, to gyves, in dungeons, perpetual thraldom, than all which thou art richer, thou art more
happy, to whom thou art able to give an alms, a lord in respect,
a petty prince! Be contented then, I say, repine and mutter
no more, "for thou art not poor indeed but in opinion." [4]

Yea, but this is very good counsel, and rightly applied to
such as have it and will not use it, that have a competency,
that are able to work and get their living by the sweat of their
brows, by their trade, that have something yet; he that hath
birds may catch birds; but what shall we do that are slaves by
nature, impotent, and unable to help ourselves, mere beggars,
that languish and pine away, that have no means at all, no hope
of means, no trust of delivery, or of better success? As those
old Britons complained to their lords and masters the Romans,
oppressed by the Picts, *mare ad barbaros, barbari ad mare*,
the barbarians drove them to the sea, the sea drove them back
to the barbarians: our present misery compels us to cry out
and howl, to make our moan to rich men; they turn us back
with a scornful answer to our misfortune again, and will take no
pity of us; they commonly overlook their poor friends in adversity; if they chance to meet them, they voluntarily forget and
will take no notice of them; they will not, they cannot help us.
Instead of comfort they threaten us, miscall, scoff at us, to
aggravate our misery, give us bad language, or if they do give
good words, what's that to relieve us? According to that of
Thales, *facile est alios monere*; who cannot give good counsel?
'tis cheap, it costs them nothing. It is an easy matter when

one's belly is full to declaim against feasting; *Qui satur est pleno laudat jejunia ventre.*   "Doth the wild ass bray when he hath grass, or loweth the ox when he hath fodder?" (Job vi, 5). *Neque enim populo Romano quidquam potest esse lætius,*[1] no man living so jocund, so merry as the people of Rome when they had plenty; but when they came to want, to be hunger-starved, "neither shame, nor laws, nor arms, nor magistrates could keep them in obedience."   Seneca pleadeth hard for poverty, and so did those lazy philosophers: but in the meantime he was rich,[2] they had wherewithal to maintain themselves; but doth any poor man extol it?   "There are those" (saith Bernard [3]) "that approve of a mean estate, but on that condition they never want themselves; and some again are meek so long as they may say or do what they list; but if occasion be offered, how far are they from all patience!"   I would to God (as he said) "no man should commend poverty, but he that is poor,"[4] or he that so much admires it would relieve, help, or ease others.

> *Nunc si nos audis, atque es divinus Apollo,*
> *Dic mihi, qui nummos non habet, unde petat:* [5]

> Now if thou hear'st us, and art a good man,
> Tell him that wants, to get means, if you can.

But no man hears us, we are most miserably dejected, the scum of the world.   *Vix habet in nobis jam nova plaga locum* [our bodies have scarce room for a new stripe].[6]   We can get no relief, no comfort, no succour, *Et nihil inveni quod mihi ferret opem.*[7] We have tried all means, yet find no remedy: no man living can express the anguish and bitterness of our souls, but we that endure it; we are distressed, forsaken, in torture of body and mind, in another hell: and what shall we do?   When Crassus [8] the Roman consul warred against the Parthians, after an unlucky battle fought, he fled away in the night, and left four thousand men, sore sick and wounded in his tents, to the fury of the enemy, which when the poor men perceived, *clamoribus et ululatibus omnia complerunt,* they made lamentable moan, and roared downright, as loud as Homer's Mars when he was hurt, which the noise of ten thousand men could not drown, and all for fear of present death.   But our estate is far more tragical and miserable, much more to be deplored, and far greater cause have we to lament; the devil and the world persecute us, all good fortune hath forsaken us, we are left to the rage of beggary, cold, hunger, thirst, nastiness, sickness, irksomeness, to continual torment, labour and pain, to derision

and contempt, bitter enemies all, and far worse than any death;
death alone we desire, death we seek, yet cannot have it, and
what shall we do? *Quod male fers, assuesce; feres bene:* accustom
thyself to it, and it will be tolerable at last. Yea, but I may not,
I cannot, *In me consumpsit vires fortuna nocendo* [Fortune hath
consumed all her arrows upon me], I am in the extremity of
human adversity; and as a shadow leaves the body when the
sun is gone, I am now left and lost, and quite forsaken of the
world. *Qui jacet in terra, non habet unde cadat* [he that is on
the ground can fall no farther]; comfort thyself with this yet,
thou art at the worst, and before it be long it will either overcome thee or thou it. If it be violent, it cannot endure, *aut
solvetur, aut solvet*: let the devil himself and all the plagues of
Egypt come upon thee at once, *Ne tu cede malis, sed contra
audentior ito,* be of good courage; misery is virtue's whetstone.

> *Serpens, sitis, ardor, arenæ,*
> *Dulcia virtuti,*[1]

as Cato told his soldiers marching in the deserts of Libya, thirst,
heat, sands, serpents, were pleasant to a valiant man; honourable enterprises are accompanied with dangers and damages,
as experience evinceth; they will make the rest of thy life relish
the better. But put case they continue; thou art not so poor
as thou wast born, and, as some hold, much better to be pitied
than envied. But be it so thou hast lost all, poor thou art,
dejected, in pain of body, grief of mind, thine enemies insult
over thee, thou art as bad as Job; "yet tell me" (saith Chrysostom), "was Job or the devil the greater conqueror? surely
Job. The devil had his goods, he sat on the muck-hill and kept
his good name; he lost his children, health, friends, but he kept
his innocency; he lost his money, but he kept his confidence in
God, which was better than any treasure."[2] Do thou then as
Job did, triumph as Job did, ánd be not molested as every fool
is.[3] *Sed qua ratione potero?* How shall this be done? Chrysostom answers, *Facile, si cœlum cogitaveris,* with great facility,
if thou shalt but meditate on heaven. Hannah wept sore,
and, troubled in mind, could not eat; "But why weepest thou?"
said Elkanah her husband, "and why eatest thou not? why is
thine heart troubled? am not I better to thee than ten sons?"[4]
and she was quiet. Thou art here vexed in this world;[5] but
say to thyself, "Why art thou troubled, O my soul?" Is not
God better to thee than all temporalities, and momentany
pleasures of the world? be then pacified. And though thou

beest now peradventure in extreme want, it may be 'tis for thy
further good,[1] to try thy patience, as it did Job's, and exercise
thee in this life: trust in God, and rely upon Him, and thou shalt
be crowned in the end.[2] What's this life to eternity? The
world hath forsaken thee, thy friends and fortunes all are gone:
yet know this, that the very hairs of thine head are numbered,
that God is a spectator of all thy miseries, He sees thy wrongs,
woes, and wants. "'Tis His good will and pleasure it should
be so, and He knows better what is for thy good than thou
thyself."[3] "His providence is over all, at all times; he hath
set a guard of angels over us, and keeps us as the apple of his
eye" (Ps. xvii, 8). Some He doth exalt, prefer, bless with
wordly riches, honours, offices, and preferments, as so many
glistering stars He makes to shine above the rest: some He
doth miraculously protect from thieves, incursions, sword, fire,
and all violent mischances, and, as the poet[4] feigns of that
Lycian Pandarus, Lycaon's son, when he shot at Menelaus the
Grecian with a strong arm and deadly arrow, Pallas, as a good
mother keeps flies from her child's face asleep, turned by the
shaft, and made it hit on the buckle of his girdle; so some He
solicitously defends, others He exposeth to danger, poverty,
sickness, want, misery, He chastiseth and corrects, as to Him
seems best, in His deep, unsearchable, and secret judgment,
and all for our good. "The tyrant took the city" (saith
Chrysostom[5]), "God did not hinder it; led them away captives,
so God would have it; he bound them, God yielded to it: flung
them into the furnace, God permitted it: heat the oven hotter,
it was granted: and when the tyrant had done his worst, God
showed His power, and the children's patience"; He freed them:
so can He thee, and can help in an instant, when it seems to
Him good.[6] "Rejoice not against me, O my enemy; for though
I fall, I shall rise: when I sit in darkness, the Lord shall lighten
me."[7] Remember all those martyrs, what they have endured,
the utmost that human rage and fury could invent, with what
patience they have borne, with what willingness embraced it.[8]
"Though he kill me," saith Job, "I will trust in him." *Justus
inexpugnabilis*,[9] as Chrysostom holds, a just man is impregnable, and not to be overcome. The gout may hurt his hands,
lameness his feet, convulsions may torture his joints, but not
rectam mentem [his upright mind], his soul is free.

> *Nempe pecus, rem,*
> *Lectos, argentum tollas licet ; in manicis, et*
> *Compedibus sævo teneas custode.*[10]

[Perhaps, you mean,
My cattle, money, movables or land,
Then take them all.—But, slave, if I command,
A cruel jailer shall thy freedom seize.]

"Take away his money, his treasure is in heaven: banish him
his country, he is an inhabitant of that heavenly Jerusalem:
cast him into bands, his conscience is free; kill his body, it shall
rise again; he fights with a shadow that contends with an
upright man": [1] he will not be moved.

> *Si fractus illabatur orbis,*
> *Impavidum ferient ruinæ:*

though heaven itself should fall on his head, he will not be
offended. He is impenetrable, as an anvil hard, as constant
as Job.

> *Ipse deus simul atque volet me solvet, opinor.*

[God can deliver me when He will, I ween.]

Be thou such a one; let thy misery be what it will, what it can,
with patience endure it; thou mayst be restored as he was.
*Terris proscriptus, ad cœlum propera; ab hominibus desertus,
ad Deum fuge* [when proscribed from the earth, haste to heaven;
when deserted by men, turn to God]. "The poor shall not
always be forgotten, the patient abiding of the meek shall not
perish for ever" (Ps. ix, 18). "The Lord will be a refuge of the
oppressed, and a defence in the time of trouble" (verse 9).

> *Servus Epictetus, mutilati corporis, Irus*
> *Pauper; at hæc inter carus erat superis.* [2]

> Lame was Epictetus, and poor Irus,
> Yet to them both God was propitious.

Lodovicus Vertomannus, that famous traveller, endured much
misery, yet surely, saith Scaliger, he was *vir Deo carus*, in that
he did escape so many dangers. God especially protected him,
he was dear unto Him. *Modo in egestate, tribulatione, convalle
deplorationis,* etc. "Thou art now in the vale of misery, in
poverty, in agony, in temptation; rest, eternity, happiness,
immortality, shall be thy reward," [3] as Chrysostom pleads,
"if thou trust in God, and keep thine innocency." *Non si
male nunc, et olim sic erit semper* [if things are bad now, they
will not always be so], a good hour may come upon a sudden;
expect a little. [4]

Yea, but this expectation is it which tortures me in the
meantime; *futura expectans præsentibus angor* [5] [while waiting

for the future, I am tortured by the present], whilst the grass grows the horse starves: despair not, but hope well.[1]

> *Spera, Batte, tibi melius lux crastina ducet;*
> *Dum spiras spera.*[2]

> [Hope on, Battus, to-morrow will bring thee better hap; while thou breathest, hope.]

Cheer up, I say, be not dismayed; *Spes alit agricolas* [hope bears up the farmers]; "he that sows in tears, shall reap in joy" (Ps. cxxvi, 7).

> *Si fortune me tormente,*
> *Esperance me contente.*

> [If fortune torments me, hope contents me.]

Hope refresheth, as much as misery depresseth; hard beginnings have many times prosperous events, and that may happen at last which never was yet. "A desire accomplished delights the soul" (Prov. xiii, 19).

> *Grata superveniet quæ non sperabitur hora:* [3]

> Which makes m' enjoy my joys long wish'd at last,
> Welcome that hour shall come when hope is past:

a lowering morning may turn to a fair afternoon, *Nube solet pulsa candidus ire dies.*[4] "The hope that is deferred is the fainting of the heart, but when the desire cometh, it is a tree of life" (Prov. xiii, 12), *suavissimum est voti compos fieri*[5] [it is most sweet to have one's wish fulfilled]. Many men are both wretched and miserable at first, but afterwards most happy; and oftentimes it so falls out, as Machiavel[6] relates of Cosmus Medices, that fortunate and renowned citizen of Europe, "that all his youth was full of perplexity, danger, and misery, till forty years were past, and then upon a sudden the sun of his honour broke out as through a cloud." Huniades was fetched out of prison, and Henry the Third of Portugal out of a poor monastery, to be crowned kings.

> *Multa cadunt inter calicem supremaque labra,*

> [There 's many a slip 'twixt the cup and the lip,]

beyond all hope and expectation many things fall out, and who knows what may happen? *Nondum omnium dierum soles occiderunt,* as Philippus said, all the suns are not yet set, a day may come to make amends for all. "Though my father

and mother forsake me, yet the Lord will gather me up"
(Ps. xxvii, 10). "Wait patiently on the Lord, and hope in
him" (Ps. xxxvii, 7). "Be strong, hope and trust in the Lord,
and he will comfort thee, and give thee thine heart's desire"
(Ps. xxvii, 14).

Sperate, et vosmet rebus servate secundis.

[Hope, and reserve yourselves for better days.]

Fret not thyself because thou art poor, contemned, or not so
well for the present as thou wouldest be, not respected as thou
oughtest to be, by birth, place, worth; or that which is a double
corrosive, thou hast been happy, honourable, and rich, art now
distressed and poor, a scorn of men, a burden to the world,
irksome to thyself and others, thou hast lost all. *Miserum est
fuisse felicem* [it is most sad to have known happiness and lost
it], and, as Boethius calls it, *infelicissimum genus infortunii;*
[the saddest kind of misfortune]; this made Timon half mad
with melancholy, to think of his former fortunes and present
misfortunes: this alone makes many miserable wretches discontent. I confess it is a great misery to have been happy,
the quintessence of infelicity to have been honourable and
rich, but yet easily to be endured: security succeeds,[1] and to
a judicious man a far better estate. The loss of thy goods and
money is no loss; "thou hast lost them, they would otherwise
have lost thee."[2] If thy money be gone, "thou art so much
the lighter,"[3] and, as St. Hierome persuades Rusticus the
monk to forsake all and follow Christ: "Gold and silver are too
heavy metals for him to carry that seeks heaven."

*Vel nos in mare proximum,
Gemmas et lapides, aurum et inutile,
Summi materiam mali
Mittamus, scelerum si bene pœnitet.*[4]

[Let us cast into the sea our jewels and gems and
worthless gold, if we truly repent of our sins.]

Zeno the philosopher lost all his goods by shipwreck, he made
light of it, fortune had done him a good turn;[5] *Opes a me, animum auferre non potest:* she can take away my means, but not
my mind. He set her at defiance ever after, for she could not
rob him that had naught to lose: for he was able to contemn
more than they could possess or desire. Alexander sent an
hundred talents of gold to Phocion of Athens for a present,
because he heard he was a good man: but Phocion returned his

talents back again with a *Permitte me in posterum virum bonum esse*, [permit me] to be a good man still; let me be as I am: *Non mi aurum posco, nec mi pretium* [I ask not gold nor rich reward]. That Theban Crates flung of his own accord his money into the sea, *Abite nummi, ego vos mergam, ne mergar a vobis*, I had rather drown you than you should drown me. Can Stoics and Epicures thus contemn wealth, and shall not we that are Christians? It was *mascula vox et præclara*, a generous speech of Cotta in Sallust,[1] "Many miseries have happened unto me at home, and in the wars abroad, of which by the help of God some I have endured, some I have repelled, and by mine own valour overcome: courage was never wanting to my designs, nor industry to my intents: prosperity or adversity could never alter my disposition." A wise man's mind, as Seneca holds, "is like the state of the world above the moon, ever serene."[2] Come then what can come, befall what may befall, *infractum invictumque animum opponas*[3] [meet it with mind undismayed and unbroken]; *rebus augustis animosus atque fortis appare* [show thyself in adversity spirited and bold] (Hor. *Od.* 11, *lib.* 2). Hope and patience are two sovereign remedies for all, the surest reposals, the softest cushions to lean on in adversity:

> *Durum : sed levius fit patientia,*
> *Quicquid corrigere est nefas.*[4]

> ['Tis hard: but patience must endure,
> And soothe the woes it cannot cure.]

If it cannot be helped, or amended, make the best of it;[5] *necessitati qui se accommodat, sapit*,[6] he is wise that suits himself to the time. As at a game at tables, so do by all such inevitable accidents:

> *Ita vita est hominum quasi cum ludas tesseris,*
> *Si illud quod est maxime opus jactu non cadit,*
> *Illud quod cecidit forte, id arte ut corrigas;*[7]

if thou canst not fling what thou wouldst, play thy cast as well as thou canst. Everything, saith Epictetus, hath two handles, the one to be held by, the other not: 'tis in our choice to take and leave whether we will[8] (all which Simplicius, his commentator, hath illustrated by many examples), and 'tis in our power, as they say, to make or mar ourselves. Conform thyself then to thy present fortune, and cut thy coat according to thy cloth; *Ut quimus (quod aiunt) quando quod volumus non licet*[9] [let us do as we can (as the proverb is) since we may not as we will]; be

contented with thy lot, state, and calling, whatsoever it is, and
rest as well satisfied with thy present condition in this life.

> *Esto quod es ; quod sunt alii, sine quemlibet esse ;*
> *Quod non es, nolis ; quod potes esse, velis.*

> Be as thou art: and as they are, so let
> Others be still; what is and may be covet.

And as he that is invited to a feast eats what is set before him
and looks for no other, enjoy that thou hast, and ask no more
of God than what He thinks fit to bestow upon thee.[1] *Non
cuivis contingit adire Corinthum* [not every one is privileged to
visit Corinth], we may not be all gentlemen, all Catos, or Lælii,
as Tully telleth us, all honourable, illustrious, and serene, all
rich; but because mortal men want many things, "therefore,"
saith Theodoret,[2] "hath God diversely distributed His gifts,
wealth to one, skill to another, that rich men might encourage
and set poor men at work, poor men might learn several trades
to the common good." As a piece of arras is composed of
several parcels, some wrought of silk, some of gold, silver,
crewel of divers colours, all to serve for the exornation of the
whole; music is made of divers discords and keys; a total sum
of many small numbers; so is a commonwealth of several
inequal trades and callings. If all should be Crœsi and Darii,
all idle, all in fortunes equal, who should till the land?[3] as
Menenius Agrippa well satisfied the tumultuous rout of Rome,
in his elegant apologue of the belly and the rest of the members.[4]
Who should build houses, make our several stuffs for raiments?
We should all be starved for company, as Poverty declared at
large in Aristophanes' *Plutus*, and sue at last to be as we were at
first. And therefore God hath appointed this inequality of
states, orders, and degrees, a subordination, as in all other
things. The earth yields nourishment to vegetals, sensible
creatures feed on vegetals, both are substitutes to reasonable
souls, and men are subject amongst themselves, and all to
higher powers, so God would have it. All things then being
rightly examined and duly considered as they ought, there is
no such cause of so general discontent, 'tis not in the matter
itself, but in our mind, as we moderate our passions and esteem
of things. *Nihil aliud necessarium ut sis miser* (saith Cardan [5])
quam ut te miserum credas: let thy fortune be what it will, 'tis
thy mind alone that makes thee poor or rich, miserable or happy.
Vidi ego (saith divine Seneca) *in villa hilari et amœna mœstos,
et media solitudine occupatos ; non locus sed animus facit ad*

tranquillitatem: "I have seen men miserably dejected in a pleasant village, and some again well occupied and at good ease in a solitary desert; 'tis the mind, not the place, causeth tranquillity, and that gives true content." I will yet add a word or two for a corollary. Many rich men, I dare boldly say it, that lie on down beds, with delicacies pampered every day, in their well-furnished houses, live at less heart's ease, with more anguish, more bodily pain, and through their intemperance more bitter hours, than many a prisoner or galley-slave; *Mæcenas in pluma æque vigilat ac Regulus in dolio* [1] [Mæcenas can no more sleep on his feather-bed than Regulus in his cask]: those poor starved Hollanders, whom Bartison their captain left in Nova Zembla, *anno* 1596,[2] or those eight miserable Englishmen that were lately left behind to winter in a stove in Greenland in 77 degrees of latitude, 1630,[3] so pitifully forsaken, and forced to shift for themselves in a vast, dark, and desert place, to strive and struggle with hunger, cold, desperation, and death itself. 'Tis a patient and quiet mind (I say it again and again) gives true peace and content. So for all other things, they are, as old Chremes told us,[4] as we use them.

> *Parentes, patriam, amicos, genus, cognatos, divitias,*
> *Hæc perinde sunt ac illius animus qui ea possidet;*
> *Qui uti scit, ei bona; qui utitur non recte, mala.*

Parents, friends, fortunes, country, birth, alliance, etc., ebb and flow with our conceit; please or displease, as we accept and construe them, or apply them to ourselves. *Faber quisque fortunæ suæ* [every one is the architect of his own fortune], and in some sort I may truly say, prosperity and adversity are in our own hands. *Nemo læditur nisi a seipso* [no one is injured except by himself], and, which Seneca confirms out of his judgment and experience, "Every man's mind is stronger than fortune, and leads him to what side he will; a cause to himself each one is of his good or bad life." [5] But will we, or nill we, make the worst of it, and suppose a man in the greatest extremity, 'tis a fortune which some indefinitely prefer before prosperity; of two extremes it is the best. *Luxuriant animi rebus plerumque secundis*, men in prosperity forget God and themselves, they are besotted with their wealth as birds with henbane:[6] miserable if fortune forsake them, but more miserable if she tarry and overwhelm them:[7] for when they come to be in great place, rich, they that were most temperate, sober, and discreet in their private fortunes, as Nero, Otho, Vitellius,

Heliogabalus (*optimi imperatores nisi imperassent* [excellent
rulers till they were put to the test]), degenerate on a sudden
into brute beasts, so prodigious in lust, such tyrannical oppressors,
etc., they cannot moderate themselves, they become monsters,
odious, harpies, what not? *Cum triumphos, opes, honores adepti
sunt, ad voluptatem et otium deinceps se convertunt* [when they
attain to triumphs, wealth, and honours, they give themselves
up to pleasure and sloth]: 'twas Cato's note,[1] they cannot
contain. For that cause belike,

> *Eutrapelus cuicunque nocere volebat,*
> *Vestimenta dabat pretiosa : beatus enim jam,*
> *Cum pulchris tunicis sumet nova consilia et spes,*
> *Dormiet in lucem, scorto postponet honestum*
> *Officium.*[2]

Eutrapelus, when he would hurt a knave,
Gave him gay clothes and wealth to make him brave:
Because now rich, he would quite change his mind,
Keep whores, fly out, set honesty behind.

On the other side, in adversity many mutter and repine, despair,
etc.; both bad, I confess:

> *Ut calceus olim ;*
> *Si pede major erit, subvertet : si minor, uret,*[3]

as a shoe too big or too little, one pincheth, the other sets the
foot awry, *sed e malis minimum* [but of evils choose the least].
If adversity hath killed his thousand, prosperity hath killed his
ten thousand: therefore adversity is to be preferred; *hæc fræno
indiget, illa solatio*; [the one needs a curb, the other a solace]
illa fallit, hæc instruit [4]: the one deceives, the other instructs; the
one miserably happy, the other happily miserable; and therefore many philosophers have voluntarily sought adversity, and
so much commend it in their precepts. Demetrius, in Seneca,
esteemed it a great infelicity, that in his lifetime he had no misfortune, *miserum cui nihil unquam accidisset adversi*. Adversity
then is not so heavily to be taken, and we ought not in such
cases so much to macerate ourselves: there is no such odds in
poverty and riches. To conclude in Hierome's words,[5] "I will
ask our magnificoes, that build with marble and bestow a whole
manor on a thread, what difference between them and Paul the
Eremite, that bare old man? They drink in jewels, he in his
hand: he is poor and goes to heaven, they are rich and go
to hell."

MEMB. IV.

Against Servitude, Loss of Liberty, Imprisonment, Banishment

SERVITUDE, loss of liberty, imprisonment, are no such miseries as they are held to be: we are slaves and servants the best of us all: as we do reverence our masters, so do our masters their superiors: gentlemen serve nobles, and nobles subordinate to kings, *omne sub regno graviore regnum* [every throne is subject to a greater], princes themselves are God's servants, *reges in ipsos imperium est Jovis*. They are subject to their own laws, and, as the kings of China, endure more than slavish imprisonment, to maintain their state and greatness, they never come abroad. Alexander was a slave to fear, Cæsar of pride, Vespasian to his money (*nihil enim refert, rerum sis servus an hominum* [it makes no difference whether one is a slave of persons or of things]), Heliogabalus to his gut, and so of the rest. Lovers are slaves to their mistresses, rich men to their gold, courtiers generally to lust and ambition, and all slaves to our affections, as Evangelus well discourseth in Macrobius,[1] and Seneca [2] the philosopher, *assiduam servitutem extremam et ineluctabilem* he calls it, a continual slavery, to be so captivated by vices; and who is free? Why then dost thou repine? *Satis est potens*, Hierome saith, *qui servire non cogitur* [he is powerful enough who is not forced to do servile work]. Thou carriest no burdens, thou art no prisoner, no drudge, and thousands want that liberty, those pleasures which thou hast. Thou art not sick, and what wouldst thou have? But *nitimur in vetitum*, we must all eat of the forbidden fruit. Were we enjoined to go to such and such places, we would not willingly go: but being barred of our liberty, this alone torments our wandering soul that we may not go. A citizen of ours, saith Cardan,[3] was sixty years of age, and had never been forth of the walls of the city of Milan; the prince hearing of it, commanded him not to stir out: being now forbidden that which all his life he had neglected, he earnestly desired, and being denied, *dolore confectus mortem obiit*, he died for grief.

What I have said of servitude, I say again of imprisonment. We are all prisoners. What is our life but a prison? [4] We are all imprisoned in an island. The world itself to some men is a prison, our narrow seas as so many ditches, and when they have compassed the globe of the earth, they would fain go see what is done in the moon. In Muscovy and many other northern

parts, all over Scandia, they are imprisoned half the year in
stoves, they dare not peep out for cold.[1] At Aden in Arabia
they are penned in all day long with that other extreme of
heat, and keep their markets in the night.[2] What is a ship
but a prison? And so many cities are but as so many hives of
bees, ant-hills; but that which thou abhorrest, many seek:
women keep in all winter, and most part of summer, to preserve their beauties; some for love of study: Demosthenes shaved
his beard because he would cut off all occasion from going
abroad; how many monks and friars, anchorites, abandon the
world! *Monachus in urbe, piscis in arido* [a monk in town is
like a fish out of water]. Art in prison? Make right use of it,
and mortify thyself; "Where may a man contemplate better
than in solitariness, or study more than in quietness?"[3] Many
worthy men have been imprisoned all their lives, and it hath
been occasion of great honour and glory to them, much public
good by their excellent meditation. Ptolemæus, King of
Egypt, *cum viribus attenuatis infirma valetudine laboraret, miro
discendi studio affectus*, etc., now being taken with a grievous
infirmity of body that he could not stir abroad, became Strato's
scholar, fell hard to his book, and gave himself wholly to contemplation, and upon that occasion (as mine author[4] adds),
pulcherrimum regiæ opulentiæ monumentum [as the fairest monument of his wealth and power], etc., to his great honour built
that renowned library at Alexandria, wherein were 40,000
volumes. Severinus Boethius never writ so elegantly as in
prison, Paul so devoutly, for most of his Epistles were dictated
in his bands. "Joseph," saith Austin,[5] "got more credit in
prison than when he distributed corn, and was lord of Pharaoh's
house." It brings many a lewd, riotous fellow home, many
wandering rogues it settles, that would otherwise have been
like raving tigers, ruined themselves and others.

Banishment is no grievance at all, *Omne solum forti patria*
[every soil is a fatherland to the brave], etc., *et patria est ubicunque bene est*, that's a man's country where he is well at
ease. "Many travel for pleasure to that city," saith Seneca,
"to which thou art banished, and what a part of the citizens
are strangers born in other places!" *Incolentibus patria*,[6] 'tis
their country that are born in it, and they would think themselves banished to go to the place which thou leavest, and
from which thou art so loath to depart. 'Tis no disparagement
to be a stranger, or so irksome to be an exile. "The rain is a
stranger to the earth, rivers to the sea, Jupiter in Egypt, the

sun to us all. The soul is an alien to the body, a nightingale to the air, a swallow in a house, and Ganymede in heaven, an elephant at Rome, a phœnix in India"; [1] and such things commonly please us best which are most strange and come farthest off. Those old Hebrews esteemed the whole world Gentiles; the Greeks held all barbarians but themselves; our modern Italians account of us as dull Transalpines by way of reproach, they scorn thee and thy country which thou so much admirest. 'Tis a childish humour to hone after home, to be discontent at that which others seek; to prefer, as base Icelanders and Norwegians do, their own ragged island before Italy or Greece, the gardens of the world. There is a base nation in the north, saith Pliny,[2] called Chauci, that live amongst rocks and sands by the seaside, feed on fish, drink water: and yet these base people account themselves slaves in respect when they come to Rome. *Ita est profecto* (as he concludes), *multis fortuna parcit in pœnam;* so it is, fortune favours some to live at home, to their further punishment: 'tis want of judgment. All places are distant from heaven alike, the sun shines haply as warm in one city as in another, and to a wise man there is no difference of climes; friends are everywhere to him that behaves himself well, and a prophet is not esteemed in his own country. Alexander, Cæsar, Trajan, Hadrian, were as so many land-leapers, now in the east, now in the west, little at home, and Poluo Venetus, Lod. Vertomannus, Pinzonus, Cadamustus, Columbus, Americus Vespuccius, Vascus Gama, Drake, Candish, Oliver à Nort, Schouten, got all their honour by voluntary expeditions. But you say such men's travel is voluntary; we are compelled, and as malefactors must depart: yet know this of Plato [3] to be true, *ultori Deo summa cura peregrinus est,* God hath an especial care of strangers, "and when he wants friends and allies, he shall deserve better and find more favour with God and men." Besides, the pleasure of peregrination, variety of objects will make amends; and so many nobles, Tully, Aristides, Themistocles, Theseus, Codrus, etc., as have been banished, will give sufficient credit unto it. Read Peter Alcionius his two books of this subject.

MEMB. V.

Against Sorrow for Death of Friends or otherwise, vain Fear, etc.

DEATH and departure of friends are things generally grievous, *Omnium quæ in humana vita contingunt, luctus atque mors sunt acerbissima,*[1] the most austere and bitter accidents that can happen to a man in this life; *in æternum valedicere,* to part for ever, to forsake the world and all our friends, 'tis *ultimum terribilium,* the last and the greatest terror, most irksome and troublesome unto us, *Homo toties moritur, quoties amittit suos* [2] [a man dies every time he loses his dear ones]. And though we hope for a better life, eternal happiness, after these painful and miserable days, yet we cannot compose ourselves willingly to die; the remembrance of it is most grievous unto us, especially to such who are fortunate and rich: they start at the name of death, as an horse at a rotten post. Say what you can of that other world, with Metezuma that Indian prince,[3] *Bonum est esse hic,* they had rather be here. Nay, many generous spirits, and grave staid men otherwise, are so tender in this, that at the loss of a dear friend they will cry out, roar, and tear their hair, lamenting some months after, howling "Ohone," as those Irish women, and Greeks at their graves,[4] commit many undecent actions, and almost go besides themselves. "My dear father, my sweet husband, mine only brother's dead; to whom shall I make my moan?" *O me miserum! Quis dabit in lacrimas fontem?* [Woe is me! who shall ope the fount of tears?], etc. "What shall I do?"

> *Sed totum hoc studium luctu fraterna mihi mors*
> *Abstulit, hei misero frater adempte mihi!* [5]

> My brother's death my study hath undone,
> Woe 's me, alas, my brother he is gone!

Mezentius would not live after his son:

> *Nunc vivo, nec adhuc homines lucemque relinquo,*
> *Sed linquam.* [6]

> [I still live, nor yet have left the world of the living,
> but I shall leave it.]

And Pompey's wife cried out at the news of her husband's death,

> *Turpe mori post te solo non posse dolore,* [7]

> ['Twere shame that I should not die from sheer grief
> for thee,]

violenta luctu [carried away by the violence of her grief] *et nescia tolerandi*, as Tacitus [1] of Agrippina, [and] not able to moderate her passions. So when she heard her son was slain, she abruptly broke off her work, changed countenance and colour, tore her hair, and fell a-roaring downright:

> *Subitus miseræ color ossa reliquit,*
> *Excussi manibus radii, revolutaque pensa:*
> *Evolat infelix et femineo ululatu*
> *Scissa comam.*

[Quick fled the colour from her cheeks, her hands
Let fall the distaff and unroll the reel.
With locks dishevelled and with piercing shrieks
She rushed abroad.]

Another would needs run upon the sword's point after Euryalus' departure:

> *Figite me, si qua est pietas, in me omnia tela*
> *Conjicite, o Rutili;* [2]

[O pierce me through, if ye have any hearts,
Rutulians, at me cast all your darts;]

"O let me die, some good man or other make an end of me!" How did Achilles take on for Patroclus' departure! A black cloud of sorrows overshadowed him, saith Homer. Jacob rent his clothes, put sackcloth about his loins, sorrowed for his son a long season, and could not be comforted, but would needs go down into the grave unto his son (Gen. xxxvii, 35). Many years after, the remembrance of such friends, of such accidents, is most grievous unto us, to see or hear of it, though it concern not ourselves but others. Scaliger saith of himself, that he never read Socrates' death in Plato's *Phædo* but he wept: Austin shed tears when he read the destruction of Troy.[3] But howsoever this passion of sorrow be violent, bitter, and seizeth familiarly on wise, valiant, discreet men, yet it may surely be withstood, it may be diverted. For what is there in this life, that it should be so dear unto us? or that we should so much deplore the departure of a friend? The greatest pleasures are common society, to enjoy one another's presence, feasting, hawking, hunting, brooks, woods, hills, music, dancing, etc.; all this is but vanity and loss of time, as I have sufficiently declared.

> *Dum bibimus, dum serta, unguenta, puellas*
> *Poscimus, obrepit non intellecta senectus.*[4]

Whilst we drink, prank ourselves, with wenches dally,
Old age upon 's at unawares doth sally.

As alchemists spend that small modicum they have to get
gold, and never find it, we lose and neglect eternity, for a
little momentany pleasure which we cannot enjoy, nor shall
ever attain to in this life. We abhor death, pain, and grief,
all, and yet we will do nothing of that which should vindicate
us from, but rather voluntarily thrust ourselves upon it. "The
lascivious prefers his whore before his life or good estate; an
angry man his revenge: a parasite his gut; ambitious, honours;
covetous, wealth; a thief his booty; a soldier his spoil; we
abhor diseases, and yet we pull them upon us." [1] We are never
better or freer from cares than when we sleep, and yet, which
we so much avoid and lament, death is but a perpetual sleep;
and why should it, as Epicurus argues, so much affright us?
"When we are, death is not: but when death is, then we are
not": [2] our life is tedious and troublesome unto him that lives
best; "'tis a misery to be born, a pain to live, a trouble to
die": [3] death makes an end of our miseries, and yet we cannot
consider of it; a little before Socrates drank his potion of
cicuta [hemlock], he bid the citizens of Athens cheerfully farewell, and concluded his speech with this short sentence: "My
time is now come to be gone, I to my death, you to live on;
but which of these is best, God alone knows." [4] For there is
no pleasure here but sorrow is annexed to it, repentance follows
it. "If I feed liberally, I am likely sick, or surfeit: if I live
sparingly, my hunger and thirst is not allayed; I am well neither
full nor fasting; if I live honest, I burn in lust"; if I take my
pleasure, I tire and starve myself, and do injury to my body
and soul.[5] "Of so small a quantity of mirth, how much
sorrow! after so little pleasure, how great misery!" [6] 'Tis both
ways troublesome to me, to rise and go to bed, to eat and
provide my meat; cares and contentions attend me all day
long, fears and suspicions all my life. I am discontented, and
why should I desire so much to live? But an happy death will
make an end of all our woes and miseries; *omnibus una meis
certa medela malis* [it is the one sure remedy for all my ills];
why shouldst not thou then say with old Simeon, since thou art
so well affected, "Lord, now let thy servant depart in peace"?
or with Paul, "I desire to be dissolved, and to be with Christ"?
Beata mors quæ ad beatam vitam aditum aperit, 'tis a blessed
hour that leads us to a blessed life,[7] and blessed are they that
die in the Lord. But life is sweet, and death is not so terrible
in itself as the concomitants of it, a loathsome disease, pain,
horror, etc., and many times the manner of it, to be hanged,

to be broken on the wheel, to be burned alive. Servetus [1] the heretic, that suffered in Geneva, when he was brought to the stake, and saw the executioner come with fire in his hand, *homo viso igne tam horrendum exclamavit, ut universum populum perterrefecerit,* roared so loud, that he terrified the people. An old Stoic would have scorned this. It troubles some to be unburied, or so:

> *Non te optima mater*
> *Condet humi, patriove onerabit membra sepulchro;*
> *Alitibus linquere feris, aut gurgite mersum*
> *Unda feret, piscesque impasti vulnera lambent.*

> Thy gentle parents shall not bury thee,
> Amongst thine ancestors entomb'd to be,
> But feral fowl thy carcass shall devour,
> Or drowned corpse hungry fish-maws shall scour.

As Socrates told Crito, it concerns me not what is done with me when I am dead; *facilis jactura sepulchri* [small sacrifice to lose a grave]: I care not so long as I feel it not; let them set mine head on the pike of Teneriffe, and my quarters in the four parts of the world, *pascam licet in cruce corvos* [on the cross let me feed the crows], let wolves or bears devour me; *cœlo tegitur qui non habet urnam,* [2] the canopy of heaven covers him that hath no tomb. So likewise for our friends, why should their departure so much trouble us? They are better as we hope, and for what then dost thou lament, as those do whom Paul taxed in his time (1 Thess. iv, 13), "that have no hope"? 'Tis fit there should be some solemnity:

> *Sed sepelire decet defunctum, pectore forti,*
> *Constantes, unumque diem fletui indulgentes.* [3]

> ['Tis fitting to bury the dead, relaxing naught of our
> fortitude, yet giving up one day to mourning.]

Job's friends said not a word to him the first seven days, but let sorrow and discontent take their course, themselves sitting sad and silent by him. When Jupiter himself wept for Sarpedon, what else did the poet insinuate, but that some sorrow is good?

> *Quis matrem nisi mentis inops in funere nati*
> *Flere vetat?* [4]

Who can blame a tender mother if she weep for her children? Beside, as Plutarch [5] holds, 'tis not in our power not to lament, *indolentia non cuivis contingit,* it takes away mercy and pity not to be sad; 'tis a natural passion to weep for our friends, an

irresistible passion to lament and grieve. "I know not how"
(saith Seneca), "but sometimes 'tis good to be miserable in
misery: and for the most part all grief evacuates itself by tears ":

Est quædam flere voluptas,
Expletur lacrimis egeriturque dolor ; [1]

"yet after a day's mourning or two, comfort thyself for thy
heaviness" (Eccles. xxxviii, 17). *Non decet defunctum ignavo
quæstu prosequi* [2] [it is not becoming to follow the dead with
unmanly wailing]; 'twas Germanicus' advice of old, that we
should not dwell too long upon our passions, to be desperately
sad, immoderate grievers, to let them tyrannize, there 's *indo-
lentiæ ars* [an art in suppressing grief], a medium to be kept:
we do not (saith Austin [3]) forbid men to grieve, but to grieve
overmuch. "I forbid not a man to be angry, but I ask for
what cause he is so. Not to be sad, but why is he sad? Not
to fear, but wherefore is he afraid?" I require a moderation
as well as a just reason. The Romans and most civil commonwealths have set a time to such solemnities, they must not mourn
after a set day, "or if in a family a child be born, a daughter or
son married, some state or honour be conferred, a brother be
redeemed from his bands, a friend from his enemies," or the
like, they must lament no more.[4] And 'tis fit it should be so;
to what end is all their funeral pomp, complaints, and tears?
When Socrates was dying, his friends Apollodorus and Crito,
with some others, were weeping by him, which he perceiving,
asked them what they meant: "for that very cause he put all
the women out of the room; upon which words of his they
were abashed, and ceased from their tears." [5] Lodovicus
Cortesius, a rich lawyer of Padua (as Bernardinus Scardeonius
relates [6]), commanded by his last will, and a great mulct if
otherwise to his heir, that no funeral should be kept for him,
no man should lament: but as at a wedding, music and minstrels
to be provided; and instead of black mourners, he took order
"that twelve virgins clad in green should carry him to the
church." [7] His will and testament was accordingly performed,
and he buried in St. Sophia's Church. Tully [8] was much grieved
for his daughter Tulliola's death at first, until such time that he
had confirmed his mind with some philosophical precepts; "then
he began to triumph over fortune and grief, and for her reception
into heaven to be much more joyed than before he was troubled
for her loss." [9] If an heathen man could so fortify himself
from philosophy, what shall a Christian from divinity? Why

dost thou so macerate thyself? 'Tis an inevitable chance, the
first statute in Magna Charta, an everlasting Act of Parliament,
all must die.[1]

Constat æterna positumque lege est,
Ut constet genitum nihil.[2]

['Tis a fixed and eternal law that nothing is immortal.]

It cannot be revoked, we are all mortal, and these all commanding gods and princes "die like men": *involvit humile pariter
et celsum caput, æquatque summis infima* [it includeth the lofty
and the humble, it levels the highest with the lowest].[3] "O
weak condition of human estate!" Sylvius exclaims: Ladislaus,
King of Bohemia,[4] eighteen years of age, in the flower of his
youth, so potent, rich, fortunate and happy, in the midst of all
his friends, amongst so many physicians,[5] now ready to be
married,[6] in thirty-six hours sickened and died. We must
so be gone sooner or later all, and as Calliopius in the comedy
took his leave of his spectators and auditors, *Vos valete et plaudite*
[I bid you farewell; clap me when I am gone], *Calliopius recensui,*
must we bid the world farewell (*exit* Calliopius), and having now
played our parts, for ever be gone. Tombs and monuments
have the like fate, *data sunt ipsis quoque fata sepulchris,* kingdoms, provinces, towns, and cities have their periods, and are
consumed. In those flourishing times of Troy, Mycenæ was
the fairest city in Greece, *Græciæ cunctæ imperitabat* [it ruled
over the whole of Greece], but it, alas, and that Assyrian Nineveh
are quite overthrown;[7] the like fate hath that Egyptian and
Bœotian Thebes, Delos, *commune Græciæ conciliabulum,* the
common council-house of Greece; and Babylon, the greatest
city that ever the sun shone on,[8] hath now nothing but walls
and rubbish left. *Quid Pandioniæ restat nisi nomen Athenæ?*[9]
[What remains of ancient Athens save the name?] Thus
Pausanias[10] complained in his times. And where is Troy itself
now, Persepolis, Carthage, Cyzicum, Sparta, Argos, and all those
Grecian cities? Syracuse and Agrigentum, the fairest towns
in Sicily, which had sometime 700,000 inhabitants, are now
decayed: the names of Hiero, Empedocles, etc., of those mighty
numbers of people, only left. One Anacharsis is remembered
amongst the Scythians; the world itself must have an end, and
every part of it. *Cæteræ igitur urbes sunt mortales* [other cities
are mortal], as Peter Gillius[11] concludes of Constantinople,
hæc sane, quamdiu erunt homines, futura mihi videtur immortalis
[but this one methinks will be immortal as long as men exist];

but 'tis not so: nor site, nor strength, nor sea, nor land can
vindicate a city, but it and all must vanish at last. And as to
a traveller great mountains seem plains afar off, at last are not
discerned at all; cities, men, monuments decay, *nec solidis
prodest sua machina terris* [nor is the earth saved by its solid
structure], the names are only left, those at length forgotten,
and are involved in perpetual night.

"Returning out of Asia, when I sailed from Ægina toward
Megara, I began" (saith Servius Sulpicius, in a consolatory
epistle of his to Tully [1]) "to view the country round about.
Ægina was behind me, Megara before, Piræus on the right hand,
Corinth on the left, what flourishing towns heretofore, now
prostrate and overwhelmed before mine eyes! I began to think
with myself, Alas! why are we men so much disquieted with the
departure of a friend, whose life is much shorter, when so many
goodly cities lie buried before us? [2] Remember, O Servius,
thou art a man; and with that I was much confirmed, and
corrected myself." Correct then likewise, and comfort thyself
in this, that we must necessarily die, and all die, that we shall
rise again; as Tully held: *Jucundiorque multo congressus noster
futurus, quam insuavis et acerbus digressus*, our second meeting
shall be much more pleasant than our departure was grievous.

Ay, but he was my most dear and loving friend, my sole
friend:

> *Quis desiderio sit pudor aut modus
> Tam cari capitis?* [3]

> And who can blame my woe?

Thou mayst be ashamed, I say with Seneca, [4] to confess it,
"in such a tempest as this to have but one anchor," [5] go seek
another; and for his part thou dost him great injury to desire
his longer life. "Wilt thou have him crazed and sickly still,"
like a tired traveller that comes weary to his inn, begin his
journey afresh, "or to be freed from his miseries? Thou hast
more need rejoice that he is gone." [6] Another complains of a
most sweet wife, a young wife, *Nondum sustulerat flavum
Proserpina crinem* [not yet had Proserpina tied up her golden
hair], such a wife as no mortal man ever had, so good a wife,
but she is now dead and gone, *Lethæoque jacet condita sarcophago*
[she lies buried in the silent tomb]. I reply to him in Seneca's
words, if such a woman at least ever was to be had, "he did
either so find or make her; if he found her, he may as happily
find another"; [7] if he made her, as Critobulus in Xenophon did

by his, he may as good cheap inform another, *et bona tam sequitur,*
quam bona prima fuit; he need not despair so long as the same
master is to be had.   But was she good?   Had she been so
tried peradventure as that Ephesian widow in Petronius, by
some swaggering soldier, she might not have held out.   Many
a man would have been willingly rid of his: before thou wast
bound, now thou art free; "and 'tis but a folly to love thy
fetters, though they be of gold." [1]   Come into a third place,
you shall have an aged father sighing for a son, a pretty child;

> *Impube pectus quale vel impia*
> *Molliret Thracum pectora :* [2]

> He now lies asleep,
> Would make an impious Thracian weep;

or some fine daughter that died young, *Nondum experta novi*
gaudia prima tori [not having yet tasted the joys of wedlock];
or a forlorn son for his deceased father.   But why?   *Prior exiit,*
prior intravit, he came first, and he must go first.   *Tu frustra*
pius, heu [3] [in vain art thou pious], etc.   What, wouldst thou
have the laws of nature altered, and him to live always?   Julius
Cæsar, Augustus, Alcibiades, Galen, Aristotle, lost their fathers
young.   And why on the other side shouldst thou so heavily
take the death of thy little son?

> *Nam quia nec fato, merita nec morte peribat,*
> *Sed miser ante diem,* [4]

he died before his time, perhaps, not yet come to the solstice of
his age, yet was he not mortal?   Hear that divine Epictetus,[1]
"If thou covet thy wife, friends, children should live always,
thou art a fool."   He was a fine child indeed, *dignus Apollineis*
lacrimis [worthy to be wept by Apollo], a sweet, a loving, a fair,
a witty child, of great hope, another Eteoneus, whom Pindarus
the poet and Aristides the rhetorician so much lament; but who
can tell whether he would have been an honest man?   He might
have proved a thief, a rogue, a spendthrift, a disobedient son,
vexed and galled thee more than all the world beside, he might
have wrangled with thee and disagreed, or with his brothers, as
Eteocles and Polynices, and broke thy heart; he is now gone to
eternity, as another Ganymede, in the flower of his youth,[6]
"as if he had risen," said Plutarch,[7] "from the midst of a feast,"
before he was drunk; "the longer he had lived, the worse he
would have been," *et quo vita longior* (Ambrose thinks), *culpa*
numerosior, more sinful, more to answer he would have had.
If he was naught, thou mayst be glad he is gone; if good, be

glad thou hadst such a son. Or art thou sure he was good?
It may be he was an hypocrite, as many are, and howsoever he
spake thee fair, peradventure he prayed, amongst the rest that
Icaromenippus heard at Jupiter's whispering-place in Lucian,
for his father's death, because he now kept him short, he was to
inherit much goods and many fair manors after his decease.
Or put case he was very good, suppose the best, may not thy
dead son expostulate with thee, as he did in the same Lucian,[1]
"Why dost thou lament my death, or call me miserable that
am much more happy than thyself? What misfortune is befallen me? Is it because I am not bald, crooked, old, rotten,
as thou art? What have I lost? some of your good cheer, gay
clothes, music, singing, dancing, kissing, merry meetings,
thalami lubentias, etc., is that it? Is it not much better not to
hunger at all than to eat? not to thirst than to drink to satisfy
thirst? not to be cold than to put on clothes to drive away cold?
You had more need rejoice that I am freed from diseases,
agues, cares, anxieties, livor, love, covetousness, hatred, envy,
malice, that I fear no more thieves, tyrants, enemies, as you
do." *Id cinerem et manes credis curare sepultos?*[2] Do they
concern us at all, think you, when we are once dead? Condole
not others then overmuch, wish not or fear thine own death,
Summum nec optes diem nec metuas,[3] 'tis to no purpose.

> *Excessi e vitæ ærumnis facilisque lubensque,*
> *Ne pejora ipsa morte dehinc videam.*

> I left this irksome life with all mine heart,
> Lest worse than death should happen to my part.

Cardinal Brundusinus[4] caused this epitaph in Rome to be
inscribed on his tomb, to show his willingness to die, and tax
those that were so loath to depart. Weep and howl no more
then, 'tis to small purpose; and as Tully adviseth us in the like
case, *Non quos amisimus, sed quantum lugere par sit, cogitemus:*
think what we do, not whom we have lost. So David did
(2 Sam. xii, 22): "While the child was yet alive, I fasted and
wept; but being now dead, why should I fast? Can I bring
him again? I shall go to him, but he cannot return to me."
He that doth otherwise is an intemperate, a weak, a silly, and
undiscreet man. Though Aristotle deny any part of intemperance to be conversant about sorrow, I am of Seneca's mind,[5]
"He that is wise is temperate, and he that is temperate is
constant, free from passion, and he that is such a one, is without
sorrow," as all wise men should be. The Thracians wept still

when a child was born, feasted and made mirth when any man was buried:[1] and so should we rather be glad for such as die well, that they are so happily freed from the miseries of this life. When Eteoneus, that noble young Greek, was so generally lamented by his friends, Pindarus the poet feigns some god saying, *Silete homines, non enim miser est*, etc., Be quiet good folks, this young man is not so miserable as you think; he is neither gone to Styx nor Acheron, *sed gloriosus et senii expers heros*, he lives for ever in the Elysian Fields. He now enjoys that happiness which your great kings so earnestly seek, and wears that garland for which ye contend. If our present weakness is such, we cannot moderate our passions in this behalf, we must divert them by all means, by doing something else, thinking of another subject. The Italians most part sleep away care and grief, if it unseasonably seize upon them; Danes, Dutchmen, Polanders, and Bohemians drink it down; our countrymen go to plays. Do something or other, let it not transpose thee, or "by premeditation make such accidents familiar,"[2] as Ulysses that wept for his dog, but not for his wife, *quod paratus esset animo obfirmato* [because he had prepared himself for the blow beforehand] (Plut. *de anim. tranq.*), accustom thyself, and harden beforehand by seeing other men's calamities, and applying them to thy present estate; *Prævisum est levius quod fuit ante malum* [an evil foreseen is easier to bear]. I will conclude with Epictetus,[3] "If thou lovest a pot, remember 'tis but a pot thou lovest, and thou wilt not be troubled when 'tis broken: if thou lovest a son or wife, remember they were mortal, and thou wilt not be so impatient." And so for false fears and all other fortuite inconveniences, mischances, calamities, to resist and prepare ourselves, not to faint is best: *Stultum est timere quod vitari non potest*,[4] 'tis a folly to fear that which cannot be avoided, or to be discouraged at all.

> *Nam quisquis trepidus pavet vel optat,*
> *Abjecit clypeum, locoque motus*
> *Nectit qua valeat trahi catenam.*[5]

For he that so faints or fears, and yields to his passion, flings away his own weapons, makes a cord to bind himself, and pulls a beam upon his own head.

MEMB. VI.

Against Envy, Livor, Emulation, Hatred, Ambition, Self-love, and all other Affections

AGAINST those other passions and affections,[1] there is no better remedy than, as mariners when they go to sea provide all things necessary to resist a tempest, to furnish ourselves with philosophical and divine precepts, other men's examples, *periculum ex aliis facere, sibi quod ex usu siet* [2] [to make trial on others of what is good for ourselves], to balance our hearts with love, charity, meekness, patience, and counterpoise those irregular motions of envy, livor, spleen, hatred, with their opposite virtues, as we bend a crooked staff another way; to oppose "sufferance to labour, patience to reproach," [3] bounty to covetousness, fortitude to pusillanimity, meekness to anger, humility to pride; to examine ourselves for what cause we are so much disquieted, on what ground, what occasion, is it just or feigned; and then either to pacify ourselves by reason, to divert by some other object, contrary passion, or premeditation: *Meditari secum oportet quo pacto adversam ærumnam ferat, pericla, damna, exilia; peregre rediens semper cogitet, aut filii peccatum, aut uxoris mortem, aut morbum filiæ; communia esse hæc* [4] [he should always be thinking how he can bear misfortune, danger, loss, exile; on entering his house he should always be prepared to find his son in mischief, his wife dead, his daughter ill; to reflect that such things are common to all]; *fieri posse, ut ne quid animo sit novum,* [that it is possible] to make them familiar, even all kind of calamities, that when they happen they may be less troublesome unto us; *in secundis meditare, quo pacto feras adversa* [in good fortune to meditate how to bear adversity]; or out of mature judgment to avoid the effect, or disannul the cause, as they do that are troubled with toothache, pull them quite out.

> *Ut vivat castor, sibi testes amputat ipse;*
> *Tu quoque, siqua nocent, abjice, tutus eris.* [5]

> The beaver bites off 's stones to save the rest:
> Do thou the like with that thou art opprest.

Or, as they that play at wasters exercise themselves by a few cudgels how to avoid an enemy's blows, let us arm ourselves against all such violent incursions which may invade our minds. A little experience and practice will inure us to it; *vetula vulpes,* as the proverb saith, *laqueo haud capitur,* an old fox is not so easily taken in a snare; an old soldier in the world methinks should not be disquieted, but ready to receive all fortunes, encounters, and, with that resolute captain, come what may come, to make answer:

> *Non ulla laborum,*
> *O virgo, nova mi facies inopinaque surgit,*
> *Omnia præcepi atque animo mecum ante peregi.*[1]

> No labour comes at unawares to me,
> For I have long before cast what may be.

> *Non hoc primum mea pectora vulnus*
> *Senserunt, graviora tuli.*

> [Not the first wound this my breast has felt; I have
> endured worse.]

The commonwealth of Venice in their armoury have this inscription, "Happy is that city which in time of peace thinks of war,"[2] a fit motto for every man's private house; happy is the man that provides for a future assault. But many times we complain, repine, and mutter without a cause, we give way to passions we may resist and will not. Socrates was bad by nature, envious, as he confessed to Zopyrus the physiognomer accusing him of it, froward and lascivious: but as he was Socrates, he did correct and amend himself. Thou art malicious, envious, covetous, impatient, no doubt, and lascivious, yet, as thou art a Christian, correct and moderate thyself. 'Tis something, I confess, and able to move any man, to see himself contemned, obscure, neglected, disgraced, undervalued, "left behind";[3] some cannot endure it, no, not constant Lipsius, a man discreet otherwise, yet too weak and passionate in this, as his words express: *Collegas olim, quos ego sine fremitu non intueor, nuper terræ filios, nunc Mæcenates et Agrippas habeo—summo jam monte potitos*[4] [my former colleagues whom I cannot behold without indignation; lately nobodies, now Mæcenases and Agrippas, at the top of the tree]. But he was much to blame for it; to a wise staid man this is nothing, we cannot all be honoured and rich, all Cæsars; if we will be content, our present state is good, and in some men's opinion to be preferred. Let them go on, get wealth, offices, titles, honours, preferments, and what they will themselves, by chance, fraud, imposture, simony, and indirect means, as too many do, by bribery, flattery, and parasitical insinuation, by impudence and time-serving, let them climb up to advancement in despite of virtue, let them "go before, cross me

on every side," *me non offendunt, modo non in oculos incurrant,*[1]
as he said, correcting his former error, they do not offend me,
so long as they run not into mine eyes. I am inglorious and
poor, *composita paupertate,* but I live secure and quiet: they
are dignified, have great means, pomp, and state, they are
glorious; but what have they with it? "Envy, trouble, anxiety,
as much labour to maintain their place with credit as to get it
at first."[2] I am contented with my fortunes, *spectator e
longinquo* [a spectator from a distance], and love *Neptunum procul
a terra spectare furentem* [to behold the raging sea from a safe spot
on shore]: he is ambitious, and not satisfied with his: "but what
gets he by it? to have all his life laid open, his reproaches seen:
not one of a thousand but he hath done more worthy of dispraise
and animadversion than commendation; no better means to help
this than to be private."[3] Let them run, ride, strive as so many
fishes for a crumb, scrape, climb, catch, snatch, cozen, collogue,
temporize and fleer, take all amongst them, wealth, honour, and
get what they can,[4] it offends me not:

> *Me mea tellus*
> *Lare secreto tutoque tegat;*[5]

[May I find in my own plot of land a safe and snug retreat;]

I am well pleased with my fortunes, *Vivo et regno simul ista
relinquens*[6] [though relinquishing all this, I live like a king].
I have learned "in what state soever I am, therewith to be
contented" (Phil. iv, 11). Come what can come, I am prepared. *Nave fera magna an parva* [whether I sail in a big or
a little ship], *ferar unus et idem,* I am the same. I was once
so mad to bustle abroad, and seek about for preferment, tire
myself, and trouble all my friends, *sed nihil labor tantus profecit;
nam dum alios amicorum mors avocat, aliis ignotus sum, his
invisus, alii large promittunt, intercedunt illi mecum solliciti, hi
vana spe lactant; dum alios ambio, hos capto, illis innotesco,
ætas perit, anni defluunt, amici fatigantur, ego deferor, et jam,
mundi tæsus, humanæque satur infidelitatis, acquiesco* [but I
gained nothing from all my labour. Some of my friends died,
others would no longer know me, others even hated me; some
made liberal promises and even pretended to intercede actively
on my behalf and fed me with false hopes; so while I paid
court to some and won over others and made myself known,
I began to get on in years, time flowed on, my friends grew
tired and I was constantly put off, until, weary of the world and
sick of the faithlessness of men, I gave up the struggle]. And

so I say still; although I may not deny but that I have had some bountiful patrons [1] and noble benefactors, *ne sim interim ingratus* [not to lay myself open to the charge of ingratitude], and I do thankfully acknowledge it, I have received some kindness, *quod Deus illis beneficium rependat* [for which may God repay them], *si non pro votis, fortasse pro meritis*, more peradventure than I deserve, though not to my desire, more of them than I did expect, yet not of others to my desert; neither am I ambitious or covetous all this while, or a Suffenus [2] to myself; what I have said, without prejudice or alteration shall stand. And now as a mired horse that struggles at first with all his might and main to get out, but when he sees no remedy, that his beating will not serve, lies still, I have laboured in vain, rest satisfied, and if I may usurp that of Prudentius,[3]

> *Inveni portum; spes et fortuna valete,*
> *Nil mihi vobiscum, ludite nunc alios.*

> Mine haven's found; fortune and hope adieu,
> Mock others now, for I have done with you.

MEMB. VII.

Against Repulse, Abuses, Injuries, Contempts, Disgraces, Contumelies, Slanders, Scoffs, etc.

I MAY not yet conclude, think to appease passions or quiet the mind, till such time as I have likewise removed some other of their more eminent and ordinary causes, which produce so grievous tortures and discontents. To divert all I cannot hope; to point alone at some few of the chiefest is that which I aim at.

Repulse and disgrace are two main causes of discontent, but to an understanding man not so hardly to be taken. Cæsar himself hath been denied, and when two stand equal in fortune, birth, and all other qualities alike, one of necessity must lose.[4] Why shouldst thou take it so grievously? It hath been a familiar thing for thee thyself to deny others. If every man might have what he would, we should all be deified, emperors, kings, princes; if whatsoever vain hope suggests, unsatiable appetite affects, our preposterous judgment thinks fit were granted, we should have another chaos in an instant, a mere confusion. It is some satisfaction to him that is repelled, that

dignities, honours, offices, are not always given by desert or
worth, but for love, affinity, friendship, affection, great men's
letters, or as commonly they are bought and sold.[1]   "Honours
in court are bestowed not according to men's virtues and good
conditions" (as an old courtier observes), "but as every man
hath means, or more potent friends, so he is preferred." [2] "With
us in France" (for so their own countryman relates [3]) "most
part the matter is carried by favour and grace; he that can get
a great man to be his mediator, runs away with all the preferment." *Indignissimus plerumque præfertur, Vatinius Catoni,
illaudatus laudatissimo* [the most unworthy are usually preferred, Vatinius to Cato, a man with no credentials to the
most highly recommended]:

> *Servi dominantur; aselli*
> *Ornantur phaleris, dephalerantur equi.*

[Slaves rule; asses are decked with trappings, horses
    go without.]

An illiterate fool sits in a man's seat, and the common people
hold him learned, grave, and wise. "One professeth" (Cardan
well notes [4]) "for a thousand crowns, but he deserves not ten,
whenas he that deserves a thousand cannot get ten." *Salarium
non dat multis salem* [many do not get salt from their salary].
As good horses draw in carts as coaches. And oftentimes,
which Machiavel seconds, *principes non sunt qui ob insignem
virtutem principatu digni sunt* [5] [those are not princes who for
their distinguished merit should be such], he that is most
worthy wants employment; he that hath skill to be a pilot
wants a ship, and he that could govern a commonwealth, a world
itself, a king in conceit, wants means to exercise his worth,
hath not a poor office to manage. And yet all this while he is
a better man that is fit to reign, *etsi careat regno*, though he want
a kingdom, "than he that hath one, and knows not how to
rule it." [6] A lion serves not always his keeper, but oftentimes
the keeper the lion, and as Polydore Virgil hath it,[7] *multi reges
ut pupilli ob inscitiam non regunt sed reguntur* [many kings, on
account of their ignorance, have to be ruled, like schoolboys,
instead of ruling]. Hiero of Syracuse was a brave king, but
wanted a kingdom; Perseus of Macedon had nothing of a king
but the bare name and title, for he could not govern it: so great
places are often ill bestowed, worthy persons unrespected. Many
times, too, the servants have more means than the masters
whom they serve, which Epictetus [8] counts an eye-sore and

inconvenient. But who can help it? It is an ordinary thing
in these days to see a base impudent ass, illiterate, unworthy,
unsufficient, to be preferred before his betters, because he can
put himself forward, because he looks big, can bustle in the
world, hath a fair outside, can temporize, collogue, insinuate,
or hath good store of friends and money, whereas a more
discreet, modest, and better-deserving man shall lie hid or have
a repulse. 'Twas so of old, and ever will be, and which Tiresias
advised Ulysses in the poet,[1] *Accipe qua ratione queas ditescere*
[hear how you can make yourself rich], etc., is still in use; lie,
flatter, and dissemble: if not, as he concludes, *Ergo pauper eris*,
then go like a beggar, as thou art. Erasmus, Melancthon,
Lipsius, Budæus, Cardan, lived and died poor. Gesner was a
silly old man, *baculo innixus* [leaning on his stick], amongst all
those huffing cardinals, swelling bishops, that flourished in his
time and rode on foot-clothes. It is not honesty, learning,
worth, wisdom, that prefers men. "The race is not to the
swift, nor the battle to the strong," but, as the wise man[2] said,
chance, and sometimes a ridiculous chance. *Casus plerumque
ridiculus multos elevavit.*[3] 'Tis fortune's doings, as they say,
which made Brutus now dying exclaim, *O misera virtus! ergo
nihil quam verba eras, atqui ego te tanquam rem excercebam, sed
tu serviebas fortunæ* [Out on thee, virtue! Thou wast, then,
nothing but a name. I practised thee as something real, and
thou wast but the slave of fortune]. Believe it hereafter, O my
friends! virtue serves fortune. Yet be not discouraged (O my
well-deserving spirits) with this which I have said, it may be
otherwise, though seldom I confess, yet sometimes it is. But
to your further content, I 'll tell you a tale.[4] In Moronia Pia,
or Moronia Felix,[5] I know not whether, nor how long since, nor
in what cathedral church, a fat prebend fell void. The carcass
scarce cold, many suitors were up in an instant. The first
had rich friends, a good purse, and he was resolved to outbid
any man before he would lose it, every man supposed he should
carry it. The second was my lord bishop's chaplain (in whose
gift it was), and he thought it his due to have it. The third
was nobly born, and he meant to get it by his great parents,
patrons, and allies. The fourth stood upon his worth, he had
newly found out strange mysteries in chemistry, and other rare
inventions, which he would detect to the public good. The
fifth was a painful preacher, and he was commended by the
whole parish where he dwelt, he had all their hands to his
certificate. The sixth was the prebendary's son lately deceased,

his father died in debt (for it, as they say), left a wife and many
poor children.   The seventh stood upon fair promises, which
to him and his noble friends had been formerly made for the
next place in his lordship's gift.   The eighth pretended great
losses, and what he had suffered for the Church, what pains he
had taken at home and abroad, and besides, he brought noblemen's letters.   The ninth had married a kinswoman, and he
sent his wife to sue for him.   The tenth was a foreign doctor, a
late convert, and wanted means.   The eleventh would exchange
for another, he did not like the former's site, could not agree
with his neighbours and fellows upon any terms, he would be
gone.   The twelfth and last was (a suitor in conceit) a right
honest, civil, sober man, an excellent scholar, and such a one
as lived private in the university, but he had neither means nor
money to compass it; besides he hated all such courses, he
could not speak for himself, neither had he any friends to
solicit his cause, and therefore made no suit, could not expect,
neither did he hope for, or look after it.   The good bishop,
amongst a jury of competitors thus perplexed, and not yet
resolved what to do or on whom to bestow it, at the last, of his
own accord, mere motion, and bountiful nature, gave it freely
to the university student, altogether unknown to him but by
fame; and to be brief, the academical scholar had the prebend
sent him for a present.   The news was no sooner published
abroad, but all good students rejoiced, and were much cheered
up with it, though some would not believe it; others, as men
amazed, said it was a miracle; but one amongst the rest thanked
God for it, and said, *Nunc juvat tandem studiosum esse, et Deo
integro corde servire* [now at length it proves worth while to
be studious, and to serve God whole-heartedly].   You have
heard my tale: but alas! it is but a tale, a mere fiction, 'twas
never so, never like to be, and so let it rest.   Well, be it so
then; they have wealth and honour, fortune and preferment,
every man (there's no remedy) must scamble as he may, and
shift as he can; yet Cardan comforted himself with this, "the
star Fomalhaut would make him immortal,"[1] and that after
his decease his books should be found in ladies' studies.[2]   *Dignum
laude virum Musa vetat mori*[3] [the Muse suffers not to die the
man deserving of fame].   But why shouldst thou take thy
neglect, thy canvas, so to heart?   It may be thou art not fit;
but as a child that puts on his father's shoes, hat, headpiece,
breastplate, breeches, or holds his spear, but is neither able
to wield the one or wear the other,[4] so wouldst thou do by

such an office, place, or magistracy: thou art unfit. "And what is dignity to an unworthy man, but" (as Salvianus holds [1]) "a gold ring in a swine's snout?" Thou art a brute. Like a bad actor (so Plutarch compares such men [2]) in a tragedy, *diadema fert, at vox non auditur:* thou wouldst play a king's part, but actest a clown, speakest like an ass. *Magna petis, Phaethon, et quœ non viribus istis* [3] [a great thing is this thou aimest at, Phaethon, something beyond thy strength], etc., as James and John, the sons of Zebedee, did ask they knew not what; *nescis, temerarie, nescis:* thou dost, as another Suffenus, overween thyself; thou art wise in thine own conceit, but in other more mature judgment altogether unfit to manage such a business.   Or be it thou art more deserving than any of thy rank, God in His providence hath reserved thee for some other fortunes, *sic superis visum* [so the gods have willed].   Thou art humble as thou art, it may be; hadst thou been preferred, thou wouldst have forgotten God and thyself, insulted over others, contemned thy friends, been a block, a tyrant, or a demi-god,[4] *sequiturque superbia formam* [and beauty inspires pride]. "Therefore," saith Chrysostom, "good men do not always find grace and favour, lest they should be puffed up with turgent titles, grow insolent and proud." [5]

Injuries, abuses, are very offensive, and so much the more in that they think *veterem ferendo invitant novam,* by taking one they provoke another: but it is an erroneous opinion, for if that were true, there would be no end of abusing each other; *lis litem generat* [one quarrel provokes another]; 'tis much better with patience to bear, or quietly to put it up.   If an ass kick me, saith Socrates, shall I strike him again?   And when his wife Xantippe struck and misused him,[6] to some friends that would have had him strike her again, he replied that he would not make them sport, or that they should stand by and say, *Eia Socrates! eia Xantippe!* [Go it, Socrates! go it, Xantippe!] as we do when dogs fight, animate them the more by clapping of hands.   Many men spend themselves, their goods, friends, fortunes, upon small quarrels, and sometimes at other men's procurements, with much vexation of spirit and anguish of mind, all which with good advice or mediation of friends might have been happily composed, or if patience had taken place. Patience in such cases is a most sovereign remedy, to put up, conceal, or dissemble it, to forget and forgive,[7] "not seven, but seventy-seven times," [8] "as often as he repents forgive him" (Luke xvii, 3), as our Saviour enjoins us, stroken, "to turn the other side": [1] as our Apostle persuades us,[2] "to recompense no man evil for evil, but as much as is possible to have peace with all men: not to avenge ourselves, and we shall heap burning coals upon our adversary's head." "For if you put up wrong" (as Chrysostom comments), "you get the victory; he that loseth his money loseth not the conquest in this our philosophy." [3] If he contend with thee, submit thyself unto him first, yield to him. *Durum et durum non faciunt murum,* as the diverb is, two refractory spirits will never agree, the only means to overcome is to relent, *obsequio vinces* [you will conquer by giving way]. Euclid in Plutarch, when his brother had angered him, swore he would be revenged; but he gently replied, "Let me not live if I do not make thee to love me again," [4] upon which meek answer he was pacified.

> *Flectitur obsequio curvatus ab arbore ramus,*
> *Frangis si vires experiare tuas.*[5]

> A branch if easily bended yields to thee,
> Pull hard it breaks: the difference you see.

The noble family of the Columni [6] in Rome, when they were expelled the city by that furious Alexander the Sixth, gave the bending branch therefore as an impress, with this motto, *Flecti potest, frangi non potest,* to signify that he might break them by force, but so never make them stoop, for they fled in the midst of their hard usage to the kingdom of Naples, and were honourably entertained by Frederick the king, according to their callings. Gentleness in this case might have done much more, and let thine adversary be never so perverse, it may be by that means thou mayst win him; *favore et benevolentia etiam immanis animus mansuescit,*[7] soft words pacify wrath, and the fiercest spirits are so soonest overcome; a generous lion will not hurt a beast that lies prostrate, nor an elephant an innocuous creature, but is *infestus infestis,* a terror and scourge alone to such as are stubborn and make resistance.[8] It was the symbol of Emanuel Philibert, Duke of Savoy, and he was not mistaken in it, for

> *Quo quisque est major, magis est placabilis iræ,*
> *Et faciles motus mens generosa capit.*[9]

> A greater man is soonest pacified,
> A noble spirit quickly satisfied.

It is reported by Gualter Mapes,[10] an old historiographer of ours (who lived 400 years since), that King Edward senior, and

Leolin, Prince of Wales, being at an interview near Aust upon
Severn, in Gloucestershire, and the prince, sent for, refused to
come to the king; he would needs go over to him: which Leolin
perceiving, "went up to the arms in water, and embracing his
boat, would have carried him out upon his shoulders, adding
that his humility and wisdom had triumphed over his pride and
folly"; [1] and thereupon was reconciled unto him and did his
homage.   If thou canst not so win him, put it up; if thou beest
a true Christian, a good divine, an imitator of Christ, ("for he
was reviled and put it up, whipped and sought no revenge" [2]),
thou wilt pray for thine enemies, "and bless them that persecute thee"; [3] be patient, meek, humble, etc.   An honest man
will not offer thee injury, *probus non vult*; if he were a brangling
knave, 'tis his fashion so to do; where is least heart is most
tongue; *quo quisque stultior, eo magis insolescit*, the more sottish
he is, still the more insolent.   "Do not answer a fool according
to his folly." [4]   If he be thy superior, bear it by all means,
grieve not at it, let him take his course; [5] Anytus and Meletus
"may kill me,[6] they cannot hurt me," as that generous Socrates
made answer in like case.   *Mens immota manet*, though the
body be torn in pieces with wild horses, broken on the wheel,
pinched with fiery tongs, the soul cannot be distracted.   'Tis
an ordinary thing for great men to vilify and insult, oppress,
injure, tyrannize, to take what liberty they list, and who dare
speak against?   *Miserum est ab eo lædi, a quo non possis queri,*
a miserable thing 'tis to be injured of him from whom is no
appeal: and not safe to write against him that can proscribe
and punish a man at his pleasure,[7] which Asinius Pollio was ware
of, when Octavianus provoked him.   'Tis hard, I confess, to
be so injured: one of Chilo's three difficult things: "To keep
counsel, spend his time well, put up injuries"; [8] but be thou
patient, and leave revenge unto the Lord.   "Vengeance is
mine, and I will repay, saith the Lord." [9]   "I know the Lord,"
saith David,[10] "will avenge the afflicted and judge the poor."
"No man" (as Plato further adds) "can so severely punish his
adversary, as God will such as oppress miserable men." [11]

> *Iterum ille rem judicatam judicat,*
> *Majoreque mulcta mulctat.*[12]

[He tries once more the case after it has been decided,
and inflicts a heavier penalty.]

If there be any religion, any God, and that God be just, it shall
be so; if thou believest the one, believe the other: *erit, erit,* it

shall be so. Nemesis comes after, *sero sed serio* [slowly but surely], stay but a little and thou shalt see God's just judgment overtake him.

Raro antecedentem scelestum
Deseruit pede pœna claudo.[1]

[Yet with sure steps, though lame and slow,
Vengeance o'ertakes the trembling villain's speed.]

Thou shalt perceive that verified of Samuel to Agag (1 Sam. xv, 33): "Thy sword hath made many women childless, so shall thy mother be childless amongst other women." It shall be done to them as they have done to others. Conradinus, that brave Suevian prince, came with a well-prepared army into the kingdom of Naples, was taken prisoner by King Charles, and put to death in the flower of his youth; a little after (*ultionem Conradini mortis* [a nemesis for the death of Conradinus], Pandulphus Collinutius, *Hist. Neap. lib.* 5, calls it), King Charles his own son, with two hundred nobles, was so taken prisoner, and beheaded in like sort. Not in this only, but in all other offences, *quo quisque peccat in eo punietur*,[2] they shall be punished in the same kind, in the same part, like nature, eye with or in the eye, head with or in the head, persecution with persecution, lust with effects of lust; let them march on with ensigns displayed, let drums beat on, trumpets sound taratantarra, let them sack cities, take the spoil of countries, murder infants, deflower virgins, destroy, burn, persecute, and tyrannize, they shall be fully rewarded at last in the same measure, they and theirs, and that to their desert.

Ad generum Cereris sine cæde et sanguine pauci
Descendunt reges et sicca morte tyranni.[3]

Few tyrants in their beds do die,
But stabb'd or maim'd to hell they hie.

Oftentimes too a base contemptible fellow is the instrument of God's justice to punish, to torture, and vex them, as an ichneumon doth a crocodile. They shall be recompensed according to the works of their hands, as Haman was hanged on the gallows he provided for Mordecai. "They shall have sorrow of heart, and be destroyed from under the heaven" (Lam. iii, 64, 65, 66). Only be thou patient: *vincit qui patitur*[4] [he who suffers conquers]: and in the end thou shalt be crowned. Yea, but 'tis a hard matter to do this, flesh and blood may not abide it; 'tis *grave, grave!* No (Chrysostom replies), *non est grave, o homo!* 'tis not so grievous, "neither had God commanded it,

if it had been so difficult." But how shall it be done? "Easily,"
as he follows it, "if thou shalt look to heaven, behold the beauty
of it, and what God hath promised to such as put up injuries." [1]
But if thou resist and go about *vim vi repellere* [to repel force
with force], as the custom of the world is, to right thyself, or
hast given just cause of offence, 'tis no injury then, but a condign
punishment; thou hast deserved as much: *A te principium, in te
recidit crimen quod a te fuit; peccasti, quiesce* [thou didst commence; the crime thou didst commit has recoiled on thine own
head; thou hast sinned, hold thy peace], as Ambrose expostulates with Cain, *lib. 3 de Abel et Cain.* Dionysius of Syracuse, [2]
in his exile, was made to stand without door, *patienter ferendum,
fortasse nos tale quid fecimus, quum in honore essemus* [we must
endure patiently; perhaps we did something of the same kind
when we were great], he wisely put it up, and laid the fault
where it was, on his own pride and scorn, which in his prosperity he had formerly showed others. 'Tis Tully's axiom, [3]
*ferre ea molestissime homines non debent, quæ ipsorum culpa
contracta sunt* [men should not chafe at sufferings which they
have brought on themselves by their own fault]; self do, self
have, as the saying is, they may thank themselves. For he
that doth wrong must look to be wronged again; *habet et musca
splenem, et formicæ sua bilis inest*; the least fly hath a spleen,
and a little bee a sting. An ass overwhelmed a thistlewarp's
nest, the little bird pecked his galled back in revenge; [4] and the
humble-bee in the fable flung down the eagle's eggs out of
Jupiter's lap. Bracides, in Plutarch, put his hand into a mouse's
nest and hurt her young ones, she bit him by the finger: "I see
now" (saith he), "there is no creature so contemptible that will
not be revenged." [5] 'Tis *lex talionis*, and the nature of all things
so to do: if thou wilt live quietly thyself, do no wrong to others; [6]
if any be done thee, put it up, with patience endure it, for
"this is thankworthy," saith our Apostle, [7] "if any man for
conscience towards God endure grief, and suffer wrong unde-
served; for what praise is it, if when ye be buffeted for your
faults, ye take it patiently? But if when you do well, ye suffer
wrong, and take it patiently, there is thanks with God; for
hereunto verily we are called." *Qui mala non fert, ipse sibi
testis est per impatientiam quod bonus non est,* he that cannot bear
injuries witnesseth against himself that he is no good man, as
Gregory holds. "'Tis the nature of wicked men to do injuries,
as it is the property of all honest men patiently to bear them." [8]
Improbitas nullo flectitur obsequio [wickedness is swayed by no

concession]. The wolf in the emblem [1] sucked the goat (so the
shepherd would have it), but he kept nevertheless a wolf's
nature; a knave will be a knave.[2] Injury is on the other side
a good man's footboy, his *fidus Achates*, and as a lackey follows
him wheresoever he goes. Besides, *misera est fortuna quæ caret
inimico*, he is in a miserable estate that wants enemies; it is a
thing not to be avoided, and therefore with more patience to
be endured.[3] Cato Censorius, that upright Cato of whom
Paterculus gives that honourable *elogium* [encomium], *Bene
fecit quod aliter facere non potuit* [he acted uprightly because
he could not act otherwise], was fifty times indicted and accused
by his fellow-citizens,[4] and, as Ammianus well hath it,[5] *Quis
erit innocens si clam vel palam accusasse sufficiat?* if it be sufficient
to accuse a man openly or in private, who shall be free? If there
were no other respect than that of Christianity, religion, and
the like, to induce men to be long-suffering and patient, yet
methinks the nature of injury itself is sufficient to keep them
quiet; the tumults, uproars, miseries, discontents, anguish, loss,
dangers that attend upon it might restrain the calamities of
contention: for as it is with ordinary gamesters, the gains go to
the box, so falls it out to such as contend; the lawyers get all;
and therefore if they would consider of it, *aliena pericula cautos*,
other men's misfortunes in this kind, and common experience,
might detain them. The more they contend, the more they are
involved in a labyrinth of woes,[6] and the catastrophe is to
consume one another, like the elephant and dragon's conflict
in Pliny;[7] the dragon got under the elephant's belly, and sucked
his blood so long, till he fell down dead upon the dragon, and
killed him with the fall, so both were ruined. 'Tis an hydra's
head, contention; the more they strive, the more they may: and
as Praxiteles did by his glass, when he saw a scurvy face in it,
brake it in pieces; but for that one he saw many more as bad in
a moment: for one injury done they provoke another *cum
fænore* [with interest], and twenty enemies for one. *Noli
irritare crabrones* [don't stir up a hornet's nest], oppose not
thyself to a multitude: but if thou hast received a wrong, wisely
consider of it, and if thou canst possibly, compose thyself with
patience to bear it. This is the safest course, and thou shalt
find greatest ease to be quiet.

I say the same of scoffs, slanders, contumelies, obloquies,
defamations, detractions, pasquilling libels, and the like, which
may tend anyway to our disgrace: 'tis but opinion; if we could
neglect, contemn, or with patience digest them, they would

reflect on them that offered them at first.[1] A wise citizen,
I know not whence, had a scold to his wife: when she brawled,
he played on his drum, and by that means madded her more,
because she saw that he would not be moved. Diogenes in a
crowd, when one called him back and told him how the boys
laughed him to scorn, *Ego, inquit, non rideor* [I, he said, am not
being laughed at], took no notice of it. Socrates was brought
upon the stage by Aristophanes, and misused to his face, but he
laughed as if it concerned him not: and as Ælian relates of him,
whatsoever good or bad accident or fortune befell him, going in
or coming out, Socrates still kept the same countenance; even
so should a Christian soldier do, as Hierome describes him, *per
infamiam et bonam famam grassari ad immortalitatem*, march on
through good and bad reports to immortality, not to be moved:[2]
for honesty is a sufficient reward, *probitas sibi præmium*, and
in our times the sole recompense to do well, is to do well: but
naughtiness will punish itself at last, *improbis ipsa nequitia
supplicium*.[3] As the diverb is,

> *Qui bene fecerunt, illi sua facta sequentur;*
> *Qui male fecerunt, facta sequentur eos:*

> They that do well, shall have reward at last:
> But they that ill, shall suffer for that's past.

Yea, but I am ashamed, disgraced, dishonoured, degraded,
exploded: my notorious crimes and villainies are come to light
(*deprendi miserum est* [it is a wretched thing to be caught]), my
filthy lust, abominable oppression and avarice lies open, my
good name's lost, my fortune's gone, I have been stigmatized,
whipped at post, arraigned and condemned, I am a common
obloquy, I have lost my ears, odious, execrable, abhorred of
God and men. Be content, 'tis but a nine days' wonder, and as
one sorrow drives out another, one passion another, one cloud
another, one rumour is expelled by another; every day almost
come new news unto our ears, as how the sun was eclipsed,
meteors seen i' th' air, monsters born, prodigies, how the Turks
were overthrown in Persia, an earthquake in Helvetia, Calabria,
Japan, or China, an inundation in Holland, a great plague in
Constantinople, a fire at Prague, a dearth in Germany, such a
man is made a lord, a bishop, another hanged, deposed, pressed
to death, for some murder, treason, rape, theft, oppression, all
which we do hear at first with a kind of admiration, detestation,
consternation, but by and by they are buried in silence: thy
father's dead, thy brother robbed, wife runs mad, neighbour

hath killed himself; 'tis heavy, ghastly, fearful news at first, in
every man's mouth, table talk; but after a while who speaks or
thinks of it? It will be so with thee and thine offence, it will
be forgotten in an instant, be it theft, rape, sodomy, murder,
incest, treason, etc.; thou art not the first offender, nor shalt
not be the last, 'tis no wonder, every hour such malefactors are
called in question, nothing so common, *Quocunque in populo,
quocunque sub axe* [in every people, in every clime]. Comfort
thyself, thou art not the sole man. If he that were guiltless
himself should fling the first stone at thee, and he alone should
accuse thee that were faultless, how many executioners, how
many accusers wouldst thou have? If every man's sins were
written in his forehead, and secret faults known, how many
thousands would parallel, if not exceed, thine offence! It may
be the judge that gave sentence, the jury that condemned thee,
the spectators that gazed on thee, deserved much more, and
were far more guilty than thou thyself. But it is thine infelicity
to be taken, to be made a public example of justice, to be a
terror to the rest; yet should every man have his desert, thou
wouldst peradventure be a saint in comparison; *vexat censura
columbas* [even the doves are criticized], poor souls are punished;
the great ones do twenty thousand times worse, and are not so
much as spoken of.

> *Non rete accipitri tenditur neque milvio,*
> *Qui male faciunt nobis; illis qui nil faciunt tenditur.*[1]

> The net 's not laid for kites or birds of prey,
> But for the harmless still our gins we lay.

Be not dismayed then, *humanum est errare*, we are all sinners,
daily and hourly subject to temptations, the best of us is a
hypocrite, a grievous offender in God's sight; Noah, Lot, David,
Peter, etc., how many mortal sins do we commit! Shall I say,
be penitent, ask forgiveness, and make amends by the sequel
of thy life for that foul offence thou hast committed? recover thy
credit by some noble exploit, as Themistocles did, for he was a
most deboshed and vicious youth, *sed juventæ maculas præclaris
factis delevit*, but made the world amends by brave exploits; at
last become a new man, and seek to be reformed. He that
runs away in a battle, as Demosthenes said, may fight again;
and he that hath a fall may stand as upright as ever he did
before. *Nemo desperet meliora lapsus* [let no man despair of
making good a lapse], a wicked liver may be reclaimed, and
prove an honest man; he that is odious in present, hissed out,

an exile, may be received again with all men's favours, and singular applause; so Tully was in Rome, Alcibiades in Athens. Let thy disgrace then be what it will, *quod fit, infectum non potest esse*, that which is past cannot be recalled; trouble not thyself, vex and grieve thyself no more, be it obloquy, disgrace, etc.   No better way than to neglect, contemn, or seem not to regard it, to make no reckoning of it, *Deesse robur arguit dicacitas* [too much talking indicates a lack of strength]: if thou be guiltless it concerns thee not.

> *Irrita vaniloquæ quid curas spicula linguæ?*
> *Latrantem curatne alta Diana canem?* [1]

[What carest thou for the vain shafts of a slanderous tongue?] Doth the moon care for the barking of a dog?   They detract, scoff and rail, saith one,[2] and bark at me on every side, but I, like that Albanian dog sometime given to Alexander for a present, *vindico me ab illis solo contemptu*, I lie still and sleep, vindicate myself by contempt alone.   *Expers terroris Achilles armatus*[3] [Achilles armed knows not fear]: as a tortoise in his shell, *virtutue mea me involvo*[4] [I wrap myself in my own virtue], or an urchin round, *nil moror ictus* [I heed not their blows], a lizard in camomile,[5] I decline their fury and am safe.

> *Integritas virtusque suo munimine tuta,*
> *Non patet adversæ morsibus invidiæ:*

Virtue and integrity are their own fence,
Care not for envy or what comes from thence.

Let them rail then, scoff, and slander, *sapiens contumelia non afficitur*, a wise man, Seneca thinks, is not moved, because he knows, *contra sycophantæ morsum non est remedium*, there is no remedy for it: kings and princes, wise, grave, prudent, holy, good men, divine, all are so served alike.   *O Jane, a tergo quem nulla ciconia pinsit*[6] [O Janus, who hast never been caricatured from behind], Antevorta and Postvorta, Jupiter's guardians, may not help in this case, they cannot protect; Moses had a Dathan, a Corah, David a Shimei, God Himself is blasphemed: *nondum felix es si te nondum turba deridet* [thou art not yet fortunate if the crowd has not yet mocked thee].   It is an ordinary thing so to be misused.   *Regium est cum bene feceris male audire*[7] [it is a royal privilege to act well and yet be ill spoken of], the chiefest men and most understanding are so vilified; let him take his course.[8]   And as that lusty courser in Æsop, that contemned the poor ass, came by and by after with

his bowels burst, a pack on his back, and was derided of the
same ass: *contemnentur ab iis quos ipsi prius contempsere, et
irridebuntur ab iis quos ipsi prius irrisere,* they shall be contemned
and laughed to scorn of those whom they have formerly derided.
Let them contemn, defame, or undervalue, insult, oppress, scoff,
slander, abuse, wrong, curse and swear, feign and lie, do thou
comfort thyself with a good conscience, *in sinu gaudeas* [rejoice
in your own heart], when they have all done, "a good conscience
is a continual feast," [1] innocency will vindicate itself: and which
the poet gave out of Hercules, *Diis fruitur iratis* [he enjoys the
anger of the gods], enjoy thyself, though all the world be set
against thee, contemn and say with him, *Elogium mihi præ
foribus* [my epitaph is writ large], my posy is, "not to be moved;
that my palladium, my breast-plate, my buckler, with which
I ward all injuries, offences, lies, slanders; I lean upon that
stake of modesty, so receive and break asunder all that foolish
force of livor and spleen." [2]   And whosoever he is that shall
observe these short instructions, without all question he shall
much ease and benefit himself.

In fine, if princes would do justice, judges be upright, clergymen truly devout, and so live as they teach, if great men would
not be so insolent, if soldiers would quietly defend us, the
poor would be patient, rich men would be liberal and humble,
citizens honest, magistrates meek, superiors would give good
example, subjects peaceable, young men would stand in awe:
if parents would be kind to their children, and they again
obedient to their parents, brethren agree amongst themselves,
enemies be reconciled, servants trusty to their masters, virgins
chaste, wives modest, husbands would be loving and less
jealous: if we could imitate Christ and His apostles, live after
God's laws, these mischiefs would not so frequently happen
amongst us; but being most part so irreconcilable as we are,
perverse, proud, insolent, factious, and malicious, prone to contention, anger and revenge, of such fiery spirits, so captious,
impious, irreligious, so opposite to virtue, void of grace, how
should it otherwise be?   Many men are very testy by nature,
apt to mistake, apt to quarrel, apt to provoke and misinterpret
to the worst everything that is said or done, and thereupon
heap unto themselves a great deal of trouble, and disquietness
to others; smatterers in other men's matters, tale-bearers,
whisperers, liars, they cannot speak in season, or hold their
tongues when they should, *et suam partem itidem tacere, cum
aliena est oratio:* [3] they will speak more than comes to their

shares, in all companies, and by those bad courses accumulate much evil to their own souls (*qui contendit, sibi convicium facit* [he who quarrels brings reproach upon himself]), their life is a perpetual brawl, they snarl like so many dogs, with their wives, children, servants, neighbours, and all the rest of their friends, they can agree with nobody. But to such as are judicious, meek, submiss, and quiet, these matters are easily remedied; they will forbear upon all such occasions, neglect, contemn, or take no notice of them, dissemble, or wisely turn it off. If it be a natural impediment, as a red nose, squint eyes, crooked legs, or any such imperfection, infirmity, disgrace, reproach, the best way is to speak of it first thyself,[1] and so thou shalt surely take away all occasions from others to jest at, or contemn, that they may perceive thee to be careless of it; Vatinius was wont to scoff at his own deformed feet, to prevent his enemies' obloquies and sarcasms in that kind; or else by prevention, as Cotys, King of Thrace, that brake a company of fine glasses presented to him, with his own hands, lest he should be overmuch moved when they were broken by chance. And sometimes again, so that it be discreetly and moderately done, it shall not be amiss to make resistance, to take down such a saucy companion; no better means to vindicate himself to purchase final peace: for he that suffers himself to be ridden, or through pusillanimity or sottishness will let every man baffle him, shall be a common laughing-stock for all to flout at. As a cur that goes through a village, if he clap his tail between his legs and run away, every cur will insult over him; but if he bristle up himself and stand to it, give but a counter-snarl, there's not a dog dares meddle with him: much is in a man's courage and discreet carriage of himself.

Many other grievances there are, which happen to mortals in this life, from friends, wives, children, servants, masters, companions, neighbours, our own defaults, ignorance, errors, intemperance, indiscretion, infirmities, etc., and many good remedies to mitigate and oppose them, many divine precepts to counterpoise our hearts, special antidotes both in Scripture and human authors, which whoso will observe shall purchase much ease and quietness unto himself. I will point at a few. Those prophetical, apostolical admonitions are well known to all; what Solomon, Siracides, our Saviour Christ Himself hath said tending to this purpose, as, "Fear God: obey the prince: be sober and watch: pray continually: be angry, but sin not: remember thy last: fashion not yourselves to this world, etc.:

apply yourselves to the times: strive not with a mighty man:
recompense good for evil: let nothing be done through contention or vainglory, but with meekness of mind, every man
esteeming of others better than himself: love one another";
or that epitome of the law and the prophets, which our Saviour
inculcates, "Love God above all, thy neighbour as thyself":
and "Whatsoever you would that men should do unto you, so
do unto them," which Alexander Severus writ in letters of gold
and used as a motto, Hierome commends to Celantia as an
excellent way,[1] amongst so many enticements and worldly
provocations, to rectify her life. Out of human authors take
these few cautions: "Know thyself.[2] Be contented with thy
lot.[3] Trust not wealth, beauty, nor parasites, they will bring
thee to destruction.[4] Have peace with all men, war with vice.[5]
Be not idle.[6] Look before you leap.[7] Beware of Had I wist.[8]
Honour thy parents, speak well of friends.[9] Be temperate in
four things, *lingua, locis, oculis, et poculis* [in speech, in going
about, in looking, and in drinking]. Watch thine eye. Moderate
thine expenses. Hear much, speak little.[10] *Sustine et abstine* [11]
[bear and refrain]. If thou seest aught amiss in another, mend
it in thyself. Keep thine own counsel, reveal not thy secrets,
be silent in thine intentions. Give not ear to tale-tellers,
babblers,[12] be not scurrilous in conversation. Jest without
bitterness:[13] give no man cause of offence: set thine house in
order: take heed of suretyship.[14] *Fide et diffide* [15] [trust and
mistrust], as a fox on the ice, take heed whom you trust. Live
not beyond thy means.[16] Give cheerfully.[17] Pay thy dues
willingly. Be not a slave to thy money. Omit not occasion,
embrace opportunity, lose no time.[18] Be humble to thy superiors,
respective to thine equals, affable to all, but not familiar.[19]
Flatter no man. Lie not, dissemble not.[20] Keep thy word and
promise, be constant in a good resolution. Speak truth. Be
not opinative, maintain no factions. Lay no wagers, make no
comparisons. Find no faults, meddle not with other men's
matters.[21] Admire not thyself. Be not proud or popular.[22]
Insult not. *Fortunam reverenter habe* [bear fortune modestly].
Fear not that which cannot be avoided.[23] Grieve not for that
which cannot be recalled.[24] Undervalue not thyself.[25] Accuse
no man, commend no man rashly.[26] Go not to law without
great cause. Strive not with a greater man. Cast not off an
old friend. Take heed of a reconciled enemy. If thou come
as a guest, stay not too long.[27] Be not unthankful. Be meek,
merciful, and patient. Do good to all. Be not fond of fair

words. Be not a neuter in a faction.[1] Moderate thy passions. Think no place without a witness.[2] Admonish thy friend in secret, commend him in public.[3] Keep good company. Love others, to be beloved thyself.[4] *Ama tanquam osurus* [in loving remember that you may one day hate]. *Amicus tardo fias* [form friendships slowly]. Provide for a tempest. *Noli irritare crabrones* [do not stir up a hornet's nest]. Do not prostitute thy soul for gain. Make not a fool of thyself to make others merry. Marry not an old crone or a fool for money. Be not over solicitous or curious. Seek that which may be found. Seem not greater than thou art. Take thy pleasure soberly. *Ocymum ne terito* [do not grind clover]. Live merrily as thou canst.[5] Take heed by other men's examples.[6] Go as thou wouldst be met, sit as thou wouldst be found. Yield to the time, follow the stream.[7] Wilt thou live free from fears and cares? Live innocently, keep thyself upright, thou needest no other keeper," [8] etc. Look for more in Isocrates, Seneca, Plutarch, Epictetus, etc., and for defect, consult with cheese-trenchers and painted cloths.

MEMB. VIII.

Against Melancholy itself

"EVERY man," saith Seneca, "thinks his own burthen the heaviest," [9] and a melancholy man above all others complains most; weariness of life, abhorring all company and light, fear, sorrow, suspicion, anguish of mind, bashfulness, and those other dread symptoms of body and mind, must needs aggravate this misery; yet, conferred to other maladies, they are not so heinous as they be taken. For first, this disease is either in habit or disposition, curable or incurable. If new and in disposition, 'tis commonly pleasant, and it may be helped. If inveterate, or a habit, yet they have *lucida intervalla* [lucid intervals], sometimes well, and sometimes ill; or if more continuate, as the Veientes were to the Romans,[10] 'tis *hostis magis assiduus quam gravis*, a more durable enemy than dangerous: and amongst many inconveniences, some comforts are annexed to it. First, it is not catching, and, as Erasmus comforted himself when he was grievously sick of the stone, though it was most trouble-some, and an intolerable pain to him, yet it was no whit offensive to others, not loathsome to the spectators, ghastly, fulsome, terrible, as plagues, apoplexies, leprosies,- wounds, sores, tetters, pox, pestilent agues are, which either admit of no company, terrify or offend those that are present. In this malady, that which is is wholly to themselves, and those symptoms not so dreadful, if they be compared to the opposite extremes. They are most part bashful, suspicious, solitary, etc., therefore no such ambitious, impudent intruders as some are, no sharkers, no cony-catchers, no prowlers, no smell-feasts, praters, panders, parasites, bawds, drunkards, whoremasters; necessity and defect compel them to be honest; as Micio told Demea in the comedy,[1]

> *Hæc si neque ego neque tu fecimus,*
> *Non sinit egestas facere nos ;*

if we be honest 'twas poverty made us so: if we melancholy men be not as bad as he that is worst, 'tis our dame Melancholy kept us so: *Non deerat voluntas sed facultas* [not the will but the power was wanting].

Besides, they are freed in this from many other infirmities, solitariness makes them more apt to contemplate, suspicion wary, which is a necessary humour in these times, *nam pol qui maxime cavet, is sæpe cautor captus est,*[2] he that takes most heed is often circumvented and overtaken. Fear and sorrow keep them temperate and sober, and free them from many dissolute acts, which jollity and boldness thrust men upon: they are therefore no *sicarii*, roaring boys, thieves, or assassinates. As they are soon dejected, so they are as soon, by soft words and good persuasions, reared. Wearisomeness of life makes them they arc not so besotted on the transitory vain pleasures of the world. If they dote in one thing, they are wise and well understanding in most other. If it be inveterate, they are *insensati*, most part doting, or quite mad, insensible to any wrongs, ridiculous to others, but most happy and secure to themselves. Dotage is a state which many much magnify and commend: so is simplicity, and folly, as he said, *Hic furor, o superi, sit mihi perpetuus*[3] [with this madness I pray the gods I may ever be afflicted]. Some think fools and dizzards live the merriest lives, as Ajax in Sophocles, *Nihil scire vita jucundissima,* 'tis the pleasantest life to know nothing; *iners malorum remedium ignorantia,* ignorance is a downright remedy of evils. These curious arts and laborious sciences, Galen's, Tully's, Aristotle's, Justinian's, do but trouble the world, some think; we might

live better with that illiterate Virginian simplicity, and gross
ignorance; entire idiots do best, they are not macerated with
cares, tormented with fears, and anxiety, as other wise men
are: for, as he said,[1] if folly were a pain, you should hear them
howl, roar, and cry out in every house, as you go by in the
street, but they are most free, jocund, and merry, and in some
countries, as amongst the Turks,[2] honoured for saints, and
abundantly maintained out of the common stock.[3] They are
no dissemblers, liars, hypocrites, for fools and madmen tell
commonly truth. In a word, as they are distressed, so are they
pitied, which some hold better than to be envied, better to be
sad than merry, better to be foolish and quiet, *quam sapere et
ringi*, [than] to be wise and still vexed; better to be miserable
than happy: of two extremes it is the best.

SECT. IV. MEMB. I.

SUBSECT. I.—*Of Physic which cureth with Medicines*

AFTER a long and tedious discourse of these six non-natural
things and their several rectifications, all which are comprehended in diet, I am come now at last to *Pharmaceutice*, or that
kind of physic which cureth by medicines, which apothecaries
most part make, mingle, or sell in their shops. Many cavil at
this kind of physic, and hold it unnecessary, unprofitable to this
or any other disease, because those countries which use it least
live longest and are best in health, as Hector Boethius [4] relates
of the isles of Orcades, the people are still sound of body and
mind, without any use of physic, they live commonly 120
years; and Ortelius in his Itinerary of the inhabitants of the
Forest of Arden, "they are very painful, long-lived, sound,"
etc.[5] Martianus Capella,[6] speaking of the Indians of his time,
saith they were (much like our western Indians now) "bigger
than ordinary men, bred coarsely, very long-lived, insomuch
that he that died at an hundred years of age went before his
time," etc. Damianus à Goes, Saxo Grammaticus, Aubanus
Bohemus, say the like of them that live in Norway, Lapland,
Finmark, Biarmia,[7] Carelia, all over Scandia, and those northern
countries, they are most healthful and very long-lived, in which
places there is no use at all of physic, the name of it is not
once heard. Dithmarus Bleskenius, in his accurate description

of Iceland, 1607, makes mention amongst other matters of the
inhabitants and their manner of living, "which is dried fish
instead of bread, butter, cheese, and salt meats; most part
they drink water and whey, and yet without physic or physician
they live many of them 250 years." [1] I find the same relation
by Lerius, and some other writers, of Indians in America.
Paulus Jovius, in his description of Britain, and Levinus
Lemnius, observe as much of this our island, that there was of
old no use of physic amongst us,[2] and but little at this day,
except it be for a few nice idle citizens, surfeiting courtiers, and
stall-fed gentlemen lubbers. The country people use kitchen
physic, and common experience tells us that they live freest
from all manner of infirmities that make least use of apothecaries' physic. Many are overthrown by preposterous use of
it, and thereby get their bane, that might otherwise have
escaped; some think physicians kill as many as they save,[3] and
who can tell *quot Themison ægros autumno occiderit uno* [4] [how
many patients Themison has killed in one autumn]? how many
murders they make in a year, *quibus impune licet hominem
occidere*, that may freely kill folks, and have a reward for it?
and, according to the Dutch proverb, a new physician must
have a new churchyard; and who daily observes it not? Many
that did ill under physicians' hands have happily escaped when
they have been given over by them, left to God and nature and
themselves; 'twas Pliny's dilemma of old, "Every disease is
either curable or incurable, a man recovers of it or is killed
by it; both ways physic is to be rejected. If it be deadly, it
cannot be cured; if it may be helped, it requires no physician,
nature will expel it of itself." [5] Plato made it a great sign of
an intemperate and corrupt commonwealth, where lawyers and
physicians did abound; and the Romans distasted them so much
that they were often banished out of their city, as Pliny and
Celsus relate, for 600 years not admitted. It is no art at all,
as some hold, no, not worthy the name of a liberal science (nor
law neither), as Pet. And. Canonherius,[6] a patrician of Rome
and a great doctor himself, "one of their own tribe," proves
by sixteen arguments, because it is mercenary as now used,
base, and as fiddlers play for a reward. *Juridicis, medicis,
fisco, fas vivere rapto* [lawyers, doctors, and the Treasury are
licensed to live on robbery]; 'tis a corrupt trade, no science,
art, no profession; the beginning, practice, and progress of it,
all is naught, full of imposture, incertainty, and doth generally
more harm than good. The devil himself was the first inventor

of it: *Inventum est medicina meum* [medicine is my invention],
said Apollo; and what was Apollo, but the devil? The Greeks
first made an art of it, and they were all deluded by Apollo's
sons, priests, oracles. If we may believe Varro, Pliny, Columella, most of their best medicines were derived from his
oracles. Æsculapius his son had his temples erected to his
deity, and did many famous cures; but, as Lactantius holds,
he was a magician, a mere impostor, and as his successors,
Phaon, Podalirius, Melampus, Menecrates (another god), by
charms, spells, and ministry of bad spirits, performed most of
their cures. The first that ever wrote in physic to any purpose
was Hippocrates, and his disciple and commentator Galen,
whom Scaliger calls *fimbriam Hippocratis* [the fringe of Hippo-
crates]; but, as Cardan [1] censures them, both immethodical and
obscure, as all those old ones are, their precepts confused, their
medicines obsolete, and now most part rejected. Those cures
which they did, Paracelsus holds, were rather done out of their
patients' confidence, and good opinion they had of them,[2] than
out of any skill of theirs, which was very small, he saith, they
themselves idiots and infants, as are all their academical
followers. The Arabians received it from the Greeks, and so
the Latins, adding new precepts and medicines of their own,
but so imperfect still, that through ignorance of professors, impostors, mountebanks, empirics, disagreeing of sectaries (which
are as many almost as there be diseases), envy, covetousness,
and the like, they do much harm amongst us. They are so
different in their consultations, prescriptions, mistaking many
times the party's constitution, disease, and causes of it, they
give quite contrary physic.[3] "One saith this, another that,"[4]
out of singularity or opposition, as he said of Hadrian, *multitudo
medicorum principem interfecit*, a multitude of physicians hath
killed the emperor; *plus a medico quam a morbo periculi*, more
danger there is from the physician than from the disease.
Besides, there is much imposture and malice amongst them.
"All arts" (saith Cardan [5]) "admit of cozening, physic amongst
the rest doth appropriate it to herself;" and tells a story of one
Curtius, a physician in Venice; because he was a stranger, and
practised amongst them, the rest of the physicians did still
cross him in all his precepts. If he prescribed hot medicines
they would prescribe cold, *miscentes pro calidis frigida, pro
frigidis humida, pro purgantibus astringentia*, binders for purgatives, *omnia perturbabant* [they altered everything]. If the
party miscarried, *Curtium damnabant*, Curtius killed him, that

disagreed from them; if he recovered, then they cured him
themselves.[1] Much emulation, imposture, malice, there is
amongst them: if they be honest and mean well, yet a knave
apothecary that administers the physic and makes the medicine
may do infinite harm by his old obsolete doses, adulterine drugs,
bad mixtures, *quid pro quo*, etc. See Fuchsius, *lib.* i, *sect.* i,
cap. 8, Cordus' Dispensatory, and Brassavola's *Examen simpl.*,
etc. But it is their ignorance that doth more harm than
rashness; their art is wholly conjectural, if it be an art, uncertain, imperfect, and got by killing of men, they are a kind
of butchers, leeches, men-slayers; chirurgeons and apothecaries
especially, that are indeed the physicians' hangmen, *carnifices*,
and common executioners; though to say truth, physicians
themselves come not far behind; for according to that facete
epigram of Maximilianus Urentius, what's the difference?

> *Chirurgicus medico quo differt? scilicet isto,*
> *Enecat hic succis, enecat ille manu :*
> *Carnifice hoc ambo tantum differre videntur,*
> *Tardius hi faciunt, quod facit ille cito.*

> [Wherein differs the surgeon from the doctor?   In this
> way, that the one kills with his drugs, the other
> with his knife.   Both differ from the hangman
> only in doing slowly what he does quickly.]

But I return to their skill; many diseases they cannot cure at
all, as apoplexy, epilepsy, stone, strangury, gout (*tollere nodosam
nescit medicina podagram* [the medical art cannot cure the gout]);
quartan agues, a common ague sometimes stumbles them all;
they cannot so much as ease, they know not how to judge of it.
If by pulses, that doctrine, some hold, is wholly superstitious,
and I dare boldly say with Andrew Dudith,[2] "that variety of
pulses, described by Galen, is neither observed nor understood
of any." And for urine, that is *meretrix medicorum*, the most
deceitful thing of all, as Forestus and some other physicians
have proved at large. I say nothing of critic days, errors in
indications, etc. The most rational of them, and skilful, are
so often deceived, that as Tholosanus infers,[3] "I had rather
believe and commit myself to a mere empiric than to a mere
doctor, and I cannot sufficiently commend that custom of the
Babylonians, that have no professed physicians, but bring all
their patients to the market to be cured": which Herodotus
relates of the Egyptians, Strabo, Sardus, and Aubanus Bohemus
of many other nations. And those that prescribed physic

amongst them, did not so arrogantly take upon them to cure all diseases as our professors do, but some one, some another, as their skill and experience did serve. "One cured the eyes, a second the teeth, a third the head, another the lower parts,"[1] etc., not for gain, but in charity, to do good; they made neither art, profession, nor trade of it, which in other places was accustomed: and therefore Cambyses in Xenophon[2] told Cyrus that, to his thinking, physicians "were like tailors and cobblers, the one mended our sick bodies as the other did our clothes." But I will urge these cavilling and contumelious arguments no farther, lest some physician should mistake me, and deny me physic when I am sick: for my part, I am well persuaded of physic: I can distinguish the abuse from the use, in this and many other arts and sciences; *Aliud vinum, aliud ebrietas*,[3] wine and drunkenness are two distinct things. I acknowledge it a most noble and divine science, insomuch that Apollo, Æsculapius, and the first founders of it *merito pro diis habiti*, were worthily counted gods by succeeding ages, for the excellency of their invention. And whereas Apollo at Delos, Venus at Cyprus, Diana at Ephesus, and those other gods, were confined and adored alone in some peculiar places, Æsculapius had his temple and altars everywhere, in Corinth, Lacedæmon, Athens, Thebes, Epidaurus, etc., as Pausanius records, for the latitude of his art, deity, worth, and necessity. With all virtuous and wise men therefore I honour the name and calling, as I am enjoined "to honour the physician for necessity's sake. The knowledge of the physician lifteth up his head, and in the sight of great men he shall be admired. The Lord hath created medicines of the earth, and he that is wise will not abhor them" (Ecclus. xxxviii. 1). But of this noble subject how many panegyrics are worthily written! For my part, as Sallust said of Carthage, *præstat silere quam pauca dicere* [it is better to say nothing than too little]; I have said, yet one thing I will add, that this kind of physic is very moderately and advisedly to be used, upon good occasion, when the former of diet will not take place. And 'tis no other which I say, than that which Arnoldus prescribes in his eighth Aphorism: "A discreet and godly physician doth first endeavour to expel a disease by medicinal diet, then by pure medicine";[4] and in his ninth, "He that may be cured by diet, must not meddle with physic."[5] So in [his] eleventh Aphorism: "A modest and wise physician will never hasten to use medicines, but upon urgent necessity, and that sparingly too":[6] because (as he adds in his thirteenth Aphorism) "Who-

soever takes much physic in his youth, shall soon bewail it in
his old age": [1] purgative physic especially, which doth much
debilitate nature. For which causes some physicians refrain
from the use of purgatives, or else sparingly use them. Henricus
Ayrerus,[2] in a consultation for a melancholy person, would
have him take as few purges as he could, "because there be no
such medicines which do not steal away some of our strength,
and rob the parts of our body," weaken nature, and cause that
cacochymia (which Celsus [3] and others observe) or ill digestion,
and bad juice through all the parts of it. Galen himself confesseth [4] "that purgative physic is contrary to nature, takes
away some of our best spirits, and consumes the very substance
of our bodies." But this, without question, is to be understood
of such purges as are unseasonably or immoderately taken;
they have their excellent use in this, as well as most other
infirmities. Of alteratives and cordials no man doubts, be
they simples or compounds. I will, amongst that infinite variety
of medicines which I find in every pharmacopœia, every
physician, herbalist, etc., single out some of the chiefest.

SUBSECT. II.—*Simples proper to Melancholy, against
Exotic Simples*

Medicines properly applied to melancholy, are either simple
or compound. Simples are alterative or purgative. Alteratives
are such as correct, strengthen nature, alter, anyway hinder or
resist the disease; and they be herbs, stones, minerals, etc., all
proper to this humour. For as there be divers distinct infirmities continually vexing us:

Νοῦσοι δ' ἀνθρώποισιν ἐφ' ἡμέρῃ ἠδ' ἐπὶ νυκτὶ
Αὐτόματοι φοιτῶσι, κακὰ θνητοῖσι φέρουσαι
Σιγῇ, ἐπεὶ φωνὴν ἐξείλετο μητίετα Ζεύς·[5]

Diseases steal both day and night on men,
For Jupiter hath taken voice from them:

so there be several remedies, as he [6] saith, "each disease a
medicine, for every humour; and as some hold, every clime, every
country, and more than that, every private place, hath his
proper remedies growing in it, peculiar almost to the domineering and most frequent maladies of it. As one discourseth,[7]
"Wormwood grows sparingly in Italy, because most part there
they be misaffected with hot diseases; but henbane, poppy,

and such cold herbs: with us in Germany and Poland great store
of it in every waste." Baracellus, *Horto geniali,* and Baptista
Porta, *Physiognomicæ lib.* 6, *cap.* 23, give many instances and
examples of it, and bring many other proofs. For that cause
belike that learned Fuchsius of Nuremberg, "when he came into
a village, considered always what herbs did grow most frequently
about it, and those he distilled in a silver limbec,"[1] making use
of others amongst them as occasion served. I know that many
are of opinion our northern simples are weak, unperfect, not so
well concocted, of such force, as those in the southern parts,
not so fit to be used in physic, and will therefore fetch their
drugs afar off: senna, cassia out of Egypt, rhubarb from Barbary, aloes from Zocotora, turbith, agaric, myrobolanes, hermo-
dactyls, from the East Indies, tobacco from the West, and some
as far as China, hellebore from the Anticyræ, or that of Austria
which bears the purple flower, which Matthiolus so much
approves, and so of the rest. In the kingdom of Valencia in
Spain, Maginus commends two mountains, Mariola and Rena-
golosa, famous for simples;[2] Leander Albertus, Baldus,[3] a
mountain near the Lake Benacus in the territory of Verona, to
which all the herbalists in the country continually flock; Ortelius
one in Apulia,[4] Munster Mons Major in Istria: others Montpelier in France;[5] Prosper Alpinus prefers Egyptian simples,
Garcias ab Horto Indian before the rest, another those of Italy,
Crete, etc. Many times they are over-curious in this kind, whom
Fuchsius taxeth, *Instit. lib.* 1, *sec.* 1, *cap.* 1, "that think they do
nothing, except they rake all over India, Arabia, Ethiopia for
remedies, and fetch their physic from the three quarters of the
world, and from beyond the Garamantes. Many an old wife
or country woman doth often more good with a few known and
common garden herbs than our bombast physicians with all their
prodigious, sumptuous, far-fetched, rare, conjectural medicines."[6]
Without all question, if we have not these rare exotic simples,
we hold that at home which is in virtue equivalent unto them;
ours will serve as well as theirs, if they be taken in proportion-
able quantity, fitted and qualified aright, if not much better,
and more proper to our constitutions. But so 'tis for the most
part, as Pliny writes to Gallus, "We are careless of that which
is near us, and follow that which is afar off, to know which we
will travel and sail beyond the seas, wholly neglecting that which
is under our eyes."[7] Opium in Turkey doth scarce offend, with
us in a small quantity it stupefies: cicuta, or hemlock, is a strong
poison in Greece, but with us it hath no such violent effects:

I conclude with J. Voschius, who, as he much inveighs against
those exotic medicines, so he promiseth by our European a
full cure and absolute of all diseases; *a capite ad calcem* [from
head to heel], *nostræ regionis herbæ nostris corporibus magis
conducunt,* our own simples agree best with us. It was a thing
that Fernelius much laboured in his French practice, to reduce
all his cure to our proper and domestic physic: so did Janus
Cornarius,[1] and Martin Rulandus in Germany, T[imothy]
B[right] with us, as appeareth by a treatise of his divulged in
our tongue, 1615, to prove the sufficiency of English medicines
to the cure of all manner of diseases. If our simples be not
altogether of such force, or so apposite, it may be, if like industry
were used, those far-fetched drugs would prosper as well with
us as in those countries whence now we have them, as well as
cherries, artichokes, tobacco, and many such. There have been
divers worthy physicians which have tried excellent conclusions
in this kind, and many diligent, painful apothecaries, as Gesner,
Besler, Gerard, etc.; but amongst the rest those famous public
gardens of Padua in Italy, Nuremberg in Germany, Leyden in
Holland, Montpelier in France (and ours in Oxford now in
fieri [course of construction], at the cost and charges of the
Right Honourable the Lord Danvers, Earl of Danby), are much
to be commended, wherein all exotic plants almost are to be
seen, and liberal allowance yearly made for their better maintenance, that young students may be the sooner informed in the
knowledge of them: which as Fuchsius holds,[2] "is most necessary for that exquisite manner of curing," and as great a shame
for a physician not to observe them as for a workman not to
know his axe, saw, square, or any other tool which he must of
necessity use.

SUBSECT. III.—*Alteratives, Herbs, other Vegetals, etc.*

Amongst those 800 simples, which Galeottus reckons up,
lib. 3 de promisc. doctor. cap. 3, and many exquisite herbalists
have written of, these few following alone I find appropriated to
this humour: of which some be alteratives; "which by a secret
force," [3] saith Renodeus, "and special quality expel future
diseases, perfectly cure those which are, and many such incurable effects." This is as well observed in other plants, stones,
minerals, and creatures as in herbs, in other maladies as in this.
How many things are related of a man's skull! What several

virtues of corns in a horse's leg, of a wolf's liver,[1] etc.! Of
divers excrements of beasts, all good against several diseases![2]
What extraordinary virtues are ascribed unto plants! *Satyrium
et eruca* [3] *penem erigunt, vitex et nymphæa semen extinguunt,*
some herbs provoke lust, some again, as agnus castus, water-
lily, quite extinguish seed;[4] poppy causeth sleep, cabbage
resisteth drunkenness, etc., and that which is more to be admired,
that such and such plants should have a peculiar virtue to such
particular parts,[5] as to the head aniseeds, foalfoot, betony,
calamint, eye-bright, lavender, bays, roses, rue, sage, marjoram, peony, etc.; for the lungs, calamint, liquorice, enula
campana, hyssop, horehound, water germander, etc.; for the
heart, borage, bugloss, saffron, balm, basil, rosemary, violet,
roses, etc.; for the stomach, wormwood, mints, betony, balm,
centaury, sorrel, purslane; for the liver, earth-pine or chamæ-
pitys, germander, agrimony, fennel, endive, succory, liverwort,
barberries; for the spleen, maiden hair, finger-fern, dodder of
thyme, hop, the rind of ash, betony; for the kidneys, gromwell,
parsley, saxifrage, plantain, mallow; for the womb, mugwort,
pennyroyal, featherfew, savin, etc.; for the joints, camomile,
St. John's wort, origan, rue, cowslips, centaury the less, etc.;
and so to peculiar diseases. To this of melancholy you shall
find a catalogue of herbs proper, and that in every part. See
more in Wecker, Renodeus, Heurnius, *lib. 2, cap.* 19, etc. I will
briefly speak of some of them, as first of alteratives, which Galen,
in his third book of diseased parts, prefers before diminutives, and
Trallianus brags that he hath done more cures on melancholy
men by moistening than by purging of them.[6]

In this catalogue, borage and bugloss may challenge the
chiefest place, whether in substance, juice, roots, seeds, flowers,
leaves, decoctions, distilled waters, extracts, oils, etc., for such
kind of herbs be diversely varied. Bugloss is hot and moist,
and therefore worthily reckoned up amongst those herbs which
expel melancholy and exhilarate the heart [7] (Galen, *lib.* 6,
cap. 80, *de simpl. med.*, Dioscorides, *lib.* 4, *cap.* 123). Pliny
much magnifies this plant. It may be diversely used; as in
broth, in wine,[8] in conserves, syrups, etc. It is an excellent
cordial, and against this malady most frequently prescribed; a
herb indeed of such sovereignty, that, as Diodorus, *lib.* 7 *Bibl.*,
Plinius, *lib.* 25, *cap.* 2, *et lib.* 21, *cap.* 22, Plutarch, *Sympos.*
lib. 1, *cap.* 1, Dioscorides, *lib.* 5, *cap.* 40, Cælius, *lib.* 19, *cap.* 3,
suppose, it was that famous nepenthes of Homer,[9] which
Polydamna, Thon's wife (then King of Thebes in Egypt), sent

Helena for a token, of such rare virtue, that if taken steeped in
wine, if wife and children, father and mother, brother and
sister, and all thy dearest friends should die before thy face,
thou couldst not grieve or shed a tear for them.

> *Qui semel id patera mistum Nepenthes Iaccho*
> *Hauserit, lacrimam, non si suavissima proles,*
> *Si germanus ei carus, materque paterque*
> *Oppetat, ante oculos ferro confossus atroci.*

Helena's commended bowl to exhilarate the heart had no other
ingredient, as most of our critics conjecture, than this of borage.

Melissa, balm, hath an admirable virtue to alter melancholy,
be it steeped in our ordinary drink, extracted, or otherwise
taken.   Cardan, *lib*. 8, much admires this herb.   It heats and
dries, saith Heurnius,[1] in the second degree, with a wonderful
virtue comforts the heart, and purgeth all melancholy vapours
from the spirits (Matthiol. *in lib*. 3, *cap*. 10, *in Dioscoridem*).
Besides they ascribe other virtues to it, "as to help concoction,
to cleanse the brain, expel all careful thoughts and anxious
imaginations." [2]   The same words in effect are in Avicenna,
Pliny, Simon Sethi, Fuchsius, Lobel, Delacampius, and every
herbalist.   Nothing better for him that is melancholy than to
steep this and borage in his ordinary drink.

Matthiolus, in his fifth book of Medicinal Epistles, reckons up
scorzonera, "not against poison only, falling sickness, and such
as are vertiginous, but to this malady; the root of it taken by
itself expels sorrow, causeth mirth and lightness of heart." [3]

Antonius Musa, that renowned physician to Cæsar Augustus,
in his book which he writ of the virtues of betony, *cap*. 6,
wonderfully commends that herb, *animas hominum et corpora
custodit, securas de metu reddit*, it preserves both body and mind
from fears, cares, griefs, cures falling sickness, this and many
other diseases; to whom Galen subscribes, *lib*. 7 *Simpl. med.*,
Dioscorides, *lib*. 4, *cap*. 1, etc.

Marigold is much approved against melancholy, and often
used therefore in our ordinary broth, as good against this and
many other diseases.

Lupulus, hop, is a sovereign remedy; Fuchsius, *cap*. 58
Plant. hist., much extols it; "it purgeth all choler, and purifies
the blood." [4]   Matthiolus, *cap*. 140, *in* 4 *Dioscor*. wonders the
physicians of his time made no more use of it, because it rarefies
and cleanseth: we use it to this purpose in our ordinary beer,
which before was thick and fulsome.

Wormwood, centaury, pennyroyal, are likewise magnified and much prescribed (as I shall after show), especially in hypochondriac melancholy, daily to be used, sod in whey; and, as Ruffus Ephesius, Aretæus,[1] relate, by breaking wind, helping concoction, many melancholy men have been cured with the frequent use of them alone.

And because the spleen and blood are often misaffected in melancholy, I may not omit endive, succory, dandelion, fumitory, etc., which cleanse the blood; scolopendria, cuscuta, ceterach, mugwort, liverwort, ash, tamarisk, genist, maidenhair, etc., which much help and ease the spleen.

To these I may add roses, violets, capers, featherfew, scordium, stœchas, rosemary, *ros solis* [sundew], saffron, ocyme, sweet apples, wine, tobacco, sanders, etc., that Peruvian chamico, *monstrosa facultate* [of extraordinary powers], etc., Linschoten's datura; and to such as are cold, the decoction of guiacum,[2] China sarsaparilla, sassafras, the flowers of carduus benedictus, which I find much used by Montanus in his consultations, Julius Alexandrinus, Lælius Eugubinus, and others.   Bernardus Penottus [3] prefers his *herba solis*, or Dutch sundew, before all the rest in this disease, "and will admit of no herb upon the earth to be comparable to it."   It excells Homer's moly, cures this, falling sickness, and almost all other infirmities.   The same Penottus speaks of an excellent balm out of Aponensis, which, taken to the quantity of three drops in a cup of wine, "will cause a sudden alteration, drive away dumps, and cheer up the heart." [4] Ant. Guianerius, in his Antidotary, hath many such.[5]   Jacobus de Dondis the Aggregator repeats ambergrease, nutmegs, and allspice amongst the rest.   But that cannot be general; amber and spice will make a hot brain mad, good for cold and moist. Garcias ab Horto hath many Indian plants, whose virtues he much magnifies in this disease.   Lemnius, *Instit. cap.* 58, admires rue, and commends it to have excellent virtue, "to expel vain imaginations, devils, and to ease afflicted souls." [6]   Other things are much magnified by writers,[7] as an old cock, a ram's head, a wolf's heart borne or eaten, which Mercurialis approves; Prosper Alpinus the water of Nilus; Gomesius all sea-water, and at seasonable times to be sea-sick: goat's milk, whey, etc.

Precious stones are diversely censured; many explode the use
of them or any minerals in physic, of whom Thomas Erastus is
the chief, in his tract against Paracelsus, and in an epistle of
his to Peter Monavius. "That stones can work any wonders,
let them believe that list, no man shall persuade me; for my
part, I have found by experience there is no virtue in them." [1]
But Matthiolus, in his Comment upon Dioscorides,[2] is as profuse on the other side in their commendation; so is Cardan,
Renodeus, Alardus, Rueus, Encelius, Marbodeus, etc. Matthiolus
specifies in coral,[3] and Oswaldus Crollius, *Basil. Chym.*, prefers
the salt of coral.   Christoph. Encelius,[4] *lib.* 3, *cap.* 131, will have
them to be as so many several medicines against melancholy,
sorrow, fear, dullness, and the like; Renodeus admires them,[5]
"besides they adorn kings' crowns, grace the fingers, enrich
our household stuff, defend us from enchantments, preserve
health, cure diseases, they drive away grief, cares, and exhilarate
the mind."   The particulars be these.

Granatus [the garnet], a precious stone so called because it is
like the kernels of a pomegranate, an unperfect kind of ruby,
it comes from Calicut; "if hung about the neck or taken in
drink, it much resisteth sorrow and recreates the heart." [6]   The
same properties I find ascribed to the jacinth and topaz; they
allay anger, grief, diminish madness, much delight and exhilarate
the mind.[7]   "If it be either carried about or taken in a potion,
it will increase wisdom," saith Cardan, "expel fear"; [8] he brags
that he hath cured many madmen with it, which, when they
laid by the stone, were as mad again as ever they were at first.
Petrus Bayerus, *lib.* 2, *cap.* 13, *Veni mecum*, Fran. Rueus,
cap. 19 *de gemmis*, say as much of the chrysolite, a friend of
wisdom, an enemy to folly.[9]   Pliny, *lib.* 37, Solinus, *cap.* 52,
Albertus, *de lapid.*, Cardan, Encelius, *lib.* 3, *cap.* 66, highly
magnifies the virtue of the beryl; "it much avails to a good
understanding, repressesth vain conceits, evil thoughts, causeth
mirth," etc.[10]   In the belly of a swallow there is a stone found
called chelidonius, "which if it be lapped in a fair cloth, and tied
to the right arm, will cure lunatics, madmen, make them amiable
and merry." [11]

There is a kind of onyx called a chalcedony, which hath the
same qualities, "avails much against phantastic illusions which
proceed from melancholy," [12] preserves the vigour and good
estate of the whole body.

The eban stone, which goldsmiths use to sleeken their gold with, borne about or given to drink, hath the same properties, or not much unlike.[1]

Levinus Lemnius, *Institut. ad vit. cap.* 58, amongst other jewels, makes mention of two more notable, carbuncle and coral, "which drive away childish fears, devils, overcome sorrow, and hung about the neck repress troublesome dreams," [2] which properties almost Cardan gives to that green-coloured emmetris [3] if it be carried about, or worn in a ring; Rueus to the diamond.

Nicholas Cabeus, a Jesuit of Ferrara, in the first book of his Magnetical Philosophy, *cap.* 3, speaking of the virtues of a loadstone, recites many several opinions; some say that if it be taken in parcels inward, *si quis per frusta voret, juventutem restituet*, it will, like viper's wine, restore one to his youth; and yet if carried about them, others will have it to cause melancholy; let experience determine.

Mercurialis admires the emerald for his virtues in pacifying all affections of the mind; others the sapphire, which is "the fairest of all precious stones, of sky-colour, and a great enemy to black choler, frees the mind, mends manners," [4] etc.   Jacobus de Dondis, in his catalogue of simples, hath ambergrease, *os in corde cervi*, the bone in a stag's heart,[5] a monocerot's horn, bezoar's stone (of which elsewhere [6]), it is found in the belly of a little beast in the East Indies, brought into Europe by Hollanders and our countrymen merchants.   Renodeus, *cap.* 22, *lib.* 3, *de ment. med.*, saith he saw two of these beasts alive, in the castle of the Lord of Vitry at Coubert.

Lapis lazuli and Armenus, because they purge, shall be mentioned in their place.

Of the rest in brief thus much I will add out of Cardan, Renodeus, *cap.* 23, *lib.* 3, Rondeletius, *lib.* 1 *de Testat. cap.* 15, etc., "that almost all jewels and precious stones have excellent virtues to pacify the affections of the mind, for which cause rich men so much covet to have them": [7] and "those smaller unions which are found in shells amongst the Persians and Indians," by the consent of all writers, "are very cordial," [8] and most part avail to the exhilaration of the heart.

Most men say as much of gold and some other minerals as these have done of precious stones.   Erastus still maintains the opposite part. *Disput. in Paracelsum, cap.* 4, *fol.* 196, he confesseth of gold, "that it makes the heart merry, but in no other sense but as it is in a miser's chest": [9] *at mihi plaudo simul ac nummos contemplor in arca* [I am well pleased with myself as.

soon as I see the money in my chest], as he said in the poet,
it so revives the spirits, and is an excellent receipt against
melancholy.

> For gold in physic is a cordial,
> Therefore he loved gold in special.[1]

Aurum potabile [potable gold] he discommends, and inveighs
against it, by reason of the corrosive waters which are used in
it:[2] which argument our Dr. Gwinne urgeth against Dr.
Antonius. Erastus[3] concludes their philosophical stones and
potable gold, etc., "to be no better than poison," a mere imposture, a *non ens*; digged out of that broody hill belike this
golden stone is, *ubi nascetur ridiculus mus* [whence the absurd
little mouse is to be born]. Paracelsus and his chemistical
followers, as so many Promethei, will fetch fire from heaven,
will cure all manner of diseases with minerals, accounting them
the only physic on the other side. Paracelsus[4] calls Galen,
Hippocrates, and all their adherents, infants, idiots, sophisters,
etc.: *Apage sis istos qui Vulcanias istas metamorphoses sugillant,
inscitiæ soboles, supinæ pertinaciæ alumnos, etc.* [away with
those who cavil at these fiery transformations, rank ignoramuses,
obstinate fools, etc.], not worthy the name of physicians, for
want of these remedies; and brags that by them he can make
a man live 160 years, or to the world's end; with their alexiphar-
macums, panaceas, mummias, *unguentum armarium*, and such
magnetical cures, *Lampas vitæ et mortis, Balneum Dianæ,
Balsamum, Electrum Magico-physicum, Amuleta Martialia*, etc.,[5]
what will not he and his followers effect? He brags, moreover,
that he was *primus medicorum* [the first of physicians], and did
more famous cures than all the physicians in Europe besides,
"a drop of his preparations should go farther than a dram or
ounce of theirs,"[6] those loathsome and fulsome filthy potions,
heteroclitical pills (so he calls them), horse medicines, *ad
quorum aspectum Cyclops Polyphemus exhorresceret* [at the sight
of which the Cyclops Polyphemus would shudder]. And though
some condemn their skill and magnetical cures as tending to
magical superstition, witchery, charms, etc., yet they admire,
stiffly vindicate nevertheless, and infinitely prefer them. But
these are both in extremes; the middle sort approve of minerals,
though not in so high a degree. Lemnius, *lib.* 3, *cap.* 6, *de occult.
nat. mir.*, commends gold inwardly and outwardly used, as in
rings, excellent good in medicines; and such mixtures as are made
for melancholy men, saith Wecker, *Antid. spec. lib.* 1, to whom
Renodeus subscribes, *lib.* 2, *cap.* 2; Ficinus, *lib.* 2, *cap.* 1

Fernelius, *Meth. med. lib.* 5, *cap.* 21, *de cardiacis*; Daniel Sennertus, *lib.* 1, *part.* 2, *cap.* 9; Audernacus, Libavius, Quercetanus,
Oswaldus Crollius, Euonymus, Rubeus, and Matthiolus in the
fourth book of his Epistles, Andreas à Blawen, *Epist. ad Matthiolum*, as commended and formerly used by Avicenna, Arnoldus,
and many others.   Matthiolus in the same place approves of
potable gold, mercury, with many such chemical confections,[1]
and goes so far in approbation of them that he holds "no man
can be an excellent physician that hath not some skill in
chemistical distillations, and that chronic diseases can hardly
be cured without mineral medicines." [2]   Look for antimony
among purgers.

SUBSECT. V.—*Compound Alteratives; Censure of Compounds
and Mixed Physic*

Pliny, *lib.* 24, *cap.* 1, bitterly taxeth all compound medicines,
"Men's knavery, imposture, and captious wits have invented
these shops, in which every man's life is set to sale: and by and
by came in those compositions and inexplicable mixtures, far-
fetched out of India and Arabia; a medicine for a botch must
be had as far as the Red Sea," [3] etc.   And 'tis not without cause
which he saith, for out of question they are much to blame in
their compositions. [4]   "Whilst they make infinite variety of
mixtures," as Fuchsius notes,[5] "they think they get themselves great credit, excel others, and to be more learned than
the rest, because they make many variations"; but he accounts
them fools, and "whilst they brag of their skill, and think to
get themselves a name, they become ridiculous, betray their
ignorance and error."   A few simples, well prepared and understood, are better than such an heap of nonsense-confused compounds, which are in apothecaries' shops ordinarily sold; in
which many vain, superfluous, corrupt, exolete things out of
date are to be had" (saith Cornarius), "a company of barbarous
names given to syrups, juleps, an unnecessary company of
mixed medicines"; *rudis indigestaque moles* [a strange chaotic
mass].   Many times (as Agrippa taxeth) there is by this means
"more danger from the medicine than from the disease"; [6]
when they put together they know not what, or leave it to an
illiterate apothecary to be made, they cause death and horror
for health.   Those old physicians had no such mixtures; a
simple potion of hellebore in Hippocrates' time was the ordinary

purge; and at this day, saith Mat. Riccius,[1] in that flourishing
commonwealth of China, "their physicians give precepts quite
opposite to ours, not unhappy in their physic; they use altogether
roots, herbs, and simples in their medicines, and all their physic
in a manner is comprehended in an herbal: no science, no
school, no art, no degree, but, like a trade, every man in private
is instructed of his master." Cardan [2] cracks that he can cure
all diseases with water alone, as Hippocrates of old did most
infirmities with one medicine. Let the best of our rational
physicians demonstrate and give a sufficient reason for those
intricate mixtures, why just so many simples in mithridate or
treacle, why such and such quantity; may they not be reduced
to half or a quarter? *Frustra fit per plura* (as the saying is)
quod fieri potest per pauciora [it is idle to use much where little
will do]; 300 simples in a julep, potion, or a little pill, to
what end or purpose? I know what Alkindus,[3] Capivaccius,
Montagna, and Simon è Tover, the best of them all and most
rational, have said in this kind; but neither he, they, nor any
one of them gives his reader, to my judgment, that satisfaction
which he ought; why such, so many simples? Roger Bacon
hath taxed many errors in his tract *de graduationibus*, explained
some things, but not cleared. Mercurialis, in his book *de
composit. medicin.*, gives instance in *hamech*, and *philonium
Romanum*, which Hamech, an Arabian, and Philonius, a Roman,
long since composed, but *crasse* [coarsely] as the rest. If they
be so exact, as by him it seems they were, and those mixtures
so perfect, why doth Fernelius alter the one, and why is the
other obsolete? Cardan [4] taxeth Galen for presuming out of
his ambition to correct *theriacum Andromachi*, and we as justly
may carp at all the rest. Galen's medicines are now exploded
and rejected; what Nicholas Meripsa, Mesue, Celsus, Scribanius,
Actuarius, etc., writ of old are most part contemned. Mellichius,
Cordus, Wecker, Quercetan, Renodeus, the Venetian, Florentine
states, have their several receipts and magistrals; they of
Nuremberg have theirs, and *Augustana Pharmacopœia*, peculiar
medicines to the meridian of the city; London hers; every city,
town, almost every private man hath his own mixtures, compositions, receipts, magistrals, precepts, as if he scorned antiquity,
and all others, in respect of himself. But each man must
correct and alter to show his skill, every opinative fellow must
maintain his own paradox, be it what it will; *Delirant reges,
plectuntur Achivi*: they dote, and in the meantime the poor
patients pay for their new experiments, the commonalty rue it.

Thus others object, thus I may conceive out of the weakness of my apprehension; but to say truth, there is no such fault, no such ambition, no novelty or ostentation, as some suppose; but as one answers,[1] this of compound medicines "is a most noble and profitable invention, found out and brought into physic with great judgment, wisdom, counsel, and discretion." Mixed diseases must have mixed remedies, and such simples are commonly mixed as have reference to the part affected, some to qualify, the rest to comfort, some one part, some another. Cardan and Brassavola both hold that *nullum simplex medicamentum sine noxa*, no simple medicine is without hurt or offence; and although Hippocrates, Erasistratus, Diocles, of old, in the infancy of this art, were content with ordinary simples, yet now, saith Aetius,[2] "necessity compelleth to seek for new remedies, and to make compounds of simples, as well to correct their harms if cold, dry, hot, thick, thin, insipid, noisome to smell, to make them savoury to the palate, pleasant to taste and take, and to preserve them for continuance, by admixtion of sugar, honey, to make them last months and years for several uses." In such cases, compound medicines may be approved, and Arnoldus in his eighteenth Aphorism doth allow of it: "If simples cannot, necessity compels us to use compounds";[3] so for receipts and magistrals, *dies diem docet*, one day teacheth another, and they are as so many words or phrases, *Quæ nunc sunt in honore vocabula, si volet usus* [which are now in fashion], ebb and flow with the season, and as wits vary, so they may be infinitely varied. *Quisque suum placitum quo capiatur habet:* every man as he likes; so many men so many minds; and yet all tending to good purpose, though not the same way. As arts and sciences, so physic is still perfected amongst the rest. *Horæ Musarum nutrices* [the Hours are the nurses of the Muses], and experience teacheth us every day many things which our predecessors knew not of.[4] Nature is not effete, as he saith, or so lavish to bestow all her gifts upon an age, but hath reserved some for posterity, to show her power, that she is still the same, and not old or consumed. Birds and beasts can cure themselves by nature, *naturæ usu ea plerumque cognoscunt, quæ homines vix longo labore et doctrina assequuntur,*[5] but men must use much labour and industry to find it out. But I digress.

Compound medicines are inwardly taken, or outwardly applied. Inwardly taken, be either liquid or solid; liquid, are fluid or consisting. Fluid, as wines and syrups. The wines ordinarily used to this disease are wormwood wine, tamarisk, and *buglossatum*, wine made of borage and bugloss; the composition of which is specified in Arnoldus Villanovanus, *lib. de vinis*, of borage, balm, bugloss, cinnamon, etc., and highly commended for his virtues: "it drives away leprosy, scabs, clears the blood, recreates the spirits, exhilarates the mind, purgeth the brain of those anxious black melancholy fumes, and cleanseth the whole body of that black humour by urine. To which I add," saith Villanovanus, "that it will bring madmen, and such raging bedlams as are tied in chains, to the use of their reason again. My conscience bears me witness that I do not lie, I saw a grave matron helped by this means; she was so choleric, and so furious sometimes, that she was almost mad and beside herself; she said and did she knew not what, scolded, beat her maids, and was now ready to be bound, till she drank of this borage wine, and by this excellent remedy was cured, which a poor foreigner, a silly beggar, taught her by chance, that came to crave an alms from door to door." [1] The juice of borage, if it be clarified and drunk in wine, will do as much, the roots sliced and steeped, etc., saith Ant. Mizaldus, *Art. med.*, who cites this story verbatim out of Villanovanus, and so doth Magninus, a physician of Milan, in his Regiment of Health. Such another excellent compound water I find in Rubeus, *de distill. sect. 3*, which he highly magnifies out of Savonarola, "for such as are solitary, dull, heavy or sad without a cause, or be troubled with trembling of heart." [2] Other excellent compound waters for melancholy he cites in the same place, "if their melancholy be not inflamed, or their temperature over-hot." [3] Euonymus hath a precious *aquavitæ* to this purpose, for such as are cold. But he and most commend *aurum potabile* [potable gold], and every writer prescribes clarified whey, with borage, bugloss, endive, succory, etc., of goat's milk especially, some indefinitely at all times, some thirty days together in the spring, every morning fasting, a good draught. Syrups are very good, and often used to digest this humour in the heart, spleen, liver, etc. As syrup of borage (there is a famous syrup of borage highly commended by Laurentius to this purpose in his tract of melancholy), *de pomis* [of apples] of King Sabor, now obsolete, of thyme and epithyme, hops, scolopendria, fumitory, maidenhair, byzantine, etc. These are most used for preparatives to other physic, mixed with distilled waters of like nature, or in juleps otherwise.

Consisting, are conserves or confections: conserves of borage, bugloss, balm, fumitory, succory, maidenhair, violets, roses, wormwood, etc.; confections, treacle, mithridate, eclegms or linctures, etc.; solid, as aromatical confections; hot, *diambra, diamargaritum calidum, dianthus, diamoschum dulce, electuarium de gemmis, lætificans Galeni et Rhasis, diagalinga, diacyminum, dianisum, diatrion piperion, diazinziber, diacapers, diacinnamomum*; cold, as *diamargaritum frigidum, diacoralli, diarrhodon abbatis, diacodion*, etc., as every pharmacopœia will show you, with their tables or losings [1] that are made out of them; with condites and the like.

Outwardly used as occasion serves, as amulets, oils hot and cold, as of camomile, stœchados, violets, roses, almonds, poppy, nymphæa, mandrake, etc., to be used after bathing, or to procure sleep.

Ointments composed of the said species, oils and wax, etc., as *alabastritum, populeum*, some hot, some cold, to moisten, procure sleep, and correct other accidents.

Liniments are made of the same matter to the like purpose: emplasters of herbs, flowers, roots, etc., with oils and other liquors mixed and boiled together.

Cataplasms, salves, or poultices, made of green herbs, pounded, or sod in water till they be soft, which are applied to the hypochondries, and other parts, when the body is empty.

Cerotes are applied to several parts, and frontals, to take away pain, grief, heat, procure sleep. Fomentations or sponges, wet in some decoctions, etc., epithemata, or those moist medicines, laid on linen, to bathe and cool several parts misaffected.

Sacculi, or little bags of herbs, flowers, seeds, roots, and the like, applied to the head, heart, stomach, etc.; odoraments, balls, perfumes, posies to smell to, all which have their several uses in melancholy, as shall be showed when I treat of the cure of the distinct species by themselves.

MEMB. II.

SUBSECT. I.—*Purging Simples upward*

MELANAGOGA, or melancholy - purging medicines, are either simple or compound, and that gently, or violently, purging upward or downward. These following purge upward. Asarum, or asarabacca, which, as Mesue saith, is hot in the second degree and dry in the third; "it is commonly taken in wine, whey," [2] or, as with us, the juice of two or three leaves, or more some-times, pounded in posset drink qualified with a little liquorice or aniseed, to avoid the fulsomeness of the taste, or as *diasarum Fernelii*.   Brassavola, *in Cathart.*, reckons it up amongst those simples that only purge melancholy, and Ruellius confirms as much out of his experience, that it purgeth black choler, like hellebore itself.[1]   Galen, *lib.* 6 *Simplic.*, and Matthiolus ascribe other virtues to it, and will have it purge other humours as well as this.[2]

Laurel, by Heurnius, *Method. ad prax. liv.* 2, *cap.* 24, is put amongst the strong purgers of melancholy; it is hot and dry in the fourth degree.   Dioscorides, *lib.* 11, *cap.* 114, adds other effects to it.[3]   Pliny sets down fifteen berries in drink for a sufficient potion: it is commonly corrected with his opposites, cold and moist, as juice of endive, purslane, and is taken in a potion to seven grains and a half.   But this, and asarabacca, every gentlewoman in the country knows how to give; they are two common vomits.

Scilla, or sea-onion, is hot and dry in the third degree.   Brassa-vola, *in Cathart.*, out of Mesue, others, and his own experience, will have this simple to purge melancholy alone.[4]   It is an ordinary vomit, *vinum scilliticum*, mixed with rubel in a little white wine.

White hellebore, which some call sneezing-powder, a strong purger upward, which many reject, as being too violent: Mesue and Averroes will not admit of it, "by reason of danger of suffocation,"[5] "great pain and trouble it puts the poor patient to," saith Dodonæus.[6]   Yet Galen, *lib.* 6 *Simpl. med.* and Dioscorides, *cap.* 145, allow of it.   It was indeed "terrible in former times,"[7] as Pliny notes, but now familiar, insomuch that many took it in those days, "that were students, to quicken their wits,"[8] which Persius, *Sat.* 1, objects to Accius the poet, *Ilias Acci ebria veratro* [the Iliad of Accius is drunk with helle-bore].   "It helps melancholy, the falling sickness, madness, gout, etc., but not to be taken of old men, youths, such as are weaklings, nice, or effeminate, troubled with headache, high-coloured, or fear strangling,"[9] saith Dioscorides.   Oribasius, an old physician, hath written very copiously, and approves of it, "in such affections which can otherwise hardly be cured."[10] Heurnius, *lib.* 2 *Prax. med. de vomitoriis*, will not have it used "but with great caution, by reason of its strength, and then when antimony will do no good,"[11] which caused Hermophilus to compare it to a stout captain (as Codronchus observes,

cap. 7, *Comment. de helleb.*) that will see all his soldiers go before
him and come *post principia* [after the first ranks], like the
bragging soldier, last himself; when other helps fail in inveterate
melancholy, in a desperate case, this vomit is to be taken.[1]
And yet for all this, if it be well prepared, it may be securely
given at first.[2] Matthiolus[3] brags that he hath often, to the
good of many, made use of it, and Heurnius, "that he hath
happily used it, prepared after his own prescript,"[4] and with
good success. Christophorus à Vega, *lib.* 3, *cap.* 41, is of the
same opinion, that it may be lawfully given; and our country
gentlewomen find it by their common practice that there is no
such great danger in it.   Dr. Turner, speaking of this plant in
his Herbal, telleth us that in his time it was an ordinary receipt
among goodwives, to give hellebore in powder, to ii[d] weight,
and he is not much against it.   But they do commonly exceed,
for who so bold as blind Bayard? and prescribe it by penny-
worths, and such irrational ways, as I have heard myself market
folks ask for it in an apothecary's shop: but with what success
God knows; they smart often for their rash boldness and folly,
break a vein, make their eyes ready to start out of their heads,
or kill themselves.   So that the fault is not in the physic, but
in the rude and undiscreet handling of it.   He that will know,
therefore, when to use, how to prepare it aright, and in what
dose, let him read Heurnius, *lib.* 2 *Prax. med.*, Brassavola *de
Cathart.*, Godefridus Stegius, the Emperor Rudolphus' physician,
cap. 16, Matthiolus *in Dioscor.*, and that excellent commentary
of Baptista Codronchus, which is *instar omnium* [worth all the
rest], *de helleb. alb.*, where he shall find great diversity of
examples and receipts.

   Antimony, or stibium, which our chemists so much magnify,
is either taken in substance or infusion, etc., and frequently
prescribed in this disease. "It helps all infirmities," saith
Matthiolus,[5] "which proceed from black choler, falling sickness,
and hypochondriacal passions"; and for farther proof of his
assertion, he gives several instances of such as have been freed
with it: one of Andrew Gallus, a physician of Trent, that after
many other essays, "imputes the recovery of his health, next
after God, to this remedy alone";[6] another of George Hantshius,
that in like sort, when other medicines failed, "was by this
restored to his former health, and which of his knowledge others
have likewise tried, and by the help of this admirable medicine,
been recovered";[7] a third of a parish priest at Prague in
Bohemia, "that was so far gone with melancholy, that he

doted, and spake he knew not what; but after he had taken twelve grains of stibium (as I myself saw, and can witness, for I was called to see this miraculous accident), he was purged of a deal of black choler, like little gobbets of flesh, and all his excrements were as black blood" [1] (a medicine fitter for a horse than a man), "yet it did him so much good, that the next day he was perfectly cured." This very story of the Bohemian priest Sckenkius relates verbatim, *Exoter. experiment. ad. var. morb. cent.* 6, *observ.* 6, with great approbation of it. Hercules de Saxonia calls it a profitable medicine, if it be taken after meat to six or eight grains, of such as are apt to vomit. Rodericus à Fonseca, the Spaniard, and late professor of Padua in Italy, extols it to this disease, *tom.* 2, *consul.* 85; so doth Lod. Mercatus, *de inter. morb. cur. lib.* 1, *cap.* 17, with many others. Jacobus Gervinus, a French physician, on the other side, *lib.* 2 *de venenis confut.*, explodes all this, and saith he took three grains only upon Matthiolus' and some others' commendation, but it almost killed him, whereupon he concludes, "Antimony is rather poison than a medicine." [2] Th. Erastus concurs with him in his opinon, and so doth Ælian Montaltus, *cap.* 30 *de melan.* But what do I talk? 'tis the subject of whole books; I might cite a century of authors pro and con. I will conclude with Zuinger,[3] antimony is like Scanderbeg's sword, which is either good or bad, strong or weak, as the party is that prescribes or useth it; "a worthy medicine if it be rightly applied to a strong man, otherwise poison." For the preparing of it, look in *Euonymi Thesaurus*, Quercetan, Oswaldus Crollius, *Basil. Chym.*, Basil. Valentinus, etc.

Tobacco, divine, rare, superexcellent tobacco, which goes far beyond all the panaceas, potable gold, and philosophers' stones, a sovereign remedy to all diseases. A good vomit, I confess, a virtuous herb, if it be well qualified, opportunely taken, and medicinally used; but as it is commonly abused by most men, which take it as tinkers do ale, 'tis a plague, a mischief, a violent purger of goods, lands, health; hellish, devilish, and damned tobacco, the ruin and overthrow of body and soul.

Subsect. II.—*Simples purging Melancholy downward*

Polypody and epithyme are, without all exceptions, gentle purgers of melancholy. Dioscorides will have them void

phlegm; but Brassavola, out of his experience, averreth that they
purge this humour; they are used in decoction, infusion, etc.,
simple, mixed, etc.

Myrobalanes, all five kinds, are happily prescribed against
melancholy and quartan agues;[1] Brassavola speaks out of "a
thousand experiences,"[2] he gave them in pills, decoctions, etc.;
look for peculiar receipts in him.

Stœchas, fumitory, dodder, herb mercury, roots of capers,
genista or broom, pennyroyal, and half-boiled cabbage, I find in
this catalogue of purgers of black choler, origan, featherfew,
ammoniac salt, saltpetre;[3] but these are very gentle; alypus,
dragon root, centaury, dittany, colutea, which Fuchsius,
cap. 168, and others take for senna, but most distinguish.
Senna is in the middle of violent and gentle purgers downward,
hot in the second degree, dry in the first. Brassavola calls it
"a wonderful herb against melancholy, it scours the blood,
illightens the spirits, shakes off sorrow";[4] "a most profitable
medicine," as Dodonæus terms it,[5] invented by the Arabians,
and not heard of before. It is taken divers ways, in powder,
infusion, but most commonly in the infusion, with ginger or
some cordial flowers added to correct it. Actuarius commends
it sod in broth, with an old cock, or in whey, which is the
common conveyer of all such things as purge black choler;
or steeped in wine, which Heurnius accounts sufficient, without
any farther correction.

Aloes by most is said to purge choler, but Aurelianus, *lib. 2,
cap. 6, de morb. chron.*, Arculanus, *cap.* 6 *in* 9 *Rhasis*, Julius
Alexandrinus, *consil.* 185 *Scoltz.*, Crato, *consil.* 189 *Scoltz.*, prescribe it to this disease; as good for the stomach and to open
the hemrods, out of Mesue, Rhasis, Serapio, Avicenna: Menardus,
Ep. lib. 1, *epist.* 1, opposeth it; aloes "doth not open the veins,"[6]
or move the hemrods, which Leonhartus Fuchsius, *Paradox.
lib.* 1, likewise affirms; but Brassavola and Dodonæus defend
Mesue out of their experience; let Valesius[7] end the controversy.

Lapis Armenus and lazuli are much magnified by Alexander,
lib. 1, *cap.* 16,[8] Avicenna, Aetius, and Actuarius, if they be
well washed, that the water be no more coloured, fifty times
some say. "That good Alexander" (saith Guianerus) "puts
such confidence in this one medicine, that he thought all melancholy passions might be cured by it; and I for my part have
oftentimes happily used it, and was never deceived in the
operation of it."[9] The like may be said of lapis lazuli, though
it be somewhat weaker than the other. Garcias ab Horto,

Hist. lib. 1, *cap.* 65, relates that the physicians of the Moors familiarly prescribe it to all melancholy passions,[1] and Matthiolus, *Ep. lib.* 3, brags of that happy success which he still had in the administration of it.[2] Nicholas Meripsa puts it amongst the best remedies, *sect.* 1, *cap.* 12, *in Antidotis*; "and if this will not serve" (saith Rhasis) "then there remains nothing but lapis Armenus and hellebore itself."[3] Valescus and Jason Pratensis much commend *pulvis hali*, which is made of it. Janus Damascen, 2, *cap.* 12, Hercules de Saxonia, etc., speak well of it. Crato will not approve this; it and both hellebores, he saith, are no better than poison. Victor Trincavellius, *lib.* 2, *cap.* 14, found it in his experience "to be very noisome, to trouble the stomach, and hurt their bodies that take it overmuch."[4]

Black hellebore, that most renowned plant, and famous purger of melancholy, which all antiquity so much used and admired, was first found out by Melanpodius [5] a shepherd, as Pliny records, *lib.* 25, *cap.* 5, who, seeing it to purge his goats when they raved,[6] practised it upon Elige and Calene, King Prœtus' daughters, that ruled in Arcadia, near the fountain Clitorius, and restored them to their former health. In Hippocrates' time it was in only request, insomuch that he writ a book of it, a fragment of which remains yet. Theophrastus, Galen,[7] Pliny; Cælius Aurelianus, as ancient as Galen, *lib.* 1, *cap.* 6; Aretæus, *lib.* 1, *cap.* 5; Oribasius, *lib.* 7 *collect.*, a famous Greek; Aetius, *ser.* 3, *cap.* 112 *et* 113; P. Ægineta, Galen's ape, *lib.* 7, *cap.* 4; Actuarius; Trallianus, *lib.* 5, *cap.* 15; Cornelius Celsus, only remaining of the old Latins, *lib.* 3, *cap.* 23, extol and admire this excellent plant; and it was generally so much esteemed of the ancients for this disease amongst the rest, that they sent all such as were crazed, or that doted, to the Anticyræ, or to Phocis in Achaia, to be purged, where this plant was in abundance to be had. In Strabo's time it was an ordinary voyage; *Naviget Anticyras* [let him sail to Anticyra]: a common proverb among the Greeks and Latins, to bid a dizzard or a madman go take hellebore; as in Lucian, Menippus to Tantalus, *Tantale, desipis, helleboro epoto tibi opus est, eoque sane meraco*, Thou art out of thy little wit, O Tantalus, and must needs drink hellebore, and that without mixture. Aristophanes, *in Vespis*, "Drink hellebore," etc., and Harpax, in the comedian,[8] told Simo and Ballio, two doting fellows, that they had need to be purged with this plant. When that proud Menacrates ὁ Ζεὺς [surnamed Zeus], had writ an arrogant letter to Philip of Macedon, he sent back no other answer but this, *Consulo tibi ut ad Anticyram te con-feras* [I advise you to pay a visit to Anticyra], noting thereby that he was crazed, *atque helleboro indigere*, [and] had much need of a good purge. Lilius Giraldus saith that Hercules, after all his mad pranks upon his wife and children, was per-fectly cured by a purge of hellebore, which an Anticyrian administered unto him. They that were sound commonly took it to quicken their wits (as Ennius of old, *Qui non nisi potus ad arma prosiluit dicenda* [1] [who never essayed to write of war-like deeds save in his cups], and as our poets drink sack to improve their inventions); I find it so registered by A. Gellius, *lib.* 17, *cap.* 15. Carneades the Academic, when he was to write against Zeno the Stoic, purged himself with hellebore first, which Petronius [2] puts upon Chrysippus. In such esteem it continued for many ages, till at length Mesue and some other Arabians began to reject and reprehend it, upon whose authority for many following lustres it was much debased and quite out of request, held to be poison and no medicine; and is still oppugned to this day by Crato [3] and some junior physicians. Their reasons are, because Aristotle, *lib.* 1 *de plant. cap.* 3, said henbane and hellebore were poison; and Alexander Aphrodisiæus, in the preface of his Problems, gave out, that (speaking of hellebore) "quails fed on that which was poison to men." [4] Galen, *lib.* 6 *Epid. com.* 5, *text.* 35, confirms as much; Constan-tine the emperor, in his Geoponics, [5] attributes no other virtue to it than to kill mice and rats, flies and mouldwarps; and so Mizaldus, Nicander of old, Gervinus, Sckenkius, and some other neoterics that have written of poisons, speak of hellebore in a chief place. Nicholas Leonicus [6] hath a story of Solon, that, besieging I know not what city, steeped hellebore in a spring of water, which by pipes was conveyed into the middle of the town, and so either poisoned, or else made them so feeble and weak by purging, that they were not able to bear arms. Not-withstanding all these cavils and objections, most of our late writers do much approve of it: Gariopontus, *lib.* 1, *cap.* 13,[7] Codronchus, *Com. de helleb.*, Fallopius, *lib. de med. purg. simpl. cap.* 69, *et consil.* 15 *Trincavellii*, Montanus, 239, Frisimelica, *consil.* 14, Hercules de Saxonia, so that it be opportunely given. Jacobus de Dondis, Agg.; Amatus Lusit. *cent.* 66; Godef. Stegius, *cap.* 13; Hollerius, and all our herbalists subscribe. Fernelius, *Meth. med. lib.* 5, *cap.* 16, confesseth it to be "a terrible purge and hard to take, yet well given to strong men, and such as have able bodies." [8] P. Forestus and Capivaccius

forbid it to be taken in substance, but allow it in decoction or
infusion, both which ways P. Monavius approves above all
others, *Epist.* 231 *Scoltzii*; Jacchinus, *in* 9 *Rhasis*, commends a
receipt of his own preparing; Penottus another of his chemically
prepared, Euonymus another. Hildesheim, *Spicil.* 2 *de mel.*,
hath many examples how it should be used, with diversity of
receipts. Heurnius, *lib.* 7 *Prax. med. cap.* 14, calls it "an
innocent medicine howsoever, if it be well prepared."[1]   The
root of it is only in use, which may be kept many years, and
by some given in substance, as by Fallopius and Brassavola
amongst the rest, who brags that he was the first that restored
it again to its use,[2] and tells a story how he cured one Malatesta,
a madman, that was thought to be possessed, in the Duke of
Ferrara's court, with one purge of black hellebore in substance:
the receipt is there to be seen; his excrements were like ink,
he perfectly healed at once;[3] Vidus Vidius, a Dutch physician,
will not admit of it in substance, to whom most subscribe, but
as before in the decoction, infusion, or, which is all in all, in
the extract, which he prefers before the rest, and calls *suave
medicamentum,* a sweet medicine, an easy, that may be securely
given to women, children, and weaklings.   Baracellus, *Horto
Geniali,* terms it *maximæ præstantiæ medicamentum,* a medicine
of great worth and note.   Quercetan, in his *Spagir. Phar.,* and
many others, tell wonders of the extract.   Paracelsus above all
the rest is the greatest admirer of this plant; and especially the
extract; he calls it *theriacum, terrestre balsamum,* another treacle,
a terrestrial balm, *instar omnium,* "all in all, the sole and last
refuge to cure this malady, the gout, epilepsy, leprosy, etc."[4]
If this will not help, no physic in the world can but mineral, it
is the upshot of all.   Matthiolus laughs at those that except
against it, and though some abhor it out of the authority of
Mesue, and dare not adventure to prescribe it, "yet I" (saith
he) "have happily used it six hundred times without offence,
and communicated it to divers worthy physicians, who have
given me great thanks for it."[5]   Look for receipts, dose,
preparation, and other cautions concerning this simple, in him,
Brassavola, Baracellus, Codronchus, and the rest.

Subsect. III.—*Compound Purgers*

Compound medicines which purge melancholy are either taken
in the superior or inferior parts: superior at mouth or nostrils.
At the mouth, swallowed or not swallowed: if swallowed, liquid

or solid: liquid, as compound wine of hellebore, scilla or sea-
onion, senna, *vinum scilliticum, helleboratum,* which Quercetan
so much applauds [1] "for melancholy and madness, either inwardly taken, or outwardly applied to the head, with little
pieces of linen dipped warm in it." *Oxymel scilliticum, syrupus
helleboratus major* and *minor* in Quercetan, and *syrupus genistæ*
for hypochondriacal melancholy in the same author, compound
syrup of succory, of fumitory, polypody, etc., Heurnius his
purging cock-broth.   Some except against these syrups, as
appears by Udalrinus Leonorus his Epistle to Matthiolus,[2] as
most pernicious, and that out of Hippocrates, *cocta movere, et
medicari, non cruda,* no raw things to be used in physic; but
this in the following epistle is exploded and soundly confuted
by Matthiolus: many juleps, potions, receipts, are composed of
these, as you shall find in Hildesheim, *Spicil.* 2, Heurnius, *lib.* 2,
cap. 14, George Sckenkius, *Ital. med. prax.,* etc.
   Solid purges are confections, electuaries, pills by themselves,
or compound with others, as *de lapide lazuli, Armeno, pil.
Indæ,* of fumitory, etc.; confection of hamech, which, though
most approve, Solenander, *sec.* 5, *consil.* 22, bitterly inveighs
against, so doth Rondeletius, *Pharmacop. officina,* Fernelius,
and others; diasenna, diapolypodium, diacassia, diacatholicon,
Wecker's electuary *de epithymo,* Ptolemy's hierologadium, of
which divers receipts are daily made.
   Aetius, 22, 23, commends *hieram Ruffi.* Trincavellius, *consil.*
12, *lib.* 4, approves of hiera; *Non, inquit, invenio melius medicamentum,* I find no better medicine, he saith. Heurnius adds
pil. aggregat., pills *de epithymo, pil. Ind.* Mesue describes in
the Florentine Antidotary, *pilulæ sine quibus esse nolo, pilulæ
cochiæ cum helleboro, pil. Arabicæ, fœtidæ, de quinque generibus
myrobalanorum,* etc., more proper to melancholy, not excluding
in the meantime turbith, manna, rhubarb, agaric, elescophe,
etc. which are not so proper to this humour.   For, as Montaltus
holds, *cap.* 30, and Montanus, *cholera etiam purganda, quod
atræ sit pabulum,* choler is to be purged because it feeds the
other: and some are of an opinion, as Erasistratus and Asclepiades maintained of old, against whom Galen disputes, "that
no physic doth purge one humour alone, but all alike or what is
next." [3] Most therefore in their receipts and magistrals which are
coined here, make a mixture of several simples and compounds to
purge all humours in general as well as this.   Some rather use
potions than pills to purge this humour, because that, as Heurnius
and Crato observe, *hic succus a sicco remedio ægre trahitur,* this

juice is not so easily drawn by dry remedies, and, as Montanus adviseth, *cons*. 25, "All drying medicines are to be repelled, as aloe, hiera, and all pills whatsoever,"[1] because the disease is dry of itself.

I might here insert many receipts of prescribed potions, boles, etc., the doses of these, but that they are common in every good physician, and that I am loath to incur the censure of Forestus, *lib*. 3, *cap*. 6, *de urinis*, "against those that divulge and publish medicines in their mother-tongue,"[2] and lest I should give occasion thereby to some ignorant reader to practise on himself, without the consent of a good physician.

Such as are not swallowed, but only kept in the mouth, are gargarisms, used commonly after a purge, when the body is soluble and loose. Or apophlegmatisms, masticatories, to be held and chewed in the mouth, which are gentle, as hyssop, origan, pennyroyal, thyme, mustard; strong, as pellitory, pepper, ginger, etc.

Such as are taken into the nostrils, *errhina*, are liquid or dry, juice of pimpernel, onions, etc., castor, pepper, white hellebore, etc. To these you may add odoraments, perfumes, and suffumigations, etc.

Taken into the inferior parts are clysters strong or weak, suppositories of Castilian soap, honey boiled to a consistence; or stronger of scammony, hellebore, etc.

These are all used, and prescribed to this malady upon several occasions, as shall be showed in its place.

MEMB. III.

Chirurgical Remedies

In letting of blood three main circumstances are to be considered, "Who, how much, when?"[3] That is, that it be done to such a one as may endure it, or to whom it may belong, that he be of a competent age, not too young, nor too old, overweak, fat, or lean, sore laboured, but to such as have need, are full of bad blood, noxious humours, and may be eased by it.

The quantity depends upon the party's habit of body, as he is strong or weak, full or empty, may spare more or less.

In the morning is the fittest time: some doubt whether it be best fasting or full, whether the moon's motion or aspect of planets be to be observed; some affirm, some deny, some grant in acute, but not in chronic diseases, whether before or after physic. 'Tis Heurnius' aphorism, *a phlebotomia auspicandam esse curationem, non a pharmacia*, you must begin with blood-letting and not physic; some except this peculiar malady. But what do I? Horatius Augenius, a physician of Padua, hath lately writ seventeen books of this subject, Jobertus, etc.

Particular kinds of blood-letting in use are three;[1] first is that opening a vein in the arm with a sharp knife, or in the head, knees, or any other parts, as shall be thought fit.

Cupping-glasses, with or without scarification, *ocissime compescunt*, saith Fernelius, they work presently, and are applied to several parts, to divert humours, aches, winds, etc.

Horse-leeches are much used in melancholy, applied especially to the hemrods. Horatius Augenius, *lib.* 10, *cap.* 10, Platerus, *de mentis alienat. cap.* 3, Altomarus, Piso, and many others, prefer them before any evacuations in this kind.

Cauteries[2] or searing with hot irons, combustions, borings, lancings, which, because they are terrible, *dropax* and *sinapismus* are invented, by plasters to raise blisters, and eating medicines of pitch, mustard-seed, and the like.

Issues still to be kept open, made as the former, and applied in and to several parts, have their use here on divers occasions, as shall be showed.

SECT. V.   MEMB. I.

SUBSECT. I.—*Particular Cure of the three several Kinds;*
of Head-Melancholy

THE general cures thus briefly examined and discussed, it remains now to apply these medicines to the three particular species or kinds, that, according to the several parts affected, each man may tell in some sort how to help or ease himself. I will treat of head-melancholy first, in which, as in all other good cures, we must begin with diet, as a matter of most moment, able oftentimes of itself to work this effect. "I have read," saith Laurentius, *cap.* 8 *de melanch.*, "that in old diseases which have gotten the upper hand or an habit, the manner of living is to more purpose than whatsoever can be drawn out of the most precious boxes of the apothecaries." This diet, as I have said, is not only in choice of meat and drink, but of all

those other non-natural things. Let air be clear and moist
most part: diet moistening, of good juice, easy of digestion, and
not windy: drink clear, and well brewed, not too strong, nor too
small. "Make a melancholy man fat," as Rhasis saith,[1] "and
thou hast finished the cure." Exercise not too remiss, nor too
violent. Sleep a little more than ordinary. Excrements daily
to be voided by art or nature;[2] and, which Fernelius enjoins
his patient, *consil.* 44, above the rest, to avoid all passions and
perturbations of the mind. Let him not be alone or idle (in
any kind of melancholy), but still accompanied with such friends
and familiars he most affects, neatly dressed, washed, and
combed, according to his ability at least, in clean sweet linen,
spruce, handsome, decent, and good apparel; for nothing sooner
dejects a man than want, squalor, and nastiness, foul or old
clothes out of fashion. Concerning the medicinal part, he that
will satisfy himself at large (in this precedent of diet) and see
all at once, the whole cure and manner of it in every distinct
species, let him consult with Gordonius, Valescus, with Prosper
Calenius, *lib. de atra bile ad Card. Cæsium*; Laurentius, *cap.* 8
et 9 *de melan.*; Ælian Montaltus, *de mel. cap.* 26, 27, 28, 29, 30;
Donatus ab Altomari, *cap.* 7 *Artis med.*; Hercules de Saxonia,
in Panth. cap. 7, *et tract. ejus peculiar. de melan. per Bolzettam
edit. Venetiis*, 1620, *cap.* 17, 18, 19; Savonarola, *rub.* 82, *tract.* 8,
cap. 1; Sckenkius, *in Prax. curat. Ital. med.*; Heurnius, *cap.* 12
de morb.; Victorius Faventinus, *Pract. Magn. et Empir.*; Hildesheim, *Spicil.* 2 *de man. et mel.*; Fel. Plater, Stockerus, Bruel,
P. Bayerus, Forestus, Fuchsius, Capivaccius, Rondeletius, Jason
Pratensis; Sallust. Salvian. *de remed. lib.* 2, *cap.* 1; Jacchinus,
iu 9 *Rhasis*; Lod. Mercatus, *de inter. morb. cur. lib.* 1, *cap.* 17;
Alexan. Messaria, *Pract. med. lib.* 1, *cap.* 21, *de mel.*; Piso, Hollerius, etc., that have culled out of those old Greeks, Arabians,
and Latins whatsoever is observable or fit to be used. Or let
him read those counsels and consultations of Hugo Senensis,
consil. 13 *et* 14; Reinerus Solenander, *consil.* 6, *sec.* 1, *et consil.* 3,
sec. 3; Crato, *consil.* 16, *lib.* 1; Montanus, 20, 22, and his
following counsels; Lælius à Fonte Eugubinus, *consult.* 44, 69,
77, 125, 129, 142; Fernelius, *consil.* 44, 45, 46; Jul. Cæsar
Claudinus, Mercurialis, Frambesarius, Sennertus, etc.; wherein
he shall find particular receipts, the whole method, preparatives,
purgers, correctors, averters, cordials in great variety and
abundance: out of which, because every man cannot attend to
read or peruse them, I will collect, for the benefit of the reader,
some few more notable medicines.

SUBSECT. II.—*Blood-letting*

Phlebotomy is promiscuously used before and after physic, commonly before, and upon occasion is often reiterated, if there be any need at least of it. For Galen and many others make a doubt of bleeding at all in this kind of head-melancholy. If the malady, saith Piso, *cap.* 23, and Altomarus, *cap.* 7, Fuchsius, *cap.* 33, "shall proceed primarily from the misaffected brain, the patient in such case shall not need at all to bleed, except the blood otherwise abound, the veins be full, inflamed blood, and the party ready to run mad." [1] In immaterial melancholy, which especially comes from a cold distemperature of spirits, Hercules de Saxonia, *cap.* 17, will not admit of phlebotomy; Laurentius, *cap.* 9, approves it out of the authority of the Arabians; but as Mesue, Rhasis, Alexander appoint, "especially in the head," [2] to open the veins of the forehead, nose, and ears is good. They commonly set cupping-glasses on the party's shoulders, having first scarified the place; they apply horse-leeches on the head, and in all melancholy diseases, whether essential or accidental, they cause the hemrods to be opened, having the eleventh aphorism of the sixth book of Hippocrates for their ground and warrant, which saith, "That in melancholy and mad men, the varicose tumour or hæmorrhoides appearing doth heal the same." Valescus prescribes blood-letting in all three kinds, whom Sallustus Salvianus follows. "If the blood abound, which is discerned by the fullness of the veins, his precedent diet, the party's laughter, age, etc., begin with the median or middle vein of the arm: if the blood be ruddy and clear, stop it, but if black in the spring-time, or a good season, or thick, let it run, according to the party's strength: and some eight or twelve days after, open the head-vein, and the veins in the forehead, or provoke it out of the nostrils, or cupping-glasses," etc. [3] Trallianus allows of this, "If there have been any suppression or stopping of blood at nose, or hemrods, or women's months, then to open a vein in the head or about the ankles." [4] Yet he doth hardly approve of this course, if melancholy be sited in the head alone, or in any other dotage, "except it primarily proceed from blood, or that the malady be increased by it; for blood-letting refrigerates and dries up, except the body be very full of blood, and a kind of ruddiness in the face." [5] Therefore I conclude with Aretæus, "Before you let blood, deliberate of it," [6] and well consider all circumstances belonging to it.

Subsect. III.—*Preparatives and Purgers*

After blood-letting we must proceed to other medicines; first prepare, and then purge, *Augeæ stabulum purgare*, make the body clean before we hope to do any good. Gualter Bruel would have a practitioner begin first with a clyster of his, which he prescribes before blood-letting: the common sort, as Mercurialis, Montaltus, *cap.* 30, etc., proceed from lenitives to preparatives, and so to purgers. Lenitives are well known, *electuarium lenitivum, diaphænicum, diacatholicon*, etc. Preparatives are usually syrups of borage, bugloss, apples, fumitory, thyme, and epithyme, with double as much of the same decoction or distilled water, or of the waters of bugloss, balm, hops, endive, scolopendry, fumitory, etc., or these sod in whey, which must be reiterated and used for many days together. Purges come last, "which must not be used at all, if the malady may be otherwise helped," because they weaken nature and dry so much; and in giving of them, "we must begin with the gentlest first."[1] Some forbid all hot medicines, as Alexander and Salvianus, etc., *ne insaniores inde fiant* [lest it make them more crazy]; hot medicines increase the disease "by drying too much."[2] Purge downward rather than upward, use potions rather than pills, and when you begin physic, persevere and continue in a course; for as one observes, *movere et non educere in omnibus malum est:*[3] to stir up the humour (as one purge commonly doth), and not to prosecute, doth more harm than good. They must continue in a course of physic, yet not so that they tire and oppress nature, *danda quies naturæ*, they must now and then remit, and let nature have some rest. The most gentle purges to begin with, are senna,[4] cassia, epithyme, myrobalanes, catholicon: if these prevail not, we may proceed to stronger, as the confection of hamech, *pil. Indæ, fumitoriæ, de assaieret*, of lapis Armenus and lazuli, diasenna. Or if pills be too dry, some prescribe both hellebores in the last place,[5] amongst the rest Aretæus, "because this disease will resist a gentle medicine."[6] Laurentius and Hercules de Saxonia would have antimony tried last, "if the party be strong, and it warily given."[7] Trincavellius[8] prefers hierologodium, to whom Francis Alexander, in his *Apol. rad.* 5, subscribes; a very good medicine they account it. But Crato, in a counsel of his for the Duke of Bavaria's chancellor, wholly rejects it.

I find a vast chaos of medicines, a confusion of receipts and magistrals, amongst writers, appropriated to this disease; some

of the chiefest I will rehearse.   To be sea-sick first is very good
at seasonable times.[1]   *Helleborismus Matthioli*, with which he
vaunts and boasts he did so many several cures, "I never gave
it" (saith he), "but, after once or twice, by the help of God,
they were happily cured." [2]   The manner of making it he sets
down at large in his third book of Epistles to George Hantshius,
a physician.   Gualter Bruel and Heurnius make mention of it
with great approbation; so doth Sckenkius in his memorable
cures, and experimental medicines, *cent. 6, observ.* 37 that
famous helleborism of Montanus, which he so often repeats in
his consultations and counsels, as 28, *pro melan. sacerdote*, and
consil. 148, *pro hypochondriaco*, and cracks "to be a most
sovereign remedy for all melancholy persons, which he hath
often given without offence, and found by long experience and
observations to be such." [3]

Quercetan prefers a syrup of hellebore in his *Spagirica Phar-
mac.*, and hellebore's extract, *cap.* 5, of his invention likewise
("a most safe medicine and not unfit to be given children" [4]),
before all remedies whatsoever.

Paracelsus, in his book of black hellebore, admits this medicine,
but as it is prepared by him.   "It is most certain" (saith he)
"that the virtue of this herb is great, and admirable in effect,
and little differing from balm itself; and he that knows well how
to make use of it hath more art than all their books contain,
or all the doctors in Germany can show." [5]

Ælianus Montaltus, in his exquisite work *de morb. capitis*,
cap. 31, *de mel.*, sets a special receipt of his own, which in his
practice "he fortunately used"; [6] because it is but short I will
set it down.

> R syrupi de pomis ʒij, aquæ borag. ʒiiij,
> ellebori nigri per noctem infusi in ligatura
> 6 vel 8 gr. mane facta colatura exhibe.

Other receipts of the same to this purpose you shall find in
him.   Valescus admires *pulvis hali*, and Jason Pratensis after
him: the confection of which our new London Pharmacopœia
hath lately revived.   "Put case" (saith he) "all other medicines
fail, by the help of God this alone shall do it, and 'tis a crowned
medicine which must be kept in secret." [7]

> R epithymi semunc., lapidis lazuli, agarici ana ʒij,
> scammonii, ʒj, caryophyllorum numero 20 ; pulverisentur
> omnia, et ipsius pulveris scrup. 4 singulis septimanis assumat.

To these I may add *Arnoldi vinum buglossatum*, or borage

wine before mentioned, which Mizaldus [8] calls *vinum mirabile*,
a wonderful wine, and Stockerus vouchsafes to repeat verbatim
amongst other receipts; Rubeus his compound water out of
Savonarola; [1] Pinetus his balm; Cardan's *pulvis hyacinthi*, with
which, in his book *de curis admirandis*, he boasts that he had
cured many melancholy persons in eight days, which Sckenkius
puts amongst his observable medicines; [2] Altomarus his syrup,
with which, he calls God so solemnly to witness, he hath in his
kind done many excellent cures,[3] and which Sckenkius, *cent. 7,
observ.* 80, mentioneth, Daniel Sennertus, *lib. 1, part. 2, cap. 12,*
so much commends; Rulandus' admirable water for melancholy,
which, *cent. 2, cap.* 96, he names *spiritum vitæ aureum, panaceam,*
what not? and his absolute medicine of 50 eggs, *Curat. Empir.
cent. 1, cur.* 5, to be taken three in a morning, with a powder
of his.   Faventinus, *Prac. Empir.*, doubles this number of eggs,
and will have 101,[4] to be taken by three and three in like sort,
which Sallustius Salvianus approves, *de red. med. lib. 2, cap. 1,*
with some of the same powder, till all be spent, a most excellent
remedy for all melancholy and mad men.

> ℞ *epithymi, thymi, ana drachmas duas, sacchari albi unciam
>   unam, croci grana tria,*
> *cinnamomi drachmam unam; misce, fiat pulvis.*

All these yet are nothing to those chemical preparatives of
aqua chelidonia, quintessence of hellebore, salts, extracts,
distillations, oils, *aurum potabile,* etc.[5] Dr. Anthony, in his
book *de auro potab., edit.* 1600, is all in all for it.   "And though
all the school of Galenists, with a wicked and unthankful
pride and scorn, detest it in their practice, yet in more grievous
diseases, when their vegetals will do no good," they are compelled to seek the help of minerals, though they "use them rashly,
unprofitably, slackly, and to no purpose." [6]   Rhenanus, a Dutch
chemist, in his book *de sale e puteo emergente,* takes upon him to
apologize for Anthony, and sets light by all that speak against
him.   But what do I meddle with this great controversy, which
is the subject of many volumes?   Let Paracelsus, Quercetan,
Crollius, and the brethren of the Rosy Cross defend themselves
as they may.   Crato, Erastus, and the Galenists oppugn Paracelsus; he brags on the other side, he did more famous cures
by this means than all the Galenists in Europe, and calls himself a monarch; Galen, Hippocrates, infants, illiterate, etc.   As
Thessalus of old railed against those ancient Asclepiadean
writers, "he condemns others, insults, triumphs, overcomes all

antiquity" (saith Galen as if he spake to him), "declares himself a conqueror, and crowns his own doings." [1] "One drop of their chemical preparatives shall do more good than all their fulsome potions." [2] Erastus and the rest of the Galenists vilify them on the other side, as heretics in physic: "Paracelsus did that in physic, which Luther in divinity." [3] "A drunken rogue he was, a base fellow, a magician, he had the devil for his master, devils his familiar companions, and what he did was done by the help of the devil." [4] Thus they contend and rail, and every mart write books pro and con, *et adhuc sub judice lis est* [and the case is still proceeding]: let them agree as they will, I proceed.

SUBSECT. IV.—*Averters*

Averters and purgers must go together, as tending all to the same purpose, to divert this rebellious humour, and turn it another way. In this range, clysters and suppositories challenge a chief place, to draw this humour from the brain and heart to the more ignoble parts. Some would have them still used a few days between, and those to be made with the boiled seeds of anise, fennel, and bastard saffron, hops, thyme, epithyme, mallows, fumitory, bugloss, polypody, senna, diasenna, hamech, cassia, diacatholicon, hierologodium, oil of violets, sweet almonds, etc. For without question a clyster, opportunely used, cannot choose in this, as most other maladies, but to do very much good; *clysteres nutriunt*, sometimes clysters nourish, as they may be prepared, as I was informed not long since by a learned lecture of our Natural Philosophy Reader,[5] which he handled by way of discourse, out of some other noted physicians. Such things as provoke urine most commend, but not sweat. Trincavellius, *consil.* 16, *cap.* 1, in head-melancholy forbids it. P. Bayerus and others approve frictions of the outward parts, and to bathe them with warm water. Instead of ordinary frictions, Cardan prescribes rubbing with nettles till they blister the skin, which likewise Bassardus Visontinus so much magnifies.[6]

Sneezing, masticatories, and nasals are generally received. Montaltus, *cap.* 34, Hildesheim, *Spicil.* 2, *fol.* 136 and 138, give several receipts of all three. Hercules de Saxonia relates of an empiric in Venice "that had a strong water to purge by the mouth and nostrils, which he still used in head-melancholy, and would sell for no gold." [7]

To open months and hemrods is very good physic, "if they

have been formerly stopped." [1]   Faventinus would have them
opened with horse-leeches, so would Hercules de Saxonia.
Julius Alexandrinus, *consil.* 185 *Scoltzii*, thinks aloes fitter:
most [2] approve horse-leeches in this case, to be applied to the
forehead, nostrils,[3] and other places.

Montaltus, *cap.* 29, out of Alexander and others, prescribes
"cupping-glasses, and issues in the left thigh." [4]   Aretæus,
lib. 7, *cap.* 5, Paulus Regolinus, Sylvius, will have them without scarification, "applied to the shoulders and back, thighs
and feet": [5] Montaltus, *cap.* 34, bids "open an issue in the arm,
or hinder part of the head." [6]   Piso enjoins ligatures, frictions,
suppositories, and cupping-glasses, still without scarification,
and the rest.[7]

Cauteries and hot irons are to be used "in the suture of the
crown, and the seared or ulcerated place suffered to run a good
while. 'Tis not amiss to bore the skull with an instrument,
to let out the fuliginous vapours." [8]   Sallust. Salvianus, *de re
medic. lib.* 2, *cap.* 1, "because this humour hardly yields to other
physic, would have the leg cauterized, or the left leg, below the
knee,[9] and the head bored in two or three places," [10] for that it
much avails to the exhalation of the vapours. "I saw" (saith
he) "a melancholy man at Rome, that by no remedies could be
healed, but when by chance he was wounded in the head, and
the skull broken, he was excellently cured." [11]   Another, to the
admiration of the beholders, "breaking his head with a fall
from on high, was instantly recovered of his dotage." [12]   Gordonius, *cap.* 13, *part.* 2, would have these cauteries tried last,
when no other physic will serve. "The head to be shaved and
bored to let out fumes, which without doubt will do much good.
I saw a melancholy man wounded in the head with a sword,
his brain-pan broken; so long as the wound was open he was
well, but when his wound was healed his dotage returned again." [13]
But Alexander Messaria, a professor in Padua, *lib.* 1 *Pract.
med. cap.* 21, *de melanchol.*, will allow no cauteries at all, 'tis too
stiff an humour and too thick, as he holds, to be so evaporated.

Guianerius, *cap.* 8, *tract.* 15, cured a nobleman in Savoy, by
boring alone, "leaving the hole open a month together," [14] by
means of which, after two years' melancholy and madness, he
was delivered. All approve of this remedy in the suture of the
crown; but Arculanus would have the cautery to be made with
gold. In many other parts these cauteries are prescribed for
melancholy men, as in the thighs (Mercurialis, *consil.* 86), arms,
legs (*idem, consil.* 6, *et* 19, *et* 25), Montanus, 86, Rodericus à

Fonseca, *tom. 2, consult.* 84, *pro hypochond., coxa dextra* [in
the right thigh], etc., but most in the head, "if other physic
will do no good."

SUBSECT. V.—*Alteratives and Cordials, corroborating, resolving
the Relics, and mending the Temperament*

Because this humour is so malign of itself, and so hard to be
removed, the relics are to be cleansed, by alteratives, cordials,
and such means: the temper is to be altered and amended,
with such things as fortify and strengthen the heart and brain,
"which are commonly both affected in this malady, and do
mutually misaffect one another":[1] which are still to be given
every other day, or some few days inserted after a purge or
like physic, as occasion serves, and are of such force that many
times they help alone, and as Arnoldus holds in his Aphorisms,
are to be "preferred before all other medicines, in what kind
soever."[2]

Amongst this number of cordials and alteratives I do not find
a more present remedy than a cup of wine or strong drink, if
it be soberly and opportunely used. It makes a man bold,
hardy, courageous, "whetteth the wit,"[3] if moderately taken,
and (as Plutarch saith, *Symp.* 7, *quæst.* 12) "it makes those which
are otherwise dull to exhale and evaporate like frankincense,"[4]
or quicken (Xenophon adds) as oil doth fire.[5] "A famous cordial"
Matthiolus, *in Dioscoridem,* calls it, "an excellent nutriment to
refresh the body, it makes a good colour, a flourishing age,
helps concoction, fortifies the stomach, takes away obstructions,
provokes urine, drives out excrements, procures sleep, clears
the blood, expels wind and cold poisons, attenuates, concocts,
dissipates all thick vapours and fuliginous humours."[6] And
that which is all in all to my purpose, it takes away fear and
sorrow. *Curas edaces dissipat Evius*[7] [the God of Wine dissolves
heart-eating care]. "It glads the heart of man" (Ps. civ, 15),
hilaritatis dulce seminarium [a sweet nursery of cheerfulness].
Helena's bowl, the sole nectar of the gods, or that true nepenthes
in Homer,[8] which puts away care and grief, as Oribasius,
5 *Collect. cap.* 7, and some others will, was naught else but a
cup of good wine. "It makes the mind of the king and of the
fatherless both one, of the bond and freeman, poor and rich;
it turneth all his thoughts to joy and mirth, makes him remember
no sorrow or debt, but enricheth his heart, and makes him speak

by talents" (Esdras iii, 19, 20, 21). It gives life itself, spirits,
wit, etc. For which cause the ancients called Bacchus *Liber
pater a liberando* [Father Liber, because he liberated], and
sacrificed to Bacchus and Pallas still upon an altar.[1] "Wine
measurably drunk, and in time, brings gladness and cheerful-
ness of mind," [2] it "cheereth God and men" (Judges ix, 13);
lætitiæ Bacchus dator [Bacchus the giver of joy], it makes an old
wife dance, and such as are in misery to forget evil, and be
merry.[3]

> *Bacchus et afflictis requiem mortalibus affert,*
> *Crura licet duro compede vincta forent.*

> Wine makes a troubled soul to rest,
> Though feet with fetters be opprest.

Demetrius in Plutarch, when he fell into Seleucus' hands, and
was prisoner in Syria, "spent his time with dice and drink that
he might so ease his discontented mind, and avoid those continual cogitations of his present condition wherewith he was
tormented." [4] Therefore Solomon, Prov. xxxi, 6, bids "wine
be given to him that is ready to perish,[5] and to him that hath
grief of heart; let him drink that he forget his poverty, and
remember his misery no more." *Sollicitis animis onus eximit*,
it easeth a burdened soul, nothing speedier, nothing better;
which the prophet Zachary perceived, when he said, "that in
the time of Messias they of Ephraim should be glad, and their
heart should rejoice as through wine." All which makes me
very well approve of that pretty description of a feast in Bartholomæus Anglicus; [6] when grace was said, their hands washed,
and the guests sufficiently exhilarated with good discourse,
sweet music, dainty fare, *exhilarationis gratia, pocula iterum
atque iterum offeruntur:* as a corollary to conclude the feast
and continue their mirth, a grace-cup came in to cheer their
hearts, and they drank healths to one another again and again.
Which (as J. Fredericus Matenesius, *Crit. Christ. lib. 2, cap. 5,
6, et 7*) was an old custom in all ages in every commonwealth,
so as they be not enforced *bibere per violentiam* [to drink by
violent means], but as in that royal feast of Assuerus,[7] which
lasted 180 days, "without compulsion they drank by order in
golden vessels," when and what they would themselves. This
of drink is a most easy and parable remedy, a common, a cheap,
still ready against fear, sorrow, and such troublesome thoughts
that molest the mind; as brimstone with fire, the spirits on a
sudden are enlightened by it. "No better physic" (saith

Rhasis [1]) "for a melancholy man: and he that can keep company, and carouse, needs no other medicines," 'tis enough. His countryman Avicenna, 31 *Doct. 2, cap.* 8, proceeds farther yet, and will have him that is troubled in mind, or melancholy, not to drink only, but now and then to be drunk: excellent good physic it is for this and many other diseases. Magninus, *Reg. san. part.* 3, *cap.* 31, will have them to be so once a month at least, and gives his reasons for it, "because it scours the body by vomit, urine, sweat, of all manner of superfluities, and keeps it clean." [2]　Of the same mind is Seneca the philosopher, in his book *de tranquil. lib.* 1, *cap.* 15: *Nonnunquam ut in aliis morbis ad ebrietatem usque veniendum; curas deprimit, tristitiæ medetur,* it is good sometimes to be drunk, it helps sorrow, depresseth cares; and so concludes his tract with a cup of wine: *Habes, Serene carissime, quæ ad tranquillitatem animæ pertinent* [Here, my dear Serenus, you have what is required for peace of mind]. But these are Epicureal tenents, tending to looseness of life, luxury, and atheism, maintained alone by some heathens, dissolute Arabians, profane Christians, and are exploded by Rabbi Moses, *tract.* 4, Guliel. Placentius, *lib.* 1, *cap.* 8, Valescus de Taranta, and most accurately ventilated by Jo. Sylvaticus, a late writer and physician of Milan, *Med. cont. cap.* 14, where you shall find this tenent copiously confuted.

Howsoever you say, if this be true that wine and strong drink have such virtue to expel fear and sorrow and to exhilarate the mind, ever hereafter let's drink and be merry.

> *Prome reconditum, Lyde strenua, Cæcubum*
> *Capaciores puer huc affer scyphos,*
> *Et Chia vina aut Lesbia.* [3]

> Come, lusty, Lyda, fill's a cup of sack,
> And, sirrah drawer, bigger pots we lack,
> And Scio wines that have so good a smack.

I say with him in A. Gellius, [4] "let us maintain the vigour of our souls with a moderate cup of wine," *Natis in usum lætitiæ scyphis* [5] [cups made for joy], "and drink to refresh our mind; if there be any cold sorrow in it, or torpid bashfulness, let's wash it all away." *Nunc vino pellite curas* [now banish care with wine]; so saith Horace, [6] so saith Anacreon:

> Μεθύοντα γάρ με κεῖσθαι
> Πολὺ κρεῖσσον ἢ θανόντα. [7]

['Tis much better that I should lie drunk than dead.]

Let's drive down care with a cup of wine: and so say I too
(though I drink none myself), for all this may be done, so that
it be modestly, soberly, opportunely used: so that "they be not
drunk with wine, wherein is excess," which our Apostle fore-
warns; for, as Chrysostom well comments on that place,[1] *ad
lætitiam datum est vinum, non ad ebrietatem*, 'tis for mirth, wine,
but not for madness: and will you know where, when, and how
that is to be understood? *Vis discere ubi bonum sit vinum?
Audi quid dicat Scriptura*, hear the Scriptures, "Give wine to
them that are in sorrow," or, as Paul bid Timothy drink wine
for his stomach's sake, for concoction, health, or some such
honest occasion.   Otherwise, as Pliny telleth us,[2] if singular
moderation be not had, "nothing so pernicious, 'tis mere
vinegar, *blandus dæmon* [a seductive demon], poison itself."
But hear a more fearful doom (Hab. ii, 15 and 16): "Woe be
to him that makes his neighbour drunk, shameful spewing shall
be upon his glory."   Let not good fellows triumph therefore
(saith Matthiolus) that I have so much commended wine; if it
be immoderately taken, "instead of making glad, it confounds
both body and soul, it makes a giddy head, a sorrowful heart."
And 'twas well said of the poet of old, "Wine causeth mirth and
grief," [3] nothing so good for some, so bad for others,[4] especially,
as one observes,[5] *qui a causa calida male habent*, that are hot or
inflamed (and so of spices, they alone, as I have showed,
cause head-melancholy themselves); they must not use wine as
an ordinary drink, or in their diet.[6]   But to determine with
Laurentius, *cap. 8 de melan.*, wine is bad for madmen, and
such as are troubled with heat in their inner parts or brains;
but to melancholy which is cold (as most is), wine, soberly
used, may be very good.

I may say the same of the decoction of china-roots, sassafras,
sarsaparilla, guaiacum: china, saith Manardus, makes a good
colour in the face, takes away melancholy, and all infirmities
proceeding from cold; even so sarsaparilla provokes sweat
mightily, guaiacum dries.   Claudinus, *consult*. 89 *et* 46, Montanus, Capivaccius, *consult*. 188 *Scoltzii*, make frequent and good
use of guaiacum and china, "so that the liver be not incensed," [7]
good for such as are cold, as most melancholy men are, but by
no means to be mentioned in hot.

The Turks have a drink called coffa (for they use no wine),
so named of a berry as black as soot, and as bitter (like that
black drink which was in use amongst the Lacedæmonians, and
perhaps the same), which they sip still of, and sup as warm as

they can suffer; they spend much time in those coffa-houses,
which are somewhat like our alehouses or taverns, and there
they sit chatting and drinking to drive away the time, and to
be merry together, because they find by experience that kind
of drink, so used, helpeth digestion, and procureth alacrity.
Some of them take opium to this purpose.

Borage, balm, saffron, gold, I have spoken of; Montaltus,
cap. 23, commends scorzonera roots condite. Garcias ab Horto,
Plant. hist. lib. 2, cap. 25, makes mention of an herb called
datura, "which, if it be eaten for twenty-four hours following,
takes away all sense of grief, makes them incline to laughter and
mirth": [1] and another called bang, like in effect to opium,
"which puts them for a time into a kind of ecstasis," and
makes them gently to laugh. One of the Roman emperors
had a seed, which he did ordinarily eat to exhilarate himself.
Christophorus Ayrerus [2] prefers bezoar stone, and the confection of alkermes, before other cordials, and amber in some
cases. "Alkermes comforts the inner parts"; [3] and bezoar
stone hath an especial virtue against all melancholy affections,
"it refresheth the heart, and corroborates the whole body." [4]
Amber provokes urine, helps the body, breaks wind, etc.[5] After
a purge, three or four grains of bezoar stone and three grain of
ambergrease, drunk or taken in borage or bugloss water in which
gold hot hath been quenched, will do much good, and the purge
shall diminish less (the heart so refreshed) of the strength and
substance of the body.

> R confect. alkermes ℥ss. lap. bezoar. Ɖj,
> *succini albi subtiliss. pulverisat. Ɖjj, cum*
> *syrup. de cort. citri ; fiat electuarium.*

To bezoar's stone most subscribe, Manardus, and many
others; [6] "it takes away sadness, and makes him merry that
useth it; I have seen some that have been much diseased with
faintness, swooning, and melancholy, that, taking the weight
of three grains of this stone in the water of ox-tongue, have
been cured." Garcias ab Horto brags how many desperate
cures he hath done upon melancholy men by this alone, when
all physicians had forsaken them. But alkermes many except
against; in some cases it may help, if it be good and of the
best, such as that of Montpelier in France, which Jodocus
Sincerus, *Itinerario Galliæ,*[7] so much magnifies, and would have
no traveller omit to see it made. But it is not so general a
medicine as the other. Fernelius, *consil.* 49, suspects alkermes,

by reason of its heat; "Nothing" (saith he) "sooner exasperates this disease than the use of hot working meats and medicines"; and would have them for that cause warily taken.[1] I conclude, therefore, of this and all other medicines, as Thucydides of the plague at Athens, no remedy could be prescribed for it, *nam quod uni profuit, hoc aliis erat exitio*: there is no catholic medicine to be had: that which helps one, is pernicious to another.

Diamargaritum frigidum, diambra, diaboraginatum, electuarium lætificans Galeni et Rhasis, de gemmis, dianthos, diamoschum dulce et amarum, electuarium conciliatoris, syrup. cydoniorum de pomis, conserves of roses, violets, fumitory, *enula campana*, satyrion, lemons, orange-peels condite, etc., have their good use.

> ℞ *diamoschi dulcis et amari, ana ʒjj ;
> diabuglossati, diaboraginati, sacchari violacei,
> ana ʒj ; misce cum syrupo de pomis.*[2]

Every physician is full of such receipts: one only I will add for the rareness of it, which I find recorded by many learned authors, as an approved medicine against dotage, head-melancholy, and such diseases of the brain. Take a ram's head [3] that never meddled with an ewe, cut off at a blow, and the horns only taken away, boil it well, skin and wool together; after it is well sod, take out the brains, and put these spices to it, cinnamon, ginger, nutmeg, mace, cloves, *ana ʒss*, mingle the powder of these spices with it, and heat them in a platter upon a chafing-dish of coals together, stirring them well, that they do not burn; take heed it be not overmuch dried, or drier than a calf's brains ready to be eaten. Keep it so prepared, and for three days give it the patient fasting, so that he fast two hours after it. It may be eaten with bread in an egg or broth, or any way, so it be taken. For fourteen days let him use this diet, drink no wine, etc. Gesner, *Hist. animal. lib.* 1, *pag.* 917; Caricterius, *Pract.* 13, *in Nich. de metri. pag.* 129; *Iatro. Wittenberg. edit. Tubing. pag.* 62, mention this medicine, though with some variation; he that list may try it, and many such.[4]

Odoraments to smell to, of rose-water, violet flowers, balm, rose-cakes, vinegar, etc., do much recreate the brains and spirits; according to Solomon, Prov. xxvii, 9, "They rejoice the heart," and as some say, nourish: 'tis a question commonly controverted in our schools, *an odores nutriant* [whether scents nourish]; let Ficinus, *lib.* 2, *cap.* 18, decide it; many arguments he brings to prove it: [5] as of Democritus, that lived by the smell of bread alone, applied to his nostrils, for some few days, when for old age he could eat no meat. Ferrerius, *lib. 2 Meth.*, speaks of an excellent confection of his making, of wine, saffron, etc., which he prescribed to dull, weak, feeble, and dying men to smell to, and by it to have done very much good, *æque fere profuisse olfactu et potu*, as if he had given them drink. Our noble and learned Lord Verulam,[1] in his book *de vita et morte*, commends therefore all such cold smells as any way serve to refrigerate the spirits. Montanus, *consil.* 31, prescribes a form which he would have his melancholy patient never to have out of his hands. If you will have them spagirically prepared, look in Oswaldus Crollius, *Basil. Chymica.*

Irrigations of the head shaven, "of the flowers of water-lilies, lettuce, violets, camomile, wild mallows, wether's-head, etc.,"[2] must be used many mornings together. Montanus, *consil.* 31, would have the head so washed once a week. Lælius à Fonte Eugubinus, *consult.* 44, for an Italian count troubled with head-melancholy, repeats many medicines which he tried, "but two alone which did the cure: use of whey made of goat's milk, with the extract of hellebore, and irrigations of the head with water-lilies, lettuce, violets, camomile, etc., upon the suture of the crown."[3] Piso commends a ram's lungs applied hot to the fore-part of the head, or a young lamb divided in the back, exenterated, etc.;[4] all acknowledge the chief cure to consist in moistening throughout. Some, saith Laurentius, use powders, and caps to the brain; but forasmuch as such aromatical things are hot and dry, they must be sparingly administered.

Unto the heart we may do well to apply bags, epithemes, ointments, of which Laurentius, *cap.* 9 *de melan.*, gives examples. Bruel prescribes an epitheme for the heart, of bugloss, borage, water-lily, violet waters, sweet wine, balm leaves, nutmegs, cloves, etc.

For the belly, make a fomentation of oil, in which the seeds of cummin, rue, carrots, dill, have been boiled.[5]

Baths are of wonderful great force in this malady, much admired by Galen,[6] Aetius,[7] Rhasis, etc., of sweet water, in which is boiled the leaves of mallows, roses, violets, water-lilies, wether's-head, flowers of bugloss, camomile, melilot, etc. Guianerius, *cap.* 8, *tract.* 15, would have them used twice a day, and when they come forth of the baths, their backbones to be anointed with oil of almonds, violets, nymphæa, fresh capon-grease, etc.

Amulets and things to be borne about, I find prescribed, taxed by some, approved by Renodeus, Platerus (*Amuleta, inquit,*

non negligenda [he says that amulets should not be neglected]),
and others; look for them in Mizaldus, Porta, Albertus, etc.
Bassardus Visontinus, *Ant. philos.*, commends hypericon, or
St. John's wort, gathered on a Friday in the hour of Jupiter,
"when it comes to his effectual operation (that is about the
full moon in July); so gathered and borne, or hung about the
neck, it mightily helps this affection, and drives away all
phantastical spirits." [1]   Philes, a Greek author that flourished
in the time of Michael Palæologus, writes [2] that a sheep or kid's
skin, whom a wolf worried, *Hædus inhumani raptus ab ore
lupi* [3] [a kid snatched from the jaws of a cruel wolf], ought not
at all to be worn about a man, "because it causeth palpitation
of the heart," not for any fear, but a secret virtue which amulets
have.   A ring made of the hoof of an ass's right fore-foot carried
about, etc.: I say with Renodeus,[4] they are not altogether to
be rejected.   Peony doth cure epilepsy; precious stones most
diseases; a wolf's dung borne with one helps the colic,[5] a spider
an ague,[6] etc.   Being in the country in the vacation time not
many years since, at Lindley in Leicestershire, my father's
house, I first observed this amulet of a spider in a nut-shell
lapped in silk, etc., so applied for an ague by my mother; [7]
whom although I knew to have excellent skill in chirurgery,
sore eyes, aches, etc., and such experimental medicines, as all
the country where she dwelt can witness, to have done many
famous and good cures upon divers poor folks, that were otherwise destitute of help, yet, among all other experiments, this
methought was most absurd and ridiculous, I could see no
warrant for it.   *Quid aranea cum febre?* [What has a spider to
do with fever?]   For what antipathy? till at length, rambling
amongst authors (as often I do), I found this very medicine in
Dioscorides, approved by Matthiolus, repeated by Aldrovandus,
cap. de aranea, lib. de insectis; I began to have a better opinion
of it, and to give more credit to amulets, when I saw it in
some parties answer to experience.   Some medicines are to be
exploded, that consist of words, characters, spells, and charms,
which can do no good at all, but out of a strong conceit, as
Pomponatius proves; or the devil's policy, who is the first
founder and teacher of them.

SUBSECT. VI.—*Correctors of Accidents to Procure Sleep. Against
fearful Dreams, Redness, etc.*

When you have used all good means and helps of alteratives,
averters, diminutives, yet there will be still certain accidents
to be corrected and amended, as waking, fearful dreams, flushing
in the face to some, ruddiness, etc.

Waking, by reason of their continual cares, fears, sorrows,
dry brains, is a symptom that much crucifies melancholy men,
and must therefore be speedily helped, and sleep by all means
procured, which sometimes is a sufficient remedy of itself without any other physic.[1] Sckenkius, in his Observations, hath
an example of a woman that was so cured. The means to
procure it are inward or outward. Inwardly taken, are
simples, or compounds; simples, as poppy, nymphæa, violets,
roses, lettuce, mandrake, henbane, nightshade or solanum,
saffron, hemp-seed, nutmegs, willows with their seeds, juice,
decoctions, distilled waters, etc. Compounds are syrups, or
opiates, syrup of poppy, violets, verbasco, which are commonly
taken with distilled waters.

> ℞ *diacodii ʒj, diascordii ʒss, aquæ lactucæ ʒiij ss;
> mista fiat potio ad horam somni sumenda.*

*Requies Nicholai, Philonium Romanum, Triphera magna, pilulæ
de cynoglossa,* diascordium, *laudanum Paracelsi,* opium, are in
use, etc. Country folks commonly make a posset of hemp-
seed, which Fuchsius in his Herbal so much discommends; yet
I have seen the good effect, and it may be used where better
medicines are not to be had.

Laudanum Paracelsi is prescribed in two or three grains,
with a dram of diascordium, which Oswald. Crollius commends.
Opium itself is most part used outwardly, to smell to in a ball,
though commonly so taken by the Turks to the same quantity
for a cordial,[2] and at Goa in the Indies: the dose forty or
fifty grains.

Rulandus calls *Requiem Nicholai, ultimum refugium,* the last
refuge; but of this and the rest look for peculiar receipts in
Victorius Faventinus, *cap. de phrenesi,* Heurnius, *cap. de mania,*
Hildesheim, *Spicil. 4, de somno et vigil.,* etc. Outwardly used,
as oil of nutmegs by extraction or expression with rosewater
to anoint the temples, oils of poppy, nenuphar, mandrake,
purslane, violets, all to the same purpose.

Montan., *consil.* 24 and 25, much commends odoraments of

opium, vinegar, and rose-water. Laurentius, *cap.* 9, prescribes pomanders and nodules; see the receipts in him; Codronchus, wormwood to smell to.[1]

Unguentum alabastritum, populeum, are used to anoint the temples, nostrils, or, if they be too weak, they mix saffron and opium. Take a grain or two of opium, and dissolve it with three or four drops of rose-water in a spoon, and after mingle with it as much *unguentum populeum* as a nut, use it as before: or else take half a dram of opium, *unguentum populeum,* oil of nenuphar, rose-water, rose-vinegar, of each half an ounce, with as much virgin wax as a nut, anoint your temples with some of it, *ad horam somni* [at bed-time].

Sacks of wormwood, mandrake,[2] henbane,[3] roses made like pillows and laid under the patient's head, are mentioned by Cardan and Mizaldus; "to anoint the soles of the feet with the fat of a dormouse, the teeth with ear-wax of a dog, swine's gall, hare's ears":[4] charms, etc.

Frontlets are well known to every goodwife: rose-water and vinegar, with a little woman's milk, and nutmegs grated upon a rose-cake applied to both temples.

For an emplaster, take of castorium a dram and a half, of opium half a scruple, mixed both together with a little water of life, make two small plasters thereof, and apply them to the temples.

Rulandus, *cent.* 1, *cur.* 17, *cent.* 3, *cur.* 94, prescribes epithemes and lotions of the head, with the decoction of flowers of nymphæa, violet-leaves, mandrake roots, henbane, white poppy; Herc. de Saxonia, *stillicidia,* or droppings, etc. Lotions of the feet do much avail of the said herbs: by these means, saith Laurentius, I think you may procure sleep to the most melancholy man in the world. Some use horse-leeches behind the ears, and apply opium to the place.

Bayerus,[5] *lib.* 2, *cap.* 13, sets down some remedies against fearful dreams, and such as walk and talk in their sleep. Baptista Porta, *Mag. nat. lib.* 2, *cap.* 6, to procure pleasant dreams and quiet rest, would have you take hippoglossa, or the herb horse-tongue, balm, to use them or their distilled waters after supper, etc. Such men must not eat beans, pease, garlic, onions, cabbage, venison, hare, use black wines, or any meat hard of digestion at supper, or lie on their backs, etc.

Rusticus pudor, bashfulness, flushing in the face, high colour, ruddiness, are common grievances, which much torture many melancholy men, when they meet a man, or come in company

of their betters, strangers, after a meal,[1] or if they drink a cup
of wine or strong drink, they are as red and flect, and sweat,
as if they had been at a mayor's feast, *præsertim si metus
accesserit* [especially if at the same time they are in fear], it
exceeds, they think every man observes, takes notice of it: and
fear alone will effect it, suspicion without any other cause.[2]
Sckenkius, *Observ. med. lib.* 1, speaks of a waiting-gentlewoman
in the Duke of Savoy's court, that was so much offended with
it, that she kneeled down to him, and offered Biarus, a physician,
all that she had to be cured of it. And 'tis most true, that
Antony Lodovicus [3] saith in his book *de pudore*, "bashfulness
either hurts or helps"; such men I am sure it hurts. If it
proceed from suspicion or fear, Felix Plater [4] prescribes no other
remedy but to reject and contemn it: *Id populus curat scilicet*
[to be sure, people take note of it], as a worthy physician [5] in
our town said to a friend of mine in like case, complaining
without a cause; suppose one look red, what matter is it?
make light of it, who observes it?

If it trouble at or after meals (as Jobertus observes, *Med.
pract. lib.* 1, *cap.* 7 [6]), after a little exercise or stirring, for many
are then hot and red in the face, or if they do nothing at all,
especially women; he would have them let blood in both arms,
first one, then another, two or three days between, if blood
abound; to use frictions of the other parts, feet especially, and
washing of them, because of that consent which is between the
head and the feet. And withal to refrigerate the face, by
washing it often with rose, violet, nenuphar, lettuce, lovage
waters, and the like: [7] but the best of all is that *lac virginale*,
or strained liquor of litargy: it is diversely prepared; by Jobertus
thus: R *lithar. argent. unc.* j, *cerussæ candidissimæ* ʒ jjj, *caphuræ*
Ə jj; *dissolvantur aquarum solani, lactucæ, et nenupharis ana
unc.* jjj, *aceti vini albi unc.* jj; *aliquot horas resideat, deinde trans-
mittatur per philt., aqua servetur in vase vitreo, ac ea bis terve
facies quotidie irroretur.* Quercetan, *Spagir. phar. cap.* 6, commends the water of frogs' spawn for ruddiness in the face.[8]
Crato, *consil.* 283 *Scoltzii,* would fain have them use all summer
the condite flowers of succory, strawberry-water, roses [9] (cupping-
glasses are good for the time), *consil.* 285 *et* 286, and to defecate
impure blood with the infusion of senna, savory, balm-water.
Hollerius knew one cured alone with the use of succory boiled,[10]
and drunk for five months, every morning in the summer.

It is good overnight to anoint the face with hare's blood, and
in the morning to wash it with strawberry and cowslip water,

the juice of distilled lemons,[1] juice of cucumbers, or to use the
seeds of melons, or kernels of peaches beaten small, or the roots
of arum, and mixed with wheat-bran to bake it in an oven,
and to crumble it in strawberry-water, or to put fresh cheese-
curds to a red face.[2]

If it trouble them at meal-times that flushing, as oft it doth,
with sweating or the like, they must avoid all violent passions
and actions, as laughing, etc., strong drink, and drink very
little, one draught, saith Crato,[3] and that about the midst of
their meal; avoid at all times indurate salt, and especially
spice and windy meat.

Crato prescribes the condite fruit of wild rose to a nobleman
his patient, to be taken before dinner or supper, to the quantity
of a chestnut. It is made of sugar, as that of quinces. The
decoction of the roots of sow-thistle before meat, by the same
author is much approved.[4] To eat of a baked apple some
advise, or of a preserved quince, cummin-seed prepared with
meat instead of salt, to keep down fumes; not to study or to
be intentive after meals.

> ℞ *nucleorum persic. seminis melonum ana unc.* ℈*ss*
> *aquæ fragorum l. ij; misce, utatur mane.*

To apply cupping-glasses to the shoulders [5] is very good. For
the other kind of ruddiness which is settled in the face with
pimples, etc., because it pertains not to my subject, I will not
meddle with it. I refer you to Crato's Counsels, Arnoldus,
lib. 1 *Breviar. cap.* 39, 1, Ruland, Peter Forestus, *de fuco, lib.* 31,
obser. 2, to Platerus, Mercurialis, Ulmus, Rondeletius, Heurnius,
Manardus, and others that have written largely of it.

Those other grievances and symptoms of headache, palpitation of heart, vertigo, deliquium, etc., which trouble many
melancholy men, because they are copiously handled apart in
every physician, I do voluntarily omit.

MEMB. II.

Cure of Melancholy over all the Body

WHERE the melancholy blood possesseth the whole body with
the brain, it is best to begin with blood-letting.[6] The Greeks
prescribe the median or middle vein to be opened,[7] and so much
blood to be taken away as the patient may well spare, and the

cut that is made must be wide enough.   The Arabians hold it
fittest to be taken from that arm on which side there is more pain
and heaviness in the head: if black blood issue forth, bleed on;
if it be clear and good, let it be instantly suppressed, "because
the malice of melancholy is much corrected by the goodness of
the blood." [1]   If the party's strength will not admit much
evacuation in this kind at once, it must be assayed again and
again: if it may not be conveniently taken from the arm, it
must be taken from the knees and ankles, especially to such
men or women whose hemrods or months have been stopped.
If the malady continue, it is not amiss to evacuate in a part
in the forehead,[2] and to virgins in the ankles, who are melancholy for love matters; so to widows that are much grieved and
troubled with sorrow and cares: for bad blood flows in the
heart, and so crucifies the mind.   The hemrods are to be opened
with an instrument or horse-lecches, etc.   See more in Montaltus, *cap.* 29.   Sckenkius hath an example of one that was
cured by an accidental wound in his thigh; much bleeding freed
him from melancholy.[3]   Diet, diminutives, alteratives, cordials,
correctors as before, intermixed as occasion serves, "all their
study must be to make a melancholy man fat, and then the
cure is ended." [4]   *Diuretica,* or medicines to procure urine, are
prescribed by some in this kind, hot and cold: hot where the
heat of the liver doth not forbid; cold where the heat of the
liver is very great: amongst hot are parsley roots, lovage, fennel,
etc.: cold, melon-seeds, etc., with whey of goat's milk, which
is the common conveyer.[5]

To purge and purify the blood, use sow-thistle, succory,
senna, endive, carduus benedictus, dandelion, hop, maidenhair,
fumitory, bugloss, borage, etc., with their juice, decoctions,
distilled waters, syrups, etc.[6]

Oswaldus Crollius, *Basil. Chym.*, much admires salt of corals
in this case, and Aetius, *Tetrabib. ser. 2, cap.* 114, *hieram Archi-
genis,* which is an excellent medicine to purify the blood, "for
all melancholy affections, falling sickness, none to be compared
to it."

MEMB. III.

SUBSECT. I.—*Cure of Hypochondriacal Melancholy*

IN this cure, as in the rest, is especially required the rectification of those six non-natural things above all, as good diet, which Montanus, *consil.* 27, enjoins a French nobleman, "to have an especial care of it, without which all other remedies are in vain." Blood-letting is not to be used, except the patient's body be very full of blood, and that it be derived from the liver and spleen to the stomach and his vessels, then to draw it back, to cut the inner vein of either arm,[1] some say the *salvatella*, and if the malady be continuate, to open a vein in the forehead.[2]

Preparatives and alteratives may be used as before, saving that there must be respect had as well to the liver, spleen, stomach, hypochondries, as to the heart and brain. To comfort the stomach [3] and inner parts against wind and obstructions, by Aretæus, Galen, Aetius, Aurelianus, etc., and many latter writers, are still prescribed the decoctions of wormwood, centaury, pennyroyal, betony, sod in whey and daily drunk: many have been cured by this medicine alone.

Prosper Alpinus and some others as much magnify the water of Nilus against this malady, an especial good remedy for windy melancholy. For which reason belike Ptolemæus Philadelphus, when he married his daughter Berenice to the King of Assyria (as Celsus, *lib.* 2, records), *magnis impensis Nili aquam afferri jussit,* to his great charge caused the water of Nilus to be carried with her, and gave command that during her life she should use no other drink. I find those that commend use of apples, in splenetic and this kind of melancholy (lamb's-wool some call it), which, howsoever approved, must certainly be corrected of cold rawness and wind.

Codronchus, in his book *de sale absin.*, magnifies the oil and salt of wormwood above all other remedies, "which works better and speedier than any simple whatsoever, and much to be preferred before all those fulsome decoctions and infusions, which must offend by reason of their quantity; this alone, in a small measure taken, expels wind, and that most forcibly, moves urine, cleanseth the stomach of all gross humours, crudities, helps appetite," etc.[4] Arnoldus hath a wormwood wine which he would have used, which every pharmacopœia speaks of.

Diminutives and purgers' may be taken as before,[1] of hiera,
manna, cassia, which Montanus, *consil.* 230, for an Italian abbot,
in this kind prefers before all other simples, "And these must
be often used, still abstaining from those which are more violent
lest they do exasperate the stomach, etc., and the mischief by
that means be increased;"[2] though in some physicians I find
very strong purgers, hellebore itself, prescribed in this affection.
If it long continue, vomits may be taken after meat, or otherwise gently procured with warm water, oxymel, etc., now and
then. Fuchsius, *cap.* 33, prescribes hellebore; but still take
heed in this malady, which I have often warned, of hot medicines,
"because" (as Salvianus adds) "drought follows heat, which
increaseth the disease":[3] and yet Baptista Sylvaticus, *controv.*
32, forbids cold medicines, "because they increase obstructions
and other bad symptoms."[4] But this varies as the parties do,
and 'tis not easy to determine which to use. "The stomach
most part in this infirmity is cold, the liver hot; scarce therefore" (which Montanus insinuates, *consil.* 229, for the Earl of
Montfort) "can you help the one and not hurt the other":[5]
much discretion must be used; take no physic at all, he concludes, without great need. Lælius Eugubinus, *consil.* 77 for an
hypochondriacal German prince, used many medicines; "but
it was after signified to him in letters, that the decoction of
china and sassafras, and salt of sassafras, wrought him an
incredible good."[6] In his 108th *consult.* he used as happily
the same remedies; this to a third might have been poison,
by overheating his liver and blood.

For the other parts look for remedies in Savonarola, Gordonius, Massaria, Mercatus, Johnson, etc. One for the spleen,
amongst many other, I will not omit, cited by Hildesheim,
Spicil. 2, prescribed by Mat. Flaccus, and out of the authority
of Benevenius. Antony Benevenius in a hypochondriacal
passion "cured an exceeding great swelling of the spleen with
capers alone, a meat befitting that infirmity, and frequent use
of the water of a smith's forge; by this physic he helped a sick
man whom all other physicians had forsaken, that for seven
years had been splenetic."[7] And of such force is this water,
"that those creatures as drink of it have commonly little or no
spleen."[8] See more excellent medicines for the spleen in him
and Lod. Mercatus,[9] who is a great magnifier of this medicine.
This *chalybs præparatus*, or steel-drink, is much likewise commended to this disease by Daniel Sennertus, *lib.* 1, *part.* 2, cap. 12,
and admired by J. Cæsar Claudinus, *Respons.* 29; he calls steel

the proper alexipharmacum of this malady,[1] and much magnifies
it; look for receipts in them.   Averters must be used to the
liver and spleen, and to scour the meseraic veins; and they are
either to open, or provoke urine.   You can open no place better
than the hemrods, "which if by horse-leeches they be made to
flow, there may not be again such an excellent remedy," as Plater
holds.[2]   Sallustius Salvianus will admit no other phlebotomy
but this; and by his experience in an hospital which he kept,
he found all mad and melancholy men worse for other blood-
letting.   Laurentius, *cap.* 15, calls this of horse-leeches a sure
remedy to empty the spleen and meseraic membrane.   Only
Montanus, *consil.* 241, is against it; "To other men" (saith he)
"this opening of the hemrods seems to be a profitable remedy;
for my part I do not approve of it, because it draws away the
thinnest blood, and leaves the thickest behind."[3]

Aetius, Vidus Vidius, Mercurialis, Fuchsius, recommend
diuretics, or such things as provoke urine, as aniseeds, dill,
fennel, germander, ground-pine, sod in water, or drunk in
powder; and yet P. Bayerus [4] is against them, and so is Hollerius;
"All melancholy men" (saith he) "must avoid such things as
provoke urine, because by them the subtile or thinnest is
evacuated, the thicker matter remains."

Clysters are in good request.   Trincavellius, *lib.* 3, *cap.* 38,
for a young nobleman, esteems of them in the first place, and
Hercules de Saxonia, *Panth. lib.* 1, *cap.* 16, is a great approver
of them.   "I have found" (saith he) "by experience that many
hypochondriacal melancholy men have been cured by the sole
use of clysters." [5]   Receipts are to be had in him.

Besides those fomentations, irrigations, inunctions, odoraments, prescribed for the head, there must be the like used for
the liver, spleen, stomach, hypochondries, etc.   "In crudity"
(saith Piso) "'tis good to bind the stomach hard," [6] to hinder
wind and to help concoction.

Of inward medicines I need not speak; use the same cordials
as before.   In this kind of melancholy, some prescribe treacle
in winter, especially before or after purges, or in the spring, as
Avicenna; [7] Trincavellius,[8] mithridate; Montaltus,[9] peony seeds,
unicorn's horn, *os de corde cervi* [a bone from a deer's heart], etc.

Amongst topics or outward medicines, none are more precious
than baths, but of them I have spoken.   Fomentations to the
hypochondries are very good, of wine and water in which are
sod southernwood, melilot, epithyme, mugwort, senna, polypody,
as also cerotes,[10] plasters,[11] liniments, ointments for the spleen,

liver, and hypochondries, of which look for examples in Laurentius, Jobertus, *lib.* 3, *cap.* 1, *Pra. med.*, Montanus, *consil.* 231,
Montaltus, *cap.* 33, Hercules de Saxonia, Faventinus.   And so of
epithemes, digestive powders, bags, oils.   Octavius Horatianus,
lib. 2, *cap.* 5, prescribes chalastic cataplasms, or dry purging
medicines; Piso dropaces of pitch and oil of rue, applied at
certain times to the stomach, to the metaphrene, or part of the
back which is over against the heart; [1] Aetius sinapisms; Montaltus, *cap.* 35, would have the thighs to be cauterized,[2] Mercurialis prescribes beneath the knees; Lælius Eugubinus, *consil.* 77, for an hypochondriacal Dutchman, will have the cautery
made in the right thigh, and so Montanus, *consil.* 55.   The same
Montanus, *consil.* 34, approves of issues in the arms or hinder
part of the head.   Bernardus Paternus, in Hildesheim, *Spicil.* 2,
would have issues made in both the thighs; [3] Lod. Mercatus [4]
prescribes them near the spleen, *aut prope ventriculi regimen*
[or near the region of the belly], or in either of the thighs.
Ligatures, frictions, and cupping-glasses above or about the
belly, without scarification, which Felix Platerus so much
approves,[5] may be used as before.

SUBSECT. II.—*Correctors to expel Wind.   Against Costiveness, etc.*

In this kind of melancholy one of the most offensive symptoms
is wind, which, as in the other species, so in this, hath great need
to be corrected and expelled.

The medicines to expel it are either inwardly taken, or outwardly.   Inwardly to expel wind, are simples or compounds:
simples are herbs, roots, etc., as galanga, gentian, angelica,
enula, calamus aromaticus, valerian, zedoary, iris, condite
ginger, aristolochy, cicliminus, china, dittander, pennyroyal,
rue, calamint, bay-berries and bay-leaves, betony, rosemary,
hyssop, sabine, centaury, mint, camomile, stœchas, ugnus
castus, broom-flowers, origan, orange-peels, etc.; spices, as
saffron, cinnamon, bezoar stone, myrrh, mace, nutmegs, pepper,
cloves, ginger, seeds of anise, fennel, ammi, cari, nettle, rue, etc.,
juniper berries, grana Paradisi; compounds, dianisum, diagalanga, diacyminum, diacalaminth, *electuarium de baccis lauri,
benedicta laxativa, pulvis ad flatus, antid. Florent., pulvis carminativus, aromaticum rosatum*, treacle, mithridate, etc.   This
one caution of Gualter Bruel is to be observed in the administering of these hot medicines and dry, "that whilst they covet to

expel wind, they do not inflame the blood and increase the disease. Sometimes" (as he saith) "medicines must more decline to heat, sometimes more to cold, as the circumstances require, and as the parties are inclined to heat or cold." [1]

Outwardly taken to expel winds, are oils, as of camomile, rue, bays, etc.; fomentations of the hypochondries, with the decoctions of dill, pennyroyal, rue, bay-leaves, cummin, etc., bags of camomile-flowers, aniseed, cummin, bays, rue, worm-wood, ointments of the oil of spikenard, wormwood, rue, etc. Aretæus [2] prescribes cataplasms of camomile flowers, fennel, aniseeds, cummin, rosemary, wormwood leaves, etc.

Cupping-glasses applied to the hypochondries, without scari-fication, do wonderfully resolve wind.[3] Fernelius, *consil.* 43, much approves of them at the lower end of the belly; Lod. Mercatus calls them a powerful remedy, and testifies moreover out of his own knowledge how many he hath seen suddenly eased by them.[4] Julius Cæsar Claudinus, *Respons. med. resp.* 33, admires these cupping-glasses, which he calls, out of Galen, "a kind of enchantment, they cause such present help." [5]

Empirics have a myriad of medicines, as to swallow a bullet of lead, etc., which I voluntarily omit. Amatus Lusitanus, *cent.* 4, *curat.* 54, for an hypochondriacal person that was extremely tormented with wind, prescribes a strange remedy. Put a pair of bellows' end into a clyster pipe, and applying it into the fundament, open the bowels, so draw forth the wind, *natura non admittit vacuum* [nature does not allow a vacuum]. He vaunts he was the first invented this remedy, and by means of it speedily eased a melancholy man. Of the cure of this flatuous melancholy, read more in Fienus, *de flatibus, cap.* 26, *et passim alias* [and elsewhere *passim*].

Against headache, vertigo, vapours which ascend forth of the stomach to molest the head, read Hercules de Saxonia and others.

If costiveness offend in this, or any other of the three species, it is to be corrected with suppositories, clysters, or lenitives, powder of senna, condite prunes, etc.

$\qquad$ ℞ *elect. lenit. e succo rosar. ana ℥j ; misce.*

Take as much as a nutmeg at a time, half an hour before dinner or supper, or *pil. mastichin.* ℥j, in six pills, a pill or two at a time. See more in Montanus, *consil.* 229, Hildesheim, *Spicil.* 2. P. Cnemander and Montanus commend "Cyprian turpentine, which they would have familiarly taken, to the quantity of a

small nut, two or three hours before dinner and supper, twice
or thrice a week if need be; for, besides that it keeps the belly
soluble, it clears the stomach, opens obstructions, cleanseth the
liver, provokes urine." [1]

These in brief are the ordinary medicines which belong to
the cure of melancholy, which, if they be used aright, no doubt
may do much good. *Si non levando, saltem leniendo valent
peculiaria bene selecta*, saith Bessardus; a good choice of particular receipts must needs ease, if not quite cure, not one,
but all or most, as occasion serves. *Et quæ non prosunt singula,
multa juvant* [and where they do not help singly, they may
together].

NOTES

PAGE 5

[1] Consil. 235, pro Abbate Italo.
[2] Consil. 23. Aut curabitur, aut certe minus afficietur, si volet.

PAGE 6

[1] Vide Renatum Morey, Animad. in Scholam Salernit. cap. 38. Si ad 40 annos possent producere vitam, cur non ad centum? si ad centum, cur non ad mille?
[2] Hist. Chinensium.
[3] Alii dubitant an dæmon possit morbos curare quos non fecit, alii negant, sed quotidiana experientia confirmat, magos magno multorum stupore morbos curare, singulas corporis parte citra impedimentum permeare, et mediis nobis ignotis curare.
[4] Agentia cum patientibus conjugunt.
[5] Cap. 11 de Servat.

PAGE 7

[1] Hæc alii rident, sed vereor ne, dum nolumus esse creduli, vitium non effugiamus incredulitatis.
[2] Refert Solomonem mentis morbos curasse, et dæmones abegisse ipsos carminibus, quod et coram Vespasiano fecit Eleazar.
[3] Spirituales morbi spiritualiter curari debent.
[4] Sigillum ex auro peculiari ad melancholiam, etc.
[5] Lib. 1 de occult. Philos. Nihil refert an Deus an diabolus, angeli an immundi spiritus ægro opem ferant, modo morbus curetur.
[6] Magus minister et vicarius Dei.   [7] [Ps. lxxxii, 6.]
[8] Utere forti imaginatione et experieris effectum, dicant in adversum quicquid volunt theologi.

PAGE 8

[1] Idem Plinius contendit quosdam esse morbos qui incantationibus solum curentur.
[2] Qui talibus credunt, aut ad eorum domos euntes, aut suis domibus introducunt, aut interrogant, sciant se fidem Christianam et baptismum prævaricasse, et apostatas esse.—Austin de superstit. observ. Hoc pacto a Deo deficitur ad diabolum.—P. Mart.
[3] Mori præstat quam superstitiose sanari. Disquis. mag. lib. 2, cap. 2, sect. 1, quæst. 1, tom. 3.
[4] P. Lombard.   [5] Suffitus, gladiorum ictus, etc.
[6] The Lord hath created medicines of the earth, and he that is wise will not abhor them. Ecclus. xxxviii, 4.

PAGE 9

[1] My son, fail not in thy sickness, but pray unto the Lord, and he will make thee whole. Ecclus. xxxviii, 9.
[2] Huc omne principium, huc refer exitum.—Hor. carm. 3, od. 6.
[3] Music and fine fare can do no good.
[4] Hor. lib. 1, ep. 2.
[5] Sint Crœsi et Crassi licet, non hos Pactolus aureas undas agens eripiet unquam e miseriis.

⁶ Scientia de Deo debet in medico infixa esse.—Mesue Arabs. Sanat omnes languores Deus. For you shall pray to your Lord, that he would prosper that which is given for ease, and then use physic for the prolonging of life.—Ecclus. xxxviii, 4.

PAGE 10

¹ Omnes optant quandam in medicina felicitatem, sed hanc non est quod expectent, nisi Deum vera fide invocent, atque ægros similiter ad ardentem vocationem excitent.

² Lemnius e Gregor. exhor. ad vitam opt. instit. cap. 48. Quicquid meditaris aggredi aut perficere. Deum in consilium adhibeto.

³ Commentar. lib. 5. Ob infelicem pugnam contristatus, in ægritudinem incidit, ita ut a medicis curari non posset.

⁴ In his animi malis princeps imprimis ad Deum precetur, et peccatis veniam exoret, inde ad medicinam, etc.

⁵ Greg. Tholos. tom. 2, lib. 28, cap. 7, Syntax. In vestibulo templi Solomonis liber remediorum cujusque morbi fuit, quem revulsit Ezechias, quod populus, neglecto Deo nec invocato, sanitatem inde peteret.

⁶ Livius, lib. 22. Strepunt aures clamoribus plorantium sociorum, sæpius nos quam deorum invocantium opem.

PAGE 11

¹ Rulandus adjungit optimam orationem ad finem Empiricorum. Mercurialis, consil. 25, ita concludit. Montanus passim, etc., et plures alii, etc.

² Lipsius. ³ Cap. 26.

PAGE 12

¹ Lib. 2, cap. 7, de Deo. Morbisque in genera descriptis deos reperimus.

² Selden, prolog. cap. 3, de diis Syris. Rosinus.

³ See Lilii Giraldi syntagma de diis, etc.

⁴ 12 Cal. Januarii ferias celebrant, ut angores et animi solicitudines propitiata depellat.

⁵ Hanc divæ pennam consecravi.—Lipsius.

PAGE 13

¹ Jodocus Sincerus, Itin. Galliæ, 1617. Huc mente captos deducunt, et statis orationibus, sacrisque peractis, in illum lectum dormitum ponunt, etc.

² In Gallia Narbonensi.

³ Lib. de orig. festorum. Collo suspensa et pergameno inscripta, cum signo crucis, etc.

⁴ Em. Acosta, Com. rerum in Oriente gest. a societat. Jesu, anno 1568. Epist. Gonsalvi Fernandis, anno 1560, e Japonia.

⁵ Spicil. de morbis dæmoniacis. Sic a sacrificulis parati unguentis magicis corpori illitis, ut stultæ plebeculæ persuadeant tales curari a Sancto Antonio.

⁶ Printed at London, 4to by J. Roberts, 1605.

⁷ Greg. lib. 8. Cujus fanum ægrotantium multitudine refertum undiquaque, et tabellis pendentibus, in quibus sanati languores erant inscripti.

PAGE 14

¹ Hor. lib. 1, od. 5.

² Mali angeli sumpserunt olim nomen Jovis, Junonis, Apollinis, etc., quos Gentiles deos credebant, nunc S. Sebastiani, Barbaræ, etc., nomen habent, et aliorum.

³ Part. 2, cap. 9, de spect. Veneri substituunt Virginem Mariam.

⁴ Ad hæc ludibria Deus connivet frequentur; ubi relicto verbo Dei, ad Satanam curritur, quales hi sunt, qui aquam lustralem, crucem, etc., lubricæ fidei hominibus offerunt.

⁵ Carior est ipsi homo quam sibi. ⁶ Bernard. ⁷ Austin.

[1] Ecclus. xxxviii.   In the sight of great men he shall be in admiration.
[2] Tom. 4, tract. 3, de morbis amentium.   Horum multi non nisi a **magis**
curandi et astrologis, quoniam origo ejus a cœlis petenda est.
[3] Lib. de Podagra.   [4] Sect. 5.
[5] Langius, J. Cæsar Claudinus, consult.

PAGE 16

[1] Prædestinatum ad hunc curandum.
[2] Helleborus curat, sed quod ab omni datus medico vanum est.
[3] Antid. gen. lib. 3, cap. 2.
[4] Quod sæpe evenit, lib. 3, cap. 1, cum non sit necessitas.   Frustra
fatigant remediis ægros, qui victus ratione curari possunt.—Heurnius.
[5] Modestus et sapiens medicus nunquam properabit ad pharmacum,
nisi cogente necessitate.   41 Aphor. Prudens et pius medicus cibis prius
medicinalibus quam medicinis puris morbum expellere satagat.
[6] Brev. 1, cap. 18.
[7] Similitudo sæpe bonis medicis imponit.
[8] Qui melancholicis præbent remedia non satis valida.   Longiores morbi
imprimis solertiam medici postulant et fidelitatem, qui enim tumultuario
hos tractant, vires absque ullo commodo lædunt et frangunt, etc.

PAGE 17

[1] Naturæ remissionem dare oportet.
[2] Plerique hoc morbo medicina nihil profecisse visi sunt, et sibi demissi
invaluerunt.
[3] Abderitani, ep. Hippoc.
[4] Quicquid auri apud nos est, libenter persolvemus, etiamsi tota urbs
nostra aurum esset.

PAGE 18

[1] Seneca.   [2] Pers. Sat. 3.
[3] De anima.   Barbara tamen immanitate et deploranda inscitia contemnunt præcepta sanitatis, mortem et morbos ultro accersunt.
[4] Consul. 173, e Scoltzio, Melanch.   Ægrorum hoc fere proprium est,
ut graviora dicant esse symptomata, quam revera sunt.
[5] Melancholici plerumque medicis sunt molesti, ut alia aliis adjungant.

PAGE 19

[1] Oportet infirmo imprimere salutem, utcunque promittere, etsi ipse
desperet.   Nullum medicamentum efficax, nisi medicus etiam fuerit fortis
imaginationis.
[2] De promisc. doct. cap. 15.   Quoniam sanitatis formam animi medici
continent.
[3] Spes et confidentia plus valent quam medicina.
[4] Felicior in medicina ob fidem ethnicorum.
[5] Aphoris. 89.   Æger, qui plurimos consulit medicos, plerumque in
errorem singulorum cadit.
[6] Nihil ita sanitatem impedit, ac remediorum crebra mutatio, nec venit
vulnus ad cicatricem in quo diversa medicamenta tentantur.
[7] Melancholicorum proprium, quum ex eorum arbitrio non fit subita
mutatio in melius, alterare medicos, qui quidvis, etc.
[8] Consil. 31.   Dum ad varia se conferunt, nullo prosunt.
[9] Imprimis hoc statuere oportet, requiri perseverantiam, et tolerantiam.
Exiguo enim tempore nihil ex, etc.
[10] Si curari vult, opus est pertinaci perseverantia, fideli obedientia, et
patientia singulari; si tædet aut desperet, nullum habebit effectum.

[11] Ægritudine amittunt patientiam, et inde morbi incurabiles.
[12] Non ad mensem aut annum, sed oportet toto vitæ curriculo curationi operam dare.

PAGE 20

[1] Camerarius, Emb. 55, cent. 2.
[2] Præfat. de nar. med.   In libellis quæ vulgo versantur apud literatos, incautiores multa legunt, a quibus decipiuntur, eximia illis, sed portentosum hauriunt venenum.
[3] Operari ex libris, absque cognitione et solerti ingenio, periculosum est. Unde monemur, quam insipidum scriptis auctoribus credere, quod hic suo didicit periculo.
[4] Consil. 23.   Hæc omnia si quo ordine decet, egerit, vel curabitur, vel certe minus afficietur.

PAGE 21

[1] Fuchsius, cap. 2, lib. 1.
[2] In pract. med. Hæc affectio nostris temporibus frequentissima, ergo maxime pertinet ad nos hujus curationem intelligere.
[3] Si aliquis horum morborum summus sanatur, sanantur omnes inferiores.
[4] Instit. cap. 8, sect. 1.   Victus nomine non tam cibus et potus, sed aer, exercitatio, somnus, vigilia, et reliquæ res sex non-naturales continentur.
[5] Sufficit plerumque regimen rerum sex non-naturalium.

PAGE 22

[1] Et in his potissima sanitas consistit.
[2] Nihil hic agendum sine exquisita vivendi ratione, etc.
[3] Si recens malum sit, ad pristinum habitum recuperandum, alia medela non est opus.
[4] Consil. 99, lib. 2.   Si celsitudo tua, rectam victus rationem, etc.
[5] Moneo, Domine, ut sis prudens ad victum, sine quo cætera remedia frustra adhibentur.
[6] Omnia remedia irrita et vana sine his. Novistis me plerosque ita laborantes victu potius quam medicamentis curasse.
[7] Lib. 1 de finibus. Tarentinis et Siculis.
[8] Modo non multum elongentur.
[9] Lib. 1 de melan. cap. 7.   Calidus et humidus cibus concoctu facilis, flatus exortes, elixi non assi, neque sibi frixi sint.
[10] Si interna tantum pulpa devoretur, non superficies torrida ab igne.
[11] Bene nutrientes cibi, tenella ætas multum valet, carnes non virosæ, nec pingues.
[12] Hodœpor. peregr. Hierosol.

PAGE 23

[1] Inimica stomacho.   [2] Not fried or buttered, but potched.
[3] Consil. 16.   Non improbatur butyrum et oleum, si tamen plus quam par sit, non profundatur: sacchari et mellis usus, utiliter ad ciborum condimenta comprobatur.
[4] Mercurialis consil. 88.   Acerba omnia evitentur.
[5] Ovid. Met. lib. 15.

PAGE 24

[1] Peregr. Hier.
[2] The Dukes of Venice were then permitted to marry.   [3] De Legibus.
[4] Lib. 4, cap. 10.   Magna urbis utilitas cum perennes fontes muris includuntur, quod si natura non præstat, effodiendi, etc.
[5] Opera gigantum dicit aliquis.   [6] De aquæduct.
[7] Curtius Fons a quadragesimo lapide in urbem opere arcuato perductus.
—Plin. 36, 15.
[8] Quæque domus Romæ fistulas habebat et canales, etc.

II—S 887

Page 25

[1] Lib. 2, cap. 20. Jod. à Meggen, cap. 15, pereg. Hier. Bellonius.
[2] Cypr. Echovius, Delic. Hisp. Aqua profluens inde in omnes fere domos ducitur, in puteis quoque æstivo tempore frigidissima conservatur.
[3] Sir Hugh Middleton, Baronet.
[4] De quæsitis med. cent. fol. 354.
[5] De piscibus lib. Habent omnes in lautitiis, modo non sint e cœnoso loco.
[6] De pisc. cap. 2, lib. 7. Plurimum præstat ad utilitatem et jucunditatem. Idem Trallianus lib. 1, cap. 16. Pisces petrosi, et molles carne.
[7] Etsi omnes putredini sunt obnoxii, ubi secundis mensis, incepto jam priore, devorentur, commodi succi prosunt, qui dulcedine sunt præditi, ut dulcia cerasa, poma, etc.
[8] Lib. 2, cap. 1. [9] Montanus, consil. 24.
[10] Pyra quæ grato sunt sapore, cocta mala, poma tosta, et saccharo vel anisi semine conspersa, utiliter statim a prandio vel a cœna sumi possunt, eo quod ventriculum roborent et vapores caput petentes reprimant.—Mont.

Page 26

[1] Punica mala aurantia commode permittuntur modo non sint austera et acida.
[2] Olera omnia præter boraginem, buglossum, intybum, feniculum, anisum, melissum vitari debent.
[3] Mercurialis, Pract. Med.
[4] Lib. 2 de com. Solus homo edit bibitque, etc.
[5] Consil. 21, 18. Si plus ingeratur quam par est, et ventriculus tolerare posset, nocet, et cruditates generat, etc.
[6] Observat. lib. 1. Assuescat bis in die cibos, sumere, certa semper hora.
[7] Ne plus ingerat cavendum quam ventriculus ferre potest, semperque surgat a mensa non satur.

Page 27

[1] Siquidem qui semimansum velociter ingerunt cibum, ventriculo laborem inferunt, et flatus maximos promovent.—Crato.
[2] Quidam maxime comedere nituntur, putantes ea ratione se vires refecturos; ignorantes, non ea quæ ingerunt posse vires reficere, sed quæ probe concoquunt.
[3] Multa appetunt, pauca digerunt.
[4] Saturnal. lib. 7, cap. 4.
[5] Modicus et temperatus cibus et carni et animæ utilis est.
[6] Hygiasticon, reg. 14. 16 unciæ per diem sufficiant, computato pane, carne ovis, vel aliis obsoniis, et totidem vel paulo plures unciæ potus.
[7] Idem, reg. 27. Plures in domibus suis brevi tempore pascentes extinguuntur, qui si triremibus vincti fuissent, aut gregario pane pasti, sani et incolumes in longam ætatem vitam prorogassent.
[8] Nihil deterius quam diversa nutrientia simul adjungere, et comedendi tempus prorogare.
[9] Lib. 1. hist. [10] Hor. Od. lib. 1, ode ult.
[11] Ciborum varietate et copia in eadem mensa nihil nocentius homini ad salutem.—Fr. Valleriola, Observ. lib. 2, cap. 6.
[12] Tull. orat. pro M. Marcello.

Page 28

[1] Nullus cibum sumere debet, nisi stomachus sit vacuus. Gordon., lib. med. lib. 1, cap. 11.
[2] E multis eduliis unum elige, relictisque cæteris ex eo comede.
[3] Lib. de atra bile. Simplex sit cibus et non varius: quod licet dignitati tuæ ob convivas difficile videatur, etc.
[4] Celsitudo tua prandeat sola, absque apparatu aulico; contentus sit

illustrissimus princeps duobus tantum ferculis, vinoque Rhenano solum in mensa utatur.
[5] Semper intra satietatem a mensa recedat, uno ferculo contentus.
[6] Lib. de Hel. et Jejunio. Multo melius in terram vina fudisses.
[7] Crato. Multum refert non ignorare qui cibi priores, etc.; liquida præcedant carnium jura, pisces, fructus, etc.
[8] Cœna brevior sit prandio.

PAGE 29

[1] Tract. 6, contradict. 1, lib. 1.
[2] Super omnia quotidianum leporem habuit, et pomis indulsit.
[3] Annal. 6. Ridere solebat eos, qui post tricesimum ætatis annum, ad cognoscenda corpori suo noxia vel utilia, alicujus consilii indigerent.
[4] A Lessio edit. 1614.
[5] Ægyptii olim omnes morbos curabant vomitu et jejunio.—Bohemus, lib. 1, cap. 5.
[6] Cat. Major: Melior conditio senis viventis ex præscripto artis medicæ, quam adolescentis luxuriosi.

PAGE 30

[1] Debet per amœna exerceri, et loca viridia, excretis prius arte vel natura alvi excrementis.
[2] Hildesheim, Spicil. 2, de mel. Primum omnium operam dabis ut singulis diebus habeas beneficium ventris, semper cavendo ne alvus sit diutius astricta.
[3] Si non sponte, clysteribus purgetur.
[4] Balneorum usus dulcium, siquid aliud, ipsis opitulatur. Credo hæc dici cum aliqua jactantia, inquit Montanus, consil. 26.

PAGE 31

[1] In quibus jejunus diu sedeat eo tempore, ne sudorem excitent aut manifestum teporem, sed quadam refrigeratione humectent.
[2] Aqua non sit calida, sed tepida, ne sudor sequatur.
[3] Lotiones capitis ex lixivio, in quo herbas capitales coxerint.
[4] Cap. 8 de mel.   [5] Aut axungia pulli.—Piso.
[6] Thermæ Nympheæ.
[7] Sandys, lib. 1, saith that women go twice a week to the baths at least.
[8] Epist. 3.
[9] Nec alvum excernunt, quin aquam secum portent qua partes obscænas lavent.—Busbequius, ep. 3, Leg. Turciæ.

PAGE 32

[1] Hildesheim, Spicil. 2 de mel. hypochon. Si non adesset jecoris caliditas, thermas laudarem, et si non nimia humoris exsiccatio esset metuenda.
[2] Fol. 141.
[3] Thermas Luccenses adeat, ibique aquas ejus per 15 dies potet, et calidarum aquarum stillicidiis tum caput tum ventriculum de more subjiciat.
[4] In Panth.   [5] Aquæ Porrectanæ.   [6] Aquæ Aquariæ.
[7] Ad aquas Aponenses velut ad sacram anchoram confugiat.
[8] Joh. Bauhinus, lib. 3, cap. 14 Hist. admir. fontis Bollensis in ducat. Wittenberg., laudat aquas Bollenses ad melancholicos morbos, mærorem, fascinationem, aliaque animi pathemata.
[9] Balnea Chalderina.   [10] Hepar externe ungatur ne calefiat.
[11] Nocent calidis et siccis, cholericis, et omnibus morbis ex cholera, hepatis, splenisque affectionibus.

Page 33

[1] Lib. de aqua. Qui breve hoc vitæ curriculum cupiunt sani transigere, frigidis aquis sæpe lavare debent, nulli ætati cum sit incongrua, calidis imprimis utilis.

[2] Solvit Venus rationis vim impeditam, ingentes iras remittit, etc.

[3] Multi comitiales, melancholici, insani, hujus usu solo sanati.

[4] Si omittatur coitus, contristat, et plurimum gravat corpus et animum.

[5] Nisi certo constet nimium semen aut sanguinem causam esse, aut amor præcesserit, aut, etc.

[6] Athletis, arthriticis, podagricis nocet, nec opportuna prodest, nisi fortibus et qui multo sanguine abundant. Idem Scaliger, exerc. 269. Turcis ideo luctatoribus prohibitum.

[7] De sanit. tuend. lib. 1.

[8] Lib. 1, cap. 7. Exhaurit enim spiritus animumque debilitat.

Page 34

[1] Frigidis et siccis corporibus inimicissima.

[2] Vesci intra satietatem, impigrum esse ad laborem, vitale semen, conservare.

[3] Nequitia est quæ te non sinit esse senem.

[4] Vide Montanum, Pet. Godefridum, Amorum lib. 2, cap. 6. Curiosum de his, nam et numerum definite Talimudistis, unicuique sciatis assignari suum tempus, etc.

[5] Thespiadas genuit.   [6] Vide Lampridium, vit. ejus.

[7] Et lassata viris, etc.

[8] Vid. Mizald. cent. 8, 11, Lemnium, lib. 2, cap. 16, Catullum ad Ipsithillam, etc., Ovid. Eleg. lib. 3 et 6, etc. Quot itinera una nocte confecissent, tot coronas ludicro deo puta Triphallo, Marsiæ, Hermæ, Priapo donarent. Cingemus tibi mentulam coronis, etc.

[9] Pornoboscodid. Gasp. Barthii.

Page 35

[1] Nich. de Lynna, cited by Mercator in his Map.

[2] Mons Sloto. Some call it the highest hill in the world, next Teneriffe in the Canaries. Lat. 81.

[3] Cap. 26, in his Treatise of Magnetic Bodies.

[4] Lege lib. 1, cap. 23 et 24, de magnetica philosophia, et lib. 3, cap. 4.

[5] 1612.   [6] Mr. Briggs his map, and North-west Fox.

[7] Lib. 2, cap. 64, de nob. civitat. Quinsay, et cap. 10, de Cambalu.

Page 36

[1] Lib. 4 Exped. ad Sinas, cap. 3, et lib. 5, cap. 18.

[2] M. Polus in Asia Presb. Joh. meminit, lib. 2, cap. 30.

[3] Alluaresius et alii.   [4] Lat. 10 gr. Aust.

[5] Ferdinando de Quir., anno 1612.

[6] Alarum pennæ continent in longitudine 12 passus, elephantem in sublime tollere potest.—Polus, lib. 3, cap. 40.

[7] Lib. 2 Descript. Terræ Sanctæ.   [8] Natur. quæst. lib. 4, cap. 2.

[9] Lib. de reg. Congo.   [10] Exercit. 47.

[11] See Mr. Carpenter's Geography, lib. 2, cap. 6, et Bern. Telesius, lib de mari.

Page 37

[1] Exercit. 52, de maris motu causæ investigandæ: prima reciprocationis, secunda varietatis, tertia celeritatis, quarta cessationis, quinta privationis, sexta contrarietatis. [Moabar = Coromandel.]

[2] Patricius saith fifty-two miles in height.

[3] Lib. de explicatione locorum mathem. Aristot.

[4] Laet. lib. 17, cap. 18, descrip. occid. Ind.

[5] Luge [? Teyde] alii vocant.

[6] Geor. Wernerus. Aquæ tanta celeritate erumpunt et absorbentur, ut expedito equiti aditum intercludant.

[7] Boissardus de Magis, cap. de Pilapiis.

Page 38

[1] In campis Lovicen. solum visuntur in nive; et ubinam vere, æstate, autumno se occultant?—Hermes, Polit. lib. 1. Jul. Bellius.

[2] Statim ineunte vere silvæ strepunt eorum cantilenis.—Muscovit. comment.

[3] Immergunt se fluminibus lacubusque per hiemem totam, etc.

[4] Cæterasque volucres Pontum hieme adveniente e nostris regionibus Europæis transvolantes.

[5] Survey of Cornwall.

[6] Porro ciconiæ quonam e loco veniant, quo se conferant, incompertum adhuc; agmen venientium, descendentium, ut gruum venisse cernimus, nocturnis opinor temporibus. In patentibus Asiæ campis certo die congregant se, eam quæ novissime advenit lacerant, inde avolant.— Cosmog. lib. 4, cap. 126.

Page 39

[1] Comment. Muscov. [Agnus Scythicus, the rhizome of a fern, which is covered with silky hairs and bears a fanciful resemblance to a lamb.]

[2] Hist. Scot. lib. 1. [The barnacle goose was supposed to grow out of barnacles attached to pieces of timber, or on trees overhanging the water.]

[3] Vertomannus, lib. 5, cap. 16, mentioneth a tree that bears fruits to eat, wood to burn, bark to make ropes, wine and water to drink, oil and sugar, and leaves as tiles to cover houses, flowers, for clothes, etc.

[4] Animal insectum Cusino, ut quis legere vel scribere possit sine alterius ope lumulus.

[5] Cosmog. lib. 1, cap. 435, et lib. 3, cap. 1. Habent ollas a natura formatas e terra extractas, similes illis a figulis factis, coronas, pisces, aves, et omnes animantium species.

[6] Ut solent hirundines et ranæ præ frigoris magnitudine mori, et postea redeunte vere 24 Aprilis reviviscere.

[7] Vid. Pererium in Gen. Cor. a Lapide, et alios.

Page 40

[1] In Necyomantia, tom. 2.

[2] [The Cave of Trophonius, an underground oracle at Lehadea in Bœotia].

[3] Fracastorius, lib. de simp.; Georgius Merula, lib. de mem.; Julius Billius, etc.

[4] Simlerus, Ortelius. Brachiis centum sub terra reperta est, in qua quadraginta octo cadavera inerant, anchoræ, etc.

[5] Pisces et conchæ in montibus reperiuntur.

[6] Lib. de locis mathemat. Aristot.

[7] Or plane as Patricius holds, which Austin, Lactantius, and some others held of old as round as a trencher.

[8] Lib. de Zilphis et Pygmæis. They penetrate the earth as we do the air.

Page 41

[1] Lib. 2, cap. 112.

[2] Commentar. ad annum 1537. Quicquid dicunt philosophi, quædam sunt Tartari ostia, et loca puniendis animis destinata, ut Hecla mons, etc., ubi mortuorum spiritus visuntur, etc. Voluit Deus extare talia loca, ut discant mortales.

³ Ubi miserabiles ejulantium voces audiuntur, qui auditoribus horrorem incutiunt haud vulgarem, etc.

⁴ Ex sepulchris apparent mense Martio, et rursus sub terram se abscondunt, etc.

PAGE 42

¹ Descript. Græc. lib. 6, de Pelop.

² Conclave Ignatii [an allusion to Donne's book, Ignatius his Conclave].

³ Melius dubitare de occultis, quam litigare de incertis, ubi flamma inferni, etc.

⁴ See Dr. Rainolds, prælect. 55 in Apoc.

PAGE 43

¹ As they come from the sea, so they return to the sea again by secret passages, as in all likelihood the Caspian Sea vents itself into the Euxine or ocean.

² Seneca, Quæst. lib. capp. 3, 4, 5, 6, 7, 8, 9, 10, 11, 12, de causis aquarum perpetuis.

³ In iis nec pullos hirundines excludunt, neque, etc.

⁴ Th. Ravennas, lib. de vit. hom. prærog. cap. ult.

⁵ At Quito in Peru plus auri quam terræ foditur in aurifodinis.

PAGE 44

¹ Ad Caput Bonæ Spei incolæ sunt nigerrimi. Si sol causa, cur non Hispani et Itali æque nigri, in eadem latitudine, æque distantes ab Æquatore, hi ad Austrum, illi ad Boream? qui sub Presbytero Johan. habitant subfusci sunt, in Zeilan et Malabar nigri, æque distantes ab Æquatore, eodemque cœli parallelo: sed hoc magis mirari quis possit, in tota America nusquam nigros inveniri, præter paucos in loco Quareno illis dicto: quæ hujus coloris causa efficiens, cœlive an terræ qualitas, an soli proprietas, aut ipsorum hominum innata ratio, aut omnia?—Ortelius in Africa, Theat.

² Regio quocunque anni tempore temperatissima.—Ortel. Multas Galliæ et Italiæ regiones, molli tepore, et benigna quadam temperie, prorsus antecellit.—Jovius.

³ Lat. 45 Danubii.   ⁴ Quevira, lat. 40.

⁵ In Sir Fra. Drake's voyage. [See Hakluyt, Everyman ed., vol. vi., pp. 240–5.]

⁶ [Newfoundland].   ⁷ Lansius, Orat. contra Hungaros.

PAGE 45

¹ Lisbon, lat. 38.   ² Dantzic, lat. 54.

³ De nat. novi orbis, lib. 1, cap. 9.   Suavissimus omnium locus, etc.

⁴ The same variety of weather Lod. Guicciardine observes betwixt Liège and Aix not far distant (Descript. Belg.).

⁵ Magin. Quadus.   ⁶ Hist. lib. 5.

PAGE 46

¹ Lib. 11, cap. 7.

² Lib. 2, cap. 9. Cur Potosi et Plata, urbes in tam tenui intervallo, utraque montosa, etc.

PAGE 47

¹ Terra malos homines nunc educat atque pusillos.

² Nav. lib. 1, cap. 5.   ³ Strabo.

⁴ As under the Equator in many parts, showers here at such a time, winds at such a time, the brise they call it.

PAGE 48

[1] Ferd. Cortesius [Hernando Cortes], lib. Novus orbis inscript.
[2] Lapidatum est.—Livy.
[3] Cosmog. lib. 4, cap. 22. Hæ tempestatibus decidunt e nubibus æculentis, depascunturque more locustorum omnia virentia.
[4] Hort. Genial. An a terra sursum rapiuntur a solo iterumque cum pluviis præcipitantur? etc.
[5] Tam ominosus proventus in naturales causas referri vix potest.
[6] Cosmog. cap. 6.
[7] Cardan saith vapours rise 288 miles from the earth, Eratosthenes 48 miles.
[8] De subtil. lib. 2.   [9] In Progymnas.
[10] Præfat. ad Euclid. Catop.

PAGE 49

[1] Manucodiatæ, birds that live continually in the air, and are never seen on ground but dead: see Ulysses Aldrovand. Ornithol., Scal. Exerc. cap. 229.
[2] Laet. Descrip. Amer.
[3] Epist. lib. 1, p. 83. Ex quibus constat nec diversa aeris et æthcris diaphana esse, nec refractiones aliunde quam a crasso aere causari. Non dura aut impervia, sed liquida, subtilis, motuique planetarum facile cedens.
[4] In Progymn. lib. 2, exempl. quinque.
[5] In Theoria nova met. cœlestium, 1578.
[6] Epit. Astron. lib. 4.
[7] Multa sane hinc consequuntur absurda, et si nihil aliud, tot cometæ in æthere animadversi, qui nullius orbis ductum comitantur, id ipsum sufficienter refellunt.—Tycho, Astr. epist. pag. 107.

PAGE 50

[1] In Theoricis planetarum; three above the firmament, which all wise men reject.
[2] Theor. nova cœlest. meteor.   [3] Lib. de fabrica mundi.

PAGE 51

[1] Lib. de cometis.
[2] An sit crux et nubecula in cœlis ad Polum Antarcticum, quod ex Corsalio refert Patricius.
[3] Gilbertus Origanus.
[4] See this discussed in Sir Walter Raleigh's History, in Zanch. ad Casman.
[5] Vid. Fromundum de Meteoris, lib. 5, artic. 5, et Lansbergium.

PAGE 52

[1] Peculiari libello.
[2] Comment. in motum terræ, Middlebergi, 1630, 4.
[3] Peculiari libello.
[4] See Mr. Carpenter's Geogr. cap. 4, lib. 1, Campanella, et Origanus, præf. Ephemer., where Scripture places are answered.
[5] De Magnete.   [6] Comment. in 2 cap. Sphær. Jo. de Sacr. Boşc.
[7] Dist. 3 gr. 1 a Polo.

PAGE 53

[1] Præf. Ephem.
[2] Which may be full of planets, perhaps, to us unseen, as those about Jupiter, etc.
[3] Luna circumterrestris planeta quum sit, consentaneum est esse in Luna viventes creaturas, et singulis planetarum globis sui serviunt circulatores, ex qua consideratione de eorum incolis summa probabilitate concludimus, quod et Tychoni Braheo, e sola consideratione vastitatis eorum, visum fuit.—Kepl. Dissert. cum nun. sid. f. 29.

PAGE 54

[1] Temperare non possum quin ex inventis tuis hoc moneam, veri non absimile, non tam in Luna, sed etiam in Jove, et reliquis planetis incolas esse.—Kepl. fo. 26. Si non sint accolæ in Jovis globo, qui notent admirandam hanc varietatem oculis, cui bono quatuor illi planetæ Jovem circum cursitant?

[2] Some of those above Jupiter I have seen myself by the help of a glass eight feet long.

[3] Rerum Angl. lib. 1, cap. 27, de viridibus pueris. [Nubrigensis is William of Newburgh, the twelfth-century historian.]

[4] Infiniti alii mundi, vel, ut Brunus, terræ huic nostræ similes.

[5] Libro cont. philos. cap. 29.

PAGE 55

[1] Kepler, fol. 2 Dissert. Quid impedit quin credamus ex his initiis, plures alios mundos detegendos, vel (ut Democrito placuit) infinitos?

[2] Lege Somnium Kepleri, edit. 1635.

[3] Quid igitur inquies, si sint in cœlo plures globi, similes nostræ telluris, an cum illis certabimus, quis meliorem mundi plagam teneat? Si nobiliores illorum globi, nos non sumus creaturarum rationalium nobilissimi: quomodo igitur omnia propter hominem? quomodo nos domini operum Dei?—Kepler, fol. 29.

[4] Francofort. quarto, 1620; ibid. quarto, 1622.

[5] Præfat. in Comment. in Genesin. Modo suadent theologos, summa ignoratione versari, veras scientias admittere nolle, et tyrannidem exercere, ut eos falsis dogmatibus, superstitionibus, et religione Catholica detineant.

PAGE 56

[1] Theat. Biblico.

[2] His argumentis plane satisfecisti, do maculas in luna esse maria, do lucidas partes esse terram.—Kepler, fol. 16.   [3] Anno 1616.

PAGE 57

[1] In Hypothes. de mundo, edit. 1597.   [2] Lugduni, 1633.

[3] Jo. Fabricius de maculis in sole. Witenb. 1611.

[4] In Burboniis sideribus.

[5] Lib. de Burboniis sid. Stellæ sunt erraticæ, quæ propriis orbibus feruntur, non longe a sole dissitis, sed juxta solem.

[6] Braccini fol. 1630, lib. 4, cap. 52, 55, 59, etc.

PAGE 58

[1] Lugdun. Bat. an. 1612.

[2] Ne se subducant, et relicta statione decessum parent, ut curiositatis finem faciant.

[3] Hercules, tuam fidem! Satira Menip. edit. 1608.

[4] Sardi venales. Satira Menip. an. 1612.

[5] Puteani Comus sic incipit, or as Lipsius' Satire in a dream.

PAGE 59

[1] Trithemius, lib .de 7 secundis.

[2] They have fetched Trajanus' soul out of hell, and canonize for saints whom they list.

[3] In Minucius. Sine delectu tempestates tangunt loca sacra et profana, bonorum et malorum fata juxta, nullo ordine res fiunt; soluta legibus fortuna dominatur.

[4] Vel malus vel impotens, qui peccatum permittit, etc.; unde hæc superstitio?

[5] Quid fecit Deus ante mundum creatum? ubi vixit otiosus a suo subjecto, etc.

[6] Lib. 3 Recog. Pet. cap. 3.   Peter answers by the simile of an egg-shell, which is cunningly made, yet of necessity to be broken; so is the world, etc., that the excellent state of heaven might be made manifest.

PAGE 60

[1] Ut me pluma levat, sic grave mergit onus.
[2] Exercit. 184.   [3] Laet. descrip. occid. Indiæ.
[4] Daniel, principio Historiæ.

PAGE 61

[1] Veniant ad me audituri quo esculento, quo item poculento uti debeant, et præter alimentum ipsum potumque, ventos ipsos docebo, item aeris ambientis temperiem, insuper regiones quas eligere, quas vitare ex usu sit.
[2] Leo Afer, Maginus, etc.   [3] Lib. 1 Scot. hist.
[4] Lib. 1 de rer. var.   [5] Horat.   [6] Maginus.

PAGE 62

[1] Haitonus de Tartaris.
[2] Cyropæd. lib. 8.   Perpetuum inde ver.
[3] The air so clear, it never breeds the plague.
[4] Leander Albertus in Campania, e Plutarcho, vita Luculli. Cum Cn. Pompeius, Marcus Cicero, multique nobiles viri L. Lucullum æstivo tempore convenissent, Pompeius inter cœnandum familiariter jocatus est, eam villam imprimis sibi sumptuosam et elegantem videri, fenestris, porticibus, etc.
[5] Godwin, vita Jo. Voysey, al. Harman.
[6] Descript. Brit.   [7] In Oxfordshire.
[8] Leander Albertus.   [9] Cap. 21 de vit. hom. prorog.

PAGE 63

[1] The possession of Robert Bradshaw, Esq.   [Orton-on-the-Hill.]
[2] Of George Purefey, Esq.
[3] The possession of William Purefey, Esq.   [Caulcutt.]
[4] The seat of Sir John Reppington, Kt.
[5] Sir Henry Goodier's, lately deceased.
[6] The dwelling-house of Hum. Adderly, Esq.
[7] Sir John Harpar's, lately deceased.
[8] Sir George Gresley's, Kt.
[9] Lib. 1, cap. 2.   [10] The seat of G. Purefey, Esq.

PAGE 64

[1] For I am now incumbent of that rectory, presented thereto by my right honourable patron the Lord Berkley.
[2] Sir Francis Willoughby.
[3] Montani et maritimi salubriores, acclives, et ad boream vergentes.
[4] The dwelling of Sir To. Burdet, Knight Baronet.
[5] [Now known as Mount Edgecombe.]
[6] In his Survey of Cornwall, book 2.
[7] Prope paludes, stagna, et loca concava, vel ad austrum, vel ad occidentem inclinatæ, domus sunt morbosæ.
[8] Oportet igitur ad sanitatem domus in altioribus ædificare, et ad speculationem.
[9] By John Bancroft, Dr. of Divinity, my quondam tutor in Christ Church, Oxon, now the Right Reverend Lord Bishop of Oxon, who built this house for himself and his successors.

[10] Hieme erit vehementer frigida, et æstate non salubris: paludes enim faciunt crassum aerem, et difficiles morbos.
[11] Vendas quot assibus possis, et si nequeas, relinquas.
[12] Lib. 1, cap. 2. In Orco habitat.
[13] Aurora musis amica.—Vitruv.

PAGE 65

[1] Ædes orientem spectantes vir nobilissimus inhabitet, et curet ut sit aer clarus, lucidus, odoriferus. Eligat habitationem optimo aere jucundam.
[2] Quoniam angustiæ itinerum et altitudo tectorum, non perinde solis calorem admittit.   [3] [Chester.]
[4] Consil. 21, lib. 2. Frigidus aer, nubilosus, densus, vitandus, æque ac venti septentrionales, etc.
[5] Consil. 24.   [6] Fenestram non aperiat.

PAGE 66

[1] Discutit sol horrorem crassi spiritus, mentem exhilarat, non enim tam corpora, quam et animi mutationem inde subeunt, pro cœli et ventorum ratione, et sani aliter affecti sini cœlo nubilo, aliter sereno. De natura ventorum, see Pliny, lib. 2, cap. 26, 27, 28, Strabo, lib. 7, etc.
[2] Fynes Moryson, part. 1, cap. 4.
[3] Altomarus, cap. 7; Bruel. Aer sit lucidus, bene olens, humidus. Montaltus idem, cap. 26. Olfactus rerum suavium.—Laurentius, cap. 8.
[4] Ant. Philos., cap de melanc.
[5] Tract. 15, cap. 9. Ex redolentibus herbis et foliis vitis viniferæ, salicis, etc.
[6] Pavimentum aceto et aqua rosacea irrorare.—Laurent. cap. 8.

PAGE 67

[1] Lib. 1, cap. de morb. Afrorum. In Nigritarum regione tanta aeris temperies, ut siquis alibi morbosus eo advehatur, optimæ statim sanitati restituatur; quod multis accidisse, ipse meis oculis vidi.
[2] Lib. de peregrinat.
[3] Epist. 2, cen. 1. Nec quisquam tam lapis aut frutex, quem non titillat amœna illa variaque spectio locorum, urbium, gentium, etc.
[4] Epist. 86.   [5] Lib. 2 de legibus.
[6] Lib. 45.   [7] Keckerman, præfat. Polit.
[8] Fynes Moryson, cap. 3, part. 1.
[9] Mutatio de loco in locum, itinera, et voiagia longa et indeterminata, et hospitare in diversis diversoriis.

PAGE 68

[1] Modo ruri esse, modo in urbe, sæpius in agro venari, etc.
[2] [Barcelona] in Catalonia in Spain.
[3] Laudaturque domus longos quæ prospicit agros.
[4] Many towns there are of that name, saith Adricomius, all high-sited.
[5] Lately resigned for some special reasons.
[6] At Lindley in Leicestershire, the possession and dwelling-place of Ralph Burton, Esquire, my late deceased father.
[7] In Icon animorum.

PAGE 69

[1] Ægrotantes oves in alium locum transportandæ sunt, ut, alium aerem et aquam participantes, coalescant et corroborentur.
[2] Alia utilia, sed ex mutatione aeris potissimum curatus.
[3] Ne te dæmon otiosum inveniat.
[4] Præstat aliud agere quam nihil.

PAGE 70

[1] Lib. 1 de dictis Socratis. Qui tesseris et risui excitando vacant, aliquid faciunt, et si liceret his meliora agere.

[2] Amasis compelled every man once a year to tell how he lived.

[3] Nostra memoria Mahometes Othomannus qui Græciæ imperium subvertit, cum oratorum postulata audiret exterarum gentium, cochlearia lignea assidue cælabat, aut aliquid in tabula affingebat.

[4] Sandys, fol. 37 of his Voyage to Jerusalem.

[5] Perkins, Cases of Conscience, lib. 3, cap. 4, q. 3.

[6] Luscinius Grunnio.

PAGE 71

[1] Non est cura melior quam injungere iis necessaria, et opportuna; operum administratio illis magnum sanitatis incrementum, et quæ repleant animos eorum, et incutiant iis diversas cogitationes.—Cont. 1, tract. 9.

[2] Ante exercitium, leves toto corpore fricationes conveniunt. Ad hunc morbum exercitationes, quum recte et suo tempore fiunt, mirifice conducunt, et sanitatem tuentur, etc.—Crato.

[3] Lib. 1 de san. tuend.

[4] Exercitium naturæ dormientis stimulatio, membrorum solatium, morborum medela, fuga vitiorum, medicina languorum, destructio omnium malorum.

[5] Alimentis in ventriculo probe concoctis.

[6] Jejuno ventre, vesica et alvo ab excrementis purgato, fricatis membris, lotis manibus et oculis, etc.—Lib de atra bile.

[7] Quousque corpus universum intumescat, et floridum appareat, sudoreque, etc.

[8] Omnino sudorem vitent.—Valescus de Tar. cap. 7, lib. 1.

[9] Exercitium si excedat, valde periculosum.—Sallust. Salvianus, de remed. lib. 2, cap. 1.

PAGE 72

[1] Camden, in Staffordshire.

[2] Fridevallius, lib. 1, cap. 2. Optima omnium exercitationum; multi ab hac solummodo morbis liberati.

[3] Josephus Quercetanus, Dialect. polit. sect. 2, cap. 11. Inter omnia exercitia præstantiæ laudem meretur.

[4] Chiron in monte Pelio, præceptor heroum, eos a morbis animi venationibus et puris cibis tuebatur.—M. Tyrius.

[5] Nobilitas omnis fere urbes fastidit, castellis, et liberiore cœlo gaudet, generisque dignitatem una maxime venatione et falconum aucupiis tuetur.

[6] Jos. Scaliger, commen. in Cir. in fol. 344; Salmuth, 23 de nov. repert. com. in Pancir.

[7] Demetrius Constantinop. de re accipitraria liber, a P. Gillio Latine redditus; Ælius; Epist. Aquilæ, Symmachi, et Theodotionis ad Ptolemæum, etc.

[8] Lonicerus, Geffreus, Jovius.

PAGE 73

[1] Sir Antony Shirley's Relations.   [2] Hakluyt.

[3] Coturnicum aucupio.   [4] Fynes Moryson, part. 3, cap. 8.

[5] Non minorem voluptatem animo capiunt, quam qui feras insectantur, aut missis canibus, comprehendunt, quum, retia trahentes, squamosas pecudes in ripas adducunt.

[6] More piscatorum cruribus ocreatus.

[7] Si principibus venatio leporis non sit inhonesta, nescio quomodo piscatio cyprinorum videri debeat pudenda.

PAGE 74

[1] Omnino turpis piscatio, nullo studio digna, illiberalis credita est, quod nullum habet ingenium, nullam perspicaciam.

[2] Præcipua hinc Anglis gloria, crebræ victoriæ partæ.—Jovius.

[3] Cap. 7.   [4] Fracastorius.

[5] Ambulationes subdiales, quas hortenses auræ ministrant, sub fornice viridi, pampinis virentibus concameratæ.

PAGE 75

[1] Theophylact.   [2] Itinerar. Ital.

[3] Sedet ægrotus cæspite viridi, et cum inclementia canicularis terras excoquit, et siccat flumina, ipse securus sedet sub arborea fronde, et, ad doloris sui solatium, naribus suis gramineas redolet species; pascit oculos herbarum amœna viriditas, aures suavi modulamine demulcet pictarum concentus avium, etc. Deus bone, quanta pauperibus procuras solatia!

[4] Diod. Siculus, lib. 2.

[5] Lib. 13 de animal. cap. 13.

[6] Pet. Gillius; Paul Hentznerus, Itinerar. Italiæ, 1617; Jod. Sincerus, Itinerar. Galliæ, 1617; Simp. lib. 1, quest. 4.

[7] Jucundissima deambulatio juxta mare, et navigatio prope terram. In utraque fluminis ripa.

[8] Aurei panes, aurea obsonia, vis margaritarum aceto subacta, etc.

PAGE 76

[1] Lucan.

[2] 300 pellices, pocillatores, et pincernæ innumeri, pueri loti purpura induti, etc. ex omnium pulchritudine delecti.

[3] Ubi omnia cantu strepunt.

[4] Odyss. 4.   [5] Lucan, lib. 10.

PAGE 77

[1] Iliad 22.   [2] Between Ardres and Guines, 1519.

[3] [Bois-le-Duc, or 'S Hertogenbosch.]

[4] Swertius, in Deliciis, fol. 487. Veteri Horatiorum exemplo, virtute et successu admirabili, cæsis hostibus 17 in conspectu patriæ, etc.

[5] Paterculus, vol. post.

[6] Quos antea audivi, inquit, hodie vidi deos.

PAGE 78

[1] Pandectæ Triumph. fol.   [2] Lib. 6, cap. 14, de bello Jud.

[3] Procopius.   [4] Laet. lib. 10 Amer. descript.

[5] Romulus Amasæus, præfat. Pausan.   [6] Virg. Georg. 1.

PAGE 79

[1] Boterus, lib. 3 Polit. cap. 1.

[2] See Athenæus, Deipnosoph.

[3] Ludi votivi, sacri, ludicri, Megalenses, Cereales, Florales, Martiales, etc. Rosinus, 5, 12.

[4] See Lipsius, Amphitheatrum; Rosinus, lib. 5; Meursius de ludis Græcorum.

[5] 1500 men at once, tigers, lions, elephants, horses, dogs, bears, etc.

PAGE 80

[1] Lib. ult. et lib. 1 ad finem. Consuetudine non minus laudabili quam veteri. Contubernia rhetorum, rhythmorum in urbibus et municipiis, certisque diebus exercebant se sagittarii, gladiatores, etc. Alia ingenii animique exercitia, quorum præcipuum studium, principem populum tragœdiis, comœdiis, fabulis scenicis, aliisque id genus ludis recreare.

² Orbis terræ descript. part 3.
³ Lampridius.   ⁴ Spartian.
⁵ Delectatus lusis catulorum, porcellorum, ut perdices inter se pugnarent;
aut ut aves parvulæ sursum et deorsum volitarent, his maxime delectatus,
ut sollicitudines publicas sublevaret.

PAGE 81

¹ Brumales læte ut possint producere noctes.   ² Miles. 4.
³ O dii! similibus sæpe conviviis date ut ipse videndo delectetur, et
postmodum narrando delectet.—Theod. Prodromus, Amaranto dial.
interpret. Gilberto Gaulmino.
⁴ Epist. lib. 8, Ruffino.   ⁵ Hor.
⁶ Lib. 4.   Gallicæ consuetudinis est ut viatores etiam invitos consistere
cogant, et quid quisque eorum audierit aut cognorit de qua re quærunt.

PAGE 82

¹ Vitæ ejus, lib. ult.   ² Juven. [Persius.]
³ They account them unlawful because sortilegious.
⁴ Instit. cap. 44.   In his ludis plerumque non ars aut peritia viget, sed
fraus, fallacia, dolus, astutia, casus, fortuna, temeritas locum habent,
non ratio, consilium, sapientia, etc.
⁵ Abusus tam frequens hodie in Europa ut plerique crebro harum usu
patrimonium profundant, exhaustisque facultatibus ad inopiam redigantur.
⁶ Ubi semel prurigo ista animum occupat ægre discuti potest, sollici-
tantibus undique ejusdem farinæ hominibus, damnosas illas voluptates
repetunt, quod et scortatoribus insitum, etc.

PAGE 83

¹ Instituitur ista exercitatio, non lucri sed valetudinis et oblectamenti
ratione, et quo animus defatigatus respiret, novasque vires ad subeundos
labores denuo concipiat.
² Latrunculorum ludus inventus est a duce, ut cum miles intolerabili
fame laboraret, altero die edens, altero ludens, famis obliviceretur.—
Bellonius. See more of this game in Daniel Souter's Palamedes, vel de
variis ludis, lib. 3.
³ Dr. [Sir John] Hayward in vita ejus.
⁴ Muscovit. commentarium.
⁵ Inter cives Fessanos latrunculorum ludus est usitatissimus.—Lib. 3,
de Africa.

PAGE 84

¹ Tullius.   ² [James the First's, in his Book of Sports (1618).]
³ De mor. gent.   ⁴ Polycrat. lib. 1, cap. 8.
⁵ Idem Sarisburiensis.   ⁶ Hist. lib. 1.

PAGE 85

¹ Nemo desidet otiosus, ita nemo asinino more ad seram noctem laborat;
nam ea plusquam servilis ærumna, quæ opificum vita est, exceptis
Utopiensibus, qui diem in 24 horas dividunt, sex duntaxat operi deputant,
reliquum somno et cibo cujusque arbitrio permittitur.
² Rurum Burgund. lib. 4.

PAGE 86

¹ Jussit hominem deferri ad palatium et lecto ducali collocari, etc.
Mirari homo ubi se eo loci videt.
² Quid interest, inquit Lodovicus Vives (epist. ad Francisc. Barducem),
inter diem illius et nostros aliquot annos? nihil penitus, nisi quod, etc.
³ Hen. Stephan. præfat. Herodoti.

[4] Orat. 12. Siquis animo fuerit afflictus aut æger, nec somnum admittens, is mihi videtur e regione stans talis imaginis, oblivisci omnium posse, quæ humanæ vitæ atrocia et difficilia accidere solent.

Page 87

[1] 3 de anima.   [2] Iliad 19.   [3] Topogr. Rom. part. 1.

Page 88

[1] Quod heroum conviviis legi solitæ.
[2] Melancthon de Heliodoro.
[3] Pluvines.   [4] Thibault.
[5] As in travelling the rest go forward and look before them, an antiquary alone looks round about him, seeing things past, etc., hath a complete horizon.—Janus Bifrons.   [6] Cardan.

Page 89

[1] Hondius, præfat. Mercatoris.   [2] Atlas Geog.
[3] [The Polish duke, Radzivilius.]

Page 90

[1] Cardan.   [2] Lib. de cupid. divitiarum.
[3] Leon. Digges, præfat. ad Perpet. prognost.
[4] Plus capio voluptatis, etc.   [5] In Hyperchen. divis. 3.
[6] Cardan, præfat. Rerum variet.   [7] Poetices lib.
[8] Lib. 3, ode 9. Donec gratus eram tibi, etc.
[9] De Peloponnes. lib. 6 descript. Græc.
[10] Quos si integros haberemus, Dii boni, quas opes, quos thesauros teneremus!

Page 91

[1] Isaac Wake, Musæ Regnantes.
[2] Si unquam mihi in fatis sit, ut captivus ducar, si mihi daretur optio, hoc cuperem carcere concludi, his catenis illigari, cum hisce captivis concatenatis ætatem agere.
[3] Epist. Primerio. Plerumque in qua simul ac pedem posui, foribus pessulum abdo; ambitionem autem, amorem, libidinem, etc., excludo, quorum parens est ignavia, imperitia nutrix, et in ipso æternitatis gremio, inter tot illustres animas sedem mihi sumo, cum ingenti quidem animo, ut subinde magnatum me misereat, qui felicitatem hanc ignorant.

Page 92

[1] Chil. 2, cent. 1, adag. 1.   [2] Virg. Eclog. 1.
[3] Founder of our public library in Oxon.
[4] Ours in Christ Church, Oxon.

Page 93

[1] Animus levatur inde a curis multa quiete et tranquillitate fruens.
[2] Ser. 38, ad Fratres Erem.
[3] Hom. 4, de pœnitentia. Nam neque arborum comæ pro pecorum tuguriis factæ, meridie per æstatem, optabilem exhibentes umbram oves ita reficiunt, ac Scripturarum lectio afflictas angore animas solatur et recreat.
[4] Otium sine literis mors est, et vivi hominis sepultura.—Seneca.
[5] Cap. 99, lib. 57, de rer. var.
[6] Fortem reddunt animum et constantem; et pium colloquium non permittit animum absurda cogitatione torqueri.

¹ Altercationibus utantur, quæ non permittunt animum submergi profundis cogitationibus, de quibus otiose cogitat et tristatur in iis.
² Bodin. prefat. ad Meth. hist.　　³ Operum subcis. cap. 15.
⁴ [Lorenzo de' Medici.]　　⁵ Hor.
⁵ Fatendum est cacumine Olympi constitutus supra ventos et procellas, et omnes res humanas.
⁷ In Ps. xxxvi. Omnis morbus animi in Scriptura habet medicinam; tantum opus est ut qui sit æger non recuset potionem quam Deus temperavit.
⁸ In Moral. Speculum quo nos intueri possimus.
⁹ Hom. 28. Ut incantatione viris fugatur, ita lectione malum.
¹⁰ Iterum atque iterum moneo, ut animam sacræ scripturæ lectione occupes. Masticat divinum pabulum meditatio.

¹ Ad 2 definit. 2 elem. In disciplinis humanis nihil præstantius reperitur: quippe miracula quædam numerorum eruit tam abstrusa et recondita, tanta nihilo minus facilitate et voluptate, ut, etc.
² Which contained 1,080,000 weights of brass.
³ Vide Clavium in com. de Sacrobosco.
⁴ Distantias cœlorum sola optica dijudicat.

¹ Cap. 4 et 5.　　　　² [Rosicrucians.]

¹ Printed at London, Anno 1620.
² Once Astronomy Reader at Gresham College.
³ Printed at London by William Jones, 1623.
⁴ Præfat. Meth. Astrol.
⁵ [Palindromes, lines that read the same forwards and backwards.]

¹ [A celebrated enigmatical epitaph.]
² Tot tibi sunt dotes virgo, quot sidera cœlo.
³ Da pie Christe, urbi bona; sit pax tempore nostro.
⁴ Chaloncrus, lib. 9 de Rep. Angl.
⁵ Hortus coronarius, medicus, et culinarius, etc.

¹ Tom. 1, de sanit. tuend. Qui rationem corporis non habent, sed cogunt mortalem immortali, terrestrem æthereæ æqualem præstare industriam. Cæterum ut camelo usu venit, quod ei bos prædixerat, cum eidem servirent domino et parte oneris levare illum camelus recusasset, paulo post et ipsius cutem, et totum onus cogeretur gestare (quod mortuo bove impletum), ita animo quoque contingit, dum defatigato corpori, etc.
² Ut pulchram illam et amabilem sanitatem præstemus.
³ Interdicendæ vigiliæ, somni paulo longiores conciliandi.—Altomarus, cap. 7. Somnus supra modum prodest, quovismodo conciliandus.—Piso.
⁴ Ovid.　　　　　⁵ In Hippoc. Aphorism.

¹ Crato, cons. 21, lib. 2. Duabus aut tribus horis post cœnam, quum jam cibus ad fundum ventriculi resederit, primum super latere dextro quiescendum, quod in tali decubitu jecur sub ventriculo quiescat, non

gravans sed cibum calefaciens, perinde ac ignis lebetem qui illi admovetur; post primum somnum quiescendum latere sinistro. etc.

[5] Sæpius accidit melancholicis, ut nimium exsiccato cerebro vigiliis attenuentur.—Ficinus, lib. 1, cap. 29.

[5] Ter.   [6] Ut sis nocte levis, sit tibi cœna brevis.
[6] Juven, Sat. 3.   [6] Hor. Ser. lib. 1, Sat. 5.
[7] Sepositis curis omnibus quantum fieri potest, una cum vestibus, etc.—Kirkst.

PAGE 101

[1] Ad horam somni aures suavibus cantibus et sonis delenire.

[2] Lectio jucunda, aut sermo, ad quem attentior animus convertitur, aut aqua ab alto in subjectam pelvim delabatur, etc.

[3] Ovid..   [4] Aceti sorbitio.
[5] Attenuat melancholiam, et ad conciliandum somnum juvat.
[6] Quod lieni acetum conveniat.
[7] Cont. 1, tract. 9.   Meditandum de aceto.
[8] Sect. 5, memb. 1, subsect. 6.   [9] Lib. de sanit. tuenda.
[10] In Som. Scip. Fit enim fere ut cogitationes nostræ et sermones pariant aliquid in somno, quale de Homero scribit Ennius, de quo videlicet sæpissime vigilans solebat cogitare et loqui.

PAGE 102

[1] Aristeæ hist.
[2] Optimum de cœlestibus et honestis meditari, et ea facere.
[3] Lib. 3, de causis corr. art.   Tam mira monstra quæstionum sæpe nascuntur inter eos, ut mirer eos interdum in somniis non terreri, aut de illis in tenebris audere verba facere, adeo res sunt monstrosæ.
[4] Icon. lib. 1.   [5] Sect. 5, memb. 1, subs. 6.

PAGE 103

[1] Animi perturbationes summe fugiendæ, metus potissimum et tristitia: eorumque loco animus demulcendus hilaritate, animi constantia, bona spe; removendi terrores, et eorum consortium quos non probant.

[2] Phantasiæ eorum placide subvertendæ, terrores ab animo removendi.
[3] Ab omni fixa cogitatione quovismodo avertantur.
[4] Cuncta mala corporis ab animo procedunt, quæ nisi curentur, corpus curari minime potest.—Charmides.
[5] Dissertat. An morbi graviores corporis an animi? Renoldo interpret. Ut parum absit a furore, rapitur a Lyceo in concionem, a concione ad mare. a mari in Siciliam, etc.
[6] Ira bilem movet, sanguinem adurit, vitales spiritus accendit, mœstitia universum corpus infrigidat, calorem innatum extinguit, appetitum destruit, concoctionem impedit, corpus exsiccat, intellectum pervertit. Quamobrem hæc omnia prorsus vitanda sunt, et pro virili fugienda.
[7] De mel. cap. 26. Ex illis solum remedium; multi ex visis, auditis, etc., sanati sunt.

PAGE 104

[1] Pro viribus annitendum in prædictis, tum in aliis, a quibus malum velut a primaria causa occasionem nactum est; imaginationes absurdæ falsæque et mœstitia quæcunque subierit propulsetur, aut aliud agendo, aut ratione persuadendo earum mutationem subito facere.

[2] Lib. 2, cap. 16, de occult. nat. Quisquis huic malo obnoxius est, acriter obsistat, et summa cura obluctetur, nec ullo modo foveat imaginationes tacite obrepentes animo, blandas ab initio et amabiles, sed quæ adeo convalescunt, ut nulla ratione excuti queant.

PAGE 105

[1] 3 Tusc.; Ad Apollonium.   [2] Fracastorius.

[3] Epist. de secretis artis et naturæ, cap. 7, de retard. sen.   Remedium esset contra corruptionem propriam, si quilibet exerceret regimen sanitatis, quod consistit in rebus sex non naturalibus.

[4] Pro aliquo vituperio non indigneris, nec pro amissione alicujus rei, pro morte alicujus, nec pro carcere, nec pro exilio, nec pro alia re, nec irascaris, nec timeas, nec doleas, sed cum summa præsentia hæc sustineas.

[5] Quodsi incommoda adversitatis infortunia hoc malum invexerint, his infractum animum opponas, Dei verbo ejusque fiducia te suffulcias, etc.— Lemnius, lib. 1, cap. 16.

PAGE 106

[1] Lib. 2 de ira.

PAGE 107

[1] Cap. 3 de affect. anim.   Ut in civitatibus contumaces qui non cedunt politico imperio vi coercendi sunt; ita Deus nobis indidit alteram imperii formam; si cor non deponit vitiosum affectum, membra foras coercenda sunt, ne ruant in quod affectus impellat; et locomotiva, quæ herili imperio obtemperat, alteri resistat.

[2] Imaginatio impellit spiritus, et inde nervi moventur, etc., et obtemperant imaginationi et appetitui mirabili fœdere, ad exsequendum quod jubent.   [3] Ovid. Trist. lib. 5.

[4] Participes inde calamitatis nostræ sunt, et velut exonerata in eos sarcina onere levamur.—Arist. Eth. lib. 9.

[5] Camerarius, Embl. 26, cent. 2.   [6] Sympos. lib. 6, cap. 10.

[7] Epist. 8, lib. 3.   Adversa fortuna habet in querelis levamentum; et malorum relatio, etc.

[8] Alloquium cari juvat, et solamen amici.

PAGE 108

[1] Emblem. 54, cent. 1.

[2] As David did to Jonathan, 1 Sam. xx.

[3] Seneca, Epist. 67.

[4] Hic in civitate magna et turba magna neminem reperire possumus quocum suspirare familiariter aut jocari libere possimus.   Quare te expectamus, te desideramus, te arcessimus.   Multa sunt enim quæ me sollicitant et angunt, quæ mihi videor, aures tuas nactus, unius ambulationis exhaurire sermone posse.

[5] Ovid.   [6] De amicitia.

[7] De tranquil. cap. 7.   Optimum est amicum fidelem nancisci in quem secreta nostra infundamus; nihil æque oblectat animum, quam ubi sint præparata pectora, in quæ tuto secreta descendant, quorum conscientia æque ac tua: quorum sermo solitudinem leniat, sententia consilium expediat, hilaritas tristitiam dissipet, conspectusque ipse delectet.

PAGE 109

[1] Comment. lib. 5.   Ad Deum confugiamus, et peccatis veniam precemur, inde ad amicos, et cui plurimum tribuimus, nos patefaciamus totos, et animi vulnus quo affligimur: nihil ad reficiendum animum efficacius.

[2] Ep. Q. frat.   [3] Aphor. prim.   [4] Epist. 10.

PAGE 110

[1] Observando motus, gestus, manus, pedes, oculos, phantasiam.—Piso.

[2] Mulier melancholia correpta ex longa viri peregrinatione, et iracunde omnibus respondens, quum maritus domum reversus, præter spem, etc.

³ Præ dolore moriturus, quum nunciatum esset uxorem peperisse filium, subito recuperavit.

⁴ Nisi affectus longo tempore infestaverit, tali artificio imaginationes curare oportet, præsertim ubi malum ab his velut a primaria causa occasionem habuerit.

⁵ Lib. 1, cap. 16. Si ex tristitia aut alio affectu cœperit, speciem considera, aut aliud quid eorum, quæ subitam alterationem facere possunt.

⁶ Evitandi monstrifici aspectus, etc.

⁷ Neque enim tam actio, aut recordatio rerum hujusmodi displicet, sed iis vel gestus alterius imaginationi adumbrare, vehementer molestum.—Galat. de mor. cap. 7.

⁸ Tranquil. Præcipue vitentur tristes, et omnia deplorantes; tranquillitati inimicus est comes perturbatus, omnia gemens.

Page iii

¹ Illorum quoque hominum, a quorum consortio abhorrent, præsentia amovenda, nec sermonibus ingratis obtundendi; si quis insaniam ab insania sic curari æstimet, et proterve utitur, magis quam æger insanit.—Crato, consil. 184 Scoltzii.

² Molliter ac suaviter æger tractetur, nec ad ea adigatur quæ non curat.

³ Ob suspiciones, curas, æmulationem, ambitionem, iras, etc., quas locus ille ministrat, et quæ fecissent melancholicum.

Page 112

¹ Nisi prius animum turbatissimum curasset; oculi sine capite, nec corpus sine anima curari potest.

² E Græco.

³ Et nos non paucos sanavimus, animi motibus ad debitum revocatis.—Lib. 1 de sanit. tuend.

⁴ Consol. ad Apollonium. Si quis sapienter et suo tempore adhibeat, remedia morbis diversis diversa sunt; dolentem sermo benignus sublevat.

Page 113

¹ Lib. 12 Epist.

² De nat. deorum. Consolatur afflictos, deducit perterritos a timore, cupiditates imprimis et iracundias comprimit.

³ Heauton. Act. 1, scen. 1. Ne metue, ne verere, crede inquam mihi, aut consolando, aut consilio, aut re juvero.

⁴ Novi fœneratorem avarum apud meos sic curatum, qui multam pecuniam amiserat.

⁵ Lib. 1, consil. 12. Incredibile dictu quantum juvent.

⁶ Nemo istiusmodi conditionis hominibus insultet, aut in illos sit severior, verum miseriæ potius indolescat, vicemque deploret.—Lib. 2, cap. 16.

Page 114

¹ Cap. 7. Idem Piso, Laurentius, cap. 8.

² Quod timet nihil est, ubi cogitur et videt.

³ Una vice blandiantur, una vice iisdem terrorem incutiant.

⁴ Si vero fuerit ex novo malo audito, vel ex animi accidente, aut de amissione mercium, aut morte amici, introducantur nova contraria his quæ ipsum ad gaudia moveant; de hoc semper niti debemus, etc.

⁵ Lib. 3, cap. 14.

⁶ Cap. 3. Castratio olim a veteribus usa in morbis desperatis, etc.

⁷ Lib. 1, cap. 5. Sic morbum morbo, ut clavum clavo, retundimus, et malo nodo malum cuneum adhibemus. Novi ego qui ex subito hostium incursu et inopinato timore quartanam depulerat.

[8] Lib. 7, cap. 50. In acie pugnans febre quartana liberatus est.
[9] Jacchinus, cap. 15, in 9 Rhasis. Mont. cap. 26.
[10] Lib. 1, cap. 16. Aversantur eos qui eorum affectus rident, contemnunt. Si ranas et viperas comedisse se putant, concedere debemus, et spem de cura facere.
[11] Cap. 8 de mel.

PAGE 115

[1] Cistam posuit ex medicorum consilio prope eum, in quem alium se mortuum fingentem posuit; hic in cista jacens, etc.
[2] Serres, 1550.
[3] In 9 Rhasis. Magnam vim habet musica.
[4] Cap. de mania. Admiranda profecto res est, et digna expensione, quod sonorum concinnitas mentem emolliat, sistatque procellosas ipsius affectiones.
[5] Languens animus inde erigitur et reviviscit, nec tam aures afficit,, sed et sonitu per arterias undique diffuso, spiritus tum vitales tum animales excitat, mentem reddens agilem, etc.
[6] Musica venustate sua mentes severiores capit, etc.
[7] Animos tristes subito exhilarat, nubilos vultus serenat, austeritatem reponit, jucunditatem exponit, barbariemque facit deponere gentes, mores instituit, iracundiam mitigat.

PAGE 116

[1] Cithara tristitiam jucundat, timidos furores attenuat, cruentam sævitiam blande reficit, languorem, etc.
[2] Pet. Aretine.   [3] Castilio, de aulic. lib. 1, fol. 27.
[4] Lib. de natali, cap. 12.
[5] Quod spiritus qui in corde agitant tremulum et subsaltantem recipiunt aerem in pectus, et inde excitantur, a spiritu musculi moventur, etc.
[6] Arbores radicibus avulsæ, etc.

PAGE 117

[1] Mr. Carew of Anthony, in Descript. Cornwall, saith of whales, that they will come and show themselves dancing at the sound of a trumpet (fol. 35, 1, et fol. 154, 2 book).
[2] De cervo, equo, cane, urso idem compertum; musica afficiuntur.
[3] Numen inest numeris.
[4] Sæpe graves morbos modulatum carmen abegit, Et desperatis conciliavit opem.
[5] Lib. 5, cap. 7. Mœrentibus mœrorem adimam, lætantem vero seipso reddam hilariorem, amantem calidiorem, religiosum divino numine correptum, et ad deos colendos paratiorem.
[6] Natalis Comes, Myth. lib. 4, cap. 12.
[7] Lib. 5 de rep. Curat musica furorem Sancti Viti.
[8] Exilire e convivio.—Cardan, Subtil. lib. 13.   [9] Iliad 1.
[10] Lib. 9, cap. 1. Psaltrias sambucistrasque, et convivalia ludorum oblectamenta addita epulis, ex Asia invexit in urbem.

PAGE 118

[1] Comineus.
[2] Ista libenter et magna cum voluptate spectare soleo. Et scio te illecebris hisce captum iri et insuper tripudiaturum, haud dubie demulcebere.
[3] In musicis supra omnem fidem capior et oblector; choreas libentissime aspicio, pulchrarum feminarum venustate detineor, otiari inter has solutus curis possum.   [4] 2 de legibus.

Page 119

[1] Sympos. quæst. 5. Musica multos magis dementat quam vinum.
[2] Animi morbi vel a musica curantur vel inferuntur.
[3] Lib. 3 de anima. Lætitia purgat sanguinem, valetudinem conservat, colorem inducit florentem, nitidum, gratum.
[4] Spiritus temperat, calorem excitat, naturalem virtutem corroborat, juvenile corpus diu servat, vitam prorogat, ingenium acuit, et hominum negotiis quibuslibet aptiorem reddit.—Schola Salern.
[5] Dum contumelia vacant et festiva lenitate mordent, mediocres animi ægritudines sanari solent, etc.
[6] De mor. fol. 57. Amamus ideo eos qui sunt faceti et jucundi.
[7] Regim. sanit. part. 2. Nota quod amicus bonus et dilectus socius narrationibus suis jucundis superat omnem melodiam.
[8] Lib. 21, cap. 27.   [9] Comment. in 4 Odyss.
[10] Lib. 26, cap. 15.
[11] Homericum illud Nepenthes, quod mœrorem tollit, et euthymiam et hilaritatem parit.   [12] Plaut. Bacch.

Page 120

[1] De ægritud. capitis. Omni modo generet lætitiam in iis, de iis quæ audiuntur et videntur, aut odorantur, aut gustantur, aut quocunque modo sentiri possunt, et aspectu formarum multi decoris et ornatus, et negotiatione jucunda, et blandientibus ludis, et promissis distrahantur eorum animi, de re aliqua quam timent et dolent.
[2] Utantur venationibus, ludis, jocis, amicorum consortiis, quæ non sinunt animum turbari, vino et cantu et loci mutatione, et biberia, et gaudio, ex quibus præcipue delectantur.
[3] Piso. Ex fabulis et ludis quærenda delectatio. His versetur qui maxime grati sunt; cantus et chorea ad lætitiam prosunt.
[4] Præcipue valet ad expellendam melancholiam stare in cantibus, ludis, et sonis, et habitare cum familiaribus, et præcipue cum puellis jucundis.
[5] Par. 5 de avocamentis, lib. de absolvendo luctu.
[6] Corporum complexus, cantus, ludi, formæ, etc.
[7] Circa hortos Epicuri frequentes.
[8] Deipnosoph. lib. 10. Coronavit florido serto incendens odores, in culcita plumea collocavit, dulciculam potionem propinans, psaltriam adduxit, etc.
[9] Ut reclinata suaviter in lectum puella, etc.

Page 121

[1] Tom. 2, consult. 85.
[2] Epist. fam. lib. 7, 22 epist. Heri domum bene potus, seroque redieram.
[3] Valer. Max. cap. 8, lib. 8. Interposita arundine cruribus suis, cum filiis ludens, ab Alcibiade risus est .
[4] Hor.   [5] [Cosmo de' Medici.]
[6] Hominibus facetis et ludis puerilibus ultra modum deditus adeo ut si cui in eo tam gravitatem quam levitatem considerare liceret, duas personas distinctas in eo esse diceret.
[7] De nugis curial. lib. 1, cap. 4. Magistratus et viri graves, a ludis levioribus arcendi.

Page 122

[1] Machiavel, vita ejus. Ab amico reprehensus, quod præter dignitatem tripudiis operam daret, respondet, etc.
[2] There is a time for all things, to weep, laugh, mourn, dance.—Eccles. iii, 4.
[3] Hor.   [4] Sir John Harington, Epigr.
[5] Lucretia toto sis licet usque die, Thaida nocte volo.
[6] Lil. Giraldus, Hist. deor. syntag. 1.   [7] Lib. 3 de aur. asin.

NOTES

8 Eo quod risus esset laboris et modesti victus condimentum.
9 Calcag. epig.
10 Cap. 61.   In deliciis habuit scurras et adulatores.

PAGE 123

1 Universa gens supra mortales cæteros conviviorum studiosissima. Ea enim per varias et exquisitas dapes, interpositis musicis et joculatoribus, in multas sæpius horas extrahunt, ac subinde productis choreis et amoribus feminarum indulgent, etc.
2 Syntag. de Musis.
3 Athenæus, lib. 12 et 14. Assiduis mulierum vocibus cantuque symphoniæ palatium Persarum regis totum personabat.—Jovius, Hist. lib. 18.
4 Eobanus Hessus.   5 Fracastorius.
6 Vivite ergo læti, O amici, procul ab angustia, vivite læti.
7 Iterum precor et obtestor, vivite læti: illud quod cor urit, negligite.
8 Lætus in præsens animus quod ultra Oderit curare.—Hor. He was both sacerdos and medicus.

PAGE 124

1 Hæc autem non tam ut sacerdos, amici, mando vobis, quam ut medicus; nam absque hac una tanquam medicinarum vita, medicinæ omnes ad vitam producendam adhibitæ moriuntur: vivite læti.
2 Lœchæus, Anacreon.   3 Lucian. Necyomantia, tom. 2.
4 Omnia mundana nugas æstima. Hoc solum tota vita persequere, ut præsentibus bene compositis, minime curiosus, aut ulla in re sollicitus, quam plurimum potes vitam hilarem traducas.
5 Hildesheim, Spicil. 2 de mania, fol. 161. Studia literarum et animi perturbationes fugiat, et quantum potest jucunde vivat.
6 Lib. de atra bile. Gravioribus curis ludos et facetias aliquando interpone, jocos, et quæ solent animum relaxare.
7 Consil. 30. Mala valetudo aucta et contracta est tristitia, ac propterea exhilaratione animi removenda.
8 Athen. Deipnosoph. lib. 1.

PAGE 125

1 Juven. Sat. 8.   2 Hor.
3 Froissart, Hist. lib. 1. Hispani cum Anglorum vires ferre non possent, in fugam se dederunt, etc. Præcipites in fluvium se dederunt, ne in hostium manus venirent.
4 Ter.   5 Hor.

PAGE 126

1 Ἢ πίθι ἢ ἄπιθι. [Either drink or depart].
2 Lib. de libris propriis. Hos libros scio multos spernere, nam felices his se non indigere putant, infelices ad solationem miseriæ non sufficere. Et tamen felicibus moderationem, dum inconstantiam humanæ felicitatis docent, præstant; infelices si omnia recte æstimare velint, felices reddere possunt.

PAGE 127

1 Nullum medicamentum omnes sanare potest; sunt affectus animi qui prorsus sunt insanabiles; non tamen artis opus sperni debet, aut medicinæ, aut philosophiæ.
2 [These are the crazy consolations of a foolish mind.]
3 Sallust. Verba virtutem non addunt, nec imperatoris oratio facile timido fortem.
4 Job, cap. 16.   5 Epist. 13, lib. 1.
6 Hor.   7 Lib. 2, Essays, cap. 6.

Page 128

[1] Alium paupertas, alium orbitas, hunc morbi, illum timor, alium injuriæ, hunc insidiæ, illum uxor, filii distrahunt.—Cardan.

[2] Boethius, lib. 1, met. 5.

[3] Apuleius, 4 Florid. Nihil homini tam prospere datum divinitus, quin ei admixtum sit aliquid difficultatis, in amplissima quaque lætitia subest quædam querimonia, conjugatione quadam mellis et fellis.

[4] Si omnes premantur, quis tu es qui solus evadere cupis ab ea lege quæ neminem præterit? cur te non mortalem factum et universi orbis regem fieri non doles?

[5] Puteanus, Ep. 75. Neque cuiquam præcipue dolendum eo quod accidit universis.

[6] Lorchan. Gallobelgicus, lib. 3, anno 1598, de Belgis. Euge! sed eheu! inquis, quid agemus? ubi pro epithalamio Bellonæ flagellum, pro musica harmonia terribilem lituorum et tubarum audias clangorem, pro tædis nuptialibus, villarum, pagorum, urbium videas incendia; ubi pro jubilo lamenta, pro risu fletus aerem complent.

[7] Ita est profecto, et quisquis hæc videre abnuis, huic sæculo parum aptus es, aut potius nostrorum omnium conditionem ignoras, quibus reciproco quodam nexu læta tristibus, tristia lætis invicem succedunt.

[8] In Tusc. e vetere poeta.

[9] Cardan, lib. 1 de consol. Est consolationis genus non leve, quod a necessitate fit; sive feras, sive non feras, ferendum est tamen.

[10] Seneca.

[11] Omni dolori tempus est medicina; ipsum luctum extinguit, injurias delet, omnis mali oblivionem adfert.

Page 129

[1] Habet hoc quoque commodum omnis infelicitas, suaviorem vitam cum abierit relinquit.

[2] Virg.   [3] Ovid.

[4] Lorchan. Sunt namque infera superis, humana terrenis longe disparia. Etenim beatæ mentes feruntur libere, et sine ullo impedimento, stellæ, æthereique orbes cursus et conversiones suas jam sæculis innumerabilibus constantissime conficiunt; verum homines magnis angustiis. Neque hac naturæ lege est quisquam mortalium solutus.

[5] Dionysius Halicar. lib. 8. Non enim unquam contigit, nec post homines natos invenies quemquam, cui omnia ex animi sententia successerint, ita ut nulla in re fortuna sit ei adversata.

[6] Vit. Gonsalvi, lib. ult. Ut ducibus fatale sit clarissimis a culpa sua, secus circumveniri cum malitia et invidia, imminutaque dignitate per contumeliam mori.

[7] In terris purum illum ætherem non invenies, et ventos serenos; nimbos potius, procellas, calumnias. Lips. Cent. misc. ep. 8.

Page 130

[1] Si omnes homines sua mala suasque curas in unum cumulum conferrent, æquis divisuri portionibus, etc.

[2] Hor. Ser. lib. 1.

[3] Quod unusquisque propria mala novit, aliorum nesciat, in causa est, ut se inter alios miserum putet. Cardan, lib. 3 de consol. Plutarch de consol. ad Apollonium.

[4] Quam multos putas qui se cœlo proximos putarent, totidem regulos, si de fortunæ tuæ reliquiis pars iis minima contingat.—Boeth. de consol. lib. 2, pros. 4.

PAGE 131

[1] Hesiod. Esto quod es; quod sunt alii, sine quemlibet esse; Quod non es, nolis; quod potes esse, velis.
[2] Æsopi fab.   [3] Seneca.
[4] Si dormirent semper omnes, nullus alio felicior esset.—Cardan.
[5] Seneca, de ira.
[6] Plato, Axiocho. An ignoras vitam hanc peregrinationem, etc., quam sapientes cum gaudio percurrunt.
[7] Sic expedit; medicus non dat quod patiens vult, sed quod ipse bonum scit.

PAGE 132

[1] Frumentum non egreditur nisi trituratum, etc.
[2] Non est poena damnantis sed flagellum corrigentis.
[3] Ad hæreditatem æternam sic erudimur.
[4] Confess. 6.
[5] Nauclerum tempestas, athletam stadium, ducem pugna, magnanimum calamitas, Christianum vero tentatio probat et examinat.
[6] Sen. Herc. Fur.
[7] Ideo Deus asperum fecit iter, ne dum delectantur in via, obliviscantur eorum quæ sunt in patria.
[8] Boethius, lib. 5, met. 4.
[9] Boeth. pros. ult. Manet spectator cunctorum desuper præscius deus, bonis præmia, malis supplicia dispensans.
[10] Lib. de provid. Voluptatem capiunt dii siquando magnos viros colluctantes cum calamitate vident.

PAGE 133

[1] Ecce spectaculum Deo dignum, vir fortis cum mala fortuna compositus.
[2] 1 Pet. v. 7; Ps. lv, 22.
[3] Raro sub eodem lare honestas et forma habitant.
[4] Josephus Mussus, vita ejus.
[5] Homuncio brevis, macilentus, umbra hominis, etc. Ad stuporem ejus eruditionem et eloquentiam admirati sunt.

PAGE 134

[1] [Muley Hassan.]   [2] Nox habet suas voluptates.
[3] Lib. 5, ad finem. Cæcus potest esse sapiens et beatus, etc.
[4] In Convivio, lib. 25.   [5] Joachimus Camerarius, vit. ejus.
[6] Riber. vit. ejus.   [7] Macrobius.   [8] Sueton, cap. 7, 9.
[9] Lib. 1. Corpore exili et despecto, sed ingenio et prudentia longe ante se reges cæteros præveniens.
[10] Alexander Gaguinus, Hist. Polandiæ. Corpore parvus eram, cubito vix altior uno, Sed tamen in parvo corpore magnus eram.

PAGE 135

[1] Ovid.   [2] Vir. Æneid. 10.   [3] [See Deut. ii, 20.]
[4] Lib. 2, cap. 20. Oneri est illis corporis moles, et spiritus minus vividi.
[5] Corpore breves prudentiores quum coarctata sit anima. Ingenio pollet cui vim natura negavit.
[6] Multis ad salutem animæ profuit corporis ægritudo.—Petrarch.
[7] Lib. 7. Summa est totius philosophiæ, si tales, etc.

PAGE 136

[1] Plinius, Epist. lib. 7. Quem infirmum libido sollicitat, aut avaritia, aut honores? nemini invidet, neminem miratur, neminem despicit, sermone maligno non alitur. [The letter (ep. 26), is addressed to Maximus, not Rufus.]

² Non terret princeps, magister, parens, judex; at ægritudo superveniens omnia correxit.
³ Nat. Chytræus, Europ. deliciis. Labor, dolor, ægritudo, luctus, servire superbis dominis, jugum ferre superstitionis, quos habet caros sepelire, etc., condimenta vitæ sunt.
⁴ Non tam mari quam prœlio virtus, etiam lecto exhibetur: vincetur aut vincet; aut tu febrem relinques, aut ipsa te.—Seneca.
⁵ [Wilibald Pirckheimer.]
⁶ Tullius [de fin. 2, 30]. Vesicæ morbo laborans, et urinæ mittendæ difficultate tanta, ut vix incrementum caperet; repellebat hæc omnia animi gaudium ob memoriam inventorum.
⁷ Boeth. lib. 2, pr. 4. Huic sensus exuberat, sed est pudori degener sanguis.

PAGE 137

¹ Gaspar Ens, Polit. thes.
² Alii pro pecunia emunt nobilitatem, alii illam lenocinio, alii veneficiis, alii parricidiis; multis perditio nobilitate conciliat, plerique adulatione, detractione, calumniis, etc.—Agrip. de vanit. scien.
³ Ex homicidio sæpe orta nobilitas et strenua carnificina.
⁴ Plures ob prostitutas filias, uxores, nobiles facti; multos venationes, rapinæ, cædes, præstigia, etc.   ⁵ Sat. Menip.

PAGE 138

¹ Cum enim hos dici nobiles videmus, qui divitiis abundant, divitiæ vero raro virtutis sunt comites, quis non videt ortum nobilitatis degenerem? hunc usuræ ditarunt, illum spolia, proditiones; hic veneficiis ditatus, ille adulationibus, huic adulteria lucrum præbent, nonullis mendacia, quidam ex conjuge quæstum faciunt, plerique ex natis, etc.—Florent. Hist. lib. 3.
² Juven.
³ Robusta improbitas a tyrannide incepta, etc.
⁴ Gaspar Ens, Thesauro polit.
⁵ Gresserus, Itinerar. fol. 266.   ⁶ Hor.
⁷ Syl. nup. lib. 4, num. 111.   ⁸ Exod. xxxii.

PAGE 139

¹ Omnium nobilium sufficientia in eo probatur si venatica noverint, si aleam, si corporis vires ingentibus poculis commonstrent, si naturæ robur numerosa venere probent, etc.
² Difficile est, ut non sit superbus dives.—Austin, ser. 24.
³ Nobilitas nihil aliud nisi improbitas, furor, rapina, latrocinium, homicidium, luxus, venatio, violentia, etc.
⁴ The fool took away my lord in the mask, 'twas apposite.
⁵ De miser. curial. Miseri sunt, inepti sunt, turpes sunt, multi ut parietes ædium suarum speciosi.
⁶ Miraris aureas vestes, equos, canes, ordinem famulorum, lautas mensas, ædes, villas, prædia, piscinas, silvas, etc., hæc omnia stultus assequi potest. Pandarus noster lenocinio nobilitatus est.—Æneas Sylvius.
⁷ Bellonius, Observ. lib. 2.

PAGE 140

¹ Mat. Riccius, lib. 1, cap. 3. Ad regendam remp. soli doctores aut licentiati adsciscuntur, etc.
² Lib. 1 Hist. Conditione servus, cæterum acer bello, et animi magnitudine maximorum regum nemini secundus: ob hæc a Mameluchis in regem electus.

[2] Olaus Magnus, lib. 18. Saxo Grammaticus. A quo rex Sueno et cætera Danorum regum stemmata.
[4] Seneca, de Contro. Philos. epist.
[5] Corpore sunt et animo fortiores spurii, plerumque ob amoris vehementiam, seminis crass., etc.

PAGE 141

[1] Vita Castruccii. Nec præter rationem mirum videri debet, si quis rem considerare velit, omnes eos vel saltem maximam partem, qui in hoc terrarum orbe res præstantiores aggressi sunt, atque inter cæteros ævi sui heroas excelluerunt, aut obscuro aut abjecto loco editos, et prognatos fuisse abjectis parentibus. Eorum ego catalogum infinitum recensere possem.   [2] Exercit. 265.
[3] Flor. Hist. lib. 3. Quod si nudos nos conspici contingat, omnium una eademque erit facies; nam si ipsi nostras, nos eorum vestes induamus, nos, etc.
[4] Ut merito dicam, quod simpliciter sentiam, Paulum Schalichium scriptorem, et doctorem, pluris facio quam comitem Hunnorum, et Baronem Skradinum. Encyclopædiam tuam et orbem disciplinarum omnibus provinciis antefero.—Balæus, Epist. nuncupat. ad 5 cent. ultimam script. Brit.
[5] Præfat Hist. lib. 1. Virtute tua major, quam aut Etrusci imperii fortuna, aut numerosa et decora prolis felicitate beatior evadis.
[6] Curtius.   [7] Bodine, de rep. lib. 3, cap. 8.

PAGE 142

[1] Æneas Sylvius, lib. 2, cap. 29.
[2] If children be proud, haughty, foolish, they defile the nobility of their kindred.—Eccl. xxii, 8.
[3] Cujus possessio nec furto eripi, nec incendio absumi, nec aquarum voragine absorberi, vel vi morbi destrui potest.
[4] Send them both to some strange place naked, ad ignotos, as Aristippus said, you shall see the difference. Bacon's Essays.
[5] Familiæ splendor nihil opis attulit, etc.
[6] Fluvius hic illustris, humanarum rerum imago, quæ parvis ductæ sub initiis, in immensum crescunt, et subito evanescunt. Exilis hic primo fluvius, in admirandam magnitudinem excrescit, tandemque in mari Euxino evanescit.—J. Stuckius, Pereg. mar. Euxini.

PAGE 143

[1] Sabinus, in 6 Ovid. Met. fab. 4.
[2] Lib. 1, de 4 complexionibus.   [3] Hor. Epod. 4.
[4] Lib. 2, ep. 15. Natus sordido turguriolo et paupere domo, qui vix milio rugientem ventrem, etc.

PAGE 144

[1] Nihil fortunato insipiente intolerabilius.
[2] Claud. lib. 1, in Eutrop.
[3] Lib. 1 de Rep. Gal. Quoniam et commodiore utuntur conditione, et honestiore loco nati, jam inde a parvulis ad morum civilitatem educati sunt, et assuefacti.

PAGE 145

[1] Nullum paupertate gravius onus.
[2] Ne quis iræ divinæ judicium putaret, aut paupertas exosa foret.—Gualt. in cap. 2, ver. 18 Lucæ.

[3] Inter proceres Thebanos numeratus, lectum habuit genus, frequens familitium, domus amplas, etc.—Apuleius, Florid. lib. 4.

[4] P. Blesensis, ep. 72 et 232. Oblatos respui honores, ex onere metiens motus ambitiosos; rogatus non ivi, etc.

Page 146

[1] Sudat pauper foras in opere, dives in cogitatione; hic os aperit oscitatione, ille ructatione; gravius ille fastidio, quam hic inedia cruciatur.—Ber. ser.

[2] In Hyperchen. Natura æqua est, puerosque videmus mendicorum nulla ex parte regum filiis dissimiles, plerumque saniores.

[3] Gallo, tom. 2.

[4] Et e contubernio fœdi atque olidi ventris mors tandem educit.—Seneca, ep. 103.

[5] Divitiarum sequela, luxus, intemperies, arrogantia, superbia, furor injustus, omnisque irrationibilis motus.

[6] Juven. Sat. 6.   [7] Saturn. Epist.

[8] Vos quidem divites putatis felices, sed nescitis eorum miserias.

[9] Et quota pars hæc eorum quæ istos discruciant? si nossetis metus et curas, quibus obnoxii sunt, plane fugiendas vobis divitias existimaretis.

[10] Seneca in Herc. Œtæo.

Page 147

[1] Et diis similes stulta cogitatio facit.

[2] Flamma simul libidinis ingreditur; ita, furor et superbia, divitiarum sequela.—Chrys.

[3] Omnium oculis, odio, insidiis expositus, semper sollicitus, fortunæ ludibrium.

[4] Hor. lib. 2, Od. 10.

[5] Quid me felicem toties jactastis amici? Qui cecidit, stabili non fuit ille loco.—Boeth.

[6] Ut postquam impinguati fuerint, devorentur.   [7] Hor.

Page 148

[1] Cap. 6 de curat. Græc. affect. cap. de providentia. Quotiescunque divitiis affluentem hominem videmus, eumque pessimum, ne quæso hunc beatissimum putemus, sed infelicem censeamus, etc.

[2] Hor. lib. 4, Od. 9.   [3] Hor. lib. 2.

Page 149

[1] Florid. lib. 4. Dives ille cibo interdicitur, et in omni copia sua cibum non accipit, cum interea totum ejus servitium hilare sit, atque epuletur.

[2] Epist. 115.

[3] Hor. Et mihi curto Ire licet mulo vel si libet usque Tarentum.

[4] Brisonius.

Page 150

[1] Si modum excesseris, suavissima sunt molesta.

[2] Et in cupidiis gulæ, coquus et pueri illotis manibus ab exoneratione ventris omnia tractant, etc.—Cardan, lib. 8, cap. 46, de rerum varietate.

[3] Epist.

[4] Plin. lib. 57, cap. 6.   [5] Zonaras, Annal. 3.

[6] Plutarch. vit. ejus.   [7] Hor. Ser. lib. 1, Sat. 2.

[8] Cap. 30. Nullam vestem bis induit.

PAGE 151

[1] Ad generum Cereris sine cæde et sanguine pauci Descendunt reges, et sicca morte tyranni.
[2] "God shall deliver his soul from the power of the grave."—Ps. xlix, 15.
[3] Contempl. Idiot. cap. 37. Divitiarum acquisitio magni laboris, possessio magni timoris, amissio magni doloris.
[4] Boethius de consol. phil. lib. 3.

PAGE 152

[1] Austin in Ps. lxxvi. Omnis philosophiæ magistra, ad cœlum via.
[2] Bonæ mentis soror paupertas.
[3] Pædagoga pietatis sobria, pia mater, cultu simplex, habitu secura, consilio benesuada.—Apul.
[4] Cardan. Opprobrium non est paupertas: quod latro eripit, aut pater non reliquit, cur mihi vitio daretur, si fortuna divitias invidit? non aquilæ, non, etc. [5] Tully.
[6] Epist. 74. Servus, summe homo; servus sum, immo contubernalis, servus sum, at humilis amicus, immo conservus si cogitaveris.
[7] Epist. 66 et 90.

PAGE 153

[1] Panormitan, rebus gestis Alph.
[2] Lib. 4, num. 218. Quidam deprehensus quod sederet loco nobilium, mea nobilitas, ait, est circa caput, vestra declinat ad caudam.
[3] Tanto beatior es, quanto collectior.
[4] Non amoribus inservit, non appetit honores, et qualitercunque relictus satis habet, hominem se esse meminit, invidet nemini, neminem despicit, neminem miratur, sermonibus malignis non attendit aut alitur.—Plinius.
[5] Politianus, in Rustico.
[6] Gyges regno Lydiæ inflatus sciscitatum misit Apollinem an quis mortalium se felicior esset. Aglaium Arcadum pauperrimum Apollo prætulit, qui terminos agri sui nunquam excesserat, rure suo contentus.— Val. lib. 1, cap. 7.

PAGE 154

[1] Hor. Hæc est Vita solutorum misera ambitione, gravique.
[2] Amos vi.
[3] Præfat. lib. 7. Odit naturam quod infra deos sit; irascitur diis quod quis illi antecedat.
[4] De ira, cap. 31, lib. 3. Et si multum acceperit, injuriam putat plura non accepisse; non agit pro tribunatu gratias, sed queritur quod non sit ad præturam perductus; neque hæc grata, si desit consulatus.
[5] Lips. admir. [6] Of some 90,000 inhabitants now.

PAGE 155

[1] Read the story at large in John Fox, his Acts and Monuments.
[2] Hor. Sat. 2, Ser. lib. 2.
[3] 5 Florent. Hist. Virtus quietem parat, quies otium, otium porro luxum generat, luxus interitum, a quo iterum ad saluberrimas, etc.

PAGE 156

[1] Guicciard. in Hiponest. Nulla infelicitas subjectum esse legi naturæ, etc. [2] Persius.

PAGE 157

[1] Omnes divites qui cœlo et terra frui possunt.
[2] Hor. lib. 1, epist. 12.
[3] Seneca, epist. 15. Panem et aquam natura desiderat, et hæc qui

habet, ipso cum Jove de felicitate contendat. Cibus simplex famem sedat, vestis tenuis frigus arcet.—Senec. epist. 8.

[4] Boethius.   [5] Muffæus et alii.
[6] Brisonius.   [7] Ps. civ, 15.
[8] Si recte philosophemini, quicquid aptam moderationem supergreditur, oneri potius quam usui est. [Madaurensis =Apuleius, a native of Madaura.]
[9] Lib. 7, 16.   Cereris munus et aquæ poculum mortales quærunt habere, et quorum saties nunquam est; luxus autem, sunt cætera, non epulæ.
[10] Satis est dives qui pane non indiget; nimium potens qui servire non cogitur. Ambitiosa non est fames, etc.
[11] Euripides, Menalip. O fili, mediocres divitiæ hominibus conveniunt, nimia vero moles perniciosa.

PAGE 158

[1] Hor.   [2] O noctes cœnæque deum.
[3] Per mille fraudes doctosque dolos ejicitur, apud sociam paupertatem ejusque cultores divertens in eorum sinu et tutela deliciatur.
[4] Lucan.   [5] Lips. Miscell. ep. 40.
[6] Sat. 6, lib. 2.   [7] Hor. Sat. 4.   [8] Apuleius.

PAGE 159

[1] Chytræus, in Europæ deliciis.   Accipite, cives Veneti, quod est optimum in rebus humanis, res humanas contemnere.
[2] Vah, vivere etiam nunc lubet, as Demea said, Adelph. Act. 3.   Quam multis non egeo, quam multa non desidero, ut Socrates in pompa, ille in nundinis.
[3] Epictetus, cap. 77.   Quo sum destinatus, et sequar alacriter.
[4] Puteanus, Ep. 62.   [5] Marullus.
[6] Hoc erat in votis, modus agri non ita parvus, Hortus ubi et tecto vicinus jugis aquæ fons, et paulum silvæ, etc.—Hor. Sat. 6, lib. 2 Ser.
[7] Hieronym.
[8] Seneca, Consil. ad Albinum, cap. 11.   Qui continet se intra naturæ limites, paupertatem non sentit; qui excedit, eum in opibus paupertas sequitur.

PAGE 160

[1] Hom. 12.   Pro his quæ accepisti gratias age, noli indignare pro his quæ non accepisti.
[2] Nat. Chytræus, Deliciis Europ. Gustonii in ædibus Hubianis in cœnaculo e regione mensæ.
[3] Quid non habet melius pauper quam dives? vitam, valetudinem, cibum, somnum, libertatem, etc.—Cardan.
[4] Martial. lib. 10, epig. 47.   Read it out thyself in the author.
[5] Confess. lib. 6.   Transiens per vicum quendam Mediolanensem, animadverti pauperem quendam mendicum, jam credo saturum, jocantem atque ridentem, et ingemui et locutus sum cum amicis qui mecum erant, etc.
[6] Et certe ille lætabatur, ego anxius; securus ille, ego trepidus.   Et si percontaretur me quispiam an exultare mallem, an metuere, responderem, exultare: et si rursus interrogaret an ego talis essem, an qualis nunc sum, me ipsis curis confectum eligerem; sed perversitate, non veritate.

PAGE 161

[1] Hor.   [2] Hor. Ep. lib. 1.
[3] O si nunc morerer, inquit, quanta et qualia mihi imperfect a manerent: sed si mensibus decem vel octo super vixero, omnia redigam ad libellum, ab omni debito creditoque me explicabo; prætereunt interim menses decem et octo et cum illis anni, et adhuc restant plura quam prius; quid

igitur speras, O insane, finem quem rebus tuis non inveneras in juventa, in senecta impositurum? O dementiam, quum ob curas et negotia tuo judicio sis infelix, quid putas futurum quum plura supererint?—Cardan, lib. 8, cap. 40, de rer. var.
[4] Plutarch.

PAGE 162

[1] Lib. de natali, cap. 1.
[2] Apud Stobæum, ser. 17. [3] Hom. 12, in 2 Cor. vi.
[4] Non in paupertate, sed in paupere (Senec.), non re, sed opinione labores.

PAGE 163

[1] Vopiscus, Aureliano. Sed si populus famelicus inedia laboret, nec arma, leges, pudor, magistratus, coercere valent.
[2] One of the richest men in Rome.
[3] Serm. Quidam sunt qui pauperes esse volunt ita ut nihil illis desit; sic commendant ut nullam patiantur inopiam; sunt et alii mites, quamdiu dicitur et agitur ad eorum arbitrium, etc.
[4] Nemo paupertatem commendaret nisi pauper.
[5] Petronius, Catalec. [6] Ovid.
[7] Ovid. [8] Plutarch. vit. Crassi.

PAGE 164

[1] Lucan, lib. 9.
[2] An quum super fimo sedit Job, an eum omnia abstulit diabolus, etc., pecuniis privatus fiduciam Deo habuit, omni thesauro pretiosiorem.
[3] Hæc videntes sponte philosophemini, nec insipientum affectibus agitemur. [4] 1 Sam. i, 8.
[5] James i, 2. "My brethren, count it an exceeding joy, when you fall into divers temptations."

PAGE 165

[1] Afflictio dat intellectum. Quos Deus diligit, castigat. Deus optimum quemque aut mala valetudine aut luctu afficit.—Seneca.
[2] Quam sordet mihi terra quum cœlum intueor.
[3] Senec. de providentia, cap. 2. Diis ita visum, dii melius norunt quid sit in commodum meum.
[4] Hom. Iliad 4.
[5] Hom. 9. Voluit urbem tyrannus evertere, et Deus non prohibuit; voluit captivos ducere, non impedivit; voluit ligare, concessit, etc.
[6] Ps. cxliii. De terra inopem, de stercore erigit pauperem.
[7] Micah vii, 7.
[8] Preme, preme, ego cum Pindaro, ἀβάπτιστός εἰμι φέλλος ὡς ὑπὲρ ἕρκος ἅλμας, immersibilis sum sicut suber super maris septum.—Lipsius.
[9] Hic ure, hic seca, ut in æternum parcas.—Austin. Diis fruitur iratis, superat et crescit malis. Mucium ignis, Fabricium paupertas, Regulum tormenta, Socratem venenum superare non potuit.
[10] Hor. Epist. 16, lib. 1.

PAGE 166

[1] Hom. 5. Auferet pecunias? at habet in cœlis: patria dejiciet? at in cœlestem civitatem mittet: vincula injiciet? at habet solutam conscientiam: corpus interficiet, at iterum resurget; cum umbra pugnat qui cum justo pugnat.
[2] Leonides.
[3] Modo in pressura, in tentationibus, erit postea bonum tuum requies, æternitas, immortalitas.
[4] Dabit Deus his quoque finem. [5] [Cic. de fin. 1, 18.]

PAGE 167

[1] Nemo desperet meliora lapsus.   [2] Theocritus.
[3] Hor.   [4] Ovid.   [5] Thales.
[6] Lib. 7 Flor. Hist. Omnium felicissimus, et locupletissimus, etc.,
incarceratus sæpe adolescentiam periculo mortis habuit sollicitudinis et
discriminis plenam, etc.

PAGE 168

[1] Lætior successit securitas quæ simul cum divitiis cohabitare nescit.—
Camden.
[2] Pecuniam perdidisti, fortassis illa te perderet manens.—Seneca.
[3] Expeditior es ob pecuniarum jacturam. Fortuna opes auferre, non
animum potest.—Seneca.
[4] Hor.   [5] Jubet me posthac fortuna expeditius philosophari.

PAGE 169

[1] In frag. Quirites, multa mihi pericula domi, militiæ multa adversa
fuere, quorum alia toleravi, alia deorum auxilio repuli et virtute mea;
nunquam animus negotio defuit, nec decretis labor; nullæ res nec pros-
peræ nec adversæ ingenium mutabant.
[2] Qualis mundi status supra lunam semper serenus.
[3] Bona mens nullum tristioris fortunæ recipit incursum (Val. lib. 4,
cap. 1). Qui nil potest sperare, desperet nihil.   [4] Hor.
[5] Æquam memento rebus in arduis servare mentem.—Lib. 2, Od. 3.
[6] Epict. cap. 18.   [7] Ter. Adel. Act. 4, sc. 7.
[8] Unaquæque res duas habet ansas, alteram quæ teneri, alteram quæ
non potest; in manu nostra quam volumus accipere.
[9] Ter. And. Act. 4, sc. 6.

PAGE 170

[1] Epictetus. Invitatus ad convivium, quæ apponuntur comedis, non
quæris ultra; in mundo multa rogitas quæ dii negant.
[2] Cap. 6 de providentia. Mortales cum sint rerum omnium indigi, ideo
Deus aliis divitias, aliis paupertatem distribuit, ut qui opibus pollent,
materiam subministrent; qui vero inopes, exercitatas artibus manus
admoveant.
[3] Si sint omnes æquales, necesse est ut omnes fame pereant; quis aratro
terram sulcaret, quis sementem faceret, quis plantas sereret, quis vinum
exprimeret?
[4] Liv. lib. 2.   [5] Lib. 3, de cons.

PAGE 171

[1] Seneca.
[2] Vide Isaacum Pontanum, Descript. Amsterdam. lib. 2, cap. 22.
[3] Vide Ed. Pelham's book, edit. 1630.
[4] Heautontim. Act. 1, sc. 2.
[5] Epist. 98. Omni fortuna valentior ipse animus, in utramque partem
res suas ducit, beatæque ac miseræ vitæ sibi causa est.
[6] Fortuna quem nimium fovet stultum facit.—Pub. Syrus.
[7] Seneca de beat. vit. cap. 14. Miseri si deserantur ab ea, miseriores si
obruantur.

PAGE 172

[1] Plutarch, vit. ejus.   [2] Hor. Epist. lib. 1, ep. 18.
[3] Hor.   [4] Boeth. 2.
[5] Epist. lib. 3, vit. Paul. Eremit. Libet eos nunc interrogare qui domus
marmoribus vestiunt, qui uno filo villarum ponunt pretia, huic seni modo
quid unquam defuit? vos gemma bibitis, ille concavis manibus naturæ
satisfecit; ille pauper Paradisum capit, vos avaros Gehenna suscipiet.

PAGE 173

[1] Satur. lib. 11. Alius libidini servit, alius ambitioni, omnes spei, omnes timori.
[2] Nat. lib. 3.   [3] Consol. lib. 3.
[4] O generose, quid est vita nisi carcer animi?

PAGE 174

[1] Herbastein.
[2] Vertomannus, Navig. lib. 2, cap. 4. Commercia in nundinis noctu hora secunda ob nimios qui sæviunt interdiu æstus exercent.
[3] Ubi verior contemplatio quam in solitudine? ubi studium solidius quam in quiete?
[4] Alex. ab Alex. Gen. dier. lib. 1, cap. 2.
[5] In Ps. lxxvi. Non ita laudatur Joseph cum frumenta distribueret, ac quum carcerem habitaret.   [6] Boethius.

PAGE 175

[1] Philostratus in Deliciis. Peregrini sunt imbres in terra et fluvii in mari, Jupiter apud Ægyptos, sol apud omnes; hospes anima in corpore, luscinia in aere, hirundo in domo, Ganymedes cœlo, etc.
[2] Lib. 16, cap. 1. Nullam frugem habent, potus ex imbre: et hæ gentes si vincantur, etc.
[3] Lib. 5 de legibus. Cumque cognatis careat et amicis, majorem apud deos et apud homines misericordiam meretur.

PAGE 176

[1] Cardan. de consol. lib. 2.   [2] [Publius Syrus.]   [3] Benzo.
[4] Summo mane ululatum oriuntur, pectora percutientes, etc., miserabile spectaculum exhibentes.—Ortelius, in Græcia.
[5] Catullus.   [6] Virgil.   [7] Lucan.

PAGE 177

[1] 3 Annal.   [2] Virg. Æn. 9.   [3] Confess. lib. 1.   [4] Juvenalis.

PAGE 178

[1] Amator scortum vitæ præponit, iracundus vindictam, parasitus gulam, ambitiosus honores, avarus opes, miles rapinam, fur prædam; morbos odimus et accersimus.—Cardan.
[2] Seneca. Quum nos sumus, mors non adest; cum vero mors adest, tum nos non sumus.
[3] Bernard. cap. 3 Med. Nasci miserum, vivere pœna, angustia mori.
[4] Plato, Apol. Socratis. Sed jam hora est hinc abire, etc.
[5] Comedi ad satietatem, gravitas me offendit; parcius edi, non est expletum desiderium; venereas delicias sequor, hinc morbus, lassitudo, etc.
[6] Bern. cap. 3 Med. De tantilla lætitia quanta tristitia; post tantam voluptatem quam gravis miseria!
[7] Est enim mors piorum felix transitus de labore ad refrigerium, de expectatione ad præmium, de agone ad brabeum.

PAGE 179

[1] Vaticanus, vita ejus.   [2] Luc.   [3] Il. 19 Homer.   [4] Ovid.
[5] Consol. ad Apollon. Non est libertate nostra positum non dolere, misericordiam abolet, etc.

PAGE 180

[1] Ovid. 4 Trist.   [2] Tacitus, lib. 2.
[3] Lib. 9, cap. 9, de Civitate Dei. Non quæro cum irascatur sed cur, non utrum sit tristis sed unde, non utrum timeat sed quid timeat.

[4] Festus, verbo minuitur. Luctui dies indicebatur cum liberi nascantur. cum frater aut, amicus ab hospite captivus domum redeat, puella desponsetur.

[5] Ob hanc causam mulieres ablegaram ne talia facerent; nos hæc audientes erubuimus et destitimus a lacrimis.

[6] Lib. 1, class. 8, de claris. jurisconsultis Patavinis.

[7] 12 innuptæ puellæ amictæ viridibus pannis, etc.

[8] Lib. de consol.

[9] Præceptis philosophiæ confirmatus adversus omnem fortunæ vim, et te consecrata in cœlumque recepta, tanta affectus lætitia sum ac voluptate, quantam animo capere possum, ac exultare plane mihi videor, victorque de omni dolore et fortuna triumphare.

PAGE 181

[1] Ut lignum uri natum, arista secari, sic homines mori.

[2] Boeth. lib. 2, met. 3.   [3] Boeth.

[4] Nic. Hensel. Breslagr. fol. 47.

[5] Twenty then present.

[6] To Magdalen, the daughter of Charles the Seventh of France. Obeunt noctesque diesque, etc.

[7] Assyriorum regio funditus deleta.

[8] Omnium quot unquam sol aspexit urbium maxima.

[9] Ovid.   [10] Arcad. lib. 8.

[11] Præfat. Topogr. Constantinop.

PAGE 182

[1] Epist. Tull. lib. 4.

[2] Quum tot oppidorum cadavera ante oculos projecta jacent.

[3] Hor. lib. 1, Od. 24.

[4] De remed. fortuit.

[5] Erubesce tanta tempestate quod ad unam anchoram stabas.

[6] Vis ægrum, et morbidum, sitibundum?—gaude potius quod his malis liberatus sit.

[7] Uxorem bonam aut invenisti, aut sic fecisti; si inveneris, aliam habere te posse ex hoc intelligamus: si feceris, bene speres, salvus est artifex.

PAGE 183

[1] Stulti est compedes licet aureas amare.

[2] Hor.   [3] Hor. lib. 1, Od. 24.   [4] Virg. Æn. 4.

[5] Cap. 19.   Si id studes ut uxor, amici, liberi perpetuo vivant, stultus es.

[6] Deus quos diligit juvenes rapit.—Menander.

[7] Consol. ad Apoll.   Apollonius filius tuus in flore decessit, ante nos ad æternitatem digressus, tanquam e convivio abiens, priusquam in errorem aliquem e temulentia incideret, quales in longa senecta accidere solent.

PAGE 184

[1] Tom. 1, Tract. de luctu.   Quid me mortuum miserum vocas, qui te sum multo felicior? aut quid acerbi mihi putas contigisse? an quia non sum malus senex, ut tu facie rugosus, incurvus, etc.   O demens, quid tibi videtur in vita boni? nimirum amicitias, cœnas, etc.   Longe melius non esurire quam edere; non sitire, etc.—Gaude potius quod morbos et febres effugerim, angorem animi, etc.   Ejulatus quid prodest, quid lachrymæ, etc.

[2] Virgil.   [3] [Martial.]

[4] Chytræus, Deliciis Europæ.   [5] Epist. 85.

PAGE 185

[1] Sardus, de mor. gen.
[2] Præmeditatione facilem reddere quemque casum.—Plutarchus, consolatione ad Apollonium. Assuefacere nos casibus debemus.—Tull. lib. 3 Tusculan. Quæst.
[3] Cap. 8. Si ollam diligas, memento te ollam diligere, non perturbaberis ea confracta; si filium aut uxorem, memento hominem a te diligi, etc.
[4] Seneca.   [5] Boeth. lib. 1, pros. 4.

PAGE 186

[1] Qui invidiam ferre non potest, ferre contemptum cogitur.
[2] Ter. Heautont.
[3] Epictetus, cap. 14. Si labor objectus fuerit tolerantiæ, convicium patientiæ, etc., si ita consueveris, vitiis non obtemperabis.
[4] Ter. Phor.   [5] Alciat. Embl.

PAGE 187

[1] Virg. Æn.
[2] Nat. Chytræus, Deliciis Europæ. Felix civitas quæ tempore pacis de bello cogitat.
[3] Occupet extremum scabies; mihi turpe relinqui est.—Hor.
[4] Lipsius, Epist. quæst. lib. 1, ep. 7.

PAGE 188

[1] Lipsius, Epist. lib. 1, epist. 7.
[2] Gloria comitem habet invidiam, pari onere premitur retinendo ac acquirendo.
[3] Quid aliud ambitiosus sibi parat quam ut probra ejus pateant? nemo vivens qui non habet in vita plura vituperatione quam laude digna; his malis non melius occurritur, quam si bene latueris.
[4] Et omnes fama per urbes garrula laudet.
[5] Sen. Her. Fur.   [6] Hor.

PAGE 189

[1] The right honourable Lady Frances, Countess Dowager of Exeter. The Lord Berkley.
[2] [A bad poet in Catullus (22), who had a high opinion of himself.]
[3] Distichon ejus in militem Christianum e Græco. Engraven on the tomb of Fr. Puccius the Florentine in Rome. Chytræus in Deliciis.
[4] Pædaretus in 300 Lacedæmoniorum numerum non electus risit, gratulari se diocns civitatem habere 300 cives se meliores.

PAGE 190

[1] Kissing goes by favour.
[2] Æneas Syl. de miser. curial. Dantur honores in curiis non secundum honores et virtutes, sed ut quisque ditior est atque potentior, eo magis honoratur.
[3] Sesellius, lib. 2 de repub. Gallorum. Favore apud nos et gratia plerumque res agitur; et qui commodum aliquem nacti sunt intercessorem, aditum fere habent ad omnes præfecturas.
[4] Imperiti periti munus occupat, et sic apud vulgus habetur. Ille profitetur mille coronatis, cum nec decem mereatur; alius e diverso mille dignus, vix decem consequi potest.
[5] Epist. dedic. disput. Zeubbeo Bondemontio et Cosmo Ruccelaio.
[6] Quam is qui regnat, et regnandi sit imperitus.
[7] Lib. 22 Hist.
[8] Ministri locupletiores sunt iis quibus ministratur.

II—U 887

PAGE 191

[1] Hor. lib. 2, Sat. 5.   [2] Solomon, Eccles. ix, 11.   [3] Sat. Menip.
[4] Tale quid est apud Valent. Andream, Apolog. manip. 5, apol. 39.

PAGE 192

[1] Stella Fomalhaut immortalitatem dabit.
[2] Lib. de lib. propriis.   [3] Hor.
[4] Qui induit thoracem aut galeam, etc.
[5] [Two provinces of Moronia (Foolsland), in Joseph Hall's Mundus
Alter et Idem].

PAGE 193

[1] Lib. 4 de guber. Dei. Quid est dignitas indigno nisi circulus aureus
in naribus suis?
[2] In Lysandro.   [3] Ovid. Met.
[4] Magistratus virum indicat.
[5] Ideo boni viri aliquando gratiam non accipiunt, ne in superbiam
eleventur ventositate jactantiæ, ne altitudo muneris negligentiores efficiat.
[6] Ælian.   [7] Injuriarum remedium est oblivio.   [8] Matt. xviii, 22.

PAGE 194

[1] Matt. v, 39.   [2] Rom. xii, 18.
[3] Si toleras injuriam, victor evadis; qui enim pecuniis privatus est, non
est privatus victoria in hac philosophia.
[4] Dispeream nisi te ultus fuero: dispeream nisi ut me deinceps ames
effecero.
[5] Joach. Camerarius, Embl. 21, cent. 1.
[6] [The Colonnas.]   [7] Heliodorus.
[8] Reipsa reperi nihil esse homini melius facilitate et clementia.—Ter.
Adelp.   [9] Ovid.   [10] Camden, in Glouc.

PAGE 195

[1] Usque ad pectus ingressus est, aquam, etc.; cymbam amplectens,
Sapientissime rex, ait, tua humilitas meam vicit superbiam, et sapientia
triumphavit ineptiam; collum ascende quod contra te fatuus erexi, intrabis
terram quam hodie fecit tuam benignitas, etc.
[2] Chrysostom.   Contumeliis affectus est et eas pertulit; opprobriis, nec
ultus est; verberibus cæsus, nec vicem reddidit.
[3] Rom. xii, 14.   [4] Prov.
[5] Contend not with a greater man.—[Eccles. vi, 10].
[6] Occidere possunt.
[7] Non facile aut tutum in eum scribere qui potest proscribere.
[8] Arcana tacere, otium recte collocare ,injuriam posse ferre, difficillimum.
[9] Rom. xii.   [10] Ps. xiii, 12.
[11] Nullus tam severe inimicum suum ulcisci potest, quam Deus solet
miserorum oppressores.
[12] Arcturus in Plaut.

PAGE 196

[1] Hor. Od. 3, 2.   [2] Wisd. xi, 16.   [3] Juvenal.
[4] Apud Christianos non qui patitur, sed qui facit injuriam miser est.—
Leo, Ser.

PAGE 197

[1] Neque præcepisset Deus si grave fuisset; sed qua ratione potero?
facile si cœlum suspexeris, et ejus pulchritudine, et quod pollicetur Deus,
etc.

² Valer. lib. 4, cap. 1.   ³ Ep. Q. frat.
⁴ Camerarius, Emb. 75, cent. 2.
⁵ Papæ, inquit: nullum animal tam pusillum quod non cupiat ulcisci.
⁶ Quod tibi fieri non vis, alteri ne feceris.   ⁷ 1 Pet. ii.
⁸ Siquidem malorum proprium est inferre damna, et bonorum pedissequa est injuria.

PAGE 198

¹ Alciat. Emb.
² Naturam expellas furca licet usque recurret.
³ By many indignities we come to dignities. Tibi subjicito quæ fiunt aliis, furtum convicia, etc. Et in iis in te admissis non excandesces.—Epictetus.
⁴ Plutarch. Quinquagies Catoni dies dicta ab inimicis.
⁵ Lib. 18.
⁶ Hoc scio pro certo quod si cum stercore certo, Vinco seu vincor, semper ego maculor.   ⁷ Lib. 8, cap. 2.

PAGE 199

¹ Obloquutus est, probrumque tibi intulit quispiam, sive vera is dixerit, sive falsa, maximam tibi coronam texueris si mansuete convicium tuleris.—Chrys. in 6 cap. ad Rom. ser. 10.
² Tullius, epist. Dolabellæ. Tu forti sis animo; et tua moderatio, constantia, eorum infamet injuriam.
³ Boethius, Consol. lib. 4, pros. 3.

PAGE 200

¹ Ter. Phor.

PAGE 201

¹ Camerar. Emb. 61, cent. 3.
² Lipsius, Elect. lib. 3, ult. Latrant me; jaceo, ac taceo, etc.
³ Catullus.
⁴ The symbol of J. Kevenheder, a Carinthian baron, saith Sambucus.
⁵ The symbol of Gonzaga, Duke of Mantua.   ⁶ Pers. Sat. 1.
⁷ Magni animi est injurias despicere.—Seneca de ira, cap. 31.
⁸ Quid turpius quam sapientis vitam ex insipientis sermone pendere?—Tullius, 2 de finibus.

PAGE 202

¹ Tua te conscientia salvare, in cubiculum ingredere, ubi secure requiescas. Minuit se quodammodo proba bonitas conscientiæ secretum.—Boethius, lib. 1, pros. 4.
² Ringantur licet et maledicant; Palladium illud pectori oppono, non moveri: consisto modestiæ veluti sudi innitens, excipio et frango stultissimum impetum livoris.—Putean. lib. 2, epist. 58.
³ Mil. Glor. Act. 3, Plautus.

PAGE 203

¹ Bion said his father was a rogue, his mother a whore, to prevent obloquy, and to show that naught belonged to him but goods of the mind.

PAGE 204

¹ Lib. 2, ep. 25.   ² Nosce teipsum.   ³ Contentus abi.
⁴ Ne fidas opibus, neque parasitis, trahunt in præcipitium.
⁵ Pacem cum hominibus habe, bellum cum vitiis. Otho. 2 imperat. symb.

⁶ Dæmon te nunquam otiosum inveniat.—Hieron.
⁷ Diu deliberandum quod statuendum est semel.
⁸ Insipientis est dicere Non putaram.
⁹ Ames parentem, si æquum; aliter, feras; præstes parentibus pietatem, amicis dilectionem.
¹⁰ Comprime linguam. Quid de quoque viro et cui dicas sæpe caveto. Libentius audias quam loquaris; vive ut vivas.
¹¹ Epictetus. Optime feceris si ea fugeris quæ in alio reprehendis. Nemini dixeris quæ nolis efferri.
¹² Fuge susurrones. Percontatorem fugito, etc.
¹³ Sint sales sine vilitate.—Sen.   ¹⁴ Sponde, presto noxa.
¹⁵ Camerar. Emb. 55, cent. 2. Cave cui credas, vel nemini fidas.—Epicharmus.
¹⁶ Tecum habita.   ¹⁷ Bis dat qui cito dat.
¹⁸ Post est occasio calva.   ¹⁹ Nimia familiaritas parit contemptum.
²⁰ Mendacium servile vitium.
²¹ Arcanum neque tu scrutaberis ullius unquam, Commissumque teges.—Hor. lib. 1, Ep. 19.   Nec tua laudabis studia aut aliena reprendes.—Hor. lib. 1, Ep. 18.
²² Ne te quæsiveris extra.
²³ Stultum est timere, quod vitari non potest.
²⁴ De re amissa irreparabili ne doleas.
²⁵ Tanti eris aliis quanti tibi fueris.
²⁶ Neminem cito laudes vel accuses.
²⁷ Nullius hospitis grata est mora longa.

Page 205

¹ Solonis lex apud Aristotelem; Gellius, lib. 2, cap. 12.
² Nullum locum putes sine teste, semper adesse Deum cogita.
³ Secreto amicos admone, lauda palam.
⁴ Ut ameris amabilis esto. Eros et Anteros gemelli Veneris, amatio et redamatio. Plat.
⁵ Dum fata sinunt vivite læti.—Seneca.
⁶ Id apprime in vita utile, ex aliis observare sibi quod ex usu siet.—Ter.
⁷ Dum furor in cursu currenti cede furori. Cretizandum cum Crete. Temporibus servi, nec contra flamina flato.
⁸ Nulla certior custodia innocentia: inexpugnabile munimentum munimento non egere.
⁹ Unicuique suum onus intolerabile videtur.   ¹⁰ Livius.

Page 206

¹ Ter. scen. 2, Adelphi.   ² Plautus.   ³ Petronius, Catal.

Page 207

¹ Parmeno Cælestinæ, Act. 8. Si stultitia dolor esset, in nulla non domo ejulatus audires.
² Busbequius; Sandys, lib. 1, fol. 89.
³ Quis hodie beatior, quam cui licet stultum esse, et eorundam immunitatibus frui?—Sat. Menip.   ⁴ Lib. Hist.
⁵ Parvo viventes laboriosi, longævi, suo contenti, ad centum annos vivunt.
⁶ Lib. 6 de Nup. Philol. Ultra humanam fragilitatem prolixi, ut immature pereat qui centenarius moriatur, etc.   ⁷ [Perm.]

Page 208

¹ Victus eorum caseo et lacte consistit, potus aqua et serum ; pisces loco panis habent; ita multos annos sæpe 250 absque medico et medicina vivunt.

² Lib. de 4 complex.
³ Per mortes agunt experimenta et animas nostras negotiantur; et quod aliis exitiale hominem occidere, iis impunitas summa.—Plinius.
⁴ Juven.
⁵ Omnis morbus lethalis aut curabilis, in vitam desinit aut in mortem. Utroque igitur modo medicina inutilis; si lethalis, curari non potest; si curabilis, non requirit medicum: natura expellet.
⁶ In Interpretationes politico-morales in 7 Aphorism. Hippoc. libros.

PAGE 209

¹ Præfat. de contrad. med.
² Opinio facit medicos: a fair gown, a velvet cap, the name of a doctor is all in all.
³ Morbus alius pro alio curatur; aliud remedium pro alio.
⁴ Contrarias proferunt sententias.—Card.
⁵ Lib. 3 de sap. Omnes artes fraudem admittunt, sola medicina sponte eam accersit.

PAGE 210

¹ Omnis ægrotus propria culpa perit, sed nemo nisi medici beneficio restituitur.—Agrippa.
² Lib. 3, Crat. ep. Winceslao Raphæno. Ausim dicere, tot pulsuum differentias, quæ describuntur a Galeno, nec a quoquam intelligi, nec observari posse.
³ Lib. 28, cap. 7, Syntax. art. mirab. Mallem ego expertis credere solum, quam mere ratiocinantibus: neque satis laudare possum institutum Babylonicum, etc.

PAGE 211

¹ Herod. Euterpe, de Ægyptiis. Apud eos singulorum morborum sunt singuli medici; alius curat oculos, alius dentes, alius caput, partes occultas alius.
² Cyrop. lib. 1. Velut vestium fractarum resarcinatores, etc.
³ Chrys. Hom.
⁴ Prudens et pius medicus morbum ante expellere satagit, cibis medicinalibus, quam puris medicinis.
⁵ Cuicunque potest per alimenta restitui sanitas, fugiendus est penitus usus medicamentorum.
⁶ Modestus et sapiens medicus nunquam properabit ad pharmaciam, nisi cogente necessitate.

PAGE 212

¹ Quicunque pharmacatur in juventute, deflebit in senectute.
² Hildesh. Spic. 2 de mel. fol. 276. Nulla est ferme medicina purgans, quæ non aliquam de viribus et partibus corporis deprædatur.
³ Lib. 1, et Bart. lib. 8, cap. 12.
⁴ De vict. acut. Omne purgans medicamentum, corpori purgato contrarium, etc., succos et spiritus abducit, substantiam corporis aufert.
⁵ Hesiod. Op.
⁶ Heurnius, præf. pra. med. Quot morborum sunt ideæ, tot remediorum genera variis potentiis decorata.
⁷ Penottus, Denar. med. Quæcunque regio producit simplicia, pro morbis regionis; crescit raro absinthium in Italia, quod ibi plerumque morbi calidi, sed cicuta, papaver, et herbæ frigidæ; apud nos Germanos et Polonos ubique provenit absinthium.

PAGE 213

[1] Quum in villam venit, consideravit quæ ibi crescebant medicamenta, simplicia frequentiora, et iis plerumque usus distillatis, et aliter, alimbacum ideo argenteum circumferens.
[2] Geog. Ad quos magnus herbariorum numerus undique confluit.
[3] Baldus mons [Monte Baldo] prope Benacum herbilegis maxime notus.
[4] Herbæ medicis utiles omnium in Apulia feracissimæ.
[5] Sincerus, Itiner. Gallia.
[6] Qui se nihil effecisse arbitrantur, nisi Indiam, Æthiopiam, Arabiam, et ultra Garamantas a tribus mundi partibus exquisita remedia corradunt. Tutius sæpe medetur rustica anus una, etc.
[7] Ep. lib. 8. Proximorum incuriosi longinqua sectamur, et ad ea cognoscenda iter ingredi et mare transmittere solemus; at quæ sub oculis posita negligimus.

PAGE 214

[1] Exotica rejecit, domesticis solum nos contentos esse voluit.—Melch. Adamus, vit. ejus.
[2] Instit. lib. 1, cap. 8, sec. 1. Ad exquisitam curandi rationem, quorum cognitio imprimis necessaria est.
[3] Quæ cæca vi ac specifica qualitate morbos futuros arcent.—Lib. 1, cap. 10, Instit. Phar.

PAGE 215

[1] Galen, lib. Hepar lupi hepaticos curat.
[2] Stercus pecoris ad epilepsiam, etc.
[3] Priestpintle, rocket.   [4] Sabina fetum educit.
[5] Wecker. Vide Oswaldum Crollium, lib. de internis rerum signaturis, de herbis particularibus parti cuique convenientibus.
[6] Idem Laurentius, cap. 9.
[7] Dicor borago, gaudia semper ago.
[8] Vino infusum hilaritatem facit.   [9] Odyss. 4.

PAGE 216

[1] Lib. 2, cap. 2, Prax. med. Mira vi lætitiam præbet et cor confirmat, vapores melancholicos purgat a spiritibus.
[2] Proprium est ejus animum hilarem reddere, concoctionem juvare, cerebri obstructiones resecare, sollicitudines fugare, sollicitas imaginationes tollere.
[3] Non solum ad viperarum morsus, comitiales, vertiginosos; sed per se accommodata radix tristitiam discutit, hilaritatemque conciliat.
[4] Bilem utramque detrahit, sanguinem purgat.

PAGE 217

[1] Lib. 7, cap. 5. Laet, Occid. Indiæ descrip. lib. 10, cap. 2.
[2] Heurnius, lib. 2, consil. 185, Scoltzii consil. 77.
[3] Præf. Denar. med. Omnes capitis dolores et phantasmata tollit; scias nullam herbam in terris huic comparandam viribus et bonitate nasci.
[4] Optimum medicamentum in celeri cordis confortatione, et ad omnes qui tristantur, etc.
[5] Rondeletius helenium, quod vim habet miram ad hilaritatem et multi pro secreto habent. Sckenkius, Observ. med. cent. 5, observ. 86.
[6] Afflictas mentes relevat, animi imaginationes et dæmones expellit.
[7] Sckenkius, Mizaldus, Rhasis.

PAGE 218

[1] Cratonis Ep. vol. 1. Credat qui vult gemmas mirabilia efficere; mihi, qui et ratione et experientia didici aliter rem habere, nullus facile persuadebit falsum esse verum.   [2] Lib. de gemmis.
[3] Margaritæ et corallum ad melancholiam præcipue valent.
[4] Margaritæ et gemmæ spiritus confortant et cor, melancholiam fugant.
[5] Præfat. ad Lap. prec. lib. 2, sect. 2, de mat. med. Regum coronas ornant, digitos illustrant, supellectilem ditant, e fascino tuentur, morbis medentur, sanitatem conservant, mentem exhilarant, tristitiam pellunt.
[6] Encelius, lib. 3, cap. 4. Suspensus vel ebibitus tristitiæ multum resistit, et cor recreat.
[7] Idem, cap. 5 et cap. 6, de hyacintho et topazio. Iram sedat, et animi tristitiam pellit.
[8] Lapis hic gestatus aut ebibitus prudentiam auget, nocturnos timores pellit; insanos hac sanavi, et quum lapidem abjecerint, erupit iterum stultitia.
[9] Inducit sapientiam, fugat stultitiam. Idem Cardanus, lunaticos juvat.
[10] Confert ad bonum intellectum, comprimit malas cogitationes, etc. Alacres reddit.
[11] Albertus; Encelius, cap. 44, lib. 3; Plin. lib. 37, cap. 10; Jacobus de Dondis: Dextro brachio alligatus sanat lunaticos, insanos, facit amabiles, jucundos.
[12] Valet contra phantasticas illusiones ex melancholia.

PAGE 219

[1] Amentes sanat, tristitiam pellit, iram, etc.
[2] Valet ad fugandos timores et dæmones, turbulenta somnia abigit, et nocturnos puerorum timores compescit.
[3] Somnia læta facit argenteo annulo gestatus.
[4] Atræ bili adversatur, omnium gemmarum pulcherrima, cœli colorem refert, animum ab errore liberat, mores in melius mutat.
[5] Longis mœroribus feliciter medetur, deliquiis, etc.
[6] Sec. 5, memb. 1, subs. 5.
[7] Gestamen lapidum et gemmarum maximum fert auxilium et juvamen; unde qui dites sunt gemmas secum ferre student.
[8] Margaritæ et uniones quæ a conchis et piscibus apud Persas et Indos, valde cordiales sunt, etc.
[9] Aurum lætitiam generat, non in corde, sed in arca virorum.

PAGE 220

[1] Chaucer.
[2] Aurum non aurum. Noxium ob aquas rodentes.
[3] Ep. ad Monavium. Metallica omnia in universum quovismodo parata, nec tuto nec commode intra corpus sumi.
[4] In Parag. Stultissimus pilus occipitis mei plus scit quam omnes vestri doctores, et calceorum meorum annuli doctiores sunt quam vester Galenus et Avicenna, barba mea plus experta est quam vestræ omnes academiæ.
[5] Vide Ernestum Burgravium, edit. Franaker [? Frankfurt], 8vo, 1611, Crollius, and others.
[6] Plus proficiet gutta mea quam tot eorum drachmæ et unciæ.

PAGE 221

[1] Nonnulli huic supra modum indulgent, usum etsi non adeo magnum, non tamen abjiciendum censeo.

[2] Ausim dicere neminem medicum excellentem qui non in hac distillatione chymica sit versatus. Morbi chronici devinci citra metallica vix possint, aut ubi sanguis corrumpitur.

[3] Fraudes hominum et ingeniorum capturæ, officinas invenere istas, in quibus sua cuique venalis promittitur vita; statim compositiones et mixturæ inexplicabiles ex Arabia et India, ulceri parvo medicina a Rubro Mari importatur.

[4] Arnoldus, Aphor. 15. Fallax medicus qui, potens mederi simplicibus, composita dolose aut frustra quærit.

[5] Lib. 1, sect. 1, cap. 8. Dum infinita medicamenta miscent, laudem sibi comparare student, et in hoc studio alter alterum superare conatur, dum quisque quo plura miscuerit, eo se doctiorem putat; inde fit ut suam prodant inscitiam, dum ostentant peritiam, et se ridiculos exhibeant, etc.

[6] Multo plus periculi a medicamento quam a morbo, etc.

Page 222

[1] Expedit. in Sinas, lib. 1, cap. 5. Præcepta medici dant nostris diversa, in medendo non infelices; pharmacis utuntur simplicibus, herbis, radicibus, etc.; tota eorum medicina nostræ herbariæ præceptis continetur; nullus ludus hujus artis, quisque privatus a quolibet magistro eruditur.

[2] Lib. de aqua.   [3] Opusc. de dos.

[4] Subtil. cap. de scientiis.

Page 223

[1] Quercetan, Pharmacop. restitut. cap. 2. Nobilissimum et utilissimum inventum summa cum necessitate adinventum et introductum.

[2] Cap. 25, Tetrabib. 4, ser. 2. Necessitas nunc cogit aliquando noxia quærere remedia, et ex simplicibus compositas facere, tum ad saporem, odorem, palati gratiam, ad correctionem simplicium, tum ad futuros usus, conservationem, etc.

[3] Cum simplicia non possunt necessitas cogit ad composita.

[4] Lips. Epist.   [5] Theod. Prodromus, Amor. lib. 9.

Page 224

[1] Sanguinem corruptum emaculat, scabiem abolet, lepram curat, spiritus recreat, et animum exhilarat. Melancholicos humores per urinam educit, et cerebrum a crassis, ærumnosis melancholiæ fumis purgat, quibus addo dementes et furiosos vinculis retinendos plurimum juvat, et ad rationis usum ducit. Testis est mihi conscientia, quod viderim matronam quandam hinc liberatam, quæ frequentius ex iracundia demens, et impos animi dicenda tacenda loquebatur, adeo furens ut ligari cogeretur. Fuit ei præstantissimo remedio vini istius usus, indicatus a peregrino homine mendico, eleemosynam præ foribus dictæ matronæ implorante.

[2] Iis qui tristantur sine causa, et vitant amicorum societatem et tremunt corde.

[3] Modo non inflammetur melancholia, aut calidiore temperamento sint.

Page 225

[1] [Lozenges].   [2] Heurnius. Datur in sero lactis, aut vino.

Page 226

[1] Veratri modo expurgat cerebrum, roborat memoriam.—Fuchsius.

[2] Crassos et biliosos humores per vomitum educit.

[3] Vomitum et menses ciet; valet ad hydrop., etc.

[4] Materias atras educit.

[5] Ab arte ideo rejiciendum, ob periculum suffocationis.

[6] Cap. 16. Magna vi educit, et molestia cum summa.
[7] Quondam terribile.
[8] Multi studiorum gratia ad providenda acrius quæ commentabantur.
[9] Medetur comitialibus melancholicis, podagricis; vetatur senibus, pueris, mollibus, et effeminatis.
[10] Collect. lib. 8, cap. 3. In affectionibus iis quæ difficulter curantur, helleborum damus.
[11] Non sine summa cautione hoc remedio utemur; est enim validissimum, et quum vires antimonii contemnit morbus, in auxilium evocatur, modo valide vires efflorescant.

PAGE 227

[1] Aetius, Tetrab. cap. 1, ser. 2. Iis solum dari vult helleborum album, qui secus spem non habent, non iis qui syncopem timent, etc.
[2] Cum salute multorum.   [3] Cap. 12 de morbis cap.
[4] Nos facillime utimur nostro præparato helleboro albo.
[5] In lib. 5 Dioscor. cap. 3. Omnibus opitulatur morbis, quos atra bilis excitavit, comitialibus, iisque præsertim qui hypocondriacas obtinent passiones.
[6] Andreas Gallus, Tridentinus medicus, salutem huic medicamento post Deum debet.
[7] Integræ sanitati brevi restitutus; id quod aliis accidisse scio, qui hoc mirabili medicamento usi sunt.

PAGE 228

[1] Qui melancholicus factus plane desipiebat, multaque stulte loquebatur, huic exhibitum 12 gr. stibium, quod paulo post atram bilem ex alvo eduxit (ut ego vidi, qui vocatus tanquam ad miraculum adfui testari possum), et ramenta tanquam carnis dissecta in partes; totum excrementum tanquam sanguinem nigerrimum repræsentabat.
[2] Antimonium venenum, non medicamentum.
[3] Cratonis ep. sect. vel ad Monavium ep. In utramque partem dignissimum medicamentum, si recte utentur, secus venenum.

PAGE 229

[1] Mærores fugant; utilissime dantur melancholicis et quaternariis.
[2] Millies horum vires expertus sum.
[3] Sal nitrum, sal ammoniacum, dracontii radix, dictamnum.
[4] Calet ordine secundo, siccat primo, adversus omnia vitia atræ bilis valet, sanguinem mundat, spiritus illustrat, mœrorem discutit herba mirifica.
[5] Cap. 4, lib. 2.   [6] Recentiores negant ora venarum resecare.
[7] An aloe aperiat ora venarum, lib. 9, cont. 3.
[8] Vapores abstergit a vitalibus partibus.
[9] Tract. 15, cap. 6. Bonus Alexander, tantam lapide Armeno confidentiam habuit, ut omnes melancholicas passiones ab eo curari posse crederet, et ego inde sæpissime usus sum, et in ejus exhibitione nunquam fraudatus fui.

PAGE 230

[1] Maurorum medici hoc lapide plerumque purgant melancholiam, etc.
[2] Quo ego sæpe feliciter usus sum, et magno cum auxilio.
[3] Si non hoc, nihil restat nisi helleborus, et lapis Armenus.—Consil. 184 Scoltzii.
[4] Multa corpora vidi gravissime hinc agitata, et stomacho multum obfuisse.

⁵ [Melampus.]   ⁶ Cum vidisset ab eo curari capras furentes, etc.
⁷ Lib 6 Simpl. med.
⁸ Pseudolo, Act. 4. scen. ult.   Helleboro hisce hominibus opus est.

Page 231

¹ Hor.   ² In Satyr.
³ Crato, consil. 16, lib. 2.   Etsi multi magni viri probent, in bonam partem accipiant medici, non probem.
⁴ Vescuntur veratro coturnices quod hominibus toxicum est.
⁵ Lib. 23, cap. 7, 12, 14.   ⁶ De var. hist.
⁷ Corpus incolume reddit, et juvenile efficit.
⁸ Veteres non sine causa usi sunt: Difficilis ex helleboro purgatio, et
terroris plena, sed robustis datur tamen, etc.

Page 232

¹ Innocens medicamentum, modo rite paretur.
² Absit jactantia, ego primus præbere cœpi, etc.
³ In Cathart.   Ex una sola evacuatione furor cessavit et quietus inde
vixit.   Tale exemplum apud Sckenkium et apud Scoltzium, ep. 231.
P. Monavius se stolidum curasse jactat hoc epoto tribus aut quatuor vicibus.
⁴ Ultimum refugium, extremum medicamentum, quod cætera omnia
claudit; quæcunque cæteris laxativis pelli non possunt ad hunc pertinent;
si non huic, nulli cedunt.
⁵ Testari possum me sexcentis hominibus helleborum nigrum exhibuisse,
nullo prorsus incommodo, etc.

Page 233

¹ Pharmacop.   Optimum est ad maniam et omnes melancholicos
affectus, tum intra assumptum, tum extra, secus capiti cum linteolis in eo
madefactis tepide admotum.
² Epist. Matth. lib. 3.   Tales syrupi nocentissimi et omnibus modis
extirpandi.
³ Purgantia censebant medicamenta, non unum humorem attrahere,
sed quemcunque attigerint in suam naturam convertere.

Page 234

¹ Religantur omnes exsiccantes medicinæ, ut aloe, hiera, pilulæ quæcunque.
² Contra eos qui lingua vulgari et vernacula remedia et medicamenta
præscribunt, et quibusvis communia faciunt.
³ Quis, quantum, quando?

Page 235

¹ Fernelius, lib. 2, cap. 19.
² Renodeus, lib. 5, cap. 21.   De his Mercurialis, lib. 3 de composit.
med. cap. 24, Heurnius, lib. 1 Prax. med., Wecker, etc.

Page 236

¹ Cont. lib. 1, cap. 9.   Festines ad impinguationem, et cum impinguantur,
removetur malum.   ² Beneficium ventris.

Page 237

¹ Si ex primario cerebri affectu melancholici evaserint, sanguinis detractione non indigent, nisi ob alias causas sanguis mittatur, si multus in
vasis, etc., frustra enim fatigatur corpus, etc.
² Competit iis phlebotomia frontis.

[3] Si sanguis abundet, quod scitur ex venarum repletione, victus ratione præcedente, risu ægri, ætate, et aliis, tundatur mediana; et si sanguis apparet clarus et ruber, supprimatur; aut si vere, si niger aut crassus, permittatur fluere pro viribus ægri, dein post 8 vel. 12 diem aperiatur cephalica partis magis affectæ, et vena frontis, aut sanguis provocetur setis per nares, etc.

[4] Si quibus consuetæ suæ suppressæ sunt menses, etc., talo secare oportet, aut vena frontis si sanguis peccet cerebro.

[5] Nisi ortum ducat a sanguine, ne morbus inde augeatur: phlebotomia refrigerat et exsiccat, nisi corpus sit valde sanguineum, rubicundum.

[6] Cum sanguinem detrahere oportet, deliberatione indiget.—Aretæus, lib. 7, cap. 5.

Page 238

[1] A lenioribus auspicandum (Valescus, Piso, Bruel), rariusque medicamentis purgantibus utendum, ni sit opus.

[2] Quia corpus exsiccant, morbum augent.

[3] Guianerius, Tract. 15, cap. 6.

[4] Piso.   [5] Rhasis.   Sæpe valent ex helleboro.

[6] Lib. 7.   Exiguis medicamentis morbus non obsequitur.

[7] Modo caute detur et robustis.   [8] Consil. 10, lib. 1.

Page 239

[1] Plin. lib. 31, cap. 6.   Navigationes ob vomitionem prosunt plurimis morbis capitis, et omnibus ob quos helleborum bibitur.   Idem Dioscorides, lib. 5, cap. 13; Avicenna tertia imprimis.

[2] Nunquam dedimus, quin ex una aut altera assumptione, Deo juvante, fuerint ad salutem restituti.

[3] Lib. 2.   Inter composita purgantia melancholiam.

[4] Longo experimento a se observatum esse, melancholicos sine offensa egregie curandos valere.   Idem, responsione ad Aubertum, veratrum nigrum, alias timidum et periculosum, vini spiritu etiam et oleo commodum sic usui redditur ut etiam pueris tuto administrari possit.

[5] Certum est hujus herbæ virtutem maximam et mirabilem esse, parumque distare a balsamo.   Et qui norit eo recte uti, plus habet artis quam tota scribentium cohors aut omnes doctores in Germania.

[6] Quo feliciter usus sum.

[7] Hoc posito quod aliæ medicina non valeant, ista tunc Dei misericordia valebit, et est medicina coronata, quæ secretissime teneatur.

[8] Lib. de artif. med.

Page 240

[1] Sect. 3.   Optimum remedium aqua composita Savonarola.

[2] Sckenkius, observ. 31.

[3] Donatus ab Altomari, cap. 7.   Testor Deum, me multos melancholicos hujus solius syrupi usu curasse, facta prius purgatione.

[4] Centum ova et unum.   Quolibet mane sumant ova sorbilia, cum sequenti pulvere supra ovum aspersa, et contineant quousque assumpserint centum et unum, maniacis et melancholicis utilissimum remedium.

[5] Quercetan, cap. 4 Phar.; Oswaldus Crollius.

[6] Cap. 1.   Licet tota Galenistarum schola, mineralia non sine impio et ingrato fastu a sua practica detestentur; tamen in gravioribus morbis omni vegetabilium derelicto subsidio, ad mineralia confugiunt, licet ea temere, ignaviter, et inutiliter usurpent.   Ad finem libri.

Page 241

[1] Veteres maledictis incessit, vincit, et contra omnem antiquitatem coronatur, ipseque a se victor declaratur.—Gal. lib. 1 Meth. cap. 2.

[2] Codronchus, de sale absinthii.

[3] Idem Paracelsus in medicina, quod Lutherus in theologia.

[4] Disput. in eundem, parte 1. Magus ebrius, illiteratus, dæmonem præceptorem habuit, dæmones familiares, etc.

[5] Master D. Lapworth.

[6] Ant. Philos. cap. de melan. Frictio vertice, etc.

[7] Aqua fortissima purgans os, nares, quam non vult auro vendere.

PAGE 242

[1] Mercurialis, consil. 6 et 30. Hæmorrhoidum et mensium provocatio juvat, modo ex eorum suppressione ortum habuerit.

[2] Laurentius, Bruel, etc.

[3] P. Bayerus, lib. 2, cap. 13. Naribus, etc.

[4] Cucurbitulæ siccæ, et fontanellæ crure sinistro.

[5] Hildesheim, Spicil. 2. Vapores a cerebro trahendi sunt frictionibus universi, cucurbitulis siccis, humeris ac dorso affixis, circa pedes et crura.

[6] Fontanellam aperi juxta occipitum, aut brachium.

[7] Balani, ligaturæ, frictiones, etc.

[8] Cauterium fiat sutura coronali, diu fluere permittantur loca ulcerosa. Trepano etiam cranii densitas imminui poterit, ut vaporibus fuliginosis exitus pateat.

[9] Quoniam difficulter cedit aliis medicamentis, ideo fiat in vertice cauterium, aut crure sinistro infra genu.

[10] Fiant duo aut tria cauteria, cum ossis perforatione.

[11] Vidi Romæ melancholicum qui, adhibitis multis remediis, sanari non poterat; sed cum cranium gladio fractum esset, optime sanatus est.

[12] Et alterum vidi melancholicum, qui ex alto cadens, non sine astantium admiratione liberatus est.

[13] Radatur caput et fiat cauterium in capite; procul dubio ista faciunt ad fumorum exhalationem; vidi melancholicum a fortuna gladio vulneratum, et cranium fractum; quamdiu vulnus apertum, curatus optime; at cum vulnus sanatum, reversa est mania.

[14] Usque ad duram matrem trepanari feci, et per mensem aperte stetit.

PAGE 243

[1] Cordis ratio semper habenda quod cerebro compatitur, et esse invicem officiunt.

[2] Aphor. 38. Medicina theriacalis præ cæteris eligenda.

[3] Galen. de temp. lib. 3, cap. 3. Moderate vinum sumptum acuit ingenium.

[4] Tardos aliter et tristes thuris in modum exhalare facit.

[5] Hilaritatem ut oleum flammam excitat.

[6] Viribus retinendis cardiacum eximium, nutriendo corpori alimentum optimum, ætatem floridam facit, calorem innatum fovet, concoctionem juvat, stomachum roborat, excrementis viam parat, urinam movet, somnum conciliat, venena, frigidos flatus dissipat, crassos humores attenuat, coquit, discutit, etc.

[7] Hor. lib. 2, od. 11.   [8] Odyss. 4.

PAGE 244

[1] Pausanias.   [2] Siracides [Ecclus.] xxxiv, 28.

[3] Legitur et prisci Catonis, Sæpe mero caluisse virtus.

[4] In pocula et aleam se præcipitavit, et iis fere tempus traduxit, ut ægram crapula mentem levaret, et conditionis præsentis cogitationes quibus agitabatur sobrius vitaret.

[5] So did the Athenians of old, as Suidas relates, and so do the Germans at this day.

[6] Lib. 6, cap. 23 et 24, de rerum proprietat.   [7] Esther i, 8.

[1] Tract. 1, Cont. lib. 1. Non est res laudabilior eo, vel cura melior; qui melancholicus, utatur societate hominum et biberia; et qui potest sustinere usum vini, non indiget alia medicina, quod eo sunt omnia ad usum necessaria hujus passionis.

[2] Tum quod sequatur inde sudor, vomitio, urina, a quibus superfluitates a corpore removentur et remanet corpus mundum.   [3] Hor.

[4] Lib. 15, 2, Noct. Att. Vigorem animi moderato vini usu tueamur, et calefacto simul refotoque animo, si quid in eo vel frigidæ tristitiæ, vel torpentis verecundiæ fuerit, diluamus.

[5] Hor. lib. 1, Od. 27.   [6] Od. 7, lib. 1, 31.

[7] Nam præstat ebrium me quam mortuum jacere.

[1] Ephes. v, 18. ser. 19, in cap. 5.

[2] Lib. 14, 5. Nihil perniciosius viribus si modus absit, venenum.

[3] Theocritus, Idyl. 13. Vino dari lætitiam et dolorem.

[4] Renodeus.

[5] Mercurialis, consil. 25. Vinum frigidis optimum, et pessimum ferina melancholia.

[6] Fernelius, consil. 44 et 45, vinum prohibet assiduum, et aromata.

[7] Modo jecur non incendatur.

[1] Per 24 horas sensum doloris omnem tollit, et ridere facit.

[2] Hildesheim, Spicil. 2.

[3] Alkermes omnia vitalia viscera mire confortat.

[4] Contra omnes melancholicos affectus confert, ac certum est ipsius usu omnes cordis et corporis vires mirum in modum refici.

[5] Succinum vero albissimum confortat ventriculum, flatum discutit, urinam movet, etc.

[6] Garcias ab Horto, Aromatum lib. 1, cap. 15. Adversus omnes morbos melancholicos conducit, et venenum. Ego (inquit) utor in morbis melancholicis, etc., et deploratos hujus usu ad pristinam sanitatem restitui. See more in Bauhinus' book de lap. bezoar, cap. 45.

[7] Edit. 1617. Monspelii electuarium fit pretiosissimum alkerm., etc.

[1] Nihil morbum hunc æque exasperat, ac alimentorum vel calidiorum usus. Alkermes ideo suspectus, et quod semel moneam, caute adhibenda calida medicamenta.

[2] Sckenkius, lib. 1 Observat. de mania. Ad mentis alienationem, et desipientiam vitio cerebri obortam, in manuscripto codice Germanico, tale medicamentum reperi.

[3] Caput arietis nondum experti venerem, uno ictu amputatum, cornibus tantum demotis, integrum cum lana et pelle bene elixabis, tum aperto cerebrum eximes, et addens aromata, etc.

[4] Cinis testudinis ustus, et vino potus, melancholiam curat, et rasura cornu rhinocerotis, etc.—Sckenkius.

[5] Instat in matrice, quod sursum et deorsum ad odoris sensum præcipitatur.

[1] Viscount St. Albans.

[2] Ex decocto florum nymphææ, lactucæ, violarum, chamomilæ, althæææ, capitis vervecum, etc.

³ Inter auxilia multa adhibita, duo visa sunt remedium adferre, usus seri caprini cum extracto hellebori, et irrigatio ex lacte nymphææ, violarum, etc., suturæ coronali adhibita; his remediis sanitatem pristinam adeptus est.

⁴ Confert et pulmo arietis, calidus agnus per dorsum divisus, exenteratus, admotus sincipiti.

⁵ Semina cumini, rutæ, dauci, anethi cocta.

⁶ Lib. 3 de locis affect. ⁷ Tetrab. 2, ser. 1, cap. 10.

Page 250

¹ Cap. de mel. Collectum die Vener. hora Jovis cum ad energiam venit, i.e. ad plenilunium Julii, inde gesta et collo appensa hunc affectum apprime juvat et fanaticos spiritus expellit.

² Lib. de proprietat. animal. Ovis a lupo correptæ pellem non esse pro indumento corporis usurpandam, cordis enim palpitationem excitat, etc.

³ Mart. ⁴ Phar. lib. 1, cap. 12.

⁵ Aetius, cap. 31, Tet. 3, ser. 4.

⁶ Dioscorides, Ulysses Aldrovandus de aranea.

⁷ Mistress Dorothy Burton; she died 1629.

Page 251

¹ Solo somno curata est citra medici auxilium, fol. 154.

² Bellonius, Observat. lib. 3, cap. 15. Lassitudinem et labores animi tollunt; inde Garcias ab Horto, lib. 1, cap. 4, Simp. med.

Page 252

¹ Absinthium somnos allicit olfactu.

² Read Lemnius, lib. her. bib. cap. 2, of mandrake.

³ Hyoscyamus sub cervicali viridis.

⁴ Plantam pedis inungere pinguedine gliris dicunt efficacissimum, et quod vix credi potest, dentes inunctos ex sorditie aurium canis somnum profundum conciliare, etc.—Cardan, de rerum varietat.

⁵ Veni mecum lib.

Page 253

¹ Aut si quid incautius exciderit, aut, etc.

² Nam qua parte pavor simul est pudor additus illi.—Statius.

³ Olisiponensis medicus; pudor aut juvat aut lædit.

⁴ De mentis alienat. ⁵ Mr. Doctor Ashworth.

⁶ Facies nonnullis maxime calet rubetque, si se paululum exercuerint; nonnullis quiescentibus idem accidit, feminis præsertim; causa quicquid fervidum aut halituosum sanguinem facit.

⁷ Interim faciei prospiciendum ut ipsa refrigeretur; utrumque præstabit frequens potio ex aqua rosarum, violarum, nenupharis, etc.

⁸ Ad faciei ruborem aqua spermatis ranarum.

⁹ Recte utantur in æstate floribus cichorii saccharo conditis vel saccharo rosaceo, etc.

¹⁰ Solo usu decocti cichorii.

Page 254

¹ Utile imprimis noctu faciem illinire sanguine leporino, et mane aqua fragrorum vel aqua floribus verbasci cum succo limonum distillato abluere.

² Utile rubenti faciei caseum recentem imponere.

³ Consil. 21. lib. Unico vini haustu sit contentus.

⁴ Idem, consil. 283 Scoltzii. Laudatur conditus rosæ caninæ fructus ante prandium et cænam ad magnitudinem castaneæ. Decoctum radium sonchi, si ante cibum sumatur, valet plurimum.

⁵ Cucurbit. ad scapulas appositæ.

⁶ Piso. ⁷ Mediana præ cæteris.

NOTES
311

Page 255

[1] Succi melancholici malitia a sanguinis bonitate corrigitur.
[2] Perseverante malo, ex quacunque parte sanguinis detrahi debet.
[3] Observat. fol. 154. Curatus ex vulnere in crure ob cruorem amissum.
[4] Studium sit omne ut melancholicus impinguetur: ex quo enim pingues et carnosi, illico sani sunt.
[5] Hildesheim, Spicil. 2. Inter calida radix petroselini, apii, feniculi; inter frigida emulsio seminis melonum cum sero caprino, quod est commune vehiculum.
[6] Hoc unum præmoneo, domine, ut sis diligens circa victum, sine quo cætera remedia frustra adhibentur.

Page 256

[1] Laurentius, cap. 15. Evulsionis gratia venam internam alterius brachii secamus.
[2] Si pertinax morbus, venam fronte secabis.—Bruel.
[3] Ego maximam curam stomacho delegabo.—Octa. Horatianus, lib. 2, cap. 7.
[4] Citius et efficacius suas vires exercet quam solent decocta ac diluta in quantitate multa, et magna cum assumentium molestia desumpta. Flatus hic sal efficaciter dissipat, urinam movet, humores crassos abstergit, stomachum egregie confortat, cruditatem, nauseam, appetentiam mirum in modum renovat, etc.

Page 257

[1] Piso, Altomarus, Laurentius, cap. 15.
[2] His utendum sæpius iteratis: a vehementioribus semper abstinendum, ne ventrem exasperent.
[3] Lib. 2, cap. 1. Quoniam caliditate conjuncta est siccitas quæ malum auget.
[4] Quisquis frigidis auxiliis hoc morbo usus fuerit, is obstructionem aliaque symptomata augebit.
[5] Ventriculus plerumque frigidus, hepar calidum; quomodo ergo ventriculum calefaciet, vel refrigerabit hepar, sine alterius maximo detrimento?
[6] Significatum per literas, incredibilem utilitatem ex decocto chinæ, et sassafras percepisse.
[7] Tumorem splenis incurabilem sola cappari curavit, cibo tali ægritudine aptissimo: soloque usu aquæ, in qua faber ferrarius sæpe candens ferrum extinxerat, etc.
[8] Animalia quæ apud hos fabros educantur, exiguos habent lienes.
[9] Lib. 1, cap. 17.

Page 258

[1] Continuus ejus usus semper felicem in ægris finem est assecutus.
[2] Si hæmorrhoides fluxerint, nullum præstantius esset remedium, quæ sanguisugis admotis provocari poterunt.—Observat. lib. 1, pro hypoc. leguleio.
[3] Aliis apertio hæc in hoc morbo videtur utilissima; mihi non admodum probatur, quia sanguinem tenuem attrahit et crassum relinquit.
[4] Lib. 2, cap. 13. Omnes melancholici debent omittere urinam provocantia, quoniam per ea educitur subtile, et remanet crassum.
[5] Ego experientia probavi, multos hypocondriacos solo usu clysterum fuisse sanatos.
[6] In cruditate optimum, ventriculum arctius alligari.
[7] ℥j theriacæ, vere præsertim et æstate.
[8] Cons. 12, lib. 1.   [9] Cap. 33.
[10] Trincavellius, consil. 15. Cerotum pro sene melancholico ad jecur optimum.
[11] Emplastra pro splene.—Fernel. consil. 45.

PAGE 259

[1] Dropax e pice navali et oleo rutaceo affigatur ventriculo, et toti metaphreni.
[2] Cauteria cruribus inusta.
[3] Fontanellæ sint in utroque crure   [4] Lib. 1, cap. 17.
[5] De mentis alienat. cap. 3. Flatus egregie discutiunt materiamque evocant.

PAGE 260

[1] Cavendum hic diligenter a multum calefacientibus atque exsiccantibus, sive alimenta fuerint hæc, sive medicamenta: nonnulli enim, ut ventositates et rugitus compescant, hujusmodi utentes medicamentis, plurimum peccant, morbum sic augentes: debent enim medicamenta declinare ad calidum vel frigidum secundum exigentiam circumstantiarum, vel ut patiens inclinat ad cal. et frigid.
[2] Cap. 5, lib. 7.   [3] Piso, Bruel. Mire flatus resolvit.
[4] Lib. 1, cap. 17. Nonnullos præ tensione ventris deploratos illico restitutos his videmus.
[5] Velut incantamentum quoddam ex flatuoso spiritu, dolorem ortum levant.

PAGE 261

[1] Terebinthinam Cypriam habeant familiarem, ad quantitatem deglutiant nucis parvæ, tribus horis ante prandium vel cœnam, ter singulis septimanis prout expedire videbitur; nam præterquam quod alvum mollem efficit, obstructiones aperit, ventriculum purgat, urinam provocat, hepar mundificat.

THE THIRD PARTITION

THE SYNOPSIS OF THE THIRD PARTITION

Preface or Introduction. *Subsect.* 1.

Love and Love-Melancholy, *Memb.* 1, *Sect.* 1.

Love's definition, pedigree, object, fair, amiable, gracious, and pleasant, from which comes beauty, grace, which all desire and love, parts affected.

Division or kinds, *Subs.* 2.

Natural, in things without life, as love and hatred of elements; and with life, as vegetal, vine and elm, sympathy, antipathy, etc.

Sensible, as of beasts, for pleasure, preservation of kind, mutual agreement, custom, bringing up together, etc.

Rational,

Simple, which hath three objects, as *M.* 1,

Profitable, *Subs.* 1. — Health, wealth, honour, we love our benefactors, nothing so amiable as profit, or that which hath a show of commodity.

Pleasant, *Subs.* 2. — Things without life, made by art, pictures, sports, games, sensible objects, as hawks, hounds, horses; Or men themselves for similitude of manners, natural affection, as to friends, children, kinsmen, etc., for glory, such as commend us.

Of women, as — Before marriage, as heroical melancholy, *Sect.* 2, *vide* ♈. Or after marriage, as jealousy, *Sect.* 3, *vide* ♉.

Honest, *Subs.* 3. — Fucate in show, by some error or hypocrisy; some seem and are not; or truly for virtue, honesty, good parts, learning, eloquence, etc.

Mixed of all three, which extends to *M.* 3, — Common good, our neighbour, country, friends, which is charity; the defect of which is cause of much discontent and melancholy. or God, *Sect.* 4. In excess, *vide* ♊. In defect, *vide* ♋.

♈ Heroical or love-Melancholy, in which consider,

Memb. 1.

His pedigree, power, extent to vegetals and sensible creatures, as well as men, to spirits, devils, etc.

His name, definition, object, part affected, tyranny.

Causes, *Memb.* 2.

Stars, temperature, full diet, place, country, clime, condition, idleness, *Subs.* 1.

Natural allurements, and causes of love, as beauty, its praise, how it allureth.

Comeliness, grace, resulting from the whole or some parts, as face, eyes, hair, hands, etc. *Subs.* 2.

Artificial allurements, and provocations of lust and love, gestures, apparel, dowry, money, etc.

Quest. Whether beauty owe more to art or nature? *Subs.* 3.

Opportunity of time and place, conference, discourse, music, singing, dancing, amorous tales, lascivious objects, familiarity, gifts, promises, etc. *Subs.* 4.

Bawds and philters, *Subs.* 5.

Symptoms or signs, *Memb.* 3.

Of body — Dryness, paleness, leanness, waking, sighing, etc. *Quest. An detur pulsus amatorius?*

Of mind.

Bad, as — Fear, sorrow, suspicion, anxiety, etc. A hell, torment, fire, blindness, etc. Dotage, slavery, neglect of business.

Good, as — Spruceness, neatness, courage, aptness to learn music, singing, dancing, poetry, etc.

Prognostics; despair, madness, frenzy, death, *Memb.* 4.

Cures, *Memb.* 5.

By labour, diet, physic, abstinence, *Subs.* 1.

To withstand the beginnings, avoid occasions, fair and foul means, change of place, contrary passion, witty inventions, discommend the former, bring in another, *Subs.* 2.

By good counsel, persuasion, from future miseries, inconveniences. etc. By philters, magical and poetical cures, *Subs.* 4. [*Subs.* 3.

To let them have their desire disputed pro and con. Impediments removed, reasons for it. *Subs.* 5.

His name, definition, extent, power, tyranny, *Memb.* 1.

8 Jealousy, *Sect.* 3.

Division, Equivocations, kinds, *Subs.* 1.

Improper or Proper
- To many beasts; as swans, cocks, bulls.
- To kings and princes, of their subjects, successors.
- To friends, parents, tutors over their children, or otherwise.
- Before marriage, corrivals, etc. [wise.
- After, as in this place our present subject.

Causes, *Sect.* 2.

In the parties themselves or from others.
- Idleness, impotency in one party, melancholy, long absence.
- They have been naught themselves. Hard usage, unkindness, wantonness, inequality of years, persons, fortunes, etc.
- Outward enticements and provocations of others.

Symptoms, *Memb.* 2. — Fear, sorrow, suspicion, anguish of mind, strange actions, gestures, looks, speeches, locking up, outrages, severe laws, prodigious trials, etc.

Prognostics, *Memb.* 3. — Despair, madness, to make away themselves, and others.

Cures, *Memb.* 4.
- By avoiding occasions, always busy, never to be idle.
- By good counsel, advice of friends, to contemn or dissemble it. *Subs.* 1.
- By prevention before marriage. Plato's communion.
- To marry such as are equal in years, birth, fortunes, beauty, of like conditions, etc.
- Of a good family, good education. To use them well.

II Religious melancholy, *Sect.* 4.

In excess of such as do that which is not required, *Memb.* 1.

A proof that there is such a species of melancholy, name, object God, what his beauty is, how it allureth, part and parties affected, superstitious, idolaters, prophets, heretics, etc. *Subs.* 1.

Causes, *Subs.* 2.

From others or from themselves.
- The devil's allurements, false miracles, priests for their gain. Politicians to keep men in obedience, bad instructors, blind guides.
- Simplicity, fear, ignorance, solitariness, melancholy, curiosity, pride, vainglory, decayed image of God.

Symptoms, *Subs.* 3.

General
- Zeal without knowledge, obstinacy, superstition, strange devotion, stupidity, confidence, stiff defence of their tenents, mutual love and hate of other sects, belief of incredibilities, impossibilities.
- Of heretics, pride, contumacy, contempt of others, wilfulness, vainglory, singularity, prodigious paradoxes.

Particular.
- In superstitious blind zeal, obedience, strange works, fasting, sacrifices, oblations, prayers, vows, pseudo-martyrdom, mad and ridiculous customs, ceremonies, observations.
- In pseudo-prophets, visions, revelations, dreams, prophecies, new doctrines, etc., of Jews, Gentiles, Mahometans, etc.

Prognostics, *Subs.* 4. — New doctrines, paradoxes, blasphemies, madness, stupidity, despair, damnation.

Cures, *Subs.* 5. — By physic, if need be, conference, good counsel, persuasion, compulsion, correction, punishment. *Quæritur an cogi debent? Affir.*

In defect, as *Memb.* 2.

Secure, void of grace and fears. — Epicures, atheists, magicians, hypocrites, such as have cauterized consciences, or else are in a reprobate sense, worldly-secure, some philosophers, impenitent sinners, *Subs.* 1.

or

Distrustful, or too timorous, as desperate. In despair consider,

Causes, *Subs.* 2.
- The devil and his allurements, rigid preachers that wound their consciences, melancholy, contemplation, solitariness.
- How melancholy and despair differ. Distrust, weakness of faith. Guilty conscience for offence committed, misunderstanding Scripture.

Symptoms, *Subs.* 3. — Fear, sorrow, anguish of mind, extreme tortures and horror of conscience, fearful dreams, conceits, visions, etc.

Prognostics. Blasphemy, violent death, *Subs.* 4.

Cures, *Subs.* 5. — Physic, as occasion serves, conference, not to be idle or alone. Good counsel, good company, all comforts and contents, etc.

THE THIRD PARTITION

LOVE-MELANCHOLY

THE FIRST SECTION, MEMBER, SUBSECTION

The Preface

THERE will not be wanting, I presume, one or other that will much discommend some part of this treatise of love-melancholy, and object (which Erasmus in his preface to Sir Thomas More [1] suspects of his) "that it is too light for a divine, too comical a subject" to speak of love-symptoms, too phantastical, and fit alone for a wanton poet, a feeling young lovesick gallant, an effeminate courtier, or some such idle person.   And 'tis true they say: for by the naughtiness of men it is so come to pass, as Caussinus observes,[2] *ut castis auribus vox amoris suspecta sit, et invisa,* the very name of love is odious to chaster ears; and therefore some again, out of an affected gravity, will dislike all for the name's sake before they read a word, dissembling with him in Petronius,[3] and seem to be angry that their ears are violated with such obscene speeches, that so they may be admired 'for grave philosophers and staid carriage.   They cannot abide to hear talk of love-toys, or amorous discourses, *vultu, gestu, oculis* [in expression, gestures, glances], in their outward actions averse, and yet in their cogitations they are all out as bad, if not worse than others.

> *Erubuit, posuitque meum Lucretia librum,*
> *Sed coram Bruto ; Brute recede, legit.*[4]

> [When Brutus came, she blushed and hid my book;
> She 'll read again when Brutus does not look.]

But let these cavillers and counterfeit Catos know, that, as the Lord John answered the queen in that Italian Guazzo,[5] an old, a grave, discreet man is fittest to discourse of love matters, because he hath likely more experience, observed more, hath a more staid judgment, can better discern, resolve, discuss,

3

advise, give better cautions and more solid precepts, better
inform his auditors in such a subject, and by reason of his
riper years sooner divert. Besides, *nihil in hac amoris voce
subtimendum*, there is nothing here to be excepted at; love is a
species of melancholy, and a necessary part of this my treatise,
which I may not omit; *operi suscepto inserviendum fuit:* so
Jacobus Micyllus pleadeth for himself in his translation of
Lucian's Dialogues, and so do I; I must and will perform my
task. And that short excuse of Mercerus for his edition of
Aristænetus shall be mine: "If I have spent my time ill to
write, let not them be so idle as to read." [1]   But I am persuaded
it is not so ill spent, I ought not to excuse or repent myself of
this subject, on which many grave and worthy men have written
whole volumes, Plato, Plutarch, Plotinus, Maximus Tyrius,
Alcinous, Avicenna, Leon Hebræus in three large dialogues,
Xenophon, *Sympos.*, Theophrastus, if we may believe Athenæus,
lib. 13, *cap.* 9, Picus Mirandula, Marius Æquicola, both in
Italian, Kornmannus, *de linea Amoris, lib.* 3, Petrus Godefridus
hath handled in three books, P. Hædus, and which almost every
physician, as Arnoldus Villanovanus, Valleriola, *Observat. med.
lib.* 2, *observ.* 7, Ælian Montaltus and Laurentius in their treatises
of melancholy, Jason Pratensis, *de morb. cap.*, Valescus de
Taranta, Gordonius, Hercules de Saxonia, Savonarola, Langius,
etc., have treated of apart, and in their works. I excuse
myself, therefore, with Peter Godefridus, Valleriola, Ficinus,
and in Langius' words: "Cadmus Milesius writ fourteen books
of love, and why should I be ashamed to write an epistle in
favour of young men, of this subject?" [2]   A company of stern
readers dislike the second of the Æneids, and Virgil's gravity,
for inserting such amorous passions in an heroical subject; but
Servius,[3] his commentator, justly vindicates the poet's worth,
wisdom, and discretion in doing as he did. Castalio would not
have young men read the Canticles,[4] because to his thinking it
was too light and amorous a tract, a ballad of ballads, as our
old English translation hath it. He might as well forbid the
reading of Genesis, because of the loves of Jacob and Rachel,
the stories of Sichem and Dinah, Judah and Tamar; reject
the Book of Numbers, for the fornications of the people of
Israel with the Moabites; that of Judges for Samson and
Dalilah's embracings; that of the Kings, for David and Bathsheba's adulteries, the incest of Amnon and Tamar, Solomon's
concubines, etc., the stories of Esther, Judith, Susanna, and
many such. Dicæarchus, and some other, carp at Plato's

majesty, that he would vouchsafe to indite such love-toys:
amongst the rest, for that dalliance with Agatho:

Suavia dans Agathoni, animam ipse in labra tenebam;
Ægra etenim properans tanquam abitura fuit.

[When kissing Agathon, I held my very soul upon my
lips, for it rushed thither as though it meant to
leave me.]

For my part, saith Maximus Tyrius,[1] a great Platonist himself, *me non tantum admiratio habet, sed etiam stupor,* I do not
only admire, but stand amazed to read that Plato and Socrates
both should expel Homer from their city because he writ of such
light and wanton subjects, *quod Junonem cum Jove in Ida con-*
cumbentes inducit, ab immortali nube contectos, Vulcan's net,
Mars' and Venus' fopperies before all the gods; because Apollo
fled when he was persecuted by Achilles, the gods were wounded
and ran whining away,[2] as Mars that roared louder than Stentor,
and covered nine acres of ground with his fall; Vulcan was a
summer's day falling down from heaven, and in Lemnos Isle
brake his leg, etc., with such ridiculous passages; whenas both
Socrates and Plato, by his testimony, writ lighter themselves:
Quid enim tam distat (as he follows it) *quam amans a temperante,*
formarum admirator a demente? [What greater contrast can
there be than between a lover and a man of self-restraint, an
admirer of beauty and a madman?], what can be more absurd
than for grave philosophers to treat of such fooleries, to admire
Autolycus, Alcibiades, for their beauties as they did, to run
after, to gaze, to dote on fair Phædrus, delicate Agatho, young
Lysis, fine Charmides, *hæccine philosophum decent?* Doth this
become grave philosophers? Thus peradventure Callias, Thrasy-
machus, Polus, Aristophanes, or some of his adversaries and
emulators might object; but neither they nor Anytus and
Meletus, his bitter enemies, that condemned him for teaching
Critias to tyrannize, his impiety for swearing by dogs and
plane-trees, for his juggling sophistry, etc., never so much as
upbraided him with impure love, writing or speaking of that
subject; and therefore without question, as he concludes, both
Socrates and Plato in this are justly to be excused.[3] But
suppose they had been a little overseen, should divine Plato be
defamed? No; rather, as he said of Cato's drunkenness, if
Cato were drunk, it should be no vice at all to be drunk. They
reprove Plato then, but without cause (as Ficinus pleads);

"for all love is honest and good, and they are worthy to be loved that speak well of love."[1] "Being to speak of this admirable affection of love" (saith Valleriola [2]), "there lies open a vast and philosophical field to my discourse, by which many lovers become mad: let me leave my more serious meditations, wander in these philosophical fields, and look into those pleasant groves of the Muses, where with unspeakable variety of flowers we may make garlands to ourselves, not to adorn us only, but with their pleasant smell and juice to nourish our souls, and fill our minds desirous of knowledge," etc. After a harsh and unpleasing discourse of melancholy, which hath hitherto molested your patience and tired the author, give him leave with Godefridus the lawyer,[3] and Laurentius (*cap.* 5), to recreate himself in this kind after his laborious studies, "since so many grave divines and worthy men have without offence to manners, to help themselves and others, voluntarily written of it." Heliodorus, a bishop, penned a love story of Theagenes and Chariclea, and when some Catos of his time reprehended him for it, chose rather, saith Nicephorus,[4] to leave his bishopric than his book. Æneas Sylvius, an ancient divine, and past forty years of age, as he confesseth himself [5] (after Pope Pius Secundus), indited that wanton history of Euryalus and Lucretia. And how many superintendents of learning could I reckon up, that have written of light phantastical subjects! Beroaldus, Erasmus; Alpheratius,[6] twenty-four times printed in Spanish, etc. Give me leave then to refresh my Muse a little, and my weary readers, to expatiate in this delightsome field, *hoc deliciarum campo*, as Fonseca terms it, to season a surly discourse with a more pleasing aspersion of love matters.[7] *Edulcare vitam convenit*, as the poet invites us, *curas nugis*, etc., 'tis good to sweeten our life with some pleasing toys to relish it, and, as Pliny tells us, *magna pars studiosorum amœnitates quærimus*, most of our students love such pleasant subjects.[8] Though Macrobius teach us otherwise, "that those old sages banished all such light tracts from their studies to nurses' cradles, to please only the ear";[9] yet out of Apuleius I will oppose as honourable patrons, Solon, Plato, Xenophon, Hadrian, etc.,[10] that as highly approve of these treatises. On the other side methinks they are not to be disliked, they are not so unfit. I will not peremptorily say, as one did,[11] *tam suavia dicam facinora, ut male sit ei qui talibus non delectetur*, I will tell you such pretty stories, that foul befall him that is not pleased with them; *neque dicam ea quæ vobis usui sit audivisse, et voluptati meminisse* [nor will I say things which you will hear with profit and remember with pleasure], with that confidence as Beroaldus doth his enarrations on Propertius. I will not expect or hope for that approbation which Lipsius gives to his Epictetus: *Pluris facio quum relego; semper ut novum, et quum repetivi, repetendum*, the more I read, the more shall I covet to read. I will not press you with my pamphlets, or beg attention, but if you like them you may. Pliny holds it expedient, and most fit, *severitatem jucunditate etiam in scriptis condire*, to season our works with some pleasant discourse; Synesius approves it, *licet in ludicris ludere* [it is permissible to trifle with trifles]; the poet [1] admires it:

> *Omne tulit punctum qui miscuit utile dulci;*
>
> [All votes to him the first place shall assign
> Who with the sweet the useful can combine;]

and there be those, without question, that are more willing to read such toys than I am to write.[2] "Let me not live," saith Aretine's Antonia, "if I had not rather hear thy discourse than see a play!"[3] No doubt but there be more of her mind, ever have been, ever will be, as Hierome[4] bears me witness: "A far greater part had rather read Apuleius than Plato." Tully himself confesseth he could not understand Plato's *Timæus*, and therefore cared less for it; but every schoolboy hath that famous testament of Grunnius Corocotta Porcellus at his fingers' ends. The comical poet

> *Id sibi negoti credidit solum dari,*
> *Populo ut placerent quas fecisset fabulas,*

made this his only care and sole study, to please the people, tickle the ear, and to delight; but mine earnest intent is as much to profit as to please, *non tam ut populo placerem, quam ut populum juvarem*; and these my writings, I hope, shall take like gilded pills, which are so composed as well to tempt the appetite and deceive the palate, as to help and medicinally work upon the whole body; my lines shall not only recreate but rectify the mind. I think I have said enough; if not, let him that is otherwise minded remember that of Madaurensis; "he was in his life a philosopher" (as Ausonius apologizeth for him), "in his epigrams a lover, in his precepts most severe;[5] in his epistle to Cærellia a wanton." Annianus, Sulpicius, Evenus, Menander, and many old poets besides, did *in scriptis prurire*, write Fescennines, Atellanes, and lascivious songs, *lætam materiam*; yet they had *in moribus censuram et severitatem,* they were chaste, severe, and upright livers.

> *Castum esse decet pium poetam*
> *Ipsum, versiculos nihil necesse est,*
> *Qui tum denique habent salem et leporem.*

> ['Tis true, the poet should be chaste;
> But need his lines, so they be graced
> With wit, and captivate the taste?]

I am of Catullus' opinion, and make the same apology in mine own behalf: *Hoc etiam quod scribo, pendet plerumque ex aliorum sententia et auctoritate; nec ipse forsan insanio, sed insanientes sequor. Atqui detur hoc insanire me; semel insanivimus omnes, et tute ipse opinor insanis aliquando, et is, et ille, et ego scilicet* [I write for the most part to satisfy the taste and judgment of others; I am not mad myself, but I follow those who are. Yet grant that this shows me mad; we have all raved once, and you yourself, I think, dote sometimes, and he, and he, and of course I too]. *Homo sum, humani a me nihil alienum puto* [I am a human being, I count nothing human foreign to myself]: and, which he urgeth for himself, accused of the like fault, I as justly plead, *Lasciva est nobis pagina, vita proba est;*[1] howsoever my lines err, my life is honest, *Vita verecunda est, musa jocosa mihi.*[2] But I presume I need no such apologies; I need not, as Socrates in Plato, cover his face when he spake of love, or blush and hide mine eyes, as Pallas did in her hood, when she was consulted by Jupiter about Mercury's marriage, *quod super nuptiis virgo consulitur;*[3] it is no such lascivious, obscene, or wanton discourse; I have not offended your chaster ears with anything that is here written, as many French and Italian authors in their modern language of late have done, nay, some of our Latin pontifical writers, Zanchius, Asorius, Abulensis, Burchardus, etc., whom Rivet[4] accuseth to be more lascivious than Virgil in *Priapeiis,* Petronius in *Catalectis,* Aristophanes in *Lysistrata,* Martialis, or any other pagan profane writer, *qui tam atrociter* (one notes[5]) *hoc genere peccarunt, ut multa ingeniosissime scripta obscœnitatum gratia castœ mentes abhorreant* [who have erred so grossly in this sort that much of their most ingenious writing repels pure minds by its obscenity]. 'Tis not scurrile this, but chaste, honest, most part serious, and even of religion itself. "Incensed" (as he said) "with the love of finding love, we have sought it, and found it."[6] More yet, I have augmented and added something to this light treatise (if light) which was not in the former editions, I am not ashamed to confess it, with a good author,[1] *quod extendi et locupletari hoc subjectum plerique postulabant, et eorum importunitate victus, animum utcunque renitentem eo adegi, ut jam sexta vice calamum in manum sumerem, scriptionique longe et a studiis et professione mea alienæ me accingerem, horas aliquas a seriis meis occupationibus interim suffuratus, easque veluti ludo cuidam ac recreationi destinans* [yielding to the solicitations of many who begged me to dwell at greater length on this topic, I overcame my reluctance and for the sixth time took the pen in my hand for a kind of composition very foreign to my studies and profession, stealing from my serious occupations a few hours to devote to lighter pursuits]:

> *Cogor . . . retrorsum*
> *Vela dare, atque iterare cursus*
> *Olim relictos,*[2]

[I am compelled to reverse my direction and retrace my course,]

etsi non ignorarem novos fortasse detractores novis hisce interpolationibus meis minime defuturos [although well aware that these additions would procure me fresh detractors].

And thus much I have thought good to say by way of preface, lest any man (which Godefridus feared in his book [3]) should blame in me lightness, wantonness, rashness, in speaking of love's causes, enticements, symptoms, remedies, lawful and unlawful loves, and lust itself. "I speak it only to tax and deter others from it, not to teach, but to show the vanities and fopperies of this heroical or herculean love," and to "apply remedies unto it." [4] I will treat of this with like liberty as of the rest.

> *Sed dicam vobis, vos porro dicite multis*
> *Millibus, et facite hæc charta loquatur anus.*[5]

[I will tell you, and do you go and tell thousands more,
so that this page shall chatter like an old woman.]

Condemn me not, good reader, then, or censure me hardly, if some part of this treatise to thy thinking as yet be too light; but consider better of it. *Omnia munda mundis* [to the pure all things are pure], a naked man to a modest woman is no otherwise than a picture, as Augusta Livia truly said,[6] and *mala mens, malus animus* [7] [to construe it ill shows an evil will], 'tis as 'tis taken. If in thy censure it be too light, I advise thee as Lipsius did his reader for some places of Plautus, *Istos quasi Sirenum scopulos prætervehare* [to pass them by like rocks

of the Sirens], if they like thee not, let them pass; or oppose
that which is good to that which is bad, and reject not therefore all. For to invert that verse of Martial, and with Hierome
Wolfius to apply it to my present purpose, *sunt mala, sunt
quædam mediocria, sunt bona plura*; some is good, some bad,
some is indifferent. I say farther with him yet, I have inserted
(*levicula quædam et ridicula ascribere non sum gravatus, circum-
foranea quædam e theatris, a plateis, etiam e popinis* [1] [I have not
refrained from putting down certain levities and absurdities,
such as are current in the theatres, the market-places, and
even the cook-shops]) some things more homely, light, or
comical, *litans Gratiis* [sacrificing to the Graces], etc., which I
would request every man to interpret to the best, and, as
Julius Cæsar Scaliger besought Cardan, *Si quid urbaniuscule
lusum a nobis, per deos immortales te oro, Hieronyme Cardane,
ne me male capias* [if I have written anything in lighter vein,
please do not take it amiss], I beseech thee, good reader, not to
mistake me, or misconstrue what is here written; *per Musas et
Charites, et omnia poetarum numina, benigne lector, oro te ne me
male capias*. 'Tis a comical subject; in sober sadness I crave
pardon of what is amiss, and desire thee to suspend thy judgment, wink at small faults, or to be silent at least; but if thou
likest, speak well of it, and wish me good success. *Extremum
hunc, Arethusa, mihi concede laborem* [grant me, Arethusa, to
achieve this last labour].

I am resolved howsoever, *velis, nolis, audacter stadium intrare*,
[whether thou wilt or not, to enter the arena boldly], in the
Olympics, with those Eliensian wrestlers in Philostratus, boldly
to show myself in this common stage, and in this tragi-comedy
of love to act several parts, some satirically, some comically,
some in a mixed tone, as the subject I have in hand gives occasion,
and present scene shall require or offer itself.

SUBSECT. II.—*Love's Beginning, Object, Definition, Division*

"Love's limits are ample and great, and a spacious walk it
hath, beset with thorns," and for that cause, which Scaliger [2]
reprehends in Cardan, "not lightly to be passed over." Lest
I incur the same censure, I will examine all the kinds of love,
his nature, beginning, difference, objects, how it is honest or
dishonest, a virtue or vice, a natural passion or a disease, his
power and effects, how far it extends: of which, although

something has been said in the first partition, in those sections
of perturbations ("for love and hatred are the first and most
common passions, from which all the rest arise, and are attendant," as Piccolomineus holds,[1] or, as Nich. Caussinus, the
primum mobile [first mover] of all other affections, which carry
them all about them), I will now more copiously dilate, through
all his parts and several branches, that so it may better appear
what love is, and how it varies with the objects, how in defect,
or (which is most ordinary and common) immoderate and in
excess, causeth melancholy.

Love, universally taken, is defined to be a desire, as a word
of more ample signification; and though Leon Hebræus, the
most copious writer of this subject, in his third dialogue makes
no difference, yet in his first he distinguisheth them again, and
defines love by desire. "Love is a voluntary affection, and
desire to enjoy that which is good.[1] Desire wisheth, love enjoys;
the end of the one is the beginning of the other; that which we
love is present; that which we desire is absent."[3] "It is worth
the labour," saith Plotinus,[4] "to consider well of love, whether
it be a god or a devil, or passion of the mind, or partly god,
partly devil, partly passion." He concludes love to participate
of all three, to arise from desire of that which is beautiful and
fair, and defines it to be "an action of the mind desiring that
which is good." Plato calls it the great devil,[5] for its vehemency,
and sovereignty over all other passions, and defines it an appetite
"by which we desire some good to be present."[6] Ficinus in
his comment adds the word fair to this definition: "Love is a
desire of enjoying that which is good and fair." Austin dilates
this common definition, and will have love to be a delectation
of the heart, "for something which we seek to win, or joy to have,
coveting by desire, resting in joy."[7] Scaliger, *Exerc.* 301, taxeth
these former definitions, and will not have love to be defined
by desire or appetite; "for when we enjoy the things we desire,
there remains no more appetite": as he defines it, "Love is an
affection by which we are either united to the thing we love, or
perpetuate our union";[8] which agrees in part with Leon
Hebræus.

Now this love varies as his object varies, which is always
good, amiable, fair, gracious, and pleasant. "All things desire
that which is good,"[9] as we are taught in the Ethics, or at least
that which to them seems to be good; *quid enim vis mali* (as
Austin well infers), *dic mihi? puto nihil in omnibus actionibus*;
thou wilt wish no harm, I suppose, no ill in all thine actions,

thoughts, or desires, *nihil mali vis*; thou wilt not have bad corn, bad soil, a naughty tree, but all good: a good servant, a good horse, a good son, a good friend, a good neighbour, a good wife.[1] From this goodness comes beauty; from beauty, grace and comeliness, which result as so many rays from their good parts, make us to love, and so to covet it: for were it not pleasing and gracious in our eyes, we should not seek. "No man loves," saith Aristotle, 9 *Mor. cap.* 5, "but he that was first delighted with comeliness and beauty."[2] As this fair object varies, so doth our love; for, as Proclus holds, *omne pulchrum amabile*, every fair thing is amiable, and what we love is fair and gracious in our eyes, or at least we do so apprehend and still esteem of it. "Amiableness is the object of love, the scope and end is to obtain it, for whose sake we love, and which our mind covets to enjoy."[3] And it seems to us especially fair and good; for good, fair, and unity cannot be separated. Beauty shines, Plato saith, and by reason of its splendour and shining causeth admiration; and the fairer the object is, the more eagerly it is sought. For, as the same Plato defines it, "Beauty is a lively shining or glittering brightness, resulting from effused good by ideas, seeds, reasons, shadows, stirring up our minds that by this good they may be united and made one."[4] Others will have beauty to be the perfection of the whole composition, "caused out of the congruous symmetry, measure, order and manner of parts; and that comeliness which proceeds from this beauty is called grace, and from thence all fair things are gracious."[5] For grace and beauty are so wonderfully annexed, "so sweetly and gently win our souls, and strongly allure, that they confound our judgment and cannot be distinguished. Beauty and grace are like those beams and shinings that come from the glorious and divine sun,"[6] which are diverse, as they proceed from the diverse objects, to please and affect our several senses; as "the species of beauty are taken at our eyes, ears, or conceived in our inner soul,"[7] as Plato disputes at large in his dialogue *de Pulchro, Phædrus, Hippias*, and, after many sophistical errors confuted, concludes that beauty is a grace in all things, delighting the eyes, ears, and soul itself; so that, as Valesius infers hence, whatsoever pleaseth our ears, eyes, and soul, must needs be beautiful, fair, and delightsome to us. "And nothing can more please our ears than music, or pacify our minds."[8] Fair houses, pictures, orchards, gardens, fields, a fair hawk, a fair horse is most acceptable unto us; whatsoever pleaseth our eyes and ears, we call beautiful and

fair; "Pleasure belongeth to the rest of the senses, but grace
and beauty to these two alone." [1] As the objects vary and
are diverse, so they diversely affect our eyes, ears, and soul
itself; which gives occasion to some to make so many several
kinds of love as there be objects: one beauty ariseth from God,
of which and divine love St. Dionysius, [2] with many Fathers and
neoterics, have written just volumes, *de amore dei* [concerning
the love of God], as they term it, many parænetical discourses;
another from His creatures: there is a beauty of the body, a
beauty of the soul, a beauty from virtue, *formam martyrum*
[a beauty of martyrs], Austin calls it, *quam videmus oculis
animi*, which we see with the eyes of our mind; which beauty,
as Tully saith, if we could discern with these corporal eyes,
admirabiles sui amores excitaret, would cause admirable affections,
and ravish our souls. This other beauty, which ariseth from
those extreme parts, and graces which proceed from gestures,
speeches, several motions, and proportions of creatures, men
and women (especially from women, which made those old
poets put the three Graces still in Venus' company, as
attending on her and holding up her train), are infinite almost,
and vary their names with their objects, as love of money,
covetousness, love of beauty, lust, immoderate desire of any
pleasure, concupiscence, friendship, love, good will, etc., and is
either virtue or vice, honest, dishonest, in excess, defect, as
shall be showed in his place; heroical love, religious love, etc.,
which may be reduced to a twofold division, according to the
principal parts which are affected, the brain and liver: *amor
et amicitia* [love and friendship], which Scaliger, *Exercitat*. 301,
Valesius, and Melancthon warrant out of Plato, φιλεῖν and
ἐρᾶν, from that speech of Pausanias, belike, that makes two
Veneres and two loves. "One Venus is ancient without a
mother, and descended from heaven, whom we call celestial;
the younger, begotten of Jupiter and Dione, whom commonly
we call Venus." [3] Ficinus, in his comment upon this place,
cap. 8, following Plato, calls these two loves two devils, or good
and bad angels according to us, which are still hovering about
our souls. "The one rears to heaven, the other depresseth us
to hell; [4] the one good, which stirs us up to the contemplation
of that divine beauty for whose sake we perform justice and
all godly offices, study philosophy, etc.; [5] the other base, and
though bad yet to be respected; for indeed both are good in their
own natures: procreation of children is as necessary as that
finding out of truth, but therefore called bad, because it is

abused, and withdraws our soul from the speculation of that
other to viler objects." So far Ficinus. St. Austin, *lib.* 15 *de
Civ. Dei, et sup. Ps. lxiv*, hath delivered as much in effect:
"Every creature is good, and may be loved well or ill": [1] and
"Two cities make two loves, Jerusalem and Babylon, the love
of God the one, the love of the world the other; of these two
cities we all are citizens, as by examination of ourselves we
may soon find, and of which." [2] The one love is the root of
all mischief, the other of all good. So, in his 15th *cap. lib. de
amor. Ecclesiæ*, he will have those four cardinal virtues to be
naught else but love rightly composed; in his 15th book *de
Civ. Dei, cap.* 22, he calls virtue the order of love, whom Thomas
following, 1, *part.* 2, *quæst.* 55, *art.* 1, and *quæst.* 56, 3, *quæst.* 62,
art. 2, confirms as much, and amplifies in many words. Lucian,
to the same purpose, hath a division of his own: "One love was
born in the sea, which is as various and raging in young men's
breasts as the sea itself, and causeth burning lust: the other is
that golden chain which was let down from heaven, and with
a divine fury ravisheth our souls, made to the image of God,
and stirs us up to comprehend the innate and incorruptible
beauty to which we were once created." [3] Beroaldus hath
expressed all this in an epigram of his:

> *Dogmata divini memorant si vera Platonis,*
>   *Sunt geminæ Veneres, et geminatus amor.*
> *Cælestis Venus est nullo gencrata parente,*
>   *Quæ casto sanctos nectit amore viros.*
> *Altera sed Venus est totum vulgata per orbem,*
>   *Quæ divum mentes alligat, atque hominum ;*
> *Improba, seductrix, petulans,* etc.

> If divine Plato's tenents they be true,
>   Two Veneres, two loves there be;
> The one from heaven, unbegotten still,
>   Which knits our souls in unity.
> The other famous over all the world,
>   Binding the hearts of gods and men;
> Dishonest, wanton, and seducing she,
>   Rules whom she will, both where and when.

This twofold division of love Origen likewise follows, in his
Comment on the Canticles, one from God, the other from the
devil, as he holds (understanding it in the worse sense), which
many others repeat and imitate. Both which (to omit all subdivisions) in excess or defect, as they are abused, or degenerate,
cause melancholy in a particular kind, as shall be showed in his
place. Austin, in another tract, makes a threefold division of

this love, which we may use well or ill: "God, our neighbour,
and the world: God above us, our neighbour next us, the world
beneath us. In the course of our desires, God hath three
things, the world one, our neighbour two.[1] Our desire to God
is either from God, with God, or to God, and ordinarily so runs.
From God, when it receives from Him, whence, and for which
it should love Him: with God, when it contradicts His will in
nothing: to God, when it seeks to repose and rest itself in Him.
Our love to our neighbour may proceed from him, and run
with him, not to him: from him, as when we rejoice of his
good safety and well doing: with him, when we desire to have
him a fellow and companion of our journey in the way of the
Lord: not in him, because there is no aid, hope, or confidence
in man. From the world our love comes, when we begin to
admire the Creator in His works, and glorify God in His creatures:
with the world it should run, if, according to the mutability of
all temporalities, it should be dejected in adversity, or over-
elevated in prosperity: to the world, if it would settle itself in
his vain delights and studies." Many such partitions of love
I could repeat, and subdivisions, but lest (which Scaliger objects
to Cardan, *Exercitat* 501) "I confound filthy burning lust with
pure and divine love,"[2] I will follow that accurate division of
Leon Hebræus, *dial.* 2, betwixt Sophia and Philo, where he
speaks of natural, sensible, and rational love, and handleth
each apart. Natural love or hatred is that sympathy or antipathy which is to be seen in animate and inanimate creatures,
in the four elements, metals, stones, *gravia tendunt deorsum*
[heavy bodies tend downwards], as a stone to his centre, fire
upward, and rivers to the sea. The sun, moon, and stars go
still round, *amantes naturæ debita exercere*,[3] for love of perfection.
This love is manifest, I say, in inanimate creatures. How
comes a loadstone to draw iron to it? jet chaff? the ground to
covet showers, but for love? No creature, St. Hierome concludes, is to be found, *quod non aliquid amat* [that doth not
love something], no stock, no stone, that hath not some feeling
of love. 'Tis more eminent in plants, herbs, and is especially
observed in vegetals; as between the vine and elm a great
sympathy; between the vine and the cabbage, between the vine
and the olive (*Virgo fugit Bromium*[4] [the virgin shuns Bacchus]),
between the vine and bays a great antipathy; "the vine loves not
the bay, nor his smell, and will kill him, if he grow near him";[5]
the bur and the lentil cannot endure one another, the olive and
the myrtle embrace each other in roots and branches if they

grow near.[1] Read more of this in Piccolomineus, *grad.* 7, *cap.* 1;
Crescentius, *lib.* 5 *de agric.*; Baptista Porta, *de mag. lib.* 1, *cap.*
de plant. odio et element. sym.; Fracastorius *de sym. et antip.* Of
the love and hatred of planets, consult with every astrologer:
Leon Hebræus gives many fabulous reasons, and moralizeth
them withal.

Sensible love is that of brute beasts, of which the same Leon
Hebræus, *dial.* 2, assigns these causes. First, for the pleasure
they take in the act of generation, male and female love one
another. Secondly, for the preservation of the species, and
desire of young brood. Thirdly, for the mutual agreement, as
being of the same kind: *Sus sui, canis cani, bos bovi, et asinus*
asino pulcherrimus videtur [pig appears most beautiful to pig,
ass to ass, ox to ox, dog to dog], as Epicharmus held, and
according to that adage of Diogenianus, *Adsidet usque graculus*
apud graculum [one daw sits by another], they much delight in
one another's company, *Formicæ grata est formica, cicada cicadæ* [2]
[ant likes ant and grasshopper grasshopper], and birds of a
feather will gather together. Fourthly, for custom, use, and
familiarity, as if a dog be trained up with a lion and a bear,
contrary to their natures, they will love each other. Hawks,
dogs, horses, love their masters and keepers: many stories I
could relate in this kind, but see Gillius, *de hist. anim. lib.* 3,
cap. 14, those two Epistles of Lipsius, of dogs and horses,
A. Gellius, etc. Fifthly, for bringing up, as if a bitch bring up
a kid, a hen ducklings, an hedge-sparrow a cuckoo, etc.

The third kind is *amor cognitionis*, as Leon calls it, rational
love, *intellectivus amor*, and is proper to men, on which I must
insist. This appears in God, angels, men. God is love itself,
the fountain of love, the disciple of love, as Plato styles Him;
the servant of peace, the God of love and peace; have peace
with all men and God is with you.

> *Quisquis veneratur Olympum,*
> *Ipse sibi mundum subjicit atque Deum.* [3]

> [Whoever reveres heaven subjects to himself the world
> and God.]

"By this love" (saith Gerson) "we purchase heaven," [4] and
buy the kingdom of God. This love is either in the Trinity
itself (for the Holy Ghost is the love of the Father and the
Son, etc., John iii, 35, and v, 20, and xiv, 31), or towards us
His creatures, as in making the world.[5] *Amor mundum fecit*,
love built cities, *mundi anima* [the soul of the world], invented

arts, sciences, and all good things, incites us to virtue and
humanity, combines and quickens; keeps peace on earth, quietness by sea, mirth in the winds and elements, expels all fear,
anger, and rusticity; [1] *circulus a bono in bonum*, a round circle
still from good to good; for love is the beginner and end of all
our actions, the efficient and instrumental cause, as our poets
in their symbols, impresses, emblems [2] of rings, squares, etc.,
shadow unto us.

> *Si rerum quæris fuerit quis finis et ortus,*
> *Desine ; nam causa est unica solus amor.*

> If first and last of anything you wit,
> Cease; love 's the sole and only cause of it.

Love, saith Leo,[3] made the world, and afterwards, in redeeming
of it, "God so loved the world, that he gave his only begotten
son for it" (John iii, 16), "Behold what love the Father hath
showed on us, that we should be called the sons of God" (1 John
iii, 1). Or by His sweet Providence, in protecting of it; either
all in general, or His saints elect and Church in particular, whom
He keeps as the apple of His eye, whom He loves freely, as
Hosea, xiv. 5, speaks, and dearly respects, *Carior est ipsis homo
quam sibi* [4] [man is dearer to them than to himself]. Not that
we are fair, nor for any merit or grace of ours, for we are most
vile and base; but out of His incomparable love and goodness,
out of His Divine Nature. And this is that Homer's golden
chain, which reacheth down from heaven to earth, by which
every creature is annexed, and depends on his Creator. He made
all, saith Moses,[5] "and it was good," and He loves it as good.

The love of angels and living souls is mutual amongst themselves, towards us militant in the Church, and all such as love
God; as the sunbeams irradiate the earth from those celestial
thrones, they by their well-wishes reflect on us, *in salute hominum
promovenda alacres, et constantes administri* [6] [they are alert to
promote the salvation of men, and are their constant supports],
there is joy in heaven for every sinner that repenteth; they pray
for us, are solicitous for our good, *casti genii* [7] [pure guardian
angels].

> *Ubi regnat caritas, suave desiderium,*
> *Lætitiaque e' amor Deo conjunctus.*

> [Where reigneth charity, sweet desire, joy, and love
> that unites with God.]

Love proper to mortal men is the third member of this subdivision, and the subject of my following discourse.

MEMB. II.

SUBSECT. I.—*Love of Men, which varies as his Objects,*
Profitable, Pleasant, Honest

VALESIUS, *lib.* 3, *contr.* 13, defines this love which is in men,
"to be an affection of both powers, appetite and reason."[1]
The rational resides in the brain, the other in the liver (as before
hath been said out of Plato and others); the heart is diversely
affected of both, and carried a thousand ways by consent.
The sensitive faculty most part overrules reason, the soul is
carried hoodwinked, and the understanding captive like a beast.
"The heart is variously inclined, sometimes they are merry,
sometimes sad, and from love arise hope and fear, jealousy,
fury, desperation."[2] Now this love of men is diverse, and
varies as the object varies by which they are enticed, as virtue,
wisdom, eloquence, profit, wealth, money, fame, honour, or
comeliness of person, etc. Leon Hebræus, in his first Dialogue,
reduceth them all to these three, *utile, jucundum, honestum,*
profitable, pleasant, honest (out of Aristotle, belike, 8 *Moral.*);
of which he discourseth at large, and whatsoever is beautiful
and fair is referred to them, or anyway to be desired. "To
profitable is ascribed health, wealth, honour, etc., which is
rather ambition, desire, covetousness, than love."[3] Friends,
children, love of women, all delightful and pleasant objects,
are referred to the second.[4] The love of honest things consists
in virtue and wisdom, and is preferred before that which is
profitable and pleasant: intellectual, about that which is honest.
St. Austin calls "profitable, worldly; pleasant, carnal; honest,
spiritual.[5] Of and from all three, result charity, friendship,
and true love, which respects God and our neighbour."[6] Of
each of these I will briefly dilate, and show in what sort they
cause melancholy.

Amongst all these fair enticing objects, which procure love
and bewitch the soul of man, there is none so moving, so forcible
as profit, and that which carrieth with it a show of commodity.
Health indeed is a precious thing, to recover and preserve
which we will undergo any misery, drink bitter potions, freely
give our goods: restore a man to his health, his purse lies open
to thee, bountiful he is, thankful and beholding to thee; but
give him wealth and honour, give him gold, or what shall be for
his advantage and preferment, and thou shalt command his
affections, oblige him eternally to thee; heart, hand, life, and

all is at thy service, thou art his dear and loving friend, good
and gracious lord and master, his Mæcenas; he is thy slave, thy
vassal, most devote, affectioned, and bound in all duty: tell
him good tidings in this kind, there spoke an angel, a blessed
hour that brings in gain, he is thy creature, and thou his creator,
he hugs and admires thee; he is thine for ever. No loadstone
so attractive as that of profit, none so fair an object as this of
gold; nothing wins a man sooner than a good turn; bounty
and liberality command body and soul: [1]

>*Munera (crede mihi) placant hominesque deosque ;*
>*Placatur donis Jupiter ipse datis.*

>Good turns doth pacify both God and men,
>And Jupiter himself is won by them.

Gold of all other is a most delicious object; a sweet light, a
goodly lustre it hath; *gratius aurum quam solem intuemur*, saith
Austin, and we had rather see it than the sun. Sweet and
pleasant in getting, in keeping; it seasons all our labours,
intolerable pains we take for it, base employments, endure bitter
flouts and taunts, long journeys, heavy burdens, all are made
light and easy by this hope of gain; *At mihi plaudo ipse domi,
simul ac nummos contemplor in arca* [I am well pleased with
myself at home as soon as I set eyes on the money in my strong-
box]. The sight of gold refresheth our spirits and ravisheth
our hearts, as that Babylonian garment and golden wedge did
Achan in the camp,[2] the very sight and hearing sets on fire his
soul with desire of it. It will make a man run to the antipodes,
or tarry at home and turn parasite, lie, flatter, prostitute himself, swear and bear false witness; he will venture his body,
kill a king, murder his father, and damn his soul to come at it.
Formosior auri massa, as he [3] well observed, the mass of gold
is fairer than all your Grecian pictures, that Apelles, Phidias, or
any doting painter could ever make: we are enamoured with it.

>*Prima fere vota, et cunctis notissima templis,*
>*Divitiæ ut crescant.*[4]

>[Our first prayer, with which all the temples are
>familiar, is for an increase in wealth.]

All our labours, studies, endeavours, vows, prayers and wishes,
are to get, how to compass it.

>*Hæc est illa cui famulatur maximus orbis,*
>*Diva potens rerum, domitrixque pecunia fati.*[5]

>[This is she on whom the whole world waits hand and
>foot, the all-powerful and all-ruling goddess Money.

This is the great goddess we adore and worship; this is the sole object of our desire. If we have it, as we think, we are made for ever, thrice happy, princes, lords, etc. If we lose it, we are dull, heavy, dejected, discontent, miserable, desperate, and mad. Our estate and *bene esse* [well-being] ebbs and flows with our commodity; and as we are endowed or enriched, so are we beloved and esteemed: it lasts no longer than our wealth; when that is gone, and the object removed, farewell friendship; as long as bounty, good cheer, and rewards were to be hoped, friends enough; they were tied to thee by the teeth, and would follow thee as crows do a carcass: but when thy goods are gone and spent, the lamp of their love is out, and thou shalt be contemned, scorned, hated, injured. Lucian's Timon,[1] when he lived in prosperity, was the sole spectacle of Greece, only admired; who but Timon? Everybody loved, honoured, applauded him, each man offered him his service, and sought to be kin to him; but when his gold was spent, his fair possessions gone, farewell Timon: none so ugly, none so deformed, so odious an object as Timon, no man so ridiculous on a sudden, they gave him a penny to buy a rope, no man would know him.

'Tis the general humour of the world, commodity steers our affections throughout, we love those that are fortunate and rich, that thrive, or by whom we may receive mutual kindness, hope for like courtesies, get any good, gain, or profit; hate those, and abhor on the other side, which are poor and miserable, or by whom we may sustain loss or inconvenience. And even those that were now familiar and dear unto us, our loving and long friends, neighbours, kinsmen, allies, with whom we have conversed and lived as so many Geryons [2] for some years past, striving still to give one another all good content and entertainment, with mutual invitations, feastings, disports, offices, for whom we would ride, run, spend ourselves, and of whom we have so freely and honourably spoken, to whom we have given all those turgent titles and magnificent elogiums, most excellent and most noble, worthy, wise, grave, learned, valiant, etc., and magnified beyond measure: if any controversy arise between us, some trespass, injury, abuse, some part of our goods be detained, a piece of land come to be litigious, if they cross us in our suit, or touch the string of our commodity, we detest and depress them upon a sudden: neither affinity, consanguinity, or old acquaintance can contain us, but *rupto jecore exierit caprificus* [3] [the wild fig-tree breaks out from the shattered breast]. A golden apple sets all together by the ears, as if a marrow-

bone or honeycomb were flung amongst bears: father and son,
brother and sister, kinsmen are at odds: and look what malice,
deadly hatred can invent, that shall be done, *Terribile, dirum,
pestilens, atrox, ferum* [terrible, dreadful, destructive, cruel,
fierce], mutual injuries, desire of revenge, and how to hurt
them, him and his, are all our studies. If our pleasures be
interrupt, we can tolerate it; our bodies hurt, we can put it up
and be reconciled; but touch our commodities, we are most
impatient: fair becomes foul, the Graces are turned to Harpies,
friendly salutations to bitter imprecations, mutual· feastings to
plotting villainies, minings and counterminings; good words to
satires and invectives, we revile *e contra*, naught but his imperfections are in our eyes, he is a base knave, a devil, a monster,
a caterpillar, a viper, an hog-rubber, etc. *Desinit in piscem
mulier formosa superne* [the beauteous woman tails off into a
fish]; the scene is altered on a sudden, love is turned to hate,
mirth to melancholy: so furiously are we most part bent, our
affections fixed upon this object of commodity, and upon
money, the desire of which in excess is covetousness: ambition
tyrannizeth over our souls, as I have showed,[1] and in defect
crucifies as much as if a man by negligence, ill husbandry,
improvidence, prodigality, waste and consume his goods and
fortunes, beggary follows, and melancholy, he becomes an
abject, odious and "worse than an infidel, in not providing
for his family."[2]

SUBSECT. II.—*Pleasant Objects of Love*

Pleasant objects are infinite, whether they be such as have
life, or be without life. Inanimate are countries, provinces,
towers, towns, cities, as he said, *Pulcherrimam insulam videmus,
etiam cum non videmus*,[3] we see a fair island by description,
when we see it not. The sun never saw a fairer city,[4] *Thessala
Tempe* [another Tempe in Thessaly], orchards, gardens, pleasant
walks, groves, fountains, etc. The heaven itself is said to be
fair or foul;[5] fair buildings, fair pictures,[6] all artificial, elaborate,
and curious works, clothes, give an admirable lustre; we admire,
and gaze upon them, *ut pueri Junonis avem*, as children do on a
peacock; a fair dog, a fair horse and hawk, etc.: *Thessalus
amat equum pullinum, buculum Ægyptius, Lacedæmonius catalum*[7]
[the Thessalian is fond of a colt, the Egyptian of a bullock, the
Lacedæmonian of a whelp], etc.; such things we love, are most
gracious in our sight, acceptable unto us, and whatsoever else

may cause this passion, if it be superfluous or immoderately loved, as Guianerius observes. These things in themselves are pleasing and good, singular ornaments, necessary, comely, and fit to be had; but when we fix an immoderate eye, and dote on them overmuch, this pleasure may turn to pain, bring much sorrow and discontent unto us, work our final overthrow, and cause melancholy in the end. Many are carried away with those bewitching sports of gaming, hawking, hunting, and such vain pleasures, as I have said:[1] some with immoderate desire of fame, to be crowned in the Olympics, knighted in the field, etc., and by these means ruinate themselves. The lascivious dotes on his fair mistress, the glutton on his dishes, which are infinitely varied to please the palate, the epicure on his several pleasures, the superstitious on his idol, and fats himself with future joys, as Turks feed themselves with an imaginary persuasion of a sensual paradise: so several pleasant objects diversely affect divers men. But the fairest objects and enticings proceed from men themselves, which most frequently captivate, allure, and make them dote beyond all measure upon one another, and that for many respects. First, as some suppose, by that secret force of stars (*Quod me tibi temperat astrum?* [Which star fits me for thee?]). They do singularly dote on such a man, hate such again, and can give no reason for it. *Non amo te, Sabidi*[2] [Sabidius, I love thee not], etc. Alexander admired Hephæstion, Hadrian Antinous, Nero Sporus, etc. The physicians refer this to their temperament, astrologers to trine and sextile aspects, or opposite of their several ascendants, lords of their genitures, love and hatred of planets; Cicogna[3] to concord and discord of spirits; but most to outward graces. A merry companion is welcome and acceptable to all men, and therefore, saith Gomesius,[4] princes and great men entertain jesters and players commonly in their courts. But *Pares cum paribus facillime congregantur*,[5] 'tis that similitude of manners which ties most men in an inseparable link,[6] as if they be addicted to the same studies or disports, they delight in one another's companies, "birds of a feather will gather together": if they be of diverse inclinations, or opposite in manners, they can seldom agree. Secondly, affability, custom, and familiarity may convert nature many times,[7] though they be different in manners, as if they be countrymen, fellow-students, colleagues, or have been fellow-soldiers, brethren in affliction[8] (*acerba calamitatum societas diversi etiam ingenii homines conjugit*[9]), affinity, or some such accidental occasion, though they cannot agree amongst themselves, they will stick together like burs, and hold against a third; so after some discontinuance, or death, enmity ceaseth:

Pascitur in vivis livor, post fata quiescit ;
[Envy feeds on the living, after death 'tis still;]

or in a foreign place. *Et cecidere odia, et tristes mors obruit iras* [and hatred vanished, and anger was extinguished in death]. A third cause of love and hate may be mutual offices, *acceptum beneficium*; commend him, use him kindly, take his part in a quarrel, relieve him in his misery, thou winnest him for ever; do the opposite, and be sure of a perpetual enemy.[1] Praise and dispraise of each other do as much, though unknown, as Scioppius [2] by Scaliger and Casaubonus: *mulus mulum scabit* [mule scratches mule]; who but Scaliger with him? what encomiums, epithets, elogiums? *Antistes sapientiæ, perpetuus dictator, literarum ornamentum, Europæ miraculum* [the high priest and perpetual dictator of wisdom, the ornament of letters, the wonder of Europe], noble Scaliger, *incredibilis ingenii præstantia, etc., diis potius quam hominibus per omnia comparandus, scripta ejus aurea ancilia de cœlo delapsa poplitibus veneramur flexis* [this incredible genius, comparable to gods rather than to men, we venerate his writings on bended knees, like the shield that fell from heaven], etc., but when they began to vary, none so absurd as Scaliger, so vile and base, as his books *de Burdonum familia*, and other satirical invectives, may witness. Ovid *in Ibin* [against Ibis], Archilochus himself, was not so bitter. Another great tie or cause of love is consanguinity: parents are dear to their children, children to their parents, brothers and sisters, cousins of all sorts, as a hen and chickens, all of a knot: every crow thinks her own bird fairest. Many memorable examples are in this kind, and 'tis *portenti simile* [monstrous] if they do not: "a mother cannot forget her child;" [3] Solomon so found out the true owner; love of parents may not be concealed, 'tis natural, descends, and they that are inhuman in this kind are unworthy of that air they breathe, and of the four elements; yet many unnatural examples we have in this rank, of hard-hearted parents, disobedient children, of disagreeing brothers,[4] nothing so common. The love of kinsmen is grown cold, "many kinsmen" (as the saying is), "few friends;" if thine estate be good, and thou able *par pari referre*, to requite their kindness, there will be mutual correspondence, otherwise thou art a burden, most odious to them above all others. The last object that ties man and man, is comeliness of person, and beauty alone, as men love women with a wanton eye: which κατ' ἐξοχὴν [*par excellence*] is termed heroical, or love-melancholy. Other loves (saith Piccolomineus[1]) are so called with some contraction, as the love of wine, gold, etc., but this of women is predominant in a higher strain, whose part affected is the liver, and this love deserves a longer explication, and shall be dilated apart in the next section.

Subsect. III.—*Honest Objects of Love*

Beauty is the common object of all love, "as jet draws a straw, so doth beauty love":[2] virtue and honesty are great motives, and give as fair a lustre as the rest, especially if they be sincere and right, not fucate, but proceeding from true form and an incorrupt judgment; those two Venus' twins, Eros and Anteros, are then most firm and fast. For many times otherwise men are deceived by their flattering Gnathos,[3] dissembling chameleons, outsides, hypocrites that make a show of great love, learning, pretend honesty, virtue, zeal, modesty, with affected looks and counterfeit gestures: feigned protestations often steal away the hearts and favours of men, and deceive them, *specie virtutis et umbra* [by the outward show of merit], whenas, *revera* and indeed, there is no worth or honesty at all in them, no truth, but mere hypocrisy, subtilty, knavery, and the like. As true friends they are, as he that Cælius Secundus met by the highway side; and hard it is in this temporizing age to distinguish such companions, or to find them out. Such Gnathos as these for the most part belong to great men, and by this glozing flattery, affability, and such-like philters, so dive and insinuate into their favours, that they are taken for men of excellent worth, wisdom, learning, demi-gods, and so screw themselves into dignities, honours, offices; but these men cause harsh confusion often, and as many stirs as Rehoboam's counsellors in a commonwealth, overthrow themselves and others. Tandlerus and some authors make a doubt whether love and hatred may be compelled by philters or characters; Cardan and Marbodius by precious stones and amulets; astrologers by election of times, etc., as I shall elsewhere discuss.[4] The true object of this honest love is virtue, wisdom, honesty, real worth,[5] *interna forma* [the internal character], and this love cannot deceive or be compelled; *ut ameris amabilis esto* [to be loved

you must be lovable], love itself is the most potent *philtrum*,
virtue and wisdom, *gratia gratum faciens*, the sole and only
grace, not counterfeit, but open, honest, simple, naked, "descending from heaven," [1] as our Apostle hath it, an infused habit
from God, which hath given several gifts, as wit, learning,
tongues, for which they shall be amiable and gracious (Eph.
iv, 11), as to Saul stature and a goodly presence (1 Sam. ix, 1).
Joseph found favour in Pharaoh's court (Gen. xxxix) for his
person; [2] and Daniel with the princes of the eunuchs (Dan. i, 9).
Christ was gracious with God and men (Luke ii, 52).   There
is still some peculiar grace, as of good discourse, eloquence, wit,
honesty, which is the *primum mobile*, first mover, and a most
forcible loadstone to draw the favours and good wills of men's
eyes, ears, and affections unto them.   When Jesus spake, "they
were all astonied at his answers" (Luke ii, 47), "and wondered
at his gracious words which proceeded from his mouth."   An
orator steals away the hearts of men, and as another Orpheus,
quo vult, unde vult [whither he will and whence he will], he pulls
them to him by speech alone: a sweet voice causeth admiration; and he that can utter himself in good words, in our
ordinary phrase, is called a proper man, a divine spirit.   For
which cause belike, our old poets, *senatus populusque poetarum*
[the poets' assembly], made Mercury the gentleman-usher to
the Graces, captain of eloquence, and those *Charites* to be
Jupiter's and Eurymone's daughters, descended from above.
Though they be otherwise deformed, crooked, ugly to behold,
those good parts of the mind denominate them fair.   Plato
commends the beauty of Socrates; yet who was more grim of
countenance, stern and ghastly to look upon?   So are and have
been many great philosophers, as Gregory Nazianzen observes,[3]
"deformed most part in that which is to be seen with the eyes,
but most elegant in that which is not to be seen."   *Sæpe sub
attrita latitat sapientia veste* [wisdom oft lurks beneath a shabby
coat].   Æsop, Democritus, Aristotle, Politianus, Melancthon,
Gesner, etc., withered old men, *Sileni Alcibiadis* [4] [Silenuses
of Alcibiades], very harsh and impolite to the eye; but who were
so terse, polite, eloquent, generally learned, temperate and
modest?   No man then living was so fair as Alcibiades, so lovely
quoad superficiem, to the eye, as Boethius observes,[5] but he
had *corpus turpissimum interne*, a most deformed soul.   Honesty,
virtue, fair conditions, are great enticers to such as are well
given, and much avail to get the favour and good will of men.
Abdolonymus in Curtius, a poor man (but, which mine author

notes, "the cause of this poverty was his honesty"[1]), for his
modesty and continency from a private person (for they found
him digging in his garden) was saluted king, and preferred before
all the magnificoes of his time, *injecta ei vestis purpura auroque
distincta*, "a purple embroidered garment was put upon him,
and they bade him wash himself, and, as he was worthy, take
upon him the style and spirit of a king," [2] continue his continency and the rest of his good parts.   Titus Pomponius Atticus,
that noble citizen of Rome, was so fair conditioned, of so sweet
a carriage, that he was generally beloved of all good men, of
Cæsar, Pompey, Antony, Tully, of divers sects, etc., *multas
hæreditates* (Cornelius Nepos writes [3]) *sola bonitate consecutus* [he
obtained many legacies solely as a tribute to his good dis-
position]. *Operæ pretium audire*, etc., it is worthy of your
attention, Livy cries, "you that scorn all but riches, and give
no esteem to virtue, except they be wealthy withal, Q. Cincinnatus had but four acres, and by the consent of the senate
was chosen dictator of Rome." [4]   Of such account were Cato,
Fabricius, Aristides, Antonius, Probus, for their eminent worth:
so Cæsar, Trajan, Alexander, admired for valour, Hephæstion
loved Alexander, but Parmenio the king: [5] *Titus, deliciæ humani
generis*, and which Aurelius Victor hath of Vespasian, the
dilling of his time, as Edgar Etheling was in England,[6] for his
excellent virtues: their memory is yet fresh, sweet, and we
love them many ages after, though they be dead:[7] *Suavem
memoriam sui reliquit* [he left behind a pleasant memory],
saith Lipsius of his friend, living and dead they are all one.
"I have ever loved, as thou knowest" (so Tully wrote to Dola-
bella [8]), "Marcus Brutus for his great wit, singular honesty,
constancy, sweet conditions; and believe it, there is nothing
so amiable and fair as virtue." [9]   "I do mightily love Cal-
visinus" (so Pliny writes to Sossius), "a most industrious, eloquent, upright man, which is all in all with me":[10] the affection
came from his good parts.   And, as St. Austin comments on
the 84th Psalm, "there is a peculiar beauty of justice," and
inward beauty, "which we see with the eyes of our hearts, love,
and are enamoured with, as in martyrs, though their bodies
be torn in pieces with wild beasts, yet this beauty shines, and
we love their virtues." [11]   The Stoics are of opinion that a wise
man is only fair; [12] and Cato in Tully, 3 *de Finibus*, contends the
same, that the lineaments of the mind are far fairer than those
of the body, incomparably beyond them: wisdom and valour,
according to Xenophon, especially deserve the name of beauty,[13]

and denominate one fair, *et incomparabiliter pulchrior est* (as
Austin holds) *veritas Christianorum quam Helena Græcorum*
[Christian truth is incomparably fairer than Grecian Helen].
"Wine is strong, the king is strong, women are strong, but truth
overcometh all things" (1 Esdras iii, 10, 11, 12). "Blessed is
the man that findeth wisdom, and getteth understanding; for
the merchandise thereof is better than silver, and the gain
thereof better than gold; it is more precious than pearls, and
all the things thou canst desire are not to be compared to her"
(Prov. ii, 13, 14, 15). A wise, true, just, upright, and good
man, I say it again, is only fair: it is reported [1] of Magdalen,
Queen of France, and wife to Louis XI, a Scottish woman by
birth, that walking forth in an evening with her ladies, she
spied M. Alanus, one of the king's chaplains, a silly, old, hard-
favoured man,[2] fast asleep in a bower, and kissed him sweetly;
when the young ladies laughed at her for it, she replied, that it
was not his person that she did embrace and reverence, but,
with a Platonic love, the divine beauty of his soul.[3] Thus in
all ages virtue hath been adored, admired, a singular lustre
hath proceeded from it: and the more virtuous he is, the more
gracious, the more admired. No man so much followed upon
earth as Christ Himself; and as the Psalmist saith, xlv, 2,
"He was fairer than the sons of men." Chrysostom, *Hom.* 8
in Mat.; Bernard, *Ser.* 1, *de omnibus sanctis*; Austin, Cassiodore,
Hierome, *in* 9 *Mat.*, interpret it of the beauty of His person;[4]
there was a divine majesty in His looks, it shined like lightning
and drew all men to it: but Basil, Cyril, *lib.* 6 *super* 55 *Esaiæ*,
Theodoret, Arnobius, etc., of the beauty of His divinity, justice,
grace, eloquence, etc., Thomas, *in Ps. xliv*, of both; and so
doth Baradius, and Peter Morales, *lib. de pulchritud. Jesu et
Mariæ*, adding as much of Joseph and the Virgin Mary: *Hæc
alios forma præcesserit omnes* [this one shall excel all others in
beauty], according to that prediction of *Sibylla Cumæa* [the
Sibyl of Cumæ]. Be they present or absent, near us or afar
off, this beauty shines, and will attract men many miles to
come and visit it. Plato and Pythagoras left their country to
see those wise Egyptian priests: Apollonius travelled into
Ethiopia, Persia, to consult with the Magi, Brachmanni, gymnosophists. The Queen of Sheba came to visit Solomon; and many,
saith Hierome,[5] went out of Spain and remote places a thousand
miles, to behold that eloquent Livy: *Multi Romam non ut urbem
pulcherrimam, aut urbis et orbis dominum Octavianum, sed ut
hunc unum inviserent audirentque, a Gadibus profecti sunt* [6] [many

went from Gades to Rome, not to behold the beauties of the
city or Octavian the lord of the world, but to enjoy the company
and conversation of this man alone]. No beauty leaves such
an impression, strikes so deep, or links the souls of men closer
than virtue.[1]

> *Non per deos aut pictor posset,*
> *Aut statuarius ullus fingere*
> *Talem pulchritudinem qualem virtus habet;* [2]

no painter, no graver, no carver can express virtue's lustre, or
those admirable rays that come from it, those enchanting rays
that enamour posterity, those everlasting rays that continue
to the world's end. Many, saith Favorinus, that loved and
admired Alcibiades in his youth, knew not, cared not for Alcibiades a man, *nunc intuentes quærebant Alcibiadem;* but the
beauty of Socrates is still the same; virtue's lustre never fades,[3]
is ever fresh and green, *semper viva* to all succeeding ages, and
a most attractive loadstone, to draw and combine such as are
present. For that reason, belike, Homer feigns the three Graces
to be linked and tied hand in hand, because the hearts of men
are so firmly united with such graces. "O sweet bands"
(Seneca exclaims), "which so happily combine, that those
which are bound by them love their binders, desiring withal
much more harder to be bound," [4] and as so many Geryons to
be united into one. For the nature of true friendship is to
combine, to be like affected, of one mind,

> *Velle et nolle ambobus idem, satiataque toto*
> *Mens ævo,* [5]

as the poet saith, still to continue one and the same. And
where this love takes place there is peace and quietness, a true
correspondence, perfect amity, a diapason of vows and wishes,
the same opinions, as between David and Jonathan,[6] Damon
and Pythias, Pylades and Orestes, Nisus and Euryalus,[7] Theseus
and Pirithous, they will live and die together, and prosecute
one another with good turns [8] (*nam vinci in amore turpissimum
putant* [9] [for they think it the greatest reproach to be surpassed
in the display of affection]), not only living, but when their
friends are dead, with tombs and monuments, *nænias* [funeral
songs), epitaphs, elegies, inscriptions, pyramids, obelisks,
statues, images, pictures, histories, poems, annals, feasts, anni-
versaries, many ages after (as Plato's scholars did) they will
parentare still, omit no good office that may tend to the preservation of their names, honours, and eternal memory. *Illum*

coloribus, illum cera, illum ære, etc.,[1] "He did express his
friends in colours, in wax, in brass, in ivory, marble, gold, and
silver" (as Pliny reports of a citizen in Rome), "and in a great
auditory not long since recited a just volume of his life." In
another place, speaking of an epigram which Martial had composed in praise of him,[2] "He gave me as much as he might, and
would have done more if he could: though what can a man
give more than honour, glory, and eternity? But that which
he wrote, peradventure, will not continue, yet he wrote it to
continue."[3] 'Tis all the recompense a poor scholar can make
his well-deserving patron, Mæcenas, friend, to mention him in
his works, to dedicate a book to his name, to write his life, etc.,
as all our poets, orators, historiographers have ever done, and
the greatest revenge such men take of their adversaries, to
persecute them with satires, invectives, etc.,[4] and 'tis both
ways of great moment, as Plato gives us to understand.[5] Paulus
Jovius, in the fourth book of the life and deeds of Pope Leo
Decimus, his noble patron, concludes in these words: "Because
I cannot honour him as other, rich men do, with like endeavour,
affection, and piety I have undertaken to write his life; since
my fortunes will not give me leave to make a more sumptuous
monument, I will perform those rites to his sacred ashes, which
a small, perhaps, but a liberal wit can afford."[6] But I rove.
Where this true love is wanting, there can be no firm peace,
friendship from teeth outward, counterfeit, or, for some by-
respects, so long dissembled till they have satisfied their own
ends, which upon every small occasion breaks out into enmity,
open war, defiance, heart-burnings, whispering, calumnies, contentions, and all manner of bitter melancholy discontents. And
those men which have no other object of their love than greatness, wealth, authority, etc., are rather feared than beloved;
nec amant quemquam, nec amantur ab ullo [they neither love
nor are loved]; and howsoever borne with for a time, yet for
their tyranny and oppression, griping, covetousness, currish
hardness, folly, intemperance, imprudence, and such-like vices,
they are generally odious, abhorred of all, both God and men.

> *Non uxor salvum te vult, non filius, omnes*
> *Vicini oderunt;*

wife and children, friends, neighbours, all the world forsakes
them, would fain be rid of them, and are compelled many
times to lay violent hands on them, or else God's judgments
overtake them: instead of Graces, come Furies. So when fair

Abigail, a woman of singular wisdom, was acceptable to David,
Nabal was churlish and evil-conditioned;[1] and therefore Mordecai was received when Haman was executed, Haman the
favourite, "that had his seat above the other princes, to whom
all the king's servants that stood in the gates bowed their
knees and reverenced."[2] Though they flourish many times, such
hypocrites, such temporizing foxes, and blear the world's eyes
by flattery, bribery, dissembling their natures, or other men's
weakness, that cannot so apprehend their tricks, yet in the
end they will be discerned, and precipitated in a moment:
"Surely," saith David, "thou hast set them in slippery places"
(Ps. lxxiii, 18); as so many Sejani, they will come down to the
Gemonian scales;[3] and, as Eusebius in Ammianus,[4] that was in
such authority, *ad jubendum imperatorem*, be cast down headlong on a sudden. Or put case they escape, and rest unmasked
to their lives' end, yet after their death their memory stinks as
a snuff of a candle put out, and those that durst not so much
as mutter against them in their lives, will prosecute their name
with satires, libels, and bitter imprecations, they shall *male
audire* [be in ill repute] in all succeeding ages, and be odious
to the world's end.

MEMB. III.

Charity composed of all three Kinds, Pleasant, Profitable, Honest

BESIDES this love that comes from profit, pleasant, honest (for
one good turn asks another in equity), that which proceeds from
the law of nature, or from discipline and philosophy, there is
yet another love compounded of all these three, which is charity,
and includes piety, dilection, benevolence, friendship, even all
those virtuous habits; for love is the circle equant of all other
affections, of which Aristotle dilates at large in his Ethics, and
is commanded by God, which no man can well perform, but he
that is a Christian, and a true regenerate man. This is "to
love God above all, and our neighbour as ourself";[5] for this
love is *lychnus accendens et accensus*, a communicating light,
apt to illuminate itself as well as others. All other objects are
fair, and very beautiful, I confess; kindred, alliance, friendship,
the love that we owe to our country, nature, wealth, pleasure,
honour, and such moral respects, etc., of which read copious

Aristotle in his Morals; [1] a man is beloved of a man, in that he
is a man; but all these are far more eminent and great, when
they shall proceed from a sanctified spirit, that hath a true
touch of religion and a reference to God. Nature binds all
creatures to love their young ones; an hen to preserve her brood
will run upon a lion, an hind will fight with a bull, a sow with a
bear, a silly sheep with a fox. So the same nature urgeth a
man to love his parents (*Dii me, pater, omnes oderint, ni te magis
quam oculos amem meos!* [2] [O father, may all the gods hate me
if I love thee not more than my eyes!]), and this love cannot
be dissolved, as Tully holds, "without detestable offence": [3]
but much more God's commandment, which enjoins a filial
love, and an obedience in this kind. "The love of brethren is
great, and like an arch of stones, where if one be displaced, all
comes down," [4] no love so forcible and strong, honest, to the
combination of which, nature, fortune, virtue, happily concur;
yet this love comes short of it. *Dulce et decorum pro patria
mori* ['tis sweet and honourable to die for one's country], "it
cannot be expressed, what a deal of charity that one name of
country contains." [5] *Amor laudis et patriæ pro stipendio est*
[love of praise and country can take the place of pay]; the Decii
did *se devovere*, Horatii, Curii, Scævola, Regulus, Codrus, sacrifice
themselves for their country's peace and good.

> *Una dies Fabios ad bellum miserat omnes,*
> *Ad bellum missos perdidit una dies.* [6]

> One day the Fabii stoutly warred,
> One day the Fabii were destroyed.

Fifty thousand Englishmen lost their lives willingly near Battle
Abbey, in defence of their country. P. Æmilius, *lib.* 6, speaks
of six senators of Calais, that came with halters in their hands
to the King of England, to die for the rest. [7] This love makes
so many writers take such pains, so many historiographers,
physicians, etc., or at least as they pretend, for common safety,
and their country's benefit. *Sanctum nomen amicitiæ, sociorum
communio sacra:* [8] friendship is a holy name, and a sacred
communion of friends. "As the sun is in the firmament, so is
friendship in the world," [9] a most divine and heavenly band.
As nuptial love makes, this perfects mankind, and is to be preferred (if you will stand to the judgment of Cornelius Nepos [10])
before affinity or consanguinity; *plus in amicitia valet similitudo
morum, quam affinitas*, etc., the cords of love bind faster than
any other wreath whatsoever. Take this away, and take all

pleasure, joy, comfort, happiness, and true content out of the
world; 'tis the greatest tie, the surest indenture, strongest band,
and, as our modern Maro [1] decides it, is much to be preferred
before the rest.

> Hard is the doubt, and difficult to deem,
> When all three kinds of love together meet;
> And do dispart the heart with power extreme,
> Whether shall weigh the balance down; to wit,
> The dear affection unto kindred sweet,
> Or raging fire of love to women kind,
> Or zeal of friends, combin'd by virtues meet;
> But of them all the band of virtuous mind,
> Methinks the gentle heart should most assured bind.
>
> For natural affection soon doth cease,
> And quenched is with Cupid's greater flame;
> But faithful friendship doth them both suppress,
> And them with mastering discipline doth tame,
> Through thoughts aspiring to eternal fame.
> For as the soul doth rule the earthly mass,
> And all the service of the body frame,
> So love of soul doth love of body pass,
> No less than perfect gold surmounts the meanest brass.

A faithful friend is better than gold,[2][3] a medicine of misery,
an only possession;[4] yet this love of friends, nuptial, heroical,
profitable, pleasant, honest, all three loves put together, are
little worth, if they proceed not from a true Christian illuminated
soul, if it be not done *in ordine ad Deum*, for God's sake.
"Though I had the gift of prophecy, spake with tongues of men
and angels, though I feed the poor with all my goods, give my
body to be burned, and have not this love, it profiteth me
nothing" (1 Cor. xiii, 1, 2, 3); 'tis *splendidum peccatum* [a splendid
sin], without charity. This is an all-apprehending love, a
deifying love, a refined, pure, divine love, the quintessence of
all love, the true philosopher's stone, *Non potest enim*, as Austin
infers,[5] *veraciter amicus esse hominis, nisi fuerit ipsius primitus
veritatis*, he is no true friend that loves not God's truth. And
therefore this is true love indeed, the cause of all good to mortal
men, that reconciles all creatures, and glues them together in
perpetual amity and firm league, and can no more abide bitterness, hate, malice, than fair and foul weather, light and darkness,
sterility and plenty may be together. As the sun in the firmament (I say), so is love in the world; and for this cause 'tis love
without an addition, love κατ' ἐξοχὴν [*par excellence*], love of
God, and love of men. "The love of God begets the love of

man; and by this love of our neighbour the love of God is nourished and increased." [1] By this happy union of love, "all well-governed families and cities are combined, the heavens annexed, and divine souls complicated, the world itself composed, and all that is in it conjoined in God, and reduced to one." [2] "This love causeth true and absolute virtues, the life, spirit, and root of every virtuous action," [3] it finisheth prosperity, easeth adversity, corrects all natural encumbrances, inconveniences, sustained by faith and hope, which with this our love make an indissoluble twist, a Gordian knot, an equilateral triangle, "and yet the greatest of them is love" (1 Cor. xiii, 13), "which inflames our souls with a divine heat, and being so inflamed, purged, and so purgeth, elevates to God, makes an atonement, and reconciles us unto Him." [4] "That other love infects the soul of man, this cleanseth; that depresses, this rears; that causeth cares and troubles, this quietness of mind; this informs, that deforms our life; that leads to repentance, this to heaven." [5] For if once we be truly linked and touched with this charity, we shall love God above all, our neighbour as ourself, as we are enjoined (Mark xii, 31, Matt. xix, 19), perform those duties and exercises, even all the operations of a good Christian.

"This love suffereth long, it is bountiful, envieth not, boasteth not itself, is not puffed up, it deceiveth not, it seeketh not his own things, is not provoked to anger, it thinketh not evil, it rejoiceth not in iniquity, but in truth. It suffereth all things, believeth all things, hopeth all things" (1 Cor. xiii, 4, 5, 6, 7); "it covereth all trespasses" (Prov. x, 12); "a multitude of sins" (1 Pet. 4); as our Saviour told the woman in the Gospel, that washed His feet, "many sins were forgiven her, for she loved much" (Luke vii, 47); "it will defend the fatherless and the widow" (Isa. i, 17); "will seek no revenge, or be mindful of wrong" (Levit. xix, 18); "will bring home his brother's ox if he go astray, as it is commanded" (Deut. xxii, 1); "will resist evil, give to him that asketh, and not turn from him that borroweth, bless them that curse him, love his enemy" (Matt. v); "bear his brother's burthen" (Gal. vi, 7). He that so loves will be hospitable, and distribute to the necessities of the saints; he will, if it be possible, have peace with all men, "feed his enemy if he be hungry, if he be athirst give him drink"; he will perform those seven works of mercy, "he will make himself equal to them of the lower sort, rejoice with them that rejoice, weep with them that weep" (Rom. xii); he will speak

truth to his neighbour, be courteous and tender-hearted, "for-
giving others for Christ's sake, as God forgave him" (Eph. iv, 32);
he will be "like-minded" (Phil. ii, 2), "of one judgment; be
humble, meek, long-suffering" (Col. iii), "forbear, forget and
forgive" (vv. 12, 13, 23), and what he doth shall be heartily
done to God, and not to men; "Be pitiful and courteous"
(1 Pet. iii), "seek peace and follow it." He will love his brother,
not in word and tongue, but in deed and truth (1 John iii, 18),
"and he that loves God, Christ will love him that is begotten
of him" (1 John v, 1), etc. Thus should we willingly do, if we
had a true touch of this charity, of this divine love, if we could
perform this which we are enjoined, forget and forgive, and
compose ourselves to those Christian laws of love.

> *O felix hominum genus,*
> *Si vestros animos amor*
> *Quo cœlum regitur regat !* [1]

> [O happy race of men, did but love which rules the
> heaven rule your souls !]

Angelical souls, how blessed, how happy should we be, so
loving, how might we triumph over the devil, and have another
heaven upon earth!

But this we cannot do; and which is the cause of all our woes,
miseries, discontent, melancholy, want of this charity.[2] We
do *invicem angariare* [constrain one another by turns], contemn, insult, vex, torture, molest, and hold one another's noses
to the grindstone hard, provoke, rail, scoff, calumniate, challenge,
hate, abuse (hardhearted, implacable, malicious, peevish,
inexorable as we are), to satisfy our lust or private spleen, for
toys, trifles, and impertinent occasions,[3] spend ourselves, goods,
friends, fortunes, to be revenged on our adversary, to ruin him
and his. 'Tis all our study, practice, and business how to plot
mischief, mine, countermine, defend and offend, ward ourselves,
injure others, hurt all; as if we were born to do mischief, and
that with such eagerness and bitterness, with such rancour,
malice, rage, and fury, we prosecute our intended designs, that
neither affinity or consanguinity, love or fear of God or men
can contain us: no satisfaction, no composition will be accepted,
no offices will serve, no submission; though he shall upon his
knees, as Sarpedon did to Glaucus in Homer, acknowledging
his error, yield himself with tears in his eyes, beg his pardon, we
will not relent, forgive, or forget, till we have confounded him
and his, "made dice of his bones," as they say, see him rot in

prison, banish his friends, followers, *et omne invisum genus*
[and the whole hated tribe], rooted him out and all his
posterity. Monsters of men as we are, dogs, wolves, tigers,[1]
fiends, incarnate devils, we do not only contend, oppress, and
tyrannize ourselves, but as so many firebrands we set on and
animate others: our whole life is a perpetual combat, a conflict, a
set battle, a snarling fit. *Eris dea* [the goddess Strife] is settled
in our tents, *Omnia de lite*[2] [all things arose from strife], opposing
wit to wit, wealth to wealth, strength to strength, fortunes to
fortunes, friends to friends; as at a sea-fight we turn our broad-
sides, or [as] two millstones with continual attrition we fire
ourselves, or break [one] another's backs, and both are ruined
and consumed in the end. Miserable wretches, to fat and
enrich ourselves, we care not how we get it—*Quocunque modo
rem*—how many thousands we undo, whom we oppress, by whose
ruin and downfall we arise, whom we injure, fatherless children,
widows, common societies, to satisfy our own private lust.
Though we have myriads, abundance of wealth and treasure
(pitiless, merciless, remorseless, and uncharitable in the highest
degree), and our poor brother in need, sickness, in great extremity,
and now ready to be starved for want of food, we had rather,
as the fox told the ape, his tail should sweep the ground still,
than cover his buttocks; rather spend it idly, consume it with
dogs, hawks, hounds, unnecessary buildings, in riotous apparel,
ingurgitate, or let it be lost, than he should have part of it;
rather take from him that little which he hath than relieve him.[3]

Like the dog in the manger, we neither use it ourselves, let
others make use of or enjoy it; part with nothing while we live;
for want of disposing our household and setting things in order,
set all the world together by the ears after our death. Poor
Lazarus lies howling at his gates for a few crumbs, he only
seeks chippings, offals; let him roar and howl, famish, and eat
his own flesh, he respects him not. A poor decayed kinsman
of his sets upon him by the way in all his jollity, and runs
begging bareheaded by him, conjuring by those former bonds
of friendship, alliance, consanguinity, etc., uncle, cousin,
brother, father,

> *Per ego has lachrymas, dextramque tuam te,*
> *Si quidquam de te merui, fuit aut tibi quidquam.*
> *Dulce meum, miserere mei.*

[By these tears, by thy right hand, I beseech thee, if
ever I did thee a service or gave thee pleasure,
pity me.]

"Show some pity for Christ's sake, pity a sick man, an old man," etc., he cares not, ride on: pretend sickness, inevitable loss of limbs, goods, plead suretyship, or shipwreck, fires, common calamities, show thy wants and imperfections,

> *Et si per sanctum juratus dicat Osirim,*
> *Credite, non ludo, crudeles tollite claudum.*

> [And if he swear by Osiris, "I jest not, believe me,
> be not so cruel, pick up a lame man."]

Swear, protest, take God and all His angels to witness, *Quære peregrinum* [tell that to the marines], thou art a counterfeit crank, a cheater, he is not touched with it, *pauper ubique jacet* [there are beggars everywhere], ride on, he takes no notice of it. Put up a supplication to him in the name of a thousand orphans, an hospital, a spital, a prison, as he goes by, they cry out to him for aid, ride on, *surdo narras* [you speak to deaf ears], he cares not, let them eat stones, devour themselves with vermin, rot in their own dung, he cares not. Show him a decayed haven, a bridge, a school, a fortification, etc., or some public work, ride on; "Good your worship, your honour, for God's sake, your country's sake," ride on. But show him a roll wherein his name shall be registered in golden letters and commended to all posterity, his arms set up, with his devices to be seen, then peradventure he will stay and contribute; or if thou canst thunder upon him, as papists do, with satisfactory and meritorious works, or persuade him by this means he shall save his soul out of hell, and free it from purgatory (if he be of any religion), then in all likelihood he will listen and stay; or that he have no children, no near kinsman, heir, he cares for at least, or cannot well tell otherwise how or where to bestow his possessions (for carry them with him he cannot), it may be then he will build some school or hospital in his life, or be induced to give liberally to pious uses after his death. For I dare boldly say, vainglory, that opinion of merit, and this enforced necessity, when they know not otherwise how to leave, or what better to do with them, is the main cause of most of our good works. I will not urge this to derogate from any man's charitable devotion, or bounty in this kind, to censure any good work; no doubt there be many sanctified, heroical, and worthy-minded men, that in true zeal and for virtue's sake (divine spirits), that out of commiseration and pity extend their liberality, and as much as in them lies do good to all men, clothe the naked, feed the hungry, comfort the sick and needy, relieve all, forget

and forgive injuries, as true charity requires; yet most part
there is *simulatum quid*, a deal of hypocrisy in this kind, much
default and defect. Cosmus Medices,[1] that rich citizen of
Florence, ingenuously confessed to a near friend of his, that
would know of him why he built so many public and magnificent palaces and bestowed so liberally on scholars, not that
he loved learning more than others, "but to eternize his own
name, to be immortal by the benefit of scholars; for when his
friends were dead, walls decayed, and all inscriptions gone,
books would remain to the world's end." [2] The lanthorn in
Athens was built by Xenocles, the theatre by Pericles,[3] the
famous port Piræus by Musicles, Pallas' Palladium by Phidias,
the Pantheon by Callicrates; but these brave monuments are
decayed all, and ruined long since, their builders' names alone
flourish by mediation of writers. And as he [4] said of that Marian
oak, now cut down and dead, *nullius agricolæ manu culta stirps
tam diuturna, quam quæ poetæ versu seminari potest*, no plant
can grow so long as that which is *ingenio sata*, set and manured
by those ever-living wits. Allon-bachuth, that weeping oak,
under which Deborah, Rebecca's nurse, died and was buried,[5]
may not survive the memory of such everlasting monuments.
Vainglory and emulation (as to most men) was the cause
efficient, and to be a trumpeter of his own fame Cosmus' sole
intent, so to do good that all the world might take notice of it.
Such for the most part is the charity of our times, such our
benefactors, Mæcenates and patrons. Show me amongst so
many myriads a truly devout, a right, honest, upright, meek,
humble, a patient, innocuous, innocent, a merciful, a loving, a
charitable man! *Probus quis nobiscum vivit?* [6] [What honest
man lives among us?] Show me a Caleb or a Joshua! *Dic
mihi, Musa, virum!* Show a virtuous woman, a constant wife,
a good neighbour, a trusty servant, an obedient child, a true
friend, etc. Crows in Africa are not so scant. He that shall
examine this iron age wherein we live,[7] where love is cold,
et jam terras Astræa reliquit, Justice fled with her assistants,
virtue expelled,

Justitiæ soror,
Incorrupta fides, nudaque veritas,

[Uncorrupted Honesty, sister of Justice, and naked Truth,]

all goodness, gone, where vice abounds, the devil is loose, and
see one man vilify and insult over his brother, as if he were
an innocent or a block, oppress, tyrannize, prey upon, torture

him, vex, gall, torment and crucify him, starve him, where is
charity?　He that shall see men swear and forswear,[2] lie and
bear false witness, to advantage themselves, prejudice others,
hazard goods, lives, fortunes, credit, all, to be revenged on
their enemies, men so unspeakable in their lusts, unnatural in
malice, such bloody designments, Italian blaspheming, Spanish
renouncing, etc., may well ask where is charity?　He that
shall observe so many lawsuits, such endless contentions, such
plotting, undermining, so much money spent with such eagerness and fury, every man for himself his own ends, the devil
for all; so many distressed souls, such lamentable complaints,
so many factions, conspiracies, seditions, oppressions, abuses,
injuries, such grudging, repining, discontent, so much emulation,
envy, so many brawls, quarrels, monomachies, etc., may well
require what is become of charity? when we see and read of such
cruel wars, tumults, uproars, bloody battles, so many men
slain,[2] so many cities ruinated, etc. (for what else is the subject
of all our stories almost, but bills, bows, and guns?), so many
murders and massacres, etc., where is charity?　Or see men
wholly devote to God, churchmen, professed divines, holy men,
"to make the trumpet of the gospel the trumpet of war," [3] a
company of hell-born Jesuits, and fiery-spirited friars, *facem
præferre* [apply the torch] to all seditions, as so many firebrands
set all the world by the ears (I say nothing of their contentious
and railing books, whole ages spent in writing one against
another, and that with such virulency and bitterness, *Bioneis
sermonibus et sale nigro*), and by their bloody inquisitions, that
in thirty years, Bale saith, consumed 39 princes, 148 earls,
235 barons, 14,755 commons, worse than those ten persecutions,
may justly doubt where is charity?　*Obsecro vos quales hi
demum Christiani!*　Are these Christians? I beseech you, tell
me.　He that shall observe and see these things may say to
them as Cato to Cæsar, *Credo quæ de inferis dicuntur falsa
existimas,* Sure I think thou art of opinion there is neither
heaven nor hell.　Let them pretend religion, zeal, make what
shows they will, give alms, peace-makers, frequent sermons if
we may guess at the tree by the fruit, they are no better than
hypocrites, epicures, atheists; with the "fool in their hearts
they say there is no God." [4]　'Tis no marvel then if being so
uncharitable, hard-hearted as we are, we have so frequent
and so many discontents, such melancholy fits, so many
bitter pangs, mutual discords, all in a combustion, often
complaints, so common grievances, general mischiefs, *si tantæ*

in terris tragœdiæ, quibus labefactatur et misere laceratur humanum genus [if there are so many calamities to shake and rend the human race], so many pestilences, wars, uproars, losses, deluges, fires, inundations, God's vengeance, and all the plagues of Egypt come not upon us, since we are so currish one towards another, so respectless of God and our neighbours, and by our crying sins pull these miseries upon our own heads. Nay more, 'tis justly to be feared, which Josephus once said of his countrymen Jews,[1] "If the Romans had not come when they did to sack their city, surely it had been swallowed up with some earthquake, deluge, or fired from heaven as Sodom and Gomorrah; their desperate malice, wickedness, and peevishness was such." 'Tis to be suspected, if we continue these wretched ways, we may look for the like heavy visitations to come upon us. If we had any sense or feeling of these things, surely we should not go on as we do, in such irregular courses, practise all manner of impieties; our whole carriage would not be so averse from God. If a man would but consider, when he is in the midst and full career of such prodigious and uncharitable actions, how displeasing they are in God's sight, how noxious to himself, as Solomon told Joab (1 Kings, ii), "The Lord shall bring this blood upon their heads"; Prov. i, 27: "Sudden desolation and destruction shall come like a whirlwind upon them, affliction, anguish"; "The reward of his hand shall be given him" (Isa. iii, 11), etc.; "They shall fall into the pit they have digged for others," and when they are scraping, tyrannizing, getting, wallowing in their wealth, "This night, O fool, I will take away thy soul," what a severe account they must make; and how gracious on the other side a charitable man is in God's eyes,[2] *haurit sibi gratiam* [he draws to himself grace]; Matt. v, 7: "Blessed are the merciful, for they shall obtain mercy"; "He that lendeth to the poor, gives to God"; and how it shall be restored to them again, how "by their patience and long-suffering they shall heap coals on their enemies' heads" (Rom. xii), "and he that followeth after righteousness and mercy shall find righteousness and glory"; surely they would check their desires, curb in their unnatural, inordinate affections, agree amongst themselves, abstain from doing evil, amend their lives, and learn to do well. "Behold how comely and good a thing it is for brethren to live together in union:[3] it is like the precious ointment," etc. How odious to contend one with the other! *Miseri quid luctatiunculis hisce volumus? ecce mors supra caput est, et supremum illus tribunal, ubi et dicta et facta nostra*

examinanda sunt. Sapiamus! [1] Why do we contend and vex
one another? behold, death is over our heads, and we must
shortly give an account of all our uncharitable words and
actions; think upon it, and be wise.

SECT. II. MEMB. I.

SUBSECT. I.—*Heroical Love causing Melancholy. His Pedigree,
Power, and Extent*

IN the precedent section mention was made, amongst other
pleasant objects, of this comeliness and beauty which proceeds
from women, that causeth heroical, or love-melancholy, is more
eminent above the rest, and properly called love. The part
affected in men is the liver, and therefore called heroical,
because commonly gallants, noblemen, and the most generous
spirits are possessed with it. His power and extent is very
large, and in that twofold division of love,[2] φιλεῖν and ἐρᾶν,[3]
those two *Veneres* which Plato and some other make mention
of, it is most eminent, and κατ᾽ ἐξοχὴν [*par excellence*] called
Venus, as I have said, or love itself. Which although it be
denominated from men, and most evident in them, yet it extends
and shows itself in vegetal and sensible creatures, those incorporeal substances (as shall be specified), and hath a large
dominion of sovereignty over them. His pedigree is very
ancient, derived from the beginning of the world, as Phædrus
contends,[4] and his parentage of such antiquity, that no poet
could ever find it out.[5] Hesiod makes Terra and Chaos to be
Love's parents, before the gods were born:[6] *Ante deos omnes
primum generavit Amorem.* Some think it is the self-same fire
Prometheus fetched from heaven. Plutarch, *Amator. libello,*
will have Love to be the son of Iris and Favonius; but Socrates
in that pleasant dialogue of Plato, when it came to his turn
to speak of love (of which subject Agatho the rhetorician,
magniloquus Agatho, that chanter Agatho, had newly given
occasion), in a poetical strain, telleth this tale: When Venus
was born, all the gods were invited to a banquet, and amongst
the rest, Porus the god of bounty and wealth;[7] Penia or Poverty
came a-begging to the door; Porus, well whittled with nectar
(for there was no wine in those days), walking in Jupiter's

garden, in a bower met with Penia, and in his drink got her with
child, of whom was born Love; and because he was begotten
on Venus' birthday, Venus still attends upon him.   The moral
of this is in Ficinus.[1]   Another tale is there borrowed out of
Aristophanes: In the beginning of the world, men had four
arms and four feet, but for their pride, because they compared
themselves with the gods, were parted into halves, and now
peradventure by love they hope to be united again and made
one.[2]   Otherwise thus: Vulcan met two lovers, and bid them
ask what they would and they should have it; but they made
answer, *O Vulcane faber Deorum,* etc., "O Vulcan the gods'
great smith, we beseech thee to work us anew in thy furnace,
and of two make us one; which he presently did, and ever
since true lovers are either all one, or else desire to be united."[3]
Many such tales you shall find in Leon Hebræus, *Dial.* 3, and
their moral to them.   The reason why Love was still painted
young, (as Phornutus and others will[4]) "is because young men
are most apt to love; soft, fair, and fat, because such folks are
soonest taken; naked, because all true affection is simple and
open; he smiles, because merry and given to delights; hath a
quiver, to show his power, none can escape; is blind, because
he sees not where he strikes, whom he hits," etc.[5]   His power
and sovereignty is expressed by the poets, in that he is held to
be a god, and a great commanding god, above Jupiter himself;[6]
magnus dæmon [a mighty spirit], as Plato calls him, the strongest
and merriest of all the gods according to Alcinous and Athenæus.[7]
Amor virorum rex, Amor rex et deum, as Euripides, [Love is]
the god of gods and governor of men; for we must all do homage
to him, keep an holiday for his deity, adore in his temples,
worship his image (*numen enim hoc non est nudum nomen* [for
this is a deity and not merely a name]), and sacrifice to his altar,
that conquers all, and rules all:[8]

> *Mallem cum icone, cervo et apro Æolico,*
> *Cum Antæo et Stymphalicis avibus luctari*
> *Quam cum amore,*[3]

I had rather contend with bulls, lions, bears, and giants, than
with Love; he is so powerful, enforceth all to pay tribute to him,
domineers over all, and can make mad and sober whom he
list; insomuch that Cæcilius, in Tully's Tusculans, holds him to
be no better than a fool or an idiot that doth not acknowledge
Love to be a great god,

> *Cui in manu sit quem esse dementem velit,*
> *Quem sapere, quem sanari, quem in morbum injici,* etc.[4]

[that can make mad whom he will, or sane], that can make sick
and cure whom he list. Homer and Stesichorus were both
made blind, if you will believe Leon Hebræus,[1] for speaking
against his godhead: and though Aristophanes degrade him,
and say that he was scornfully rejected from the council of
the gods, had his wings clipped besides, that he might come no
more amongst them, and to his farther disgrace banished heaven
for ever, and confined to dwell on earth,[2] yet he is of that
power, majesty, omnipotency, and dominion, that no creature
can withstand him.[3]

> *Imperat Cupido etiam diis pro arbitrio,*
> *Et ipsum arcere ne armipotens potest Jupiter.*[4]

> [Cupid rules over the gods too as he listeth, and not
> even Jupiter can keep him at bay.]

He is more than quarter master with the gods;

> *Tenet*
> *Thetide æquor, umbras Æaco, cœlum Jove,*

> ⌜He shares the empire of the sea with Thetis, of the
> shades with Æacus, of the sky with Jove,⌝

and hath not so much possession as dominion. Jupiter himself
was turned into a satyr, shepherd, a bull, a swan, a golden
shower, and what not, for love; that as Lucian's[5] Juno right
well objected to him, *Ludus amoris tu es*, Thou art Cupid
whirligig. How did he insult over all the other gods, Mars,
Neptune, Pan, Mercury, Bacchus, and the rest! Lucian[6] brings
in Jupiter complaining of Cupid that he could not be quiet
for him, and the Moon lamenting that she was so impotently
besotted on Endymion, even Venus herself confessing as much,
how rudely and in what sort her own son Cupid had used her,
being his mother, "now drawing her to Mount Ida, for the love
of that Trojan Anchises, now to Libanus for that Assyrian
youth's sake.[7] And although she threatened to break his bow
and arrows, to clip his wings, and whipped him besides on the
bare buttocks with her pantofle,[8] yet all would not serve, he was
too headstrong and unruly." That monster-conquering Hercules
was tamed by him:

> *Quem non mille feræ, quem non Stheneleius hostis,*
> *Nec potuit Juno vincere, vicit amor.*

> Whom neither beasts nor enemies could tame,
> Nor Juno's might subdue, Love quell'd the same.

Your bravest soldiers and most generous spirits are enervated with it, *ubi muliebribus blanditiis permittunt se, et inquinantur amplexibus*.[1] Apollo, that took upon him to cure all diseases, could not help himself of this;[2] and therefore Socrates calls Love a tyrant,[3] and brings him triumphing in a chariot, whom Petrarch imitates in his Triumph of Love, and Fracastorius in an elegant poem expresseth at large, Cupid riding, Mars and Apollo following his chariot, Psyche weeping, etc.

In vegetal creatures what sovereignty love hath, by many pregnant proofs and familiar examples may be proved, especially of palm-trees, which are both he and she, and express not a sympathy but a love-passion, as by many observations have been confirmed.

> *Vivunt in venerem frondes, omnisque vicissim*
> *Felix arbor amat, nutant et mutua palmæ*
> *Fœdera, populeo suspirat populus ictu,*
> *Et platano platanus, alnoque assibilat alnus.*[4]

> [Boughs live for love, every tree in turn grows amorous,
>   they nod their troth, poplar sighs to poplar and
>   plane to plane, and alder whispers to alder.]

Constantine, *de agric. lib.* 10, *cap.* 4, gives an instance out of Florentius his Georgics, of a palm-tree that loved most fervently, "and would not be comforted until such time her love applied herself unto her; you might see the two trees bend, and of their own accords stretch out their boughs to embrace and kiss each other: they will give manifest signs of mutual love."[5] Ammianus Marcellinus, *lib.* 24, reports that they marry one another, and fall in love if they grow in sight; and when the wind brings the smell to them they are marvellously affected. Philostratus, *in Imaginibus*, observes as much, and Galen, *lib.* 6 *de locis affectis, cap.* 5; they will be sick for love, ready to die and pine away, which the husbandmen perceiving, saith Constantine, "stroke many palms that grow together, and so stroking again the palm that is enamoured, they carry kisses from the one to the other";[6] or tying the leaves and branches of the one to the stem of the other, will make them both flourish and prosper a great deal better: "which are enamoured, they can perceive by the bending of boughs and inclination of their bodies."[7] If any man think this which I say to be a tale, let him read that story of two palm-trees in Italy, the male growing at Brundusium, the female at Otranto (related by Jovianus Pontanus in an excellent poem, sometime tutor to Alphonsus Junior, King of Naples, his secretary of state, and a great philosopher), "which were barren, and so continued a long time," till they

came to see one another growing up higher, though many
stadiums asunder. Pierius, in his Hieroglyphics, and Melchior
Guilandinus, *mem.* 3, *tract. de papyro,* cites this story of Pontanus for a truth. See more in Salmuth, *Comment. in Pancirol.
de nova repert. tit.* 1, *de novo orbe,* Mizaldus, *Arcanorum lib.* 2,
Sandys' Voyages, *lib.* 2, *fol.* 103, etc.

If such fury be in vegetals, what shall we think of sensible
creatures? how much more violent and apparent shall it be in
them!

> *Omne adeo genus in terris hominumque ferarumque,*
> *Et genus æquoreum, pecudes, pictæque volucres*
> *In furias ignemque ruunt; amor omnibus idem.*[1]

> All kinds of creatures in the earth,
> 　And fishes of the sea,
> And painted birds do rage alike;
> 　This love bears equal sway.

> *Hic deus et terras et maria alta domat.*[2]

> [This deity subdues both land and sea.]

Common experience and our sense will inform us how violently
brute beasts are carried away with this passion, horses above
the rest, *furor est insignis equarum.* Cupid in Lucian bids
Venus his mother be of good cheer, for he was now familiar
with lions, and oftentimes did get on their backs, hold them
by the mane, and ride them about like horses, and they would
fawn upon him with their tails.[3] Bulls, bears, and boars are
so furious in this kind, they kill one another: but especially
cocks, lions,[4] and harts, which are so fierce that you may hear
them fight half a mile off, saith Turberville,[5] and many times kill
each other, or compel them to abandon the rut, that they may
remain masters in their places; "and when one hath driven
his corrival away, he raiseth his nose up into the air, and looks
aloft, as though he gave thanks to nature," which affords him
such great delight. How birds are affected in this kind, appears
out of Aristotle; he will have them to sing *ob futuram venerem,*
for joy or in hope of their venery which is to come.

> *Aeriæ primum volucres te, diva, tuumque*
> *Significant initum, perculsæ corda tua vi.*[6]

> [First the birds of the air welcome Venus and proclaim
> 　her approach, smitten deep with her passion.]

"Fishes pine away for love and wax lean," if Gomesius'[7] authority
may be taken, and are rampant too, some of them: Peter Gillius,

lib. 10 *de hist. animal.*, tells wonders of a triton in Epirus: there
was a well not far from the shore, where the country wenches
fetched water; the triton, *stupri causa*, would set upon them
and carry them to the sea, and there drown them if they would
not yield;[1] so love tyrannizeth in dumb creatures.   Yet this is
natural for one beast to dote upon another of the same kind;
but what strange fury is that, when a beast shall dote upon a
man?   Saxo Grammaticus, *lib.* 10 *Dan. Hist.*, hath a story of
a bear that loved a woman, kept her in his den a long time and
begot a son of her, out of whose loins proceeded many northern
kings: this is the original belike of that common tale of Valentine
and Orson.   Ælian, Pliny, Peter Gillius, are full of such relations.
A peacock in Leucadia loved a maid, and when she died the
peacock pined.   "A dolphin loved a boy called Hernias, and
when he died, the fish came on land, and so perished."[2]   The
like adds Gillius, *lib.* 10, *cap.* 22, out of Apion, *Ægypt. lib.* 15;
a dolphin at Puteoli loved a child, would come often to him,
let him get on his back, and carry him about, "and when by
sickness the child was taken away, the dolphin died."[3]   "Every
book is full" (saith Busbequius, the emperor's orator with the
Grand Signior, not long since, *ep.* 3, *Legat. Turc.*), "and yields
such instances, to believe which I was always afraid, lest I
should be thought to give credit to fables, until I saw a lynx,
which I had from Assyria, so affected towards one of my men,
that it cannot be denied but that he was in love with him.[4]
When my man was present, the beast would use many notable
enticements and pleasant motions, and when he was going, hold
him back, and look after him when he was gone, very sad in his
absence, but most jocund when he returned: and when my man
went from me, the beast expressed his love with continual
sickness, and after he had pined away some few days, died."
Such another story he hath of a crane of Majorca, that loved a
Spaniard, that would walk any way with him, and in his
absence seek about for him, make a noise that he might hear
her, and knock at his door, "and when he took his last farewell, famished herself."[5]   Such pretty pranks can love play
with birds, fishes, beasts:

> *Cælestis ætheris, ponti, terræ claves habet Venus,*
> *Solaque istorum omnium imperium obtinet :*[6]

> [Venus hath the keys of sky, sea, and earth, and is
>   sole mistress of them all:]

and, if all be certain that is credibly reported, with the spirits of the air, and devils of hell themselves, who are as much enamoured and dote (if I may use that word) as any other creatures whatsoever. For if those stories be true that are written of incubus and succubus, of nymphs, lascivious fauns, satyrs, and those heathen gods which were devils, those lascivious Telchines, of whom the Platonists tell so many fables, or those familiar meetings in our days, and company of witches and devils, there is some probability for it. I know that Biarmannus, Wierus, *lib.* 1, *cap.* 19 *et* 24, and some others stoutly deny it, that the devil hath any carnal copulation with women, that the devil takes no pleasure in such facts, they be mere phantasies, all such relations of incubi, succubi, lies and tales; but Austin, *lib.* 15 *de Civit.* *Dei,* doth acknowledge it; Erastus, *de lamiis;* Jacobus Sprenger and his colleagues, etc.; Zanchius, *cap.* 16, *lib.* 4, *de oper. Dei;* [1] Dandinus, *in Arist. de anima, lib.* 2, *text.* 29, *com.* 30; Bodine, *lib.* 2, *cap.* 7, and Paracelsus, a great champion of this tenent amongst the rest, which give sundry peculiar instances, by many testimonies, proofs, and confessions evince it. Hector Boethius, in his Scottish History, hath three or four such examples, which Cardan confirms out of him, *lib.* 16, *cap.* 43, of such as have had familiar company many years with them, and that in the habit of men and women. Philostratus, in his fourth book *de vita Apollonii,* hath a memorable instance in this kind, which I may not omit, of one Menippus Lycius, a young man twenty - five years of age, that going between Cenchreas and Corinth, met such a phantasm in the habit of a fair gentlewoman, which, taking him by the hand, carried him home to her house in the suburbs of Corinth, and told him she was a Phœnician by birth, and if he would tarry with her, "he should hear her sing and play, and drink such wine as never any drank, and no man should molest him; but she being fair and lovely would live and die with him, that was fair and lovely to behold." [2] The young man, a philosopher, otherwise staid and discreet, able to moderate his passions, though not this of love, tarried with her awhile to his great content, and at last married her, to whose wedding, amongst other guests, came Apollonius, who, by some probable conjectures, found her out to be a serpent, a lamia, and that all her furniture was like Tantalus' gold described by Homer, no substance, but mere illusions. When she saw herself descried, she wept, and desired Apollonius to be silent, but he would not be moved, and thereupon she, plate, house, and all that was in it, vanished in an instant: "many thousands took notice of this

fact, for it was done in the midst of Greece."[1] Sabine, in his
Comment on the tenth of Ovid's Metamorphoses, at the tale
of Orpheus, telleth us of a gentleman of Bavaria, that for many
months together bewailed the loss of his dear wife; at length
the devil in her habit came and comforted him, and told him,
because he was so importunate for her, that she would come and
live with him again, on that condition he would be new married,
never swear and blaspheme as he used formerly to do; for if
he did, she should be gone: "he vowed it, married, and lived
with her, she brought him children, and governed his house,
but was still pale and sad,[2] and so continued, till one day falling
out with him, he fell a-swearing; she vanished thereupon, and
was never after seen. This I have heard," saith Sabine, "from
persons of good credit, which told me that the Duke of Bavaria
did tell it for a certainty to the Duke of Saxony."[3] One more
I will relate out of Florilegus, *ad annum* 1058, an honest historian
of our nation, because he telleth it so confidently, as a thing in
those days talked of all over Europe. A young gentleman of
Rome, the same day that he was married, after dinner with the
bride and his friends went a-walking into the fields, and towards
evening to the tennis-court to recreate himself; whilst he played,
he put his ring upon the finger of Venus' statua, which was
thereby, made in brass; after he had sufficiently played, and
now made an end of his sport, he came to fetch his ring, but
Venus had bowed her finger in, and he could not get it off;
whereupon, loath to make his company tarry, at the present
there left it, intending to fetch it the next day or at some more
convenient time, went thence to supper, and so to bed. In
the night, when he should come to perform those nuptial rites,
Venus steps between him and his wife (unseen or felt of her),
and told her that she was his wife, that he had betrothed himself unto her by that ring which he put upon her finger: she
troubled him for some following nights. He, not knowing how
to help himself, made his moan to one Palumbus, a learned
magician in those days, who gave him a letter, and bid him
at such a time of the night, in such a cross-way, at the town's
end, where old Saturn would pass by with his associates in procession, as commonly he did, deliver that script with his own
hands to Saturn himself; the young man, of a bold spirit,
accordingly did it; and when the old fiend had read it, he
called Venus to him, who rode before him, and commanded
her to deliver his ring, which forthwith she did, and so the
gentleman was freed. Many such stories I find in several

authors [1] to confirm this which I have said; as that more
notable amongst the rest, of Philinium and Machates in Phlegon's
tract *de rebus mirabilibus*,[2] and though many be against it,
yet I, for my part, will subscribe to Lactantius, *lib.* 14, *cap.* 15,
"God sent angels to the tuition of men; but whilst they lived
amongst us, that mischievous all-commander of the earth, and
hot in lust, enticed them by little and little to this vice, and
defiled them with the company of women;" [3] and to Anaxagoras,
de Resurrect., "Many of those spiritual bodies, overcome by the
love of maids, and lust, failed, of whom those were born we
call giants." [4]   Justin Martyr, Clemens Alexandrinus, Sulpicius
Severus, Eusebius, etc., to this sense make a twofold fall of
angels, one from the beginning of the world, another a little
before the deluge, as Moses teacheth us, openly professing that
these genii can beget, and have carnal copulation with women.[5]
At Japan in the East Indies, at this present (if we may believe
the relation of travellers [6]), there is an idol called Teuchedy, to
whom one of the fairest virgins in the country is monthly
brought, and left in a private room, in the *fotoqui*, or church,
where she sits alone to be deflowered.   At certain times the
Teuchedy (which is thought to be the devil) appears to her,
and knoweth her carnally.   Every month a fair virgin is taken
in; but what becomes of the old, no man can tell.   In that
goodly temple of Jupiter Belus in Babylon, there was a fair
chapel, saith Herodotus,[7] an eye-witness of it, in which was
splendide stratus lectus et apposita mensa aurea, a brave bed, a
table of gold, etc., into which no creature came but one only
woman, which their god made choice of, as the Chaldean priests
told him, and that their god lay with her himself,[8] as at Thebes
in Egypt was the like done of old.   So that you see this is no
news; the devils themselves, or their juggling priests, have
played such pranks in all ages.   Many divines stiffly contradict
this; but I will conclude with Lipsius, that since "examples,
testimonies, and confessions of those unhappy women are so
manifest on the other side, and many even in this our town
of Louvain, that it is likely to be so.[9]   One thing I will add, that
I suppose that in no age past, I know not by what destiny of
this unhappy time, have there ever appeared or showed themselves so many lecherous devils, satyrs, and genii, as in this of
ours, as appears by the daily narrations and judicial sentences
upon record." [10]   Read more of this question in Plutarch, *vit.
Numæ*; Austin, *de Civ. Dei, lib.* 15; Wierus, *lib.* 3 *de præstig.
Dæm.*; Giraldus Cambrensis, *Itinerar. Camb. lib.* 1; *Malleus*

malefic. quæst. 5, *part.* 1; Jacobus Reussus, *lib.* 5, *cap.* 6, *fol.* 54;
Godelman, *lib.* 2, *cap.* 4; Erastus; Valesius, *de sacra philo. cap.* 40;
John Nider, *Formicar. lib.* 5, *cap.* 9; Stroz. Cicogna, *lib.* 3, *cap.* 3;
Delrio; Lipsius; Bodine, *Dæmonol. lib.* 2, *cap.* 7; Pererius, *in
Gen. lib.* 8, *in* 6 *cap. ver.* 2; King James, etc.

SUBSECT. II.—*How Love tyrannizeth over men. Love, or Heroical
Melancholy, his definition, part affected*

You have heard how this tyrant Love rageth with brute beasts
and spirits; now let us consider what passions it causeth
amongst men.

Improbe amor, quid non mortalia pectora cogis?[1] [Cruel Love,
to what dost thou not force the hearts of men?] How it
tickles the hearts of mortal men, *horresco referens*, I am almost
afraid to relate, amazed, and ashamed,[2] it hath wrought such
stupend and prodigious effects, such foul offences. Love
indeed (I may not deny) first united provinces, built cities, and
by a perpetual generation makes and preserves mankind, propa-
gates the Church; but if it rage, it is no more love, but burning
lust, a disease, frenzy, madness, hell. *Est orcus ille, vis est
immedicabilis, est rabies insana;*[3] 'tis no virtuous habit this, but
a vehement perturbation of the mind, a monster of nature, wit,
and art, as Alexis in Athenæus[4] sets it out, *viriliter audax,
muliebriter timidum, furore præceps, labore infractum, mel
felleum, blanda percussio* [of masculine boldness and female
timidity, headstrong and untamed, bitter honey, pleasant
punishment], etc. It subverts kingdoms, overthrows cities,
towns, families, mars, corrupts, and makes a massacre of men;
thunder and lightning, wars, fires, plagues, have not done that
mischief to mankind, as this burning lust, this brutish passion.
Let Sodom and Gomorrah, Troy (which Dares Phrygius and
Dictys Cretensis will make good), and I know not how many
cities bear record, *et fuit ante Helenam* [and these were also
before Helen], etc.; all succeeding ages will subscribe: Joanna
of Naples in Italy, Fredegunde and Brunhalt in France, all
histories are full of these basilisks. Besides those daily monomachies, murders, effusion of blood, rapes, riot, and immoderate
expense, to satisfy their lusts, beggary, shame, loss, torture,
punishment, disgrace, loathsome diseases that proceed from
thence, worse than calentures and pestilent fevers, those often

gouts, pox, arthritis, palsies, cramps, sciatica, convulsions, aches, combustions, etc., which torment the body, that feral melancholy which crucifies the soul in this life, and everlastingly torments in the world to come.

Notwithstanding they know these and many such miseries, threats, tortures, will surely come upon them, rewards, exhortations, *e contra* [on the other hand]; yet either out of their own weakness, a depraved nature, or love's tyranny, which so furiously rageth, they suffer themselves to be led like an ox to the slaughter; (*Facilis descensus Averni*) they go down headlong to their own perdition, they will commit folly with beasts, men "leaving the natural use of women," as Paul saith,[1] "burned in lust one towards another, and man with man wrought filthiness."

Semiramis equo, Pasiphae tauro, Aristo Ephesius asinæ se commiscuit, Fulvius equæ, alii canibus, capris, etc., unde monstra nascuntur aliquando, Centauri, Sylvani, et ad terrorem hominum prodigiosa spectra. Nec cum brutis, sed ipsis hominibus rem habent, quod peccatum Sodomiæ vulgo dicitur; et frequens olim vitium apud Orientalis illos fuit, Græcos nimirum, Italos, Afros, Asianos: Hercules Hylam habuit, Polycletum, Dionem, Perithoonta, Abderum et Phryga;[2] alii et Euristium ab Hercule amatum tradunt. Socrates pulchrorum adolescentum causa frequens gymnasium adibat, flagitiosoque spectaculo pascebat oculos, quod et Philebus et Phædo rivales, Charmides et reliqui Platonis dialogi satis superque testatum faciunt:[3] quod vero Alcibiades de eodem Socrate loquatur, lubens conticesco, sed et abhorreo; tantum incitamentum præbet libidini. At hunc perstrinxit Theodoretus, lib. de curat. Græc. affect. cap. ultimo. Quin et ipse Plato suum demiratur Agathonem, Xenophon Cliniam, Virgilius Alexin, Anacreon Bathyllum. Quod autem de Nerone, Claudio, cæterorumque portentosa libidine memoriæ proditum, mallem a Petronio, Suetonio, cæterisque petatis, quando omnem fidem excedat, quam a me expectetis; sed vetera querimur. Apud Asianos, Turcas,[4] Italos, nunquam frequentius hoc quam hodierno die vitium; Diana Romanorum Sodomia; officinæ horum alicubi apud Turcas, qui saxis semina mandant, *arenas arantes; et frequentes querelæ, etiam inter ipsos conjuges hac de re*, quæ virorum concubitum illicitum calceo in oppositam partem verso magistratui indicant; *nullum apud Italos familiare magis peccatum, qui et post Lucianum[5] et Tatium,[6] scriptis voluminibus defendunt. Johannes de la Casa, Beventinus Episcopus, divinum opus vocat, suave scelus, adeoque jactat se non alia usum Venere.*

*Nihil usitatius apud monachos, cardinales, sacrificulos, etiam
furor hic ad mortem, ad insaniam.*[1] *Angelus Politianus,*[2] *ob pueri
amorem, violentas sibi manus injecit. Et horrendum sane dictu,
quantum apud nos patrum memoria, scelus detestandum hoc
sævierit! Quum enim, anno* 1538, prudentissimus Rex Henricus
Octavus cucullatorum cœnobia, et sacrificorum collegia,
votariorum, per venerabiles legum Doctores Thomam Leum,
Richardum Laytonum visitari fecerat, etc., tanto numero reperti
sunt apud eos scortatores, cinædi, ganeones, pædicones, puerarii,
pæderastæ, Sodomitæ (*Balei*[3] *verbis utor*), Ganymedes, etc., ut in
unoquoque eorum novam credideris Gomorrham. *Sed vide si lubet
eorundem catalogum apud eundem Baleum;* Puellæ (*inquit*) in lectis
dormire non poterant ob fratres necromanticos. *Hæc si apud
votarios,monachos,sanctos scilicet homunciones,quid in foro, quid in
aula factum suspiceris? quid apud nobiles, quid inter fornices, quam
non fœditatem, quam non spurcitiem? Sileo interim turpes illas,
et ne nominandas quidem, monachorum mastrupationes, mastur-
batores.*[4] *Rodericus a Castro*[5] *vocat, tum et eos qui se invicem ad
Venerem excitandam flagris cædunt, spintrias,succubas, ambubeias,
et lasciviente lumbo tribadas illas mulierculas, quæ se invicem
fricant, et præter eunuchos etiam ad Venerem explendam, artificiosa
illa veretra habent. Immo quod magis mirere, femina feminam Con-
stantinopoli non ita pridem deperiit, ausa rem plane incredibilem,
mutato cultu mentita virum de nuptiis sermonem init, et brevi
nupta est: sed auctorem ipsum consule, Busbequium. Omitto
salinarios illos Ægyptiacos, qui cum formosarum cadaveribus
concumbunt;*[6] *et eorum vesanam libidinem, qui etiam idola et
imagines depereunt. Nota est fabula Pygmalionis apud Ovidium;*[7]
Mundi et Paulini apud Hegesippum, Belli Jud. lib. 2, *cap.* 4;
Pontius, C. Cæsaris legatus, referente Plinio, lib. 35, *cap.* 3, *quem
suspicor eum esse qui Christum crucifixit, picturis Ataluntæ et
Helenæ adeo libidine incensus, ut tollere eas vellet si natura tectorii
permisisset; alius statuam Bonæ Fortunæ deperiit (Ælianus,
lib.* 9, *cap.* 37), *alius Bonæ Deæ, et ne qua pars probro vacet,*
raptus ad stupra (*quod ait ille*[8]) et ne os quidem a libidine
exceptum.[9] *Heliogabalus per omnia cava corporis libidinem
recepit (Lamprid. vita ejus). Hostius*[10] *quidam specula fecit, et
ita disposuit, ut quum virum ipse pateretur, aversus omnes admis-
sarii motus in speculo videret, ac deinde falsa magnitudine ipsius
membri tanquam vera gauderet, simul virum et feminam passus,
quod dictu fœdum et abominandum. Ut veram plane sit, quod
apud Plutarchum*[11] *Gryllus Ulyssi objecit.* Ad hunc usque diem
apud nos neque mas marem, neque femina feminam amavit,

qualia multa apud vos memorabiles et præclari viri fecerunt:
ut viles missos faciam, Hercules imberbem sectans socium,
amicos deseruit, etc. Vestræ libidines intra suos naturæ fines
coerceri non possunt, quin instar fluvii exundantis atrocem
fœditatem, tumultum, confusionemque naturæ gignant in re
venerea: nam et capras, porcos, equos inierunt viri, et feminæ
insano bestiarum amore exarserunt, unde Minotauri, Centauri,
Sylvani, Sphinges, etc. *Sed ne confutando doceam, aut ea foras
efferam, quæ non omnes scire convenit (hæc enim doctis solummodo, quod causa non absimili Rodericus,*[1] *scripta velim) ne
levissimis ingeniis et depravatis mentibus fœdissimi sceleris
notitiam, etc., nolo quem diutius hisce sordibus inquinare.*

I come at last to that heroical love, which is proper to men
and women, is a frequent cause of melancholy, and deserves
much rather to be called burning lust, than by such an honourable title. There is an honest love, I confess, which is natural,
*laqueus occultus captivans corda hominum, ut a mulieribus non
possint separari,* a secret snare to captivate the hearts of men,
as Christopher Fonseca proves,[2] a strong allurement, of a most
attractive, occult, adamantine property and powerful virtue,
and no man living can avoid it. *Et qui vim non sensit amoris,
aut lapis est, aut bellua*[3] [he who does not feel the power of love
is either a stone or an animal]. He is not a man but a block,
a very stone, *aut numen, aut Nebuchadnezzar*[4] [either a god or
Nebuchadnezzar], he hath a gourd for his head, a *pepon* [pump-
kin] for his heart, that hath not felt the power of it, and a
rare creature to be found, one in an age, *Qui nunquam visæ
flagravit amore puellæ* [in whom the sight of a maiden has never
kindled love]; for *semel insanivimus omnes,* dote we either young
or old, as he[5] said, and none are excepted but Minerva and the
Muses: so Cupid in Lucian[6] complains to his mother Venus,
that amongst all the rest his arrows could not pierce them.
But this nuptial love is a common passion, an honest, for men
to love in the way of marriage; *ut materia appetit formam, sic
mulier virum* [as matter seeks form, so does woman man]. You
know marriage is honourable, a blessed calling, appointed by
God Himself in Paradise; it breeds true peace, tranquillity,
content, and happiness, *qua nulla est aut fuit unquam sanctior
conjunctio* [than which there is not nor ever has been any
holier union], as Daphnæus in Plutarch[7] could well prove,
et quæ generi humano immortalitatem parat [which makes the
human race immortal], when they live without jarring, scolding,
lovingly as they should do.

Felices ter et amplius
Quos irrupta tenent copula, nec ullis
Divulsus querimoniis
Suprema citius solvit amor die.[1]

Thrice happy they, and more than that,
  Whom bond of love so firmly ties,
That without brawls till death them part,
  'Tis undissolv'd and never dies.

As Seneca lived with his Paulina, Abraham and Sarah, Orpheus
and Eurydice, Arria and Pætus, Artemisia and Mausolus,
Rubenius Celer, that would needs have it engraven on his
tomb, he had led his life with Ennea, his dear wife, forty-three
years eight months, and never fell out. There is no pleasure
in this world comparable to it, 'tis *summum mortalitatis bonum*
[the highest good of humanity], *hominum divumque voluptas,
Alma Venus* [2] [the delight of men and gods, bountiful Venus];
*latet enim in muliere aliquid majus potentiusque omnibus aliis
humanis voluptatibus*, as one [3] holds, there's something in a
woman beyond all human delight; a magnetic virtue, a charming
quality, an occult and powerful motive. The husband rules
her as head, but she again commands his heart, he is her servant,
she his only joy and content: no happiness is like unto it, no love
so great as this of man and wife, no such comfort as *placens
uxor*,[4] a sweet wife:

Omnis amor magnus, sed aperto in conjuge major; [5]

[Love is ever great,
But greatest in the wedded state;]

when they love at last as fresh as they did at first, *caraque caro
consenescit conjugi* [6] [still dear companions as the years go on],
as Homer brings Paris kissing Helen, after they had been married
ten years, protesting withal that he loved her as dear as he did
the first hour that he was betrothed. And in their old age,
when they make much of one another, saying, as he did to
his wife in the poet,

Uxor, vivamus quod viximus, et moriamur,
Servantes nomen sumpsimus in thalamo;
Nec ferat ulla dies ut commutemur in ævo,
Quin tibi sim juvenis, tuque puella mihi.[7]

Dear wife, let's live in love, and die together,
  As hitherto we have in all good will:
Let no day change or alter our affections,
  But let's be young to one another still.

Such should conjugal love be, still the same, and as they are

one flesh, so should they be of one mind, as in an aristocratical
government, one consent, Geryon-like,[1] *coalescere in unum*,
have one heart in two bodies, will and nill the same. A good
wife, according to Plutarch, should be as a looking-glass to
represent her husband's face and passion: if he be pleasant,
she should be merry; if he laugh, she should smile; if he look
sad, she should participate of his sorrow, and bear a part with him,
and so they should continue in mutual love one towards another.

> *Et me ab amore tuo deducet nulla senectus,*
> *Sive ego Tithonus, sive ego Nestor ero.*[2]

> No age shall part my love from thee, sweet wife,
> Though I live Nestor or Tithonus' life.

And she again to him, as the bride saluted the bridegroom of
old in Rome,[3] *Ubi tu Caius, ego semper Caia*, Be thou still Caius,
I 'll be Caia.

'Tis a happy state this indeed, when the fountain is blessed
(saith Solomon, Prov. v, 18), "and he rejoiceth with the wife of
his youth, and she is to him as the loving hind and pleasant
roe, and he delights in her continually." But this love of ours
is immoderate, inordinate, and not to be comprehended in any
bounds. It will not contain itself within the union of marriage,
or apply to one object, but is a wandering, extravagant, a
domineering, a boundless, an irrefragable, a destructive passion:
sometimes this burning lust rageth after marriage, and then it
is properly called jealousy; sometimes before, and then it is
called heroical melancholy; it extends sometimes to corrivals,
etc., begets rapes, incests, murders: *Marcus Antonius compressit
Faustinam sororem, Caracalla Juliam novercam, Nero matrem,
Caligula sorores, Cinyras Myrrham filiam, etc.* But it is confined within no terms of blood, years, sex, or whatsoever else.
Some furiously rage before they come to discretion or age.
Quartilla in Petronius never remembered she was a maid;[4]
and the Wife of Bath, in Chaucer, cracks,

> Since I was twelve years old, believe,
> Husbands at kirk-door had I five.

Aretine's Lucretia sold her maidenhead a thousand times before
she was twenty-four years old, *plus millies vendiderant virginitatem, etc., neque te celabo, non deerant qui ut integram ambirent.*[5]
Rahab, that harlot, began to be a professed quean at ten years
of age, and was but fifteen when she hid the spies, as Hugh
Broughton proves,[6] to whom Serrarius the Jesuit, *quæst. 6 in
cap. 2 Josue*, subscribes. Generally women begin *pubescere*,

as they call it, or *catulire*, as Julius Pollux cites, *lib. 2, cap. 3,
Onomast.* out of Aristophanes, at fourteen years old, then they
do offer themselves, and some plainly rage.[1] Leo Afer saith,[2]
that in Africa a man shall scarce find a maid at fourteen years
of age, they are so forward, and many amongst us after they
come into the teens do not live without husbands, but linger.
What pranks in this kind the middle age have played is not to
be recorded, *Si mihi sint centum linguæ, sint oraque centum*
[if I had a hundred tongues, a hundred mouths], no tongue
can sufficiently declare, every story is full of men and women's
insatiable lust, Neros, Heliogabali, Bonosi, etc. *Cælius Aufile-
num, et Quintius Aufilenam depereunt, etc.*[3] They neigh after
other men's wives (as Jeremy, *cap.* v, 8, complaineth) like fed
horses, or range like town bulls, *raptores virginum et viduarum*
[ravishers of widows and maids], as many of our great ones do.
Solomon's wisdom was extinguished in this fire of lust, Samson's
strength enervated, piety in Lot's daughters quite forgot,
gravity of priesthood in Eli's sons, reverend old age in the
Elders that would violate Susanna, filial duty in Absalom to his
stepmother, brotherly love in Amnon towards his sister.
Human, divine laws, precepts, exhortations, fear of God and
men, fair, foul means, fame, fortunes, shame, disgrace, honour
cannot oppose, stave off, or withstand the fury of it, *omnia
vincit amor* [love subdues all], etc. No cord nor cable can so
forcibly draw, or hold so fast, as love can do with a twined
thread. The scorching beams under the equinoctial, or extremity of cold within the circle Arctic, where the very seas
are frozen, cold or torrid zone cannot avoid or expel this heat,
fury, and rage of mortal men.

> *Quo fugis? ah, demens! nulla est fuga, tu licet usque
> Ad Tanaim fugias, usque sequetur amor.*[4]

> [Whither fleest thou, poor fool?   There is no escape;
> though thou flee to farthest Tanais, love will
> still pursue thee.]

Of women's unnatural, unsatiable lust, what country, what
village doth not complain?[5]   Mother and daughter sometimes
dote on the same man; father and son, master and servant
on one woman.

> *Sed amor, sed ineffrenata libido,
> Quid castum in terris intentatumque reliquit?*[6]

> [From the assaults of love and of unbridled passion
> what upon earth has escaped chaste and inviolate?]

What breach of vows and oaths, fury, dotage, madness, might
I reckon up! Yet this is more tolerable in youth, and such as
are still in their hot blood; but for an old fool to dote, to see an
old lecher, what more odious, what can be more absurd? and yet
what so common? Who so furious? *Amare ea ætate si occe-
perint, multo insaniunt acrius* [1] [if they commence to love at that
age, they become much more crazy]. Some dote then more
than ever they did in their youth. How many decrepit, hoary,
harsh, writhen, bursten-bellied, crooked, toothless, bald, blear-
eyed, impotent, rotten old men shall you see flickering still in
every place? One gets him a young wife, another a courtesan,
and when he can scarce lift his leg over a sill, and hath one foot
already in Charon's boat, when he hath the trembling in his
joints, the gout in his feet, a perpetual rheum in his head, a
continuate cough, "his sight fails him, thick of hearing, his
breath stinks," [2] all his moisture is dried up and gone, may
not spit from him, a very child again, that cannot dress himself,
or cut his own meat, yet he will be dreaming of, and honing
after wenches; what can be more unseemly? Worse it is in
women than in men; when she is *ætate declivis, diu vidua, mater
olim, parum decore matrimonium sequi videtur*, an old widow,
a mother so long since (in Pliny's opinion [3]), she doth very unseemly seek to marry; yet whilst she is so old a crone, [4] a beldam,
she can neither see nor hear, go nor stand, a mere carcass, [5]
a witch, and scarce feel, she caterwauls, and must have a stallion,
a champion, she must and will marry again, and betroth herself
to some young man, that hates to look on [her] but for her
goods, [6] abhors the sight of her; to the prejudice of her good
name, her own undoing, grief of friends, and ruin of her children.

But to enlarge or illustrate this power and effects of love is to
set a candle in the sun. It rageth with all sorts and conditions
of men, [7] yet is most evident among such as are young and lusty,
in the flower of their years, nobly descended, high fed, such as
live idly and at ease; and for that cause (which our divines
call burning lust) this *ferinus insanus amor*, [8] this mad and
beastly passion, as I have said, is named by our physicians
heroical love, and a more honourable title put upon it, *amor
nobilis*, as Savonarola styles it, [9] because noble men and women
make a common practice of it, and are so ordinarily affected
with it. Avicenna, *lib.* 3, *fen.* 1, *tract.* 4, *cap.* 23, calleth this
passion *Ilishi*, and defines it to be "a disease or melancholy
vexation, or anguish of mind, in which a man continually
meditates of the beauty, gesture, manners of his mistress, and

troubles himself about it";[1] "desiring" (as Savonarola adds)
"with all intentions and eagerness of mind to compass or enjoy
her; as commonly hunters trouble themselves about their
sports, the covetous about their gold and goods, so is he tormented still about his mistress."[2] Arnoldus Villanovanus, in
his book of heroical love, defines it "a continual cogitation of
that which he desires, with a confidence or hope of compassing
it";[3] which definition his commentator cavils at. For continual cogitation is not the *genus*, but a symptom of love; we
continually think of that which we hate and abhor, as well as
that which we love; and many things we covet and desire, without all hope of attaining. Carolus à Lorme, in his Questions,
makes a doubt, *an amor sit morbus*, whether this heroical love
be a disease: Julius Pollux, *Onomast. lib.* 6, *cap.* 44, determines
it. They that are in love are likewise sick;[4] *lascivus, salax,
lasciviens, et qui in venerem furit, vere est ægrotus.* Arnoldus
will have it improperly so called, and a malady rather of the
body than mind. Tully, in his Tusculans, defines it a furious
disease of the mind; Plato, madness itself; Ficinus, his commentator, *cap.* 12, a species of madness, "for many have run
mad for women" (1 Esdras, iv, 26); but Rhasis, "a melancholy
passion";[5] and most physicians make it a species or kind of
melancholy (as will appear by the symptoms), and treat of it
apart; whom I mean to imitate, and to discuss it in all his
kinds, to examine his several causes, to show his symptoms,
indications, prognostics, effects, that so it may be with more
facility cured.

The part affected in the meantime, as Arnoldus supposeth,[6]
"is the former part of the head for want of moisture," which
his commentator rejects. Langius, *Med. epist. lib.* 1, *cap.* 24,
will have this passion sited in the liver, and to keep residence
in the heart, "to proceed first from the eyes so carried by our
spirits, and kindled with imagination in the liver and heart";[7]
cogit amare jecur [the liver compels to love], as the saying is.
Medium ferit per hepar [he strikes right through the liver], as
Cupid in Anacreon. For some such cause belike Homer[8] feigns
Titius' liver (who was enamoured of Latona) to be still gnawed
by two vultures day and night in hell, "for that young men's
bowels thus enamoured are so continually tormented by love."[9]
Gordonius, *cap.* 2, *part.* 2, "will have the testicles an immediate
subject or cause, the liver an antecedent."[10] Fracastorius
agrees in this with Gordonius, *inde primitus imaginatio venerea,
erectio, etc., titillatissimam partem vocat, ita ut nisi extruso*

semine gestiens voluptas non cessat, nec assidua veneris recordatio,
addit Guastavinius, Comment. 4 sect. prob. 27 Arist. But properly
it is a passion of the brain, as all other melancholy, by reason of
corrupt imagination,[1] and so doth Jason Pratensis, *cap.* 19 *de
morb. cerebri* (who writes copiously of this erotical love), place
and reckon it amongst the affections of the brain. Melancthon,
de anima,[2] confutes those that make the liver a part affected,
and Guianerius, *tract.* 15, *cap.* 13 *et* 17, though many put all
the affections in the heart, refers it to the brain. Ficinus,
cap. 7, *in Convivium Platonis,* "will have the blood to be the
part affected." Jo. Freitagius, *cap.* 14 *Noct. med.,* supposeth
all four affected, heart, liver, brain, blood; but the major part
concur upon the brain, 'tis *imaginatio læsa* [a disordered
imagination], and both imagination and reason are misaffected;
because of his corrupt judgment, and continual meditation of
that which he desires, he may truly be said to be melancholy.[3]
If it be violent, or his disease inveterate, as I have determined
in the precedent partitions, both imagination and reason are
misaffected, first one, then the other.

MEMB. II.

Subsect. I.—*Causes of Heroical Love, Temperature, full Diet,*
Idleness, Place, Climate, etc.

Of all causes the remotest are stars. Ficinus, *cap.* 19,[4] saith
they are most prone to this burning lust, that have Venus in
Leo in their horoscope, when the Moon and Venus be mutually
aspected, or such as be of Venus' complexion. Plutarch interprets astrologically that tale of Mars and Venus, "in whose
genitures ♂ and ♀ are in conjunction," they are commonly
lascivious, and if women, queans;[5] as the goodwife of Bath
confessed in Chaucer:

> I followed aye mine inclination,
> By virtue of my constellation.

But of all those astrological aphorisms which I have ever read,
that of Cardan is most memorable, for which howsoever he is
bitterly censured by Marinus Marcennus,[6] a malapert friar,
and some others (which he himself suspected [7]), yet methinks
it is free, downright, plain and ingenuous. In his eighth

geniture,[1] or example, he hath these words of himself: ☽ ♀ h *et* ☿ h
in ☿ *dignitatibus assiduam mihi venereorum cogitationem præsta-*
bunt, ita ut nunquam quiescam. Et paulo post, *Cogitatio vene-*
reorum me torquet perpetuo, et quam facto implere non licuit, aut
fecisse potentem puduit, cogitatione assidua mentitus sum volup-
tatem. Et alibi, *Ob* ☾ *et* ☿ *dominium et radiorum mixtionem,*
profundum fuit ingenium, sed lascivum, egoque turpi libidini
deditus et obscœnus. So far Cardan of himself, *quod de se fatetur*
ideo ut utilitatem adferat studiosis hujusce disciplinæ,[2] and for
this he is traduced by Marcennus, whenas in effect he saith no
more than what Gregory Nazianzen of old to Chilo his scholar,
Offerebant se mihi visendæ mulieres, quarum præcellenti elegantia
et decore spectabili tentabatur meæ integritas pudicitiæ. Et
quidem flagitium vitavi fornicationis, at munditiæ virginalis
florem arcana cordis cogitatione fœdavi. Sed ad rem. Aptiores
ad masculinam venerem sunt quorum genesi Venus est in signo
masculino, et in Saturni finibus aut oppositione, etc. Ptolemæus
in *Quadripart.* plura de his et specialia habet aphorismata, longo
procul dubio usu confirmata, et ab experientia multa perfecta,
inquit commentator ejus Cardanus. Tho. Campanella, *Astro-*
logiæ lib. 4, *cap.* 8, *articulis* 4 *et* 5, insaniam amatoriam remon-
strantia, multa præ cæteris accumulat aphorismata, quæ qui
volet, consulat. Chiromantici ex cingulo Veneris plerumque
conjecturam faciunt, et monte Veneris, de quorum decretis,
Taisnierum, Johan. de Indagine, Goclenium, ceterosque si lubet,
inspicias. Physicians divine wholly from the temperature and
complexion; phlegmatic persons are seldom taken, according
to Ficinus, *Comment. cap.* 9; naturally melancholy less than they,
but once taken they are never freed; though many are of opinion
flatuous or hypochondriacal melancholy are most subject of
all others to this infirmity. Valescus assigns their strong
imagination for a cause, Bodine abundance of wind, Gordonius
of seed, and spirits or atomi in the seed, which cause their
violent and furious passions. Sanguine thence are soon caught,
young folks most apt to love, and by their good wills, saith
Lucian,[3] "would have a bout with every one they see": the
colt's evil is common to all complexions. Theomnestus, a
young and lusty gallant, acknowledgeth (in the said author)
all this to be verified in him: "I am so amorously given, you
may sooner number the sea-sands, and snow falling from the
skies, than my several loves. Cupid had shot all his arrows
at me, I am deluded with various desires, one love succeeds
another, and that so soon, that before one is ended, I begin with

a second; she that is last is still fairest, and she that is present
pleaseth me most: as an hydra's head my loves increase, no
Iolaus can help me.   Mine eyes are so moist a refuge and
sanctuary of love, that they draw all beauties to them, and
are never satisfied.   I am in a doubt what fury of Venus this
should be.   Alas, how have I offended her so to vex me? what
Hippolytus am I?"[1]   What Telchin is my genius? or is it a
natural imperfection, an hereditary passion?   Another in
Anacreon[2] confesseth that he had twenty sweethearts in
Athens at once, fifteen at Corinth, as many at Thebes, at
Lesbos, and at Rhodes, twice as many in Ionia, thrice in Caria,
twenty thousand in all: or in a word, εἰ φύλλα πάντα, etc.:

> *Folia arborum omnium si*
> *Nosti referre cuncta,*
> *Aut computare arenas*
> *In æquore universas,*
> *Solum meorum amorum*
> *Te fecero logistam.*

> Canst count the leaves in May,
> Or sand i' th' ocean sea?
> Then count my loves I pray.

His eyes are like a balance, apt to propend each way, and to
be weighed down with every wench's looks, his heart a weather-
cock, his affection tinder, or naphtha itself, which every fair
object, sweet smile, or mistress' favour sets on fire.   Guianerius,
tract. 15 *cap.* 14, refers all this to "the hot temperature of the
testicles";[3] Ferrandus, a Frenchman, in his *Erotique Mel.* (which
book came first to my hands after the third edition[4]) to certain
atomi in the seed, "such as are very spermatic and full of
seed."   I find the same in *Aristotle, sect.* 4, *prob.* 17, *Si non
secernatur semen, cessare tentigines non possunt,* as Guastavinius
his commentator translates it: for which cause these young
men that be strong set, of able bodies, are so subject to it.
Hercules de Saxonia hath the same words in effect.   But most
part, I say, such are aptest to love that are young and lusty,
live at ease, stall-fed, free from cares, like cattle in a rank
pasture, idle and solitary persons, they must needs *hirquitallire*
[play the goat], as Guastavinius recites out of Censorinus.

> *Mens erit apta capi tum quum lætissima rerum.*
> *Ut seges in pingui luxuriabit humo.*[5]

> The mind is apt to lust, and hot or cold,
> As corn luxuriates in a better mould.

The place itself makes much wherein we live, the clime, air, and discipline if they concur. In our Mysia, saith Galen, near to Pergamus, thou shalt scarce find an adulterer, but many at Rome, by reason of the delights of the seat. It was that plenty of all things, which made Corinth [1] so infamous of old, and the opportunity of the place to entertain those foreign comers; every day strangers came in, at each gate, from all quarters. In that one temple of Venus a thousand whores did prostitute themselves, as Strabo writes, besides Lais and the rest of better note: all nations resorted thither, as to a school of Venus. Your hot and southern countries are prone to lust, and far more incontinent than those that live in the north, as Bodine discourseth at large, *Method. hist. cap. 5. Molles Asiatici* [the Orientals are amorous]; so are Turks, Greeks, Spaniards, Italians, even all that latitude; and in those tracts, such as are more fruitful, plentiful, and delicious, as Valence in Spain, Capua in Italy, *domicilium luxus* [a home of luxury] Tully terms it, and (which Hannibal's soldiers can witness) Canopus in Egypt, Sybaris, Phæacia, Baiæ, Cyprus, Lampsacus.[2] In Naples [3] the fruits of the soil and pleasant air enervate their bodies, and alter constitutions: insomuch that Florus calls it *certamen Bacchi et Veneris* [a contest between Bacchus and Venus], but Foliot [4] admires it. In Italy and Spain they have their stews in every great city, as in Rome, Venice, Florence, wherein, some say, dwell ninety thousand inhabitants, of which ten thousand are courtesans; and yet for all this, every gentleman almost hath a peculiar mistress; fornications, adulteries, are nowhere so common: *urbs est jam tota lupanar;* how should a man live honest amongst so many provocations? Now if vigour of youth, greatness, liberty I mean, and that impunity of sin which grandees take unto themselves in this kind shall meet, what a gap must it needs open to all manner of vice, with what fury will it rage! For, as Maximus Tyrius the Platonist observes,[5] *libido consecuta quum fuerit materiam improbam, et præruptam licentiam, et effrenatam audaciam* [when lust finds a vicious subject with unrestrained passion and utter shamelessness], etc., what will not lust effect in such persons? For commonly princes and great men make no scruple at all of such matters, but with that whore in Spartian, *quicquid libet licet*, they think they may do what they list, profess it publicly, and rather brag with Proculus (that writ to a friend of his in Rome, what famous exploits he had done in that kind [6]) than any way be abashed at it. Nicholas Sanders relates of Henry VIII [7]

(I know not how truly), *quod paucas vidit pulchriores quas non concupierit, et paucissimas non concupierit quas non violarit,* he saw very few [pretty] maids that he did not desire, and desired fewer whom he did not enjoy: nothing so familiar amongst them, 'tis most of their business: Sardanapalus, Messalina, and Joan of Naples are not comparable to meaner men and women[1]; Solomon of old had a thousand concubines; Ahasuerus his eunuchs and keepers; Nero his Tigellinus, panders, and bawds; the Turks, Muscovites, Mogors, Xeriffs of Barbary, and Persian Sophies, are no whit inferior to them in our times. *Delectus fit omnium puellarum toto regno forma præstantiorum* (saith Jovius[2]) *pro imperatore; et quas ille linquit, nobiles habent* [there is a levy throughout the kingdom of girls of striking beauty for the emperor; and those whom he leaves go to the nobles]; they press and muster up wenches as we do soldiers, and have their choice of the rarest beauties their countries can afford, and yet all this cannot keep them from adultery, incest, sodomy, buggery, and such prodigious lusts. We may conclude, that if they be young, fortunate, rich, high-fed, and idle withal, it is almost impossible that they should live honest, not rage, and precipitate themselves into these inconveniences of burning lust.

> *Otium et reges prius et beatas*
> *Perdidit urbes.*[3]

> [Rich kings and cities fair to naught
> By idle dalliance have been brought.]

Idleness overthrows all, *Vacuo pectore regnat amor,* love tyrannizeth in an idle person. *Amore abundas, Antipho* [thou overflowest with love, Antipho]. If thou hast nothing to do, *Invidia vel amore miser torquebere,*[4] thou shalt be haled in pieces with envy, lust, some passion or other. *Homines nihil agendo male agere discunt* [through doing nothing men learn to do ill]. 'Tis Aristotle's simile, "As match or touchwood takes fire, so doth an idle person love."[5] *Quæritur Ægisthus quare sit factus adulter,* etc., why was Ægisthus a whoremaster? You need not ask a reason of it. Ismenodora stole Baccho, a woman forced a man, as Aurora did Cephalus:[6] no marvel, saith Plutarch,[7] *luxurians opibus more hominum mulier agit:* she was rich, fortunate and jolly, and doth but as men do in that case, as Jupiter did by Europa, Neptune by Amymone. The poets therefore did well to feign all shepherds lovers, to give themselves to songs and dalliances, because they lived such idle lives. For

love, as Theophrastus defines it, is *otiosi animi affectus*,[1] an
affection of an idle mind,[2] or as Seneca describes it, *Juventa
gignitur, luxu nutritur, feriis alitur, otioque inter lætæ fortunæ
bona*, youth begets it, riot maintains it, idleness nourisheth it,
etc., which makes Gordonius the physician, *cap. 20, part. 2*,
call this disease the proper passion of nobility.[3] Now if a
weak judgment and a strong apprehension do concur, how,
saith Hercules de Saxonia, shall they resist? Savonarola
appropriates it almost to "monks, friars, and religious persons,
because they live solitarily, fare daintily, and do nothing": [4]
and well he may, for how should they otherwise choose?

Diet alone is able to cause it: a rare thing to see a young
man or a woman that lives idly and fares well, of what condition soever, not to be in love. Alcibiades [5] was still dallying
with wanton young women, immoderate in his expenses,
effeminate in his apparel, ever in love, but why? he was over-
delicate in his diet, too frequent and excessive in banquets.
Ubicunque securitas, ibi libido dominatur: lust and security
domineer together, as St. Hierome averreth. All which the
Wife of Bath in Chaucer freely justifies:

> For all to sicker, as cold engrendreth hail,
> A liquorish tongue must have a liquorish tail.

Especially if they shall further it by choice diet, as many times
those Sybarites and Phæaces do, feed liberally, and by their
good will eat nothing else but lascivious meats. *Vinum imprimis generosum,*[6] *legumen, fabas, radices omnium generum bene
conditas, et largo pipere aspersas, carduos hortulanos, lactucas,
erucas,*[7] *rapas, porros, cæpas, nucem piceam, amygdalas dulces,
electuaria, syrupos, succos, cochleas, conchus, pisces optime præ-
paratos, aviculas, testiculos animalium, ova, condimenta diver-
sorum generum, molles lectos, pulvinaria, etc. Et quicquid fere
medici impotentia rei venereæ laboranti præscribunt, hoc quasi
diasatyrion habent in deliciis, et his dapes multo delicatiores;
mulsum, exquisitas et exoticas fruges, aromata, placentas, expressos
succos multis ferculis variatos, ipsumque vinum suavitate vin-
centes, et quicquid culina, pharmacopæia, aut quæque fere officina
subministrare possit.* [First and foremost strong wine, vegetables,
beans, roots of all kinds, well seasoned and with plenty of pepper,
garden radishes, lettuces, rocket, rapes, leeks, onions, pine-nuts,
sweet almonds, electuaries, syrups, juices, snails, shell-fish, fish
tastefully cooked, poultry, testicles of animals, eggs, various
sauces, soft beds and couches, etc. Also . . . more delicate

dishes, mulled wine, choice fruits, scents, cakes, essences more tasty than wine, and all the products of the kitchen, the chemist's shop, or any other factory.] *Et hoc plerumque victu quum se ganeones infarciant, ut ille*[1] *ob Chrysidem suam, se bulbis et cochleis curavit; etiam ad Venerem se parent, et ad hanc palæstram se exerceant, qui fieri possit, ut non misere depereant, ut non penitus insaniant?*[2] Æstuans venter cito despuit in libidinem, *Hieronymus ait.* Post prandia Callyroen da.[3] *Quis enim continere se potest?* Luxuriosa res vinum,[4] *fomentum libidinis vocat Augustinus; blandum dæmonem, Bernardus; lac veneris, Aristophanes.* Non Ætna, non Vesuvius tantis ardoribus æstuant, ut juveniles medullæ vino plenæ, *addit Hieronymus*:[5] *unde ob optimum vinum Lampsacus olim Priapo sacer: et venerandi Bacchi socia, apud Orpheum*[6] *Venus audit. Hæc si vinum simplex, et per se sumptum præstare possit (nam,* Quo me, Bacche, rapis tui plenum?[7]), *quam non insaniam, quem non furorem a cæteris expectemus? Gomesius*[8] *salem enumerat inter ea quæ intempestivam libidinem provocare solent,* et salaciores fieri feminas ob esum salis contendit: Venerem ideo dicunt ab Oceano ortam.

Unde tot in Veneta scortorum millia cursant?
In promptu causa est, est Venus orta mari.[9]

Et hinc fœta mater Salacea Oceani conjux, *verbumque fortasse salax a sale effluxit. Mala Bacchica tantum olim in amoribus prævaluerunt, ut coronæ ex illis statuæ Bacchi ponerentur. Cubebis in vino maceratis utuntur Indi Orientales ad Venerem excitandum,*[10] *et Surax radice Africani.*[11] *Chinæ radix eosdem effectus habet, talisque herbæ meminit, Mag. nat. lib. 2, cap. 16, Baptista Porta ex India allatæ,*[12] *cujus mentionem facit et Theophrastus. Sed infinita his similia apud Rhasin, Matthiolum, Mizaldum, cæterosque medicos occurrunt, quorum ideo mentionem feci, ne quis imperitior in hos scopulos impingat, sed pro virili tanquam syrtes et cautes consulto effugiat.*

SUBSECT. II.—*Other causes of Love-Melancholy, Sight, Beauty from the face, eyes, other parts, and how it pierceth*

Many such causes may be reckoned up, but they cannot avail, except opportunity be offered of time, place, and those other beautiful objects, or artificial enticements, as kissing, conference, discourse, gestures, concur, with such-like lascivious

provocations. Kornmannus, in his book *de linea amoris*, makes
five degrees of lust, out of Lucian [1] belike, which he handles in
five chapters, *Visus, Colloquium, Convictus, Oscula, Tactus*
[sight, converse, companionship, kissing, touch]. Sight, of all
other, is the first step of this unruly love, though sometimes it
be prevented by relation or hearing, or rather incensed. For
there be those so apt, credulous, and facile to love, that if they
hear of a proper man, or woman, they are in love before they
see them, and that merely by relation, as Achilles Tatius
observes. "Such is their intemperance and lust, that they are
as much maimed by report as if they saw them.[2] Callisthenes,
a rich young gentleman of Byzance in Thrace, hearing of Leucippe, Sostratus' fair daughter, was far in love with her, and,
out of fame and common rumour, so much incensed, that he
would needs have her to be his wife." [3] And sometimes by
reading they are so affected, as he in Lucian confesseth of
himself, "I never read that place of Panthea in Xenophon,
but I am as much affected as if I were present with her." [4]
Such persons commonly feign a kind of beauty to themselves; [5]
and so did those three gentlewomen in Balthasar Castilio [6] fall
in love with a young man whom they never knew, but only
heard him commended: or by reading of a letter; for there is a
grace cometh from hearing, as a moral philosopher informeth
us, "as well from sight; and the species of love are received
into the phantasy by relation alone": [7] *ut cupere ab aspectu, sic
velle ab auditu,*[8] both senses affect. *Interdum et absentes amamus,*
sometimes we love those that are absent, saith Philostratus,
and gives instance in his friend Athenorodus, that loved a
maid at Corinth whom he never saw; *non oculi sed mens videt,*
we see with the eyes of our understanding.

But the most familiar and usual cause of love is that which
comes by sight, which conveys those admirable rays of beauty
and pleasing graces to the heart. Plotinus derives love from
sight, ἔρως *quasi* ὄρασις. *Si nescis, oculi sunt in amore duces,*[9]
the eyes are the harbingers of love, and the first step of love
is sight, as Lilius Giraldus proves at large, *Hist. deor. syntag.* 13; [10]
they as two sluices let in the influences of that divine, powerful,
soul-ravishing, and captivating beauty, which, as one saith,[11]
"is sharper than any dart or needle, wounds deeper into the
heart; and opens a gap through our ears to that lovely wound,
which pierceth the soul itself." "Through it love is kindled
like a fire" (Ecclus. ix, 8). This amazing, confounding, admirable, amiable beauty, "than which in all nature's treasure"

(saith Isocrates) "there is nothing so majestical and sacred, nothing so divine, lovely, precious," [1] 'tis nature's crown, gold and glory; *bonum si non summum, de summis tamen non infrequenter triumphans* [if it is not the highest good, it yet frequently triumphs over the highest], whose power hence may be discerned: we contemn and abhor generally such things as are foul and ugly to behold, account them filthy, but love and covet that which is fair. 'Tis beauty in all things which pleaseth and allureth us,[2] a fair hawk, a fine garment, a goodly building, a fair house, etc. That Persian Xerxes, when he destroyed all those temples of the gods in Greece, caused that of Diana *in integrum servari*, to be spared alone for that excellent beauty and magnificence of it. Inanimate beauty can so command. 'Tis that which painters, artificers, orators, all aim at, as Erixymachus, the physician in Plato, contends. "It was beauty first that ministered occasion to art, to find out the knowledge of carving, painting, building, to find out models, perspectives, rich furnitures, and so many rare inventions." [3] Whiteness in the lily, red in the rose, purple in the violet, a lustre in all things without life, the clear light of the moon, the bright beams of the sun, splendour of gold, purple, sparkling diamond, the excellent feature of the horse, the majesty of the lion, the colour of birds, peacocks' tails, the silver scales of fish, we behold with singular delight and admiration. "And [that] which is rich in plants, delightful in flowers, wonderful in beasts, but most glorious in men," [4] doth make us affect and earnestly desire it, as when we hear any sweet harmony, an eloquent tongue, see any excellent quality, curious work of man, elaborate art, or aught that is exquisite, there ariseth instantly in us a longing for the same. We love such men, but most part for comeliness of person; we call them gods and goddesses, divine, serene, happy, etc. And of all mortal men they alone (Calcagninus holds [5]) are free from calumny; *qui divitiis, magistratu et gloria florent, injuria lacessimus*, we backbite, wrong, hate renowned, rich, and happy men, we repine at their felicity, they are undeserving, we think, fortune is a stepmother to us, a parent to them. "We envy" (saith Isocrates [6]) "wise, just, honest men, except with mutual offices and kindnesses, some good turn or other, they extort this love from us; only fair persons we love at first sight, desire their acquaintance, and adore them as so many gods: we had rather serve them than command others, and account ourselves the more beholding to them, the more service they enjoin us," though they be otherwise vicious, unhonest; we love them, favour them, and are ready to do them any good office for their beauty's sake,[1] though they have no other good quality beside. *Dic igitur, o formose adolescens* (as that eloquent Phavorinus breaks out in Stobæus[2]), *dic, Autolyce, suavius nectare loqueris; dic, o Telemache, vehementius Ulysse dicis; dic, Alcibiades, utcunque ebrius, libentius tibi licet ebrio auscultabimus.* "Speak, fair youth, speak, Autolycus, thy words are sweeter than nectar; speak, O Telemachus, thou art more powerful than Ulysses; speak, Alcibiades, though drunk, we will willingly hear thee as thou art." Faults in such are no faults: for when the said Alcibiades[3] had stolen Anytus his gold and silver plate, he was so far from prosecuting so foul a fact (though every man else condemned his impudence and insolency) that he wished it had been more, and much better (he loved him dearly) for his sweet sake. No worth is eminent in such lovely persons, all imperfections hid; *non enim facile de his quos plurimum diligimus, turpitudinem suspicamur* [we do not readily suspect baseness in those whom we love], for hearing, sight, touch, etc., our mind and all our senses are captivated, *omnes sensus formosus delectat.* Many men have been preferred for their person alone, chosen kings, as amongst the Indians, Persians,[4] Ethiopians of old the properest man of person the country could afford was elected their sovereign lord: *Gratior est pulchro veniens e corpore virtus* [worth pleases more in a fair bearer]; and so have many other nations thought and done, as Curtius observes;[5] *ingens enim in corporis majestate veneratio est*, for there is a majestical presence in such men; and so far was beauty adored amongst them, that no man was thought fit to reign that was not in all parts complete and supereminent. Agis, King of Lacedæmon, had like to have been deposed, because he married a little wife; they would not have their royal issue degenerate. Who would ever have thought that Adrian the Fourth, an English monk's bastard (as Papirius Massovius writes in his life[6]), *inops a suis relictus, squalidus et miser*, a poor forsaken child, should ever come to be Pope of Rome? But why was it? *Erat acri ingenio, facundia expedita, eleganti corpore, facieque læta ac hilari* (as he follows it out of Nubrigensis,[7] for he ploughs with his heifer), he was wise, learned, eloquent, of a pleasant, a promising countenance, a goodly, proper man; he had, in a word, a winning look of his own, and that carried it, for that he was especially advanced. So "Saul was a goodly person and a fair." Maximinus elected

emperor, etc.   Branchus, the son of Apollo, whom he begot of
Jance, Succron's daughter (saith Lactantius), when he kept
King Admetus' herds in Thessaly, now grown a man, was an
earnest suitor to his mother to know his father; the nymph
denied him, because Apollo had conjured her to the contrary;
yet overcome by his importunity at last she sent him to his
father; when he came into Apollo's presence, *malas dei reverenter
osculatus* [having reverently kissed the cheeks of the god], he
carried himself so well, and was so fair a young man, that
Apollo was infinitely taken with the beauty of his person, he
could scarce look off him, and said he was worthy of such
parents, gave him a crown of gold, the spirit of divination, and
in conclusion made him a demigod.   *O vis superba formæ!*
[What proud strength is in beauty!], a goddess beauty is, whom
the very gods adore, *nam pulchros dii amant*; she is *amoris
domina* [love's mistress], love's harbinger, love's loadstone, a
witch, a charm, etc.   Beauty is a dower of itself, a sufficient
patrimony, an ample commendation, an accurate epistle, as
Lucian,[1] Apuleius,[2] Tiraquellus, and some others conclude.
Imperio digna forma, beauty deserves a kingdom, saith Abulensis, *Paradox. 2, cap.* 110, immortality; and "more have got
this honour and eternity for their beauty, than for all other
virtues besides":[3] and such as are fair "are worthy to be
honoured of God and men."[4]   That Idalian Ganymede was
therefore fetched by Jupiter into heaven.   Hephæstion dear to
Alexander, Antinous to Hadrian.   Plato calls beauty for that
cause a privilege of nature, *naturæ gaudentis opus*, nature's
masterpiece, a dumb comment; Theophrastus, a silent fraud;
still rhetoric, Carneades, that persuades without speech, a
kingdom without a guard, because beautiful persons command
as so many captains; Socrates, a tyranny, "which tyrannizeth
over tyrants themselves"; which made Diogenes belike call
proper women queens, *quod facerent homines quæ præciperent*,
because men were so obedient to their commands.   They will
adore, cringe, compliment, and bow to a common wench (if she
be fair) as if she were a noblewoman, a countess, a queen, or a
goddess.   Those intemperate young men of Greece erected at
Delphi a golden image with infinite cost, to the eternal memory
of Phryne the courtesan, as Ælian relates,[5] for she was a most
beautiful woman, insomuch, saith Athenæus, that Apelles and
Praxiteles drew Venus' picture from her.   Thus young men will
adore and honour beauty; nay kings themselves I say will do
it, and voluntarily submit their sovereignty to a lovely woman.

"Wine is strong, kings are strong, but a woman strongest"
(1 Esdras iii, 10), as Zorobabel proved at large to King Darius,
his princes and noblemen. "Kings sit still and command sea
and land, etc., all pay tribute to the king; but women make
kings pay tribute, and have dominion over them. When they
have got gold and silver, they submit all to a beautiful woman,
give themselves wholly to her, gape and gaze on her, and all
men desire her more than gold or silver, or any precious thing:
they will leave father and mother, and venture their lives for
her, labour and travel to get, and bring all their gains to women,
steal, fight, and spoil for their mistresses' sakes. And no king
so strong, but a fair woman is stronger than he is. All things"
(as he proceeds [1]) "fear to touch the king; yet I saw him and
Apame his concubine, the daughter of the famous Bartacus,
sitting on the right hand of the king, and she took the crown
off his head, and put it on her own, and stroke him with her left
hand; yet the king gaped and gazed on her, and when she
laughed he laughed, and when she was angry he flattered to be
reconciled to her." So beauty commands even kings themselves;
nay, whole armies and kingdoms are captivated together with
their kings. *Forma vincit armatos, ferrum pulchritudo captivat;
vincentur specie, qui non vincentur prælio* [2] [beauty conquers
warriors, grace overcomes the sword; they will be subdued by
beauty who are not subdued in battle]. And 'tis a great
matter, saith Xenophon, [3] "and of which all fair persons may
worthily brag, that a strong man must labour for his living if
he will have aught, a valiant man must fight and endanger himself
for it, a wise man speak, show himself, and toil; but a fair and
beautiful person doth all with ease, he compasseth his desire
without any painstaking": God and men, heaven and earth
conspire to honour him; every one pities him above other, if
he be in need, and all the world is willing to do him good. [4]
Chariclea fell into the hand of pirates, but when all the rest
were put to the edge of the sword, she alone was preserved for
her person. [5] When Constantinople was sacked by the Turk,
Irene escaped, and was so far from being made a captive, that
she even captivated the Grand Seignior himself. [6] So did
Rosamond insult over King Henry the Second:

> I was so fair an object;
> Whom fortune made my king, my love made subject;
> He found by proof the privilege of beauty,
> That it had power to countermand all duty. [2]

It captivates the very gods themselves, *morosiora numina*
[the more austere deities]:

> *Deus ipse deorum*
> *Factus ob hanc formam bos, equus, imber, olor.*[1]

[The king of the gods for the sake of this beauty made
himself a bull, a horse, a shower, a swan.]

And those *mali genii* [evil spirits] are taken with it, as I have
already proved.[2] *Formosam barbari verentur, et ad aspectum
pulchrum immanis animus mansuescit* (Heliodorus, *lib.* 5): the
barbarians stand in awe of a fair woman, and at a beautiful
aspect a fierce spirit is pacified. For whenas Troy was taken,
and the wars ended (as Clemens Alexandrinus[3] quotes out of
Euripides), angry Menelaus, with rage and fury armed, came
with his sword drawn, to have killed Helena with his own
hands, as being the sole cause of all those wars and miseries;
but when he saw her fair face, as one amazed at her divine
beauty, he let his weapon fall, and embraced her besides; he
had no power to strike so sweet a creature. *Ergo hebetantur
enses pulchritudine*, the edge of a sharp sword (as the saying is)
is dulled with a beautiful aspect, and severity itself is overcome. Hyperides the orator, when Phryne his client was
accused at Athens for her lewdness, used no other defence in
her cause, but tearing her upper garment, disclosed her naked
breast to the judges, with which comeliness of her body and
amiable gesture they were so moved and astonished that they
did acquit her forthwith, and let her go. O noble piece of
justice! mine author exclaims: and who is he that would not
rather lose his seat and robes, forfeit his office, than give
sentence against the majesty of beauty? Such prerogatives
have fair persons, and they alone are free from danger. Par-
thenopæus was so lovely and fair, that when he fought in the
Theban wars, if his face had been by chance bare, no enemy
would offer to strike at or hurt him, such immunities hath beauty.
Beasts themselves are moved with it. Sinalda was a woman of
such excellent feature, and a queen, that when she was to be
trodden on by wild horses for a punishment, "the wild beasts
stood in admiration of her person" (Saxo Grammaticus, *lib.* 8
Dan. Hist.) "and would not hurt her."[4] Wherefore did that
royal virgin in Apuleius,[5] when she fled from the thieves' den,
in a desert, make such an apostrophe to her ass on whom she
rode (for what knew she to the contrary, but that he was an ass?):
Si me parentibus et proco formoso reddideris, quas tibi gratias,

quos honores habebo, quos cibos exhibebo? [If you take me back
to my parents and my fair betrothed I shall be grateful to you
and honour you without end, I shall give you the finest food.]
She would comb him, dress him, feed him, and trick him every
day herself, and he should work no more, toil no more, but
rest and play, etc.   And besides, she would have a dainty
picture drawn, in perpetual remembrance, a virgin riding upon
an ass's back, with this motto, *Asino vectore regia virgo fugiens
captivitatem* [a royal maid riding upon an ass to escape cap-
tivity].   Why said she all this? why did she make such promises
to a dumb beast? but that she perceived the poor ass to be
taken with her beauty; for she did often *obliquo collo pedes
puellæ decoros basiare,* kiss her feet as she rode, *et ad delicatulas
voculas tentabat adhinnire,* offer to give consent as much as in
him was to her delicate speeches, and besides he had some
feeling, as she conceived, of her misery.   And why did Theagines'
horse in Heliodorus [1] curvet, prance, and go so proudly,
exultans alacriter et superbiens, etc., but that sure, as mine
author supposeth, he was in love with his master? *dixisses
ipsum equum pulchrum intelligere pulchram domini formam*
[you would have said that the horse itself was aware of the
beauty of its master].   A fly lighted on Malthius' cheek as
he lay asleep: [2] but why?   Not to hurt him, as a parasite of
his, standing by, well perceived, *non ut pungeret, sed ut oscu-
laretur,* but certainly to kiss him, as ravished with his divine
looks.   Inanimate creatures, I suppose, have a touch of this.
When a drop of Psyche's candle fell on Cupid's shoulder, [3] I
think sure it was to kiss it.   When Venus ran to meet her rose-
cheeked Adonis, as an elegant poet of ours [4] sets her out,

> The bushes in the way
> Some catch her neck, some kiss her face,
> Some twine about her legs to make her stay,
> And all did covet her for to embrace.

Aer ipse amore inficitur, as Heliodorus holds, the air itself is in
love: for when Hero played upon her lute,

> The wanton air in twenty sweet forms danc't
> After her fingers, [5]

and those lascivious winds stayed Daphne when she fled from
Apollo:

> *Nudabant corpora venti,*
> *Obviaque adversas vibrabant flamina vestes.* [6]

[The wind exposed her limbs as her garments fluttered
in the breeze.]

Boreas ventus [the North Wind] loved Hyacinthus, and Orithyia,
Erectheus' daughter of Athens: *vi rapuit*, etc., he took her away
by force, as she was playing with other wenches at Ilissus, and
begat Zetes and Calais his two sons of her. That seas and
waters are enamoured with this our beauty, is all out as likely
as that of the air and winds; for when Leander swimmed in the
Hellespont, Neptune with his trident did beat down the waves,
but they

> Still mounted up, intending to have kissed him,
> And fell in drops like tears because they missed him.

The river Alpheus was in love with Arethusa, as she tells the
tale herself: [1]

> *Viridesque manu siccata capillos,*
> *Fluminis Alphei veteres recitavit amores :*
> *Pars ego Nympharum, etc.*

[As with her hand she wiped the moisture from her
green tresses, she thus recounted the bygone
love of the stream Alpheus. "I was once a
nymph," etc.]

When our Thame and Isis meet,

> *Oscula mille sonant, connexu brachia pallent,*
> *Mutuaque explicitis connectunt colla lacertis.* [2]

[They exchanged a thousand kisses, and with arms
intertwined hang on each other's neck.]

Inachus and Peneus, and how many loving rivers can I reckon
up, whom beauty hath enthralled! I say nothing all this while
of idols themselves that have committed idolatry in this kind,
of looking-glasses that have been rapt in love (if you will believe
poets [3]), when their ladies and mistresses looked on to dress
them.

> *Et si non habeo sensum, tua gratia sensum*
> *Exhibet, et calidi sentio amoris onus.*
> *Dirigis huc quoties spectantia lumina, flamma*
> *Succendunt inopi saucia membra mihi.*

> Though I no sense at all of feeling have,
> Yet your sweet looks do animate and save;
> And when your speaking eyes do this way turn,
> Methinks my wounded members live and burn.

I could tell you such another story of a spindle that was fired
by a fair lady's looks,[4] or fingers, some say, I know not well
whether, but fired it was by report, and of a cold bath that
suddenly smoked and was very hot when naked Cælia came

into it: *Miramur quis sit tantus et unde vapor* [we marvel whence
comes this great steam], etc.   But of all the tales in this kind,
that is the most memorable of Death himself, when he should
have stroken a sweet young virgin with his dart, he fell in love
with the object.[1]   Many more such could I relate which are to
be believed with a poetical faith.   So dumb and dead creatures
dote, but men are mad, stupefied many times at the first sight
of beauty, amazed, as that fisherman in Aristænetus, that spied
a maid bathing herself by the sea-side: [2]

> *Soluta mihi sunt omnia membra*
> *A capite ad calcem, sensusque omnis periit*
> *De pectore, tam immensus stupor animam invasit mihi.*[3]

> [My limbs quivered, I shook from head to foot, my
> senses left me, I was utterly dazed and stupefied.]

And as Lucian, in his Images, confesses of himself, that he was
at his mistress's presence void of all sense, immovable, as if he
had seen a Gorgon's head: [4] which was no such cruel monster
(as Cælius interprets it, *lib.* 3, *cap.* 9 [5]), "but the very quintessence of beauty," some fair creature, as without doubt the
poet understood in the first fiction of it, at which the spectators
were amazed.   *Miseri quibus intentata nites,*[6] poor wretches are
compelled at the very sight of her ravishing looks to run mad,
or make away themselves.

> They wait the sentence of her scornful eyes;
> And whom she favours lives, the other dies.[7]

Heliodorus, *lib.* 1, brings in Thyamis almost besides himself,
when he saw Chariclea first, and not daring to look upon her a
second time, "for he thought it unpossible for any man living
to see her and contain himself." [8]   The very fame of beauty
will fetch them to it many miles off (such an attractive power
this loadstone hath), and they will seem but short, they will
undertake any toil or trouble, long journeys, Penia or Atalanta
shall not overgo them, through seas, deserts, mountains, and
dangerous places, as they did to gaze on Psyche: "many mortal
men came far and near to see that glorious object of her age"; [9]
Paris for Helena, Corebus to Troy,

> *Illis Trojam qui forte diebus*
> *Venerat insano Cassandræ incensus amore.*

> [Who chanced to have then arrived in Troy, drawn by
> his burning passion for Cassandra.]

King John of France, once prisoner in England, came to visit

his old friends again, crossing the seas; but the truth is, his
coming was to see the Countess of Salisbury, the nonpareil of
those times, and his dear mistress. That infernal god Plutus
came from hell itself, to steal Proserpina; Achilles left all his
friends for Polyxena's sake, his enemy's daughter; and all the
Grecian gods forsook their heavenly mansions for that fair lady,
Philo Dioneus' daughter's sake, the paragon of Greece in those
days;[1] *ea enim venustate fuit, ut eam certatim omnes dii conjugem
expeterent* [for she was of such surpassing beauty that all the
gods contended for her love]: *Formosa divis imperat puella*[2]
[the beautiful maid commands the gods]. They will not only
come to see, but as a falconer makes an hungry hawk, hover
about, follow, give attendance and service, spend goods, lives,
and all their fortunes to attain:

> Were beauty under twenty locks kept fast,
> Yet love breaks through, and picks them all at last.

When fair Hero came abroad, the eyes, hearts, and affections
of her spectators were still attendant on her.[3]

> *Et medios inter vultus supereminet omnes,*
> *Perque urbem aspiciunt venientem numinis instar.*[4]

> So far above the rest fair Hero shined,
> And stole away the enchanted gazer's mind.[5]

When Peter Aretine's Lucretia[6] came first to Rome, and that
the fame of her beauty *ad urbanarum deliciarum sectatores venerat,
nemo non ad videndam eam*, etc., was spread abroad, they came
in (as they say) "thick and threefold" to see her, and hovered
about her gates, as they did of old to Lais of Corinth, and
Phryne of Thebes, *Ad cujus jacuit Græcia tota fores*[7] [at whose
gates lay all Greece]. "Every man sought to get her love,
some with gallant and costly apparel, some with an affected
pace, some with music, others with rich gifts, pleasant discourse,
multitude of followers; others with letters, vows, and promises,
to commend themselves, and to be gracious in her eyes."[8]
Happy was he that could see her, thrice happy that enjoyed
her company. Charmides in Plato was a proper young man,
in comeliness of person, "and all good qualities, far exceeding
others; whensoever fair Charmides came abroad, they seemed
all to be in love with him" (as Critias describes their carriage),
"and were troubled at the very sight of him; many came near
him, many followed him wheresoever he went,"[9] as those
formarum spectatores [who were looking out for beauties] did

Acontius, if at any time he walked abroad:[1] the Athenian lasses stared on Alcibiades; Sappho and the Mitylenian women on Phaon the fair. Such lovely sights do not only please, entice, but ravish and amaze. Cleonymus, a delicate and tender youth, present at a feast which Androcles his uncle made *in Piræo* [in the Piræus] at Athens, when he sacrificed to Mercury, so stupefied the guests, Dineas, Aristippus, Agasthenes, and the rest (as Charidemus in Lucian[2] relates it), that they could not eat their meat, they sat all supper-time gazing, glancing at him, stealing looks, and admiring of his beauty. Many will condemn these men that are so enamoured for fools; but some again commend them for it; many reject Paris' judgment, and yet Lucian approves of it, admiring Paris for his choice; he would have done as much himself, and by good desert in his mind; beauty is to be preferred "before wealth or wisdom."[3] Athenæus, *Deipnosophist. lib.* 13, *cap.* 7, holds it not such indignity for the Trojans and Greeks to contend ten years, to spend so much labour,[4] lose so many men's lives for Helen's sake, for so fair a lady's sake:[5]

> *Ob talem uxorem cui præstantissima forma,*
> *Nil mortale refert.*

[Compared with a woman of such peerless beauty, nothing human matters.]

That one woman was worth a kingdom, an hundred thousand other women, a world itself. Well might Stesichorus be blind for carping at so fair a creature,[6] and a just punishment it was. The same testimony gives Homer of the old men of Troy, that were spectators of that single combat between Paris and Menelaus at the Scæan gate, when Helena stood in presence; they said all, the war was worthily prolonged and undertaken for her sake.[7] The very gods themselves (as Homer and Isocrates[8] record) fought more for Helena than they did against the giants. When Venus lost her son Cupid,[9] she made proclamation by Mercury, that he that could bring tidings of him should have seven kisses; a noble reward some say, and much better than so many golden talents; seven such kisses to many men were more precious than seven cities, or so many provinces. One such a kiss alone would recover a man if he were a-dying: *Suaviolum Stygia sic te de valle reducet*, etc.[10] Great Alexander married Roxane, a poor man's child, only for her person.[11] 'Twas well done of Alexander, and heroically done; I admire him for it. Orlando was mad for Angelica, and who doth not condole his mishap? Thisbe died for Pyramus, Dido for Æneas; who doth not weep, as (before his conversion) Austin did, in commiseration of her estate? [1] she died for him; "methinks" (as he said) "I could die for her."

But this is not the matter in hand; what prerogative this beauty hath, of what power and sovereignty it is, and how far such persons that so much admire and dote upon it are to be justified—no man doubts of these matters; the question is, how and by what means beauty produceth this effect? By sight: the eye betrays the soul, and is both active and passive in this business; it wounds and is wounded, is an especial cause and instrument, both in the subject and in the object. "As tears, it begins in the eyes, descends to the breast"; [2] it conveys these beauteous rays, as I have said, unto the heart. *Ut vidi, ut perii!* [I saw, I was undone]. *Mars videt hanc, visamque cupit* [3] [Mars sees her and straightway desires her]. Shechem saw Dinah the daughter of Leah, and defiled her (Gen. xxxiv, 3); Jacob, Rachel (xxix, 17), "for she was beautiful and fair"; David spied Bathsheba afar off (2 Sam. xi, 2); the Elders, Susanna, as that Orthomenian Strato saw fair Aristoclea, the daughter of Theophanes, bathing herself at that Hercyne well in Lebadea,[4] and were captivated in an instant. *Viderunt oculi, rapuerunt pectora flammæ* [the eyes beheld, the heart was straight aflame]. Amnon fell sick for Tamar's sake (2 Sam. xiii, 2). The beauty of Esther was such, that she found favour not only in the sight of Ahasuerus, "but of all those that looked upon her." Gerson, Origen, and some others contended that Christ Himself was the fairest of the sons of men, and Joseph next unto Him, *speciosus præ filiis hominum*, and they will have it literally taken; His very person was such that He found grace and favour of all those that looked upon Him. Joseph was so fair, that, as the ordinary gloss hath it, *filiæ decurrerent per murum, et ad fenestras*, they ran to the top of the walls and to the windows to gaze on him, as we do commonly to see some great personage go by: and so Matthew Paris describes Matilda the Empress going through Cologne. P. Morales the Jesuit [5] saith as much of the Virgin Mary. Antony no sooner saw Cleopatra, but, saith Appian, *lib.* 1, he was enamoured of her. Theseus at the first sight of Helen was so besotted, that he esteemed himself the happiest man in the world if he might enjoy her,[6] and to that purpose kneeled down, and made his pathetical prayers unto the gods. Charicles, by chance espying that curious picture of smiling Venus naked in her temple, stood a great while gazing, as one amazed; at length he brake into that mad passionate speech, "O fortunate god Mars, that wast bound in chains, and made ridiculous for her sake!" [1] He could not contain himself, but kissed her picture, I know not how oft, and heartily desired to be so disgraced as Mars was. And what did he that his betters had not done before him?

> Atque aliquis de dis non tristibus optat
> Sic fieri turpis.[2]

When Venus came first to heaven, her comeliness was such, that (as mine author saith) "all the gods came flocking about, and saluted her, each of them went to Jupiter, and desired he might have her to be his wife." [3] When fair Autolycus came in presence, as a candle in the dark his beauty shined,[4] all men's eyes (as Xenophon describes the manner of it) "were instantly fixed on him, and moved at the sight, insomuch that they could not conceal themselves, but in gesture or looks it was discerned and expressed." Those other senses, hearing, touching, may much penetrate and affect, but none so much, none so forcible as sight. *Forma Briseis mediis in armis movit Achillem*, Achilles was moved in the midst of a battle by fair Briseis, Ajax by Tecmessa; Judith captivated that great captain Holofernes: Delilah, Samson; Rosamund, Henry the Second;[5] Roxalana, Solyman the Magnificent, etc.

> Νικᾷ δὲ καὶ σίδηρον
> Καὶ πῦρ καλή τις οὖσα.[6]

A fair woman overcomes fire and sword.

> Naught under heaven so strongly doth allure
> The sense of man and all his mind possess,
> As beauty's loveliest bait, that doth procure
> Great warriors erst their rigour to suppress,
> And mighty hands forget their manliness,
> Driven with the power of an heart-burning eye,
> And lapt in fetters of a golden tress,
> That can with melting pleasure mollify
> Their harden'd hearts inur'd to cruelty.[7]

Clitiphon ingenuously confesseth,[8] that he no sooner came in Leucippe's presence, but that he did *corde tremere, et oculis lascivius intueri*; he was wounded at the first sight, his heart panted, and he could not possibly turn his eyes from her.[9] So doth Calasiris in Heliodorus, *lib. 2*, Isis' priest, a reverend old man, complain, who by chance at Memphis seeing that Thracian

Rhodopis, might not hold his eyes off her: "I will not conceal
it, she overcame me with her presence, and quite assaulted my
continency which I had kept unto mine old age; I resisted a
long time my bodily eyes with the eyes of my understanding;
at last I was conquered, and as in a tempest carried headlong." [1]
Xenopithes, a philosopher, railed at women downright for many
years together, scorned, hated, scoffed at them; coming at last
into Daphnis a fair maid's company (as he condoles his mishap
to his friend Demaretus), though free before, *contactus nullis
ante cupidinibus*, was far in love, and quite overcome upon a
sudden.[2] *Victus sum, fateor, a Daphnide*, etc., I confess I am
taken,

> *Sola hæc inflexit sensus, animumque labentem
> Impulit,*[3]

> [She alone hath made me waver and turned my mind,]

I could hold out no longer. Such another mishap, but worse,
had Stratocles the physician, that blear-eyed old man, *muco
plenus* (so Prodromus describes him [4]); he was a severe woman-
hater all his life, *fœda et contumeliosa semper in feminas profatus*,
a bitter persecutor of the whole sex, *humanas aspides et viperas
appellabat* [he called them asps and vipers in human shape],
he forswore them all still, and mocked them wheresoever he
came, in such vile terms, *ut matrem et sorores odisses*, that if thou
hadst heard him, thou wouldst have loathed thine own mother
and sisters for his word's sake. Yet this old doting fool was
taken at last with that celestial and divine look of Myrilla, the
daughter of Anticles the gardener, that smirking wench, that
he shaved off his bushy beard, painted his face, curled his hair,[5]
wore a laurel crown to cover his bald pate, and for her love
besides was ready to run mad. For the very day that he
married he was so furious, *ut solis occasum minus expectare
posset* (a terrible, a monstrous long day), he could not stay till
it was night, *sed omnibus insalutatis in thalamum festinans
irrupit*, the meat scarce out of his mouth, without any leave-
taking, he would needs go presently to bed. What young man,
therefore, if old men be so intemperate, can secure himself?
Who can say, I will not be taken with a beautiful object, I can,
I will contain? No, saith Lucian [6] of his mistress, she is so
fair, that if thou dost but see her, "she will stupefy thee, kill
thee straight, and, Medusa-like, turn thee to a stone; thou
canst not pull thine eyes from her, but, as an adamant doth
iron, she will carry thee bound headlong whither she will

herself," infect thee like a basilisk. It holds both in men and women. Dido was amazed at Æneas' presence: *Obstupuit primo aspectu Sidonia Dido*; and, as he feelingly verified out of his experience:

> *Quam ego postquam vidi, non ita amavi ut sani solent*
> *Homines, sed eodem pacto ut insani solent.*[1]

> I lov'd her not as others soberly,
> But as a madman rageth, so did I.

So Musæus of Leander, *nusquam lumen detorquet ab illa* [he never turned his eyes from her]; and Chaucer of Palamon,[2]

> He cast his eye upon Emilia,
> And therewith he blent and cried ha, ha,
> As though he had been stroke unto the heart.

If you desire to know more particularly what this beauty is, how it doth *influere* [influence], how it doth fascinate (for, as all hold, love is a fascination), thus in brief. "This comeliness or beauty ariseth from the due proportion of the whole, or from each several part." [3] For an exact delineation of which, I refer you to poets, historiographers, and those amorous writers, to Lucian's *Imagines* and *Charidemus*, Xenophon's description of Panthea, Petronius' *Catalecta*, Heliodorus' Chariclea, Tatius' Leucippe, Longus Sophista's Daphnis and Chloe, Theodorus Prodromus his Rhodanthe, Aristænetus' and Philostratus' Epistles, Balthasar Castilio, *lib. 4 de aulico*, Laurentius, *cap.* 10 *de melan.*, Æneas Sylvius his Lucretia, and every poet almost, which have most accurately described a perfect beauty, an absolute feature, and that through every member, both in men and women. Each part must concur to the perfection of it; for as Seneca saith, *Ep.* 33, *lib.* 4, *Non est formosa mulier cujus crus laudatur et brachium, sed illa cujus simul universa facies admirationem singulis partibus dedit:* she is no fair woman, whose arm, thigh, etc., are commended, except the face and all the other parts be correspondent. And the face especially gives a lustre to the rest: the face is it that commonly denominates fair or foul: *arx formæ facies*, the face is beauty's tower; and though the other parts be deformed, yet a good face carries it (*facies non uxor amatur* ['tis the face, not the wife, that is loved]), that alone is most part respected, principally valued, *deliciis suis ferox*, and of itself able to captivate.

> *Urit te Glyceræ nitor,*
> *Urit grata protervitas*
> *Et vultus nimium lubricus aspici.*[4]

Glycera's too fair a face was it that set him on fire, too fine to
be beheld. When Chærea [1] saw the singing-wench's sweet looks,
he was so taken, that he cried out, *O faciem pulchram, deleo
omnes dehinc ex animo mulieres, tædet quotidianarum harum
formarum!* "O fair face, I 'll never love any but her, look on
any other hereafter but her; I am weary of these ordinary
beauties, away with them!" The more he sees her, the worse
he is, *uritque videndo*; as in a burning-glass the sunbeams are
re-collected to a centre, the rays of love are projected from her
eyes. It was Æneas' countenance ravished Queen Dido, *os
humerosque deo similis*, he had an angelical face.

> *O sacros vultus Baccho vel Apolline dignos,*
> *Quos vir, quos tuto femina nulla videt!* [2]

> O sacred looks, befitting majesty,
> Which never mortal wight could safely see!

Although for the greater part this beauty be most eminent in
the face, yet many times those other members yield a most
pleasing grace, and are alone sufficient to enamour. An high
brow like unto the bright heavens, *Cæli pulcherrima plaga,
Frons ubi vivit honor, frons ubi ludit amor* [a brow where honour
dwells and love disports], white and smooth like the polished
alabaster, a pair of cheeks of vermilion colour, in which love
lodgeth: *Amor qui mollibus genis puellæ pernoctas* [love that
dallies on a maid's soft cheeks]; a coral lip, *suaviorum delubrum*
[a shrine of kisses], in which *Basia mille patent, basia mille
latent* [a thousand kisses show, a thousand lie hid], *gratiarum
sedes gratissima* [3] [sweetest abode of sweetness]; a sweet-smelling
flower, from which bees may gather honey:

> *Mellilegæ volucres, quid adhuc cava thyma rosasque,[etc.*
> *Omnes ad dominæ labra venite meæ,*
> *Illa rosas spirat, etc.* [4]

> [Ye honey-gathering bees, wherefore seek ye thyme and
> roses? Come all to the lips of my mistress, she
> breathes roses, etc.]

A white and round neck, that *via lactea* [milky way]; dimple in
the chin, black eyebrows, *Cupidinis arcus* [Cupid's bow], sweet
breath, white and even teeth; [that] which some call the sale-
piece, a fine soft round pap, gives an excellent grace, *Quale
decus tumidis Pario de marmore mammis!* [5] and make a pleasant
valley, *lacteum sinum*, between two chalky hills,[6] *sororiantes
papillulas, et ad pruritum frigidos amatores solo aspectu excitantes.*

Unde is, Forma papillarum quam fuit apta premi! [1]—Again,
Urebant oculos duræ stantesque mamillæ.

A flaxen hair: golden hair was even in great account, for
which Virgil commends Dido, *Nondum sustulerat flavum Proser-
pinina crinem* [not yet had Proserpine put up her golden hair],
Et crines nodantur in aurum [the hair is tied in a golden knot].
Apollonius (*Argonaut. lib.* 4, *Jasonis flava coma incendit cor
Medeæ*) will have Jason's golden hair to be the main cause of
Medea's dotage on him.   Castor and Pollux were both yellow-
haired; Paris, Menelaus, and most amorous young men have
been such in all ages, *molles ac suaves*, as Baptista Porta infers,
Physiog. lib. 2,[2] lovely to behold.   Homer so commends Helen,
makes Patroclus and Achilles both yellow-haired; *pulchricoma*
[fair-haired] Venus; and Cupid himself was yellow-haired, *in
aurum coruscante et crispante capillo* [with bright curly golden
locks], like that neat picture of Narcissus in Callistratus, for
so Psyche spied him asleep;[3] Briseis, Polyxena, etc., *flavicomæ
omnes* [were all yellow-haired],

> And Hero the fair,
> Whom young Apollo courted for her hair.

Leland commends Guithcra, King Arthur's wife, for a fair
flaxen hair: so Paulus Æmilius sets out Clodoveus, that lovely
king of France.   Synesius [4] holds every effeminate fellow or
adulterer is fair-haired: and Apuleius adds that Venus herself,
Goddess of Love, cannot delight, "though she come accompanied
with the Graces, and all Cupid's train to attend upon her, girt
with her own girdle, and smell of cinnamon and balm, yet if
she be bald or bad-haired, she cannot please her Vulcan." [5]
Which belike makes our Venetian ladies at this day to counterfeit yellow hair so much, great women to calamistrate and curl
it up, *vibrantes ad gratiam crines, et tot orbibus in captivitatem
flexos*, to adorn their heads with spangles, pearls, and made
flowers; and all courtiers to affect a pleasing grace in this kind.
In a word, "the hairs are Cupid's nets, to catch all comers, a
brushy wood, in which Cupid builds his nest, and under whose
shadow all loves a thousand several ways sport themselves." [6]

A little soft hand, pretty little mouth, small, fine long fingers
(*Gratia quæ digitis*, 'tis that which Apollo did admire in Daphne:
laudat digitosque manusque), a straight and slender body, a
small foot, and well-proportioned leg hath an excellent lustre,
cui totum incumbit corpus uti fundamento ædes [7] [on which the
whole body rests as a house on its foundation].   Clearchus

vowed to his friend Amynander in Aristænetus,¹ that the most
attractive part in his mistress, to make him love and like her
first, was her pretty leg and foot: a soft and white skin, etc.,
have their peculiar graces: *Nebula haud est mollior ac hujus
cutis est, edepol papillam bellulam* ² [a cloud cannot be softer
than this maid's skin; a pretty little pap, forsooth].   Though
in men these parts are not so much respected; a grim Saracen
sometimes, *nudus membra Pyracmon* [a bare-limbed Cyclops],
a martial hirsute face pleaseth best; a black man is a pearl in
a fair woman's eye, and is as acceptable as lame ³ Vulcan was to
Venus; for he, being a sweaty fuliginous blacksmith, was dearly
beloved of her, when fair Apollo, nimble Mercury were rejected,
and the rest of the sweet-faced gods forsaken.   Many women
(as Petronius observes ⁴) *sordibus calent* [fall in love with low
fellows] (as many men are more moved with kitchen-wenches,
and a poor market-maid, than all these illustrious court and city
dames), will sooner dote upon a slave, a servant, a dirt-dauber,
a Brontes, a cook, a player, if they see his naked legs or arms,
torosaque brachia [brawny arms], etc.,⁵ like that huntsman
Meleager in Philostratus, though he be all in rags, obscene and
dirty, besmeared like a ruddle-man, a gipsy, or a chimney-
sweeper, than upon a noble gallant, Nireus, Hephæstion, Alcibiades, or those embroidered courtiers full of silk and gold.
Justin's wife, a citizen of Rome, fell in love with Pylades a
player, and was ready to run mad for him, had not Galen himself helped her by chance.⁶   Faustina the empress doted on
a fencer.

Not one of a thousand falls in love, but there is some peculiar
part or other which pleaseth most, and inflames him above the
rest.   A company of young philosophers on a time fell at
variance,⁷ which part of a woman was most desirable and
pleased best? some said the forehead, some the teeth, some
the eyes, cheeks, lips, neck, chin, etc.; the controversy was
referred to Lais of Corinth to decide; but she, smiling, said they
were a company of fools; for suppose they had her where they
wished, what would they first seek? ⁸ Yet, this notwithstanding, I do easily grant, *neque quis vestrum negaverit, opinor*
[and none of you, I think, will gainsay it], all parts are attractive,
but especially the eyes,⁹

> *Videt igne micantes,*
> *Sideribus similes oculos,*

[He sees her eyes sparkling like the stars,]

which are love's fowlers, *aucupium amoris*; the shoeing-horns, "the hooks of love" (as Arandus will), "the guides, touchstone, judges, that in a moment cure madmen and make sound folks mad, the watchmen of the body; what do they not? how vex they not?" [1] All this is true, and (which Athenæus, *lib.* 13 *Deipnosoph. cap.* 5, and Tatius [2] hold) they are the chief seats of love, and as James Lernutius hath facetely expressed in an elegant ode of his: [3]

> *Amorem ocellis flammeolis heræ*
> *Vidi insidentem, credite posteri,*
> *Fratresque circum ludibundos*
> *Cum pharetra volitare et arcu, etc.*

> I saw Love sitting in my mistress' eyes
> Sparkling, believe it all posterity,
> And his attendants playing round about
> With bow and arrows ready for to fly.

Scaliger calls the eyes "Cupid's arrows; [4] the tongue, the lightning of love; the paps, the tents": Balthasar Castilio, [5] the causes, the chariots, the lamps of love:

> *Æmula lumina stellis,*
> *Lumina quæ possent sollicitare deos;*

> Eyes emulating stars in light,
> Enticing gods at the first sight;

Love's orators, Petronius:

> *O blandos oculos, et o facetos,*
> *Et quadam propria nota loquaces:*
> *Illic est Venus, et leves amores,*
> *Atque ipsa in medio sedet voluptas;*

> O sweet and pretty speaking eyes,
> Where Venus, love, and pleasure lies;

Love's torches, touch-box, naphtha, and matches, Tibullus: [6]

> *Illius ex oculis quum vult exurere divos,*
> *Accendit geminas lampadas acer amor.*

> Tart Love, when he will set the gods on fire,
> Lightens the eyes as torches to desire.

Leander, at the first sight of Hero's eyes, was incensed, saith Musæus:

> *Simul in oculorum radiis* [7] *crescebat fax amorum,*
> *Et cor fervebat invecti ignis impetu;*

Pulchritudo enim celebris immaculatæ feminæ,
Acutior hominibus est veloci sagitta.
Oculus vero via est, ab oculi ictibus
Vulnus dilabitur, et in præcordia viri manat.

Love's torches 'gan to burn first in her eyes,
And set his heart on fire which never dies:
For the fair beauty of a virgin pure
Is sharper than a dart, and doth inure
A deeper wound, which pierceth to the heart
By the eyes, and causeth such a cruel smart.

A modern poet [1] brings in Amnon complaining of Tamar:

Et me fascino
Occidit ille risus et formæ lepos,
Ille nitor, illa gratia, et verus decor,
Illæ æmulantes purpuram, et rosas genæ,[2]
Oculique vinctæque aureo nodo comæ.

It was thy beauty, 'twas thy pleasing smile,
Thy grace and comeliness did me beguile;
Thy rose-like cheeks and unto purple fair,
Thy lovely eyes and golden knotted hair.

Philostratus Lemnius [3] cries out on his mistress' basilisk eyes, *ardentes faces*, those two burning-glasses, they had so inflamed his soul, that no water could quench it. "What a tyranny" (saith he), "what a penetration of bodies is this! thou drawest with violence, and swallowest me up, as Charybdis doth sailors, with thy rocky eyes: he that falls into this gulf of love can never get out." Let this be the corollary then, the strongest beams of beauty are still darted from the eyes.

Nam quis lumina tanta, tanta
Posset luminibus suis tueri,
Non statim trepidansque, palpitansque,
Præ desiderii æstuantis aura? etc.[4]

For who such eyes with his can see,
And not forthwith enamoured be!

And as men catch dotterels by putting out a leg or an arm, with those mutual glances of the eyes they first inveigle one another. *Cynthia prima suis miserum me cepit ocellis* [5] ['twas with her eyes that Cynthia first led me captive]. Of all eyes (by the way) black are most amiable, enticing and fairest, which the poet observes in commending of his mistress, *Spectandum nigris oculis, nigroque capillo* [1] [notable for black eyes and black hair], which Hesiod admires in his Alcmena,

> *Cujus a vertice ac nigricantibus oculis,*
> *Tale quiddam spirat ac ab aurea Venere.* [2]

From her black eyes, and from her golden face,
As if from Venus came a lovely grace

and Triton in his Milane, *Nigra oculos formosa mihi* [3] [a black-eyed maid to me is beautiful]. Homer [4] useth that epithet of ox-eyed in describing Juno, because a round black eye is the best, the son of beauty, and farthest from black the worse; which Polydore Virgil [5] taxeth in our nation: *Angli ut plurimum cæsiis oculis*, we have grey eyes for the most part. Baptista Porta, *Physiognom. lib.* 3, puts grey colour upon children, they be childish eyes, dull and heavy. Many commend on the other side Spanish ladies, and those Greek dames [6] at this day, for the blackness of their eyes, as Porta doth his Neapolitan young wives. Suetonius describes Julius Cæsar to have been *nigris vegetisque oculis micantibus,* of a black quick sparkling eye: and although Averroes, in his *Colliget*, will have such persons timorous, yet without question they are most amorous.

Now, last of all, I will show you by what means beauty doth fascinate, bewitch, as some hold, and work upon the soul of a man by the eye. For certainly I am of the poet's mind, love doth bewitch and strangely change us.

> *Ludit amor sensus, oculos perstringit, et aufert*
> *Libertatem animi, mira nos fascinat arte.*
> *Credo aliquis dæmon subiens præcordia flammam*
> *Concitat, et raptam tollit de cardine mentem.* [7]

Love mocks our senses, curbs our liberties,
And doth bewitch us with his art and rings,
I think some devil gets into our entrails,
And kindles coals, and heaves our souls from th' hinges.

Heliodorus, *lib.* 3, proves at large that love is witchcraft, "it gets in at our eyes, pores, nostrils, engenders the same qualities and affections in us, as were in the party whence it came." [8] The manner of the fascination, as Ficinus, 10 *cap. Com. in Plat.*, declares it, is thus: "Mortal men are then especially bewitched, whenas by often gazing one on the other they direct sight to sight, join eye to eye, and so drink and suck in love between them; for the beginning of this disease is the eye. [9] And therefore he that hath a clear eye, though he be otherwise deformed, by often looking upon him, will make one.

mad, and tie him fast to him by the eye." [1]   Leonard. Varius,
lib. 1, *cap*. 2, *de fascinat*., telleth us that by this interview
"the purer spirits are infected," [2] the one eye pierceth through
the other with his rays, which he sends forth, and many men
have those excellent piercing eyes, that, which Suetonius
relates of Augustus, their brightness is such, they compel their
spectators to look off, and can no more endure them than the
sunbeams.   Barradius, *lib*. 6, *cap*. 10, *de Harmonia Evangel.*,
reports as much of our Saviour Christ, and Peter Morales [3] of
the Virgin Mary, whom Nicephorus [4] describes likewise to have
been yellow-haired, of a wheat colour, but of a most amiable
and piercing eye.   The rays, as some think, sent from the eyes,
carry certain spiritual vapours with them, and so infect the
other party, and that in a moment.   I know, they that hold
visio fit intra mittendo [sight comes from receiving the images]
will make a doubt of this; but Ficinus proves it from blear-
eyes, "that by sight alone make others blear-eyed; and it is
more than manifest that the vapour of the corrupt blood doth
get in together with the rays, and so by the contagion the
spectator's eyes are infected." [5]   Other arguments there are of
a basilisk, that kills afar off by sight, as that Ephesian did of
whom Philostratus speaks, [6] of so pernicious an eye, he poisoned
all he looked steadily on: and that other argument, *menstruæ
feminæ*, out of Aristotle's Problems, *morbosæ* Capivaccius adds,
and Septalius the Commentator, [7] that contaminate a looking-
glass with beholding it.   "So the beams that come from the
agent's heart, by the eyes, infect the spirits about the patients,
inwardly wound, and thence the spirits infect the blood." [8]
To this effect she complained in Apuleius, [9] "Thou art the cause
of my grief; thy eyes, piercing through mine eyes to mine inner
parts, have set my bowels on fire, and therefore pity me that
am now ready to die for thy sake."   Ficinus illustrates this
with a familiar example of that Marrhusian Phædrus and
Theban Lycias: "Lycias he stares on Phædrus' face, and Phædrus
fastens the balls of his eyes upon Lycias, and with those sparkling
rays sends out his spirits.   The beams of Phædrus' eyes are
easily mingled with the beams of Lycias', and spirits are joined
to spirits.   This vapour, begot in Phædrus' heart, enters into
Lycias' bowels: and that which is a greater wonder, Phædrus'
blood is in Lycias' heart, and thence come those ordinary love-
speeches, My sweetheart Phædrus! and mine own self, my dear
bowels!   And Phædrus again to Lycias, O my light, my joy,
my soul, my life!   Phædrus follows Lycias, because his heart

would have his spirits; and Lycias follows Phædrus, because he
loves the seat of his spirits; both follow, but Lycias the earnester
of the two: the river hath more need of the fountain than the
fountain of the river; as iron is drawn to that which is touched
with a loadstone, but draws not it again, so Lycias draws
Phædrus." [1] But how comes it to pass, then, that a blind
man loves, that never saw? We read, in the Lives of the
Fathers, a story of a child that was brought up in the wilderness, from his infancy, by an old hermit: now come to man's
estate, he saw by chance two comely women wandering in the
woods: he asked the old man what creatures they were, he
told him fairies; after a while, talking *obiter* [casually], the
hermit demanded of him, which was the pleasantest sight that
ever he saw in his life? He readily replied, the two fairies
he spied in the wilderness.[2] So that, without doubt, there is
some secret loadstone in a beautiful woman, a magnetic power,
a natural inbred affection, which moves our concupiscence;
and, as he sings,

> Methinks I have a mistress yet to come,
> And still I seek, I love, I know not whom.

'Tis true indeed of natural and chaste love, but not of this
heroical passion, or rather brutish burning lust of which we
treat; we speak of wandering, wanton, adulterous eyes, which,
as he saith,[3] "lie still in wait as so many soldiers, and when
they spy an innocent spectator fixed on them, shoot him through,
and presently bewitch him: especially when they shall gaze
and gloat, as wanton lovers do one upon another, and with
a pleasant eye-conflict participate each other's souls." Hence
you may perceive how easily and how quickly we may be taken
in love; since at the twinkling of an eye, Phædrus' spirits may
so perniciously infect Lycias' blood. "Neither is it any wonder,
if we but consider how many other diseases closely, and as
suddenly, are caught by infection, plague, itch, scabs, flux,"
etc. [4] The spirits, taken in, will not let him rest that hath
received them, but egg him on, *idque petit corpus mens unde
est saucia amore* [5] [and the mind seeks the body whence it
received its love-wound]; and we may manifestly perceive a
strange eduction of spirits, by such as bleed at nose after they
be dead, at the presence of the murderer; but read more of
this in Lemnius, *lib. 2 de occult. nat. mir. cap.* 7, Valleriola,
lib. 2 Observ. cap. 7, Valesius, *Controv.*, Ficinus, Cardan, Libanius
de cruentis cadaveribus, etc.

SUBSECT. III.—*Artificial Allurements of Love, Causes and
Provocations to Lust; Gestures, Clothes, Dower, etc.*

Natural beauty is a stronger loadstone of itself, as you have
heard, a great temptation, and pierceth to the very heart; [1]
forma verecundæ nocuit mihi visa puellæ [I am smitten with the
beauty of a modest maid whom I have seen]; but much more
when those artificial enticements and provocations of gestures,
clothes, jewels, pigments, exornations, shall be annexed unto
it; those other circumstances, opportunity of time and place,
shall concur, which of themselves alone were all-sufficient, each
one in particular, to produce this effect. It is a question much
controverted by some wise men, *forma debeat plus arti an naturæ?*
whether natural or artificial objects be more powerful? but not
decided: for my part, I am of opinion that, though beauty itself
be a great motive, and give an excellent lustre *in sordibus*, in
beggary, as a jewel on a dunghill will shine and cast his rays,
it cannot be suppressed, which Heliodorus feigns of Chariclea,
though she were in beggar's weeds: yet, as it is used, artificial
is of more force, and much to be preferred.

> *Sic dentata sibi videtur Ægle,*
> *Emptis ossibus Indicoque cornu;*
> *Sic quæ nigrior est cadente moro,*
> *Cerussata sibi placet Lycoris.* [2]

> So toothless Ægle seems a pretty one,
> Set out with new-bought teeth of Indy bone:
> So foul Lycoris blacker than berry
> Herself admires, now finer than cherry.

John Lerius the Burgundian, *cap.* 8, *Hist. navigat. in Brasil.*,
is altogether on my side. "For whereas" (saith he) "at our
coming to Brazil, we found both men and women naked as
they were born, without any covering, so much as of their
privities, and could not be persuaded, by our Frenchmen that
lived a year with them, to wear any, many will think that our
so long commerce with naked women must needs be a great
provocation to lust"; but he concludes otherwise, that their
nakedness did much less entice them to lasciviousness than
our women's clothes.[3] "And I dare boldly affirm" (saith he)
"that those glittering attires, counterfeit colours,[4] headgears,
curled hairs, plaited coats, cloaks, gowns, costly stomachers,
guarded and loose garments, and all those other accoutrements
wherewith our countrywomen counterfeit a beauty, and so

curiously set out themselves, cause more inconvenience in this kind than that barbarian homeliness, although they be no whit inferior unto them in beauty. I could evince the truth of this by many other arguments, but I appeal" (saith he) "to my companions at that present, which were all of the same mind." His countryman Montaigne, in his Essays, is of the same opinion, and so are many others; out of whose assertions thus much in brief we may conclude, that beauty is more beholding to art than nature, and stronger provocations proceed from outward ornaments than such as nature hath provided. It is true that those fair sparkling eyes, white neck, coral lips, turgent paps, rose-coloured cheeks, etc., of themselves are potent enticers; but when a comely, artificial, well-composed look, pleasing gesture, an affected carriage shall be added, it must needs be far more forcible than it was, when those curious needleworks, variety of colours, purest dyes, jewels, spangles, pendants, lawn, lace, tiffanies, fair and fine linen, embroideries, calamistrations, ointments, etc., shall be added, they will make the veriest dowdy otherwise a goddess, when nature shall be furthered by art. For it is not the eye of itself that enticeth to lust, but an "adulterous eye," as Peter terms it (2, ii, 14), a wanton, a rolling, lascivious eye: a wandering eye, which Isaiah taxeth (iii, 16). Christ Himself and the Virgin Mary had most beautiful eyes, as amiable eyes as any persons, saith Barradius,[1] that ever lived, but withal so modest, so chaste, that whosoever looked on them was freed from that passion of burning lust; if we may believe Gerson[2] and Bonaventure,[3] there was no such antidote against it as the Virgin Mary's face; 'tis not the eye, but carriage of it, as they use it, that causeth such effects. When Pallas, Juno, Venus, were to win Paris' favour for the golden apple, as it is elegantly described in that pleasant interlude of Apuleius,[3] Juno came with majesty upon the stage, Minerva [with] gravity, but Venus *dulce subridens, constitit amœne; et gratissimæ Gratiæ deam propitiantes*, etc., came in smiling with her gracious graces and exquisite music, as if she had danced, *et nonnunquam saltare solis oculis*, and which was the main matter of all, she danced with her rolling eyes: they were the brokers and harbingers of her suit. So she makes her brags in a modern poet:

> Soon could I make my brow to tyrannize,
> And force the world do homage to mine eyes.[5]

The eye is a secret orator, the first bawd, *amoris porta* [the gate of love], and with private looks, winking, glances and smiles,

as so many dialogues, they make up the match many times,
and understand one another's meanings before they come to
speak a word.   Euryalus and Lucretia [1] were so mutually enamoured by the eye, and prepared to give each other entertainment, before ever they had conference: he asked her good will
with his eyes; she did *suffragari* [favour him], and gave consent
with a pleasant look.   That Thracian Rhodopis [2] was so excellent at this dumb rhetoric, "that if she had but looked upon
any one almost" (saith Calasiris) "she would have bewitched
him, and he could not possibly escape it."   For, as Salvianus
observes,[3] "the eyes are the windows of our souls, by which as
so many channels, all dishonest concupiscence gets into our
hearts."   They reveal our thoughts, and as they say, *frons
animi index* [the face is the index to the mind], but the eye of
the countenance: *Quid procacibus intuere ocellis?*[4] [Why look'st
thou at me with forward glance?], etc.   I may say the same
of smiling, gait, nakedness of parts, plausible gestures, etc.   To
laugh is the   proper passion of a man, an ordinary thing to
smile; but those counterfeit, composed, affected, artificial, and
reciprocal, those counter-smiles are the dumb-shows and prognostics of greater matters, which they most part use to inveigle
and deceive; though many fond lovers again are so frequently
mistaken, and led into a fool's paradise.   For if they see but
a fair maid laugh, or show a pleasant countenance, use some
gracious words or gestures, they apply it all to themselves, as
done in their favour; sure she loves them, she is willing,
coming, etc.

> *Stultus quando videt quod pulchra puellula ridet,*
> *Tum fatuus credit se quod amare velit.*

> When a fool sees a fair maid for to smile,
> He thinks she loves him, 'tis but to beguile.

They make an art of it, as the poet telleth us:

> *Quis credat? discunt etiam ridere puellæ,*
> *Quæritur atque illis hac quoque parte decor.*[5]

> Who can believe? to laugh maids make an art,
> And seek a pleasant grace to that same part.

And 'tis as great an enticement as any of the rest:

> *Subrisit molle puella,*
> *Cor tibi rite salit.*[6]

She makes thine heart leap with a pleasing gentle smile of hers.[7]

> *Dulce ridentem Lalagen amabo,*
> *Dulce loquentem,*[8]

I love Lalage as much for smiling as for discoursing; *delectata illa risit tam blandum*, as he said in Petronius of his mistress; being well pleased, she gave so sweet a smile. It won Ismenius, as he confesseth,[1] *Ismene subrisit amatorium*, Ismene smiled so lovingly the second time I saw her, that I could not choose but admire her: and Galla's sweet smile quite overcame Faustus the shepherd,[2] *Me aspiciens motis blande subrisit ocellis* [as she caught sight of me, she smiled sweetly]. All other gestures of the body will enforce as much. Daphnis in Lucian[3] was a poor tattered wench when I knew her first, said Crobyle, *pannosa et lacera*, but now she is a stately piece indeed, hath her maids to attend her, brave attires, money in her purse, etc.; and will you know how this came to pass? "by setting out herself after the best fashion, by her pleasant carriage, affability, sweet smiling upon all," etc. Many women dote upon a man for his complement only, and good behaviour, they are won in an instant; too credulous to believe that every light, wanton suitor who sees or makes love to them is instantly enamoured, he certainly dotes on, admires them, will surely marry, whenas he means nothing less, 'tis his ordinary carriage in all such companies. So both delude each other by such outward shows; and amongst the rest, an upright, a comely grace, courtesies, gentle salutations, cringes, a mincing gait, a decent and an affected pace, are most powerful enticers, and which the prophet Esay, a courtier himself, and a great observer, objected to the daughters of Zion (iii, 16), "they minced as they went, and made a tinkling with their feet." To say the truth, what can they not effect by such means?

> Whilst nature decks them in their best attires
> Of youth and beauty which the world admires.

Urit
Voce, manu, gressu, pectore, fronte, oculis.[4]

[She kindles love with voice, hand, step, breast, brow, eyes.]

When art shall be annexed to beauty, when wiles and guiles shall concur; for to speak as it is, love is a kind of legerdemain; mere juggling, a fascination. When they show their fair hand, fine foot and leg withal, *magnum sui desiderium nobis relinquunt*, saith Balthasar Castilio, *lib.* 1, they set us a-longing, "and so when they pull up their petticoats and outward garments,"[5] as usually they do to show their fine stockings, and those of purest silken dye, gold fringes, laces, embroiderings (it shall go

hard but when they go to church, or to any other place, all shall
be seen), 'tis but a springe to catch woodcocks; and as Chrysostom telleth them downright,[1] "though they say nothing with
their mouths, they speak in their gait, they speak with their
eyes, they speak in the carriage of their bodies." And what
shall we say otherwise of that baring of their necks, shoulders,
naked breasts, arms and wrists? to what end are they but only
to tempt men to lust?

> *Nam quid lacteolus sinus, et ipsas*
> *Præ te fers sine linteo papillas?*
> *Hoc est dicere, posce, posce, trado;*
> *Hoc est ad Venerem vocare amantes.*[2]

> [Why do you show your milk-white breast and expose
> your bosom, as if to say, "You have but to ask
> and I deliver"? Surely this is the call to love.]

There needs nó more, as Fredericus Matenesius well observes,[3]
but a crier to go before them so dressed, to bid us look out, a
trumpet to sound, or for defect a sow-gelder to blow:

> Look out, look out and see
> What object this may be
> That doth perstringe mine eye;
> A gallant lady goes
> In rich and gaudy clothes,
> But whither away God knows,
> ...look out, etc., *et quæ sequuntur,*[4]

or to what end and purpose? But to leave all these phantastical
raptures, I 'll prosecute my intended theme. Nakedness, as I
have said, is an odious thing of itself, *remedium amoris* [a cure
for love]; yet it may be so used, in part, and at set times, that
there can be no such enticement as it is:

> *Nec mihi cincta Diana placet, nec nuda Cythere,*
> *Illa voluptatis nil habet, hæc nimium.*[5]

> [For me nor Dian draped nor Venus nude;
> One charms too much, the other is too crude.]

David so espied Bathsheba, the elders Susanna: Apelles was
enamoured with Campaspe, when he was to paint her naked.[6]
Tiberius, in Suet. *cap.* 42, supped with Sestius Gallus, an old
lecher, *libidinoso sene, ea lege ut nudæ puellæ administrarent*
[on condition that naked girls should wait on them]; some say
as much of Nero, and Pontus Heuter of Carolus Pugnax.[7]
Amongst the Babylonians, it was the custom of some lascivious
queans to dance frisking in that fashion, saith Curtius, *lib.* 5,

and Sardus, *de mor. gent. lib.* 1, writes of others to that effect.
The Tuscans at some set banquets had naked women to attend
upon them,[1] which Leonicus, *Varia hist. lib. 3, cap.* 96, confirms
of such other bawdy nations. Nero would have filthy pictures
still hanging in his chamber, which is too commonly used in
our times, and Heliogabalus, *etiam coram agentes, ut ad venerem
incitarent.* So things may be abused. A servant-maid in
Aristænetus [2] spied her master and mistress through the key-
hole merrily disposed; upon the sight she fell in love with her
master.[3] Antoninus Caracalla observed his mother-in-law with
her breasts amorously laid open; he was so much moved, that
he said, *Ah si liceret!* O that I might! which she by chance
overhearing, replied as impudently, *Quicquid libet licet,*[4] Thou
mayst do what thou wilt: and upon that temptation he married
her: this object was not in cause, not the thing itself, but that
unseemly, undecent carriage of it.

When you have all done, *veniunt a veste sagittæ*, the greatest
provocations of lust are from our apparel; God makes, they say,
man shapes, and there is no motive like unto it,

> Which doth even beauty beautify,
> And most bewitch a wretched eye.[5]

A filthy knave, a deformed quean, a crooked carcass, a maukin,
a witch, a rotten post, an hedge-stake may be set out and tricked
up that it shall make as fair a show, as much enamour, as the
rest; many a silly fellow is so taken. *Primum luxuriæ aucupium,*
one calls it, the first snare of lust; Bossus,[6] *aucupium animarum*
[a snare of souls], *lethalem arundinem,* a fatal reed, the greatest
bawd, *forte lenocinium, sanguines lacrimis deplorandum,* saith
Matenesius,[7] and with tears of blood to be deplored. Not that
comeliness of clothes is therefore to be condemned, and those
usual ornaments: there is a decency and decorum in this as
well as in other things, fit to be used, becoming several persons,
and befitting their estates; he is only phantastical that is not in
fashion, and like an old image in arras hangings, when a manner
of attire is generally received; but when they are so new-
fangled, so unstaid, so prodigious in their attires, beyond their
means and fortunes, unbefitting their age, place, quality, condition, what should we otherwise think of them? Why do they
adorn themselves with so many colours of herbs, fictitious flowers,
curious needleworks, quaint devices, sweet-smelling odours,
with those inestimable riches of precious stones, pearls, rubies,
diamonds, emeralds, etc.? Why do they crown themselves

with gold and silver, use coronets and tires of several fashions,
deck themselves with pendants, bracelets, earrings, chains,
girdles, rings, pins, spangles, embroideries, shadows, rabatoes,
versicolour ribands? Why do they make such glorious shows with
their scarfs, feathers, fans, masks, furs, laces, tiffanies, ruffs, falls,
cauls, cuffs, damasks, velvets, tinsels, cloth of gold, silver, tissue?
with colours of heavens, stars, planets: the strength of metals,
stones, odours, flowers, birds, beasts, fishes, and whatsoever Africa,
Asia, America, sea, land, art and industry of man can afford?
Why do they use and covet such novelty of inventions, such new-
fangled tires, and spend such inestimable sums on them? "To
what end are those crisped, false hairs, painted faces," as the
satirist observes,[1] "such a composed gait, not a step awry?"
Why are they like so many Sybarites, or Nero's Poppæa,
Ahasuerus' concubines, so costly, so long a-dressing as Cæsar
was marshalling his army, or an hawk in pruning? *Dum moliuntur, dum comuntur, annus est*[2] [they take a year decking and
tiring themselves]: "a gardener takes not so much delight and
pains in his garden, a horseman to dress his horse, scour his
armour, a mariner about his ship, a merchant his shop and shop-
book," as they do about their faces, and all those other parts:[3]
such setting up with corks, straitening with whalebones; why
is it but, as a day-net catcheth larks, to make young men
stoop unto them? Philocharus, a gallant in Aristænetus, advised
his friend Polyænus to take heed of such enticements, "for it
was the sweet sound and motion of his mistress's spangles and
bracelets, the smell of her ointments, that captivated him
first":[4] *Illa fuit mentis prima ruina meæ* [that was the beginning
of my infatuation]. *Quid sibi vult pyxidum turba*, saith Lucian,[5]
"to what use are pins, pots, glasses, ointments, irons, combs,
bodkins, setting-sticks? why bestow they all their patrimonies
and husbands' yearly revenues on such fooleries?" *bina patrimonia singulis auribus*;[6] "why use they dragons, wasps, snakes,
for chains," enamelled jewels on their necks, ears? *Dignum
potius foret ferro manus istas religari, atque utinam monilia vere
dracones essent* [iron bands would fit their wrists better, and
I would that their chains were real dragons]; they had more
need some of them be tied in Bedlam with iron chains, have a
whip for a fan, and hair-cloths next to their skins, and instead
of wrought smocks, have their cheeks stigmatized with a hot
iron, I say, some of our Jezebels, instead of painting, if they
were well served. But why is all this labour, all this cost,
preparation, riding, running, far-fetched and dear-bought stuff?

"Because forsooth they would be fair and fine, and where nature is defective, supply it by art";[1] *Sanguine quæ vero non rubet, arte rubet* [2] [cheeks pale by nature are made red by art]; and to that purpose they anoint and paint their faces, to make Helen of Hecuba, *parvamque extortamque puellam Europen* [and an undersized, misshapen wench into an Europa]. To this intent they crush in their feet and bodies, hurt and crucify themselves, sometimes in lax clothes, an hundred yards I think in a gown, a sleeve; and sometimes again so close, *ut nudos exprimant artus* [as to show their limbs as if unclothed]. Now long tails and trains, and then short,[3] up, down, high, low, thick, thin, etc.; now little or no bands, then as big as cart-wheels; now loose bodies, then great fardingales and close-girt, etc. Why is all this, but with the whore in the Proverbs, to intoxicate some or other? *Oculorum decipulam*, one therefore calls it,[4] *et indicem libidinis*, the trap of lust, and sure token, as an ivy-bush is to a tavern.

> *Quod pulchros, Glycere, sumas de pyxide vultus,*
> *Quod tibi compositæ nec sine lege comæ :*
> *Quod niteat digitis adamas, beryllus in aure,*
> *Non sum divinus, sed scio quid cupias.*

> O Glycere, in that you paint so much,
> Your hair is so bedeckt in order such,
> With rings on fingers, bracelets in your ear,
> Although no prophet, tell I can, I fear.

To be admired, to be gazed on, to circumvent some novice; as many times they do, that instead of a lady he loves a cap and a feather, instead of a maid that should have *verum colorem, corpus solidum et succi plenum* [a natural colour, a plump and healthy body] (as Chærea describes his mistress in the poet [5]), a painted face, a ruff-band, fair and fine linen, a coronet, a flower (*Naturæque putat quod fuit artificis* [6] [he ascribes to nature what is due to art]), a wrought waistcoat he dotes on, or a pied petticoat, a pure dye instead of a proper woman. For generally, as with rich-furred conies, their cases are far better than their bodies, and like the bark of a cinnamon tree which is dearer than the whole bulk, their outward accoutrements are far more precious than their inward endowments. 'Tis too commonly so:

> *Auferimur cultu et gemmis, auroque teguntur*
> *Omnia ; pars minima est ipsa puella sui.*[7]

> With gold and jewels all is covered,
> And with a strange tire we are won
> (While she 's the least part of herself),
> And with such baubles quite undone.

Why do they keep in so long together, a whole winter sometimes, and will not be seen but by torch- or candle-light, and
come abroad with all the preparation may be, when they have
no business, but only to show themselves? *Spectatum veniunt,
veniunt spectentur ut ipsæ* [they come to see the show, and show
themselves].

> For what is beauty if it be not seen,
> Or what is't to be seen if not admir'd,
> And though admir'd, unless in love desir'd? [1]

Why do they go with such counterfeit gait, which Philo Judæus
reprehends them for,[2] and use (I say it again) such gestures,
apish, ridiculous, indecent attires, sybaritical tricks, *fucos genis,
purpurissam venis, cerussam fronti, leges oculis*, etc., use those
sweet perfumes, powders and ointments in public, flock to hear
sermons so frequent? is it for devotion? or rather, as Basil tells
them,[3] to meet their sweethearts, and see fashions; for, as he
saith, commonly they come so provided to that place, with
such curious complements, with such gestures and tires, as if
they should go to a dancing-school, a stage-play, or bawdy-
house, fitter than a church.

> When such a she-priest comes her mass to say,
> Twenty to one they all forget to pray.

"They make those holy temples, consecrated to godly martyrs
and religious uses, the shops of impudence, dens of whores and
thieves, and little better than brothel-houses." When we shall
see these things daily done, their husbands bankrupts, if not
cornutos, their wives light huswives, daughters dishonest;
and hear of such dissolute acts, as daily we do, how should we
think otherwise? what is their end, but to deceive and inveigle
young men? As tow takes fire, such enticing objects produce
their effect, how can it be altered? When Venus stood before
Anchises (as Homer feigns in one of his hymns [4]) in her costly
robes, he was instantly taken:

> *Cum ante ipsum staret Jovis filia, videns eam
> Anchises, admirabatur formam, et stupendas vestes ;
> Erat enim induta peplo, igneis radiis splendidiore ;
> Habebat quoque torques fulgidos, flexiles helices,
> Tenerum collum ambiebant monilia pulchra,
> Aurea, variegata.*

> When Venus stood before Anchises first,
> He was amaz'd to see her in her tires;
> For she had on a hood as red as fire,

And glittering chains, and ivy-twisted spires,
About her tender neck were costly brooches,
And necklaces of gold, enamell'd ouches.

So when Medea came in presence of Jason first, attended by her
nymphs and ladies, as she is described by Apollonius,[1]

Cunctas vero ignis instar sequebatur splendor,
Tantum ab aureis fimbriis resplendebat jubar,
Accenditque in oculis dulce desiderium.

A lustre followed them like flaming fire,
And from their golden borders came such beams,
Which in his eyes provok'd a sweet desire.

Such a relation we have in Plutarch,[2] when the queens came
and offered themselves to Antony, "with divers presents, and
enticing ornaments, Asiatic allurements, with such wonderful
joy and festivity, they did so inveigle the Romans, that no
man could contain himself, all was turned to delight and pleasure.
The women transformed themselves to Bacchus shapes, the men-
children to satyrs and Pans; but Antony himself was quite
besotted with Cleopatra's sweet speeches, philters, beauty,
pleasing tires: for when she sailed along the river Cydnus, with
such incredible pomp in a gilded ship, herself dressed like
Venus, her maids like the Graces, her pages like so many Cupids,
Antony was amazed, and rapt beyond himself."[3] Heliodorus,
lib. 1, brings in Damæneta, stepmother to Cnemon, "whom
she saw in his scarfs, rings, robes, and coronet, quite mad for
the love of him."[4] It was Judith's pantofles that ravished
the eyes of Holofernes. And Cardan [5] is not ashamed to confess
that, seeing his wife the first time all in white, he did admire
and instantly love her. If these outward ornaments were not
of such force, why doth Naomi give Ruth counsel how to please
Boaz? [6] And Judith, seeking to captivate Holofernes, washed
and anointed herself with sweet ointments, dressed her hair,
and put on costly attires. [7] The riot in this kind hath been
excessive in times past; no man almost came abroad, but
curled and anointed:

Et matutino sudans Crispinus amomo,
Quantum vix redolent duo funera,[8]

[And Crispinus reeking of his morning scent as strongly
as two funerals,]

one spent as much as two funerals at once; and with perfumed
hairs, *et rosa canos adorati capillos Assyrioque nardo*[9] [his grey
hairs perfumed with roses and Assyrian nard]. What strange

things doth Suetonius [1] relate in this matter of Caligula's riot! And Pliny, *lib*. 12 and 13! Read more in Dioscorides, Ulmus, Arnoldus, Rondoletius *de fuco et decoratione*; for it is now an art, as it was of old (so Seneca records [2]), *officinæ sunt adores coquentium* [there are workshops where scent is distilled]. Women are bad and men worse, no difference at all between their and our times. "Good manners" (as Seneca complains) "are extinct with wantonness, in tricking up themselves men go beyond women, they wear harlots' colours, and do not walk, but jet and dance," [3] *hic mulier, hæc vir* [the mannish woman, the womanish man], more like players, butterflies, baboons, apes, antics, than men. So ridiculous, moreover, we are in our attires, and for cost so excessive, that, as Hierome said of old, *Uno filio villarum insunt pretia, uno lino decies sestertium inseritur;* 'tis an ordinary thing to put a thousand oaks and an hundred oxen into a suit of apparel, to wear a whole manor on his back. What with shoe-ties, hangers, points, caps and feathers, scarfs, bands, cuffs, etc., in a short space their whole patrimonies are consumed. Heliogabalus is taxed by Lampridius, and admired in his age, for wearing jewels in his shoes, a common thing in our times, not for emperors and princes, but almost for serving-men and tailors; all the flowers, stars, constellations, gold and precious stones do condescend to set out their shoes. To repress the luxury of those Roman matrons, there was Lex Valeria and Oppia, [4] and a Cato to contradict; but no laws will serve to repress the pride and insolency of our days, the prodigious riot in this kind. Lucullus' wardrobe is put down by our ordinary citizens; and a cobbler's wife in Venice, a courtesan in Florence, is no whit inferior to a queen, if our geographers say true: and why is all this? "Why do they glory in their jewels" (as he saith [5]) "or exult and triumph in the beauty of clothes? why is all this cost? to incite men the sooner to burning lust." They pretend decency and ornament; but let them take heed, lest while they set out their bodies they do not damn their souls; 'tis Bernard's counsel: [6] "shine in jewels, stink in conditions; have purple robes, and a torn conscience." Let them take heed of Esay's prophecy, that their slippers and attires be not taken from them, sweet balls, bracelets, ear-rings, veils, wimples, crisping-pins, glasses, fine linen, hoods, lawns, and sweet savours, they become not bald, burnt, and stink upon a sudden. And let maids beware, as Cyprian adviseth, [7] "lest, while they wander too loosely abroad, they lose not their virginities," and, like Egyptian temples, seem fair without, but

prove rotten carcasses within. How much better were it for
them to follow that good counsel of Tertullian! "to have
their eyes painted with chastity, the Word of God inserted into
their ears, Christ's yoke tied to the hair, to subject themselves
to their husbands. If they would do so, they should be comely
enough, clothe themselves with the silk of sanctity, damask of
devotion, purple of piety and chastity, and so painted, they shall
have God Himself to be a suitor."[1] "Let whores and queans
prank up themselves, let them paint their faces with minion and
ceruse, they are but fuels of lust, and signs of a corrupt soul:
if ye be good, honest, virtuous, and religious matrons, let
sobriety, modesty, and chastity be your honour, and God
Himself your love and desire."[2] *Mulier recte olet, ubi nihil
olet,*[3] then a woman smells best, when she hath no perfume at
all; no crown, chain, or jewel (Guevara adds) is such an ornament to a virgin or virtuous woman, *quam virgini pudor,* as
chastity is: more credit in a wise man's eye and judgment
they get by their plainness, and seem fairer than they that are
set out with baubles, as a butcher's meat is with pricks, puffed
up, and adorned like so many jays with variety of colours.
It is reported of Cornelia, that virtuous Roman lady, great
Scipio's daughter, Titus Sempronius' wife, and the mother of
the Gracchi, that being by chance in company with a companion, a strange gentlewoman (some light huswife belike, that
was dressed like a May-lady, and, as most of our gentlewomen
are, "was more solicitous of her head-tire than of her health,
that spent her time betwixt a comb and a glass, and had
rather be fair than honest," as Cato said, "and have the commonwealth turned topsy-turvy than her tires marred"[4]); and she
did naught but brag of her fine robes and jewels, and provoked
the Roman matron to show hers: Cornelia kept her in talk till
her children came from school; "And these," said she, "are
my jewels," and so deluded and put off a proud, vain, phantastical huswife. How much better were it for our matrons to
do as she did, to go civilly and decently, *Honestæ mulieris instar
quæ utitur auro pro eo quod est, ad ea tantum quibus opus est,*[5]
to use gold as it is gold, and for that use it serves, and when
they need it, than to consume it in riot, beggar their husbands,
prostitute themselves, inveigle others, and peradventure damn
their own souls! How much more would it be for their honour
and credit! Thus doing, as Hierome said of Blæsilla, "Furius
did not so triumph over the Gauls, Papirius of the Samnites,
Scipio of Numantia, as she did by her temperance";[6] *pulla*

semper veste [always in sober attire], etc., they should insult
and domineer over lust, folly, vainglory, all such inordinate,
furious, and unruly passions.

But I am over-tedious, I confess, and whilst I stand gaping
after fine clothes, there is another great allurement (in the
world's eye at least) which had like to have stolen out of sight,
and that is money; *veniunt a dote sagittæ* [Cupid's shafts come
from her dowry], money makes the match; μονὸν ἀργυρον
βλέπουσιν [4] [they only look at money]; 'tis like sauce to their
meat, *cum carne condimentum,* a good dowry with a wife. Many
men, if they do hear but of a great portion, a rich heir, are
more mad than if they had all the beauteous ornaments and
those good parts art and nature can afford; they care not for
honesty, bringing up, birth, beauty, person, but for money.[2]

> *Canes et equos (o Cyrne) quærimus*
> *Nobiles, et a bona progenie;*
> *Malam vero uxorem, malique patris filiam*
> *Ducere non curat vir bonus,*
> *Modo ei magnam dotem afferat.*[2]

> Our dogs and horses still from the best breed
> We carefully seek, and well may they speed:
> But for our wives, so they prove wealthy,
> Fair or foul, we care not what they be.

If she be rich, then she is fair, fine, absolute and perfect, then
they burn like fire, they love her dearly, like pig and pie, and
are ready to hang themselves if they may not have her. Nothing
so familiar in these days as for a young man to marry an old
wife, as they say, for a piece of good: *asinum auro onustum*
[an ass laden with gold]; and though she be an old crone, and
have never a tooth in her head, neither good conditions nor
good face, a natural fool, but only rich, she shall have twenty
young gallants to be suitors in an instant. As she said in
Suetonius, *Non me, sed mea ambiunt,* 'tis not for her sake, but
for her lands or money; and an excellent match it were (as he
added) if she were away. So, on the other side, many a young
lovely maid will cast away herself upon an old, doting, decrepit
dizzard,

> *Bis puer effeto quamvis balbutiat ore,*
> *Prima legit raræ tam culta roseta puellæ,*[4]

> [Though he chatter in second childhood, yet he plucks
> the choicest roses from so fair a maid's bower,]

that is rheumatic and gouty, hath some twenty diseases, perhaps
but one eye, one leg, never a nose, no hair on his head, wit in

his brains, nor honesty, if he have land or money,[1] she will have him before all other suitors, *Dummodo sit dives barbarus ille placet*.[2] If he be rich, he is the man, a fine man, and a proper man, she will go to Jacaktres or Tidore with him; Gelasimus de Monte Aureo, Sir Giles Goosecap, Sir Amorous La-Foole, shall have her. And as Philematium in Aristænetus[3] told Eumusus, *absque argento omnia vana*, hang him that hath no money, "'tis to no purpose to talk of marriage without means,"[4] trouble me not with such motions; let others do as they will, "I'll be sure to have one shall maintain me fine and brave." Most are of her mind; *De moribus ultima fiet quæstio*,[5] for his conditions, she shall inquire after them another time, or when all is done, the match made, and everybody gone home. Lucian's Lycia[6] was a proper young maid, and had many fine gentlemen to her suitors: Ethecles, a senator's son, Melissus, a merchant, etc.; but she forsook them all for one Passius, a base, hirsute, bald-pated knave; but why was it? "His father lately died and left him sole heir of his goods and lands." This is not amongst your dust-worms alone, poor snakes that will prostitute their souls for money, but with this bait you may catch our most potent, puissant, and illustrious princes. That proud upstart domineering Bishop of Ely, in the time of Richard the First, viceroy in his absence, as Nubrigensis relates it,[7] to fortify himself and maintain his greatness, *propinquarum suarum connubiis plurimos sibi potentes et nobiles devincire curavit* (married his poor kinswomen (which came forth of Normandy by droves) to the chiefest nobles of the land, and they were glad to accept of such matches, fair or foul, for themselves, their sons, nephews, etc. *Et quis tam præclarum affinitatem sub spe magnæ promotionis non optaret?* Who would not have done as much for money and preferment? as mine author[8] adds. Vortigern, King of Britain, married Rowena the daughter of Hengist the Saxon prince, his mortal enemy; but wherefore? she had Kent for her dowry. Iagello, the great Duke of Lithuania, 1386, was mightily enamoured on Hedenga, insomuch that he turned Christian from a Pagan, and was baptized himself by the name of Uladislaus, and all his subjects for her sake: but why was it? she was daughter and heir of Poland, and his desire was to have both kingdoms incorporated into one. Charles the Great was an earnest suitor to Irene the Empress, but, saith Zonaras,[9] *ob regnum*, to annex the empire of the East to that of the West. Yet what is the event of all such matches, that are so made for money, goods, by deceit, or for burning lust, *quos fœda libido conjunxit*, what follows? they are almost mad at first, but 'tis a mere flash; as chaff and straw soon fired, burn vehemently for a while, yet out in a moment, so are all such matches made by those allurements of burning lust; where there is no respect of honesty, parentage, virtue, religion, education, and the like, they are extinguished in an instant, and instead of love comes hate; for joy, repentance and desperation itself. Franciscus Barbarus in his first book *de re uxoria, cap.* 5, hath a story of one Philip of Padua that fell in love with a common whore, and was now ready to run mad for her; his father, having no more sons, let him enjoy her; "but after a few days, the young man began to loathe, could not so much as endure the sight of her, and from one madness fell into another." [1] Such event commonly have all these lovers; and he that so marries, or for such respects, let them look for no better success than Menelaus had with Helen, Vulcan with Venus, Theseus with Phædra, Minos with Pasiphae, and Claudius with Messalina: shame, sorrow, misery, melancholy, discontent.

SUBSECT. IV.—*Importunity and Opportunity of Time, Place, Conference, Discourse, Singing, Dancing, Music, Amorous Tales, Objects, Kissing, Familiarity, Tokens, Presents, Bribes, Promises, Protestations, Tears, etc.*

All these allurements hitherto are afar off, and at a distance; I will come nearer to those other degrees of love, which are conference, kissing, dalliance, discourse, singing, dancing, amorous tales, objects, presents, etc., which as so many sirens steal away the hearts of men and women. For, as Tatius observes, *lib.* 2, "It is no sufficient trial of a maid's affection by her eyes alone, but you must say something that shall be more available, and use such other forcible engines; therefore take her by the hand, wring her fingers hard, and sigh withal; if she accept this in good part, and seem not to be much averse, then call her mistress, take her about the neck and kiss her," [2] etc. But this cannot be done except they first get opportunity of living or coming together, ingress, egress, and regress; letters and commendations may do much, outward gestures and actions: but when they come to live near one another, in the same street, village, or together in a house, love is kindled on a sudden. Many a serving-man by reason of this opportunity and importunity inveigles his master's daughter, many a gallant loves a

dowdy, many a gentleman runs upon his wife's maids, many
ladies dote upon their men, as the queen in Ariosto did upon
the dwarf, many matches are so made in haste, and they are
compelled as it were by necessity so to love,[1] which, had they
been free, come in company of others, seen that variety which
many places afford, or compared them to a third, would never
have looked one upon another. Or had not that opportunity of
discourse and familiarity been offered, they would have loathed
and contemned those whom, for want of better choice and other
objects, they are fatally driven on, and by reason of their hot
blood, idle life, full diet, etc., are forced to dote upon them
that come next. And many times those which at the first
sight cannot fancy or affect each other, but are harsh and ready
to disagree, offended with each other's carriage, like Benedick
and Beatrice in the comedy,[2] and in whom they find many
faults, by this living together in a house, conference, kissing,
colling, and such-like allurements, begin at last to dote insensibly
one upon another.

It was the greatest motive that Potiphar's wife had to
dote upon Joseph, and Clitophon[3] upon Leucippe his uncle's
daughter, because the plague being at Byzance, it was his fortune
for a time to sojourn with her, to sit next her at the table, as
he telleth the tale himself in Tatius, *lib.* 1 (which, though it be
but a fiction, is grounded upon good observation, and doth well
express the passions of lovers), he had opportunity to take her
by the hand, and after a while to kiss, and handle her paps, etc.,
which made him almost mad.[4] Ismenius the orator makes the
like confession in Eustathius, *lib.* 1; when he came first to
Sosthenes' house, and sat at table with Cratisthenes his friend,
Ismene, Sosthenes' daughter, waiting on them "with her breasts
open, arms half bare," *Nuda pedem, discincta sinum, spoliata
lacertos* [5] after the Greek fashion in those times, *nudos media
plus parte lacertos* [6] [with arms more than half bare], as Daphne
was when she fled from Phœbus (which moved him much), was
ever ready to give attendance on him, to fill him drink, her eyes
were never off him, *rogabundi oculi*, those speaking eyes, courting
eyes, enchanting eyes; but she was still smiling on him, and
when they were risen, that she had gotten a little opportunity,
"she came and drank to him, and withal trod upon his toes,
and would come and go, and when she could not speak for the
company, she would wring his hand," and blush when she met
him: and by this means first she overcame him (*bibens amorem
hauriebam simul* [I drank in love with the draught]); she would

kiss the cup and drink to him, and smile, "and drink where he drank on that side of the cup,"[1] by which mutual compressions, kissings, wringing of hands, treading of feet, etc., *ipsam mihi videbar sorbillare virginem*, "I sipt and sipt, and sipt so long, till at length I was drunk in love upon a sudden." Philochorus, in Aristænetus,[2] met a fair maid by chance, a mere stranger to him; he looked back at her, she looked back at him again, and smiled withal.

> *Ille dies leti primus, primusque malorum*
> *Causa fuit.*[3]

> [On that day I began to die, on that day my miseries commenced.]

It was the sole cause of his farther acquaintance, and love that undid him. *O nullis tutum credere blanditiis*[4] [ah, 'tis unsafe to trust any blandishments].

This opportunity of time and place, with their circumstances, are so forcible motives, that it is unpossible almost for two young folks equal in years to live together and not be in love, especially in great houses, princes' courts, where they are idle *in summo gradu* [in their exalted position], fare well, live at ease, and cannot tell otherwise how to spend their time. *Illic Hippolytum pone, Priapus erit*[5] [place there the chaste Hippolytus, he will be as lewd as Priapus]. Achilles was sent by his mother Thetis to the island of Scyros in the Ægean Sea (where Lycomedes then reigned) in his nonage to be brought up, to avoid that hard destiny of the oracle (he should be slain at the siege of Troy): and for that cause was nurtured *in gynæceo* [in the women's apartment], amongst the king's children in a woman's habit; but see the event: he compressed Deidamia, the king's fair daughter, and had a fine son, called Pyrrhus, by her. Peter Abelhardus the philosopher, as he tells the tale himself, being set by Fulbertus her uncle to teach Helonissa his lovely niece, and to that purpose sojourned in his house, and had committed *agnam tenellam famelico lupo* [a tender lamb to a famished wolf] (I use his own words), he soon got her good will, *plura erant oscula quam sententiæ* [there were more kisses than philosophical propositions], and he read more of love than any other lecture; such pretty feats can opportunity plea; *primum domo conjuncti, inde animis* [from being in the same house, they came to love one another], etc. But when, as I say, *nox, vinum, et adolescentia*, youth, wine, and night, shall concur, *nox amoris et quietis conscia* [night, the time for

love and rest], 'tis a wonder they be not all plunged over head
and ears in love; for youth is *benigna in amorem, et prona materies*,
a very combustible matter, naphtha itself, the fuel of love's
fire, and most apt to kindle it. If there be seven servants in
an ordinary house, you shall have three couple in some good
liking at least, and amongst idle persons how should it be
otherwise? "Living at Rome," saith Aretine's Lucretia, "in
the flower of my fortunes, rich, fair, young, and so well brought
up, my conversation, age, beauty, fortune, made all the world
admire and love me." [1] Night alone, that one occasion, is
enough to set all on fire, and they are so cunning in great houses
that they make their best advantage of it. Many a gentlewoman, that is guilty to herself of her imperfections, paintings,
impostures, will not willingly be seen by day, but as Castilio
noteth,[2] in the night; *Diem ut glis odit, tædarum lucem super
omnia mavult*, she hateth the day like a dormouse, and above
all things loves torches and candle-light, and if she must come
abroad in the day, she covets, as in a mercer's shop, [3] a very
obfuscate and obscure light. And good reason she hath for it:
Nocte latent mendæ [blemishes are hidden at night], and many
an amorous gull is fetched over by that means. Gomesius,
lib. 3 de sale gen. cap. 22, gives instance in a Florentine gentleman, that was so deceived with a wife; she was so radiantly
set with rings and jewels, lawns, scarfs, laces, gold, spangles,
and gaudy devices, that the young man took her to be a goddess
(for he never saw her but by torchlight); but after the wedding
solemnities, whenas he viewed her the next morning without
her tires, and in a clear day, she was so deformed, a lean, yellow,
rivelled, etc., such a beastly creature in his eyes, that he could
not endure to look upon her. Such matches are frequently
made in Italy, where they have no other opportunity to woo
but when they go to church, or, as in Turkey,[4] see them at a
distance they must interchange few or no words till such time
they come to be married, and then, as Sardus, *lib.* 1, *cap.* 3, *de
mor. gent.*, and Bohemus relate of those old Lacedæmonians,
"the bride is brought into the chamber, with her hair girt
about her, the bridegroom comes in and unties the knot, and
must not see her at all by daylight, till such time as he is made
a father by her." [5] In those hotter countries these are ordinary
practices at this day; but in our northern parts, amongst
Germans, Danes, French, and Britons, the continent of Scandia
and the rest, we assume more liberty in such cases; we allow
them, as Bohemus saith, to kiss coming and going, *et modo*

absit lascivia, in cauponem ducere, to talk merrily, sport, play, sing, and dance, so that it be modestly done, go to the ale-house and tavern together. And 'tis not amiss, though Chryso-stom,[1] Cyprian, Hierome, and some other of the Fathers speak bitterly against it: but that is the abuse which is commonly seen at some drunken matches, dissolute meetings, or great unruly feasts. "A young, pittivanted, trim-bearded fellow," saith Hierome, "will come with a company of compliments, and hold you up by the arm as you go, and wringing your fingers, will so be enticed, or entice:[2] one drinks to you, another embraceth, a third kisseth, and all this while the fiddler plays or sings a lascivious song; a fourth singles you out to dance; one speaks by becks and signs, and that which he dares not say, signifies by passions; amongst so many and so great provocations of pleasure, lust conquers the most hard and crabbed minds, and scarce can a man live honest among feastings and sports, or at such great meetings."[3] For, as he goes on, "she walks along, and with the ruffling of her clothes makes men look at her, her shoes creak, her paps tied up, her waist pulled in to make her look small, she is strait-girded, her hairs hang loose about her ears, her upper garment sometimes falls, and some-times tarries, to show her naked shoulders, and as if she would not be seen, she covers that in all haste which voluntarily she showed."[4] And not at feasts, plays, pageants, and such assemblies, but as Chrysostom objects,[5] these tricks are put in practice "at service-time in churches, and at the communion itself." If such dumb-shows, signs, and more obscure significations of love can so move, what shall they do that have full liberty to sing, dance, kiss, coll, to use all manner of discourse and dalliance? What shall he do that is beleaguered of all sides?

Quem tot, tam roseæ petunt puellæ,
Quem cultæ cupiunt nurus, amorque
Omnis undique et undecunque et usque,
Omnis ambit Amor, Venusque Hymenque.[6]

After whom so many rosy maids inquire,
Whom dainty dames and loving wights desire,
In every place, still, and at all times sue,
Whom gods and gentle goddesses do woo.

How shall he contain? The very tone of some of their voices, a pretty pleasing speech, an affected tone they use, is able of itself to captivate a young man; but when a good wit shall concur, art and eloquence, fascinating speech, pleasant dis-course, sweet gestures, the Sirens themselves cannot so enchant.

P. Jovius [1] commends his Italian countrywomen to have an
excellent faculty in this kind, above all other nations, and
amongst them the Florentine ladies: some prefer Roman and
Venetian courtesans, they have such pleasing tongues, and such
elegancy of speech, [2] that they are able to overcome a saint,
Pro facie multis vox sua lena fuit [many attract with their voice
sooner than with their looks]. *Tanta gratia vocis famam
conciliabat*, saith Petronius in his fragment of pure impurities,
I mean his *Satyricon, tam dulcis sonus permulcebat aera, ut
putares inter auras cantare Sirenum concordiam:* she sang so
sweetly that she charmed the air, and thou wouldst have thought
thou hadst heard a consort of Sirens. "O good God, when
Lais speaks, how sweet it is!" Philocaus exclaims in Aristænetus. [3]
To hear a fair young gentlewoman play upon the virginals, lute,
viol, and sing to it, which as Gellius observes, *lib.* 1, *cap.* 11,
are *lascivientium deliciæ*, the chief delight of lovers, must needs
be a great enticement. Parthenis was so taken. *Mi vox ista
avida haurit ab aure animam* [that voice of yours draws my soul
out through my enraptured ears]; "O sister Harpedona"
(she laments) "I am undone, how sweetly he sings! I'll speak
a bold word, he is the properest man that ever I saw in my
life: O how sweetly he sings, I die for his sake, O that he would
love me again!" [4] "If thou didst but hear her sing," saith
Lucian, "thou wouldst forget father and mother, forsake all
thy friends, and follow her." [5] Helena is highly commended
by Theocritus the poet for her sweet voice and music, [6] none
could play so well as she; and Daphnis in the same Idyllion:

> *Quam tibi os dulce est, et vox amabilis, o Daphni,*
> *Jucundius est audire te canentem, quam mel lingere!*

> How sweet a face hath Daphne, how lovely a voice!
> Honey itself is not so pleasant in my choice.

A sweet voice and music are powerful enticers. Those
Samian singing wenches, Aristonica, Œnanthe and Agathoclea,
regiis diadematibus insultarunt, insulted over kings themselves,
as Plutarch contends. [7] *Centum luminibus cinctum caput Argus
habebat*, Argus had an hundred eyes, all so charmed by one
silly pipe that he lost his head. Clitiphon complains in Tatius
of Leucippe's sweet tunes; [8] "he heard her play by chance
upon the lute, and sing a pretty song to it in commendations of
a rose," out of old Anacreon belike:

> *Rosa honor decusque florum,*
> *Rosa flos odorque divum,*

Hominum rosa est voluptas,
Decus illa Gratiarum,
Florente amoris hora,
Rosa suavium Diones, et**o**.

Rose the fairest of all flowers,
Rose delight of higher powers,
Rose the joy of mortal men,
Rose the pleasure of fine women,
Rose the Graces' ornament,
Rose Dione's sweet content.

To this effect the lovely virgin, with a melodious air upon her
golden-wired harp or lute, I know not well whether, played and
sang, and that transported him beyond himself, "and that
ravished his heart." It was Jason's discourse as much as his
beauty, or any other of his good parts, which delighted Medea
so much.

Delectabatur enim
Animus simul forma dulcibusque verbis.[1]

It was Cleopatra's sweet voice and pleasant speech which inveigled
Antony, above the rest of her enticements. *Verba ligant hominem
ut taurorum cornua funes:* as bulls' horns are bound with ropes,
so are men's hearts with pleasant words. "Her words burn as
fire" (Ecclus. ix, 8). Roxalana bewitched Solyman the Magnificent, and Shore's wife by this engine overcame Edward the
Fourth: *Omnibus una omnes surripuit Veneres* [2] [this one charm
replaces all others]. The Wife of Bath in Chaucer confesseth
all this out of her experience:

Some folk desire us for riches,
Some for shape, some for fairness,
Some for that she can sing or dance,
Some for gentleness, or for dalliance.

Peter Aretine's Lucretia telleth as much and more of herself: [3]
"I counterfeited honesty, as if I had been *virgo virginissima,*
more than a vestal virgin, I looked like a wife, I was so demure
and chaste, I did add such gestures, tunes, speeches, signs and
motions upon all occasions, that my spectators and auditors
were stupefied, enchanted, fastened all to their places, like so
many stocks and stones." Many silly gentlewomen are fetched
over in like sort, by a company of gulls and swaggering companions, that frequently belie nobleman's favours, rhyming
Corybantiasmi, thrasonian Rhodomantes or Bombomachides,
that have nothing in them but a few players' ends and complements, vain braggadocians, impudent intruders, that can dis-

course at table of knights' and lords' combats, like Lucian's
Leontichus,[1] of other men's travels, brave adventures, and such
common trivial news, ride, dance, sing old ballet tunes, and
wear their clothes in fashion, with a good grace; a fine sweet
gentleman, a proper man, who could not love him? She will
have him though all her friends say no, though she beg with
him. Some again are incensed by reading amorous toys,
Amadis de Gaul, Palmerin de Oliva, the Knight of the Sun,
etc., or hearing such tales of lovers,[2] descriptions of their
persons, lascivious discourses, such as Astyanassa, Helena's
waiting-woman, by the report of Suidas, writ of old, *de variis
concubitus modis*, and after her Philænis and Elephantis, or those
light tracts of Aristides Milesius [3] (mentioned by Plutarch) and
found by the Persians in Crassus' army amongst the spoils,
Aretine's dialogues, with ditties, love-songs, etc., must needs
set them on fire, with such-like pictures as those of Aretine, or
wanton objects of what kind soever; "no stronger engine than
to hear or read of love-toys, fables and discourses" (one [4] saith),
"and many by this means are quite mad." At Abdera in
Thrace (*Andromeda*, one of Euripides' tragedies, being played),
the spectators were so much moved with the object, and those
pathetical love-speeches of Perseus (amongst the rest, "O Cupid,
prince of gods and men," etc.), that every man almost, a good
while after, spake pure iambics, and raved still on Perseus'
speech, "O Cupid, prince of gods and men." As carmen,
boys, and prentices, when a new song is published with us,
go singing that new tune still in the streets, they continually
acted that tragical part of Perseus, and in every man's mouth
was "O Cupid," in every street, "O Cupid," in every house
almost, "O Cupid, prince of gods and men," pronouncing still
like stage-players, "O Cupid"; they were so possessed all with
that rapture, and thought of that pathetical love-speech, they
could not a long time after forget, or drive it out of their minds,
but "O Cupid, prince of gods and men," was ever in their mouths.
This belike made Aristotle, *Polit. lib.* 7, *cap.* 18, forbid young
men to see comedies, or to hear amorous tales.

> *Hæc igitur juvenes nequam facilesque puellæ*
> *Inspiciant,*[5]

let not young folks meddle at all with such matters. And this
made the Romans, as Vitruvius relates,[6] put Venus' temple
in the suburbs, *extra murum, ne adolescentes venereis insuescant,*
to avoid all occasions and objects. For what will not such an

object do? Ismenius, as he walked in Sosthenes' garden, being now in love, when he saw so many lascivious pictures,[1] Thetis' Marriage, and I know not what, was almost beside himself. And to say truth, with a lascivious object who is not moved, to see others dally, kiss, dance? And much more when he shall come to be an actor himself.

To kiss and be kissed, which, amongst other lascivious provocations, is as a burden in a song, and a most forcible battery, as infectious, Xenophon thinks, as the poison of a spider;[2] a great allurement, a fire itself, *procemium aut antecenium*, the prologue of burning lust (as Apuleius adds), lust itself, *Venus quinta parte sui nectaris imbuit*[3] [which Venus hath infused with the quintessence of her own nectar], a strong assault, that conquers captains, and those all-commanding forces, (*Domasque ferro sed domaris osculo*[4] [you subdue with the sword, but are subdued with a kiss]). Aretine's Lucretia, when she would in kindness overcome a suitor of hers and have her desire of him, "took him about the neck, and kissed him again and again,"[5] and to that, which she could not otherwise effect, she made him so speedily and willingly condescend. And 'tis a continual assault, *hoc non deficit incipitque semper*,[6] always fresh, and ready to begin as at first,[7] *basium nullo fine terminatur, sed semper recens est* [kissing is never finished and is always fresh], and hath a fiery touch with it.

> *Tenta modo tangere corpus,*
> *Jam tua mellifluo membra calore fluent.*[8]

[Try but to touch her, straightway your limbs will be aglow.]

Especially when they shall be lasciviously given, as he feelingly said,[9] *et me pressulum deosculata Fotis, catenatis lacertis, obtorto valgiter labello*[10] [Fotis kissed me hard, with arms intertwined, with pursed lips].

> *Valgiis suaviis,*
> *Dum semiulco suavio*
> *Meam puellam suavior,*
> *Anima tunc ægra et saucia*
> *Concurrit ad labia mihi.*[11]

[When I shower on my sweetheart smacking kisses, my soul sore and wounded rushes to my lips.]

The soul and all is moved: *Jam pluribus osculis labra crepitabant, animarum quoque mixturam facientes, inter mutuos complexus animas anhelantes*[12] [they kissed again and again, and as they

joined their lips their souls also commingled, they breathed out
their souls in their embraces].

> *Hæsimus calentes,*
> *Et transfudimus hinc et hinc labellis*
> *Errantes animas. Valete curæ.*[1]

[Locked in warm embrace, we transferred our souls to
        one another through our lips, bidding care avaunt.]

"They breathe out their souls and spirits together with their
kisses," saith Balthasar Castilio, "change hearts and spirits,
and mingle affections as they do kisses, and it is rather a con-
nection of the mind than of the body."[2]   And although these
kisses be delightsome and pleasant, ambrosial kisses, *Suaviolum
dulci dulcius ambrosia,*[3] such as Ganymede gave Jupiter,[4]
nectare suavius, sweeter than nectar, balsam, honey,[5] *Oscula
merum amorem stillantia,*[6] love-dropping kisses; for

> The gilliflower, the rose is not so sweet,
> As sugared kisses be when lovers meet:

yet they leave an irksome impression, like that of aloes or gall:

> *Ut mi ex ambrosia mutatum jam foret illud*
> *Suaviolum tristi tristius helleboro.*[7]

> At first ambrose itself was not sweeter,
> At last black hellebore was not so bitter.

They are deceitful kisses:

> *Quid me mollibus implicas lacertis?*
> *Quid fallacibus osculis inescas?* etc.[8]

> Why dost within thine arms me lap,
> And with false kisses me entrap.

They are destructive, and the more the worse: *Et quæ me perdunt,
oscula mille dabat*[9] [she compassed my fall with a thousand
kisses]; they are the bane of these miserable lovers.   There be
honest kisses, I deny not, *osculum caritatis* [the kiss of charity],
friendly kisses, modest kisses, vestal-virgin kisses, officious and
ceremonial kisses, etc. ' *Osculi sensus, brachiorum amplexus,*
kissing and embracing are proper gifts of nature to a man;
but these are too lascivious kisses, *Implicuitque suos circum
mea colla lacertos*[10] [she folded her arms about my neck], etc.,
too continuate and too violent, *Brachia non hederæ, non vincunt
oscula conchæ,* they cling like ivy, close as an oyster, bill as
doves, meretricious kisses, biting of lips,[11] *cum additamento*
[and more besides]: *Tam impresso ore* (saith Lucian[12]) *ut vix*

labia detrahant, inter deosculandum mordicantes [with mouths so close pressed that they scarce withdraw the lips, biting as they kiss], *tum et os aperientes quoque et mammas attrectantes*, etc., such kisses as she gave to Giton, *innumera oscula dedit non repugnanti puero, cervicem invadens*, innumerable kisses, etc. More than kisses, or too homely kisses: as those that he [1] spake of, *accepturus ab ipsa venere septem suavia*, etc., with such other obscenities that vain lovers use, which are abominable and pernicious. If, as Peter de Ledesmo, *Cas. cons.*, holds, every kiss a man gives his wife after marriage be *mortale peccatum*, a mortal sin, or that of Hierome,[2] *Adulter est quisquis in uxorem suam ardentior est amator* [he is an adulterer who loves his wife too passionately]; or that of Thomas, *Secund. quæst.* 154, *artic.* 4, *Contactus et osculum sit mortale peccatum* [touching and kissing is mortal sin], or that of Durand, *Rational. lib.* 1, *cap.* 10, *Abstinere debent conjuges a complexu, toto tempore quo solennitas nuptiarum interdicitur* [married couples should abstain from embracing throughout the whole of the period during which marriages are not solemnized], what shall become of all such immodest kisses [3] and obscene actions, the forerunners of brutish lust, if not lust itself? What shall become of them that often abuse their own wives? But what have I to do with this?

That which I aim at, is to show you the progress of this burning lust; to epitomize therefore all this which I have hitherto said, with a familiar example out of that elegant Musæus, observe but with me those amorous proceedings of Leander and Hero. They began first to look one on another with a lascivious look:

Oblique intuens inde nutibus . . .
Nutibus mutuis inducens in errorem mentem puellæ.
Et illa e contra nutibus mutuis juvenis
Leandri quod amorem non renuit, etc.

Inde:

Adibat in tenebris tacite quidem stringens
Roseos puellæ digitos, ex imo suspirabat
Vehementer. . . .

Inde:

Virginis autem bene olens collum osculatus,
Tale verbum ait amoris ictus stimulo,
Preces audi et amoris miserere mei, etc.
Sic fatus recusantïs persuasit mentem puellæ.

With becks and nods he first began
    To try the wench's mind,
With becks and nods and smiles again
    An answer he did find.

> And in the dark he took her by the hand,
> And wrung it hard, and sighed grievously,
> And kiss'd her too, and woo'd her as he might,
> With Pity me, sweetheart, or else I die,
> And with such words and gestures as there past,
> He won his mistress' favour at the last.

The same proceeding is elegantly described by Apollonius in his Argonautics, between Jason and Medea, by Eustathius in the ten books of the loves of Ismenias and Ismene, Achilles Tatius between his Clitophon and Leucippe, Chaucer's neat poem of Troilus and Creseid; and in that notable tale in Petronius of a soldier and a gentlewoman of Ephesus, that was so famous all over Asia for her chastity, and that mourned for her husband: the soldier wooed her with such rhetoric as lovers use to do: *Placitone etiam pugnabis amori?* [Will you resist even a suitor that you love?], etc.; at last, *frangi pertinaciam passa est* [she allowed her obstinacy to be overcome], he got her good will, not only to satisfy his lust, but to hang her dead husband's body on the cross which he watched,[1] instead of the thief's that was newly stolen away whilst he wooed her in her cabin. These are tales, you will say, but they have most significant morals, and do well express those ordinary proceedings of doting lovers.

Many such allurements there are, nods, jests, winks, smiles, wrestlings, tokens, favours, symbols, letters, valentines, etc. For which cause belike, Godefridus, *lib. 2 de amor.*, would not have women learn to write. Many such provocations are used when they come in presence, they will and will not.[2]

> *Malo me Galatea petit lasciva puella*
> *Et fugit ad salices, et se cupit ante videri.*

> My mistress with an apple woos me,
>   And hastily to covert goes
> To hide herself, but would be seen
>   With all her heart before, God knows.

Hero so tripped away from Leander as one displeased,

> Yet as she went full often look'd behind,
> And many poor excuses did she find
> To linger by the way,[3]

but if he chance to overtake her, she is most averse, nice and coy,

> *Denegat et pugnat, sed vult super omnia vinci.*

> She seems not won, but won she is at length,
> In such wars women use but half their strength.

Sometimes they lie open and are most tractable and coming, apt, yielding, and willing to embrace, to take a green gown,

with that shepherdess in Theocritus, *Idyll*. 27, to let their coats,
etc., to play and dally, at such seasons, and to some, as they
spy their advantage; and then coy, close again, so nice, so surly,
so demure, you had much better tame a colt, catch or ride a
wild horse, than get her favour or win her love, not a look, not
a smile, not a kiss for a kingdom.　Aretine's Lucretia was an
excellent artisan in this kind, as she tells her own tale: "Though
I was by nature and art most beautiful and fair, yet by these
tricks I seemed to be far more amiable than I was, for that
which men earnestly seek and cannot attain, draws on their
affection with a most furious desire.[1]　I had a suitor loved me
dearly" (said she), "and the more he gave me, the more eagerly
he wooed me, the more I seemed to neglect, to scorn him,
and, which I commonly gave others, I would not let him see
me, converse with me, no, not have a kiss.[2]　To gull him the
more and fetch him over (for him only I aimed at), I personated
mine own servant to bring in a present from a Spanish count,
whilst he was in my company, as if he had been the count's
servant, which he did excellently well perform: *Comes de monte
Turco* [the Count of Mount Turk], my lord and master, hath
sent your ladyship a small present, and part of his hunting, a
piece of venison, a pheasant, a few partridges, etc." (all which
she bought with her own money), "commends his love and
service to you, desiring you to accept of it in good part, and he
means very shortly to come and see you." [3]　Withal she showed
him rings, gloves, scarfs, coronets which others had sent her,
when there was no such matter, but only to circumvent him.
"By these means" (as she concludes) "I made the poor gentleman so mad, that he was ready to spend himself and venture
his dearest blood for my sake." [4]　Philinna, in Lucian,[5] practised all this long before, as it shall appear unto you by her
discourse; for when Diphilus her sweetheart came to see her
(as his daily custom was), she frowned upon him, would not
vouchsafe him her company, but kissed Lamprias, his corrival,
at the same time before his face: but why was it?　To make
him (as she telleth her mother that chid her for it) more jealous;
to whetten his love, to come with a greater appetite, and to
know that her favour was not so easy to be had.[6]　Many other
tricks she used besides this (as she there confesseth), for she
would fall out with, and anger him of set purpose, pick quarrels
upon no occasion, because she would be reconciled to him again.
Amantium iræ amoris redintegratio, as the old saying is, the
falling out of lovers is the renewing of love; and according to

that of Aristænetus, *jucundiores amorum post injurias deliciæ*,
love is increased by injuries, as the sunbeams are more gracious
after a cloud.   And surely this aphorism is most true; for as
Ampelis informs Chrysis in the said Lucian, "If a lover be not
jealous, angry, waspish, apt to fall out, sigh and swear, he is no
true lover.[1]   To kiss and coll, hang about her neck, protest,
swear, and wish, are but ordinary symptoms, *incipientis adhuc et
crescentis amoris signa* [signs of a love still in its infancy]; but if
he be jealous, angry, apt to mistake, etc., *bene speres licet* [you may
have good hopes], sweet sister, he is thine own; yet if you let
him alone, humour him, please him, etc., and that he perceive
once he hath you sure, without any corrival, his love will languish,
and he will not care so much for you.   Hitherto" (saith she)
"can I speak out of experience; Demophantus, a rich fellow,
was a suitor of mine; I seemed to neglect him, and gave better
entertainment to Callides the painter before his face; *principio
abiit, verbis me insectatus*, at first he went away all in a chafe,
cursing and swearing, but at last he came submitting himself,
vowing and protesting he loved me most dearly, I should have
all he had, and that he would kill himself for my sake.   Therefore I advise thee, dear sister Chrysis, and all maids, not to use
your suitors over-kindly; *insolentes enim sunt hoc cum sentiunt*,
'twill make them proud and insolent; but now and then reject
them, estrange thyself, *et si me audies, semel atque iterum exclude*,
shut him out of doors once or twice, let him dance attendance;
follow my counsel, and by this means you shall make him mad,[2]
come off roundly, stand to any conditions, and do whatsoever
you will have him."   These are the ordinary practices; yet, in
the said Lucian, Melissa methinks had a trick beyond all this;
for when her suitor came coldly on, to stir him up, she writ
one of his corrival's names and her own in a paper, *Melissa
amat Hermotimum, Hermotimus Melissam* [Melissa loves Hermotimus, and he her], causing it to be stuck upon a post for all
gazers to behold, and lost it in the way where he used to walk;
which when the silly novice perceived, *statim ut legit credidit*,
[he] instantly apprehended it was so, came raving to me, etc.;
"and so, when I was in despair of his love, four months after
I recovered him again."[3]   Eugenia drew Timocles for her
valentine, and wore his name a long time after in her bosom:
Camæna singled out Pamphilus to dance, at Myson's wedding
(some say), for there she saw him first; Felicianus overtook
Cælia by the high-way side, offered his service, thence came
further acquaintance, and thence came love.   But who can

repeat half their devices? what Aretine experienced, what conceited Lucian, or wanton Aristænetus? They will deny and
take, stiffly refuse, and yet earnestly seek the same, repel to
make them come with more eagerness, fly from if you follow,
but if averse, as a shadow they will follow you again, *fugientem
sequitur, sequentem fugit*; with a regaining retreat, a gentle
reluctancy, a smiling threat, a pretty pleasant peevishness they
will put you off, and have a thousand such several enticements.
For as he saith,[1]

> *Non est forma satis, nec quæ vult bella videri,*
> *Debet vulgari more placere suis.*
> *Dicta, sales, lusus, sermones, gratia, risus,*
> *Vincunt naturæ candidioris opus.*

> 'Tis not enough, though she be fair of hue,
> For her to use this vulgar complement:
> But pretty toys and jests, and saws and smiles,
> As far beyond what beauty can attempt.

For this cause belike Philostratus, in his Images,[2] makes divers
loves, "some young, some of one age, some of another, some
winged, some of one sex, some of another, some with torches,
some with golden apples, some with darts, gins, snares, and
other engines in their hands," as Propertius hath prettily
painted them out, *lib. 2, El. 29*, and which some interpret, divers
enticements, or divers affections of lovers, which if not alone,
yet jointly may batter and overcome the strongest constitutions.

It is reported of Decius and Valerianus, those two notorious
persecutors of the Church, that when they could enforce a
young Christian by no means (as Hierome records [3]) to sacrifice
to their idols, by no torments or promises, they took another
course to tempt him: they put him into a fair garden, and set
a young courtesan to dally with him; "she took him about the
neck and kissed him, and that which is not to be named," [4]
manibusque attrectare, etc., and all those enticements which
might be used, that whom torments could not, love might
batter and beleaguer. But such was his constancy, she could
not overcome, and when this last engine would take no place,
they left him to his own ways. At Berkeley in Gloucestershire,[5]
there was in times past a nunnery (saith Gualterus Mapes, an
old historiographer, that lived 400 years since), "of which there
was a noble and a fair lady abbess: Godwin, that subtle Earl
of Kent, travelling that way (seeking not her but hers), leaves
a nephew of his, a proper young gallant (as if he had been
sick), with her, till he came back again, and gives the young

man charge so long to counterfeit, till he had deflowered the abbess, and as many besides of the nuns as he could, and leaves him withal rings, jewels, girdles, and such toys to give them still, when they came to visit him. The young man, willing to undergo such a business, played his part so well, that in short space he got up most of their bellies, and when he had done, told his lord how he had sped; his lord made instantly to the court, tells the king how such a nunnery was become a bawdy-house, procures a visitation, gets them to be turned out, and begs the lands to his own use." [1] This story I do therefore repeat, that you may see of what force these enticements are, if they be opportunely used, and how hard it is even for the most averse and sanctified souls to resist such allurements. John Major, in the life of John the Monk, that lived in the days of Theodosius, commends the hermit to have been a man of singular continency, and of a most austere life; but one night by chance the devil came to his cell in the habit of a young market wench that had lost her way, and desired for God's sake some lodging with him. "The old man let her in, and after some common conference of her mishap, she began to inveigle him with lascivious talk and jests, to play with his beard, to kiss him, and do worse, till at last she overcame him. As he went to address himself to that business, she vanished on a sudden, and the devils in the air laughed him to scorn." [2] Whether this be a true story, or a tale, I will not much contend; it serves to illustrate this which I have said.

Yet were it so, that these of which I have hitherto spoken, and such-like enticing baits, be not sufficient, there be many others which will of themselves intend this passion of burning lust, amongst which dancing is none of the least; and it is an engine of such force, I may not omit it. *Incitamentum libidinis*, Petrarch calls it, the spur of lust, "a circle of which the devil himself is the centre.[3] Many women that use it have come dishonest home, most indifferent, none better." [4] Another terms it "the companion of all filthy delights and enticements, and 'tis not easily told what inconveniences come by it, what scurrile talk, obscene actions," [5] and many times such monstrous gestures, such lascivious motions, such wanton tunes, meretricious kisses, homely embracings

> (*ut Gaditana canoro*
> *Incipiat prurire choro, plausuque probatæ*
> *Ad terram tremula descendant clune puellæ,*
> *Irritamentum Veneris languentis*),[6]

that it will make the spectators mad. When that epitomizer
of Trogus had to the full described and set out King Ptolemy's
riot as a chief engine and instrument of his overthrow, he adds
tympanum et tripudium, fiddling and dancing: "the king was not
a spectator only, but a principal actor himself." [1] A thing
nevertheless frequently used, and part of a gentlewoman's
bringing up, to sing, dance, and play on the lute, or some such
instrument, before she can say her paternoster or Ten Commandments. 'Tis the next way, their parents think, to get them
husbands; they are compelled to learn, and by that means
incestos amores de tenero meditantur ungue [2] [from tender years
their thoughts run on unchastity]; 'tis a great allurement as
it is often used, and many are undone by it. Thais, in Lucian,
inveigled Lamprias in a dance. Herodias so far pleased Herod
that she made him swear to give her what she would ask, John
Baptist's head in a platter. Robert Duke of Normandy, [3] riding
by Falaise, spied Arletta, a fair maid, as she danced on a
green, and was so much enamoured with the object that he
must needs lie with her that night. [4] Owen Tudor won Queen
Catherine's affection in a dance, falling by chance with his
head in her lap. Who cannot parallel these stories out of his
experience? Speucippus, a noble gallant in that Greek Aristænetus, [5] seeing Panareta a fair young gentlewoman dancing
by accident, was so far in love with her that for a long time
after he could think of nothing but Panareta; he came raving
home full of Panareta: "Who would not admire her, who
would not love her, that should but see her dance as I did?
O admirable, O divine Panareta! I have seen old and new
Rome, many fair cities, many proper women, but never any like
to Panareta, they are dross, dowdies all to Panareta! O how
she danced, how she tripped, how she turned, with what a
grace! happy is that man that shall enjoy her. O most incomparable, only, Panareta!" When Xenophon, in *Symposio,* or
Banquet, had discoursed of love, and used all the engines that
might be devised to move Socrates, amongst the rest, to stir
him the more, he shuts up all with a pleasant interlude or dance
of Dionysus and Ariadne. "First Ariadne dressed like a bride
came in and took her place; by and by Dionysus entered, dancing
to the music. The spectators did all admire the young man's
carriage; and Ariadne herself was so much affected with the
sight that she could scarce sit. After a while Dionysus, beholding Ariadne, and incensed with love, bowing to her knees,
embraced her first, and kissed her with a grace; she embraced

him again, and kissed him with like affection, etc., as the
dance required; but they that stood by and saw this, did much
applaud and commend them both for it. And when Dionysus
rose up, he raised her up with him, and many pretty gestures,
embraces, kisses, and love compliments passed between them:
which when they saw fair Bacchus and beautiful Ariadne so
sweetly and so unfeignedly kissing each other, so really embracing, they swore they loved indeed, and were so inflamed
with the object that they began to rouse up themselves, as if
they would have flown. At the last, when they saw them still
so willingly embracing, and now ready to go to the bride-
chamber, they were so ravished with it, that they that were
unmarried swore they would forthwith marry, and those that
were married called instantly for their horses, and galloped
home to their wives." [1] What greater motive can there be than
this burning lust? what so violent an oppugner? Not without
good cause therefore so many general councils condemn it, so
many Fathers abhor it, so many grave men speak against it.
"Use not the company of a woman," saith Siracides, ix, 4,
"that is a singer or a dancer; neither hear, lest thou be taken in
her craftiness." *In circo non tam cernitur quam discitur libido*,
Hædus holds,[2] lust in theatres is not seen, but learned. Gregory
Nazianzen, that eloquent divine (as he relates the story himself [3]),
when a noble friend of his solemnly invited him, with other
bishops, to his daughter Olympia's wedding, refused to come:
"For it is absurd to see an old gouty bishop sit amongst
dancers"; [4] he held it unfit to be a spectator, much less an
actor. *Nemo saltat sobrius*, Tully writes, he is not a sober man
that danceth; for some such reason (belike) Domitian forbade
the Roman senators to dance, and for that fact removed many
of them from the senate. But these, you will say, are lascivious
and pagan dances, 'tis the abuse that causeth such inconvenience,
and I do not well therefore to condemn, speak against, or
"innocently to accuse the best and pleasantest thing" (so
Lucian calls it) "that belongs to mortal men." [5] You misinterpret, I condemn it not; I hold it notwithstanding an honest
disport, a lawful recreation, if it be opportune, moderately and
soberly used: I am of Plutarch's mind, "that which respects
pleasure alone, honest recreation, or bodily exercise, ought not
to be rejected and contemned": [6] I subscribe to Lucian, "'tis
an elegant thing, which cheereth up the mind, exerciseth the
body, delights the spectators, which teacheth many comely
gestures, equally affecting the ears, eyes, and soul itself." [7]

Sallust discommends singing and dancing in Sempronia, not
that she did sing or dance, but that she did it in excess, 'tis
the abuse of it; and Gregory's refusal doth not simply condemn
it, but in some folks. Many will not allow men and women to
dance together, because it is a provocation to lust; they may
as well, with Lycurgus and Mahomet, cut down all vines, forbid
the drinking of wine, for that it makes some men drunk.

> *Nihil prodest quod non lædere posset idem;*
> *Igne quid utilius?* [1]
>
> [Naught useful is but may become a curse;
> Than fire what can better be, or worse?]

I say of this, as of all other honest recreations, they are like
fire, good and bad, and I see no such inconvenience but that they
may so dance, if it be done at due times, and by fit persons:
and conclude with Wolfongus Hider,[2] and most of our modern
divines: *Si decoræ, graves, verecundæ, plena luce bonorum virorum
et matronarum honestarum, tempestive fiant, probari possunt, et
debent* [if they are seemly, staid, and modest, and carried out
in the view of good men and honest matrons, and at proper
hours, they may be regarded with favour]. "There is a time
to mourn, a time to dance" (Eccles. iii, 4). Let them take their
pleasures then, and as he [3] said of old, "young men and maids
flourishing in their age, fair and lovely to behold, well attired,
and of comely carriage, dancing a Greek galliard, and as their
dance required, kept their time, now turning, now tracing, now
apart, now altogether, now a courtesy, then a caper," etc., and
it was a pleasant sight to see those pretty knots and swimming
figures. The sun and moon (some say) dance about the earth,
the three upper planets about the sun as their centre, now
stationary, now direct, now retrograde, now *in apogæo*, then
in perigæo, now swift, then slow, occidental, oriental, they turn
round, jump and trace, ♀ and ☿ about the sun with those
thirty-three Maculæ or Borbonian planets, *circa solem saltantes
citharœdum*, saith Fromundus. Four Medicean stars dance
about Jupiter, two Austrian about Saturn, etc., and all (belike)
to the music of the spheres. Our greatest counsellors, and staid
senators, at some times dance, as David before the ark (2 Sam.
vi, 14), Miriam (Exod. xv, 20), Judith (xv, 13) (though the
devil hence perhaps hath brought in those bawdy bacchanals),
and well may they do it. The greatest soldiers, as Quintilianus,[4]
Æmilius Probus,[5] Cælius Rhodiginus,[6] have proved at large,
still use it in Greece, Rome, and the most worthy senators,

cantare, saltare [to sing, to dance].   Lucian, Macrobius, Libanius, Plutarch, Julius Pollux, Athenæus, have written just tracts in commendation of it.   In this our age it is in much request in those countries, as in all civil commonwealths, as Alexander ab Alexandro, *lib.* 4, *cap.* 10, *et lib.* 2, *cap.* 25, hath proved at large, amongst the barbarians themselves none so precious;[1] all the world allows it.

> *Divitias contemno tuas, rex Cræse, tuamque*
> *Vendo Asiam, unguentis, flore, mero, choreis.*[2]

[I scorn your riches, Crœsus, and would sell your Asia
for scents, flowers, wine and dances.]

Plato,[3] in his Commonwealth, will have dancing-schools to be maintained, "that young folks might meet, be acquainted, see one another, and be seen"; nay more, he would have them dance naked, and scoffs at them that laugh at it.   But Eusebius, *Præpar. Evangel. lib.* 1, *cap.* 11, and Theodoret, *lib.* 9 *Curat. Græc. affect.*, worthily lash him for it; and well they might: for as one saith, "the very sight of naked parts causeth enormous, exceeding concupiscences, and stirs up both men and women to burning lust."[4]   There is a mean in all things; this is my censure in brief: dancing is a pleasant recreation of body and mind, if sober and modest (such as our Christian dances are), if tempestively used; a furious motive to burning lust, if, as by pagans heretofore, unchastely abused.   But I proceed.

   If these allurements do not take place, for Simierus,[5] that great master of dalliance, shall not behave himself better, the more effectually to move others and satisfy their lust, they will swear and lie, promise, protest, forge, counterfeit, brag, bribe, flatter and dissemble of all sides.   'Twas Lucretia's counsel in Aretine, *Si vis amica frui, promitte, finge, jura, perjura, jacta, simula, mentire* [if you want to win your mistress, promise, invent, swear, forswear, boast, pretend, lie]; and they put it well in practice, as Apollo to Daphne:

> *Mihi Delphica tellus*
> *Et Claros et Tenedos, Patareaque regia servit,*
> *Jupiter est genitor.*[6]

> Delphos, Claros, and Tenedos serve me,
> And Jupiter is known my sire to be.

The poorest swains will do as much;[7] *Mille pecus nivei sunt et mihi vallibus agni,*[8] I have a thousand sheep, good store of cattle, and they are all at her command:

> *Tibi nos, tibi nostra supellex,*
> *Ruraque servierint,*[9]

house, land, goods, are at her service, as he is himself. Dino-machus, a senator's son in Lucian,[1] in love with a wench inferior to him in birth and fortunes, the sooner to accomplish his desire, wept unto her, and swore he loved her with all his heart, and her alone, and that as soon as ever his father died (a very rich man and almost decrepit) he would make her his wife. The maid by chance made her mother acquainted with the business, who being an old fox, well experienced in such matters, told her daughter, now ready to yield to his desire, that he meant nothing less; "for dost thou think he will ever care for thee, being a poor wench, that may have his choice of all the beauties in the city, one noble by birth, with so many talents, as young, better qualified, and fairer than thyself?[2] Daughter, believe him not." The maid was abashed, and so the matter broke off. When Jupiter wooed Juno first (Lilius Giraldus relates it out of an old comment on Theocritus), the better to effect his suit, he turned himself into a cuckoo, and spying her one day walking alone, separated from the other goddesses, caused a tempest suddenly to arise, for fear of which she fled to shelter; Jupiter to avoid the storm likewise flew into her lap, *in virginis Junonis gremium devolavit,* whom Juno for pity covered in her apron.[3] But he turned himself forthwith into his own shape, began to embrace and offer violence unto her, *sed illa matris metu abnuebat,* but she by no means would yield, *donec pollicitus connubium obtinuit,* till he vowed and swore to marry her, and then she gave consent. This fact was done at Thornax Hill, which ever after was called Cuckoo Hill, and in perpetual remembrance there was a temple erected to Teleia Juno in the same place. So powerful are fair promises, vows, oaths and protestations. It is an ordinary thing too in this case to belie their age, which widows usually do, that mean to marry again, and bachelors too sometimes,

Cujus octavum trepidavit ætas
Cernere lustrum,[4]

[Whose years have come in sight of twoscore,]

to say they are younger than they are. Charmides in the said Lucian loved Philematium, an old maid of forty-five years; she swore to him she was but thirty-two next December.[5] But to dissemble in this kind is familiar of all sides, and often it takes. *Fallere credentem res est operosa puellam*[6] ['tis no great triumph to deceive a credulous maid], 'tis soon done, no such great mastery,

Egregiam vero laudem, et spolia ampla,

[A splendid distinction and a glorious booty, forsooth,]

and nothing so frequent as to belie their estates, to prefer their
suits and to advance themselves. Many men, to fetch over a
young woman, widows, or whom they love, will not stick to
crack, forge, and feign anything comes next, bid his boy fetch
his cloak, rapier, gloves, jewels, etc., in such a chest, scarlet-
golden-tissue breeches, etc., when there is no such matter; or
make any scruple to give out, as he did in Petronius, that he
was master of a ship, kept so many servants; and to personate
their part the better, take upon them to be gentlemen of good
houses, well descended and allied, hire apparel at brokers', some
scavenger or pricklouse tailors to attend upon them for the
time, swear they have great possessions,[1] bribe, lie, cog, and
foist how dearly they love, how bravely they will maintain her,
like any lady, countess, duchess, or queen; they shall have
gowns, tires, jewels, coaches, and caroches, choice diet,

> The heads of parrots, tongues of nightingales,
> The brains of peacocks, and of ostriches,
> Their bath shall be the juice of gilliflowers,
> Spirit of roses and of violets,
> The milk of unicorns, etc.,

as old Volpone courted Celia in the comedy,[2] whenas they are
no such men, not worth a groat, but mere sharkers, to make a
fortune, to get their desire, or else pretend love to spend their
idle hours, to be more welcome, and for better entertainment.
The conclusion is, they mean nothing less.

> *Nil metuunt jurare, nihil promittere curant :*
> *Sed simul ac cupidæ mentis satiata libido est,*
> *Dicta nihil meminere, nihil perjuria curant.*[3]

> Oaths, vows, promises, are much protested;
> But when their mind and lust is satisfied,
> Oaths, vows, promises, are quite neglected.

Though he solemnly swear by the genius of Cæsar, by Venus'
shrine, Hymen's deity, by Jupiter and all the other gods, give
no credit to his words. For when lovers swear, Venus laughs,
Venus hæc perjuria ridet, Jupiter himself smiles,[4] and pardons
it withal; as grave Plato gives out,[5] of all perjury, that alone
for love matters is forgiven by the gods. If promises, lies, oaths,
and protestations will not avail, they fall to bribes, tokens, gifts,
and such-like feats. *Plurimus auro conciliatur amor*[6] [love is
chiefly gained by gold]: as Jupiter corrupted Danae with a
golden shower, and Liber Ariadne with a lovely crown (which
was afterwards translated into the heavens, and there for ever

shines), they will rain chequins, florins, crowns, angels, all manner of coins and stamps in her lap. And so must he certainly do that will speed, make many feasts, banquets, invitations, send her some present or other every foot. *Summo studio parentur epulæ* (saith Hædus[1]) *et crebræ fiant largitiones*, he must be very bountiful and liberal, seek and sue, not to her only, but to all her followers, friends, familiars, fiddlers, panders, parasites, and household servants; he must insinuate himself, and surely will, to all, of all sorts, messengers, porters, carriers; no man must be unrewarded or unrespected. "I had a suitor" (saith Aretine's Lucretia) "that when he came to my house, flung gold and silver about, as if it had been chaff.[2] Another suitor I had was a very choleric fellow; but I so handled him, that for all his fuming, I brought him upon his knees.[3] If there had been an excellent bit in the market, any novelty, fish, fruit, or fowl, muscadel, or malmsey, or a cup of neat wine in all the city, it was presented presently to me; though never so dear, hard to come by, yet I had it: the poor fellow was so fond at last, that I think if I would I might have had one of his eyes out of his head.[4] A third suitor was a merchant of Rome, and his manner of wooing was with exquisite music, costly banquets, poems, etc.[5] I held him off till at length he protested, promised, and swore *pro virginitate regno me donaturum*, I should have all he had, house, goods, and lands, *pro concubitu solo*; neither was there ever any conjuror, I think, to charm his spirits that used such attention or mighty words, as he did exquisite phrases,[6] or general of any army so many stratagems to win a city, as he did tricks and devices to get the love of me." Thus men are active and passive, and women not far behind them in this kind: *Audax ad omnia femina, quæ vel amat, vel odit* [a woman will stick at nothing to gratify either her love or her hate].

> For half so boldly there can non
> Swear and lie as women can.[7]

They will crack, counterfeit, and collogue as well as the best,[8] with handkerchiefs and wrought nightcaps, purses, posies, and such toys: as he justly complained:

> *Cur mittis violas? nempe ut violentius urer;*
> *Quid violas violis me violenta tuis?* etc.[9]

> Why dost thou send me violets, my dear?
> To make me burn more violent, I fear,
> With violets too violent thou art,
> To violate and wound my gentle heart.

When nothing else will serve, the last refuge is their tears. *Hæc scripsi* (*testor amorem*) *mixta lacrimis et suspiriis*, 'twixt tears and sighs I write this (I take love to witness), saith Chelidonia to Philonius.[1] *Lumina quæ modo fulmina, jam flumina lacrimarum*, those burning torches are now turned to floods of tears. Aretine's Lucretia, when her sweetheart came to town, wept in his bosom, "that he might be persuaded those tears were shed for joy of his return." [2] Quartilla in Petronius, when naught would move, fell a-weeping, and, as Balthasar Castilio paints them out, "To these crocodile's tears they will add sobs, fiery sighs, and sorrowful countenance, pale colour, leanness, and if you do but stir abroad, these fiends are ready to meet you at every turn, with such a sluttish neglected habit, dejected look, as if they were now ready to die for your sake; [3] and how," saith he, "shall a young novice, thus beset, escape?" But believe them not.

Animam ne crede puellis,
Namque est feminea tutior unda fide.[4]

[Trust not thy soul to maids, for the sea is more constant than women's vows.]

Thou thinkest, peradventure, because of her vows, tears, smiles, and protestations, she is solely thine, thou hast her heart, hand, and affection, whenas indeed there is no such matter, as the Spanish bawd said,[5] *gaudet illa habere unum in lecto, alterum in porta, tertium qui domi suspiret*, she will have one sweetheart in bed, another in the gate, a third sighing at home, a fourth, etc. Every young man she sees and likes hath as much interest, and shall as soon enjoy, as thyself. On the other side, which I have said, men are as false, let them swear, protest, and lie; *Quod vobis dicunt, dixerunt mille puellis* [6] [what they say to you, they have said to a thousand more]. They love some of them those eleven thousand virgins at once, and make them believe, each particular, he is besotted on her; or love one till they see another, and then her alone; like Milo's wife in Apuleius, *lib.* 2, *Si quem conspexerit speciosæ formæ juvenem, venustate ejus sumitur, et in eum animum intorquet* [as soon as she sees a handsome youth, she is fascinated by him and dotes on him]. 'Tis their common compliment in that case, they care not what they swear, say, or do. One while they slight them, care not for them, rail downright and scoff at them, and then again they will run mad, hang themselves, stab and kill, if they may not enjoy them. Henceforth, therefore, *nulla viro juranti femina*

credat, let not maids believe them.   These tricks and counterfeit passions are more familiar with women, *Finem hic dolori
faciet aut vitæ dies, miserere amantis* [this day will end either
my misery or my life—pity a lover], quoth Phædra to Hippolytus.[1]   Ioessa, in Lucian,[2] told Pythias, a young man, to move
him the more, that if he would not have her, she was resolved
to make away herself.   "There is a Nemesis, and it cannot
choose but grieve and trouble thee to hear that I have either
strangled or drowned myself for thy sake."   Nothing so common
to this sex as oaths, vows, and protestations, and as I have
already said, tears, which they have at command; for they can
so weep that one would think their very hearts were dissolved
within them, and would come out in tears; their eyes are like
rocks, which still drop water, *diariæ lacrimæ et sudoris in modum
turgeri promptæ*, saith Aristænetus,[3] they wipe away their tears
like sweat, weep with one eye, laugh with the other; or as
children weep and cry, they can both together.[4]

> *Neve puellarum lacrimis moveare memento,*
>   *Ut flerent oculos erudiere suos.*[5]

> Care not for women's tears, I counsel thee,
> They teach their eyes as much to weep as see.

And as much pity is to be taken of a woman weeping, as of a
goose going barefoot.   When Venus lost her son Cupid, she sent
a crier about, to bid every one that met him take heed.

> *Si flentem aspicias, ne mox fallare, caveto;*
> *Sin arridebit, magis effuge; et oscula si fors*
> *Ferre volet, fugito; sunt oscula noxia, in ipsis*
> *Suntque venena labris,* etc.[6]

> Take heed of Cupid's tears, if cautelous,
> And of his smiles and kisses, I thee tell,
> If that he offer 't, for they be noxious,
> And very poison in his lips doth dwell.

"A thousand years," as Castilio conceives, "will scarce serve
to reckon up those allurements and guiles that men and women
use to deceive one another with." [7]

SUBSECT. V.—*Bawds, Philters, Causes*

When all other engines fail, that they can proceed no farther
of themselves, their last refuge is to fly to bawds, panders,
magical philters, and receipts; rather than fail, to the devil

himself. *Flectere si nequeunt superos, Acheronta movebunt* [if
Heaven will not hear them, they will move Hell]. And by
those indirect means many a man is overcome, and precipitated
into this malady, if he take not good heed. For these bawds
first, they are everywhere so common and so many, that, as he
said of old Croton, *omnes hic* [all here] *aut captantur, aut captant*,[1]
either inveigle or be inveigled, we may say of most of our cities,
there be so many professed, cunning bawds in them. Besides,
bawdry is become an art, or a liberal science, as Lucian calls
it; and there be such tricks and subtleties, so many nurses, old
women, panders, letter-carriers, beggars, physicians, friars, confessors, employed about it, that *nullus tradere stilus sufficiat*
[no pen could recount it], one saith,

> *Trecentis versibus*
> *Tuas impuritias traloqui nemo potest.*[2]

> [Three hundred verses would not suffice to tell the
> tale of your debaucheries.]

Such occult notes, steganography, polygraphy,[3] *Nuntius ani-
matus*,[4] or magnetical telling of their minds, which Cabeus the
Jesuit,[5] by the way, counts fabulous and false; cunning conveyances in this kind, that neither Juno's jealousy, nor Danae's
custody, nor Argo's vigilancy can keep them safe. 'Tis the
last and common refuge to use an assistant, such as that Catanean
Philippa was to Joan Queen of Naples, a bawd's help,[6] an old
woman in the business, as Myrrha [7] did when she doted on
Cinyras, and could not compass her desire, the old jade her
nurse was ready at a pinch, *Dic, inquit, opemque Me sine ferre
tibi . . . et in hoc mea (pone timorem) Sedulitas erit apta tibi*,
fear it not, if it be possible to be done, I will effect it: *non est
mulieri mulier insuperabilis*, as Cælestina said,[8] let him or her
be never so honest, watched, and reserved, 'tis hard but one of
these old women will get access: and scarce shall you find, as
Austin observes,[9] in a nunnery a maid alone; "if she cannot have
egress, before her window you shall have an old woman or some
prating gossip tell her some tales of this clerk and that monk,
describing or commending some young gentleman or other unto
her." "As I was walking in the street" (saith a good fellow
in Petronius) "to see the town served one evening, I spied an
old woman in a corner selling cabbages and roots" (as our
hucksters do plums, apples, and such-like fruits); "Mother
(quoth I), can you tell where I can dwell? She, being well
pleased with my foolish urbanity, replied, And why, sir, should

I not tell? With that she rose up and went before me; I took
her for a wise woman. And by and by she led me into a by-
lane, and told me there I should dwell; I replied again, I knew
not the house; but I perceived on a sudden, by the naked queans,
that I was now come into a bawdy-house, and then too late I
began to curse the treachery of this old jade." [1] Such tricks
you shall have in many places, and amongst the rest it is ordinary
in Venice, and in the island of Zante, for a man to be bawd to
his own wife. No sooner shall you land or come on shore, but,
as the comical poet hath it,

> *Morem hunc meretrices habent,*
> *Ad portum mittunt servulos, ancillulas,*
> *Si qua peregrina navis in portum aderit;*
> *Rogant cujatus sit, quod ei nomen siet,*
> *Post illæ extemplo sese adplicant.* [2]

These white devils have their panders, bawds, and factors in
every place, to seek about and bring in customers, to tempt
and waylay novices and silly travellers. And when they have
them once within their clutches, as Ægidius Maserius in his
comment upon Valerius Flaccus describes them, "with promises and pleasant discourse, with gifts, tokens, and taking
their opportunities, they lay nets which Lucretia cannot avoid,
and baits that Hippolytus himself would swallow; they make
such strong assaults and batteries that the Goddess of Virginity
cannot withstand them: give gifts and bribes to move Penelope,
and with threats able to terrify Susanna. How many Proser-
pinas with those catchpoles doth Pluto take! These are the
sleepy rods with which their souls touched descend to hell; this
the glue or lime with which the wings of the mind once taken
cannot fly away; the devil's ministers to allure, entice," etc. [3]
Many young men and maids, without all question, are inveigled
by these Eumenides and their associates. But these are trivial
and well known. The most sly, dangerous, and cunning bawds
are your knavish physicians, empirics, mass-priests, monks,
Jesuits, [4] and friars. Though it be against Hippocrates' oath,
some of them will give a dram, promise to restore maidenheads
and do it without danger, make an abort if need be, keep down
their paps, hinder conception, procure lust, make them able
with satyrions, and now and then step in themselves. No
monastery so close, house so private, or prison so well kept,
but these honest men are admitted to censure and ask questions,
to feel their pulse beat at their bedside, and all under pretence

of giving physic. Now as for monks, confessors, and friars, as he said,

> *Non audet Stygius Pluto tentare quod audet*
> *Effrenis monachus, plenaque fraudis anus;* [1]

> That Stygian Pluto dares not tempt or do,
> What an old hag or monk will undergo;

either for himself to satisfy his own lust, for another, if he be hired thereto, or both at once, having such excellent means. For under colour of visitation, auricular confession, comfort, and penance, they have free egress and regress, and corrupt God knows how many. They can such [2] trades, some of them, practise physic, use exorcisms, etc.

> That whereas was wont to walk an elf,
> There now walks the limiter himself,
> In every bush and under every tree,
> There needs no other incubus but he. [3]

In the mountains betwixt Dauphiné and Savoy, the friars persuaded the goodwives to counterfeit themselves possessed, that their husbands might give them free access,[4] and were so familiar in those days with some of them, that, as one observes,[5] "wenches could not sleep in their beds for necromantic friars": and the good abbess in Boccace may in some sort witness, that rising betimes, mistook and put on the friar's breeches instead of her veil or hat. You have heard the story, I presume, of Paulina,[6] a chaste matron in Hegesippus, whom one of Isis' priests did prostitute to Mundus, a young knight, and made her believe it was their god Anubis. Many such pranks are played by our Jesuits, sometimes in their own habits, sometimes in others, like soldiers, courtiers, citizens, scholars, gallants, and women themselves. Proteus-like, in all forms and disguises, they go abroad in the night, to inescate and beguile young women, or to have their pleasure of other men's wives; and, if we may believe some relations,[7] they have wardrobes of several suits in their colleges for that purpose. Howsoever in public they pretend much zeal, seem to be very holy men, and bitterly preach against adultery, fornication, there are no verier bawds or whoremasters in a country. "Whose soul they should gain to God, they sacrifice to the devil." [8] But I spare these men for the present.

The last battering engines are philters, amulets, spells, charms, images, and such unlawful means: if they cannot prevail of themselves by the help of bawds, panders, and their adherents,

,they will fly for succour to the devil himself. I know there be
those that deny the devil can do any such thing (Crato, *epist.* 2,
lib. med., and many divines), there is no other fascination than
that which comes by the eyes, of which I have formerly spoken;
and if you desire to be better informed, read Camerarius, *Oper.
subcis. cent.* 2, *cap.* 5.   It was given out of old, that a Thessalian
wench had bewitched King Philip to dote upon her, and by
philters enforced his love; but when Olympias, the queen, saw
the maid of an excellent beauty, well brought up and qualified,
these, quoth she, were the philters which inveigled King Philip;
those the true charms, as Henry to Rosamund:

> One accent from thy lips the blood more warms,
> Than all their philters, exorcisms, and charms.[1]

With this alone, Lucretia brags in Aretine,[2] she could do more
than all philosophers, astrologers, alchemists, necromancers,
witches, and the rest of the crew. "As for herbs and philters,
I could never skill of them; the sole philter that ever I used was
kissing and embracing, by which alone I made men rave like
beasts stupefied, and compelled them to worship me like an
idol."   In our times it is a common thing, saith Erastus, in his
book *de lamiis*, for witches to take upon them the making of
these philters, "to force men and women to love and hate whom
they will, to cause tempests, diseases," etc.,[3] by charms, spells,
characters, knots. *Hic Thessala vendit Philtra*[4] [this one sells
Thessalian philtres]. St. Hierome proves that they can do it;
as in Hilarion's life, *epist. lib.* 3, he hath a story of a young man,
that with a philter made a maid mad for the love of him, which
maid was after cured by Hilarion. Such instances I find in
John Nider, *Formicar. lib.* 5, *cap.* 5. Plutarch records of
Lucullus, that he died of a philter; and that Cleopatra used
philters to inveigle Antony, amongst other allurements. Eusebius reports as much of Lucretius the poet. Panormitan,
lib. 4 *de gest. Alphonsi*, hath a story of one Stephen, a Neapolitan
knight, that by a philter was forced to run mad for love.   But
of all others, that which Petrarch, *Epist. famil. lib.* 1, *ep.* 5,
relates of Charles the Great is most memorable.[5] He foolishly
doted upon a woman of mean favour and condition, many years
together, wholly delighting in her company, to the great grief
and indignation of his friends and followers. When she was
dead, he did embrace her corpse, as Apollo did the bay-tree for
his Daphne, and caused her coffin (richly embalmed and decked
with jewels) to be carried about with him, over which he still

lamented. At last a venerable bishop that followed his court, prayed earnestly to God (commiserating his lord and master's case) to know the true cause of this mad passion, and whence it proceeded; it was revealed to him, in fine, that the cause of the emperor's mad love lay under the dead woman's tongue. The bishop went hastily to the carcass, and took a small ring thence; upon the removal the emperor abhorred the corpse, and, instead of it, fell as furiously in love with the bishop, he would not suffer him to be out of his presence; [1] which when the bishop perceived, he flung the ring into the midst of a great lake, where the king then was.   From that hour the emperor neglected all his other houses, dwelt at Ache,[2] built a fair house in the midst of the marsh, to his infinite expense, and a temple by it,[3] where after he was buried, and in which city all his posterity ever since use to be crowned.   Marcus the heretic is accused by Irenæus to have inveigled a young maid by this means; and some writers speak hardly of the Lady Katherine Cobham, that by the same art she circumvented Humphrey Duke of Gloucester to be her husband. Sicinius Æmilianus summoned Apuleius to come before Cneius Maximus, proconsul of Africa, that he, being a poor fellow, "had bewitched by philters Pudentilla, an ancient rich matron, to love him," [4] and, being worth so many thousand sesterces, to be his wife.   Agrippa, *lib.* 1, *cap.* 48, *Occult. philos.*, attributes much in this kind to philters, amulets, images; and Salmuth, *Com. in Pancirol. tit.* 10, *de Horol.*   Leo Afer, *lib.* 3, saith, 'tis an ordinary practice at Fez in Africa, *præstigiatores ibi plures, qui cogunt amores et concubitus*: as skilful all out as that Hyperborean magician, of whom Cleodemus, in Lucian,[5] tells so many fine feats performed in this kind.   But Erastus, Wierus, and others are against it; they grant indeed such things may be done, but (as Wierus discourseth, *lib.* 3 *de lamiis, cap.* 37) not by charms, incantations, philters, but the devil himself; *lib.* 5, *cap.* 2, he contends as much; so doth Freitagius, *Noc. med. cap.* 74, Andreas Cisalpinus, *cap.* 5; and so much Sigismundus Scheretzius, *cap.* 9, *de hirco nocturno*, proves at large. "Unchaste women by the help of these witches, the devil's kitchen-maids, have their loves brought to them in the night, and carried back again by a phantasm flying in the air in the likeness of a goat. I have heard" (saith he) "divers confess that they have been so carried on a goat's back to their sweethearts, many miles in a night." [6]   Others are of opinion that these feats, which most suppose to be done by charms and philters, are merely effected by natural causes, as by man's

blood chemically prepared, which much avails, saith Ernestus
Burgravius, *in Lucerna vitæ et mortis Indice, ad amorem conciliandum et odium* [to cause love and hatred] (so huntsmen make
their dogs love them, and farmers their pullen); 'tis an excellent
philter, as he holds, *sed vulgo prodere grande nefas*, but not fit
to be made common: and so be *mala insana*, mandrake roots,
mandrake apples,[1] precious stones, dead men's clothes, candles,
mala Bacchica, panis porcinus, hippomanes, a certain hair in a
wolf's tail,[2] etc., of which Rhasis, Dioscorides, Porta, Wecker,
Rubeus, Mizaldus, Albertus, treat: a swallow's heart, dust of
a dove's heart, *multum valent linguæ viperarum, cerebella asinorum, tela equina, palliola quibus infantes obvoluti nascuntur,
funis strangulati hominis, lapis de nido aquilæ* [there is much
virtue in vipers' tongues, asses' brains, cauls of new-born
infants, the rope by which a man has been hanged, a stone
from an eagle's nest], etc.   See more in Sckenkius, *Observat.
medicinal. lib.* 4, etc., which are as forcible and of as much
virtue as that fountain Salmacis in Vitruvius,[3] Ovid, Strabo,
that made all such mad for love that drank of it, or that hot
bath at Aix in Germany,[4] wherein Cupid once dipt his arrows,
which ever since hath a peculiar virtue to make them lovers all
that wash in it.   But hear the poet's own description of it:

> *Unde hic fervor aquis terra erumpentibus uda?*
> *Tela olim hic ludens ignea tinxit amor;*
> *Et gaudens stridore novo, fervete perennes*
> *Inquit, et hæc pharetræ sint monumenta meæ.*
> *Ex illo fervet, rarusque hic mergitur hospes,*
> *Cui non titillet pectora blandus amor.*[5]

> [Why burst these waters from the earth so hot?
> Cupid, 'tis said, once sporting in this spot,
> His fiery arrows dipped therein,
> And, as they hissed, well tickled with the din,
> He said: "Let them boil on for ever so,
> And keep alive remembrance of my bow."
> Since then they 're hot; and therein dips no wight
> But sweet love-promptings soon his soul excite.]

These above-named remedies have haply as much power as
that bath of Aix, or Venus' enchanted girdle, in which, saith
Natalis Comes, "love-toys and dalliance, pleasantness, sweetness, persuasions, subtleties, gentle speeches, and all witchcraft
to enforce love, was contained."   Read more of these in Agrippa,
de occult. Philos. lib. 1, *cap.* 50 *et* 45; *Malleus malefic. part.* 1,
quæst. 7; Delrio, *tom.* 2, *quæst.* 3, *lib.* 3; Wierus; Pomponatius,
cap. 8 *de incantat.*; Ficinus, *lib.* 13 *Theol. Plat.*; Calcagninus, etc.

MEMB. III.

Symptoms or Signs of Love-Melancholy, in Body, Mind, good, bad, etc.

SYMPTOMS are either of body or mind; of body, paleness, leanness, dryness, etc. *Pallidus omnis amans, color hic est aptus amanti* [pale is every lover, this hue beseemeth love], as the poet [1] describes lovers; *fecit amor maciem,* love causeth leanness. Avicenna, *de Ilishi, cap.* 33, makes hollow eyes, dryness, symptoms of this disease, "to go smiling to themselves, or acting as if they saw or heard some delectable object." [2]   Valleriola, *lib.* 3 *Observat. cap.* 7; Laurentius, *cap.* 10; Ælianus Montaltus, *de her. amore*; Langius, *epist.* 24, *lib.* 1, *Epist. med.,* deliver as much, *corpus exsangue pallet, corpus gracile, oculi cavi* [the body bloodless and pale, a lean body, hollow eyes], lean, pale, *ut nudis qui pressit calcibus anguem* [as one who has trodden with naked foot upon a snake), [4] hollow-eyed, their eyes are hidden in their heads, *Tenerque nitidi corporis cecidit decor* [3] [their sleek charm falls away], they pine away, and look ill with waking, cares, sighs:

> *Et qui tenebant signa Phœbeæ facis*
> *Oculi, nihil gentile nec patrium micant,*

[And eyes that were like suns for brightness lose all their
    inherited lustre,]

with groans, griefs, sadness, dullness:

> *Nulla jam Cereris subit*
> *Cura aut salutis,* [4]

want of appetite, etc. A reason of all this Jason Pratensis gives, "because of the distraction of the spirits the liver doth not perform his part, nor turns the aliment into blood as it ought, and for that cause the members are weak for want of sustenance, they are lean and pine, as the herbs of my garden do this month of May, for want of rain." [5]   The green-sickness therefore often happeneth to young women, a cachexia or an evil habit to men, besides their ordinary sighs, complaints, and lamentations, which are too frequent. As drops from a still, *ut occluso stillat ab igne liquor,* doth Cupid's fire provoke tears from a true lover's eyes:

> The mighty Mars did oft for Venus shriek,
> Privily moistening his horrid cheek
> With womanish tears; [6]

Ignis distillat in undas,
Testis erit largus qui rigat ora liquor; [1]

[Fire distils into water, witness the copious stream
that bathes his cheeks;]

with many such-like passions. When Chariclea was enamoured
of Theagenes, as Heliodorus sets her out,[2] "she was half
distracted, and spake she knew not what, sighed to herself,
lay much awake, and was lean upon a sudden": and when
she was besotted on her son-in-law, *pallor deformis, marcentes
oculi,*[3] etc., she had ugly paleness, hollow eyes, restless thoughts,
short wind, etc. Euryalus, in an epistle sent to Lucretia his
mistress, complains amongst other grievances, *Tu mihi et somni
et cibi usum abstulisti,* Thou hast taken my stomach and my
sleep from me. So he describes it aright:

> His sleep, his meat, his drink, in him bereft,
> That lean he waxeth, and dry as a shaft,
> His eyes hollow and grisly to behold,
> His hew pale and ashen to unfold,
> And solitary he was ever alone,
> And waking all the night making mone.[4]

Theocritus, *Idyll.* 2, makes a fair maid of Delphi, in love with a
young man of Minda, confess as much:

> *Ut vidi, ut insanii, ut animus mihi male affectus est,*
> *Miseræ mihi forma tabescebat, neque amplius pompam*
> *Ullam curabam, aut quando domum redieram*
> *Novi, sed me ardens quidam morbus consumebat,*
> *Decubui in lecto dies decem, et noctes decem,*
> *Defluebant capite capilli, ipsaque sola reliqua*
> *Ossa et cutis.*

> No sooner seen I had, but mad I was,
> My beauty fail'd, and I no more did care
> For any pomp, I knew not where I was,
> But sick I was, and evil I did fare;
> I lay upon my bed ten days and nights,
> A skeleton I was in all men's sights.

All these passions are well expressed by that heroical poet [5] in
the person of Dido:

> *At non infelix animi Phœnissa, nec unquam*
> *Solvitur in somnos, oculisve ac pectore amores*
> *Accipit; ingeminant curæ, rursusque resurgens*
> *Sævit amor,* etc.

> Unhappy Dido could not sleep at all,
> But lies awake, and takes no rest:
> And up she gets again, whilst care and grief,
> And raging love torment her breast.

Accius Sannazarius, *Ecloga 2, de Galatea,* in the same manner
feigns his Lycoris tormenting herself for want of sleep, sighing,
sobbing, and lamenting;[1] and Eustathius his Ismenias much
troubled, and "panting at heart, at the sight of his mistress,"[2]
he could not sleep, his bed was thorns.   All make leanness,
want of appetite, want of sleep ordinary symptoms,[3] and by
that means they are brought often so low, so much altered and
changed, that as he jested in the comedy,[4] "one can scarce
know them to be the same men."

> *Attenuant juvenum vigilatæ corpora noctes,*
> *Curaque et immenso qui fit amore dolor.*

> [Young men grow pale and lean from the sleepless
> nights and the cares and pangs of love.]

Many such symptoms there are of the body to discern lovers
by, *quis enim bene celet amorem?* [for who can hide love?] "Can
a man," saith Solomon (Prov. vi, 27), "carry fire in his bosom
and not burn?" it will hardly be hid; though they do all they
can to hide it, it must out, *plus quam mille notis* [by more than
a thousand symptoms] it may be described, *quoque magis tegitur,
tectus magis æstuat ignis*[5] [and the more it is hidden, the more
fiercely does it burn]. 'Twas Antiphanes the comedian's observation of old, love and drunkenness cannot be concealed,
celare alia possis, hæc præter duo, vini potum, etc.; words, looks,
gestures, all will betray them; but two of the most notable
signs are observed by the pulse and countenance. When
Antiochus, the son of Seleucus, was sick for Stratonice, his
mother-in-law, and would not confess his grief, or the cause of
his disease, Erasistratus the physician found him by his pulse
and countenance to be in love with her, "because that when
she came in presence, or was named, his pulse varied, and he
blushed besides."[6]   In this very sort was the love of Charicles,
the son of Polycles, discovered by Panacius the physician, as
you may read the story at large in Aristænetus.[7]   By the same
signs Galen brags that he found out Justa, Boethius the consul's
wife, to dote on Pylades the player, because at his name still
she both altered pulse and countenance, as Poliarchus did at
the name of Argenis.[8]   Franciscus Valesius, *lib. 3, controv. 13,
Med. contr.,* denies there is any such *pulsus amatorius,* or that
love may be so discerned; but Avicenna confirms this of Galen
out of his experience, *lib. 3, fen.* 1; and Gordonius, *cap.* 20;
"Their pulse," he saith, "is inordinate and swift, if she go by
whom he loves";[9] Langius, *epist.* 24, *lib.* 1, *Med. epist.;*

Nevisanus, *lib.* 4, *numer.* 66, *Syl. nuptialis*; Valescus de Taranta;
Guianerius, *tract.* 15. Valleriola sets down this for a symptom:
"Difference of pulse, neglect of business, want of sleep, often
sighs, blushings when there is any speech of their mistress, are
manifest signs."[1] But amongst the rest, Josephus Struthius,
that Polonian, in the fifth book, *cap.* 17, of his Doctrine of
Pulses, holds that this and all other passions of the mind may
be discovered by the pulse. "And if you will know," saith he,
"whether the men suspected be such or such, touch their
arteries,"[2] etc. And in his fourth book, fourteenth chapter,
he speaks of this particular pulse, "Love makes an unequal
pulse,"[3] etc.; he gives instance of a gentlewoman, a patient of
his, whom by this means he found to be much enamoured, and
with whom:[3] he named many persons, but at the last when
his name came whom he suspected, "her pulse began to vary
and to beat swifter, and so, by often feeling her pulse, he perceived what the matter was."[5] Apollonius, *Argonaut. lib.* 4,
poetically setting down the meeting of Jason and Medea, makes
them both to blush at one another's sight, and at the first they
were not able to speak.

> *Totus, Parmeno,*
> *Tremo, horreoque, postquam aspexi hanc.*[6]
>
> [I trembled all over when I beheld her.]

Phædria trembled at the sight of Thais, others sweat, blow
short, *crura tremunt ac poplites* [their legs shake under them],
are troubled with palpitation of heart upon the like occasion,
cor proximum ori, saith Aristænetus,[7] their heart is at their
mouth, leaps, these burn and freeze (for love is fire, ice, hot,
cold, itch, fever, frenzy, pleurisy, what not?), they look pale,
red, and commonly blush at their first congress, and sometimes
through violent agitation of spirits bleed at nose, or when she
is talked of; which very sign Eustathius[8] makes an argument
of Ismene's affection, that when she met her sweetheart by
chance, she changed her countenance to a maiden-blush. 'Tis
a common thing amongst lovers, as Arnulphus,[9] that merry conceited bishop, hath well expressed in a facetious epigram of his:

> *Alterno facies sibi dat responsa rubore,*
> *Et tener affectum prodit utrique pudor,* etc.
>
> Their faces answer, and by blushing say,
> How both affected are, they do betray.

But the best conjectures are taken from such symptoms as
appear when they are both present; all their speeches, amorous

glances, actions, lascivious gestures will bewray them; they cannot contain themselves, but that they will be still kissing. Stratocles, the physician, upon his wedding-day, when he was at dinner, *nihil prius sorbillavit, quam tria basia puellæ pangeret,* could not eat his meat for kissing the bride, etc.[1] First a word, and then a kiss, then some other compliment, and then a kiss, then an idle question, then a kiss, and when he had pumped his wits dry, can say no more, kissing and colling are never out of season, *Hoc non deficit incipitque semper,*[2] 'tis never at an end, another kiss, and then another, another, and another,[3] etc.: *Huc ades, o Thelayra;* "Come, kiss me, Corinna!"

> *Centum basia centies,*
> *Centum basia millies,*
> *Mille basia millies,*
> *Et tot millia millies,*
> *Quot guttæ Siculo mari,*
>   *Quot sunt sidera cœlo,*
> *Istis purpureis genis,*
> *Istis turgidulis labris,*
> *Ocellisque loquaculis,*
> *Figam continuo impetu;*
>   *O formosa Neæra.*[4]

[Ten thousand kisses, a hundred thousand, a thousand thousand, as many thousand thousand as there are drops in the Sicilian Gulf or stars in the heavens, will I impress without pausing on those glowing cheeks, those pouting lips, those prattling eyes of thine, O lovely Neæra.]

As Catullus to Lesbia:

> *Da mihi basia mille, deinde centum,*
> *Dein mille altera, da secunda centum,*
> *Dein usque altera millia, deinde centum.*

> First give an hundred,
> Then a thousand, then another
> Hundred, then unto the other
> Add a thousand, and so more,
> Till you equal with the store
> All the grass, etc.[5]

So Venus did by her Adonis, the Moon with Endymion, they are still dallying and colling, as so many doves, *Columbatimque labra conserentes labiis,* and that with alacrity and courage:

> *Affigunt avide corpus, junguntque salivas*
> *Oris, et inspirant prensantes dentibus ora.*[6]

[Greedily they embrace, mingle the moisture of their lips, and breathe on one another as they clutch with their teeth.

Tam impresso ore ut vix inde labra detrahant, cervice reclinata [1]
[bending back her neck and pressing his mouth so closely that
they could scarce separate their lips, as Lamprias in Lucian
kissed Thais; Philippus her in Aristænetus,[2] *Amore lymphato
tam furiose adhæsit, ut vix labra solvere esset, totumque os mihi
contrivit* [crazy with passion, he fastened his lips on mine with
such fury that he could scarce loosen them, and he made my
mouth all sore]; Aretine's Lucretia by a suitor of hers was so
saluted,[3] and 'tis their ordinary fashion:

> *Dentes illidunt sæpe labellis,*
> *Atque premunt arcte adfigentes oscula.*

[Often the teeth hurt the lips, pressing them tight in
the act of kissing.]

They cannot, I say, contain themselves, they will be still not
only joining hands, kissing, but embracing, treading on their
toes, etc., diving into their bosoms, and that *libenter, et cum
delectatione* [lasciviously and voluptuously], as Philostratus confesseth to his mistress;[4] and Lamprias in Lucian, *mammillas
premens, per sinum clam dextra*, etc., feeling their paps, and that
scarce honestly sometimes: as the old man in the comedy [5]
well observed of his son, *Non ego te videbam manum huic puellæ
in sinum inserere?* "Did not I see thee put thy hand into her
bosom? Go to!" with many such love tricks. Juno in Lucian,
tom. 4, Deorum dial. 6, complains to Jupiter of Ixion, he looked
so attentively on her, and sometimes would sigh and weep in
her company;[6] "and when I drank by chance, and gave Ganymede the cup, he would desire to drink still in the very cup that
I drank of, and in the same place where I drank, and would
kiss the cup, and then look steadily on me, and sometimes sigh,
and then again smile." If it be so they cannot come near to
dally, have not that opportunity, familiarity, or acquaintance
to confer and talk together; yet, if they be in presence, their
eye will bewray them: *Ubi amor ibi oculus* [where I like I look],
as the common saying is, "Where I look I like, and where I
like I love"; but they will lose themselves in her looks.

> *Alter in alterius jactantes lumina vultus,*
> *Quærebant taiti noster ubi esset amor.*

[Eyes looking into eyes asked silently, Where is your love?]

They cannot look off whom they love, they will *impregnare eam
ipsis oculis*, deflower her with their eyes, be still gazing, staring,
stealing faces, smiling, glancing at her, as Apollo on Leuconthoe,[7]

the Moon on her Endymion, when she stood still in Caria, and at Latmos caused her chariot to be stayed.[1] They must all stand and admire, or, if she go by, look after her as long as they can see her; she is *animæ auriga* [the charioteer of their soul], as Anacreon calls her, they cannot go by her door or window but, as an adamant, she draws their eyes to it; though she be not there present, they must needs glance that way, and look back to it.   Aristænetus of Euxitheus,[2] Lucian, in his *Imagines*, of· himself, and Tatius of Clitophon say as much, *Ille oculos de Leucippe nunquam dejiciebat*[3] [he never turned his eyes away from Leucippe], and many lovers confess, when they came in their mistress' presence, they could not hold off their eyes, but looked wistly and steadily on her, *inconnivo aspectu*, with much eagerness and greediness, as if they would look through, or should never have enough sight of her: *Fixis ardens obtutibus hæret* [his eyes clung to her with fixed and burning gaze].   So she will do by him, drink to him with her eyes, nay, drink him up, devour him, swallow him, as Martial's Mamurra is remembered to have done: *Inspexit molles pueros, oculisque comedit* [he looked at the soft-skinned boys, and devoured them with his eyes], etc.   There is a pleasant story to this purpose in *Navigat. Vertom. lib. 3, cap. 5.*   The Sultan of Sana's wife in Arabia, because Vertomannus was fair and white, could not look off him, from sunrising to sunsetting; she could not desist; she made him one day come into her chamber, *et geminæ horæ spatio intuebatur, non a me unquam aciem oculorum avertebat, me observans veluti Cupidinem quendam*, for two hours' space she still gazed on him.   A young man in Lucian [4] fell in love with Venus' picture; he came every morning to her temple, and there continued all day long from sunrising to sunset, unwilling to go home at night; sitting over against the goddess' picture, he did continually look upon her, and mutter to himself I know not what.[5] If so be they cannot see them whom they love, they will still be walking and waiting about their mistress' doors, taking all opportunity to see them; as in Longus Sophista,[6] Daphnis and Chloe, two lovers, were still hovering at one another's gates, he sought all occasions to be in her company, to hunt in summer, and catch birds in the frost about her father's house in the winter, that she might see him, and he her.   "A king's palace was not so diligently attended," saith Aretine's Lucretia, "as my house was when I lay in Rome;[7] the porch and street was ever full of some, walking or riding, on set purpose to see me; their eye was still upon my window; as they

passed by, they could not choose but look back to my house
when they were past, and sometimes hem or cough, or take
some impertinent occasion to speak aloud, that I might look
out and observe them." 'Tis so in other places, 'tis common
to every lover, 'tis all his felicity to be with her, to talk with
her; he is never well but in her company, and will walk "seven
or eight times a day through the street where she dwells, and
make sleeveless errands to see her";[1] plotting still where, when,
and how to visit her,

> *Lenesque sub noctem susurri,*
> *Composita repetuntur hora.*[2]

[Faint whispers are listened for in the dark at the
  trysting hour.]

And when he is gone, he thinks every minute an hour, every
hour as long as a day, ten days a whole year, till he see her
again.

> *Tempora si numeres, bene quæ numeramus amantes.*[3]

[If thou canst count the moments which we lovers count.]

And if thou be in love, thou wilt say so too, *Et longum formosa
vale*, farewell, sweetheart, *vale carissima Argenis*, etc., farewell,
my dear Argenis, once more farewell, farewell. And though
he is to meet her by compact, and that very shortly, perchance
to-morrow, yet loath to depart, he 'll take his leave again and
again, and then come back again, look after, and shake his
hand, wave his hat afar off. Now gone, he thinks it long
till he see her again, and she him, the clocks are surely set
back, the hour 's past.

> *Hospita, Demophoon, tua te Rhodopeia Phyllis*
> *Ultra promissum tempus abesse queror.*[4]

[Beloved Demophoon, thy Thracian Phyllis complains
  that thou tarriest beyond the promised hour.]

She looks out at window still to see whether he come, and by
report Phyllis went nine times to the seaside that day, to see
if her Demophoon were approaching,[5] and Troilus to the city
gates, to look for his Creseid.[6] She is ill at ease, and sick till
she see him again, peevish in the meantime, discontent, heavy,
sad; and why comes he not? where is he? why breaks he
promise? why tarries he so long? sure he is not well; sure he hath
some mischance; sure he forgets himself and me; with infinite
such. And then, confident again, up she gets, out she looks,
listens and inquires, hearkens, kens; every man afar off is sure

he, every stirring in the street, now he is there, that 's he, *male auroræ, male soli dicit, dejeratque*, etc., the longest day that ever was, so she raves, restless and impatient; for *amor non patitur moras*, love brooks no delays: the time 's quickly gone that 's spent in her company, the miles short, the way pleasant; all weather is good whilst he goes to her house, heat or cold; though his teeth chatter in his head, he moves not; wet or dry, 'tis all one; wet to the skin, he feels it not, cares not at least for it, but will easily endure it and much more, because it is done with alacrity, and for his mistress' sweet sake; let the burden be never so heavy, love makes it light. Jacob served seven years for Rachel, and it was quickly gone because he loved her.[1]   None so merry if he may haply enjoy her company, he is in heaven for a time; and if he may not, dejected in an instant, solitary, silent, he departs weeping, lamenting, sighing, complaining.

But the symptoms of the mind in lovers are almost infinite, and so diverse that no art can comprehend them; though they be merry sometimes, and rapt beyond themselves for joy, yet most part, love is a plague, a torture, an hell, a bitter-sweet passion at last; *Amor melle et felle est fecundissimus, gustum dat dulcem et amarum*[2] [love abounds with both honey and gall, it hath both sweet and bitter taste]. 'Tis *suavis amarities, dolentia delectabilis, hilare tormentum* [a sweet bitterness, a delightful grief, a cheerful torment];

> *Et me melle beant suaviora,*
> *Et me felle necant amariora.*[3]

[Its sweetness more than honey doth delight,
Its bitterness doth worse than wormwood spite.]

Like a summer fly or sphinx's wings, or a rainbow of all colours,

> *Quæ ad solis radios conversæ aureæ erant,*
> *Adversus nubes cæruleæ, quale jubar iridis,*

[Which when turned to the sun were golden and when
turned to the clouds dark, like the colours of the
rainbow,]

fair, foul, and full of variation, though most part irksome and bad.   For, in a word, the Spanish Inquisition is not comparable to it; "a torment and execution" it is, as he calls it in the poet,[4] an unquenchable fire, and what not?   "From it," saith Austin, "arise biting cares, perturbations, passions, sorrows, fears, suspicions, discontents, contentions, discords, wars,

treacheries, enmities, flattery, cozening, riot, impudence, cruelty,
knavery," etc.[1]

> *Dolor, querelæ,*
> *Lamentatio, lacrimæ perennes,*
> *Languor, anxietas, amaritudo;*
> *Aut si triste magis potest quid esse,*
> *Hos tu das comites, Neæra, vitæ.*[2]

[Grief, quarrels, laments, perpetual tears, languor,
  anxiety, bitterness, and even worse than these—such,
  Neæra, you make the companions of my life.]

These be the companions of lovers, and the ordinary symptoms,
as the poet repeats them.

> *In amore insunt vitia,*
> *Suspiciones, inimicitiæ, audaciæ,*
> *Bellum, pax rursum,* etc.[3]

> *Insomnia, ærumna, error, terror, et fuga,*
> *Incogitantia, excors immodestia,*
> *Petulantia, cupiditas, et malevolentia;*
> *Inhæret etiam aviditas, desidia, injuria,*
> *Inopia, contumelia, et dispendium,* etc.[4]

In love these vices are: suspicions,
Peace, war, and impudence, detractions,
Dreams, cares, and errors, terrors and affrights,
Immodest pranks, devices, sleights and flights,
Heart-burnings, wants, neglects, desire of wrong,
Loss continual, expense, and hurt among.

Every poet is full of such catalogues of love-symptoms; but
fear and sorrow may justly challenge the chief place. Though
Hercules de Saxonia, *cap.* 3, *Tract. de melanch.*, will exclude
fear from love-melancholy, yet I am otherwise persuaded. *Res*
est solliciti plena timoris amor.[5] 'Tis full of fear, anxiety, doubt,
care, peevishness, suspicion; it turns a man into a woman, which
made Hesiod belike put Fear and Paleness Venus' daughters:

> *Marti clypeos atque arma secanti*
> *Alma Venus peperit Pallorem, unaque Timorem,*

because fear and love are still linked together. Moreover, they
are apt to mistake, amplify, too credulous sometimes, too full
of hope and confidence, and then again very jealous, unapt to
believe or entertain any good news. The comical poet hath
prettily painted out this passage amongst the rest in a dialogue
betwixt Micio and Æschines, a gentle father and a lovesick
son.[6] "*M.* Be of good cheer, my son, thou shalt have her to
wife. *Æ.* Ah, father, do you mock me now? *M.* I mock

thee, why? *Æ.* That which I so earnestly desire, I more suspect and fear. *M.* Get you home, and send for her to be your wife. *Æ.* What now, a wife? now, father," etc. These doubts, anxieties, suspicions are the least part of their torments; they break many times from passions to actions, speak fair, and flatter, now most obsequious and willing, by and by they are averse, wrangle, fight, swear, quarrel, laugh, weep; and he that doth not so by fits, Lucian holds,[1] is not throughly touched with this loadstone of love. So their actions and passions are intermixed, but of all other passions, sorrow hath the greatest share; love to many is bitterness itself;[2] *rem amaram* Plato calls it, a bitter potion, an agony, a plague.

> *Eripite hanc pestem perniciemque mihi;*
> *Quæ mihi subrepens imos ut torpor in artus*
> *Expulit ex omni pectore lætitias.*

> O take away this plague, this mischief from me,
> Which, as a numbness over all my body,
> Expels my joys, and makes my soul so heavy.

Phædria had a true touch of this, when he cried out:

> *O Thais, utinam esset mihi*
> *Pars æqua amoris tecum, ac pariter fieret ut*
> *Aut hoc tibi doleret itidem, ut mihi dolet.*[3]

> O Thais, would thou hadst of these my pains a part,
> Or, as it doth me now, so it would make thee smart.

So had that young man, when she roared again for discontent:

> *Jactor, crucior, agitor, stimulor,*
> *Versor in amoris rota miser,*
> *Exanimor, feror, distrahor, deripior,*
> *Ubi sum, ibi non sum; ubi non sum, ibi est animus.*[4]

> I am vext and toss'd, and rack'd on love's wheel:
> Where not, I am; but where am, do not feel.

The Moon, in Lucian,[5] made her moan to Venus, that she was almost dead for love, *Pereo equidem amore*, and after a long tale, she broke off abruptly and wept: "O Venus, thou knowest my poor heart."[6] Charmides, in Lucian,[7] was so impatient that he sobbed and sighed, and tore his hair, and said he would hang himself: "I am undone, O sister Tryphœna, I cannot endure these love pangs; what shall I do?" *Vos, o dii Averrunci, solvite me his curis!* O ye gods, free me from these cares and miseries! out of the anguish of his soul, Theocles prays.[8] Shall I say, most part of a lover's life is full of agony, anxiety, fear,

and grief, complaints, sighs, suspicions, and cares (heigh-ho,
my heart is wo), full of silence and irksome solitariness?

> Frequenting shady bowers in discontent,
> To the air his fruitless clamours he will vent,

except at such times that he hath *lucida intervalla*, pleasant
gales, or sudden alterations, as if his mistress smile upon him,
give him a good look, a kiss, or that some comfortable message
be brought him, his service is accepted, etc.

He is then too confident and rapt beyond himself, as if he had
heard the nightingale in the spring before the cuckoo, or as
Callisto was at Melibœa's presence,[1] *Quis unquam hac mortali
vita tam gloriosum corpus vidit? humanitatem transcendere videor,*
etc. Who ever saw so glorious a sight, what man ever enjoyed
such delight? More content cannot be given of the gods,
wished, had, or hoped of any mortal man. There is no happiness in the world comparable to his, no content, no joy to this,
no life to love, he is in paradise.

> *Quis me uno vivit felicior? aut magis hac est
>   Optandum vita dicere quis poterit?* [2]

> Who lives so happy as myself? what bliss
> In this our life may be compared to this?

He will not change fortune in that case with a prince:

> *Donec gratus eram tibi,
>   Persarum vigui rege beatior.* [3]

The Persian kings are not so jovial as he is. *O festus dies
hominis!* [4] O happy day! so Chærea exclaims when he came
from Pamphila his sweetheart well pleased:

> *Nunc est profecto interfici cum perpeti me possem,
>   Ne hoc gaudium contaminet vita aliqua ægritudine,*

he could find in his heart to be killed instantly, lest, if he live
longer, some sorrow or sickness should contaminate his joys.
A little after, he was so merrily set upon the same occasion
that he could not contain himself.

> *O populares, ecquis me vivit hodie fortunatior?
> Nemo hercule quisquam; nam in me di plane potestatem suam
> Omnem ostendere;* [5]

"Is 't possible (O my countrymen) for any living to be so happy
as myself? No, sure, it cannot be, for the gods have showed
all their power, all their goodness in me." Yet by and by,

when this young gallant was crossed in his wench, he laments, and cries, and roars downright: *Occidi*, I am undone,

Neque virgo est usquam, neque ego, qui e conspectu illam amisi meo.
Ubi quæram, ubi investigem, quem percuncter, quam insistam viam?

"The virgin's gone, and I am gone, she's gone, she's gone, and what shall I do? where shall I seek her, where shall I find her, whom shall I ask? what way, what course shall I take? what will become of me?" *Vitales auras invitus agebat*,[1] he was weary of his life, sick, mad, and desperate, *Utinam mihi esset aliquid hic, quo nunc me præcipitem darem* [2] [would there were some precipice here down which I might throw myself]. 'Tis not Chæreas' case this alone, but his, and his, and every lover's in the like state. If he hear ill news, have bad success in his suit, she frown upon him, or that his mistress in his presence respect another more (as Hædus observes [3]), "prefer author suitor, speak more familiarly to him, or use more kindly than himself, if by nod, smile, message she discloseth herself to another, he is instantly tormented, none so dejected as he is," utterly undone, a castaway, *in quem fortuna omnia odiorum suorum crudelissima tela exonerat* [4] [on whom Fortune discharges the most cruel missiles of her hate], a dead man, the scorn of fortune, a monster of fortune, worse than naught, the loss of a kingdom had been less. Aretine's Lucretia made very good proof of this, as she relates it herself.[5] "For when I made some of my suitors believe I would betake myself to a nunnery, they took on as if they had lost father and mother, because they were for ever after to want my company." *Omnes labores leves fuere*, all other labour was light: but this might not be endured, *Tui carendum quod erat*,[6] "for I cannot be without thy company," mournful Amyntas, painful Amyntas, careful Amyntas; better a metropolitan city were sacked, a royal army overcome, an invincible armada sunk, and twenty thousand kings should perish, than her little finger ache, so zealous are they, and so tender of her good. "They would all turn friars for my sake," as she follows it, "in hope by that means to meet or see me again, as my confessors, at stool-ball or at barley-break." And so afterwards, when an importunate suitor came, "If I had bid my maid say that I was not at leisure, not within, busy, could not speak with him, he was instantly astonished, and stood like a pillar of marble; another went swearing, chafing, cursing, foaming": [7] *Illa sibi vox ipsa Jovis violentior ira, cum tonat* [8] [that word was more terrible to him than the

wrath of Jupiter when he thunders], etc., the voice of a mandrake had been sweeter music; "but he to whom I gave entertainment was in the Elysian Fields, ravished for joy, quite
beyond himself." 'Tis the general humour of all lovers, she is
their stern, pole-star, and guide: *Deliciumque animi, deliquium-
que sui* [1] [the delight of their soul and their own eclipse]. As a
tulipant to the sun (which our herbalists call narcissus) when
it shines, is *admirandus flos ad radios solis se pandens*, a glorious
flower exposing itself; but when the sun sets, or a tempest
comes, it hides itself, pines away, and hath no pleasure left [2]
(which Carolus Gonzaga, Duke of Mantua, in a cause not unlike,
sometimes used for an impress), do all inamorates to their
mistress; she is their sun, their *primum mobile*, or *anima infor-
mans* [animating soul]; this one [3] hath elegantly expressed by
a windmill, still moved by the wind, which otherwise hath no
motion of itself: *Sic tua ni spiret gratia, truncus ero.* He is
wholly animated from her breath, his soul lives in her body,
sola claves habet interitus et salutis,[4] she keeps the keys of his
life: his fortune ebbs and flows with her favour, a gracious or
bad aspect turns him up or down: *Mens mea lucescit, Lucia,
luce tua.* Howsoever his present state be pleasing or displeasing,
'tis continuate so long as he loves,[5] he can do nothing, think of
nothing but her; desire hath no rest, she is his cynosure, *Hesperus
et Vesper*, his morning and evening star, his goddess, his mistress,
his life, his soul, his everything; dreaming, waking, she is always
in his mouth; his heart, his eyes, ears, and all his thoughts are
full of her. His Laura, his Victorina, his Columbina, Flavia,
Flaminia, Cælia, Delia, or Isabella (call her how you will), she
is the sole object of his senses, the substance of his soul, *nidulus
animæ suæ*, he magnifies her above measure, *totus in illa*, full of
her, can breathe nothing but her. "I adore Melibœa," saith
lovesick Callisto,[6] "I believe in Melibœa, I honour, admire and
love my Melibœa"; his soul was soused, imparadised, imprisoned
in his lady. When Thais took her leave of Phædria,[7] *Mi Phædria,
et nunquid aliud vis?* "Sweetheart" (she said) "will you command
me any further service?" He readily replied, and gave in this
charge:

> *Egone quid velem?*
> *Dies noctesque ames me, me desideres,*
> *Me somnies, me expectes, me cogites,*
> *Me speres, me te oblectes, mecum tota sis,*
> *Meus fac sis postremo animus, quando ego sum tuus.*

> Dost ask (my dear) what service I will have?
> To love me day and night is all I crave,

> To dream on me, to expect, to think on me,
> Depend and hope, still covet me to see,
> Delight thyself in me, be wholly mine,
> For know, my love, that I am wholly thine.

But all this needed not, you will say; if she affect once, she will
be his, settle her love on him, on him alone:

> *Illum absens absentem*
> *Auditque videtque,*[1]

[Though parted, she sees and hears but him,]

she can, she must think and dream of naught else but him,
continually of him, as did Orpheus on his Eurydice:

> *Te dulcis conjux, te solo in littore mecum,*
> *Te veniente die, te discedente canebam.*

> On thee, sweet wife, was all my song.
> Morn, evening, and all along.

And Dido upon her Æneas:

> *Et quæ me insomnia terrent,*
> *Multa viri virtus, et plurima currit imago.*

> And ever and anon she thinks upon the man
> That was so fine, so fair, so blithe, so debonair.

Clitophon, in the first book of Achilles Tatius, complaineth how
that his mistress Leucippe tormented him much more in the
night than in the day.   "For all day long he had some object
or other to distract his senses, but in the night all ran upon
her.   All night long he lay awake, and could think of nothing
else but her,[2] he could not get her out of his mind; towards
morning, sleep took a little pity on him, he slumbered awhile,
but all his dreams were of her." [3]

> *Te nocte sub atra*
> *Alloquor, amplector, falsaque in imagine somni,*
> *Gaudia sollicitam palpant evanida mentem.*[4]

> In the dark night I speak, embrace, and find
> That fading joys deceive my careful mind.

The same complaint Euryalus makes to his Lucretia: "Day
and night I think of thee, I wish for thee, I talk of thee, call
on thee, look for thee, hope for thee, delight myself in thee,
day and night I love thee." [5]

> *Nec mihi vespere*
> *Surgente decedunt amores,*
> *Nec rapidum fugiente solem.*[6]

[My love-thoughts leave me not, nor when the
evening star rises nor when it flees before the sun.]

Morning, evening, all is alike with me, I have restless thoughts. *Te vigilans oculis, animo te nocte requiro*[1] [in waking hours I seek thee with my eyes, at night with my thoughts]. Still I think on thee. *Anima non est ubi animat, sed ubi amat* [the soul is not where it breathes but where it loves]. I live and breathe in thee, I wish for thee.

> *O niveam quæ te poterit mihi reddere lucem!*
> *O mihi felicem terque quaterque diem!* [2]

O happy day that shall restore thee to my sight! In the meantime he raves on her; her sweet face, eyes, actions, gestures, hands, feet, speech, length, breadth, height, depth, and the rest of her dimensions, are so surveyed, measured, and taken by that astrolabe of phantasy, and that so violently sometimes, with such earnestness and eagerness, such continuance, so strong an imagination, that at length he thinks he sees her indeed; he talks with her, he embraceth her, Ixion-like, *pro Junone nubem*, a cloud for Juno, as he said. *Nihil præter Leucippen cerno, Leucippe mihi perpetuo in oculis et animo versatur*, I see and meditate of naught but Leucippe. Be she present or absent, all is one:

> *Et quamvis aberat placidæ præsentia formæ*
> *Quem dederat præsens forma, manebat amor.* [3]

[Though her fair form was no longer present in the flesh, the love which it had inspired remained.]

That impression of her beauty is still fixed in his mind, *hærent infixi pectore vultus* [4] [the image of her face remains fixed in his heart]; as he that is bitten with a mad dog thinks all he sees dogs, dogs in his meat, dogs in his dish, dogs in his drink, his mistress is in his eyes, ears, heart, in all his senses. Valleriola had a merchant, his patient, in the same predicament; and Ulricus Molitor,[5] out of Austin, hath a story of one that through vehemency of his love passion still thought he saw his mistress present with him; she talked with him, *et commisceri cum ea vigilans videbatur*, still embracing him.

Now if this passion of love can produce such effects if it be pleasantly intended, what bitter torments shall it breed when it is with fear and continual sorrow, suspicion, care, agony, as commonly it is, still accompanied! what an intolerable pain must it be! [6]

> *Non tam grandes*
> *Gargara culmos, quot demerso*
> *Pectore curas longa nexas*
> *Usque catena, vel quæ penitus*
> *Crudelis amor vulnera miscet.*

> Mount Gargarus hath not so many stems
> As lover's breast hath grievous wounds,
> And linked cares, which love compounds.

When the King of Babylon would have punished a courtier of his for loving of a young lady of the royal blood and far above his fortunes, Apollonius [1] in presence by all means persuaded to let him alone; "for to love and not enjoy was a most unspeakable torment," no tyrant could invent the like punishment; as a gnat at a candle, in a short space he would consume himself. For love is a perpetual flux, *angor animi* [2] [mental anguish], a warfare, *militat omnis amans* [every lover is in the wars], a grievous wound is love still, and a lover's heart is Cupid's quiver, a consuming fire [3] (*Accede ad hanc, ignem*, etc. [4]), an inextinguishable fire.

> *Alitur et crescit malum,*
> *Et ardet intus, qualis Ætnæo vapor*
> *Exundat antro.* [5]

As Ætna rageth, so doth love, and more than Ætna or any material fire.

> *Nam amor sæpe Liparæo*
> *Vulcano ardentiorem flammam incendere solet.* [6]

Vulcan's flames are but smoke to this. For fire, saith Xenophon, burns them alone that stand near it, or touch it; but this fire of love burneth and scorcheth afar off, [7] and is more hot and vehement than any material fire; *Ignis in igne furit*, [8] 'tis a fire in a fire, the quintessence of fire. For when Nero burnt Rome, as Callisto urgeth, he fired houses, consumed men's bodies and goods; but this fire devours the soul itself, "and one soul is worth an hundred thousand bodies." [9] No water can quench this wild-fire.

> *In pectus cæcos absorbuit ignes,*
> *Ignes qui nec aqua perimi potuere, nec imbre*
> *Diminui, neque graminibus, magicisque susurris.* [10]

> A fire he took into his breast,
> Which water could not quench,
> Nor herb, nor art, nor magic spells
> Could quell, nor any drench,

except it be tears and sighs, for so they may chance find a little ease.

> *Sic candentia colla, sic patens frons,*
> *Sic me blanda tui, Neæra, ocelli,*

Sic pares minio genæ perurunt,
Ut ni me lacrimæ rigent perennes,
Totus in tenues eam favillas.[1]

So thy white neck, Neæra, me poor soul
Doth scorch, thy cheeks, thy wanton eyes that roll:
Were it not for my dropping tears that hinder,
I should be quite burnt up forthwith to cinder.

This fire strikes like lightning, which made those old Grecians
paint Cupid in many of their temples with Jupiter's thunderbolts in his hands; [2] for it wounds, and cannot be perceived how,
whence it came, where it pierced:

Urimur, et cæcum pectora vulnus habent,[3]
[We are aflame, our hearts smitten by an unseen hand,]

and can hardly be discerned at first.

Est mollis flamma medullas,
Et tacitum insano vivit sub pectore vulnus.[4]

A gentle wound, an easy fire it was,
And sly at first, and secretly did pass.

But by and by it began to rage and burn amain:

Pectus insanum vapor,
Amorque torret, intus sævus vorat
Penitus medullas, atque per venas meat
Visceribus ignis mersus, et venis latens,
Ut agilis altas flamma percurrit trabes.[5]

This fiery vapour rageth in the veins,
And scorcheth entrails, as when fire burns
A house, it nimbly runs along the beams,
And at the last the whole it overturns.

Abraham Hoffmannus, *lib.* 1 *Amor. conjugal. cap.* 2, *pag.* 22,
relates out of Plato, how that Empedocles the philosopher was
present at the cutting up of one that died for love, "his heart
was combust, his liver smoky, his lungs dried up, insomuch
that he verily believed his soul was either sod or roasted through
the vehemency of love's fire." [6] Which belike made a modern
writer of amorous emblems express love's fury by a pot hanging
over the fire, and Cupid blowing the coals. As the heat consumes the water, *Sic sua consumit viscera cæcus amor,*[7] so doth
love dry up his radical moisture. Another compares love to
a melting torch, which stood too near the fire.

Sic quo quis propior suæ puellæ est,
Hoc stultus propior suæ ruinæ est. [8]

The nearer he unto his mistress is,
The nearer he unto his ruin is.

So that to say truth, as Castilio describes it,[1] "The beginning, middle, end of love is naught else but sorrow, vexation, agony, torment, irksomeness, wearisomeness; so that to be squalid, ugly, miserable, solitary, discontent, dejected, to wish for death, to complain, rave, and to be peevish, are the certain signs and ordinary actions of a lovesick person." This continual pain and torture makes them forget themselves, if they be far gone with it, in doubt, despair of obtaining, or eagerly bent, to neglect all ordinary business.

> *Pendent opera interrupta, minæque*
> *Murorum ingentes, æquataque machina cœlo.*[2]

[Half finished hang the works, the frowning wall,
The battlements to heaven rising tall.]

Lovesick Dido left her work undone, so did Phædra:[3]

> *Palladis telæ vacant*
> *Et inter ipsas pensa labuntur manus.*

[The distaff is idle, the web drops from her listless hands.]

Faustus, in Mantuan,[4] took no pleasure in anything he did:

> *Nulla quies mihi dulcis erat, nullus labor ægro*
> *Pectore, sensus iners, et mens torpore sepulta,*
> *Carminis occiderat studium.*

[I found no pleasure either in rest or work, my senses
were numb and my mind inert, my love of poetry
faded.]

And 'tis the humour of them all to be careless of their persons and their estates, as the shepherd in Theocritus,[5] *Et hæc barba inculta est, squalidique capilli*, their beards flag, and they have no more care of pranking themselves, or of any business; they care not, as they say, which end goes forward.

> *Oblitusque greges et rura domestica, totus*
> *Uritur, et noctes in luctum expendit amaras.*[6]

Forgetting flocks of sheep and country farms,
The silly shepherd always mourns and burns.

Lovesick Chærea,[7] when he came from Pamphila's house and had not so good welcome as he did expect, was all amort. Parmeno meets him: *Quid tristis es?* "Why art thou so sad, man?" *unde es?* "whence com'st, how dost?" but he sadly replies, *Ego hercle nescio neque unde eam, neque quorsum eam, ita prorsus oblitus sum mei*, "I have so forgotten myself, I

neither know where I am, nor whence I come, nor whether
I will, what I do." *P.* "How so?" *Ch.* "I am in love." [1]

> *Prudens sciens,*
> *Vivus vidensque pereo, nec quid agam scio.* [2]

[Knowingly and wittingly I perish with my eyes open,
and know not what to do.]

"He that erst had his thoughts free" (as Philostratus Lemnius,
in an epistle of his, describes this fiery passion), "and spent his
time like an hard student, in those delightsome philosophical
precepts; he that with the sun and moon wandered all over the
world, with stars themselves ranged about, and left no secret
or small mystery in nature unsearched, since he was enamoured
can do nothing now but think and meditate of love-matters,
day and night composeth himself how to please his mistress; all
his study, endeavour, is to approve himself to his mistress, to win
his mistress' favour, to compass his desire, to be counted her
servant." [3]   When Peter Abelhardus, that great scholar of his
age, *cui soli patuit scibile quicquid erat* [4] [to whom alone was
known whatever is knowable], was now in love with Helonissa,
he had no mind to visit or frequent schools and scholars any
more. *Tædiosum mihi valde fuit* (as he confesseth [5]) *ad scholas
procedere, vel in iis morari* [I had no patience to go to the schools
or to stay there], all his mind was on his new mistress.

Now to this end and purpose, if there be any hope of obtaining
his suit, to prosecute his cause, he will spend himself, goods,
fortunes for her, and though he lose and alienate all his friends,
be threatened, be cast off, and disinherited; for, as the poet
saith, *Amori quis legem det?* [6] [Who can lay down the law to
love?] though he be utterly undone by it, disgraced, go a-begging,
yet for her sweet sake, to enjoy her, he will willingly beg, hazard
all he hath, goods, lands, shame, scandal, fame, and life itself.

> *Non recedam neque quiescam, noctu et interdiu,*
> *Prius profecto quam aut ipsam, aut mortem investigavero.*

> I'll never rest or cease my suit
> Till she or death do make me mute.

Parthenis in Aristænetus [7] was fully resolved to do as much.
"I may have better matches, I confess, but farewell shame,
farewell honour, farewell honesty, farewell friends and fortunes,
etc. O Harpedona, keep my counsel, I will leave all for his
sweet sake, I will have him, say no more, *contra gentes* [in the
teeth of all the world], I am resolved, I will have him." Gobryas [8]

the captain, when he had espied Rhodanthe, the fair captive maid, fell upon his knees before Mystylus the general, with tears, vows, and all the rhetoric he could, by the scars he had formerly received, the good service he had done, or whatsoever else was dear unto him, besought his governor he might have the captive virgin to be his wife, *virtutis suæ spolium*, as a reward of his worth and service; and moreover, he would forgive him the money which was owing, and all reckonings besides due unto him, "I ask no more, no part of booty, no portion, but Rhodanthe to be my wife." And whenas he could not compass her by fair means, he fell to treachery, force and villainy, and set his life at stake at last to accomplish his desire. 'Tis a common humour this, a general passion of all lovers to be so affected, and which Æmilia told Aretine, a courtier in Castilio's discourse: "Surely, Aretine, if thou werst not so indeed, thou didst not love; ingenuously confess, for if thou hadst been throughly enamoured, thou wouldst have desired nothing more than to please thy mistress. For that is the law of love, to will and nill the same." [1] *Tantum velle et nolle, velit nolit quod amica.* [2]

Undoubtedly this may be pronounced of them all, they are very slaves, drudges for the time, madmen, fools, dizzards, *atrabilarii,* [3] beside themselves, and as blind as beetles. Their dotage is most eminent, [4] *Amare simul et sapere ipsi Jovi non datur,* as Seneca holds, Jupiter himself cannot love and be wise both together; the very best of them, if once they be overtaken with this passion, the most staid, discreet, grave, generous and wise, otherwise able to govern themselves, in this commit many absurdities, many indecorums, unbefitting their gravity and persons.

> *Quisquis amat servit, sequitur captivus amantem,*
> *Fert domita cervice jugum.* [5]

> [Whoso loves is in bondage, he follows his lady-love
> like a thrall, and bears the yoke with bowed neck.]

Samson, David, Solomon, Hercules, Socrates, etc., are justly taxed of indiscretion in this point; the middle sort are betwixt hawk and buzzard; [6] and although they do perceive and acknowledge their own dotage, weakness, fury, yet they cannot withstand it; as well may witness those expostulations and confessions of Dido in Virgil:

> *Incipit effari mediaque in voce resistit.* [7]

> [She made as if to speak, but stopped with word half
> uttered.]

Phædra in Seneca:

> *Quod ratio poscit, vincit ac regnat furor,*
> *Potensque tota mente dominatur deus.*[1]

[The claims of reason are overborne by passion, and
   the God of Love completely sways her mind.]

Myrrha in Ovid:[2]

> *Illa quidem sentit, fœdoque repugnat amori,*
> *Et secum "Quo mente feror, quid molior," inquit,*
> *"Di, precor, et pietas,"* etc.

She sees and knows her fault, and doth resist,
   Against her filthy lust she doth contend,
And "Whither go I, what am I about?"
   And "God forbid!" yet doth it in the end.

Again:

> *Pervigil igni*
> *Carpitur indomito, furiosaque vota retractat,*
> *Et modo desperat, modo vult tentare, pudetque*
> *Et cupit, et quid agat, non invenit,* etc.

With raging lust she burns, and now recalls
Her vow, and then despairs, and when 'tis past,
Her former thoughts she 'll prosecute in haste,
And what to do she knows not at the last.

She will and will not, abhors; and yet as Medea did, doth it:

> *Trahit invitam nova vis, aliudque cupido,*
> *Mens aliud suadet; video meliora, proboque,*
> *Deteriora sequor.*

Reason pulls one way, burning lust another,
She sees and knows what 's good, but she doth neither.

> *O fraus, amorque, et mentis emotæ furor,*
> *Quo me abstulistis?*[3]

[Deceitful love and headstrong passion, whither have
   ye led me?]

The major part of lovers are carried headlong like so many
brute beasts; reason counsels one way, thy friends, fortunes,
shame, disgrace, danger, and an ocean of cares that will certainly
follow; yet this furious lust precipitates, counterpoiseth, weighs
down on the other; though it be their utter undoing, perpetual
infamy, loss, yet they will do it, and become at last *insensati*,
void of sense; degenerate into dogs, hogs, asses, brutes; as
Jupiter into a bull, Apuleius an ass, Lycaon a wolf, Tereus a
lapwing, Callisto a bear,[4] Elpenor and Gryllus into swine by
Circe. For what else may we think those ingenious poets to

have shadowed in their witty fictions and poems, but that a
man once given over to his lust (as Fulgentius interprets that of
Apuleius,[1] Alciat of Tereus) is no better than a beast.

> *Rex fueram, sic crista docet, sed sordida vita*
> *Immundam e tanto culmine fecit avem.*[2]

> I was a king, my crown my witness is,
> But by my filthiness am come to this.

Their blindness is all out as great, as manifest as their weakness
and dotage, or rather an inseparable companion, an ordinary
sign of it.   Love is blind,[3] as the saying is, Cupid 's blind, and
so are all his followers. *Quisquis amat ranam, ranam putat*
esse Dianam [whoso loves a frog, thinks that frog a Dian].
Every lover admires his mistress, though she be very deformed
of herself, ill-favoured, wrinkled, pimpled, pale, red, yellow,
tanned, tallow-faced, have a swollen juggler's platter face, or
a thin, lean, chitty face, have clouds in her face, be crooked,
dry, bald, goggle-eyed, blear-eyed, or with staring eyes, she
looks like a squis'd cat, hold her head still awry, heavy, dull,
hollow-eyed, black or yellow about the eyes, or squint-eyed,
sparrow-mouthed, Persian hook-nosed, have a sharp fox-nose,
a red nose, China flat, great nose, *nare simo patuloque* [snub
and flat nose], a nose like a promontory, gubber-tushed, rotten
teeth, black, uneven, brown teeth, beetle-browed, a witch's
beard, her breath stink all over the room, her nose drop winter
and summer, with a Bavarian poke under her chin, a sharp
chin, lave-eared, with a long crane's neck, which stands awry
too, *pendulis mammis,* "her dugs like two double jugs," or else
no dugs, in that other extreme, bloody-fallen fingers, she have
filthy, long unpared nails, scabbed hands or wrists, a tanned
skin, a rotten carcass, crooked back, she stoops, is lame, splay-
footed, "as slender in the middle as a cow in the waist," gouty
legs, her ankles hang over her shoes, her feet stink, she breed
lice, a mere changeling, a very monster, an oaf imperfect, her
whole complexion savours, an harsh voice, incondite gesture,
vile gait, a vast virago, or an ugly tit, a slug, a fat fustilugs, a
truss, a long lean rawbone, a skeleton, a sneaker (*si qua latent*
meliora puta [think that what is not seen is better]), and to thy
judgment looks like a mard in a lanthorn, whom thou couldst
not fancy for a world, but hatest, loathest, and wouldest have
spit in her face, or blow thy nose in her bosom, *remedium*
amoris [a cure for love] to another man, a dowdy, a slut, a
scold, a nasty, rank, rammy, filthy, beastly quean, dishonest

peradventure, obscene, base, beggarly, rude, foolish, untaught,
peevish, Irus' daughter, Thersites' sister, Grobian's scholar; if
he love her once, he admires her for all this, he takes no notice
of any such errors or imperfections of body or mind,

Ipsa hæc
Delectant, veluti Balbinum polypus Agnæ; [1]

[These very things charm him, as Agna's polypus did
 Balbinus;]

he had rather have her than any woman in the world. If he
were a king, she alone should be his queen, his empress. O that
he had but the wealth and treasure of both the Indies to endow
her with, a carrack of diamonds, a chain of pearl, a carcanet of
jewels (a pair of calf-skin gloves of fourpence a pair were fitter),
or some such toy, to send her for a token, she should have it
with all his heart; he would spend myriads of crowns for her
sake. Venus herself, Panthea, Cleopatra, Tarquin's Tanaquil,
Herod's Mariamne, or Mary of Burgundy,[2] if she were alive,
would not match her.

(*Vincit vultus hæc Tyndaridos,*
Qui moverunt horrida bella,[3]

[Her beauty surpasseth Helen's, which caused a
 mighty war,]

let Paris himself be judge), renowned Helen comes short, that
Rhodopeian Phyllis, Larissæan Coronis, Babylonian Thisbe,
Polyxena, Laura, Lesbia, etc., your counterfeit ladies were
never so fair as she is.

Quicquid erit placidi, lepidi, grati, atque faceti,
Vivida cunctorum retines Pandora deorum.[4]

Whate'er is pretty, pleasant, facete, well,
Whate'er Pandora had, she doth excel.

Dicebam Triviæ formam nihil esse Dianæ,[5] Diana was not to be
compared to her, nor Juno, nor Minerva, nor any goddess.
Thetis' feet were as bright as silver, the ankles of Hebe clearer
than crystal, the arms of Aurora as ruddy as the rose, Juno's
breasts as white as snow, Minerva wise, Venus fair; but what of
this? Dainty, come thou to me. She is all in all:

Cælia ridens
Est Venus, incedens Juno, Minerva loquens.[6]

[Cælia is Venus laughing, Juno walking, Minerva speaking.]

Fairest of fair, that fairness doth excel.[9]

Euemerus, in Aristænetus, so far admireth his mistress' good parts that he makes proclamation of them, and challengeth all comers in her behalf. "Who ever saw the beauties of the East, or of the West, let them come from all quarters, all, and tell truth, if ever they saw such an excellent feature as this is." [1] A good fellow in Petronius cries out, no tongue can tell his lady's fine feature, or express it.[2] *Quicquid dixeris minus erit*, etc.

> No tongue can her perfections tell,
> In whose each part all tongues may dwell.

Most of your lovers are of his humour and opinion. She is *nulli secunda* [second to none], a rare creature, a phœnix, the sole commandress of his thoughts, queen of his desires, his only delight: as Triton now feelingly sings,[3] that lovesick sea-god:

> *Candida Leucothoe placet, et placet atra Melæne,*
> *Sed Galatea placet longe magis omnibus una.*

> Fair Leucothe, black Melæne please me well,
> Bat Galatea doth by odds the rest excel.

All the gracious elogies, metaphors, hyperbolical comparisons of the best things in the world, the most glorious names; whatsoever, I say, is pleasant, amiable, sweet, grateful, and delicious, are too little for her.

> *Phœbo pulchrior et sorore Phœbi.*

> His Phœbe is so fair, she is so bright,
> She dims the sun's lustre, and the moon's light.

Stars, sun, moons, metals, sweet-smelling flowers, odours, perfumes, colours, gold, silver, ivory, pearls, precious stones, snow, painted birds, doves, honey, sugar, spice, cannot express her, so soft, so tender, so radiant, sweet, so fair is she.[4] *Mollior cuniculi capillo* [softer than a rabbit's fur], etc.

> *Lydia bella, puella candida,*
> *Quæ bene superas lac, et lilium,*
> *Albamque simul rosam et rubicundam,*
> *Et expolitum obur Indicum.*[5]

> Fine Lydia, my mistress, white and fair,
> The milk, the lily do not thee come near;
> The rose so white, the rose so red to see,
> And Indian ivory comes short of thee.

Such a description our English Homer makes of a fair lady:

> That Emilia that was fairer to seen,
> Than is lily upon the stalk green:
> And fresher than May with flowers new,
> For with the rose colour strove her hue,
> I no't which was the fairer of the two.[6]

In this very phrase Polyphemus courts Galatea: [1]

> *Candidior folio nivei Galatea ligustri,*
> *Floridior prato, longa procerior alno,*
> *Splendidior vitro, tenero lascivior hædo,* etc.
> *Mollior et cygni plumis, et lacte coacto.*

> Whiter Galet than the white withy-wind,
> Fresher than a field, higher than a tree,
> Brighter than glass, more wanton than a kid,
> Softer than swan's down, or aught that may be.

So she admires him again, in that conceited dialogue of Lucian, which John Secundus, an elegant Dutch modern poet, hath translated into verse.   When Doris and those other sea-nymphs upbraided her with her ugly misshapen lover Polyphemus, she replies, they speak out of envy and malice,

> *Et plane invidia huc mera vos stimulare videtur,*
> *Quod non vos itidem ut me Polyphemus amet.*

> [Plainly 'tis envy that prompts you to this, since
> Polyphemus loves you not as he loves me.]

Say what they could, he was a proper man.   And as Helonissa writ to her sweetheart Peter Abelhardus, *Si me Augustus orbis imperator uxorem expeteret, mallem tua esse meretrix quam orbis imperatrix;* she had rather be his vassal, his quean, than the world's empress or queen; *non si me Jupiter ipse forte velit,* she would not change her love for Jupiter himself.

To thy thinking she is a most loathsome creature; and as when a country fellow discommended once that exquisite picture of Helen, made by Zeuxis, for he saw no such beauty in it,[2] Nichomachus, a lovesick spectator, replied, *Sume tibi meos oculos et deam existimabis,* take mine eyes, and thou wilt think she is a goddess, dote on her forthwith, count all her vices virtues, her imperfections infirmities, absolute and perfect: if she be flat-nosed, she is lovely; if hook-nosed, kingly; if dwarfish and little, pretty; if tall, proper and man-like, our brave British Bunduica; if crooked, wise; if monstrous, comely; her defects are no defects at all, she hath no deformities. *Immo nec ipsum amicæ stercus fœtet,* though she be nasty, fulsome, as Sostratus' bitch, or Parmeno's sow; thou hadst as lieve have a snake in thy bosom, a toad in thy dish, and callest her witch, devil, hag, with all the filthy names thou canst invent; he admires her on the other side, she is his idol, lady, mistress, *Venerilla* [3] [little Venus], queen, the quintessence of beauty, an angel, a star, a goddess.

> Thou art my Vesta, thou my goddess art,
> Thy hallowed temple only is my heart.[1]

The fragrancy of a thousand courtesans is in her face: *Nec pulchræ effigies hæc Cypridis aut Stratonices*, 'tis not Venus' picture that, nor the Spanish infanta's, as you suppose (good sir), no princess, or king's daughter; no, no, but his divine mistress forsooth, his dainty Dulcinea, his dear Antiphila, to whose service he is wholly consecrate, whom he alone adores,

> *Cui comparatus indecens erit pavo,*
> *Inamabilis sciurus, et frequens phœnix.*[2]

> To whom conferr'd a peacock's undecent,
> A squirrel's harsh, a phœnix too frequent.

All the Graces, veneries, elegancies, pleasures, attend her.   He prefers her before a myriad of court ladies.

> He that commends Phyllis or Neæra,
> Or Amaryllis, or Galatea,
> Tityrus or Melibœa, by your leave,
> Let him be mute, his love the praises have.[3]

Nay, before all the gods and goddesses themselves.   So Quintus Catulus admired his squint-eyed friend Roscius; [4]

> *Pace mihi liceat (cœlestes) dicere vestra,*
> *Mortalis visus pulchrior esse Deo.*

> By your leave, gentle gods, this I 'll say true,
> There 's none of you that have so fair a hue.

All the bombast epithets, pathetical adjuncts, incomparably fair, curiously neat, divine, sweet, dainty, delicious, etc., pretty diminutives, *corculum, suaviolum* [little heart, little kiss], etc., pleasant names may be invented, bird, mouse, lamb, puss, pigeon, pigsney, kid, honey, love, dove, chicken, etc., he puts on her:

> *Meum mel, mea suavitas, meum cor,*
> *Meum suaviolum, mei lepores,*[5]

> [My honey, my sweetest, my heart, my kiss-cuddle,
> my darling,]

my life, my light, my jewel, my glory, *Margarita speciosa, cujus respectu omnia mundi pretiosa sordent,*[6] my sweet Margaret, my sole delight and darling.   And as Rhodomant courted Isabella: [7]

> By all kind words and gestures that he might,
> He calls her his dear heart, his sole beloved,
> His joyful comfort, and his sweet delight.
> His mistress, and his goddess, and such names,
> As loving knights apply to lovely dames.

Every cloth she wears, every fashion pleaseth him above measure; her hand, *O quales digitos, quos habet illa manus!* [what fingers, what hands are hers!], pretty foot, pretty coronets, her sweet carriage, sweet voice, tone, O that pretty tone, her divine and lovely looks, her everything, lovely, sweet, amiable, and pretty, pretty, pretty! Her very name (let it be what it will) is a most pretty, pleasing name; I believe now there is some secret power and virtue in names; every action, sight, habit, gesture he admires, whether she play, sing, or dance, in what tires soever she goeth, how excellent it was! how well it became her! never the like seen or heard. *Mille habet ornatus, mille decenter habet* [1] [a thousand ornaments she hath, and all become her]. Let her wear what she will, do what she will, say what she will, *Quicquid enim dicit, seu facit, omne decet,* [2] he applauds and admires everything she wears, saith or doth.

> *Illam, quicquid agit, quoquo vestigia vertit,*
>   *Composuit furtim subsequiturque decor;*
> *Seu solvit crines, fusis decet esse capillis,*
>   *Seu compsit, comptis est reverenda comis.* [3]

> Whate'er she doth, or whither e'er she go,
>   A sweet and pleasing grace attends forsooth;
> Or loose, or bind her hair, or comb it up,
>   She 's to be honoured in what she doth.

Vestem induitur, formosa est; exuitur, tota forma est: [4] let her be dressed or undressed, all is one, she is excellent still, beautiful, fair, and lovely to behold. Women do as much by men; nay more, far fonder, weaker, and that by many parasangs. "Come to me, my dear Lysias" (saith Musarium in Aristænetus [5]), "come quickly, sweetheart, all other men are satyrs, mere clowns, blockheads to thee, nobody to thee; thy looks, words, gestures, actions, etc., are incomparably beyond all others." Venus was never so much besotted on her Adonis, Phædra so delighted in Hippolytus, Ariadne in Theseus, Thisbe in her Pyramus, as she is enamoured on her Mopsus.

> Be thou the marigold, and I will be the sun,
> Be thou the friar, and I will be the nun.

I could repeat centuries of such. Now tell me what greater dotage or blindness can there be than this in both sexes? and yet their slavery is more eminent, a greater sign of their folly than the rest.

They are commonly slaves, captives, voluntary servants, *amator amicæ mancipium,* as Castilio terms him, [6] his mistress' servant, her drudge, prisoner, bondman, what not? "He composeth himself wholly to her affections to please her, and, as Æmilia said, makes himself her lackey. All his cares, actions, all his thoughts, are subordinate to her will and commandment"; her most devote, obsequious, affectionate servant and vassal. "For love" (as Cyrus in Xenophon well observed [1]) "is a mere tyranny, worse than any disease, and they that are troubled with it desire to be free and cannot, but are harder bound than if they were in iron chains." What greater captivity or slavery can there be (as Tully expostulates [2]) than to be in love? "Is he a free man over whom a woman domineers, to whom she prescribes laws, commands, forbids what she will herself? that dares deny nothing she demands? she asks, he gives; she calls, he comes; she threatens, he fears; *nequissimum hunc servum puto*, I account this man a very drudge." And as he follows it, "Is this no small servitude for an enamorate to be every hour combing his head, stiffening his beard, perfuming his hair, washing his face with sweet waters, painting, curling, and not to come abroad but sprucely crowned, decked, and apparelled?" [3] Yet these are but toys in respect, to go to the barber, baths, theatres, etc., he must attend upon her wherever she goes, run along the streets by her doors and windows to see her, take all opportunities, sleeveless errands, disguise, counterfeit shapes, and as many forms as Jupiter himself ever took; and come every day to her house (as he will surely do if he be truly enamoured) and offer her service, and follow her up and down from room to room, as Lucretia's suitors did, he cannot contain himself but he will do it, he must and will be where she is, sit next her, still talking with her. "If I did but let my glove fall by chance" (as the said Arctine's Lucretia brags), "I had one of my suitors, nay, two or three at once, ready to stoop and take it up, and kiss it, and with a low congee deliver it unto me; if I would walk, another was ready to sustain me by the arm; a third to provide fruits, pears, plums, cherries, or whatsoever I would eat or drink." [4] All this and much more he doth in her presence, and when he comes home, as Troilus on his Creseid, 'tis all his meditation to recount with himself his actions, words, gestures, what entertainment he had, how kindly she used him in such a place, how she smiled, how she graced him, and that infinitely pleased him; and then he breaks out, "O sweet Areusa, O my dearest Antiphila, O most divine looks, O lovely graces!" and thereupon instantly he makes an epigram, or a sonnet to five or seven tunes, in her commendation,

or else he ruminates how she rejected his service, denied him a
kiss, disgraced him, etc., and that as effectually torments him.
And these are his exercises betwixt comb and glass, madrigals,
elegies, etc., these his cogitations till he see her again.   But all
this is easy and gentle, and the least part of his labour and
bondage; no hunter will take such pains for his game, fowler
for his sport, or soldier to sack a city, as he will for his mistress'
favour.

> *Ipsa comes veniam, neque me salebrosa movebunt*
> *Saxa, nec obliquo dente timendus aper;*

> [I shall myself be thy comrade, nor shall the rude rocks
> daunt me nor the boar with savage tusk;]

as Phædra to Hippolytus.   No danger shall affright, for if that
be true the poets feign, Love is the son of Mars and Venus; as
he hath delights, pleasures, elegancies from his mother, so hath
he hardness, valour, and boldness from his father.   And 'tis
true that Bernard hath: *Amore nihil mollius, nihil violentius,*
nothing so boisterous, nothing so tender as love.   If once
therefore enamoured, he will go, run, ride many a mile to meet
her, day and night, in a very dark night, endure scorching heat,
cold, wait in frost and snow, rain, tempests, till his teeth chatter
in his head, those northern winds and showers cannot cool or
quench his flames of love.   *Intempesta nocte non deterretur* [the
dangers of the night will not deter him], he will, take my word,
he will sustain hunger, thirst, *penetrabit omnia, perrumpet omnia,*
"love will find out a way," through thick and thin he will to
her, *expeditissimi montes videntur amnes tranabiles* [mountains
will seem easy to cross, rivers to swim], he will swim through
an ocean, ride post over the Alps, Apennines, or Pyrenean hills,

> *Ignem marisque fluctus, atque turbines*
> *Venti paratus est transire,*[1]

> [He is ready to go through fire and water, wind and
> storm,]

though it rain daggers with their points downward, light or dark,
all is one (*Roscida per tenebras Faunus ad antra venit* [Faunus
cometh through the darkness to the dewy caves]); for her sweet
sake he will undertake Hercules' twelve labours, endure, hazard,
etc., he feels it not.   "What shall I say," saith Hædus,[2] "of
their great dangers they undergo, single combats they undertake, how they will venture their lives, creep in at windows,
gutters, climb over walls to come to their sweethearts" (anointing

the doors and hinges with oil, because they should not creak, tread soft, swim, wade, watch, etc.), "and if they be surprised, leap out at windows, cast themselves headlong down, bruising or breaking their legs or arms, and sometimes losing life itself," as Callisto did for his lovely Melibœa. Hear some of their own confessions, protestations, complaints, proffers, expostulations, wishes, brutish attempts, labours in this kind. Hercules served Omphale, put on an apron, took a distaff and spun; Thraso the soldier was so submissive to Thais that he was resolved to do whatever she enjoined. *Ego me Thaidi dedam, et faciam quod jubet*,[1] I am at her service. Philostratus, in an epistle to his mistress: "I am ready to die, sweetheart, if it be thy will; allay his thirst whom thy star hath scorched and undone; the fountains and rivers deny no man drink that comes; the fountain doth not say, Thou shalt not drink; nor the apple, Thou shalt not eat; nor the fair meadow, Walk not in me; but thou alone wilt not let me come near thee or see thee; contemned and despised, I die for grief." [2] Polyænus, when his mistress Circe did but frown upon him in Petronius, drew his sword, and bade her kill, stab, or whip him to death, he would strip himself naked, and not resist.[3] Another will take a journey to Japan, *longæ navigationis molestis non curans* [recking nothing of the hardships of a long voyage]; a third (if she say it) will not speak a word for a twelvemonth's space, her command shall be most inviolably kept; a fourth will take Hercules' club from him, and with that centurion in the Spanish *Cælestina*,[4] will kill ten men for his mistress Areusa, for a word of her mouth, he will cut bucklers in two like pippins, and flap down men like flies, *Elige quo mortis genere illum occidi cupis* [choose by what method you wish him to be killed]. Galeatus of Mantua [5] did a little more; for when he was almost mad for love of a fair maid in the city, she, to try him, belike, what he would do for her sake, bade him in jest leap into the river Po if he loved her; he forthwith did leap headlong off the bridge and was drowned. Another at Ficinum in like passion, when his mistress by chance (thinking no harm, I dare swear) bade him go hang, the next night at her doors hanged himself. "Money" (saith Xenophon) "is a very acceptable and welcome guest, yet I had rather give it my dear Clinias than take it of others, I had rather serve him than command others, I had rather be his drudge than take my ease, undergo any danger for his sake than live in security. For I had rather see Clinias than all the world besides, and had rather want the sight of

all other things than him alone; I am angry with the night and
sleep that I may not see him, and thank the light and sun
because they show me my Clinias; I will run into the fire for
his sake, and if you did but see him, I know that you likewise
would run with me." [1] So Philostratus to his mistress: "Command me what you will, I will do it; bid me go to sea, I am gone
in an instant; take so many stripes, I am ready; run through
the fire, and lay down my life and soul at thy feet, 'tis done." [2]
So did Æolus to Juno:

> *Tuus, o regina, quod optas*
> *Explorare labor, mihi jussa capessere fas est.*

> O queen, it is thy pains to enjoin me still,
> And I am bound to execute thy will.

And Phædra to Hippolytus:

> *Me vel sororem, Hippolyte, aut famulam voca,*
> *Famulamque potius, omne servitium feram.*

> O call me sister, call me servant, choose,
> Or rather servant, I am thine to use.

> *Non me per altas ire si jubeas nives,*
> *Pigeat gelatis ingredi Pindi jugis,*
> *Non si per ignes ire aut infesta agmina*
> *Cuncter, paratus ensibus pectus dare,* [3]
> *Te tunc jubere, me decet jussa exsequi.* [4]

> It shall not grieve me to the snowy hills,
> Or frozen Pindus' tops forthwith to climb,
> Or run through fire, or through an army,
> Say but the word, for I am always thine.

Callicratides, in Lucian, [5] breaks out into this passionate speech:
"O God of Heaven, grant me this life for ever to sit over against
my mistress, and to hear her sweet voice, to go in and out with
her, to have every other business common with her; I would
labour when she labours, sail when she sails; he that hates her
should hate me; and if a tyrant kill her, he should kill me; if
she should die, I would not live, and one grave should hold us
both." *Finiet illa meos moriens morientis amores* [6] [her death
shall end my love in death]. Abrocomas in Aristænetus makes
the like petition for his Delphis. [7] *Tecum vivere amem, tecum
obeam lubens* [8] [Gladly I 'd live with thee, or gladly die]. 'Tis
the same strain which Theagenes used to his Chariclea: "So
that I may but enjoy thy love, let me die presently"; Leander
to his Hero, when he besought the sea waves to let him go

quietly to his love, and kill him coming back: *Parcite dum propero, mergite dum redeo* [1] [Spare me whilst I go, drown me as I return].   'Tis the common humour of them all, to contemn death, to wish for death, to confront death in this case; "*Quippe queis nec fera, nec ignis, neque præcipitium, nec fretum, nec ensis, neque laqueus gravia videntur* [neither wild beasts nor fire nor precipice nor sea nor sword nor noose has any terrors for them], 'tis their desire" (saith Tyrius) "to die."

> *Haud timet mortem, cupit ire in ipsos*
> *Obvius enses.*

> [He does not fear death, he desires to run upon the very swords.]

Though a thousand dragons or devils kept the gates, Cerberus himself, Sciron and Procrustes lay in wait, and the way as dangerous, as inaccessible as hell, through fiery flames and over burning coulters, he will adventure for all this.   And as Peter Abelhardus lost his testicles for his Helonissa,[2] he will (I say) not venture an incision, but life itself.   For how many gallants offered to lose their lives for a night's lodging with Cleopatra in those days!   And in the hour or moment of death, 'tis their sole comfort to remember their dear mistress, as Zerbino slain in France, and Brandimart in Barbary;[3] as Arcite did his Emily:

> When he felt death,
> Dusked been his eyes, and faded is his breath,
> But on his lady yet casteth he his eye,
> His last word was, Mercy Emely,
> His spirit chang'd, and out went there,
> Whither I cannot tell, ne where.[4]

When Captain Gobrias [5] by an unlucky accident had received his death's wound, *Heu me miserum! exclamat*, "Miserable man that I am!" (instead of other devotions), he cries out, "shall I die before I see Rhodanthe my sweetheart?" *Sic amor mortem* (saith mine author), *aut quicquid humanitus accidit, aspernatur*, so love triumphs, contemns, insults over death itself.   Thirteen proper young men lost their lives for that fair Hippodamia's sake, the daughter of Œnomaus, King of Elis: when that hard condition was proposed of death or victory, they made no account of it, but courageously for love died, till Pelops at last won her by a sleight.   As many gallants desperately adventured their dearest blood for Atalanta, the daughter of Schœneus, in hope of marriage, all vanquished and

overcame, till Hippomenes by a few golden apples happily
obtained his suit.[1] Perseus of old fought with a sea-monster
for Andromeda's sake; and our St. George freed the king's
daughter of Sabea (the Golden Legend is mine author) that
was exposed to a dragon, by a terrible combat. Our knights
errant, and the Sir Lancelots of these days, I hope will adventure as much for ladies' favours, as the Squire of Dames, Knight
of the Sun, Sir Bevis of Southampton, or that renowned
peer,

> Orlando, who long time had loved dear
> Angelica the fair, and for her sake
> About the world in nations far and near,
> Did high attempts perform and undertake; [2]

he is a very dastard, a coward, a block and a beast, that will
not do as much, but they will sure, they will; for it is an ordinary
thing for these inamoratos of our time to say and do more, to
stab their arms, carouse in blood, or as that Thessalian Thero,
that bit off his own thumb, *provocans rivalem ad hoc æmulandum*,
to make his corrival do as much.[3] 'Tis frequent with them to
challenge the field for their lady and mistress' sake, to run a tilt,

> That either bears (so furiously they meet)
> The other down under the horses' feet,[4]

and then up and to it again,

> And with their axes both so sorely pour,
> That neither plate nor mail sustain'd the stour,
> But rivell'd wreak like rotten wood asunder,
> And fire did flash like lightning after thunder;

and in her quarrel, to fight so long "till their head-piece, bucklers
be all broken, and swords hacked like so many saws," [5] for they
must not see her abused in any sort, 'tis blasphemy to speak
against her, a dishonour without all good respect to name her.
'Tis common with these creatures, to drink healths upon their
bare knees, though it were a mile to the bottom (no matter of
what mixture), off it comes.[6] If she bid them they will go
barefoot to Jerusalem, to the Great Cham's court, to the East
Indies,[7] to fetch her a bird to wear in her hat: and with Drake
and Candish sail round about the world for her sweet sake,
adversis ventis [in the teeth of the wind]; serve twice seven
years as Jacob did for Rachel; do as much as Gismunda, the
daughter of Tancredus, Prince of Salerna, did for Guiscardus,
her true love, eat his heart when he died; [8] or as Artemisia

drank her husband's bones beaten to powder, and so bury him
in herself, and endure more torments than Theseus or Paris.
Et his colitur Venus magis quam thure et victimis, with such
sacrifices as these (as Aristænetus holds [1]) Venus is well pleased.
Generally they undertake any pain, any labour, any toil, for
their mistress' sake, love and admire a servant, not to her
alone, but to all her friends and followers, they hug and embrace
them for her sake; her dog, picture, and everything she wears,
they adore it as a relic. If any man come from her, they
feast him, reward him, will not be out of his company, do him
all offices, still remembering, still talking of her:

> *Nam si abest quod aves, præsto simulacra tamen sunt*
> *Illius, et nomen dulce obversatur ad aures.* [2]

> [For though the object of your love be absent, yet
> her image is with you, and her sweet name rings in
> your ears.]

The very carrier that comes from him to her is a most welcome
guest; and if he bring a letter, she will read it twenty times
over, and as Lucretia did by Euryalus, "kiss the letter a thousand
times together, and then read it"; [3] and [as] Chelidonia by
Philonius, after many sweet kisses, put the letter in her bosom, [4]

> And kiss again, and often look thereon,
> And stay the messenger that would be gone,

and ask many pretty questions, over and over again, as how
he looked, what he did, and what he said? In a word,

> *Vult placere sese amicæ, vult mihi, vult pedissequæ,*
> *Vult famulis, vult etiam ancillis, et catulo meo.* [5]

> He strives to please his mistress, and her maid,
> Her servants, and her dog, and 's well apaid.

If he get any remnant of hers, a busk-point, a feather of her
fan, a shoe-tie, a lace, a ring, a bracelet of hair,

> *Pignusque direptum lacertis,*
> *Aut digito male pertinaci,* [6]

> [A token snatched from her arms or from her archly
> resisting finger,]

he wears it for a favour on his arm, in his hat, finger, or next
his heart. Her picture he adores twice a day, and for two
hours together will not look off it; as Laodamia did by Protesilaus, when he went to war, "sit at home with his picture before

her"; [1] a garter or a bracelet of hers is more precious than any
saint's relic, he lays it up in his casket (O blessed relic!), and
every day will kiss it; if in her presence, his eye is never off her,
and drink he will where she drank, if it be possible, in that
very place, etc. If absent, he will walk in the walk, sit under
that tree where she did use to sit, in that bower, in that very
seat, *et foribus miser oscula figit* [and to relieve his misery kisses
the very door], many years after sometimes; though she be far
distant and dwell many miles off, he loves yet to walk that
way still, to have his chamber-window look that way, to walk
by that river's side, which (though far away) runs by the house
where she dwells; he loves the wind blows to that coast:

> *O quoties dixi Zephyris properantibus illuc,*
> *Felices pulchram visuri Amaryllida venti.*[2]
>
> O happy western winds that blow that way,
> For you shall see my love's fair face to-day.

He will send a message to her by the wind:

> *Vos auræ Alpinæ, placidis de montibus auræ,*
> *Hæc illi portate.*[3]
>
> [O Alpine breezes blowing from the peaceful moun-
> tains, this message bear to my beloved.]

He desires to confer with some of her acquaintance,[4] for his
heart is still with her, to talk of her,[5] admiring and commending
her, lamenting, moaning, wishing himself anything for her sake,
to have opportunity to see her, O that he might but enjoy her
presence! So did Philostratus to his mistress, "O happy ground
on which she treads! and happy were I if she would tread upon
me. I think her countenance would make the rivers stand,
and when she comes abroad, birds will sing and come about her." [6]

> *Ridebunt valles, ridebunt obvia Tempe,*
> *In florem viridis protinus ibit humus.*
>
> The fields will laugh, the pleasant valleys burn,
> And all the grass will into flowers turn.

Omnis ambrosiam spirabit aura [every breeze shall breathe
ambrosia]. "When she is in the meadow, she is fairer than
any flower, for that lasts but for a day; the river is pleasing,
but it vanisheth on a sudden, but thy flower doth not fade,
thy stream is greater than the sea. If I look upon the heaven,
methinks I see the sun fallen down to shine below, and thee to
shine in his place, whom I desire. If I look upon the night,

methinks I see two more glorious stars, Hesperus and thyself." [1]
A little after he thus courts his mistress: "If thou goest forth
of the city, the protecting gods that keep the town will run
after to gaze upon thee: if thou sail upon the seas, as so many
small boats they will follow thee: what river would not run
into the sea?" [2]   Another, he sighs and sobs, swears he hath
cor scissum, an heart bruised to powder, dissolved and melted
within him, or quite gone from him, to his mistress' bosom
belike; he is in an oven, a salamander in the fire, so scorched
with love's heat; he wisheth himself a saddle for her to sit on,
a posy for her to smell to, and it would not grieve him to be
hanged, if he might be strangled in her garters; he would
willingly die to-morrow, so that she might kill him with her own
hands.   Ovid would be a flea, a gnat, a ring; [3] Catullus, a
sparrow:

> *O si tecum ludere sicut ipsa possem,*
> *Et tristes animi levare curas;*

> [Would I might sport with thee as she does, 'twould
>   serve to lighten my heavy care;]

Anacreon, a glass, a gown, a chain, anything: [4]

> *Sed speculum ego ipse fiam,*
> *Ut me tuum usque cernas,*
> *Et vestis ipse fiam,*
> *Ut me tuum usque gestes.*
> *Mutari et opto in undam,*
> *Lavem tuos ut artus,*
> *Nardus, puella, fiam,*
> *Ut ego teipsum inungam,*
> *Sim fascia in papillis,*
> *Tuo et monile collo,*
> *Fiamque calceus, me*
> *Saltem ut pede usque calces.*

> But I a looking-glass would be,
> Still to be lookt upon by thee,
> Or I, my love, would be thy gown,
> By thee to be worn up and down;
> Or a pure well full to the brims,
> That I might wash thy purer limbs:
> Or, I 'd be precious balm to 'noint,
> With choicest care each choicest joint;
> Or, if I might, I would be fain
> About thy neck thy happy chain,
> Or would it were my blessed hap
> To be the lawn o'er thy fair pap,
> Or would I were thy shoe, to be
> Daily trod upon by thee. [5]

O thrice happy man that shall enjoy her! as they that saw
Hero in Musæus, and Salmacis to Hermaphroditus: [1]

> *Felices, mater, etc., felix nutrix,*
> *Sed longe cunctis, longeque beatior ille,*
> *Quem fructu sponsi et socii dignabere lecti.*

> [Happy thy parents and thy nurse, but far more
>   blessed than all he whom thou wilt acknowledge
>   thy spouse.]

The same passion made her break out in the comedy, *Næ illæ
fortunatæ sunt quæ cum illo cubant,*[2] happy are his bed-fellows;
and as she said of Cyrus, *Beata quæ illi uxor futura esset,*[3] blessed
is that woman that shall be his wife, nay, thrice happy she that
shall enjoy him but a night. *Una nox Jovis sceptro æquiparanda,*[4]
such a night's lodging is worth Jupiter's sceptre.

> *Qualis nox erit illa, dii, deæque!*
> *Quam mollis torus!* [5]

O what a blissful night would it be, how soft, how sweet a bed!
She will adventure all her estate for such a night, for a nectarean,
a balsam kiss alone.

> *Qui te videt beatus est,*
> *Beatior qui te audiet,*
> *Qui te potitur est deus.*[6]

> [Happy is he who sees thee, happier still he who hears
>   thee, but he who possesses thee is a god.]

The Sultan of Sana's wife in Arabia, when she had seen Vertomannus: that comely traveller, lamented to herself in this
manner: "O God, thou hast made this man whiter than the
sun, but me, mine husband, and all my children black; I would
to God he were my husband, or that I had such a son";[7] she
fell a-weeping, and so impatient for love at last, that (as Potiphar's wife did by Joseph) she would have had him gone in with
her, she sent away Gazella, Tegeia, Galzerana, her waiting-
maids, loaded him with fair promises and gifts, and wooed
him with all the rhetoric she could: *Extremum hoc miseræ da
munus amanti* [grant this last request to a wretched lover).
But when he gave no consent, she would have gone with him,
and left all, to be his page, his servant, or his lackey, *Certa
sequi carum corpus ut umbra solet* [determined to follow him
like his shadow], so that she might enjoy him, threatening
moreover to kill herself, etc. Men will do as much and

more for women, spend goods, lands, lives, fortunes; kings
will leave their crowns, as King John for Matilda the nun at
Dunmow.

> But kings in this yet privileg'd may be,
> I 'll be a monk so I may live with thee.[1]

The very gods will endure any shame (*atque aliquis de dis non
tristibus optat*, etc.), be a spectacle as Mars and Venus were to
all the rest; so did Lucian's Mercury wish, and peradventure
so dost thou. They will adventure their lives with alacrity:
pro qua non metuam mori [2] [I would not fear to die for her],
nay more, *pro qua non metuam bis mori*, I will die twice, nay,
twenty times for her. If she die, there 's no remedy, they must
die with her, they cannot help it. A lover in Calcagninus
wrote this on his darling's tomb:

> *Quincia obiit, sed non Quincia sola obiit,*
> *Quincia obiit, sed cum Quincia et ipse obii;*
> *Risus obit, obit gratia, lusus obit,*
> *Nec mea nunc anima in pectore, at in tumulo est.*

> Quincia my dear is dead, but not alone,
> For I am dead, and with her I am gone:
> Sweet smiles, mirth, graces, all with her do rest,
> And my soul too, for 'tis not in my breast.

How many doting lovers upon the like occasion might say the
same! But these are toys in respect, they will hazard their
very souls for their mistress' sake.

> *Atque aliquis inter juvenes miratus est, et verbum dixit,*
> *Non ego in cœlo cuperem Deus esse,*
> *Nostram uxorem habens domi Hero.*

> One said, To heaven would I not desire at all to go,
> If that at mine own house I had such a fine wife as Hero.

Venus forsook heaven for Adonis' sake, *cœlo præfertur Adonis.*[3]
Old Janivere, in Chaucer, thought when he had his fair May
he should never go to heaven, he should live so merrily here
on earth; had I such a mistress, he protests,

> *Cœlum diis ego non suum inviderem,*
> *Sed sortem mihi dii meam inviderent.*[4]

> I would not envy their prosperity,
> The gods should envy my felicity.

Another as earnestly desires to behold his sweetheart, he will

adventure and leave all this, and more than this, to see her
alone.

Omnia quæ patior mala si pensare velit fors,
  Una aliqua nobis prosperitate, dii
Hoc precor, ut faciant, faciant me cernere coram,
  Cor mihi captivum quæ tenet hocce, deam.[1]

  If all my mischiefs were recompensed,
  And God would give me what I requested,
  I would my mistress' presence only seek,
  Which doth mine heart in prison captive keep.

But who can reckon upon the dotage, madness, servitude and
blindness, the foolish phantasms and vanities of lovers, their
torments, wishes, idle attempts?

  Yet for all this, amongst so many irksome, absurd, troublesome symptoms, inconveniences, phantastical fits and passions
which are usually incident to such persons, there be some good
and graceful qualities in lovers, which this affection causeth.
"As it makes wise men fools, so many times it makes fools
become wise; "it makes base fellows become generous, cowards
courageous," as Cardan notes out of Plutarch;[2] "covetous,
liberal and magnificent; clowns, civil; cruel, gentle; wicked,
profane persons to become religious; slovens, neat; churls,
merciful; and dumb dogs, eloquent; your lazy drones, quick
and nimble." *Feras mentes domat Cupido* [love subdues savage
breasts], that fierce, cruel and rude Cyclops Polyphemus sighed
and shed many a salt tear for Galatea's sake. No passion
causeth greater alterations, or more vehement of joy or discontent. Plutarch, *Sympos lib.* 5, *quæst.* 1, saith "that the soul of
a man in love is full of perfumes and sweet odours, and all
manner of pleasing tones and tunes, insomuch that it is hard to
say" (as he adds) "whether love do mortal men more harm than
good."[3] It adds spirits and makes them, otherwise soft and
silly, generous and courageous, *Audacem faciebat amor*[4] [love
made him bold]. Ariadne's love made Theseus so adventurous,
and Medea's beauty Jason so victorious; *expectorat amor timorem*
[love drives fear from the heart]. Plato[5] is of opinion that the
love of Venus made Mars so valorous: "A young man will be
much abashed to commit any foul offence that shall come to the
hearing or sight of his mistress." As he that desired of his
enemy, now dying, to lay him with his face upward, *ne amasius
videret eum a tergo vulneratum*, lest his sweetheart should say he
was a coward.[6] "And if it were possible to have an army consist
of lovers, such as love, or are beloved, they would be extra-

ordinary valiant and wise in their government, modesty would
detain them from doing amiss, emulation incite them to do that
which is good and honest, and a few of them would overcome a
great company of others." [1] There is no man so pusillanimous,
so very a dastard, whom love would not incense, make of a divine
temper and an heroical spirit. As he said in like case, *Tota
ruat cœli moles, non terreor* [2] [though the heavens fall, I am not
dismayed], etc. Nothing can terrify, nothing can dismay them;
but as Sir Blandamour and Paridell, those two brave fairy
knights, fought for the love of fair Florimell in presence:

> And drawing both their swords with rage anew,
> Like two mad mastives each other slew,
> And shields did share, and mails did rash, and helms did hew:
> So furiously each other did assail,
> As if their souls at once they would have rent
> Out of their breasts, that streams of blood did rail
> Adown as if their springs of life were spent,
> That all the ground with purple blood was sprent,
> And all their armour stain'd with bloody gore;
> Yet scarcely once to breathe would they relent.
> So mortal was their malice and so sore,
> That both resolved (than yield) to die before. [3]

Every base swain in love will dare to do as much for his dear
mistress' sake. He will fight and fetch *Argivum clypeum*,[4]
that famous buckler of Argos, to do her service, adventure at
all, undertake any enterprise. And as Serranus the Spaniard,
then Governor of Sluys, made answer to Marquess Spinola, if
the enemy brought 50,000 devils against him he would keep it.
The Nine Worthies, Oliver and Rowland, and forty dozen of
peers are all in him, he is all mettle, armour of proof, more
than a man, and in this case improved beyond himself. For
as Agatho contends,[5] a true lover is wise, just, temperate, and
valiant. "I doubt not, therefore, but if a man had such an
army of lovers" (as Castilio supposeth [6]) "he might soon conquer
all the world, except by chance he met with such another army
of inamoratos to oppose it." For so perhaps they might fight
as that fatal dog and fatal hare in the heavens, course one
another round, and never make an end.[7] Castilio thinks Ferdinand King of Spain would never have conquered Granada,
had not Queen Isabel and her ladies been present at the siege:
"It cannot be expressed what courage the Spanish knights took
when the ladies were present; a few Spaniards overcame a
multitude of Moors." [8] They will undergo any danger whatsoever, as Sir Walter Manny in Edward the Third's time, stuck

full of ladies' favours, fought like a dragon. For *soli amantes*, as Plato holds,[1] *pro amicis mori appetunt*, only lovers will die for their friends, and in their mistress' quarrel. And for that cause he would have women follow the camp, to be spectators and encouragers of noble actions: upon such an occasion, the Squire of Dames[2] himself, Sir Lancelot or Sir Tristram, Cæsar or Alexander, shall not be more resolute or go beyond them.

Not courage only doth love add, but as I said, subtlety, wit, and many pretty devices, *Namque dolos inspirat amor, fraudesque ministrat*[3] [for love suggests stratagems and wiles]. Jupiter,[4] in love with Leda, and not knowing how to compass his desire, turned himself into a swan, and got Venus to pursue him in the likeness of an eagle; which she doing, for shelter he fled to Leda's lap, *et in ejus gremio se collocavit*, Leda embraced him, and so fell fast asleep, *sed dormientem Jupiter compressit*, by which means Jupiter had his will. Infinite such tricks love can devise, such fine feats in abundance, with wisdom and wariness— *Quis fallere possit amantem?*[5] [Who can deceive a lover?]—all manner of civility, decency, complement and good behaviour, *plus salis et leporis*, polite graces and merry conceits. Boccace hath a pleasant tale to this purpose, which he borrowed from the Greeks, and which Beroaldus hath turned into Latin, Bebelius in verse, of Cymon and Iphigenia. This Cymon was a fool, a proper man of person, and the governor of Cyprus' son, but a very ass, insomuch that his father, being ashamed of him, sent him to a farm-house he had in the country, to be brought up; where by chance, as his manner was, walking alone, he espied a gallant young gentlewoman, named Iphigenia, a burgomaster's daughter of Cyprus, with her maid, by a brook-side in a little thicket, fast asleep in her smock, where she had newly bathed herself. "When Cymon saw her, he stood leaning on his staff, gaping on her immovable, and in a maze";[6] at last he fell so far in love with the glorious object that he began to rouse himself up, to bethink what he was, would needs follow her to the city, and for her sake began to be civil, to learn to sing and dance, to play on instruments, and got all those gentle-manlike qualities and complements in a short space, which his friends were most glad of. In brief, he became, from an idiot and a clown, to be one of the most complete gentlemen in Cyprus, did many valorous exploits, and all for the love of Mistress Iphigenia. In a word, I may say thus much of them all, let them be never so clownish, rude and horrid, Grobians and sluts, if once they be in love they will be most neat and

spruce; for *omnibus rebus, et nitidis nitoribus antevenit amor*[1]
[love introduces itself by all means, and especially by spruceness
and elegance], they will follow the fashion, begin to trick up,
and to have a good opinion of themselves, *venustatum enim
mater Venus* [for Venus is the mother of the graces]; a ship is
not so long a-rigging as a young gentlewoman a-trimming up
herself against her sweetheart comes. A painter's shop, a
flowery meadow, no so gracious aspect in nature's storehouse
as a young maid, *nubilis puella*, a *novitsa* [*novizia*, novice] or
Venetian bride, that looks for a husband, or a young man that
is her suitor; composed looks, composed gait, clothes, gestures,
actions, all composed; all the graces, elegancies in the world are in
her face. Their best robes, ribbons, chains, jewels, lawns, linens,
laces, spangles, must come on, *præter quam res patitur student
elegantiæ*[2] [they study elegance beyond all measure], they are
beyond all measure coy, nice, and too curious on a sudden:
'tis all their study, all their business, how to wear their clothes
neat, to be polite and terse, and to set out themselves. No
sooner doth a young man see his sweetheart coming, but he
smugs up himself, pulls up his cloak now fallen about his
shoulders, ties his garters, points, sets his band, cuffs, slicks his
hair, twires his beard, etc. When Mercury was to come before
his mistress,

> *Chlamydemque ut pendeat apte*
> *Collocat, ut limbus totumque appareat aurum.*[3]

He put his cloak in order, that the lace,
And hem, and gold-work, all might have his grace.

Salmacis would not be seen of Hermaphroditus, till she had
spruced up herself first.

> *Nec tamen ante adiit, etsi properabat adire,*
> *Quam se composuit, quam circumspexit amictus,*
> *Et finxit vultum, et meruit formosa videri.*[4]

Nor did she come, although 'twas her desire,
Till she compos'd herself, and trimm'd her tire,
And set her looks to make him to admire.

Venus had so ordered the matter, that when her son Æneas[5]
was to appear before Queen Dido, he was

> *Os humerosque deo similis (namque ipsa decoram*
> *Cæsariem nato genetrix, lumenque juventæ*
> *Purpureum et lætos oculis afflarat honores),*

like a god, for she was the tire-woman herself, to set him out
with all natural and artificial impostures, as mother Mamæa

did her son Heliogabalus,[1] new chosen emperor, when he was
to be seen of the people first. When the hirsute cyclopical
Polyphemus courted Galatea:

> *Jamque tibi formæ, jamque est tibi cura placendi,*
> *Jam rigidos pectis rastris, Polypheme, capillos,*
> *Jam libet hirsutam tibi falce recidere barbam,*
> *Et spectare feros in aqua et componere vultus.*[2]

> And then he did begin to prank himself,
> To plait and comb his head, and beard to shave,
> And look his face i' th' water as a glass,
> And to compose himself for to be brave.

He was upon a sudden now spruce, and keen as a new-ground
hatchet. He now began to have a good opinion of his own
features and good parts, now to be a gallant.

> *Jam, Galatea, veni, nec munera despice nostra,*
> *Certe ego me novi, liquidæque in imagine vidi*
> *Nuper aquæ, placuitque mihi mea forma videnti.*

> Come now, my Galatea, scorn me not,
> Nor my poor presents; for but yesterday
> I saw myself i' th' water, and methought
> Full fair I was; then scorn me not, I say.

> *Non sum adeo informis, nuper me in littore vidi,*
> *Cum placidum ventis staret mare.*[3]

> [I am not so unshapely, I late saw myself upon the
> shore in a glassy sea.]

'Tis the common humour of all suitors to trick up themselves,
to be prodigal in apparel, *pure lotus*, neat, combed and curled,
with powdered hairs, *comptus et calamistratus*, with a long love-
lock, a flower in his ear, perfumed gloves, rings, scarfs, feathers,
points, etc., as if he were a prince's Ganymede, with every day
new suits, as the fashion varies; going as if he trod upon eggs;
and, as Heinsius writ to Primerius,[4] "If once he be besotten on
a wench, he must lie awake anights, renounce his book, sigh and
lament, now and then weep for his hard hap, and mark above
all things what hats, bands, doublets, breeches, are in fashion,
how to cut his beard and wear his locks, to turn up his mushatos
and curl his head, prune his pickitivant, or if he wear it abroad,
that the east side be correspondent to the west": he may be
scoffed at otherwise, as Julian, that apostate emperor, was for
wearing a long hirsute goatish beard, fit to make ropes with,
as in his *Misopogon*, or that apologetical oration he made at
Antioch to excuse himself, he doth ironically confess it hindered

his kissing, *nam non licuit inde pura puris, eoque suavioribus labra labris adjungere* [it made it impossible to put lips to lips without impediment, which would have been more pleasant], but he did not much esteem it, as it seems by the sequel, *De accipiendis dandisve osculis non laboro* [I am not much concerned about taking and giving kisses], yet (to follow mine author) it may much concern a young lover, he must be more respectful in this behalf, "he must be in league with an excellent tailor, barber,"

> *Tonsorem puerum sed arte talem,*
> *Qualis nec Thalamus fuit Neronis ;* [1]

[A young barber, but a greater artist than Nero's Thalamus;]

"have neat shoe-ties, points, garters, speak in print, walk in print, eat and drink in print, and that which is all in all, he must be mad in print."

Amongst other good qualities an amorous fellow is endowed with, he must learn to sing and dance, play upon some instrument or other, as without all doubt he will, if he be truly touched with this loadstone of love.   For as Erasmus hath it, [2] *Musicam docet amor et poesin*, love will make them musicians, and to compose ditties, madrigals, elegies, love-sonnets, and sing them to several pretty tunes, to get all good qualities may be had.   Jupiter perceived Mercury to be in love with Philologia, [3] because he learned languages, polite speech (for Suadela [Persuasion] herself was Venus' daughter, as some write), arts and sciences, *quo virgini placeret*, all to ingratiate himself and please his mistress. 'Tis their chiefest study to sing, dance; and without question, so many gentlemen and gentlewomen would not be so well qualified in this kind, if love did not incite them. "Who," saith Castilio, [4] "would learn to play, or give his mind to music, learn to dance, or make so many rhymes, love-songs, as most do, but for women's sake, because they hope by that means to purchase their good wills and win their favour?" We see this daily verified in our young women and wives, they that being maids took so much pains to sing, play, and dance, with such cost and charge to their parents to get those graceful qualities, now being married will scarce touch an instrument, they care not for it.   Constantine, *Agricult. lib.* 11, *cap.* 18, makes Cupid himself to be a great dancer; by the same token as he was capering amongst the gods, "he flung down a bowl of nectar, which, distilling upon the white rose, ever since made it red": [5] and Callistratus, by the help of Dædalus, about Cupid's statue made a many of young wenches still a-dancing, [6] to signify

belike that Cupid was much affected with it, as without all doubt
he was. For at his and Psyche's wedding, the gods being
present to grace the feast, Ganymede filled nectar in abundance
(as Apuleius describes it [1]), Vulcan was the cook, the Hours
made all fine with roses and flowers, Apollo played on the harp,
the Muses sang to it, *sed suavi musicæ superingressa Venus
saltavit*, but his mother Venus danced to his and their sweet
content. Witty Lucian [2] in that pathetical love-passage or
pleasant description of Jupiter's stealing of Europa and
swimming from Phœnicia to Crete, makes the sea calm, the
winds hush, Neptune and Amphitrite riding in their chariot to
break the waves before them, the tritons dancing round about,
with every one a torch, the sea-nymphs half naked, keeping
time on dolphins' backs, and singing *Hymenæus* [the nuptial
song], Cupid nimbly tripping on the top of the waters, and
Venus herself coming after in a shell, strewing roses and flowers
on their heads. Praxiteles, in all his pictures of Love, feigns
Cupid ever smiling, and looking upon dancers; and in Saint
Mark's garden in Rome (whose work I know not), one of the
most delicious pieces is a many of satyrs dancing about a wench
asleep.[3] So that dancing still is, as it were, a necessary appendix
to love matters. Young lasses are never better pleased than
whenas upon an holiday, after evensong, they may meet their
sweethearts, and dance about a maypole, or in a town-green
under a shady elm. Nothing so familiar in France,[4] as for
citizens' wives and maids to dance a round in the streets, and
often too, for want of better instruments, to make good music
of their own voices, and dance after it. Yea many times this
love will make old men and women, that have more toes than
teeth, dance, "John come kiss me now," mask and mum; for
Comus and Hymen love masks and all such merriments above
measure; will allow men to put on women's apparel in some
cases, and promiscuously to dance, young and old, rich and
poor, generous and base, of all sorts. Paulus Jovius taxeth
Augustine Niphus the philosopher,[5] "for that being an old man,
and a public professor, a father of many children, he was mad
for the love of a young maid (that which many of his friends
were ashamed to see), an old gouty fellow, yet would dance
after fiddlers." Many laughed him to scorn for it, but this
omnipotent love would have it so.

> *Hyacinthino bacillo*
> *Properans amor, me adegit*
> *Violenter ad sequendum.*[6]

> Love hasty with his purple staff did make
> Me follow and the dance to undertake.

And 'tis no news this, no indecorum; for why? a good reason may be given of it.   Cupid and Death met both in an inn; and being merrily disposed, they did exchange some arrows from either quiver; ever since young men die, and oftentimes old men dote.

> *Sic moritur juvenis, sic moribundus amat.*[1]
> [So the youth dies, so dying still he loves.]

And who can then withstand it?   If once we be in love, young or old, though our teeth shake in our heads like virginal jacks, or stand parallel asunder like the arches of a bridge, there is no remedy, we must dance trenchmore for a need, over tables, chairs, and stools, etc.   And princum prancum is a fine dance. Plutarch, *Sympos.* 1, *quæst.* 5, doth in some sort excuse it, and telleth us moreover in what sense *musicam docet amor, licet prius fuerit rudis,* how love makes them that had no skill before learn to sing and dance; he concludes, 'tis only that power and prerogative love hath over us.   "Love" (as he holds) "will make a silent man speak, a modest man most officious; dull, quick; slow, nimble; and that which is most to be admired, a hard, base, untractable churl, as fire doth iron in a smith's forge, free, facile, gentle, and easy to be entreated."[2]   Nay, 'twill make him prodigal in the other extreme, and give an hundred sesterces for a night's lodging,[3] as they did of old to Lais of Corinth, or *ducenta drachmarum millia pro unica nocte*[4] [two thousand drachmas for a single night], as Mundus to Paulina, spend all his fortunes (as too many do in like case) to obtain his suit.   For which cause many compare love to wine, which makes men jovial and merry, frolic and sad, whine, sing, dance, and what not.

But above all the other symptoms of lovers, this is not lightly to be overpassed, that likely of what condition soever, if once they be in love, they turn to their ability, rhymers, ballet-makers, and poets.   For, as Plutarch saith, "They will be witnesses and trumpeters of their paramours' good parts, bedecking them with verses and commendatory songs, as we do statues with gold, that they may be remembered and admired of all."[5]   Ancient men will dote in this kind sometimes as well as the rest; the heat of love will thaw their frozen affections, dissolve the ice of age, and so far enable them, though they be sixty years of age above the girdle, to be scarce thirty beneath.

Jovianus Pontanus makes an old fool rhyme, and turn poetaster
to please his mistress.

Ne ringas, Mariana, meos ne despice canos,
De sene nam juvenem, dia, referre potes, etc.[1]

Sweet Marian, do not mine age disdain,
For thou canst make an old man young again.

They will be still singing amorous songs and ditties (if young
especially), and cannot abstain, though it be when they go to,
or should be at church.   We have a pretty story to this purpose
in Westmonasteriensis,[2] an old writer of ours (if you will believe
it).   *An. Dom.* 1012, at Colewiz in Saxony, on Christmas Eve
a company of young men and maids, whilst the priest was at
mass in the church, were singing catches and love-songs in the
churchyard; he sent to them to make less noise, but they sung
on still; and if you will, you shall have the very song itself:

Equitabat homo per silvam frondosam,
Ducebatque secum Meswinden formosam,
Quid stamus, cur non imus?

A fellow rid by the greenwood side,
And fair Meswinde was his bride,
Why stand we so, and do not go?

This they sung, he chafed, till at length, impatient as he was,
he prayed to St. Magnus, patron of the church, they might all
there sing and dance till that time twelvemonth, and so they
did, without meat and drink, wearisomeness or giving over,
till at year's end they ceased singing, and were absolved by
Herebertus, Archbishop of Cologne.[3]   They will in all places be
doing thus, young folks especially, reading love stories, talking
of this or that young man, such a fair maid, singing, telling or
hearing lasciviou stales, scurrile tunes; such objects are their
sole delight, their continual meditation, and as Guastavinius
adds, *Com. in 4 sect. 27, Prob. Arist., ob seminis abundantiam
crebræ cogitationes, veneris frequens recordatio et pruriens voluptas,*
etc., an earnest longing comes hence, *pruriens corpus, pruriens
anima,* amorous conceits, tickling thoughts, sweet and pleasant
hopes; hence it is, they can think, discourse willingly, or speak
almost of no other subject.   'Tis their only desire, if it may
be done by art, to see their husband's picture in a glass, they 'll
give anything to know when they shall be married, how many
husbands they shall have, by *crommyomantia,* a kind of divination with onions [4] laid on the altar on Christmas Eve, or by

fasting on St. Agnes' Eve or Night, to know who shall be their
first husband, or by *alphitomantia*, by beans in a cake, etc., to
burn the same.   This love is the cause of all good conceits,
neatness, exornations, plays, elegancies, delights, pleasant expressions, sweet motions and gestures, joys, comforts, exultancies,
and all the sweetness of our life; [1] *Qualis jam vita foret, aut
quid jucundi sine aurea Venere?* [2] [What would life be, what
joy would there be, without golden Aphrodite?]   *Emoriar cum
ista non amplius mihi cura fuerit,* [3] let me live no longer than I
may love, saith a mad merry fellow in Mimnermus.   This love
is that salt that seasoneth our harsh and dull labours, and
gives a pleasant relish to our other unsavoury proceedings;
Absit amor, surgunt tenebræ, torpedo, veternum, pestis, etc. [4] [when
love departs, there enter darkness, sluggishness, senility, disease,
etc.].   All our feasts almost, masques, mummings, banquets,
merry meetings, weddings, pleasing songs, fine tunes, poems,
love stories, plays, comedies, Atellanes, jigs, Fescennines, elegies,
odes, etc., proceed hence.   Danaus, the son of Belus, at his
daughter's wedding at Argos, instituted the first plays (some say)
that ever were heard of.   Symbols, emblems, impresses, devices,
if we shall believe Jovius, Contiles, Paradine, Camillus de
Camillis, may be ascribed to it. [5]   Most of our arts and sciences;
painting amongst the rest was first invented, saith Patricius, [6]
ex amoris beneficio, for love's sake.   For when the daughter of
Dibutades the Sicyonian was to take leave of her sweetheart
now going to wars, *ut desiderio ejus minus tabesceret,* to comfort
herself in his absence, she took his picture with coal upon a wall,
as the candle gave the shadow, which her father admiring
perfected afterwards, and it was the first picture by report
that ever was made. [7]   And long after, Sicyon for painting,
carving, statuary, music, and philosophy, was preferred before
all the cities in Greece.   Apollo [8] was the first inventor of
physic, divination, oracles; Minerva found out weaving, Vulcan
curious ironwork, Mercury letters; but who prompted all this
into their heads?   Love.   *Nunquam talia invenissent, nisi talia
adamassent,* they loved such things, or some party, for whose
sake they were undertaken at first.   'Tis true, Vulcan made a
most admirable brooch or necklace, which long after Axion and
Temenus, Phegeus' sons, for the singular worth of it, consecrated to Apollo at Delphi, but Pharyllus the tyrant stole it
away, and presented it to Ariston's wife, on whom he miserably
doted (Parthenius tells the story out of Phylarchus); but why
did Vulcan make this excellent ouch? to give Hermione, Cadmus'

wife, whom he dearly loved. All our tilts and tournaments, Orders of the Garter, Golden Fleece, etc.—*Nobilitas sub amore jacet*—owe their beginnings to love, and many of our histories. By this means, saith Jovius, they would express their loving minds to their mistress, and to the beholders. 'Tis the sole subject almost of poetry, all our invention tends to it, all our songs (and therefore Hesiod makes the Muses and Graces still follow Cupid, and, as Plutarch holds, Menander and the rest of the poets were Love's priests); whatever those old Anacreons, all our Greek and Latin epigrammatists, love writers, Antony Diogenes the most ancient, whose epitome we find in Photius' *Bibliotheca*, Longus Sophista, Eustathius, Achilles Tatius, Aristænetus, Heliodorus, Plato, Plutarch, Lucian, Parthenius, Theodorus Prodromus, Ovid, Catullus, Tibullus, etc., our new Ariostos, Boiardos, authors of Arcadia, Urania, Faerie Queene, etc., Marullus, Lotichius, Angerianus, Stroza, Secundus, Capellanus, etc., with the rest of those facete modern poets, have written in this kind, are but as so many symptoms of love. Their whole books are a synopsis or breviary of love, the portuous of love, legends of lovers' lives and deaths, and of their memorable adventures; nay more, *quod leguntur, quod laudantur amori debent* [they owe it to love that they are read and admired], as Nevisanus the lawyer holds,[1] "there never was any excellent poet that invented good fables, or made laudable verses, which was not in love himself"; had he not taken a quill from Cupid's wings, he could never have written so amorously as he did.

> *Cynthia te vatem fecit lascive Properti,*
>   *Ingenium Galli pulchra Lycoris habet.*
> *Fama est arguti Nemesis formosa Tibulli,*
>   *Lesbia dictavit, docte Catulle, tibi.*
> *Non me Pelignus, nec spernet Mantua vatem,*
>   *Si qua Corinna mihi, si quis Alexis erit.*[2]

> Wanton Propertius and witty Gallus,
> Subtle Tibullus, and learned Catullus,
> It was Cynthia, Lesbia, Lycoris,
> That made you poets all; and if Alexis,
> Or Corinna chance my paramour to be,
> Virgil and Ovid shall not despise me.

> *Non me carminibus vincet nec Thracius Orpheus,*
> *Nec Linus.*[3]

[Not Thracian Orpheus nor Linus shall excel my poetry.]

Petrarch's Laura made him so famous, Astrophel's Stella, and

Jovianus Pontanus' mistress was the cause of his Roses, Violets, Lilies, *Nequitiæ*, *Blanditiæ*, *Joci*, *Decor*, *Nardus*, *Ver*, *Corolla*, *Thus*, *Mars*, *Pallas*, *Venus*, *Charis*, *Crocum*, *Laurus*, *Unguentem*, *Costum*, *Lacrimæ*, *Myrrha*, *Musæ*, etc., and the rest of his poems. Why are Italians at this day generally so good poets and painters? Because every man of any fashion amongst them hath his mistress. The very rustics and hog-rubbers, Menalcas and Corydon, *qui fœtent de stercore equino* [who stink of horse-dung], those fulsome knaves, if once they taste of this love-liquor, are inspired in an instant. Instead of those accurate emblems, curious impresses, gaudy masques, tilts, tournaments, etc., they have their wakes, Whitsun-ales, shepherds' feasts, meetings on holidays, country dances, roundelays, writing their names on trees,[1] true-lovers' knots, pretty gifts.

> With tokens, hearts divided, and half rings,
> Shepherds in their loves are as coy as kings.

Choosing lords, ladies, kings, queens, and valentines, etc., they go by couples:

> Corydon's Phyllis, Nysa and Mopsus,
> With dainty Dousibel and Sir Tophus.

Instead of odes, epigrams and elegies, etc., they have their ballads, country tunes, "O the broom, the bonny, bonny broom," ditties and songs, "Bess a Bell, she doth excel"; they must write likewise and indite all in rhyme.

> Thou honeysuckle of the hawthorn hedge,
> Vouchsafe in Cupid's cup my heart to pledge;
> My heart's dear blood, sweet Cis, is thy carouse
> Worth all the ale in Gammer Gubbin's house.
> I say no more, affairs call me away,
> My father's horse for provender doth stay.
> Be thou the Lady Cressetlight to me,
> Sir Trolly Lolly will I prove to thee.
> Written in haste, farewell, my cowslip sweet,
> Pray let 's a' Sunday at the alehouse meet.[2]

Your most grim Stoics and severe philosophers will melt away with this passion, and if Athenæus[3] belie them not, Aristippus, Apollodorus, Antiphanes, etc., have made love-songs and commentaries of their mistresses' praises, orators write epistles,[4] princes give titles, honours, what not? Xerxes gave to Themistocles Lampsacus to find him wine, Magnesia for bread, and Myus for the rest of his diet.[5] The Persian kings allotted whole cities to like use, *hæc civitas mulieri redimiculum præbeat, hæc in collum, hæc in crines*,[1] one whole city served to dress her hair, another her neck, a third her hood. Ahasuerus would have given Esther half his empire,[2] and Herod bid Herodias "ask what she would, she should have it."[3] Caligula gave an 100,000 sesterces to his courtesan at first word, to buy her pins, and yet when he was solicited by the senate to bestow something to repair the decayed walls of Rome for the commonwealth's good, he would give but 6000 sesterces at most. Dionysius, that Sicilian tyrant, rejected all his privy councillors, and was so besotted on Myrrha, his favourite and mistress, that he would bestow no office, or in the most weightiest business of the kingdom do aught, without her especial advice, prefer, depose, send, entertain no man, though worthy and well-deserving, but by her consent;[4] and he again whom she commended, howsoever unfit, unworthy, was as highly approved. Kings and emperors, instead of poems, build cities; Hadrian built Antinoe in Egypt, besides constellations, temples, altars, statues, images, etc., in the honour of his Antinous. Alexander bestowed infinite sums to set out his Hephæstion to all eternity. Socrates professeth himself love's servant, ignorant in all arts and sciences, a doctor alone in love matters,[5] *et quum alienarum rerum omnium scientiam diffiteretur*, saith Maximus Tyrius,[6] *his sectator, hujus negotii professor*, etc., and this he spake openly, at home and abroad, at public feasts, in the academy, *in Piræo, Lyceo, sub platano, etc.* [in the Piræus, the Lyceum, under the plane-tree, etc.], the very blood-hound of beauty, as he is styled by others. But I conclude there is no end of love's symptoms, 'tis a bottomless pit. Love is subject to no dimensions; not to be surveyed by any art or engine: and besides, I am of Hædus' mind, "no man can discourse of love matters, or judge of them aright, that hath not made trial in his own person,"[7] or, as Æneas Sylvius adds,[8] "hath not a little doted, been mad or love-sick himself." I confess I am but a novice, a contemplator only, *Nescio quid sit amor nec amo* [I know not what is love nor am I in love], I have a tincture, for why should I lie, dissemble or excuse it? yet *homo sum*, etc., not altogether inexpert in this subject, *non sum præceptor amandi* [I am not an instructor in love], and what I say is merely reading, *ex aliorum forsan ineptiis* [perhaps from the triflings of others], by mine own observation and others' relation.

MEMB. IV.

Prognostics of Love-Melancholy

WHAT fires, torments, cares, jealousies, suspicions, fears, griefs, anxieties, accompany such as are in love, I have sufficiently said; the next question is, what will be the event of such miseries, what they foretell. Some are of opinion that this love cannot be cured, *Nullis amor est medicabilis herbis* [love can be cured by no herbs], it accompanies them to the last,[1] *Idem amor exitio est pecori pecorisque magistro* [the same passion consumes both the sheep and the shepherd], and is so continuate, that by no persuasion almost it may be relieved. "Bid me not love," said Euryalus, "bid the mountains come down into the plains, bid the rivers run back to their fountains; I can as soon leave to love, as the sun leave his course." [2]

> *Et prius æquoribus pisces, et montibus umbræ,*
> *Et volucres deerunt silvis, et murmura ventis,*
> *Quam mihi discedent formosæ Amaryllidis ignes.*[3]

First seas shall want their fish, the mountains shade,
Woods singing-birds, the wind's murmur shall fade,
Than my fair Amaryllis' love allay'd.

Bid me not love, bid a deaf man hear, a blind man see, a dumb speak, lame run, counsel can do no good, a sick man cannot relish, no physic can ease me. *Non prosunt domino quæ prosunt omnibus artes* [the arts that help all others help not him], as Apollo confessed, and Jupiter himself could not be cured.

> *Omnes humanos curat medicina dolores,*
> *Solus amor morbi non habet artificem.*[4]

Physic can soon cure every disease,
Excepting love, that can it not appease.[5]

But whether love may be cured or no, and by what means, shall be explained in his place; in the meantime, if it take his course and be not otherwise eased or amended, it breaks out into outrageous often and prodigious events. *Amor et Liber violenti dii sunt*, as Tatius observes,[6] *et eo usque animum incendunt, ut pudoris oblivisci cogant*, Love and Bacchus are so violent gods, so furiously rage in our minds, that they make us forget all honesty, shame, and common civility. For such men ordinarily as are throughly possessed with this humour, become *insensati et insani* (for it is *amor insanus* [insane love],

III—G 888

as the poet calls it [1]), beside themselves, and as I have proved,
no better than beasts, irrational, stupid, headstrong, void of
fear of God or men, they frequently forswear themselves, spend,
steal, commit incests, rapes, adulteries, murders, depopulate
towns, cities, countries, to satisfy their lust.

> A devil 'tis, and mischief such doth work,
> As never yet did Pagan, Jew, or Turk.[2]

The wars of Troy may be a sufficient witness; and as Appian,
Hist. lib. 5, saith of Antony and Cleopatra, "Their love brought
themselves and all Egypt into extreme and miserable calamities."[3]
"The end of her is as bitter as wormwood, and as sharp as a
two-edged sword. Her feet go down to death, her steps lead
on to hell" (Prov. v, 4, 5). "She is more bitter than death,
and the sinner shall be taken by her" (Eccles. vii, 26). *Qui in
amore præcipitavit, pejus perit quam qui saxo salit.*[4] He that
runs headlong from the top of a rock is not in so bad a case as
he that falls into this gulf of love.[5] "For hence," saith Platina,[6]
"comes repentance, dotage, they lose themselves, their wits,
and make shipwreck of their fortunes altogether"; madness, to
make away themselves and others, violent death. *Prognosti-
catio est talis,* saith Gordonius, *si non succurratur iis, aut in
maniam cadunt, aut moriuntur:* the prognostication is, they
will either run mad, or die.[7] "For if this passion continue,"
saith Ælian Montaltus,[8] "it makes the blood hot, thick, and
black; and if the inflammation get into the brain, with continual
meditation and waking, it so dries it up that madness follows,
or else they make away themselves." *O Corydon, Corydon,
quæ te dementia cepit?*[9] [O Corydon, Corydon, what madness
hath come over thee?] Now, as Arnoldus adds, it will speedily
work these effects if it be not presently helped; "they will pine
away, run mad, and die upon a sudden"; *Facile incidunt in
maniam,* saith Valescus, quickly mad, *nisi succurratur,*[10] if good
order be not taken:

> *Eheu triste jugum quisquis amoris habet,*
> *Is prius ac norit se periisse perit.*[11]

> Oh heavy yoke of love, which whoso bears,
> Is quite undone, and that at unawares.

So she confessed of herself in the poet:

> *Insaniam priusquam quis sentiat,*
> *Vix pili intervallo a furore absum.*[12]

> I shall be mad before it be perceived,
> A hair-breadth off scarce am I, now distracted.

As mad as Orlando for his Angelica, or Hercules for his Hylas:

> *At ille ruebat quo pedes ducebant, furibundus,*
> *Nam illi sævus deus intus jecur laniabat.*

> He went he car'd not whither, mad he was,
> The cruel god so tortured him, alas!

At the sight of Hero I cannot tell how many ran mad:

> *Alius vulnus celans insanit pulchritudine puellæ.*[1]

> And whilst he doth conceal his grief,
> Madness comes on him like a thief.

Go to Bedlam for examples. It is so well known in every village, how many have either died for love, or voluntarily made away themselves, that I need not much labour to prove it; *Nec modus aut requies nisi mors reperitur amoris* [2] [love knows no limit or escape save death]: death is the common catastrophe to such persons.

> *Mori mihi contingat, non enim alia*
> *Liberatio ab ærumnis fuerit ullo pacto istis.*[3]

> Would I were dead, for nought, God knows,
> But death can rid me of these woes.

As soon as Euryalus departed from Senes, Lucretia, his paramour, "never looked up, no jests could exhilarate her sad mind, no joys comfort her wounded and distressed soul, but a little after she fell sick and died." [4] But this is a gentle end, a natural death, such persons commonly make away themselves:

> *Proprioque in sanguine lætus,*
> *Indignantem animam vacuas effudit in auras.*

> [Shedding his life-blood with glee, he gave his disdainful
> breath to the empty air.]

So did Dido:

> *Sed moriamur, ait. Sic, sic juvat ire per umbras;*

> ["But let me die," she said. "As I am, so let me
> descend to the underworld";]

Pyramus and Thisbe, Medea, Coresus and Callirhoe,[5] Theagenes the philosopher,[6] and many myriads besides, and so will ever do:

> *Et mihi fortis*
> *Est manus, est et amor, dabit hic in vulnera vires.*[7]

> Who ever heard a story of more woe,
> Than that of Juliet and her Romeo?

Read Parthenius *in Eroticis*, and Plutarch's *amatorias*

narrationes, or love stories, all tending, almost, to this purpose.
Valleriola, *lib.* 2, *observ.* 7, hath a lamentable narration of a
merchant, his patient, "that raving through impatience of
love, had he not been watched, would every while have offered
violence to himself." [1] Amatus Lusitanus, *cent.* 3, *cur.* 56,
hath such another story,[2] and Felix Plater, *Med. observ. lib.* 1,
a third of a young gentleman that studied physic, and for the
love of a doctor's daughter, having no hope to compass his
desire, poisoned himself.[3]   *Anno* 1615, a barber in Frankfort,
because his wench was betrothed to another, cut his own
throat.[4] At Neuburg, the same year, a young man, because
he could not get her parents' consent, killed his sweetheart,
and afterward himself, desiring this of the magistrate, as he
gave up the ghost, that they might be buried in one grave,[5]
Quodque rogis superest una requiescat in urna, which Gismunda
besought of Tancredus, her father,[6] that she might be in like
sort buried with Guiscardus, her lover, that so their bodies might
lie together in the grave, as their souls wander about *campos
lugentes* [7] [the mourning meadows] in the Elysian Fields, *quos
durus amor crudeli tabe peredit* [whom pitiless love with wasting
flame consumed], in a myrtle grove:

> *Et myrtea circum*
> *Silva tegit : curæ non ipsa in morte relinquunt.*

> [A myrtle grove encompasses them; but not even in
> death are they free from the cares of love.]

You have not yet heard the worst, they do not offer violence to
themselves in this rage of lust, but unto others, their nearest
and dearest friends.   Catiline killed his only son,[8] *misitque ad
Orci pallida, lethi obnubila, obsita tenebris loca* [he sent him to
the pale, misty, dark abodes of death], for the love of Aurelia
Orestilla, *quod ejus nuptias vivo filio recusaret* [because she refused
to marry him while his son was alive].   Laodice, the sister of
Mithridates, poisoned her husband, to give content to a base
fellow whom she loved.[9]   Alexander, to please Thais, a concubine of his, set Persepolis on fire.[10]   Nereus' wife, a widow and
lady of Athens, for the love of a Venetian gentleman, betrayed
the city; and he for her sake murdered his wife, the daughter
of a nobleman in Venice.[11]   Constantine Despota made away
Catherine his wife, turned his son Michael and his other children
out of doors, for the love of a base scrivener's daughter in
Thessalonica, with whose beauty he was enamoured.[12]   Leu-
cophrye betrayed the city where she dwelt, for her sweetheart's

sake, that was in the enemies' camp.[1] Pisidice, the governor's
daughter of Methymna, for the love of Achilles, betrayed the
whole island to him, her father's enemy.[2] Diognetus did as
much in the city where he dwelt, for the love of Polycrite,[3]
Medea for the love of Jason; she taught him how to tame the
fire-breathing, brass-feeted bulls, and kill the mighty dragon
that kept the golden fleece, and tore her little brother Absyrtus
in pieces, that her father Æetes might have something to detain
him, while she ran away with her beloved Jason, etc. Such
acts and scenes hath this tragi-comedy of love.

MEMB. V.

SUBSECT. I.—*Cure of Love-Melancholy, by Labour, Diet, Physic, Fasting, etc.*

ALTHOUGH it be controverted by some, whether love-melancholy
may be cured, because it is so irresistible and violent a passion;
for as you know,

> *Facilis descensus Averni ;*
> *Sed revocare gradum, superasque evadere ad auras,*
> *Hic labor, hoc opus est ;* [4]

> It is an easy passage down to hell,
> But to come back, once there, you cannot well;

yet without question, if it be taken in time, it may be helped,
and by many good remedies amended. Avicenna, *lib.* 3, *Fen.
cap.* 23 *et* 24, sets down seven compendious ways how this
malady may be eased, altered, and expelled. Savonarola nine
principal observations, Jason Pratensis prescribes eight rules,
besides physic, how this passion may be tamed, Laurentius
two main precepts, Arnoldus, Valleriola, Montaltus, Hildesheim,
Langius, and others inform us otherwise, and yet all tending
to the same purpose. The sum of which I will briefly epitomize
(for I light my candle from their torches), and enlarge again
upon occasion, as shall seem best to me, and that after mine
own method. The first rule to be observed in this stubborn
and unbridled passion, is exercise and diet. It is an old and
well-known sentence, *Sine Cere et Baccho friget Venus* [love
grows cool without bread and wine]. As an idle sedentary life,[5]
liberal feeding, are great causes of it, so the opposite, labour,

slender and sparing diet, with continual business, are the best
and most ordinary means to prevent it.

> *Otia si tollas, periere Cupidinis artes,*
> *Contemptæque jacent, et sine luce faces.*

> Take idleness away, and put to flight
> Are Cupid's arts, his torches give no light.

Minerva, Diana, Vesta, and the nine Muses were not enamoured
at all, because they never were idle.

> *Frustra blanditiæ appulistis ad has,*
> *Frustra nequitiæ venitis ad has,*
> *Frustra deliciæ obsidebitis has,*
> *Frustra has illecebræ, et procacitates,*
> *Et suspiria, et oscula, et susurri,*
> *Et quisquis male sana corda amantum*
> *Blandis ebria fascinat venenis.*[1]

> In vain are all your flatteries,
> In vain are all your knaveries,
> Delights, deceits, procacities,
> Sighs, kisses, and conspiracies,
> And whate'er is done by art,
> To bewitch a lover's heart.

'Tis in vain to set upon those that are busy.   'Tis Savonarola's
third rule, *occupari in multis et magnis negotiis* [to busy oneself
with important affairs], and Avicenna's precept, *cap.* 24 (*Cedit
amor rebus; res age, tutus eris* [2] [love retires before business; be
busy and you will be safe]), to be busy still, and, as Guianerius
enjoins,[3] about matters of great moment, if it may be. Magninus
adds, "never to be idle but at the hours of sleep." [4]

> *Et ni*
> *Posces ante diem librum cum lumine, si non*
> *Intendes animum studiis, et rebus honestis,*
> *Invidia vel amore miser torquebere.*[5]

> For if thou dost not ply thy book,
> By candle-light to study bent,
> Employ'd about some honest thing,
> Envy or love shall thee torment.

No better physic than to be always occupied, seriously intent.

> *Cur in penates rarius tenues subit,*
> *Hæc delicatas eligens pestis domos,*
> *Mediumque sanos vulgus affectus tenet?* etc.[6]

> Why, dost thou ask, poor folks are often free,
> And dainty places still molested be?

Because poor people fare coarsely, work hard, go woolward and

bare. *Non habet unde suum paupertas pascat amorem* [poverty
hath not the wherewithal to feed its passion]. Guianerius [1]
therefore prescribes his patient "to go with hair-cloth next his
skin, to go bare-footed, and bare-legged in cold weather, to
whip himself now and then, as monks do, but above all, to
fast." Not with sweet wine, mutton and pottage, as many
of those tenter-bellies do, howsoever they put on Lenten faces,
and whatsoever they pretend, but from all manner of meat.
Fasting is an all-sufficient remedy of itself; for, as Jason
Pratensis holds, the bodies of such persons that feed liberally,
and live at ease, "are full of bad spirits and devils, devilish
thoughts; no better physic for such parties than to fast." [2]
Hildesheim, *Spicil.* 2, to this of hunger, adds "often baths, much
exercise and sweat," [3] but hunger and fasting he prescribes
before the rest. And 'tis indeed our Saviour's oracle, "This
kind of devil is not cast out but by fasting and prayer," which
makes the Fathers so immoderate in commendation of fasting.
"As hunger," saith Ambrose, [4] "is a friend of virginity, so is it
an enemy to lasciviousness, but fullness overthrows chastity
and fostereth all manner of provocations." If thine horse be
too lusty, Hierome adviseth thee to take away some of his
provender; by this means those Pauls, Hilaries, Antonies, and
famous anchorites subdued the lusts of the flesh; by this means
Hilarion "made his ass, as he called his own body, leave
kicking" (so Hierome relates of him in his life [5]), when the
devil tempted him to any such foul offence. By this means
those Indian Brachmanni kept themselves continent: [6] they lay
upon the ground covered with skins, as the redshanks do on
heather, and dieted themselves sparingly on one dish, which
Guianerius would have all young men put in practice; and if
that will not serve, Gordonius [7] would have them soundly
whipped, or, to cool their courage, kept in prison, and there
fed with bread and water till they acknowledge their error and
become of another mind. If imprisonment and hunger will not
take them down, according to the directions of that Theban
Crates, [8] "time must wear it out; if time will not, the last refuge
is an halter." But this, you will say, is comically spoken.
Howsoever, fasting by all means must be still used; and as they
must refrain from such meats formerly mentioned, which cause
venery or provoke lust, so they must use an opposite diet.
Wine must be altogether avoided of the younger sort. [9] So
Plato prescribes, [10] and would have the magistrates themselves
abstain from it, for example's sake, highly commending the

Carthaginians for their temperance in this kind. And 'twas a good edict, a commendable thing, so that it were not done for some sinister respect, as those old Egyptians abstained from wine because some fabulous poets had given out, wine sprang first from the blood of the giants, or out of superstition, as our modern Turks, but for temperance, it being *animæ virus et vitiorum fomes* [a poison of the soul and a stimulant of vice], a plague itself if immoderately taken. Women of old for that cause, in hot countries, were forbid the use of it, as severely punished for drinking of wine as for adultery;[1] and young folks, as Leonicus hath recorded, *Var. hist. lib.* 3, *cap.* 87, 88, out of Athenæus and others, and is still practised in Italy and some other countries of Europe and Asia, as Claudius Minos hath well illustrated in his comment on the 23rd Emblem of Alciat. So choice is to be made of other diet.

> *Nec minus erucas aptum est vitare salaces,*
> *Et quicquid veneri corpora nostra parat.*

> Eringos are not good for to be taken,
> And all lascivious meats must be forsaken.

Those opposite meats which ought to be used are cucumbers, melons, purslane, water-lilies, rue, woodbine, ammi, lettuce, which Lemnius so much commends, *lib.* 2, *cap.* 42, and Mizaldus, *Hort. med.*, to this purpose; vitex, or agnus castus, before the rest, which, saith Magninus,[2] hath a wonderful virtue in it. Those Athenian women, in their solemn feasts called Thesmophories, were to abstain nine days from the company of men, during which time, saith Ælian, they laid a certain herb, named hanea, in their beds, which assuaged those ardent flames of love, and freed them from the torments of that violent passion. See more in Porta, Matthiolus, Crescentius, *lib.* 5, etc., and what every herbalist almost and physician hath written, *cap. de Satyriasi et Priapismo*; Rhasis amongst the rest. In some cases again, if they be much dejected and brought low in body, and now ready to despair through anguish, grief, and too sensible a feeling of their misery, a cup of wine and full diet is not amiss, and, as Valescus adviseth, *cum alia honesta venerem sæpe exercendo*, which Langius, *Epist. med. lib.* 1, *epist.* 24, approves out of Rhasis (*ad assiduationem coitus invitat*), and Guianerius seconds it, *cap.* 16, *tract.* 16, as a very profitable remedy.[3]

> *Tument tibi quum inguina, num si*
> *Ancilla, aut verna præsto est, tentigine rumpi*
> *Malis? non ego namque*, etc.[4]

Jason Pratensis[1] subscribes to this counsel of the poet, *Excretio enim aut tollit prorsus aut lenit ægritudinem*, as it did the raging lust of Ahasuerus, *qui ad impatientiam amoris leniendam, per singulas fere noctes novas puellas devirginavit.*[2] And to be drunk too by fits; but this is mad physic, if it be at all to be permitted. If not, yet some pleasure is to be allowed, as that which Vives speaks of, *lib. 3 de anima*: "A lover that hath as it were lost himself through impotency, impatience, must be called home as a traveller, by music, feasting, good wine, if need be to drunkenness itself, which many so much commend for the easing of the mind, all kinds of sports and merriments, to see fair pictures, hangings, buildings, pleasant fields, orchards, gardens, groves, ponds, pools, rivers, fishing, fowling, hawking, hunting, to hear merry tales and pleasant discourse, reading, to use exercise till he sweat, that new spirits may succeed, or by some vehement affection or contrary passion to be diverted till he be fully weaned from anger, suspicion, cares, fears, etc., and habituated into another course."[3] *Semper tecum sit* (as Sempronius adviseth Callisto his lovesick master[4]), *qui sermones joculares moveat, conciones ridiculas, dicteria falsa, suaves historias, fabulas venustas recenseat, coram ludat, etc.*, still have a pleasant companion to sing and tell merry tales, songs and facete histories, sweet discourse, etc. And as the melody of music, merriment, singing, dancing, doth augment the passion of some lovers, as Avicenna notes,[5] so it expelleth it in others, and doth very much good. These things must be warily applied, as the parties' symptoms vary, and as they shall stand variously affected.

If there be any need of physic, that the humours be altered, or any new matter aggregated, they must be cured as melancholy men. Carolus à Lorme, amongst other questions discussed for his degree at Montpelier in France, hath this: *An amantes et amentes iisdem remediis curentur?* whether lovers and madmen be cured by the same remedies? He affirms it; for love extended is mere madness. Such physic, then, as is prescribed is either inward or outward, as hath been formerly handled in the precedent partition in the cure of melancholy. Consult with Valleriola, *Observat. lib. 2, observ. 7*; Lod. Mercatus, *lib. 2, cap. 4, de mulier. affect.*; Daniel Sennertus, *lib. 1, part. 2, cap. 10*; Jacobus Ferrandus the Frenchman,[6] in his tract *de amore erotico*; Forestus, *lib. 10, observ. 29 and 30*; Jason Pratensis, and others for peculiar receipts. Amatus Lusitanus cured a young Jew, that was almost mad for love, with the

syrup of hellebore, and such other evacuations and purges which
are usually prescribed to black choler;[1] Avicenna confirms as
much if need require, and "blood-letting above the rest,"[2]
which makes *amantes ne sint amentes*, lovers to come to themselves, and keep in their right minds.[3] 'Tis the same which
Schola Salernitana [the School of Salerno], Jason Pratensis,
Hildesheim, etc., prescribe, blood-letting to be used as a principal remedy.   Those old Scythians had a trick to cure all
appetite of burning lust, by letting themselves blood under
the ears, and to make both men and women barren,[4] as Sabellicus
in his *Enneades* relates of them.   Which Salmuth, *tit.* 10 *de
Horol. comment. in Pancirol. de nov. repert.*, Mercurialis, *var.
lec. lib.* 3, *cap.* 7, out of Hippocrates and Benzo, say still is in
use amongst the Indians, a reason of which Langius gives,
lib. 1, *epist.* 10.

Huc faciunt medicamenta venerem sopientia, *ut camphora
pudendis alligata, et in braca gestata (quidam ait) membrum
flaccidum reddit.   Laboravit hoc morbo virgo nobilis, cui inter
cætera præscripsit medicus, ut laminam plumbeam multis fora-
minibus pertusam ad dies viginti portaret in dorso; ad exsiccandum
vero sperma jussit eam quam parcissime cibari, et manducare
frequenter coriandrum præparatum, et semen lactucæ et acetosæ,
et sic eam a morbo liberavit.*   Porro impediunt et remittunt
coitum folia salicis trita et epota, et si frequentius usurpentur
ipsa in totum auferunt.   Idem præstat topazius annulo gestatus,
dexterum lupi testiculum attritum, et oleo vel aqua rosata
exhibitum veneris tædium inducere scribit Alexander Benedictus: lac butyri commestum et semen cannabis, et camphora
exhibita idem præstant.   Verbena herba gestata libidinem
extinguit, pulvisquæ ranæ decollatæ et exsiccatæ.   Ad extin-
guendum coitum, ungantur membra genitalia et renes et pecten
aqua in qua opium Thebaicum sit dissolutum; libidini maxime
contraria camphora est, et coriandrum siccum frangit coitum,
et erectionem virgæ impedit; idem efficit sinapium ebibitum.
*Da verbenam in potu et non erigetur virga sex diebus; utere
mentha sicca cum aceto, genitalia illinita succo hyoscyami aut
cicutæ, coitus appetitum sedant, etc.   ℞ seminis lactuc. portulac.
coriandri an. ʒj menthæ siccæ ʒss sacchari albiss. ʒiiij pul-
veriscentur omnia subtiliter, et post ea simul misce aqua nenupharis, f. confec. solida in morsulis.   Ex his sumat mane unum
quum surgat.*   Innumera fere his similia petas ab Hildesheimo
loco prædicto, Mizaldo, Porta, cæterisque.

SUBSECT. II.—*Withstand the beginnings, avoid occasions, change his place: fair and foul means, contrary passions, with witty inventions: to bring in another, and discommend the former*

Other good rules and precepts are enjoined by our physicians, which, if not alone, yet certainly conjoined may do much; the first of which is *obstare principiis*, to withstand the beginnings. *Quisquis in primo obstitit Pepulitque amorem, tutus ac victor fuit,*[1] he that will but resist at first, may easily be a conqueror at the last.   Balthasar Castilio, *lib.* 4, urgeth this prescript above the rest. "When he shall chance" (saith he) "to light upon a woman that hath good behaviour joined with her excellent person, and shall perceive his eyes with a kind of greediness to pull unto them this image of beauty, and carry it to the heart; shall observe himself to be somewhat incensed with this influence, which moveth within; when he shall discern those subtile spirits sparkling in her eyes to administer more fuel to the fire, he must wisely withstand the beginnings, rouse up reason, stupefied almost, fortify his heart by all means, and shut up all those passages by which it may have entrance." [2] 'Tis a precept which all concur upon.

Opprime dum nova sunt subiti mala semina morbi,
Dum licet, in primo lumine siste pedem.[3]

Thy quick disease, whilst it is fresh to-day,
By all means crush, thy feet at first step stay.

Which cannot speedier be done, than if he confess his grief and passion to some judicious friend (*qui tacitus ardet magis uritur,*[4] the more he conceals, the greater is his pain) that by his good advice may happily ease him on a sudden; and withal to avoid occasions, or any circumstance that may aggravate his disease, to remove the object by all means; for who can stand by a fire and not burn?

Sussilite, obsecro, et mittite istanc foras,
Quæ misero mihi amanti ebibit sanguinem.[5]

[Leap up, ye bolts, and send her out of doors, for the love of her has drained my very life-blood.]

'Tis good therefore to keep quite out of her company, which Hierome so much labours to Paula, to Nepotian; Chrysostom so much inculcates *in ser. in contubern.*, Cyprian, and many other Fathers of the Church, Siracides in his ninth chapter, Jason Pratensis, Savonarola, Arnoldus, Valleriola, etc., and

every physician that treats of this subject.   Not only to avoid,
as Gregory Tholosanus exhorts,[1] "kissing, dalliance, all speeches,
tokens, love-letters, and the like," or as Castilio, *lib.* 4, to
converse with them, hear them speak or sing (*tolerabilius est
audire basiliscum sibilantem,* thou hadst better hear, saith
Cyprian,[2] a serpent hiss), "those amiable smiles, admirable
graces, and sweet gestures," [3] which their presence affords,

> *Neu capita liment solitis morsiunculis,*
> *Et his papillarum oppressiunculis*
> *Abstineant :* [4]

but all talk, name, mention, or cogitation of them, and of
any other women, persons, circumstance, amorous book or tale
that may administer any occasion of remembrance.   Prosper [5]
adviseth young men not to read the Canticles, and some parts
of Genesis at other times; but for such as are enamoured they
forbid, as before, the name mentioned, etc., especially all sight,
they must not so much as come near, or look upon them.

> *Et fugitare decet simulacra et pabula amoris,*
> *Abstinere sibi atque alio convertere mentem.*[6]

> [It is well to avoid all sights that feed love, and to turn
> one's thoughts elsewhere.]

"Gaze not on a maid," saith Siracides, "turn away thine eyes
from a beautiful woman" (*cap.* 9, *v.* 5, 7, 8), *Averte oculos,*
saith David, or if thou dost see them, as Ficinus adviseth, let
not thine eye be *intentus ad libidinem,* do not intend her more
than the rest: for as Propertius holds,[7] *Ipse alimenta sibi
maxima præbet amor* [love provides its own chief nourishment],
love as a snowball enlargeth itself by sight: but as Hierome to
Nepotian, *aut æqualiter ama, aut æqualiter ignora,* either see all
alike, or let all alone; make a league with thine eyes, as Job
did,[8] and that is the safest course, let all alone, see none of
them.   Nothing sooner revives, or "waxeth sore again," as
Petrarch holds,[9] "than love doth by sight.   As pomp renews
ambition, the sight of gold covetousness, a beauteous object
sets on fire this burning lust."   *Et multum saliens incitat unda
sitim.*   The sight of drink makes one dry, and the sight of
meat increaseth appetite.   'Tis dangerous therefore to see.
A young gentleman in merriment would needs put on his
mistress' clothes, and walk abroad alone, which some of her
suitors espying, stole him away for her that he represented.[10]
So much can sight enforce.   Especially if he have been formerly

enamoured, the sight of his mistress strikes him into a new
fit, and makes him rave many days after.

Infirmis causa pusilla nocet,
Ut pene extinctum cinerem si sulphure tangas,
Vivet, et ex minimo maximus ignis erit :
Sic nisi vitabis quicquid renovabit amorem,
Flamma recrudescet, quæ modo nulla fuit.[1]

A sickly man a little thing offends,
  As brimstone doth a fire decayed renew,
And make it burn afresh, doth love's dead flames,
  If that the former object it review.

Or, as the poet compares it to embers in ashes, which the wind
blows, *ut solet a ventis*, etc.,[2] a scald head (as the saying is) is
soon broken, dry wood quickly kindles, and when they have
been formerly wounded with sight, how can they by seeing but
be inflamed? Ismenias acknowledgeth as much of himself,
when he had been long absent, and almost forgotten his mistress,
"at the first sight of her, as straw in a fire, I burned afresh, and
more than ever I did before." [3] Chariclea was as much moved
at the sight of her dear Theagenes, after he had been a great
stranger.[4] Myrtila, in Aristænetus,[5] swore she would never
love Pamphilus again, and did moderate her passion so long
as he was absent; but the next time he came in presence, she
could not contain, *effuse amplexa attrectari se sinit,* etc., she
broke her vow, and did profusely embrace him. Hermotinus,
a young man (in the said author [6]), is all out as unstaid; he had
forgot his mistress quite, and by his friends was well weaned
from her love; but seeing her by chance, *agnovit veteris vestigia*
flammæ, he raved amain, *illa tamen emergens veluti lucida stella*
cœpit elucere, etc., she did appear as a blazing star or an angel
to his sight. And it is the common passion of all lovers to
be overcome in this sort. For that cause belike, Alexander,
discerning this inconvenience and danger that comes by seeing,
"when he heard Darius' wife so much commended for her
beauty, would scarce admit her to come in his sight," [7] fore-
knowing belike that of Plutarch, *formosam videre periculosissi-*
mum, how full of danger it is to see a proper woman; and though
he was intemperate in other things, yet in this *superbe se gessit,*
he carried himself bravely. And so whenas Araspus, in Xenophon, had so much magnified that divine face of Panthea to
Cyrus, "by how much she was fairer than ordinary, by so much
he was the more unwilling to see her." [8] Scipio, a young man of
twenty-three years of age, and the most beautiful of the Romans,

equal in person to that Grecian Clinias, or Homer's Nireus, at the siege of a city in Spain, whenas a noble and most fair young gentlewoman was brought unto him, "and he had heard she was betrothed to a lord, rewarded her, and sent her back to her sweetheart." [1] St. Austin, as Gregory reports of him,[2] *ne cum sorore quidem sua putavit habitandum*, would not live in the house with his own sister. Xenocrates lay with Lais of Corinth all night, and would not touch her. Socrates, though all the city of Athens supposed him to dote upon fair Alcibiades, yet when he had an opportunity *solus cum solo*, to lie [alone] in the chamber with,[3] and was wooed by him besides, as the said Alcibiades publicly confessed,[4] *formam sprevit et superbe contempsit*, he scornfully rejected him. Petrarch, that had so magnified his Laura in several poems, when by the Pope's means she was offered unto him, would not accept of her. "It is a good happiness to be free from this passion of love, and great discretion it argues in such a man that he can so contain himself; but when thou art once in love, to moderate thyself" (as he saith [5]) "is a singular point of wisdom.

> *Nam vitare plagas in amoris ne jaciamur*
> *Non ita difficile est, quam captum retibus ipsis*
> *Exire, et validos Veneris perrumpere nodos.*[6]

> To avoid such nets is no such mastery,
> But ta'en to escape is all the victory.

But, forasmuch as few men are free, so discreet lovers, or that can contain themselves and moderate their passions, to curb their senses, as not to see them, not to look lasciviously, not to confer with them, such is the fury of this headstrong passion of raging lust, and their weakness, *ferox ille ardor a natura insitus*, as he [7] terms it, such a furious desire nature hath inscribed, such unspeakable delight,

> *Sic divæ Veneris furor,*
> *Insanis adeo mentibus incubat,*

> [Love-madness so assaulteth minds diseased,]

which neither reason, counsel, poverty, pain, misery, drudgery, *partus dolor* [pangs of childbirth], etc., can deter them from; we must use some speedy means to correct and prevent that, and all other inconveniences which come by conference and the like. The best, readiest, surest way, and which all approve, is *loci mutatio* [change of place], to send them several ways, that they may neither hear of, see, nor have an opportunity to send to one another again, or live together, *soli cum sola* [entirely by themselves], as so many Gilbertines. *Elongatio a patria* [going abroad], 'tis Savonarola's fourth rule, and Gordonius' precept, *distrahatur ad longinquas regiones*, send him to travel. 'Tis that which most run upon, as so many hounds with full cry, poets, divines, philosophers, physicians, all, *mutet patriam* [let him change his country] (Valesius); as a sick man, he must be cured with change of air (Tully, 4 *Tuscul.*).[1] The best remedy is to get thee gone (Jason Pratensis); change air and soil (Laurentius); *Fuge littus amatum* [shun the well-loved shore] (Virgil); *Utile finitimis abstinuisse locis* [it will be well to keep away from the neighbourhood] (Ovid [2]); *I procul, et longas carpere perge vias* [away, away! go far from hence]; *sed fuge, tutus eris* [in flight thou shalt find safety]. Travelling is an antidote of love:

> *Magnum iter ad doctas proficisci cogor Athenas,*
> *Ut me longa gravi solvat amore via.*[3]

For this purpose, saith Propertius,[4] my parents sent me to Athens; time and patience wear away pain and grief, as fire goes out for want of fuel. *Quantum oculis, animo tam procul ibit amor* [love banished from the eyes will leave the heart]. But so as they tarry out long enough: a whole year Xenophon prescribes Critobulus,[5] *vix enim intra hoc tempus ab amore sanari poteris* [for you can scarce be cured of love in this space]: some will hardly be weaned under. All this Heinsius merrily inculcates in an epistle to his friend Primerius: First fast, then tarry, thirdly, change thy place, fourthly, think of an halter.[6] If change of place, continuance of time, absence, will not wear it out with those precedent remedies, it will hardly be removed: but these commonly are of force. Felix Plater, *Observ. lib.* 1, had a baker to his patient, almost mad for the love of his maid, and desperate; by removing her from him, he was in a short space cured. Isæus, a philosopher of Assyria, was a most dissolute liver in his youth, *palam lasciviens*, in love with all he met; but after he betook himself by his friends' advice to his study, and left women's company, he was so changed that he cared no more for plays, nor feasts, nor masks, nor songs, nor verses, fine clothes, nor no such love-toys: he became a new man upon a sudden, *tanquam si priores oculos amisisset*, (saith mine author [7]) as if he had lost his former eyes. Peter Godefridus, in the last chapter of his third book, hath a story out of St. Ambrose, of a young man, that meeting his old love after long absence, on whom he had extremely doted, would scarce take notice of her;

she wondered at it, that he should so lightly esteem her, called
him again, *lenibat dictis animum* [began to wheedle him], and
told him who she was, *Ego sum, inquit* [I am so-and-so, said
she]; *At ego non sum ego:* but he replied, he was not the same
man; *proripuit sese tandem* [he at length tore himself from her],
as Æneas fled from Dido,[1] not vouchsafing her any farther
parley, loathing his folly, and ashamed of that which formerly
he had done.   *Non sum stultus ut ante jam Neæra:*[2] O Neæra,
put your tricks, and practise hereafter, upon somebody else,
you shall befool me no longer.   Petrarch hath such another
tale of a young gallant, that loved a wench with one eye, and
for that cause by his parents was sent to travel into far countries;
"after some years he returned, and meeting the maid for whose
sake he was sent abroad, asked her how and by what chance
she lost her eye?   No, said she, I have lost none, but you have
found yours"; signifying thereby that all lovers were blind,
as Fabius saith, *Amantes de forma judicare non possunt,* lovers
cannot judge of beauty, nor scarce of anything else, as they will
easily confess, after they return unto themselves by some discontinuance or better advice, wonder at their own folly, madness, stupidity, blindness, be much abashed, "And laugh at love,
and call 't an idle thing," condemn themselves that ever they
should be so besotted or misled, and be heartily glad they
have so happily escaped.

If so be (which is seldom) that change of place will not effect
this alteration, then other remedies are to be annexed, fair and
foul means, as to persuade, promise, threaten, terrify, or to
divert by some contrary passion, rumour, tales, news, or some
witty invention to alter his affection, "by some greater sorrow
to drive out the less,"[3] saith Gordonius, as that his house is
on fire, his best friends dead, his money stolen, "that he is
made some great governor, or hath some honour, office, some
inheritance is befallen him,"[4] he shall be a knight, a baron;
or by some false accusation, as they do to such as have the
hiccup, to make them forget it.   St. Hierome, *lib. 2, epist.* 16,
to Rusticus the monk, hath an instance of a young man of
Greece, that lived in a monastery in Egypt, "that by no labour,
no continence, no persuasion could be diverted, but at last
by this trick he was delivered.   The abbot sets one of his
convent to quarrel with him, and with some scandalous reproach
or other to defame him before company, and then to come
and complain first; the witnesses were likewise suborned for the
plaintiff.   The young man wept, and when all were against him,

the abbot cunningly took his part, lest he should be overcome with immoderate grief: but what need many words? By this invention he was cured, and alienated from his pristine love-thoughts."[1] Injuries, slanders, contempts, disgraces, *spretæque injuria formæ* [the affront of slighted beauty], are very forcible means to withdraw men's affections, *contumelia affecti amatores amare desinunt*, as Lucian saith,[2] lovers reviled or neglected, contemned or misused, turn love to hate. *Redeam? Non si me obsecret*[3] [Return? Not if she asks me on her knees], "I 'll never love thee more." *Egone illam, quæ illum, quæ me, quæ non?* [I love her, who has trifled with him, with me, with whom not?] So Zephyrus hated Hyacinthus because he scorned him, and preferred his corrival Apollo (Palæphatus, *fab. Nar.*). He will not come again though he be invited. Tell him but how he was scoffed at behind his back ('tis the counsel of Avicenna), that his love is false, and entertains another, rejects him, cares not for him, or that she is a fool, a nasty quean, a slut, a vixen, a scold, a devil, or, which Italians commonly do, that he or she hath some loathsome filthy disease, gout, stone, strangury, falling sickness, and that they are hereditary, not to be avoided, he is subject to a consumption, hath the pox, that he hath three or four incurable tetters, issues; that she is bald, her breath stinks, she is mad by inheritance, and so are all the kindred, an hare-brain, with many other secret infirmities, which I will not so much as name, belonging to women. That he is an hermaphrodite, an eunuch, imperfect, impotent, a spendthrift, a gamester, a fool, a gull, a beggar, a whoremaster, far in debt, and not able to maintain her, a common drunkard, his mother was a witch, his father hanged, that he hath a wolf in his bosom, a sore leg, he is a leper, hath some incurable disease, that he will surely beat her, he cannot hold his water, that he cries out or walks in the night, will stab his bed-fellow, tell all his secrets in his sleep, and that nobody dare lie with him, his house is haunted with spirits, with such fearful and tragical things, able to avert and terrify any man or woman living. *Gordonius, cap.* 20, *part.* 2, *hunc in modum consulit: Paretur aliqua vetula turpissima aspectu, cum turpi et vili habitu; et portet subtus gremium pannum menstrualem, et dicat quod amica sua sit ebriosa, et quod mingat in lecto, et quod est epileptica et impudica; et quod in corpore suo sunt excrescentiæ enormes, cum fœtore anhelitus, et aliæ enormitates, quibus vetulæ sunt edoctæ: si nolit his persuaderi, subito extrahat pannum menstrualem,*[4] *coram facie portando, exclamando, Talis est amica tua; et si ex his non*

*demiserit, non est homo, sed diabolus incarnatus. Idem fere
Avicenna, cap. 24, de cura Ilishi, lib. 3, fen. 1, tract. 4. Narrent
res immundas vetulæ, ex quibus abominationem incurrat, et res
sordidas, et hoc assiduent.*[1] *Idem Arculanus, cap. 16, in* 9
Rhasis, etc.

Withal, as they do discommend the old, for the better effecting
a more speedy alteration they must commend another paramour,
alteram inducere, set him or her to be wooed, or woo some other
that shall be fairer, of better note, better fortune, birth, parentage, much to be preferred: *Invenies alium, si te hic fastidit Alexis* [2]
[you will soon find another lover if Alexis here disdains you];
by this means, which Jason Pratensis wisheth, to turn the
stream of affection another way: *Successore novo truditur omnis
amor* [the old love is ever thrust out by the new]; or, as Valesius
adviseth, by subdividing to diminish it,[3] as a great river cut into
many channels runs low at last. *Hortor et ut pariter binas
habeatis amicas* [I recommend you to divide your favour between
two mistresses], etc.[4] If you suspect to be taken, be sure,
saith the poet, to have two mistresses at once, or go from one
to another: as he that goes from a good fire in cold weather is
loath to depart from it, though in the next room there be a
better which will refresh him as much; there 's as much difference
of *hæc* as *hic ignis*; or bring him to some public shows, plays,
meetings, where he may see variety, and he shall likely loathe
his first choice: carry him but to the next town, yea peradventure
to the next house, and as Paris lost Œnone's love by seeing
Helena, and Cressida forsook Troilus by conversing with Dio-
mede, he will dislike his former mistress, and leave her quite
behind him, as Theseus left Ariadne fast asleep in the island
of Dia, to seek her fortune, that was erst his loving mistress.[5]
Nunc primum Dorida vetus amator contempsi, as he said,[6] Doris
is but a dowdy to this. As he that looks himself in a glass
forgets his physiognomy forthwith, this flattering glass of love
will be diminished by remove; after a little absence it will be
remitted, the next fair object will likely alter it. A young man
in Lucian [7] was pitifully in love, he came to the theatre by
chance, and by seeing other fair objects there, *mentis sanitatem
recepit,* was fully recovered, "and went merrily home, as if he
had taken a dram of oblivion." [8] A mouse (saith an apologer)
was brought up in a chest,[9] there fed with fragments of bread
and cheese, thought there could be no better meat, till coming
forth at last, and feeding liberally of other variety of viands,
loathed his former life: moralize this fable by thyself. Plato,

in his seventh book *de legibus*, hath a pretty fiction of a city underground, to which by little holes some small store of light came;[1] the inhabitants thought there could not be a better place, and at their first coming abroad they might not endure the light, *ægerrime solem intueri*, but after they were accustomed a little to it, "they deplored their fellows' misery that lived underground."[2]   A silly lover is in like state; none so fair as his mistress at first, he cares for none but her; yet after a while, when he hath compared her with others, he abhors her name, sight, and memory.   'Tis generally true; for as he observes, *Priorem flammam novus ignis extrudit; et ea mulierum natura, ut præsentes maxime ament:*[3] one fire drives out another; and such is women's weakness, that they love commonly him that is present.   And so do many men; as he confessed, he loved Amy, till he saw Floriat, and when he saw Cynthia, forgat them both; but fair Phyllis was incomparably beyond them all, Chloris surpassed her, and yet when he espied Amaryllis, she was his sole mistress; O divine Amaryllis! *quam procera, cupressi ad instar, quam elegans, quam decens!* etc., how lovely, how tall, how comely she was (saith Polemius) till he saw another, and then she was the sole subject of his thoughts.   In conclusion, her he loves best he saw last.   Triton,[4] the sea-god, first loved Leucothoe, till he came in presence of Milæne; she was the commandress of his heart, till he saw Galatea; but (as she complains [5]) he loved another eftsoons, another, and another. 'Tis a thing which, by Hierome's report, hath been usually practised.   "Heathen philosophers drive out one love with another, as they do a peg, or pin with a pin; which those seven Persian princes did to Ahasuerus, that they might requite the desire of Queen Vashti with the love of others."[6]   Pausanias, *in Eliacis*, saith that therefore one Cupid was painted to contend with another, and to take the garland from him, because one love drives out another, *Alterius vires subtrahit alter amor* [7] and Tully, 3 *Nat. Deor.*, disputing with C. Cotta, makes mention of three several Cupids, all differing in office.   Felix Plater, in the first book of his Observations, boasts how he cured a widower in Basil, a patient of his, by this stratagem alone, that doted upon a poor servant his maid, when friends, children, no persuasion could serve to alienate his mind: they motioned him to another honest man's daughter in the town, whom he loved and lived with long after, abhorring the very name and sight of the first.   After the death of Lucretia, Euryalus "would admit of no comfort, till the

Emperor Sigismund married him to a noble lady of his court,
and so in short space he was freed." [1]

SUBSECT. III.—*By counsel and persuasion, foulness of the fact,
men's, women's faults, miseries of marriage, events of lust, etc.*

As there be divers causes of this burning lust, or heroical
love, so there be many good remedies to ease and help; amongst
which, good counsel and persuasion, which I should have
handled in the first place, are of great moment, and not to be
omitted.　Many are of opinion that in this blind headstrong
passion counsel can do no good.

> *Quæ enim res in se neque consilium neque modum
> Habet, ullo eam consilio regere non potes.* [2]

> Which thing hath neither judgment, or an end,
> How should advice or counsel it amend?

Quis enim modus adsit amori? [3] [How can bounds be set to love?]
But, without question, good counsel and advice must needs be
of great force, especially if it shall proceed from a wise, fatherly,
reverend, discreet person, a man of authority, whom the parties
do respect, stand in awe of, or from a judicious friend, of itself
alone it is able to divert and suffice.　Gordonius the physician
attributes so much to it, that he would have it by all means
used in the first place.　*Amoveatur ab illa, consilio viri quem
timet, ostendendo pericula sæculi, judicium inferni, gaudia Paradisi* [let him be kept away from his beloved, and admonished
by some man of whom he stands in awe of the dangers of the
world, the punishments of hell, the joys of Paradise].　He
would have some discreet men to dissuade them, after the fury
of passion is a little spent, or by absence allayed; for it is as
intempestive at first to give counsel, as to comfort parents
when their children are in that instant departed; to no purpose
to prescribe narcotics, cordials, nectarines, potions, Homer's
nepenthes, or Helen's bowl, etc.　*Non cessabit pectus tundere*
[she will not cease to beat her breast], she will lament and howl
for a season: let passion have his course awhile, and then he
may proceed, by foreshowing the miserable events and dangers
which will surely happen, the pains of hell, joys of Paradise,
and the like, which by their preposterous courses they shall
forfeit or incur; and 'tis a fit method, a very good means;
for what Seneca [4] said of vice, I say of love, *Sine magistro
discitur, vix sine magistro deseritur,* 'tis learned of itself, but

hardly left without a tutor.[1] 'Tis not amiss therefore to
have some such overseer, to expostulate and show them such
absurdities, inconveniences, imperfections, discontents, as usually
follow; which their blindness, fury, madness, cannot apply unto
themselves, or will not apprehend through weakness; and good
for them to disclose themselves, to give ear to friendly admonitions. "Tell me, sweetheart" (saith Tryphæna to a lovesick
Charmides in Lucian [2]), "what is it that troubles thee? peradventure I can ease thy mind, and further thee in thy suit";
and so, without question, she might, and so mayst thou, if
the patient be capable of good counsel, and will hear at least
what may be said.

If he love at all, she is either an honest woman or a whore.
If dishonest, let him read or inculcate to him that fifth of
Solomon's Proverbs, Ecclus. xxvi, Ambrose, *lib.* 1, *cap.* 4, in
his book of Abel and Cain, Philo Judæus, *de mercede mer.*,
Platina's *dial. in Amores*, Espencæus, and those three books of
Pet. Hædus *de contem. amoribus*, Æneas Sylvius' tart epistle,
which he wrote to his friend Nicholas of Wartburg, which he
calls *medelam illiciti amoris* [a cure for illicit love], etc. "For
what's a whore," as he saith,[3] "but a poller of youth, ruin of
men,[4] a destruction, a devourer of patrimonies, a downfall of
honour, fodder for the devil, the gate of death, and supplement
of hell?" *Talis amor est laqueus animæ* [such a love is a snare
for the soul], etc., a bitter honey, sweet poison, delicate destruction, a voluntary mischief, *commixtum cœnum, sterquilinium* [5]
[mere filth].   And as Pet. Aretine's Lucretia, a notable quean,
confesseth: "Gluttony, anger, envy, pride, sacrilege, theft,
slaughter, were all born that day that a whore began her profession"; for, as she follows it, "her pride is greater than a rich
churl's, she is more envious than the pox, as malicious as
melancholy, as covetous as hell.[6]   If from the beginning of the
world any were *mala, pejor, pessima*, bad in the [positive, com-
parative,] superlative degree, 'tis a whore; how many have
I undone, caused to be wounded, slain! O Antonia, thou seest
what I am without, but within, God knows, a puddle of iniquity,
a sink of sin, a pocky quean." [7]   Let him now that so dotes
meditate on this; let him see the event and success of others,
Samson, Hercules, Holofernes, etc.   Those infinite mischiefs
attend it: if she be another man's wife he loves, 'tis abominable
in the sight of God and men; adultery is expressly forbidden
in God's commandment, a mortal sin, able to endanger his soul:
if he be such a one that fears God, or have any religion, he

will eschew it, and abhor the loathsomeness of his own fact.
If he love an honest maid, 'tis to abuse or marry her: if to abuse,
'tis fornication, a foul fact (though some make light of it), and
almost equal to adultery itself.   If to marry, let him seriously
consider what he takes in hand, look before he leap, as the
proverb is, or settle his affections, and examine first the party,
and condition of his estate and hers, whether it be a fit match,
for fortunes, years, parentage, and such other circumstances,
an sit suæ Veneris, whether it be likely to proceed; if not, let
him wisely stave himself off at the first, curb in his inordinate
passion and moderate his desire, by thinking of some other
subject, divert his cogitations.   Or if it be not for his good,
as Æneas, forewarned by Mercury in a dream, left Dido's love,
and in all haste got him to sea:

> *Mnesthea Surgestumque vocat fortemque Cloanthum,*
> *Classem aptent taciti jubet;* [1]

[He calls Mnestheus, Sergestus, and brave Cloanthus,
    and bids them quietly prepare to sail;]

and although she did oppose with vows, tears, prayers, and
imprecation,
> *Nullis ille movetur*
> *Fletibus, aut illas voces tractabilis audit.*

[All her tears move him not, her words fall on deaf ears.]

Let thy Mercury-reason rule thee against all allurements,
seeming delights, pleasing inward or outward provocations.
Thou mayst do this if thou wilt, *pater non deperit filiam, nec
frater sororem*, a father dotes not on his own daughter, a brother
on a sister; and why? because it is unnatural, unlawful, unfit.
If he be sickly, soft, deformed, let him think of his deformities,
vices, infirmities; if in debt, let him ruminate how to pay his
debts: if he be in any danger, let him seek to avoid it: if he
have any lawsuit or other business, he may do well to let his
love-matters alone and follow it, labour in his vocation, whatever it is.   But if he cannot so ease himself, yet let him wisely
premeditate of both their estates; if they be unequal in years,
she young and he old, what an unfit match must it needs be, an
uneven yoke, how absurd and undecent a thing is it, as Lycinus in
Lucian[2] told Timolaus, for an old bald crook-nosed knave to marry
a young wench? how odious a thing it is to see an old lecher!
What should a bald fellow do with a comb, a dumb doter with
a pipe, a blind man with a looking-glass, and thou with such a

wife? How absurd it is for a young man to marry an old wife
for a piece of good! But put case she be equal in years, birth,
fortunes, and other qualities correspondent, he doth desire to
be coupled in marriage, which is an honourable estate, but for
what respects? Her beauty belike, and comeliness of person,
that is commonly the main object, she is a most absolute form,
in his eye at least, *Cui formam Paphia, et Charites tribuere
decorem* [to whom Venus has given beauty and the Graces
charm]; but do other men affirm as much? or is it an error
in his judgment?

> *Fallunt nos oculi vagique sensus,*
> *Oppressa ratione mentiuntur,*[1]

our eyes and other senses will commonly deceive us; it may
be, to thee thyself upon a more serious examination, or after
a little absence, she is not so fair as she seems. *Quædam
videntur et non sunt* [some things do not come up to their
appearance]; compare her to another standing by, 'tis a touchstone to try, confer hand to hand, body to body, face to face,
eye to eye, nose to nose, neck to neck, etc., examine every part
by itself, then altogether, in all postures, several sites, and tell
me how thou likest her. It may be not she that is so fair, but
her coats, or put another in her clothes, and she will seem all
out as fair; as the poet [2] then prescribes, separate her from her
clothes: suppose thou saw her in a base beggar's weed, or else
dressed in some old hirsute attires out of fashion, foul linen,
coarse raiment, besmeared with soot, colly, perfumed with
opoponax, sagapenum, asafœtida, or some such filthy gums,
dirty, about some undecent action or other; or in such a case
as Brassavola the physician [3] found Malatesta, his patient, after
a potion of hellebore which he had prescribed: *Manibus in
terram depositis, et ano versus cælum elevato (ac si videretur
Socraticus ille Aristophanes, qui geometricas figuras in terram
scribens, tubera colligere videbatur), atram bilem in album parietem
injiciebat, adeoque totam cameram, et se deturpabat, ut,* etc., all-to
bewrayed, or worse; if thou saw'st her (I say), wouldst thou
affect her as thou dost? Suppose thou beheldest her in a
frosty morning, in cold weather, in some passion or perturbation
of mind, weeping, chafing, etc., rivelled and ill-favoured to
behold.[4] She many times that in a composed look seems so
amiable and delicious, *tam scitula forma* [of so elegant an
appearance], if she do but laugh or smile, makes an ugly sparrow-
mouthed face, and shows a pair of uneven, loathsome, rotten,

foul teeth: she hath a black skin, gouty legs, a deformed crooked carcass under a fine coat. It may be for all her costly tires she is bald, and though she seem so fair by dark, by candle-light, or afar off at such a distance, as Callicratides observed in Lucian,[1] "if thou should see her near, or in a morning, she would appear more ugly than a beast"; *si diligenter consideres, quid per os et nares et cæteros corporis meatus egreditur, vilius sterquilinium nunquam vidisti* [2] [if you reflect what issues from her mouth and nostrils and the other orifices of her body you will say that you have never seen worse filth]. Follow my counsel, see her undressed, see her, if it be possible, out of her attires, *furtivis nudatam coloribus* [stripped of her stolen colours], it may be she is like Æsop's jay, or Pliny's cantharides,[3] she will be loathsome, ridiculous, thou wilt not endure her sight: or suppose thou saw'st her sick, pale, in a consumption, on her death-bed, skin and bones, or now dead, *cujus erat gratissimus amplexus* [she whose embrace was so agreeable], as Bernard saith, *erit horribilis aspectus* [her aspect will be horrible]:

> *Non redolet, sed olet, quæ redolere solet.*

As a posy she smells sweet, is most fresh and fair one day, but dried up, withered, and stinks another. Beautiful Nireus, by that Homer so much admired, once dead, is more deformed than Thersites, and Solomon deceased as ugly as Marcolphus: thy lovely mistress that was erst *caris carior ocellis*,[4] dearer to thee than thine eyes, once sick or departed, is *vili vilior æstimata cæno*, worse than any dirt or dunghill. Her embraces were not so acceptable as now her looks be terrible: thou hadst better behold a Gorgon's head than Helena's carcass.

Some are of opinion that to see a woman naked is able of itself to alter his affection; and it is worthy of consideration, saith Montaigne the Frenchman in his Essays,[5] that the skilfullest masters of amorous dalliance appoint for a remedy of venerous passions a full survey of the body; which the poet insinuates:

> *Ille quod obscænas in aperto corpore partes
> Viderat, in cursu qui fuit, hæsit amor:*[6]

> The love stood still, that ran in full career,
> When once it saw those parts should not appear.

It is reported of Seleucus, King of Syria, that seeing his wife Stratonice's bald pate, as she was undressing her by chance, he could never affect her after. Remundus Lullius, the physician, spying an ulcer or canker in his mistress' breast, whom he so

dearly loved, from that day following abhorred the looks of
her. Philip the French king, as Nubrigensis, *lib*. 4, *cap*. 24,
relates it, married the King of Denmark's daughter, "and after
he had used her as a wife one night, because her breath stunk,
they say, or for some other secret fault, sent her back again to
her father." [1]   Peter Matthæus, in the life of Louis the Eleventh,
finds fault with our English chronicles,[2] for writing how Margaret, the King of Scots' daughter, and wife to Louis the
eleventh French king, was *ob graveolentiam oris* [because her
breath stunk] rejected by her husband. Many such matches
are made for by-respects, or some seemly comeliness, which
after honeymoon's past turn to bitterness; for burning lust is
but a flash, a gunpowder passion, and hatred oft follows in
the highest degree, dislike and contempt.

> *Cum se cutis arida laxat,*
> *Fiunt obscuri dentes,*[3]

[When the skin shrivels and hangs loose, and the teeth
    blacken,]

when they wax old and ill-favoured, they may commonly no
longer abide them: *Jam gravis es nobis* [thou art distasteful to
me], *begone*; they grow stale, fulsome, loathsome, odious; thou
art a beastly filthy quean, *faciem, Phœbe, cacantis habes,*[4] thou
art *Saturni podex*, withered and dry, *insipida et vetula* [savourless
and old]; *Te quia rugæ Turpant, et capitis nives*[5] [because you are
wrinkled, ugly, and grey], (I say) begone, *portæ patent, pro-
ficiscere*[6] [there is the door, go!].

  Yea, but you will infer, your mistress is complete, of a most
absolute form in all men's opinions, no exceptions can be taken
at her, nothing may be added to her person, nothing detracted,
she is the mirror of women for her beauty, comeliness, and
pleasant grace, unimitable, *meræ deliciæ, meri lepares*, she is
Myrothecium Veneris, Gratiarum pyxis, a mere magazine of
natural perfections, she hath all the Veneres and Graces, *mille
faces et mille figuras* [a thousand torches and a thousand figures],
in each part absolute and complete, *Læta genas, læta os roseum,
vaga lumina læta*[7] [with beautiful cheeks, rosy lips, and sparkling
eyes]; to be admired for her person, a most incomparable, un-
matchable piece, *aurea proles, ad simulacrum alicujus numinis
composita* [a golden progeny, formed after the image of a god],
a phœnix, *vernantis ætatulæ Venerilla*, a nymph, a fairy, like
Venus herself when she was a maid,[8] *nulli secunda*, a mere
quintessence, *flores spirans et amaracum, feminæ prodigium* [with

breath sweet as flowers, an incomparable woman]: put case
she be, how long will she continue? *Florem decoris singuli
carpunt dies:* [1] every day detracts from her person, and this
beauty is *bonum fragile,* a mere flash, a Venice glass, quickly
broken:

> *Anceps forma bonum mortalibus,*
> *. . . exigui donum breve temporis,* [2]

[Beauty to mortals is a gift of doubtful worth—a
short-lived boon,]

it will not last. As that fair flower Adonis,[3] which we call an
anemone, flourisheth but one month, this gracious all-commanding beauty fades in an instant. It is a jewel soon lost,
the painter's goddess, *falsa veritas,* a mere picture. "Favour
is deceitful, and beauty is vanity" (Prov. xxxi, 30).

> *Vitrea gemmula, fluxaque bullula, candida forma est,*
> *Nix, rosa, ros, fumus, ventus et aura nihil.* [4]

A brittle gem, bubble, is beauty pale,
A rose, dew, snow, smoke, wind, air, naught at all.

If she be fair, as the saying is, she is commonly a fool; if proud,
scornful (*sequiturque superbia formam*), or dishonest, *rara est
concordia formæ atque pudicitiæ,* "can she be fair and honest
too?" Aristo, the son of Agasicles, married a Spartan lass,
the fairest lady in all Greece next to Helen, but for her conditions the most abominable and beastly creature of the world.[5]
So that I would wish thee to respect, with Seneca,[6] not her
person but qualities. "Will you say that's a good blade which
hath a gilded scabbard, embroidered with gold and jewels?
No, but that which hath a good edge and point, well-tempered
mettle, able to resist." This beauty is of the body alone, and
what is that but, as Gregory Nazianzen telleth us, "a mock of
time and sickness"? [7] or as Boethius, "as mutable as a flower,
and 'tis not nature so makes us, but most part the infirmity of
the beholder"? [8] For ask another, he sees no such matter:
Dic mihi per gratias qualis tibi videtur, "I pray thee tell me how
thou likest my sweetheart," as she asked her sister in Aristænetus, "whom I so much admire; methinks he is the sweetest
gentleman, the properest man that ever I saw: but I am in love,
I confess (*nec pudet fateri* [nor am I ashamed to confess it]),
and cannot therefore well judge." [9] But be she fair indeed,
golden-haired, as Anacreon his Bathyllus (to examine particulars), she have *Flammeolos oculos, collaque lacteola* [10] [sparkling
eyes, a milk-white neck], a pure sanguine complexion, little

mouth, coral lips, white teeth, soft and plump neck, body, hands, feet, all fair and lovely to behold, composed of all graces, elegancies, an absolute piece:

> *Lumina sint Melitæ Junonia, dextra Minervæ,*
> *Mamillæ Veneris, sura maris dominæ,* etc.; [1]

> [Let Melita have eyes like Juno, hands like Minerva,
> breasts like Venus, a leg like Amphitrite;]

let her head be from Prague, paps out of Austria, belly from France, back from Brabant, hands out of England, feet from Rhine, buttocks from Switzerland, let her have the Spanish gait, the Venetian tire, Italian complement and endowments: [2]

> *Candida sideriis ardescant lumina flammis,*
> *Sudent colla rosas, et cedat crinibus aurum,*
> *Mellea purpureum depromant ora ruborem;*
> *Fulgeat, ac Venerem cœlesti corpore vincat,*
> *Forma dearum omnis,* etc.; [3]

> [Let her eyes flash like the stars, her neck bloom like
> the rose, her hair be brighter than gold, her lips
> be ruddy with the sweetest hue; let her radiate
> beauty more than heavenly Venus, etc.;]

let her be such a one throughout, as Lucian deciphers in his *Imagines*, as Euphranor of old painted Venus, Aristænetus describes Lais, another Helena, Chariclea, Leucippe, Lucretia, Pandora; let her have a box of beauty to repair herself still, such a one as Venus gave Phaon, when he carried her over the ford; let her use all helps art and nature can yield; be like her, and her, and whom thou wilt, or all these in one: a little sickness, a fever, small-pox, wound, scar, loss of an eye or limb, a violent passion, a distemperature of heat or cold, mars all in an instant, disfigures all; child-bearing, old age, that tyrant time, will turn Venus to Erinnys; raging time, care, rivels her upon a sudden; after she hath been married a small while, and the black ox hath trodden on her toe,[4] she will be so much altered, and wax out of favour, thou wilt not know her. One grows too fat, another too lean, etc.; modest Matilda, pretty pleasing Peg, sweet-singing Susan, mincing merry Moll, dainty dancing Doll, neat Nancy, jolly Joan, nimble Nell, kissing Kate, bouncing Bess with black eyes, fair Phyllis with fine white hands, fiddling Frank, tall Tib, slender Sib, etc., will quickly lose their grace, grow fulsome, stale, sad, heavy, dull, sour, and all at last out of fashion. *Ubi jam vultus argutia, suavis suavitatio, blandus, risus* [Where now are the lively looks, the fondling ways, the

winning laugh], etc.?   Those fair sparkling eyes will look dull,
her soft coral lips will be pale, dry, cold, rough, and blue, her
skin rugged, that soft and tender superficies will be hard and
harsh, her whole complexion change in a moment, and as
Matilda writ to King John:[1]

> I am not now as when thou saw'st me last,
> That favour soon is vanished and past;
> That rosy blush lapt in a lily vale,
> Now is with morphew overgrown and pale,

'tis so in the rest, their beauty fades as a tree in winter, which
Deianira hath elegantly expressed in the poet:

> *Deforme solis aspicis truncis nemus?*
> *Sic nostra longum forma percurrens iter,*
> *Deperdit aliquid semper, et fulget minus,*
> *Malisque minus est quicquid in nobis fuit,*
> *Olim petitum cecidit, et partu labat,*
> *Materque multum rapuit ex illa mihi,*
> *Ætas citato senior eripuit gradu.*[2]

> And as a tree that in the greenwood grows,
> With fruit and leaves, and in the summer blows,
> In winter like a stock deformed shows:
> Our beauty takes his race and journey goes,
> And doth decrease, and lose, and come to naught,
> Admir'd of old, to this by child-birth brought:
> And mother hath bereft me of my grace,
> And crooked old age coming on apace.

To conclude with Chrysostom: "When thou seest a fair and
beautiful person, a brave bona-roba, a *bella donna, quæ salivam
moveat, lepidam puellam et quam tu facile ames* [who makes your
mouth water, a dainty maid whom you can easily fall in love
with], a comely woman, having bright eyes, a merry countenance,
a shining lustre in her look, a pleasant grace, wringing thy soul
and increasing thy concupiscence; bethink with thyself that it
is but earth thou lovest, a mere excrement which so vexeth
thee, which thou so admirest, and thy raging soul will be at
rest.   Take her skin from her face, and thou shalt see all
loathsomeness under it, that beauty is a superficial skin and
bones, nerves, sinews; suppose her sick, now rivelled, hoary-
headed, hollow-cheeked, old; within she is full of filthy phlegm,
stinking, putrid, excremental stuff: snot and snivel in her
nostrils, spittle in her mouth, water in her eyes, what filth in
her brains," etc.[3]   Or take her at best, and look narrowly upon
her in the light, stand near her, nearer yet, thou shalt perceive

almost as much, and love less, as Cardan well writes,[1] *Minus amant qui acute vident* [those with a sharp eye love less], though Scaliger deride him for it: if he see her near, or look exactly at such a posture, whosoever he is, according to the true rules of symmetry and proportion, those I mean of Albertus Durer, Lomatius and Taisnier, examine him of her. If he be *elegans formarum spectator* [a good judge of beauty], he shall find many faults in physiognomy, and ill colour: if form, one side of the face likely bigger than the other, or crooked nose, bad eyes, prominent veins, concavities about the eyes, wrinkles, pimples, red streaks, freckons, hairs, warts, næves, inequalities, roughness, scabridity, paleness, yellowness, and as many colours as are in a turkey-cock's neck, many indecorums in their other parts; *est quod desideres, est quod amputes* [you find some things lacking, others superfluous], one leers, another frowns, a third gapes, squints, etc. And 'tis true that he saith,[2] *Diligenter consideranti raro facies absoluta, et quæ vitio caret*, seldom shall you find an absolute face without fault, as I have often observed; not in the face alone is this defect or disproportion to be found, but in all the other parts, of body and mind; she is fair, indeed, but foolish; pretty, comely, and decent, of a majestical presence, but peradventure imperious, unhonest, *acerba, iniqua*, self-willed; she is rich, but deformed; hath a sweet face, but bad carriage, no bringing up, a rude and wanton flirt; a neat body she hath, but it is a nasty quean otherwise, a very slut, of a bad kind. As flowers in a garden have colour some, but no smell, others have a fragrant smell, but are unseemly to the eye; one is unsavoury to the taste as rue, as bitter as wormwood, and yet a most medicinal cordial flower, most acceptable to the stomach; so are men and women; one is well qualified, but of ill proportion, poor and base: a good eye she hath, but a bad hand and foot, *fœda pedes et fœda manus*, a fine leg, bad teeth, a vast body, etc. Examine all parts of body and mind, I advise thee to inquire of all. See her angry, merry, laugh, weep, hot, cold, sick, sullen, dressed, undressed, in all attires, sites, gestures, passions, eat her meals, etc., and in some of these you will surely dislike. Yea, not her only let him observe, but her parents, how they carry themselves: for what deformities, defects, encumbrances of body or mind be in them at such an age, they will likely be subject to, be molested in like manner, they will *patrizare* or *matrizare* [take after the father or the mother]. And withal let him take notice of her companions, *in convictu* (as Guevara prescribes), *et quibuscum conversetur*, whom she converseth with. *Noscitur ex comite, qui non cognoscitur ex se* [he is known from his company who is not known from himself]. According to Thucydides, she is commonly the best, *de quo minimus foras habetur sermo*, that is least talked of abroad. For if she be a noted reveller, a gadder, a singer, a pranker or dancer, then take heed of her. For what saith Theocritus?

> *At vos festivæ ne ne saltate puellæ,*
> *En malus hircus adest in vos saltare paratus.*

> [Ye festal maidens, haste not to your dance;
> A he-goat lies in wait on you to prance.]

"Young men will do it when they come to it," fauns and satyrs will certainly play wreeks, when they come in such wanton Bacchis' or Elenora's presence. Now when they shall perceive any such obliquity, indecency, disproportion, deformity, bad conditions, etc., let them still ruminate on that, and as Hædus adviseth out of Ovid,[1] *earum mendas notent*, note their faults, vices, errors, and think of their imperfections; 'tis the next way to divert and mitigate love's furious headstrong passions, as a peacock's feet and filthy comb, they say, make him forget his fine feathers and pride of his tail; she is lovely, fair, well-favoured, well qualified, courteous and kind, "But if she be not so to me, what care I how kind she be?" I say with Philostratus,[2] *formosa aliis, mihi superba* [beautiful to others, proud to me], she is a tyrant to me, and so let her go. Besides these outward *næves* or open faults, errors, there be many inward infirmities, secret, some private (which I will omit), and some more common to the sex, sullen fits, evil qualities, filthy diseases, in this case fit to be considered; *consideratio fœditatis mulierum, menstruæ imprimis, quam immundæ sunt, quam Savonarola proponit regula septima penitus observandam; et Platina, Dial. amoris, fuse perstringit, Lodovicus Bonacialus, Mulieb. lib. 2, cap. 2, Pet. Hædus, Albertus, et infiniti fere medici.* A lover, in Calcagninus' Apologues, wished with all his heart he were his mistress' ring, to hear, embrace, see, and do I know not what; "O thou fool," quoth the ring, "if thou wer'st in my room, thou shouldst hear, observe, and see *pudenda et pœnitenda*, that which would make thee loathe and hate her, yea, peradventure, all women for her sake."[3]

I will say nothing of the vices of their minds, their pride, envy, inconstancy, weakness, malice, self-will, lightness, insatiable lust, jealousy; "No malice to a woman's" (Ecclus.

xxv, 13), "no bitterness like to hers" (Eccles. vii, 26), and as the
same author urgeth (Prov. xxxi, 10), "Who shall find a virtuous
woman?" He makes a question of it. *Neque jus neque bonum,
neque æquum sciunt, melius, pejus, prosit, obsit, nihil vident, nisi
quod libido suggerit.* "They know neither good nor bad, be it
better or worse" (as the comical poet hath it), "beneficial or
hurtful, they will do what they list."

> *Insidiæ humani generis, querimonia vitæ,*
> *Exuviæ noctis, durissima cura diei,*
> *Pæna virum, nex et juvenum,* etc.[1]

> [A snare to humanity, the affliction of life, the spoliation
> of the night, the greatest trouble by day, the plague
> of husbands, the ruin of young men.]

And to that purpose were they first made, as Jupiter insinuates
in the poet: [2]

> The fire that bold Prometheus stole from me,
> With plagues call'd women shall revenged be,
> On whose alluring and enticing face,
> Poor mortals doting shall their death embrace.

In fine, as Diogenes concludes in Nevisanus, *Nulla est femina
quæ non habeat quid*: they have all their faults.

> Every each of them hath some vice,
> If one be full of villainy,
> Another hath a liquorish eye.
> If one be full of wantonness,
> Another is a chideress.[3]

When Leander was drowned, the inhabitants of Sestos consecrated Hero's lantern to Anteros, *Anteroti sacrum*, and he that
had good success in his love should light the candle: [4] but
never any man was found to light it; which I can refer to
naught but the inconstancy and lightness of women.

> For in a thousand, good there is not one;
> All be so proud, unthankful, and unkind,
> With flinty hearts, careless of others' moan,
> In their own lusts carried most headlong blind,
> But more herein to speak I am forbidden:
> Sometimes for speaking truth one may be chidden.[5]

I am not willing, you see, to prosecute the cause against them,
and therefore take heed you mistake me not, *matronam nullam
ego tango*,[6] I honour the sex, with all good men, and as I ought
to do, rather than displease them, I will voluntarily take the
oath which Mercurius Britannicus took, *Viragin. descript.*[7] *lib. 2,
fol.* 95: *Me nihil unquam mali nobilissimo sexui, vel verbo, vel*

facto machinaturum [I will never plot evil against the most noble sex, either by word or deed], etc. Let Simonides, Mantuan, Platina, Peter Aretine, and such women-haters bear the blame, if aught be said amiss; I have not writ a tenth of that which might be urged out of them and others; *non possunt invectivæ omnes, et satiræ in feminas scriptæ, uno volumine comprehendi* [1] [all the invectives and satires written against women could not be contained in one volume]. And that which I have said (to speak truth) no more concerns them than men, though women be more frequently named in this tract; to apologize once for all, I am neither partial against them, or therefore bitter; what is said of the one, *mutato nomine* [changing the name], may most part be understood of the other. My words are like Pauso's picture in Lucian,[2] of whom, when a good fellow had bespoke an horse to be painted with his heels upwards, tumbling on his back, he made him passant; now when the fellow came for his piece, he was very angry, and said it was quite opposite to his mind; but Pauso instantly turned the picture upside down, showed him the horse at that site which he requested, and so gave him satisfaction. If any man take exception at my words, let him alter the name, read him for her, and 'tis all one in effect.

But to my purpose: If women in general be so bad (and men worse than they), what a hazard is it to marry! where shall a man find a good wife, or a woman a good husband? A woman a man may eschew, but not a wife: wedding is undoing (some say), marrying marring, wooing woeing: "a wife is a fever hectic," as Scaliger calls her, "and not to be cured but by death," [3] as out of Menander, Athenæus adds:

In pelagus te jacis negotiorum . . .
Non Libycum, non Ægeum, ubi ex triginta non pereunt
Tria navigia : ducens uxorem servatur prorsus nemo.

Thou wadest into a sea itself of woes;
In Libyc and Ægean each man knows
Of thirty not three ships are cast away,
But on this rock not one escapes, I say.

The worldly cares, miseries, discontents, that accompany marriage, I pray you learn of them that have experience, for I have none; παῖδας ἐγὼ λόγους ἐγεννησάμην,[4] *libri mentis liberi* [my books are my offspring]. For my part I'll dissemble with him:

Este procul nymphæ, fallax genus este puellæ,
Vita jugata meo non facit ingenio ;
Me juvat, etc.;

[Keep far from me, ye maids, deceitful tribe!
To wedded life me shall ye never bribe;]

many married men exclaim at the miseries of it, and rail at
wives downright; I never tried, but as I hear some of them
say, *Mare haud mare, vos mare acerrimum*,[1] an Irish Sea is not
so turbulent and raging as a litigious wife.

> *Scylla et Charybdis Sicula contorquens freta,*
> *Minus est timenda, nulla non melior fera est.*[2]

> Scylla and Charybdis are less dangerous,
> There is no beast that is so noxious.

Which made the devil belike, as most interpreters hold, when
he had taken away Job's goods, *corporis et fortunæ bona*, health,
children, friends, to persecute him the more, leave his wicked
wife, as Pineda proves out of Tertullian, Cyprian, Austin,
Chrysostom, Prosper, Gaudentius, etc., *ut novum calamitatis
inde genus viro existeret*, to vex and gall him worse *quam totus
infernus*, than all the fiends in hell, as knowing the conditions
of a bad woman. *Jupiter non tribuit homini pestilentius malum*
[Jupiter inflicted on man no worse evil], saith Simonides;
"Better dwell with a dragon or a lion, than keep house with a
wicked wife" (Ecclus. xxv, 16); "Better dwell in a wilderness"
(Prov. xxi, 19); "No wickedness like to her" (Ecclus. xxv, 19);
"She makes a sorry heart, an heavy countenance, a wounded
mind, weak hands, and feeble knees" (verse 25); "A woman
and death are two the bitterest things in the world"; *Uxor
mihi ducenda est hodie, id mihi visus est dicere, Abi domum et
suspende te* [I am to be married to-day, which sounds to me
like saying, "Go home and hang yourself"] (*Ter. And.* 1, 5).
And yet for all this we bachelors desire to be married; with that
vestal virgin, we long for it:

> *Felices nuptæ! moriar, nisi nubere dulce est.*[3]
> [Happy are ye, brides! Upon my soul, 'tis sweet to marry.]

'Tis the sweetest thing in the world, I would I had a wife, saith he,

> For fain would I leave a single life,
> If I could get me a good wife.

Heigh-ho for a husband! cries she; a bad husband, nay, the
worst that ever was, is better than none: O blissful marriage!
O most welcome marriage! and happy are they that are so
coupled: we do earnestly seek it, and are never well till we
have effected it.   But with what fate?   Like those birds in the
emblem,[4] that fed about a cage, so long as they could fly away
at their pleasure, liked well of it; but when they were taken and

might not get loose, though they had the same meat, pined
away for sullenness, and would not eat: so we commend marriage:

> *donec miselli liberi*
> *Aspicimus dominam ; sed postquam heu janua clausa est,*
> *Fel intus est quod mel fuit.*

So long as we are wooers, may kiss and coll at our pleasure,
nothing is so sweet, we are in heaven as we think; but when we
are once tied, and have lost our liberty, marriage is an hell;
"Give me my yellow hose again"; [1] a mouse in a trap lives as
merrily, we are in a purgatory some of us, if not hell itself.
Dulce bellum inexpertis, as the proverb is, 'tis fine talking of war,
and marriage sweet in contemplation, till it be tried: and then
as wars are most dangerous, irksome, every minute at death's
door, so is, etc.   When those wild Irish peers, saith Stanihurst,[2]
were feasted by King Henry the Second (at what time he kept
his Christmas at Dublin), and had tasted of his prince-like
cheer, generous wines, dainty fare, had seen his massy plate
of silver, gold, enamelled, beset with jewels, golden candle-
sticks, goodly rich hangings, brave furniture, heard his trumpets
sound, fifes, drums, and his exquisite music in all kinds; when
they had observed his majestical presence as he sat in purple
robes, crowned, with his sceptre, etc., in his royal seat,[3] the
poor men were so amazed, enamoured, and taken with the object,
that they were *pertæsi domestici et pristini tyrotarichi*, as weary
and ashamed of their own sordidity and manner of life.   They
would all be English forthwith, who but English! but when
they had now submitted themselves, and lost their former
liberty, they began to rebel some of them, others repent of what
they had done, when it was too late.   'Tis so with us bachelors;
when we see and behold those sweet faces, those gaudy shows
that women make, observe their pleasant gestures and graces,
give ear to their siren tunes, see them dance, etc., we think
their conditions are as fine as their faces, we are taken with
dumb signs, *in amplexum ruimus* [we rush into their embraces],
we rave, we burn, and would fain be married.   But when we
feel the miseries, cares, woes, that accompany it, we make our
moan many of us, cry out at length and cannot be released.
If this be true now, as some out of experience will inform us,
farewell wiving for my part, and, as the comical poet merrily
saith:

> *Perdatur ille pessime qui feminam*
> *Duxit secundus, nam nihil primo imprecor!*
> *Ignarus ut puto mali primus fuit.*[4]

> Foul fall him that brought the second match to pass,
> The first I wish no harm, poor man, alas!
> He knew not what he did, nor what it was.[1]

What shall I say to him that marries again and again, *Stulta maritali qui porrigit ora capistro* [2] [who thrusts his foolish head into the marriage halter]? I pity him not, for the first time he must do as he may, bear it out sometimes by the head and shoulders, and let his next neighbour ride, or else run away, or as that Syracusan in a tempest, when all ponderous things were to be exonerated out of the ship, *quia maximum pondus erat* [because she was the greatest burden], fling his wife into the sea. But this I confess is comically spoken, and so I pray you take it.[3] In sober sadness, marriage is a bondage, a thraldom, a yoke, an hindrance to all good enterprises ("He hath married a wife and cannot come"), a stop to all preferments, a rock on which many are saved, many impinge and are cast away: [4] not that the thing is evil in itself or troublesome, but full of all contentment and happiness, one of the three things which please God, "when a man and his wife agree together," [5] an honourable and happy estate, who knows it not? If they be sober, wise, honest, as the poet infers,

> *Si commodos nanciscantur amores,*
> *Nullum iis abest voluptatis genus.*[6]

> If fitly match'd be man and wife,
> No pleasure 's wanting to their life.

But to undiscreet sensual persons, that as brutes are wholly led by sense, it is a feral plague, many times a hell itself, and can give little or no content, being that they are often so irregular and prodigious in their lusts, so diverse in their affections. *Uxor nomen dignitatis, non voluptatis*, as he said,[7] a wife is a name of honour, not of pleasure: she is fit to bear the office, govern a family, to bring up children, sit at board's end and carve, as some carnal men think and say; they had rather go to the stews, or have now and then a snatch as they can come by it, borrow of their neighbours, than have wives of their own; except they may, as some princes and great men do, keep as many courtesans as they will themselves, fly out *impune* [with impunity], *permolere uxores alienas* [8] [violate the wives of other men], [or except] that polygamy of Turks, Lex Julia, which Cæsar once enforced in Rome (though Levinus Torrentius and others suspect it), *uti uxores quot et quas vellent liceret*, that every great man might marry and keep as many wives as

he would, or Irish divorcement, were in use: but as it is, 'tis
hard and gives not that satisfaction to these carnal men, beastly
men as too many are.[1]   What, still the same? to be tied to one,[2]
be she never so fair, never so virtuous, is a thing they may not
endure, to love one long.   Say thy pleasure, and counterfeit
as thou wilt, as Parmeno told Thais,[3] *Neque tu uno eris contenta*,
one man will never please thee; nor one woman many men.
But as Pan replied to his father Mercury, when he asked whether
he was married, *Nequaquam pater, amator enim sum*, etc.,[4] "No,
father, no, I am a lover still, and cannot be contented with one
woman."   Pitys, Echo, [the] Mænades, and I know not how
many besides, were his mistresses, he might not abide marriage.
Varietas delectat [variety pleases], 'tis loathsome and tedious;
what, one still? [that] which the satirist said of Iberina is
verified in most:

> *Unus Iberinæ vir sufficit? ocius illud*
> *Extorquebis ut hæc oculo contenta sit uno.*[5]

'Tis not one man will serve her by her will,
As soon she 'll have one eye as one man still.

As capable of any impression as *materia prima* itself, that still
desires new forms, like the sea their affections ebb and flow.
Husband is a cloak for some to hide their villainy; once married
she may fly out at her pleasure, the name of husband is a
sanctuary to make all good.   *Eo ventum* (saith Seneca) *ut nulla
virum habeat, nisi ut irritet adulterum* [things have come to such
a pass that no woman takes a husband except to spite an
adulterer].   They are right and straight, as true Trojans as
mine host's daughter, that Spanish wench in Ariosto,[6] as good
wives as Messalina.   Many men are as constant in their choice,
and as good husbands, as Nero himself; they must have their
pleasure of all they see, and are in a word far more fickle than
any woman.

> For either they be full of jealousy,
> Or masterful, or loven novelty, etc.

Good men have often ill wives, as bad as Xantippe was to
Socrates, Elenora to St. Louis, Isabella to our Edward the
Second; and good wives are as often matched to ill husbands,
as Mariamne to Herod, Serena to Diocletian, Theodora to
Theophilus, and Thyra to Gurmunde.   But I will say nothing
of dissolute and bad husbands, of bachelors and their vices;
their good qualities are a fitter subject for a just volume, too

well known already in every village, town and city, they need
no blazon; and lest I should mar any matches, or dishearten
loving maids, for this present I will let them pass.

Being that men and women are so irreligious, depraved by
nature, so wandering in their affections, so brutish, so subject
to disagreement, so unobservant of marriage rites, what shall
I say? If thou beest such a one, or thou light on such a wife,
what concord can there be, what hope of agreement? 'tis not
conjugium [marriage] but *conjurgium* [quarrelling], as the
reed and fern in the emblem,[1] averse and opposite in nature;
'tis twenty to one thou wilt not marry to thy contentment:
but as in a lottery forty blanks were drawn commonly for one
prize, out of a multitude you shall hardly choose a good one:
a small ease hence, then, little comfort.

> *Nec integrum unquam transiges lætus diem.*[2]
> [Never shalt thou be one whole day happy.]

> If he or she be such a one,
> Thou hadst much better be alone.

If she be barren, she is not——etc. If she have children, and
thy state be not good, though thou be wary and circumspect,
thy charge will undo thee,[3] *fecunda domum tibi prole gravabit*
[a too fruitful wife will impoverish you with her offspring],
thou wilt not be able to bring them up, "and what greater
misery can there be than to beget children, to whom thou canst
leave no other inheritance but hunger and thirst?"[4] *cum fames
dominatur, strident voces rogantium panem, penetrantes patris
cor* [5] [when hunger overcomes them, they break their father's
heart with their piteous cries for bread]; what so grievous as to
turn them up to the wide world, to shift for themselves? No
plague like to want; and when thou hast good means, and art
very careful of their education, they will not be ruled. Think
but of that old proverb, ἡρώων τέκνα πήματα, *heroum filii
noxæ*, great men's sons seldom do well; *O utinam aut cœlebs
mansissem, aut prole carerem!* [would that I had either remained
single, or not had children!], Augustus exclaims in Suetonius.[6]
Jacob had his Reuben, Simeon and Levi; David an Amnon,
an Absalom, Adonijah; wise men's sons are commonly fools,
insomuch that Spartian concludes, *neminem prope magnorum
virorum optimum et utilem reliquisse filium* [scarce any great
man has left a virtuous and active son]: they had been much
better to have been childless.[7] 'Tis too common in the middle
sort; thy son's a drunkard, a gamester, a spendthrift; thy

daughter a fool, a whore; thy servants lazy drones and thieves;
thy neighbours devils, they will make thee weary of thy life.
"If thy wife be froward when she may not have her will, thou
hadst better be buried alive; she will be so impatient, raving
still, and roaring like Juno in the tragedy, there 's nothing but
tempests, all is in an uproar." [1]   If she be soft and foolish,
thou werst better have a block, she will shame thee and reveal
thy secrets; if wise and learned, well qualified, there is as much
danger on the other side, *Mulierem doctam ducere periculosis-
simum* [it is very dangerous to marry a highly educated woman],
saith Nevisanus,[2] she will be too insolent and peevish:

> *Malo Venusinam quam te, Cornelia mater.*[3]
>
> [I had rather for wife a Venusian wench than thee,
> Cornelia, mother of the Gracchi.]

Take heed; if she be a slut, thou wilt loathe her; if proud,
she 'll beggar thee, "she 'll spend thy patrimony in baubles,
all Arabia will not serve to perfume her hair," saith Lucian;[4]
if fair and wanton, she 'll make thee a cornuto; if deformed,
she will paint.   "If her face be filthy by nature, she will mend
it by art," [5] *alienis et adscititiis imposturis* [by artificial and
factitious adornments], "which who can endure?"   If she do
not paint, she will look so filthy, thou canst not love her, and
that peradventure will make thee unhonest.   Cromerus, *lib.* 12
Hist., relates of Casimirus that he was unchaste because his
wife Aleida, the daughter of Henry, Landgrave of Hesse, was
so deformed.[6]   If she be poor, she brings beggary with her
(saith Nevisanus), misery and discontent.   If you marry a maid,
it is uncertain how she proves: *Hæc forsan veniet non satis apta
tibi* [this one perhaps will prove not suitable for you].   If young,
she is likely wanton and untaught; if lusty, too lascivious; and
if she be not satisfied, you know where and when, *nil nisi
iurgia,* all is in an uproar, and there is little quietness to be
had; if an old maid, 'tis a hazard she dies in childbed; if a rich
widow, *induces te in laqueum,*[7] thou dost halter thyself, she
will make all away beforehand, to her other children, etc.:
Dominam quis possit ferre tonantem? [8] [Who can endure a
virago for a wife?], she will hit thee still in the teeth with her
first husband; if a young widow, she is often unsatiable and
immodest.   If she be rich, well descended, bring a great dowry,
or be nobly allied, thy wife's friends will eat thee out of house
and home, *dives ruinam ædibus inducit,* she will be so proud,
so high-minded, so imperious.   For *nihil est magis intolerabile*

dite, there's nothing so intolerable [as a rich wife]; thou shalt be as the tassel of a goshawk,[1] "she will ride upon thee, domineer as she list," wear the breeches in her oligarchical government, and beggar thee besides.[2] *Uxores divites servitutem exigunt* [rich wives demand submission] (as Seneca hits them, *Declam. lib. 2, declam. 6*). *Dotem accepi, imperium perdidi* [I have gotten a dowry and lost my authority]. They will have sovereignty, *pro conjuge dominam arcessis* [you bring home a tyrant for a wife], they will have attendance, they will do what they list. In taking a dowry thou losest thy liberty, *dos intrat, libertas exit*,[3] hazardest thine estate,

> *Hæ sunt atque aliæ multæ in magnis dotibus*
> *Incommoditates, sumptusque intolerabiles*, etc.,

> [These and many other inconveniences accompany
> large dowries, not to mention the intolerable
> expense, etc.,]

with many such inconveniences: say the best, she is a commanding servant; thou hadst better have taken a good huswife maid in her smock. Since then there is such hazard, if thou be wise keep thyself as thou art, 'tis good to match, much better to be free.

> *Procreare liberos lepidissimum,*
> *Hercle vero liberum esse, id multo est lepidius.*[4]

> ['Tis most pleasant to beget children, but to be free
> is much more pleasant.]

"Art thou young? then match not yet; if old, match not at all."[5]

> *Vis juvenis nubere? nondum venit tempus.*
> *Ingravescente ætate jam tempus præteriit.*

And therefore, with that philosopher,[6] still make answer to thy friends that importune thee to marry, *adhuc intempestivum*, 'tis yet unseasonable, and ever will be.

Consider withal how free, how happy, how secure, how heavenly,[7] in respect, a single man is, as he said in the comedy, *Et isti quod fortunatum esse autumant, uxorem nunquam habui*, "and that which all my neighbours admire and applaud me for, account so great a happiness, I never had a wife"; consider how contentedly, quietly, neatly, plentifully, sweetly, and how merrily he lives! he hath no man to care for but himself, none to please, no charge, none to control him, is tied to no residence, no cure to serve, may go and come, when, whither, live where he will, his own master, and do what he list himself.

Consider the excellency of virgins; *Virgo cœlum meruit* [a virgin merits heaven], marriage replenisheth the earth, but virginity Paradise; [1] Elias, Eliseus, John Baptist, were bachelors: virginity is a precious jewel, a fair garland, a never-fading flower; for why was Daphne turned to a green bay-tree, but to show that virginity is immortal? [2]

> *Ut flos in septis secretus nascitur hortis,*
> *Ignotus pecori, nullo contusus aratro,*
> *Quam mulcent auræ, firmat sol, educat imber,* etc.
> *Sic virgo dum intacta manet, dum cara suis, sed*
> *Cum castum amisit,* etc.[3]

> [Look, how a flower that close in closes grows,
> Hid from rude cattle, bruiséd with no ploughs,
> Which th' air doth stroke, sun strengthen, showers shoot
>   higher, . . .
> So a virgin, while untouched she doth remain,
> Is dear to hers; but when with body's stain
> Her chaster flower is lost, etc.] [4]

Virginity is a fine picture, as Bonaventure calls it,[5] a blessed thing in itself, and if you will believe a Papist, meritorious. And although there be some inconveniences, irksomeness, solitariness, etc., incident to such persons, want of those comforts, *quæ ægro assideat et curet ægrotum, fomentum paret, roget medicum,* [one to sit with him when he is in low spirits, attend to him when he is ill, prepare the poultice, ask the doctor], etc., embracing, dalliance, kissing, colling, etc., those furious motives and wanton pleasures a new-married wife most part enjoys; yet they are but toys in respect, easily to be endured, if conferred to those frequent encumbrances of marriage. Solitariness may be otherwise avoided with mirth, music, good company, business, employment; in a word, *Gaudebit minus, et minus dolebit* [6] [he shall have less joy and less sorrow]; for their good nights, he shall have good days. And methinks some time or other, amongst so many rich bachelors, a benefactor should be found to build a monastical college for old, decayed, deformed, or discontented maids to live together in, that have lost their first loves, or otherwise miscarried, or else are willing howsoever to lead a single life. The rest, I say, are toys in respect, and sufficiently recompensed by those innumerable contents and incomparable privileges of virginity. Think of these things, confer both lives, and consider last of all these commodious prerogatives a bachelor hath, how well he is esteemed, how heartily welcome to all his friends, *quam mentitis obsequiis,* as Tertullian observes, with what counterfeit courtesies they will

adore him, follow him, present him with gifts, *hamatis donis*
[baited gifts]; "it cannot be believed" (saith Ammianus [1])
"with what humble service he shall be worshipped," how
loved and respected. "If he want children" (and have means)
"he shall be often invited, attended on by princes, and have
advocates to plead his cause for nothing," as Plutarch adds.[2]
Wilt thou then be reverenced, and had in estimation?

> *Dominus tamen et domini rex*
> *Si tu vis fieri, nullus tibi parvulus aula*
> *Luserit Æneas, nec filia dulcior illo;*
> *Jucundum et carum sterilis facit uxor amicum.*

> [If you wish to be a lord, let no little boy or darling
> girl play in your halls; a barren wife will make
> you a friend to be sought after.]

Live a single man, marry not, and thou shalt soon perceive
how these *heredipetæ* [legacy-hunters] (for so they were called
of old) will seek after thee, bribe and flatter thee for thy favour,
to be thine heir or executor: Arruntius and Haterius, those
famous parasites in this kind, as Tacitus [3] and Seneca [4] have
recorded, shall not go beyond them. Periplectomenes, that
good personate old man, *delicium senis*, well understood this
in Plautus: for when Pleusides exhorted him to marry that he
might have children of his own, he readily replied in this sort:

> *Quando habeo multos cognatos, quid opus mihi sit liberis?*
> *Nunc bene vivo et fortunate, atque animo ut lubet.*
> *Mea bona mea morte cognatis dicam interpartiant.*
> *Illi apud me edunt, me curant, visunt quid agam, ecquid velim,*
> *Qui mihi mittunt munera, ad prandium, ad cœnam vocant.*

> Whilst I have kin, what need I brats to have?
> Now I live well, and as I will, most brave.
> And when I die, my goods I 'll give away
> To them that do invite me every day,
> That visit me, and send me pretty toys,
> And strive who shall do me most courtesies.

This respect thou shalt have in like manner, living as he did,
a single man. But if thou marry once, *cogitato in omni vita
te servum fore*,[5] bethink thyself what a slavery it is, what a
heavy burden thou shalt undertake, how hard a task thou art
tied to (for, as Hierome hath it, *qui uxorem habet, debitor est,
et uxoris servus alligatus* [he that hath a wife is a debtor, and the
bondman of his wife]), and how continuate, what squalor
attends it, what irksomeness, what charges, for wife and children
are a perpetual bill of charges; besides a myriad of cares, miseries,

and troubles; for as that comical Plautus merrily and truly
said, he that wants trouble must get to be master of a ship, or
marry a wife; and, as another seconds him, "Wife and children
have undone me"; so many and such infinite encumbrances
accompany this kind of life. Furthermore, *uxor intumuit*, etc.,
or as he said in the comedy, *Duxi uxorem, quam ibi miseriam
vidi, nati filii, alia cura* [1] [I married, that was one misery;
children were born, more trouble]. All gifts and invitations
cease, no friend will esteem thee, and thou shalt be compelled
to lament thy misery, and make thy moan with Bartholomæus
Scheræus,[2] that famous poet laureate, and professor of Hebrew
in Wittenberg: "I had finished this work long since, but that
inter alia dura et tristia quæ misero mihi pene tergum fregerunt"
(I use his own words), "amongst many miseries which almost
broke my back, ονζνγια *ob Xantippismum*, a shrew to my wife,
tormented my mind above measure, and beyond the rest." So
shalt thou be compelled to complain, and to cry out at last,
with Phoroneus the lawyer, "How happy had I been, if I had
wanted a wife!" [3] If this which I have said will not suffice,
see more in Lemnius, *lib.* 4, *cap.* 13, *de occult. nat. mir.*; Espencæus, *de continentia, lib.* 6, *cap.* 8; Kornmannus *de virginitate*;
Platina *in Amor. dial.*; *Practica artis amandi*; Barbarus *de re
uxoria*; Arnisæus *in Polit. cap.* 3, and him that is *instar omnium*
[the best of all], Nevisanus the lawyer, *Sylvæ nuptial.* almost
in every page.

Subsect. IV.—*Philters, Magical and Poetical Cures*

Where persuasions and other remedies will not take place,
many fly to unlawful means, philters, amulets, magic spells,
ligatures, characters, charms, which, as a wound with the spear
of Achilles, if so made and caused, must so be cured. If forced
by spells and philters, saith Paracelsus, it must be eased by
characters, *Mag. lib.* 2, *cap.* 28, and by incantations. Fernelius,
Path. lib. 6, *cap.* 13, Sckenkius, *lib.* 4, *Observ. med.*,[4] hath some
examples of such as have been so magically caused, and magically
cured, and by witchcraft: so saith Baptista Codronchus, *lib.* 3,
cap. 9, *de mor. ven.*; *Malleus malef. cap.* 6. 'Tis not permitted
to be done, I confess; yet often attempted: see more in Wierus,
lib. 3, *cap.* 18, *de præstig., de remediis per philtra*; Delrio, *tom.* 2,
lib. 2, *quæst.* 3, *sect.* 3 *Disquisit. magic.* Cardan, *lib.* 16, *cap.* 90,
reckons up many magnetical medicines, as to piss through a
ring, etc. Mizaldus, *cent.* 3, 30, Baptista Porta, Jason Pratensis,

Lobelius, *pag.* 87, Matthiolus, etc., prescribe many absurd remedies. *Radix mandragora ebibitæ, annuli ex ungulis asini, stercus amatæ sub cervical positum, illa nesciente, etc., quum odorem fœditatis sentit, amor solvitur. Noctuæ ovum abstemios facit comestum, ex consilio Iarchæ Indorum gymnosophistæ apud Philostratum, lib. 3. Sanguis amasiæ ebibitus omnem amoris sensum tollit: Faustinam Marci Aurelii uxorem, gladiatoris amore captam, ita penitus consilio Chaldæorum liberatam, refert Julius Capitolinus.* Some of our astrologers will effect as much by characteristical images, *ex sigillis Hermetis, Salomonis, Chælis,* etc., *mulieris imago habentis crines sparsos,* etc. Our old poets and phantastical writers have many fabulous remedies for such as are lovesick, as that of Protesilaus' tomb in Philostratus, in his dialogue between Phœnix and Vinitor: Vinitor, upon occasion discoursing of the rare virtues of that shrine, telleth him that Protesilaus' altar and tomb "cures almost all manner of diseases, consumptions, dropsies, quartan-agues, sore eyes; and amongst the rest, such as are lovesick shall there be helped." [1] But the most famous is Leucata Petra, [2] that renowned rock in Greece, of which Strabo writes, *Geog. lib.* 10, not far from St. Maure's, saith Sandys, *lib.* 1, from which rock if any lover flung himself down headlong, he was instantly cured. [3] Venus after the death of Adonis, when she could take no rest for love, *Cum vesana suas torreret flamma medullas* [4] [when a raging fire burnt in her heart], came to the temple of Apollo to know what she should do to be eased of her pain; Apollo sent her to Leucata Petra, where she precipitated herself, and was forthwith freed; and when she would needs know of him a reason of it, he told her again, that he had often observed Jupiter, when he was enamoured on Juno, thither go to ease and wash himself, [5] and after him divers others. Cephalus for the love of Pelater, Desoneius' daughter, leaped down here; that Lesbian Sappho for Phaon, on whom she miserably doted, *Cupidinis æstro percita e summo præceps ruit* [6] [stung with love-frenzy, flung herself from the height], hoping thus to ease herself, and to be freed of her love-pangs.

> *Hic se Deucalion Pyrrhæ succensus amore*
> *Mersit, et illæso corpore pressit aquas.*
> *Nec mora, fugit amor,* etc. [7]

Hither Deucalion came, when Pyrrha's love
Tormented him, and leapt down to the sea,
And had no harm at all, but by and by
His love was gone and chased quite away.

This medicine Jos. Scaliger speaks of, *Ausoniarum lectionum
lib.* 18, Salmuth *in Pancirol. de* 7 *mundi mirac.*, and other
writers. Pliny reports, that amongst the Cyziceni, there is a
well consecrated to Cupid, of which if any lover taste, his
passion is mitigated: and Anthony Verdurius, *Imag. deorum, de
Cupid.*, saith that amongst the ancients there was *Amor Lethes*
[a love-god presiding over Lethe]; "he took burning torches,
and extinguished them in the river; his statua was to be seen
in the temple of Venus Erycina," of which Ovid makes mention,
and saith "that all lovers of old went thither on pilgrimage,
that would be rid of their love-pangs." [1] Pausanias, *in Phocicis*,[2]
writes of a temple dedicated *Veneri in spelunca*, to Venus in
the vault, at Naupactus in Achaia (now Lepanto), in which
your widows that would have second husbands made their
supplications to the goddess; all manner of suits concerning
lovers were commenced, and their grievances helped. The
same author, *in Achaicis*, tells as much of the river Selemnus [3]
in Greece; if any lover washed himself in it, by a secret virtue
of that water (by reason of the extreme coldness belike) he was
healed of love's torments:

> *Amoris vulnus sanat idem qui facit;* [4]

> [He that causes love's wound also heals it;]

which if it be so, that water, as he holds, is *omni auro pretiosior*,
better than any gold. Where none of all these remedies will
take place, I know no other but that all lovers must make an
head and rebel, as they did in Ausonius,[5] and crucify Cupid
till he grant their request, or satisfy their desires.

SUBSECT. V.—*The last and best Cure of Love-Melancholy is, to
let them have their Desire*

The last refuge and surest remedy, to be put in practice in
the utmost place, when no other means will take effect, is to
let them go together, and enjoy one another: *Potissima cura
est ut heros amasia sua potiatur* [the most effective cure is to
let the lover enjoy his sweetheart], saith Guianerius, *cap.* 15,
tract. 15. Æsculapius himself, to this malady, cannot invent
a better remedy, *quam ut amanti cedat amatum* (Jason Pratensis [6]),
than that a lover have his desire.

> *Et pariter torulo bini jungantur in uno,*
> *Et pulchro detur Æneæ Lavinia conjux.*

> And let them both be joined in a bed,
> And let Æneas fair Lavinia wed.

'Tis the special cure, to let them bleed in *vena hymenæia*, for love is a pleurisy, and if it be possible, so let it be, *optataque gaudia carpant* [and let them enjoy their longed-for bliss]. Arculanus holds it the speediest and the best cure,[1] 'tis Savonarola's last precept,[2] a principal infallible remedy, the last, sole, and safest refuge.

> *Julia, sola potes nostras extinguere flammas,*
> *Non nive, non glacie, sed potes igne pari.*[3]

> Julia alone can quench my desire,
> With neither ice nor snow, but with like fire.

When you have all done, saith Avicenna,[4] "there is no speedier or safer course than to join the parties together according to their desires and wishes, the custom and form of law; and so we have seen him quickly restored to his former health, that was languished away to skin and bones; after his desire was satisfied, his discontent ceased, and we thought it strange; our opinion is therefore that in such cases nature is to be obeyed." Aretæus, an old author, *lib. 3, cap. 3*, hath an instance of a young man, when no other means could prevail, was so speedily relieved.[5] What remains then but to join them in marriage?

> *Tunc et basia morsiunculasque*
> *Surreptim dare, mutuos fovere*
> *Amplexus licet, et licet jocari;*[6]

> [Then to snatch kisses and bite playfully, to cuddle
> and play;]

they may then kiss and coll, lie and look babies in one another's eyes, as their sires before them did; they may then satiate themselves with love's pleasures, which they have so long wished and expected;

> *Atque uno simul in toro quiescant,*
> *Conjuncto simul ore suavientur,*
> *Et somnos agitent quiete in una.*

> [And they may rest together on one couch, their lips
> joined in a kiss, and so sleep peacefully together.]

Yea, but *hic labor, hoc opus* [there's the rub], this cannot conveniently be done, by reason of many and several impediments. Sometimes both parties themselves are not agreed; parents, tutors, masters, guardians, will not give consent; laws,

customs, statutes hinder; poverty, superstition, fear and suspicion; many men dote on one woman, *semel et simul* [all
together]; she dotes as much on him, or them, and in modesty
must not, cannot woo, as unwilling to confess as willing to
love; she dare not make it known, show her affection, or speak
her mind. And "hard is the choice" (as it is in Euphues)
"when one is compelled either by silence to die with grief, or
by speaking to live with shame." In this case almost was the
fair Lady Elizabeth, Edward the Fourth his daughter, when she
was enamoured on Henry the Seventh, that noble young prince,
and new saluted king, when she brake forth into that passionate
speech: "O that I were worthy of that comely prince! but my
father being dead, I want friends to motion such a matter.
What shall I say? I am all alone, and dare not open my mind
to any. What if I acquaint my mother with it? bashfulness
forbids. What if some of the lords? audacity wants. O that I
might but confer with him, perhaps in discourse I might let slip
such a word that might discover mine intention!" [1] How many
modest maids may this concern! I am a poor servant, what
shall I do? I am a fatherless child, and want means, I am
blithe and buxom, young and lusty, but I have never a suitor,
Expectant stolidi ut ego illos rogatum veniam, as she said,[2] a
company of silly fellows look belike that I should woo them and
speak first: fain they would and cannot woo, *quæ primum exordia
sumam?* [3] [how shall I make a beginning?] being merely passive
they may not make suit, with many such lets and inconveniences,
which I know not; what shall we do in such a case? sing
"Fortune my foe"?

Some are so curious in this behalf, as those old Romans,
our modern Venetians, Dutch and French, that if two parties
dearly love, the one noble, the other ignoble, they may not by
their laws match, though equal otherwise in years, fortunes,
education, and all good affection. In Germany, except they
can prove their gentility by three descents, they scorn to match
with them. A nobleman must marry a noblewoman: a baron,
a baron's daughter; a knight, a knight's; a gentleman, a gentleman's: as slaters sort their slates,[4] do they degrees and families.
If she be never so rich, fair, well qualified otherwise, they will
make him forsake her. The Spaniards abhor all widows; the
Turks repute them old women if past five-and-twenty. But
these are too severe laws, and strict customs, *dandum aliquid
amori* [something must be allowed to love], we are all the sons
of Adam, 'tis opposite to nature, it ought not to be so. Again,

he loves her most impotently, she loves not him, and so *e contra*.
Pan loved Echo, Echo Satyrus, Satyrus Lyda.

> *Quantum ipsorum aliquis amantem oderat,*
> *Tantum ipsius amans odiosus erat.*[1]

They love and loathe of all sorts, he loves her, she hates him,
and is loathed of him on whom she dotes.   Cupid hath two
darts, one to force love, all of gold, and that sharp: *Quod facit
auratum est*; another blunt, of lead, and that to hinder: *fugat
hoc, facit illud amorem.*[2]   This we see too often verified in our
common experience.   Coresus dearly loved that virgin Callir-
rhoe, but the more he loved her, the more she hated him.[3]
Œnone loved Paris, but he rejected her; they are stiff of all
sides, as if beauty were therefore created to undo or be undone.
I give her all attendance, all observance, I pray and entreat,
Alma, precor, miserere mei,[4] fair mistress, pity me, I spend
myself, my time, friends, and fortunes to win her favour (as
he complains in the eclogue [5]), I lament, sigh, weep, and make
my moan to her, but she is hard as flint, *cautibus Ismariis
immotior* [more immovable than the rocks of Ismarus], as fair
and hard as a diamond, she will not respect, *Despectus tibi
sum* [I am contemned of you], or hear me:

> *Fugit illa vocantem*
> *Nil lacrimas miserata meas, nil flexa querelis.*

> [I call her, but she flees, unmoved by my tears, deaf
> to my laments.]

What shall I do?

> I wooed her as a young man should do,
> But Sir, she said, I love not you.

> *Durior at scopulis mea Cælia, marmore, ferro,*
> *Robore, rupe, antro, cornu, adamante, gelu.*[6]

> Rock, marble, heart of oak with iron barr'd,
> Frost, flint or adamants, are not so hard.

I give, I bribe, I send presents, but they are refused,

> *Rusticus es Corydon, nec munera curat Alexis.*[7]

> [Corydon is but a lout; Alexis heeds not his gifts.]

I protest, I swear, I weep,

> *Odioque rependit amores,*
> *Irrisu lacrimas;* [8]

> [And she repays my love with hate, my tears with
> mocking laughter;]

she neglects me for all this, she derides me, contemns me, she hates me, "Phillida flouts me": *Caute, feris, quercu durior Eurydice* [Eurydice is harder than rocks, than trees, than wild beasts], stiff, churlish, rocky still.

And 'tis most true, many gentlewomen are so nice, they scorn all suitors, crucify their poor paramours, and think nobody good enough for them, as dainty to please as Daphne herself:

> *Multi illam petiere, illa aspernata petentes,*
> *Nec quid Hymen, quid amor, quid sint connubia curat.*[1]

> Many did woo her, but she scorn'd them still,
> And said she would not marry by her will.

One while they will not marry, as they say at least (whenas they intend nothing less), another while not yet, when 'tis their only desire, they rave upon it. She will marry at last, but not him: he is a proper man indeed, and well qualified, but he wants means; another of her suitors hath good means, but he wants wit; one is too old, another too young, too deformed, she likes not his carriage; a third too loosely given, he is rich, but base-born: she will be a gentlewoman, a lady, as her sister is, as her mother is; she is all out as fair, as well brought up, hath as good a portion, and she looks for as good a match, as Matilda or Dorinda: if not, she is resolved as yet to tarry, so apt are young maids to boggle at every object, so soon won or lost with every toy, so quickly diverted, so hard to be pleased. In the meantime, *quot torsit amantes!* [how many lovers has she tortured!]; one suitor pines away, languisheth in love, *mori quot denique cogit!* [how many has she forced to kill themselves!]; another sighs and grieves, she cares not; and which Stroza[2] objected to Ariadne,

> *Nec magis Euryali gemitu, lacrimisque moveris,*
> *Quam prece turbati flectitur ora sali.*
> *Tu juvenem, quo non formosior alter in urbe,*
> *Spernis, et insano cogis amore mori,*

> Is no more mov'd with those sad sighs and tears,
> Of her sweetheart, then raging sea with prayers:
> Thou scorn'st the fairest youth in all our city,
> And mak'st him almost mad for love to die.

They take a pride to prank up themselves, to make young men enamoured, *captare viros et spernere captos*[3] [to bring men to their feet and then spurn them], to dote on them, and to run mad for their sakes,

Sed nullis illa movetur
Fletibus, aut voces ullas tractabilis audit.[1]

Whilst niggardly their favours they discover.
They love to be belov'd, yet scorn the lover.

All suit and service is too little for them, presents too base:

Tormentis gaudet amantis
Et spoliis.

[She gloats over the torments of her lover—and his spoils.]

As Atalanta, they must be overrun, or not won. Many young
men are as obstinate, and as curious in their choice, as tyranni-
cally proud, insulting, deceitful, false-hearted, as irrefragable
and peevish on the other side; Narcissus-like:

Multi illum juvenes, multæ petiere puellæ,
Sed fuit in tenera tam dira superbia forma,
Nulli illum juvenes, nullæ petiere puellæ.[2]

Young men and maids did to him sue,
But in his youth, so proud, so coy was he,
Young men and maids bade him adieu.

Echo wept and wooed him by all means above the rest, "Love
me for pity, or pity me for love," but he was obstinate: *Ante,*
ait, emoriar quam sit tibi copia nostri, he would rather die than
give consent. Psyche ran whining after Cupid:

Formosum tua te Psyche formosa requirit,
Et poscit te dia deum, puerumque puella; [3]

Fair Cupid, thy fair Psyche to thee sues,
A lovely lass a fine young gallant woos;

but he rejected her nevertheless. Thus many lovers do hold
out so long, doting on themselves, stand in their own light,
till in the end they come to be scorned and rejected, as Stroza's
Gargiliana was,

Te juvenes, te odere senes desertaque langues,
Quæ fueras procerum publica cura prius,

Both young and old do hate thee scorned now,
That once was all their joy and comfort too,

as Narcissus was himself,

Who, despising many,
Died ere he could enjoy the love of any.

They begin to be contemned themselves of others, as he was of
his shadow, and take up with a poor curate, or an old serving-

man at last, that might have had their choice of right good
matches in their youth; like that generous mare in Plutarch,[1]
which would admit of none but great horses, but when her tail
was cut off and mane shorn close, and she now saw herself so
deformed in the water when she came to drink, *ab asino conscendi se passa*, she was contented at last to be covered by an
ass. Yet this is a common humour, will not be left, and
cannot be helped.

> *Hanc volo quæ non vult, illam quæ vult ego nolo:*
> *Vincere vult animos, non satiare Venus.*[2]

> I love a maid, she loves me not: full fain
> She would have me, but I not her again;
> So love to crucify men's souls is bent:
> But seldom doth it please or give content.

Their love danceth in a ring, and Cupid hunts them round
about; he dotes, is doted on again, *Dumque petit petitur, pari-
terque accedit et ardet* [he woos and is wooed, he feels and kindles
love], their affection cannot be reconciled. Oftentimes they
may and will not, 'tis their own foolish proceeding that mars
all, they are too distrustful of themselves, too soon dejected:
say she be rich, thou poor; she young, thou old; she lovely and
fair, thou most ill-favoured and deformed; she noble, thou base;
she spruce and fine, but thou an ugly clown: *nil desperandum*,
there's hope enough yet: *Mopso Nisa datur, quid non speremus
amantes?* [Nisa is affianced to Mopsus: what may not we lovers
hope for?] Put thyself forward once more, as unlikely matches
have been and are daily made, see what will be the event.
Many leave roses and gather thistles, loathe honey and love
verjuice: our likings are as various as our palates. But commonly they omit opportunities, *Oscula qui sumpsit* [he who
snatched kisses], etc., they neglect the usual means and times.

> He that will not when he may,
> When he will he shall have nay.

They look to be wooed, sought after, and sued to. Most part
they will and cannot, either for the above-named reasons, or
for that there is a multitude of suitors equally enamoured,
doting all alike; and where one alone must speed, what shall
become of the rest? Hero was beloved of many, but one did
enjoy her; Penelope had a company of suitors, yet all missed
of their aim. In such cases he or they must wisely and warily
unwind themselves, unsettle his affections by those rules above
prescribed—*Quin . . . stultos excutit ignes?*[3] [Why does he not

drive out the foolish passion?]—divert his cogitations, or else bravely bear it out (as Turnus did: *Tua sit Lavinia conjux* [let Lavinia be your wife]; when he could not get her, with a kind of heroical scorn he bid Æneas take her), or with a milder farewell, let her go, *Et Phyllida solus habeto* [have Phyllis for yourself], take her to you, God give you joy, sir.   The fox in the emblem would eat no grapes, but why? because he could not get them; care not then for that which may not be had.

Many such inconveniences, lets, and hindrances there are, which cross their projects, and crucify poor lovers, which sometimes may, sometimes again cannot, be so easily removed. But put case they be reconciled all, agreed hitherto, suppose this love or good liking be betwixt two alone, both parties well pleased, there is *mutuus amor*, mutual love and great affection, yet their parents, guardians, tutors, cannot agree; thence all is dashed, the match is unequal: one rich, another poor; *durus pater*, an hard-hearted, unnatural, a covetous father will not marry his son, except he have so much money, *ita in aurum omnes insaniunt* [every one is so mad for money], as Chrysostom notes,[1] nor join his daughter in marriage, to save her dowry, or for that he cannot spare her for the service she doth him, and is resolved to part with nothing whilst he lives, not a penny; though he may peradventure well give it, he will not till he dies, and then, as a pot of money broke, it is divided amongst them that gaped after it so earnestly.   Or else he wants means to set her out, he hath no money, and though it be to the manifest prejudice of her body and soul's health, he cares not, he will take no notice of it, she must and shall tarry. Many slack and careless parents, *iniqui patres*, measure their children's affections by their own, they are now cold and decrepit themselves, past all such youthful conceits, and they will therefore starve their children's genius, have them *a pueris illico nasci senes* [2] [be old before they are young], they must not marry, *nec earum affines esse rerum quas secum fert adolescentia: ex sua libidine moderatur quæ est nunc, non quæ olim fuit*, as he said in the comedy: they will stifle nature, their young bloods must not participate of youthful pleasures, but be as they are themselves, old on a sudden.   And 'tis a general fault amongst most parents in bestowing of their children; the father wholly respects wealth; when through his folly, riot, indiscretion, he hath embezzled his estate, to recover himself he confines and prostitutes his eldest son's love and affection to some fool, or ancient or deformed piece, for money:

Phanocratæ ducet filiam, rufam illam virginem,
Cæsiam, sparso ore, adunco naso; [1]

[He shall marry the daughter of Phanocrates, that red-
haired, blear-eyed girl with the big mouth and
hooked nose;]

and though his son utterly dislike, with Clitipho in the comedy,
Non possum, pater [Father, I cannot]: if she be rich, *Eia* (he
replies), *ut elegans est, credas animum ibi esse* [look how dainty
she is; you would think she is a spirit]; he must and shall have
her, she is fair enough, young enough; if he look or hope to
inherit his lands, he shall marry, not when or whom he loves,
Archonidis hujus filiam [the daughter of Archonides here], but
whom his father commands, when and where he likes, his
affection must dance attendance upon him. His daughter is
in the same predicament forsooth; as an empty boat she must
carry what, where, when, and whom her father will. So that
in these businesses the father is still for the best advantage;
now the mother respects good kindred, most part the son a
proper woman. All which Livy exemplifies, *dec.* 1, *lib.* 4: [2]
a gentleman and a yeoman wooed a wench in Rome (contrary
to that statute that the gentry and commonalty must not
match together); the matter was controverted: the gentleman
was preferred by the mother's voice, *quæ quam splendissimis
nuptiis jungi puellam volebat* [who desired the most brilliant
match for her daughter]; the overseers stood for him that was
most worth, etc. But parents ought not be so strict in this
behalf; beauty is a dowry of itself all-sufficient, *Virgo formosa,
etsi oppido pauper, abunde dotata est* [3] [a girl with beauty, however poor, has sufficient dowry], Rachel was so married to
Jacob,[4] and Bonaventure, *in* 4 *sent.,* "denies that he so much
as venially sins, that marries a maid for comeliness of person." [5]
The Jews (Deut. xxi, 11), if they saw amongst the captives a
beautiful woman, some small circumstances observed, might
take her to wife. They should not be too severe in that kind,
especially if there be no such urgent occasion, or grievous
impediment. 'Tis good for a commonwealth, Plato holds, that
in their contracts "young men should never avoid the affinity
of poor folks, or seek after rich." [6] Poverty and base parentage
may be sufficiently recompensed by many other good qualities,
modesty, virtue, religion, and choice bringing up. "I am poor,
I confess, but am I therefore contemptible, and an abject?
Love itself is naked, the Graces, the stars, and Hercules clad
in a lion's skin." [7] Give something to virtue, love, wisdom,

favour, beauty, person; be not all for money. Besides, you
must consider that *Amor cogi non potest,* love cannot be compelled, they must affect as they may: *Fatum est in partibus
illis quas sinus abscondit* [1] [one's fate is in that part of the
anatomy which the upper fold of the toga covers]; as the
saying is, marriage and hanging goes by destiny, matches are
made in heaven.

> It lies not in our power to love or hate,
> For will in us is overrul'd by fate.

A servant maid in Aristænetus [2] loved her mistress' minion,
which when her dame perceived, *furiosa æmulatione,* in a jealous
humour she dragged her about the house by the hair of the
head, and vexed her sore. The wench cried out, "O mistress,
fortune hath made my body your servant, but not my soul!" [3]
Affections are free, not to be commanded. Moreover, it may
be to restrain their ambition, pride, and covetousness, to correct
those hereditary diseases of a family, God in His just judgment
assigns and permits such matches to be made. For I am of
Plato and Bodine's mind,[4] that families have their bounds and
periods as well as kingdoms, beyond which for extent or continuance they shall not exceed, six or seven hundred years, as
they there illustrate by a multitude of examples, and which
Peucer and Melancthon [5] approve, but in a perpetual tenor (as
we see by many pedigrees of knights, gentlemen, yeomen)
continue as they began, for many descents with little alteration.
Howsoever, let them, I say, give something to youth, to love;
they must not think they can fancy whom they appoint; *Amor
enim non imperatur, affectus liber si quis alius et vices exigens,*[6]
this is a free passion, as Pliny said in a panegyric of his, and may
not be forced. Love craves liking, as the saying is, it requires
mutual affections, a correspondency: *invito non datur nec
aufertur* [it can neither be given nor taken away against one's
will], it may not be learned, Ovid himself cannot teach us how
to love, Solomon describe, Apelles paint, or Helena express it.
They must not therefore compel or intrude; *quis enim* (as Fabius
urgeth [7]) *amare alieno animo potest?* [for who can love against
the grain?] but consider withal the miseries of enforced marriages,
take pity upon youth; and such above the rest as have daughters
to bestow, should be very careful and provident to marry them
in due time. Siracides, *cap.* 7, *vers.* 25, calls it "a weighty
matter to perform, so to marry a daughter to a man of understanding in due time." *Virgines enim tempestive locandæ,* as
Lemnius admonisheth, *lib.* 1 *cap.* 6, virgins must be provided

for in season, to prevent many diseases, of which [1] Rodericus à
Castro, *de morbis mulierum, lib. 2, cap. 3*, and Lod. Mercatus,
lib. 2 de mulier. affect. cap. 4, de melanch. virginum et viduarum,
have both largely discoursed.[2]   And therefore as well to avoid
these feral maladies, 'tis good to get them husbands betimes,
as to prevent some other gross inconveniences, and for a thing
that I know besides; *ubi nuptiarum tempus et ætas advenerit*
[when marriageable age has been reached], as Chrysostom
adviseth, let them not defer it; they perchance will marry
themselves else, or do worse.   If Nevisanus the lawyer do not
impose, they may do it by right; for as he proves out of Curtius
and some other civilians, *Sylvæ nup. lib. 2, numer. 30*, "A maid
past twenty-five years of age, against her parents' consent may
marry such a one as is unworthy of, and inferior to her, and her
father by law must be compelled to give her a competent
dowry." [3]   Mistake me not in the meantime, or think that I
do apologize here for any headstrong, unruly, wanton flirts.
I do approve that of St. Ambrose (*Comment. in Genesis xxiv*, 51),
which he hath written touching Rebecca's spousals: "A woman
should give unto her parents the choice of her husband, lest
she be reputed to be malapert and wanton, [4] if she take upon
her to make her own choice; for she should rather seem to be
desired by a man than to desire a man herself. [5]   To those
hard parents alone I retort that of Curtius, in the behalf of
modester maids, that are too remiss and careless of their due
time and riper years.   For if they tarry longer, to say truth,
they are past date, and nobody will respect them.   "A woman
with us in Italy" (saith Aretine's Lucretia), "twenty-four years
of age, is old already, past the best, of no account." [6]   An old
fellow, as Lysistrata confesseth in Aristophanes,[7] *etsi sit canus,
cito puellam virginem ducat uxorem* [in spite of his grey hairs,
can soon marry a young girl], and 'tis no news for an old fellow
to marry a young wench; but as he follows it, *mulieris brevis
occasio est, et si hoc non apprehenderit, nemo vult ducere uxorem,
expectans vero sedet* [a woman's chance does not last long; if
she does not seize it, no one will have her, she can sit and wait];
who cares for an old maid? she may sit, etc.   A virgin, as the
poet holds, *lasciva et petulans puella virgo* [a wanton and froward
maid], is like a flower, a rose withered on a sudden.

> *Quam modo nascentem rutilus conspexit Eous,*
>   *Hanc rediens sero vespere vidit anum.*[8]

She that was erst a maid as fresh as May,
Is now an old crone, time so steals away.

Let them take time then while they may, make advantage of
youth, and as he prescribes,

> *Collige, virgo, rosas dum flos novus et nova pubes,*
> *Et memor esto ævum sic properare tuum.*[1]

> Fair maids, go gather roses in the prime,
> And think that as a flower so goes on time.

Let's all love, *dum vires annique sinunt*, while we are in the
flower of years, fit for love-matters, and while time serves; for

> *Soles occidere et redire possunt,*
> *Nobis cum semel occidit brevis lux,*
> *Nox est perpetuo una dormienda.*[2]

> Suns that set may rise again,
> But if once we lose this light,
> 'Tis with us perpetual night.[3]

Volat irrevocabile tempus, time past cannot be recalled. But
we need no such exhortation, we are all commonly too forward:
yet if there be any escape, and all be not as it should, as Diogenes
struck the father when the son swore, because he taught him
no better, if a maid or young man miscarry, I think their parents
oftentimes, guardians, overseers, governors—*Neque vos* (saith
Chrysostom[4]) *a supplicio immunes evadetis, si non statim ad
nuptias*, etc.—are in as much fault, and as severely to be
punished as their children, in providing for them no sooner.

Now for such as have free liberty to bestow themselves, I
could wish that good counsel of the comical old man were
put in practice,

> *Opulentiores pauperiorum ut filias*
> *Indotatas ducant uxores domum:*
> *Et multo fiat civitas concordior,*
> *Et invidia nos minore utamur quam utimur.*[5]

> That rich men would marry poor maidens some,
> And that without dowry, and so bring them home,
> So would much concord be in our city,
> Less envy should we have, much more pity.

If they would care less for wealth, we should have much more
content and quietness in a commonwealth. Beauty, good
bringing up, methinks, is a sufficient portion of itself, *Dos est
sua forma puellis*[6] [their beauty is the maidens' dower], and
he doth well that will accept of such a wife. Eubulides, in
Aristænetus,[7] married a poor man's child, *facie non illætabili*,
of a merry countenance and heavenly visage, in pity of her
estate, and that quickly. Acontius, coming to Delos to sacrifice

to Diana, fell in love with Cydippe, a noble lass, and wanting means to get her love, flung a golden apple into her lap, with this inscription upon it:

> *Juro tibi sane per mystica sacra Dianæ,*
> *Me tibi venturum comitem, sponsumque futurum.*

> I swear by all the rites of Diana,
> I 'll come and be thy husband if I may.

She considered of it, and upon some small inquiry of his person and estate, was married unto him.

> Blessed is the wooing,
> That is not long a-doing,

as the saying is; when the parties are sufficiently known to each other, what needs such scrupulosity, so many circumstances? dost thou know her conditions, her bringing-up, like her person? let her means be what they will, take her without any more ado. Dido and Æneas were accidentally driven by a storm both into one cave, they made a match upon it;[1] Masinissa was married to that fair captive Sophonisba, King Syphax' wife, the same day that he saw her first, to prevent Scipio and Lælius, lest they should determine otherwise of her. If thou lovest the party, do as much: good education and beauty is a competent dowry, stand not upon money. *Erant olim aurei homines* (saith Theocritus) *et adamantes redamabant*, in the golden world men did so (in the reign of Ogyges[2] belike, before staggering Ninus began to domineer), if all be true that is reported: and some few nowadays will do as much, here and there one; 'tis well done, methinks, and all happiness befall them for so doing. Leontius, a philosopher of Athens, had a fair daughter called Athenais, *multo corporis lepore ac Venere* (saith mine author), of a comely carriage, he gave her no portion but her bringing-up, *occulto formæ præsagio*, out of some secret foreknowledge of her fortune, bestowing that little which he had amongst his other children. But she, thus qualified, was preferred by some friends to Constantinople, to serve Pulcheria, the emperor's sister, of whom she was baptized and called Eudocia. Theodosius, the emperor, in short space took notice of her excellent beauty and good parts, and a little after, upon his sister's sole commendation, made her his wife:[3] 'twas nobly done of Theodosius. Rhodope was the fairest lady in her days in all Egypt; she went to wash her, and by chance (her maids meanwhile looking but carelessly to her clothes), an eagle stole

away one of her shoes, and laid it in Psammetichus the King of
Egypt's lap at Memphis; he wondered at the excellency of the
shoe and pretty foot, but more *aquilæ factum* [at what the eagle
had done], at the manner of the bringing of it, and caused
forthwith proclamation to be made, that she that owned that
shoe should come presently to his court; the virgin came, and
was forthwith married to the king.[1] I say this was heroically
done, and like a prince; I commend him for it, and all such as
have means, that will either do (as he did) themselves, or so for
love, etc., marry their children.   If he be rich, let him take
such a one as wants, if she be virtuously given; for as Siracides,
cap. 7, *ver.* 19, adviseth, "Forgo not a wife and good woman;
for her grace is above gold."   If she have fortunes of her own,
let her make a man.   Danaus of Lacedæmon had a many
daughters to bestow, and means enough for them all; he never
stood inquiring after great matches, as others used to do, but
sent for a company of brave young gallants home to his house,
and bid his daughters choose every one one, whom she liked
best, and take him for her husband, without any more ado.[2]
This act of his was much approved in those times.   But in this
iron age of ours we respect riches alone (for a maid must buy
her husband now with a great dowry, if she will have him),
covetousness and filthy lucre mars all good matches, or some
such by-respects.   Crales, a Servian prince (as Nicephorus
Gregoras, *Rom. Hist. lib.* 6, relates it), was an earnest suitor
to Eudocia, the emperor's sister; though her brother much
desired it, yet she could not abide him,[3] for he had three former
wives, all basely abused; but the emperor still, *Cralis amicitiam
magni faciens* [setting much store by the friendship of Crales],
because he was a great prince and a troublesome neighbour,
much desired his affinity, and to that end betrothed his own
daughter Simonida to him, a little girl five years of age, he being
forty-five, and five years older than the emperor himself:[4] such
disproportionable and unlikely matches can wealth and a fair
fortune make.   And yet not that alone, it is not only money,
but sometimes vainglory, pride, ambition, do as much harm as
wretched covetousness itself in another extreme.   If a yeoman
have one sole daughter, he must over-match her, above her
birth and calling, to a gentleman forsooth, because of her
great portion, too good for one of her own rank, as he
supposeth; a gentleman's daughter and heir must be married
to a knight baronet's eldest son at least; and a knight's
only daughter to a baron himself, or an earl, and so

upwards, her great dower deserves it. And thus striving
for more honour to their wealth, they undo their children,
many discontents follow, and oftentimes they ruinate their
families. Paulus Jovius [1] gives instance in Galeatius the
Second, that heroical Duke of Milan: *externas affinitates,
decoras quidem regio fastu, sed sibi et posteris damnosas et fere
exitiales quæsivit* [he contracted distinguished alliances abroad
which conferred on him a royal pomp, but which proved detri-
mental and almost ruinous to him and his descendants]; he
married his eldest son John Galeatius to Isabella the King of
France his sister, but she was *socero tam gravis, ut ducentis
millibus aureorum constiterit*, her entertainment at Milan was
so costly that it almost undid him. His daughter Violanta
was married to Lionel, Duke of Clarence, the youngest son to
Edward the Third, King of England, but, *ad ejus adventum
tantæ opes tam admirabili liberalitate profusæ sunt, ut opulentissi-
morum regum splendorem superasse videretur*, he was welcomed
with such incredible magnificence that a king's purse was
scarce able to bear it; for besides many rich presents of horses,
arms, plate, money, jewels, etc., he made one dinner for him
and his company, in which were thirty-two messes, and as much
provision left, *ut relatæ a mensa dapes decem millibus hominum
sufficerent*, as would serve ten thousand men: but a little after
Lionel died, *novæ nuptæ et intempestivis conviviis operam dans*
[through riotous living], etc., and to the duke's great loss, the
solemnity was ended. So can titles, honours, ambition, make
many brave but unfortunate matches of all sides for by-respects
(though both crazed in body and mind, most unwilling, averse,
and often unfit); so love is banished, and we feel the smart of
it in the end. But I am too lavish peradventure in this subject.
    Another let or hindrance is strict and severe discipline, laws
and rigorous customs that forbid men to marry at set times and
in some places; as prentices, servants, collegiates, states of
lives in copyholds, or in some base inferior offices, *Velle licet*
[they may desire], in such cases, *potiri non licet* [they cannot
have], as he said.[2] They see but as prisoners through a grate,
they covet and catch, but *Tantalus a labris, etc.* [Tantalus
snatches at the water, etc.]. Their love is lost, and vain it is
in such an estate to attempt. *Gravissimum est adamare nec
potiri*,[3] 'tis a grievous thing to love and not enjoy. They may
indeed, I deny not, marry if they will, and have free choice
some of them; but in the meantime their case is desperate,
lupum auribus tenent, they hold a wolf by the ears, they must

either burn or starve. 'Tis *cornutum sophisma* [a sophistical dilemma], hard to resolve: if they marry they forfeit their estates, they are undone, and starve themselves through beggary and want; if they do not marry, in this heroical passion they furiously rage, are tormented, and torn in pieces by their predominate affections. Every man hath not the gift of continence; let him pray for it then,[1] as Beza adviseth in his tract *de divortiis*, because God hath so called him to a single life, in taking away the means of marriage. Paul would have gone from Mysia to Bithynia, but the spirit suffered him not,[2] and thou wouldst peradventure be a married man with all thy will, but that protecting angel holds it not fit. The devil too sometimes may divert by his ill suggestions, and mar many good matches, as the same Paul was willing to see the Romans, but hindered of Satan he could not.[3] There be those that think they are necessitated by fate, their stars have so decreed, and therefore they grumble at their hard fortune; they are well inclined to marry, but one rub or other is ever in the way: I know what astrologers say in this behalf, what Ptolemy, *Quadripartit. tract.* 4, *cap.* 4, Schoner, *lib.* 1, *cap.* 12, what Leovitius, *Genitur. exempl.* 1, which Sextus ab Heminga takes to be the horoscope of Hieronymus Wolfius, what Pezelius, Origanus, and Leovitius his illustrator Garcæus, *cap.* 12, what Junctine, Pontarius, Campanella, what the rest (to omit those Arabian conjectures *a parte conjugii, a parte lasciviæ, triplicitates Veneris*, etc., and those resolutions upon a question, *an amica potiatur*, etc.) determine in this behalf, viz. *an sit natus conjugem habiturus, facile an difficulter sit sponsam impetraturus, quot conjuges, quo tempore, quales decernantur nato uxores, de mutuo amore conjugem* [whether from his birth he is destined to marry, whether he will get a wife easily or with difficulty, how many wives he shall marry, what they shall be like, when he shall marry them, whether they shall love one another], both in men's and women's genitures, by the examination of the seventh house, the almutens, lords, and planets there, *a* ☽^{d} *et* ☉^{a}, etc., by particular aphorisms: *Si dominus* 7^{mæ} *in* 7ma *vel secunda nobilem decernit uxorem, servam aut ignobilem si duodecima. Si Venus in* 12ma, etc.; with many such, too tedious to relate. Yet let no man be troubled, or find himself grieved with such predictions; as Hier. Wolfius well saith in his astrological dialogue,[4] *non sunt prætoriana decreta* [they are not decrees of the magistrate], they be but conjectures, the stars incline, but not enforce:

Sidera corporibus præsunt cœlestia nostris,
Sunt ea de vili condita namque luto:
Cogere sed nequeunt animum ratione fruentem,
Quippe sub imperio solius ipse dei est.

[The heavenly stars control our frames which are base
clay, but they cannot force the rational mind,
which is subject to God alone.]

Wisdom, diligence, discretion, may mitigate if not quite alter
such decrees: *Fortuna sua a cujusque fingitur moribus* [a man's
fate depends on his own character]; *Qui cauti, prudentes, voti
compotes* [1] [those who are cautious and prudent obtain their
desires], etc.; let no man then be terrified or molested with such
astrological aphorisms, or be much moved, either to vain hope
or fear, from such predictions, but let every man follow his
own free will in this case, and do as he sees cause.   Better it
is indeed to marry than burn for their souls' health, but for
their present fortunes by some other means to pacify themselves
and divert the stream of this fiery torrent, to continue as they
are, rest satisfied,[2] *lugentes virginitatis florem sic aruisse,* deploring
their misery with that eunuch in Libanius, since there is no
help or remedy, and with Jephtha's daughter to bewail their
virginities.

Of like nature is superstition, those rash vows of monks and
friars, and such as live in religious orders, but far more tyrannical
and much worse.   Nature, youth, and his furious passion
forcibly inclines, and rageth on the one side; but their order
and vow checks them on the other.   *Votoque suo sua forma
repugnat* [3] [their beauty struggles with their vows].   What
merits and indulgences they heap unto themselves by it, what
commodities, I know not; but I am sure, from such rash vows
and inhuman manner of life proceed many inconveniences,
many diseases, many vices, mastupration, satyriasis, priapismus,[4] melancholy, madness, fornication, adultery, buggery,
sodomy, theft, murder, and all manner of mischiefs: read but
Bale's catalogue of sodomites, at the visitation of abbeys here
in England, Henry Stephanus his Apology for Herodotus, that
which Ulricus writes in one of his epistles, "that Pope Gregory,
when he saw 6,000 skulls and bones of infants taken out of a fish-
pond near a nunnery, thereupon retracted that decree of priests'
marriages, which was the cause of such a slaughter, was much
grieved at it, and purged himself by repentance." [5]   Read many
such, and then ask what is to be done, is this vow to be broke
or not?   No, saith Bellarmine, *cap.* 38, *lib. de monach., melius*

est scortari et uri quam de voto cœlibatus ad nuptias transire, better burn or fly out, than to break thy vow. And Coster, in his *Enchirid. de cœlibat. sacerdotum*, saith it is absolutely *gravius peccatum*, "a greater sin for a priest to marry, than to keep a concubine at home."[1] Gregory de Valence, *cap. 6 de cœlibat.*, maintains the same, as those Essæi and Montanists of old. Insomuch that many votaries, out of a false persuasion of merit and holiness in this kind, will sooner die than marry, though it be to the saving of their lives. *Anno* 1419,[2] Pius II Pope, James Rossa, nephew to the King of Portugal, and then elect Archbishop of Lisbon, being very sick at Florence, "when his physicians told him that his disease was such, he must either lie with a wench, marry, or die, cheerfully chose to die."[3] Now they commended him for it; but St. Paul teacheth otherwise, "Better marry than burn," and as St. Hierome gravely delivers it, *Aliæ sunt leges Cæsarum, aliæ Christi, aliud Papianus, aliud Paulus noster præcipit*, there's a difference betwixt God's ordinances and men's laws: and therefore Cyprian, *Epist.* 8, boldly denounceth, *Impium est, adulterum est, sacrilegum est, quodcunque humano furore statuitur, ut dispositio divina violetur*, it is abominable, impious, adulterous, and sacrilegious, what men make and ordain after their own furies to cross God's laws. Georgius Wicelius,[4] one of their own arch-divines (*Inspect. Eccles. pag.* 18), exclaims against it, and all such rash monastical vows, and would have such persons seriously to consider what they do, whom they admit, *ne in posterum querantur de inanibus stupris*, lest they repent it at last. For either, as he follows it, you must allow them concubines or suffer them to marry, for scarce shall you find three priests of three thousand, *qui per ætatem non ament*, that are not troubled with burning lust.[5] Wherefore I conclude, it is an unnatural and impious thing to bar men of this Christian liberty, too severe and inhuman an edict.

> The silly wren, the titmouse also,
> The little redbreast have their election,
> They fly I saw and together gone,
> Whereas hem list, about environ
> As they of kind have inclination,
> And as nature impress and guide,
> Of everything list to provide.
>
> But man alone, alas, the hard stond,
> Full cruelly by kind's ordinance
> Constrained is, and by statutes bound,

And debarred from all such pleasance:
What meaneth this, what is this pretence
Of laws, I wis, against all right of kind
Without a cause, so narrow men to bind? [1]

Many laymen repine still at priests' marriages above the rest,
and not at clergymen only, but of all the meaner sort and condition; they would have none marry but such as are rich and able
to maintain wives, because their parish belike shall be pestered
with orphans, and the world full of beggars: but these are hard-
hearted, unnatural, monsters of men, shallow politicians,[2] they
do not consider that a great part of the world is not yet inhabited as it ought, how many colonies into America, Terra
Australis Incognita, Africa, may be sent.[3] Let them consult
with Sir William Alexander's Book of Colonies, Orpheus Junior's
Golden Fleece,[4] Captain Whitbourne, Mr. Hagthorpe, etc., and
they shall surely be otherwise informed.   Those politic Romans
were of another mind, they thought their city and country could
never be too populous.   Hadrian the emperor said he had rather
have men than money, *malle se hominum adjectione ampliare
imperium, quam pecunia.*[5] Augustus Cæsar made an oration
in Rome *ad cœlibes* [to the bachelors], to persuade them to
marry; some countries compelled them to marry of old, as
Jews, Turks, Indians, Chinese [6] amongst the rest in these days,
who much wonder at our discipline to suffer so many idle
persons to live in monasteries, and often marvel how they can
live honest.   In the Isle of Maragnan, the governor and petty
king there did wonder at the Frenchmen, and admire how so
many friars and the rest of their company could live without
wives, they thought it a thing unpossible, and would not believe
it.[7]   If these men should but survey our multitudes of religious
houses, observe our numbers of monasteries all over Europe,
18 nunneries in Padua, in Venice 34 cloisters of monks, 28 of
nuns, etc., *ex ungue leonem* [you can tell a lion from a claw],
'tis to this proportion in all other provinces and cities, what
would they think, do they live honest?   Let them dissemble
as they will, I am of Tertullian's mind, that few can continue
but by compulsion.   "O chastity" (saith he), "thou art a rare
goddess in the world, not so easily got, seldom continuate;
thou mayst now and then be compelled, either for defect of
nature, or if discipline persuade, decrees enforce";[8] or for some
such by-respects, sullenness, discontent, they have lost their
first loves, may not have whom they will themselves, want of
means, rash vows, etc.   But can he willingly contain?   I think

not. Therefore, either out of commiseration of human imbecility
in policy, or to prevent a far worse inconvenience, for they hold
some of them as necessary as meat and drink, and because
vigour of youth, the state and temper of most men's bodies,
do so furiously desire it, they have heretofore in some nations
liberally admitted polygamy and stews, an hundred thousand
courtesans in Grand Cairo in Egypt, as Radzivilius observes,[1]
are tolerated, besides boys: how many at Fez, Rome, Naples,
Florence, Venice, etc.? and still in many other provinces and
cities of Europe they do as much, because they think young
men, churchmen, and servants amongst the rest, can hardly
live honest. The consideration of this belike made Vibius, the
Spaniard, when his friend Crassus,[2] that rich Roman gallant,
lay hid in the cave, *ut voluptatis quam ætas illa desiderat copiam
faceret*, to gratify him the more, send two lusty lasses to accompany him all that while he was there imprisoned; [3] and Surenas,
the Parthian general, when he warred against the Romans, to
carry about with him 200 concubines, as the Swiss soldiers do
now commonly their wives. But, because this course is not
generally approved, but rather contradicted as unlawful and
abhorred, in most countries they do much encourage them to
marriage,[4] give great rewards to such as have many children,
and mulct those that will not marry, *Jus trium liberorum*, and
in A. Gellius, *lib. 2, cap.* 15, Ælian, *lib.* 6, *cap.* 5, Valerius, *lib.* 1,
cap. 9, we read that three children freed the father from painful
offices, and five from all contribution.[5] "A woman shall be
saved by bearing children." Epictetus would have all marry,[6]
and as Plato will, 6 *de legibus*, he that marrieth not before
35 years of his age, must be compelled and punished, and the
money consecrated to Juno's temple, or applied to public uses.[7]
They account him, in some countries, unfortunate that dies
without a wife, a most unhappy man, as Boethius infers,[8] and
if at all happy, yet *infortunio felix*, unhappy in his supposed
happiness. They commonly deplore his estate, and much
lament him for it: "O my sweet son," etc. See Lucian, *de
luctu*, Sandys, *fol.* 83, etc.

     Yet, notwithstanding, many with us are of the opposite part,
they are married themselves, and for others, let them burn,
fire and flame, they care not, so they be not troubled with
them. Some are too curious, and some too covetous, they may
marry when they will both for ability and means, but so nice,
that, except as Theophilus the emperor was presented by his
mother Euphrosyne with all the rarest beauties of the empire

in the great chamber of his palace at once, and bid to give a golden apple to her he liked best, if they might so take and choose whom they list out of all the fair maids their nation affords, they could happily condescend to marry; otherwise, etc. Why should a man marry? saith another Epicurean rout, what's matrimony but a matter of money? why should free nature be entrenched on, confined, or obliged to this or that man or woman, with these manacles of body and goods? etc. There are those too that dearly love, admire and follow women all their lives long, *sponsi Penelopes* [Penelope's suitors], never well but in their company, wistly gazing on their beauties, observing close, hanging after them, dallying still with them, and yet dare not, will not marry. Many poor people, and of the meaner sort, are too distrustful of God's providence, "they will not, dare not for such worldly respects," fear of want, woes, miseries, or that they shall light, as Lemnius saith, "on a scold, a slut, or a bad wife." [1] And therefore, *Tristem juventam Venere deserta colunt* [2] they are resolved to live single, as Epaminondas did: [3] *Nil ait esse prius, melius nil cœlibe vita,* [4] [he says there is nothing to surpass or excel a single life], and ready with Hippolytus to abjure all women: *Detestor omnes, horreo, fugio, execror* [5] [I detest all of them; I loathe, shun, execrate them], etc. But,

> *Hippolyte, nescis quod fugis vitæ bonum,*
> *Hippolyte, nescis,*

[Hippolytus, thou knowest not what a blessing thou losest,]

alas, poor Hippolytus, thou knowest not what thou sayest, 'tis otherwise, Hippolytus. Some [6] make a doubt, *an uxor literato sit ducenda,* whether a scholar should marry; if she be fair she will bring him back from his grammar to his horn-book, or else with kissing and dalliance she will hinder his study; if foul, with scolding; he cannot well intend to both, as Philippus Beroaldus, that great Bononian doctor, once writ, *impediri enim studia literarum* [for it interferes with study], etc., but he recanted at last, and in a solemn sort with true-conceived words he did ask the world and all women forgiveness. But you shall have the story as he relates himself, in his Commentaries on the Sixth of Apuleius. "For a long time I lived a single life, *et ab uxore ducenda semper abhorrui, nec quicquam libero lecto censui jucundius* [I always shrank from marriage and rejoiced in the freedom of a single life]. I could not abide marriage, but as a rambler, *erraticus ac volaticus amator"* (to use his own words) *"per multiplices amores discurre-bam,* I took a snatch where I could get it; nay more, I railed at marriage downright, and in a public auditory, when I did interpret that sixth Satire of Juvenal, out of Plutarch and Seneca, I did heap up all the dicteries I could against women; but now recant with Stesichorus, *palinodiam cano, nec pœnitet censeri in ordine maritorum,* I approve of marriage, I am glad I am a married man,[1] I am heartily glad I have a wife, so sweet a wife, so noble a wife, so young, so chaste a wife, so loving a wife, and I do wish and desire all other men to marry; and especially scholars, that as of old Martia did by Hortensius, Terentia by Tullius, Calphurnia to Plinius, Pudentilla to Apuleius, hold the candle whilst their husbands did meditate and write,[2] so theirs may do them, and as my dear Camilla doth to me." Let other men be averse, rail then and scoff at women, and say what they can to the contrary, *vir sine uxore malorum expers est,* etc., a single man is a happy man, etc., but this is a toy:

> *Nec dulces amores sperne, puer, neque tu choreas;*[3]

> [Reject not, boy, the sweets of love and the pleasures
> of the dance;]

these men are too distrustful, and much to blame to use such speeches:

> *Parcite paucarum diffundere crimen in omnes.*[4]

They must not condemn all for some. As there be many bad, there be some good wives; as some be vicious, some be virtuous. Read what Solomon hath said in their praises (Prov. xxxi), and Siracides (*cap.* xxvi *et* xxx), "Blessed is the man that hath a virtuous wife, for the number of his days shall be double. A virtuous woman rejoiceth her husband, and she shall fulfil the years of his life in peace. A good wife is a good portion" (*et* xxxvi, 24), "an help, a pillar of rest," *columna quietis;*

> *Qui capit uxorem, fratrem capit atque sororem.*[5]

> [Who takes a wife takes a brother and a sister.]

Et v. 25, "He that hath no wife wandereth to and fro mourning." *Minuuntur atræ conjuge curæ* [cares are lightened when shared with a wife], women are the sole, only joy, and comfort of a man's life, born *ad usum et lusum hominum, firmamenta familiæ* [for man's help and pleasure, for founding a family],

> *Deliciæ humani generis, solatia vitæ,*
> *Blanditiæ noctis, placidissima cura diei,*
> *Vota virum, juvenum spes, etc.*[1]

[The delight of mankind, the comfort of life, the
ravishment of the night, the calm joy of day, the
gratification of older men and the hope of younger.]

"A wife is a young man's mistress, a middle-age's companion,
an old man's nurse," [2] *particeps lætorum et tristium* [a partner
of his joys and sorrows], a prop, an help, etc.

> *Optima viri possessio est uxor benevola,*
> *Mitigans iram et avertens animam ejus a tristitia.*[3]

> Man's best possession is a loving wife,
> She tempers anger and diverts all strife.

There is no joy, no comfort, no sweetness, no pleasure in the
world like to that of a good wife:

> *Quam cum cara domi conjux, fidusque maritus*
> *Unanimes degunt,*

[As when a loving wife and a faithful husband live in
harmony together,]

saith our Latin Homer; she is still the same in sickness and in
health, his eye, his hand, his bosom friend, his partner at all
times, his other self, not to be separated by any calamity, but
ready to share all sorrow, discontent, and as the Indian women
do, live and die with him, nay more, to die presently for him.
Admetus, King of Thessaly, when he lay upon his death-bed,
was told by Apollo's oracle, that if he could get anybody to die
for him, he should live longer yet, but when all refused, his
parents, *etsi decrepiti* [although decrepit], friends and followers
forsook him, Alcestis his wife, though young, most willingly
undertook it; what more can be desired or expected? And
although on the other side there be an infinite number of bad
husbands (I should rail downright against some of them), able
to discourage any women; yet there be some good ones again,
and those most observant of marriage rites. An honest country
fellow (as Fulgosus relates it) in the kingdom of Naples, at
plough by the sea-side,[4] saw his wife carried away by Mauritanian pirates; he ran after in all haste, up to the chin first,
and when he could wade no longer, swam, calling to the governor
of the ship to deliver his wife, or if he must not have her restored,
to let him follow as a prisoner, for he was resolved to be a galley-
slave, his drudge, willing to endure any misery, so that he

might enjoy his dear wife.¹   The Moors, seeing the man's constancy, and relating the whole matter to their governor at
Tunis, set them both free, and gave them an honest pension to
maintain themselves during their lives.²   I could tell many
stories to this effect; but put case it often prove otherwise,
because marriage is troublesome, wholly therefore to avoid it
is no argument; "He that will avoid trouble must avoid the
world" ³ (Eusebius, *Præpar. Evangel.* 5, *cap.* 50).   Some trouble
there is in marriage, I deny not; *Etsi grave sit matrimonium*,
saith Erasmus, *edulcatur tamen multis*, etc., yet there be many
things to sweeten it, a pleasant wife,⁴ *placens uxor*, pretty
children, *dulces nati, deliciæ filiorum hominum*, the chief delight
of the sons of men (Eccles. ii, 8), etc.   And howsoever, though
it were all troubles, *utilitatis publicæ causa devorandum, grave
quid libenter subeundum*,⁵ it must willingly be undergone for
public good's sake.

> *Audite (populus) hæc, inquit Susarion,*
> *Malæ sunt mulieres, veruntamen, o populares,*
> *Hoc sine malo domum inhabitare non licet.*⁶

> Hear me, O my countrymen, saith Susarion,
> Women are naught, yet no life without one.

Malum est mulier, sed necessarium malum,⁷ they are necessary
evils, and for our own ends we must make use of them to have
issue, *Supplet Venus ac restituit humanum genus* ⁸ [conjugal
intercourse renovates the human race], and to propagate the
Church.   For to what end is a man born? why lives he, but to
increase the world? and how shall he do that well, if he do
not marry?   *Matrimonium humano generi immortalitatem tribuit*,
saith Nevisanus,⁹ matrimony makes us immortal, and, according
to Tacitus,¹⁰ 'tis *firmissimum imperii munimentum*, the sole and
chief prop of an empire.   *Indigne vivit per quem non vivit et
alter*,¹¹ which Pelopidas objected to Epaminondas,¹² he was an
unworthy member of a commonwealth that left not a child
after him to defend it; and as Trismegistus to his son Tatius,
"Have no commerce with a single man";¹³ holding belike that a
bachelor could not live honestly as he should; and with Georgius
Wicelius, a great divine and holy man, who of late by twenty-six
arguments commends marriage as a thing most necessary for all
kind of persons, most laudable and fit to be embraced: and is
persuaded withal that no man can live and die religiously and
as he ought without a wife, *persuasus neminem posse neque pie
vivere, neque bene mori citra uxorem*, he is false, an enemy to the

commonwealth, injurious to himself, destructive to the world, an apostate to nature, a rebel against heaven and earth. Let our wilful, obstinate, and stale bachelors ruminate of this. "If we could live without wives," as Marcellus Numidicus said in A. Gellius,[1] "we would all want them; but because we cannot, let all marry, and consult rather to the public good than their own private pleasure or estate." It were an happy thing, as wise Euripides hath it, if we could buy children with gold and silver,[2] and be so provided *sine mulierum congressu*, without women's company; but that may not be:

> *Orbis jacebit squalido turpis situ,*
> *Vanum sine ullis classibus stabit mare,*
> *Alesque cœlo deerit et silvis fera.*[3]

Earth, air, sea, land eftsoon would come to naught,
The world itself should be to ruin brought.

Necessity therefore compels us to marry.

But what do I trouble myself, to find arguments to persuade to, or commend marriage? behold a brief abstract of all that which I have said, and much more, succinctly, pithily, pathetically, perspicuously, and elegantly delivered in twelve motions to mitigate the miseries of marriage, by Jacobus de Voragine.[4]

1. *Res est? habes quæ tueatur et augeat.*—2. *Non est? habes quæ quærat.*—3. *Secundæ res sunt? felicitas duplicatur.*—4. *Adversæ sunt? Consolatur, adsidet, onus participat ut tolerabile fiat.*—5. *Domi es? solitudinis tædium pellit.*—6. *Foras? Discedentem visu prosequitur, absentem desiderat, redeuntem læta excipit.*—7. *Nihil jucundum absque societate? Nulla societas matrimonio suavior.*—8. *Vinculum conjugalis caritatis adamantinum.*—9. *Accrescit dulcis affinium turba, duplicatur numerus parentum, fratrum, sororum, nepotum.*—10. *Pulchra sis prole parens.*—11. *Lex Mosis sterilitatem matrimonii execratur, quanto amplius cœlibatum?*—12. *Si natura pœnam non effugit, ne voluntas quidem effugiet.*

1. Hast thou means? thou hast one to keep and increase it.—2. Hast none? thou hast one to help to get it.—3. Art in prosperity? thine happiness is doubled.—4. Art in adversity? she 'll comfort, assist, bear a part of thy burden to make it more tolerable.—5. Art at home? she 'll drive away melancholy. —6. Art abroad? she looks after thee going from home, wishes for thee in thine absence, and joyfully welcomes thy return.—7. There's nothing delightsome without society, no society so

sweet as matrimony.—8. The band of conjugal love is adamantine.—9. The sweet company of kinsmen increaseth, the number
of parents is doubled, of brothers, sisters, nephews.—10. Thou
art made a father by a fair and happy issue.—11. Moses curseth
the barrenness of matrimony, how much more a single life?
—12. If nature escape not punishment, surely thy will shall
not avoid it.

All this is true, say you, and who knows it not? but how
easy a matter is it to answer these motives, and to make an
antiparodia quite opposite unto it! To exercise myself I will
essay:

1. Hast thou means? thou hast one to spend it.—2. Hast
none? thy beggary is increased.—3. Art in prosperity? thy
happiness is ended.—4. Art in adversity? like Job's wife she'll
aggravate thy misery, vex thy soul, make thy burden intolerable.
—5. Art at home? she'll scold thee out of doors.—6. Art abroad?
If thou be wise, keep thee so, she'll perhaps graft horns in thine
absence, scowl on thee coming home.—7. Nothing gives more
content than solitariness, no solitariness like this of a single
life.—8. The band of marriage is adamantine, no hope of loosing
it, thou art undone.—9. Thy number increaseth, thou shalt be
devoured by thy wife's friends.—10.—Thou art made a cornuto
by an unchaste wife, and shalt bring up other folks' children
instead of thine own.—11. Paul commends marriage, yet he
prefers a single life—12. Is marriage honourable? What an
immortal crown belongs to virginity!

So Siracides himself speaks as much as may be for and against
women, so doth almost every philosopher plead pro and con,
every poet thus argues the case (though what cares *vulgus
hominum* [the common herd] what they say?); so can I conceive
peradventure, and so canst thou: when all is said, yet since
some be good, some bad, let's put it to the venture. I conclude
therefore with Seneca:

> *Cur toro viduo jaces?*
> *Tristem juventam solve: nunc luxus rape,*
> *Effunde habenas, optimos vitæ dies*
> *Effluere prohibe.*

Why dost thou lie alone, let thy youth and best days to pass
away? Marry whilst thou mayest, *donec virenti canities abest
morosa* [while sour old age still keeps its distance], whilst thou
art yet able, yet lusty, *Elige cui dicas, tu mihi sola places* [1] [choose
one to whom thou canst say, "Thee alone I love"], make thy

choice, and that freely forthwith, make no delay, but take thy
fortune as it falls.   'Tis true,

Calamitosus est qui inciderit
In malam uxorem, felix qui in bonam.[1]

[Unlucky is he who has struck upon a bad wife, but
happy is he who has found a good one.]

'Tis an hazard both ways I confess, to live single or to marry,
Nam et uxorem ducere, et non ducere malum est[2] [it is bad both
to marry and not to marry], it may be bad, it may be good;
as it is a cross and calamity on the one side, so 'tis a sweet
delight, an incomparable happiness, a blessed estate, a most
unspeakable benefit, a sole content, on the other; 'tis all in the
proof.   Be not then so wayward, so covetous, so distrustful,
so curious and nice, but let 's all marry, *mutuos foventes amplexus.*
"Take me to thee, and thee to me," to-morrow is St. Valentine's
Day, let 's keep it holiday for Cupid's sake, for that great god
Love's sake, for Hymen's sake, and celebrate Venus' vigil[3]
with our ancestors for company together, singing as they did:

Cras amet qui nunquam amavit, quique amavit, cras amet,
Ver novum, ver jam canorum, vere natus orbis est,
Vere concordant amores, vere nubunt alites,
Et nemus coma resolvit, etc.
Cras amet, etc.

[Let those love now who never loved before,
And those who always loved now love the more;
Sweet loves are born with every opening spring;
Birds from the tender boughs their pledges sing, etc.]

Let him that is averse from marriage read more in Barbarus,
de re uxor. lib. 1, *cap.* 1, Lemnius, *de institut. cap.* 4, P. Godefridus, *de Amor. lib.* 3, *cap.* 1, Nevisanus, *lib.* 3,[4] Alex. ab Alexandro, *lib.* 4, *cap.* 8, Tunstall, Erasmus' tracts *in laudem matrimonii,* etc., and I doubt not but in the end he will rest satisfied,
recant with Beroaldus, do penance for his former folly, singing
some penitential ditties, desire to be reconciled to the deity
of this great god Love, go a pilgrimage to his shrine, offer to
his image, sacrifice upon his altar, and be as willing at
last to embrace marriage as the rest.   There will not be found,
I hope, "no, not in that severe family of Stoics, who shall
refuse to submit his grave beard and supercilious looks to the
clipping of a wife, or disagree from his fellows in this point."[5]
"For what more willingly" (as Varro holds) "can a proper man
see than a fair wife, a sweet wife, a loving wife?"[6]   Can the

world afford a better sight, sweeter content, a fairer object, a more gracious aspect?

Since then this of marriage is the last and best refuge and cure of heroical love, all doubts are cleared, and impediments removed; I say again, what remains, but that according to both their desires they be happily joined, since it cannot otherwise be helped? God send us all good wives, every man his wish in this kind, and me mine!

> And God that all this world hath ywrought
> Send him his love that hath it so deere bought.[1]

If all parties be pleased, ask their banns, 'tis a match. *Fruitur Rhodanthe sponsa sponso Dosicle*,[2] Rhodanthe and Dosicles shall go together, Clitophon and Leucippe, Theagenes and Chariclea, Poliarchus hath his Argenis, Lysander Calista (to make up the mask), *potiturque sua puer Iphis Ianthe* [3] [and young Iphis has his own Ianthe].

> And Troilus in lust and in quiet
> Is with Creseid, his own heart sweet.[4]

And although they have hardly passed the pikes,[5] through many difficulties and delays brought the match about, yet let them take this of Aristænetus [6] (that so marry) for their comfort: "After many troubles and cares, the marriages of lovers are more sweet and pleasant." [7] As we commonly conclude a comedy with a wedding [8] and shaking of hands, let 's shut up our discourse, and end all with an epithalamium.[9]

Feliciter nuptis, God give them joy together, *Hymen o Hymenæe, Hymen ades, o Hymenæe!* [10] *Bonum factum*, 'tis well done, *Haud equidem sine mente reor, sine numine divum* [Heaven, as I deem, has willed this match], 'tis an happy conjunction, a fortunate match, an even couple,

> *Ambo animis, ambo præstantes viribus, ambo*
> *Florentes annis,*

they both excel in gifts of body and mind, are both equal in years, youth, vigour, alacrity, she is fair and lovely as Lais or Helen, he as another Clinias or Alcibiades:

> *Ludite ut lubet et brevi*
> *Liberos date.*[11]

> Then modestly go sport and toy,
> And let 's have every year a boy.

"Go give a sweet smell as incense, and bring forth flowers as the lily": [12] that we may say hereafter, *Scitus mecastor natus*

est Pamphilo puer [I' faith, a pretty boy is born to Pamphilus].
In the meantime I say,

> *Ite, agite, O juvenes, non murmura vestra columbæ,*
> *Brachia, non hederæ, neque vincant oscula conchæ.*[1]

> Gentle youths, go sport yourselves betimes,
> Let not the doves outpass your murmurings,
> Or ivy clasping arms, or oyster kissings.[2]

And in the morn betime, as those Lacedæmonian lasses saluted
Helena and Menelaus,[3] singing at their windows, and wishing
good success, do we at yours:

> *Salve o sponsa, salve felix, det vobis Latona*
> *Felicem sobolem, Venus dea det æqualem amorem*
> *Inter vos mutuo; Saturnus durabiles divitias.*
> *Dormite in pectora mutuo amorem inspirantes,*
> *Et desiderium !*

> Good morrow, master bridegroom, and mistress bride,
> Many fair lovely bairns to you betide!
> Let Venus to you mutual love procure,
> Let Saturn give you riches to endure,
> Long may you sleep in one another's arms,
> Inspiring sweet desire, and free from harms.

Even all your lives long,

> *Contingat vobis turturum concordia,*
> *Corniculæ vivacitas.*[4]

> The love of turtles hap to you,
> And ravens' years still to renew.

Let the Muses sing (as he said), the Graces dance, not at their
weddings only but all their days long; "so couple their hearts,
that no irksomeness or anger ever befall them. Let him never
call her other name than my joy, my light, or she call him otherwise than sweetheart. To this happiness of theirs let not old
age any whit detract, but as their years, so let their mutual
love and comfort increase."[5] And when they depart this life,

> *Concordes quoniam vixere tot annos,*
> *Auferat hora duos eadem, nec conjugis usquam*
> *Busta suæ videat, nec sit tumulandus ab illa.*

> Because they have so sweetly liv'd together,
> Let not one die a day before the other,
> He bury her, she him, with even fate,
> One hour their souls let jointly separate.

> *Fortunati ambo! si quid mea carmina possunt,*
> *Nulla dies unquam memori vos eximet ævo.*

> [Happy both! if my lines can aught avail, no lapse of
> time shall ever bring you into oblivion.]

Atque hæc de amore dixisse sufficiat, sub correctione, quod ait ille,[1] *cujusque melius sentientis.* *Plura qui volet de remediis amoris, legat Jasonem Pratensem, Arnoldum, Montaltum, Savonarolum, Langium, Valescum, Crimisonum, Alexandrum Benedictum, Laurentium, Valleriolam; e poetis Nasonem, e nostratibus Chaucerum* [We have now said sufficient on the subject of love, under correction, as he saith, of any one who knoweth better. He who would know more of the remedies for love may consult Jason Pratensis, etc.; among the poets, Ovid, our own Chaucer], etc., with whom I conclude.

> For my words here and every part,
> I speak hem all under correction,
> Of you that feeling have in love's art,
> And put it all in your discretion,
> To entreat or make diminution,
> Of my language, that I you beseech:
> But now to purpose of my rather speech.[2]

SECT. III.   MEMB. I.

SUBSECT. I. — *Jealousy, its Equivocations, Name, Definition, Extent, several kinds; of Princes, Parents, Friends. In Beasts, Men: before marriage, as Corrivals; or after, as in this place*

VALESCUS de Taranta, *cap. de Melanchol.*, Ælian Montaltus, Felix Platerus, Guianerius, put jealousy for a cause of melancholy, others for a symptom; because melancholy persons, amongst these passions and perturbations of the mind, are most obnoxious to it.   But methinks for the latitude it hath, and that prerogative above other ordinary symptoms, it ought to be treated of as a species apart, being of so great and eminent note, so furious a passion, and almost of as great extent as love itself, as Benedetto Varchi holds,[3] "no love without a mixture of jealousy," *qui non zelat, non amat.*   For these causes I will dilate and treat of it by itself, as a bastard branch or kind of love-melancholy, which, as heroical love goeth commonly before marriage, doth usually follow, torture, and crucify in like sort, deserves therefore to be rectified alike, requires as much care and industry in setting out the several causes of it, prognostics and cures.   Which I have more willingly done, that he that is or hath been jealous may see his error as in a glass; he that is

888

not, may learn to detest, avoid it himself, and dispossess others that are anywise affected with it.

Jealousy is described and defined to be "a certain suspicion which the lover hath of the party he chiefly loveth, lest he or she should be enamoured of another"; [1] or any eager desire to enjoy some beauty alone, to have it proper to himself only: a fear or doubt lest any foreigner should participate or share with him in his love. Or (as Scaliger adds [2]) "a fear of losing her favour whom he so earnestly affects." Cardan calls it "a zeal for love, and a kind of envy lest any man should beguile us." [3] Ludovicus Vives [4] defines it in the very same words, or little differing in sense.

There be many other jealousies, but improperly so called all; as that of parents, tutors, guardians over their children, friends whom they love, or such as are left to their wardship or protection:

> *Storax, non rediit hac nocte a cœna Æschinus,*
> *Neque servulorum quispiam qui adversum ierant,*

[Storax, Æschinus did not return from supper to-night,
nor any of the slaves who went to meet him,]

as the old man in the comedy cried out in a passion, and from a solicitous fear and care he had of his adopted son; "not of beauty, but lest they should miscarry, do amiss, or anyway discredit, disgrace" (as Vives notes) "or endanger themselves and us." [5] Ægeus was so solicitous for his son Theseus (when he went to fight with the Minotaur), of his success, lest he should be foiled. [6] *Prona est timori semper in pejus fides,* [7] we are still apt to suspect the worst in such doubtful cases, as many wives in their husbands' absence, fond mothers in their children's, lest if absent they should be misled or sick, and are continually expecting news from them, how they do fare, and what is become of them, they cannot endure to have them long out of their sight: Oh, my sweet son! oh, my dear child! etc. Paul was jealous over the Church of Corinth, as he confesseth (2 Cor. xi, 2, 3), "with a godly jealousy, to present them a pure virgin to Christ"; and he was afraid still, lest, as the serpent beguiled Eve through his subtlety, so their minds should be corrupt from the simplicity that is in Christ. God Himself, in some sense, is said to be jealous: "I am a jealous God, and will visit"; [8] so Psalm lxxix, 5: "Shall thy jealousy burn like fire for ever?" But these are improperly called jealousies, and by a metaphor, to show the care and solicitude they have of them. Although some jealousies express all the symptoms of this which we treat of, fear, sorrow, anguish, anxiety, suspicion, hatred, etc., the object only varied. That of some fathers is very eminent to their sons and heirs; for though they love them dearly being children, yet now coming towards man's estate they may not well abide them; the son and heir is commonly sick of the father, and the father again may not well brook his eldest son, *inde simultates, plerumque contentiones et inimicitiæ* [thence arise quarrels, strife and enmity]. But that of princes is most notorious, as when they fear corrivals (if I may so call them), successors, emulators, subjects, or such as they have offended. *Omnisque potestas impatiens consortis erit* [1] [to share authority is ever irksome]: "they are still suspicious, lest their authority should be diminished," as one observes; [2] and as Comineus hath it, [3] "it cannot be expressed what slender causes they have of their grief and suspicion, a secret disease, that commonly lurks and breeds in princes' families." [4] Sometimes it is for their honour only, as that of Hadrian the emperor, "that killed all his emulators." [5] Saul envied David; Domitian Agricola, because he did excel him, obscure his honour, as he thought, eclipse his fame. Juno turned Prœtus' daughters into kine, for that they contended with her for beauty; [the] Cyparissæ, King Eteocles' children, were envied of the goddesses for their excellent good parts, and dancing amongst the rest, saith Constantine, "and for that cause flung headlong from heaven, and buried in a pit, but the earth took pity of them, and brought out cypress trees to preserve their memories." [6] Niobe, Arachne, and Marsyas can testify as much. [7] But it is most grievous when it is for a kingdom itself, or matters of commodity, it produceth lamentable effects, especially amongst tyrants, *in despotico imperio*, and such as are more feared than beloved of their subjects, that get and keep their sovereignty by force and fear: *Quod civibus tenere te invitis scias* [8] [you know that you hold your position against the will of the citizens], etc., as Phalaris, Dionysius, Periander held theirs. For though fear, cowardice, and jealousy, in Plutarch's opinion, be the common causes of tyranny, as in Nero, Caligula, Tiberius, yet most take them to be symptoms. For "what slave, what hangman" (as Bodine well expresseth this passion, *lib. 2, cap. 5, de rep.*) "can so cruelly torture a condemned person as this fear and suspicion? Fear of death, infamy, torments, are those furies and vultures that vex and disquiet tyrants, and torture them day and night with perpetual terrors and affrights; envy, suspicion, fear, desire of revenge, and a thousand such disagreeing perturbations, turn and affright the soul out of the hinges of health, and more grievously wound and pierce than those cruel masters can exasperate and vex their prentices or servants with clubs, whips, chains, and tortures." [1] Many terrible examples we have in this kind, amongst the Turks especially, many jealous outrages; Selimus killed Cornutus his youngest brother, five of his nephews, Mustapha Bassa, and divers others. [2] Bajazet, the second Turk, [3] jealous of the valour and greatness of Achmet Bassa, caused him to be slain. Solyman the Magnificent murdered his own son Mustapha; [4] and 'tis an ordinary thing amongst them, to make away their brothers, or any competitors, at the first coming to the crown: 'tis all the solemnity they use at their fathers' funerals. What mad pranks in his jealous fury did Herod of old commit in Jewry, when he massacred all the children of a year old! Valens the emperor in Constantinople, whenas he left no man alive of quality in his kingdom that had his name begun with Theo! Theodoti, Theognosti, Theodosii, Theoduli, etc., [5] they went all to their long home, because a wizard told him that name should succeed in his empire. And what furious designs hath Jo. Basilius, that Muscovian tyrant, practised of late! [6] It is a wonder to read that strange suspicion which Suetonius reports of Claudius Cæsar and of Domitian, they were afraid of every man they saw; [7] and which Herodian [reports] of Antoninus and Geta, those two jealous brothers, the one could not endure so much as the other's servants, but made away him, his chiefest followers, and all that belonged to him or were his well-wishers. Maximinus, "perceiving himself to be odious to most men, because he was come to that height of honour out of base beginnings, and suspecting his mean parentage would be objected to him, caused all the senators that were nobly descended to be slain in a jealous humour, turned all the servants of Alexander his predecessor out of doors, and slew many of them, because they lamented their master's death, suspecting them to be traitors for the love they bare to him." [8] When Alexander in his fury had made Clitus his dear friend to be put to death, and saw now (saith Curtius [9]) an alienation in his subjects' hearts, none durst talk with him, he began to be jealous of himself, lest they should attempt as much on him, "and said they lived like so many wild beasts in a wilderness, one afraid of another." Our modern stories afford us many notable examples. Henry the Third of France, jealous of

Henry of Lorraine, Duke of Guise, *anno* 1588, caused him to
be murdered in his own chamber.[1]   Louis the Eleventh was so
suspicious, he durst not trust his children, every man about him
he suspected for a traitor;[2] many strange tricks Comineus
telleth of him.   How jealous was our Henry the Fourth [3] of
King Richard the Second, so long as he lived, after he was
deposed! and of his own son Henry in his later days! which the
prince well perceiving, came to visit his father in his sickness,
in a watchet velvet gown, full of oilet-holes, and with needles
sticking in them (as an emblem of jealousy), and so pacified his
suspicious father, after some speeches and protestations which
he had used to that purpose.   Perpetual imprisonment, as that
of Robert Duke of Normandy,[4] in the days of Henry the First,
forbidding of marriage to some persons, with such-like edicts
and prohibitions, are ordinary in all states.   In a word (as he
said [5]) three things cause jealousy, a mighty state, a rich
treasure, a fair wife; or where there is a cracked title, much
tyranny, and many exactions.   In our state, as being freed
from all these fears and miseries, we may be most secure and
happy under the reign of our fortunate prince.

> His fortune hath indebted him to none,
> But to all his people universally;
> And not to them but for their love alone,
> Which they account as placed worthily.
> He is so set, he hath no cause to be
> Jealous, or dreadful of disloyalty;
> The pedestal whereon his greatness stands,
> Is held of all our hearts, and all our hands.[6]

But I rove, I confess.   These equivocations, jealousies, and many
such, which crucify the souls of men, are not here properly
meant, or in this distinction of ours included, but that alone
which is for beauty, tending to love, and wherein they can
brook no corrival, or endure any participation: and this jealousy
belongs as well to brute beasts as men.   Some creatures, saith
Vives,[7] swans, doves, cocks, bulls, etc., are jealous as well as
men, and as much moved, for fear of communion.

> *Grege pro toto bella juvenci,*
> *Si conjugio timuere suo,*
> *Poscunt timidi prælia cervi,*
> *Et mugitus dant concepti signa furoris.*[8]

In Venus' cause what mighty battles make
Your raving bulls, and stirs for their herd's sake:
And harts and bucks, that are so timorous,
Will fight and roar, if once they be but jealous.

In bulls, horses, goats, this is most apparently discerned; bulls
especially: *alium in pascuis non admittit*, he will not admit
another bull to feed in the same pasture, saith Oppian:[1] which
Stephanus Bathorius, late King of Poland, used as an impress,
with that motto, *Regnum non capit duos* [the throne will not
hold two]. R. T., in his Blazon of Jealousy, telleth a story of
a swan about Windsor, that finding a strange cock with his
mate, did swim I know not how many miles after to kill him,
and when he had so done, came back and killed his hen; a
certain truth, he saith, done upon Thames, as many watermen
and neighbour gentlemen can tell. *Fidem suam liberet* [let him
vindicate his good faith]; for my part, I do believe it may be
true; for swans have ever been branded with that epithet of
jealousy.

> The jealous swanne against his death that singeth,
> And eke the owle that of death bode bringeth.[2]

Some say as much of elephants,[3] that they are more jealous than
any other creatures whatsoever; and those old Egyptians, as
Pierius informeth us,[4] express in their hieroglyphics the passion
of jealousy by a camel; because that, fearing the worst still
about matters of venery, he loves solitudes, that he may enjoy
his pleasure alone,[5] *et in quoscunque obvios insurgit, zelotypiæ
stimulis agitatus*, he will quarrel and fight with whosoever
comes next, man or beast, in his jealous fits. I have read as
much of crocodiles;[6] and if Peter Martyr's authority be
authentic, *Legat. Babylonicæ, lib.* 3, you shall have a strange
tale to that purpose confidently related. Another story of the
jealousy of dogs, see in Hieron. Fabricius, *tract.* 3, *cap.* 5, *de
loquela animalium.*

But this furious passion is most eminent in men, and is as
well amongst bachelors as married men. If it appear amongst
bachelors, we commonly call them rivals or corrivals, a metaphor
derived from a river, *rivales a rivo*;[7] for as a river, saith Acron
in Hor. Art. Poet. and Donat. *in Ter. Eunuch.*, divides a common
ground betwixt two men, and both participate of it, so is a
woman indifferent between two suitors, both likely to enjoy
her; and thence comes this emulation, which breaks out many
times into tempestuous storms, and produceth lamentable
effects, murder itself, with much cruelty, many single combats.
They cannot endure the least injury done unto them before their
mistress, and in her defence will bite off one another's noses;
they are most impatient of any flout, disgrace, least emulation

or participation in that kind. *Lacerat lacertum Largi mordax
Memmius* [1] [jealous Memmius bites the arm of Largus]. Memmius the Roman (as Tully tells the story, *de oratore lib.* 2),
being corrival with Largus at Terracina, bit him by the arm,
which fact of his was so famous, that it afterwards grew to a
proverb in those parts. Phædria could not abide his corrival
Thraso; for when Parmeno demanded, *Numquid aliud imperas?*
whether he would command him any more service: "No more"
saith he) "but to speak in his behalf, and to drive away his
corrival if he could." [2] Constantine, in the eleventh book of
his Husbandry, *cap.* 11, hath a pleasant tale of the pine-tree;
she was once a fair maid, whom Phineus and Boreas, two
corrivals, dearly sought; but jealous Boreas broke her neck,
etc.[3] And in his eighteenth chapter he telleth another tale of
Mars, that in his jealousy slew Adonis.[4] Petronius calleth this
passion *amantium furiosam æmulationem,* a furious emulation;
and their symptoms are well expressed by Sir Geoffrey Chaucer
in his first Canterbury Tale. It will make the nearest and
dearest friends fall out; they will endure all other things to be
common, goods, lands, moneys, participate of each [other's]
pleasures, and take in good part any disgraces, injuries in
another kind; but as Propertius well describes it in an elegy
of his, in this they will suffer nothing, have no corrivals.

> *Tu mihi vel ferro pectus, vel perde veneno,*
>   *A domina tantum te modo tolle mea :*
> *Te socium vitæ, te corporis esse licebit,*
>   *Te dominum admitto rebus, amice, meis.*
> *Lecto te solum, lecto te deprecor uno,*
>   *Rivalem possum non ego ferre Jovem.*

> Stab me with sword, or poison strong
>   Give me to work my bane:
> So thou court not my lass, so thou
>   From mistress mine refrain.
> Command myself, my body, purse,
>   As thine own goods take all,
> And as my ever dearest friend,
>   I ever use thee shall.
> O spare my love, to have alone
>   Her to myself I crave,
> Nay, Jove himself I'll not endure
>   My rival for to have.

This jealousy which I am to treat of, is that which belongs to
married men, in respect of their own wives; to whose estate, as
no sweetness, pleasure, happiness can be compared in the

world, if they live quietly and lovingly together; so if they
disagree or be jealous, those bitter pills of sorrow and grief,
disastrous mischiefs, mischances, tortures, gripings, discontents,
are not to be separated from them. A most violent passion it
is where it taketh place, an unspeakable torment, a hellish
torture, an infernal plague, as Ariosto calls it, "a fury, a continual fever, full of suspicion, fear, and sorrow, a martyrdom,
a mirth-marring monster." "The sorrow and grief of heart of
one woman jealous of another, is heavier than death" (Ecclus.
xxvi, 6), as Peninnah did Hannah, "vex her and upbraid her
sore."[1] 'Tis a main vexation, a most intolerable burden, a
corsive to all content, a frenzy, a madness itself; as Benedetto
Varchi proves out of that select sonnet of Giovanni de la Casa,
that reverend lord, as he styles him.[2]

SUBSECT. II.—*Causes of Jealousy. Who are most apt. Idleness, Melancholy, Impotency, long Absence, Beauty, Wantonness, naught themselves. Allurements from time, place, persons, bad usage, Causes*

Astrologers make the stars a cause or sign of this bitter
passion, and out of every man's horoscope will give a probable
conjecture whether he will be jealous or no, and at what time,
by direction of the significators to their several promissors:
their aphorisms are to be read in Albubater, Pontanus, Schoner,
Junctine, etc. Bodine, *cap.* 5 *Meth. hist.*, ascribes a great cause
to the country or clime, and discourseth largely there of this
subject, saying, that southern men are more hot, lascivious,
and jealous than such as live in the north; they can hardly
contain themselves in those hotter climes, but are most subject
to prodigious lust. Leo Afer telleth incredible things almost of
the lust and jealousy of his countrymen of Africa, and especially
such as live about Carthage, and so doth every geographer of
them in Asia, Turkey, Spaniards, Italians.[3] Germany hath not
so many drunkards, England tobacconists, France dancers,
Holland mariners, as Italy alone hath jealous husbands. And
in Italy some account them of Piacenza more jealous than the
rest.[4] In Germany, France, Britain, Scandia, Poland, Muscovy, they are not so troubled with this feral malady,[5] although
Damianus à Goes, which I do much wonder at, in his
topography of Lapland, and Herbastein of Russia, against
the stream of all other geographers, would fasten it

upon those northern inhabitants. Altomarus, Poggius, and Munster in his description of Baden, reports that men and women of all sorts go commonly into the baths together, without all suspicion; "the name of jealousy" (saith Munster) "is not so much as once heard of among them." In Friesland the women kiss him they drink to, and are kissed again of those they pledge. The virgins in Holland go hand-in-hand with young men from home, glide on the ice, such is their harmless liberty, and lodge together abroad without suspicion, which rash Sansovinus, an Italian, makes a great sign of unchastity. In France, upon small acquaintance, it is usual to court other men's wives, to come to their houses, and accompany them arm-in-arm in the streets, without imputation. In the most northern countries young men and maids familiarly dance together, men and their wives, which, Siena only excepted, Italians may not abide.[1] The Greeks, on the other side, have their private baths for men and women, where they must not come near, nor so much as see one another;[2] and as Bodine observes, *lib.* 5 *de repub.*, "the Italians could never endure this,"[3] or a Spaniard, the very conceit of it would make him mad; and for that cause they lock up their women, and will not suffer them to be near men, so much as in the church, but with a partition between.[4] He telleth, moreover, how that "when he was ambassador in England, he heard Mendoza the Spanish legate finding fault with it, as a filthy custom for men and women to sit promiscuously in churches together; but Dr. Dale, the Master of the Requests, told him again that it was indeed a filthy custom in Spain, where they could not contain themselves from lascivious thoughts in their holy places, but not with us." Baronius in his Annals, out of Eusebius, taxeth Licinius the emperor for a decree of his made to this effect, *jubens ne viri simul cum mulieribus in ecclesia interessent* [ordering that men and women should not sit together in church]: for being prodigiously naught himself, *aliorum naturam ex sua vitiosa mente spectavit* [he judged others by his own vicious mind], he so esteemed others. But we are far from any such strange conceits, and will permit our wives and daughters to go to the tavern with a friend, as Aubanus saith, *modo absit lascivia* [as long as there is no lewdness], and suspect nothing, to kiss coming and going, which, as Erasmus writes in one of his epistles, they cannot endure. England is a paradise for women, and hell for horses: Italy a paradise for horses, hell for women, as the diverb goes. Some make a question whether

this headstrong passion rage more in women than men, as
Montaigne, *lib.* 3. But sure it is more outrageous in women,
as all other melancholy is, by reason of the weakness of their
sex. Scaliger, *Poet. lib. cap.* 14, concludes against women:
"Besides their inconstancy, treachery, suspicion, dissimulation,
superstition, pride" (for all women are by nature proud), "desire
of sovereignty, if they be great women" (he gives instance in
Juno), "bitterness and jealousy are the most remarkable
affections." [1]

> *Sed neque fulvus aper media tam sævus in ira est,*
> *Fulmineo rabidos dum rotat ore canes,*
> *Nec lea,* etc. [2]

> Tiger, boar, bear, viper, lioness,
> A woman's fury cannot express.

Some say red-headed women, pale-coloured, black-eyed, and
of a shrill voice, are most subject to jealousy. [3]

> High colour in a woman choler shows,
> Naught are they, peevish, proud, malicious;
> But worst of all, red, shrill, and jealous. [4]

Comparisons are odious, I neither parallel them with others,
nor debase them any more: men and women are both bad, and
too subject to this pernicious infirmity. It is most part a
symptom and cause of melancholy, as Plater and Valescus teach
us: melancholy men are apt to be jealous, and jealous apt to
be melancholy.

> Pale jealousy, child of insatiate love,
> Of heart-sick thoughts which melancholy bred,
> A hell-tormenting fear, no faith can move,
> By discontent with deadly poison fed;
> With heedless youth and error vainly led.
> A mortal plague, a virtue-drowning flood,
> A hellish fire not quenched but with blood. [5]

If idleness concur with melancholy, such persons are most apt
to be jealous; 'tis Nevisanus' note, "An idle woman is presumed
to be lascivious, and often jealous." [6] *Mulier cum sola cogitat,
male cogitat* [when a woman is left to herself, her thoughts are
evil]: and 'tis not unlikely, for they have no other business to
trouble their heads with.

More particular causes be these which follow. Impotency
first, when a man is not able of himself to perform those dues
which he ought unto his wife: for though he be an honest liver,
hurt no man, yet Trebatius the lawyer may make a question,

an suum cuique tribuat, whether he give every one their own;
and therefore when he takes notice of his wants, and perceives
her to be more craving, clamorous, unsatiable and prone to lust
than is fit, he begins presently to suspect, that wherein he is
defective, she will satisfy herself, she will be pleased by some
other means. Cornelius Gallus hath elegantly expressed this
humour in an epigram to his Lycoris:

> *Jamque alios juvenes aliosque requirit amores,*
> *Me vocat imbellem decrepitumque senem, etc.*

[Now seeks she for her sweethearts other swains,
And calls me old and feeble for my pains.]

For this cause is most evident in old men, that are cold and
dry by nature, and married *succi plenis*, to young wanton wives;
with old doting Janivere in Chaucer, they begin to mistrust
all is not well:

> She was young and he was old,
> And therefore he feared to be a cuckold.

And how should it otherwise be? Old age is a disease of itself,
loathsome, full of suspicion and fear; when it is at best, unable,
unfit for such matters. *Tam apta nuptiis quam bruma messibus,*
as welcome to a young woman as snow in harvest, saith Nevisanus;[1] *et si capis juvenculam, faciet tibi cornua*: marry a lusty
maid and she will surely graft horns on thy head. "All women
are slippery, often unfaithful to their husbands" (as Æneas
Sylvius, *Epist.* 38, seconds him), "but to old men most treacherous":[2] they had rather *mortem amplexarier*, lie with a corse,
than such a one: *Oderunt illum pueri, contemnunt mulieres*[3]
[boys hate him, women despise him]. On the other side, many
men, said Hieronymus, are suspicious of their wives, if they be
lightly given,[4] but old folks above the rest. Insomuch that she
did not complain without a cause in Apuleius,[5] of an old bald
bedridden knave she had to her goodman: "Poor woman as
I am, what shall I do? I have an old grim sire to my husband,
as bald as a coot, as little and as unable as a child," a bedful
of bones, "he keeps all the doors barred and locked upon me,
woe is me, what shall I do?" He was jealous, and she made
him a cuckold for keeping her up: suspicion without a cause,
hard usage is able of itself to make a woman fly out, that was
otherwise honest,

> *Plerasque bonas tractatio pravas*
> *Esse facit,*[6]

bad usage aggravates the matter. *Nam quando mulieres*

cognoscunt maritum hoc advertere, licentius peccant, as Nevisanus holds,[1] when a woman thinks her husband watcheth her, she will sooner offend; *Liberius peccant, et pudor omnis abest* [2] [they sin more readily, and without shame], rough handling makes them worse: as the Goodwife of Bath in Chaucer brags,

> In his own grease I made him frie
> For anger and for very jealousie.

Of two extremes, this of hard usage is the worst. 'Tis a great fault (for some men are *uxorii* [uxorious]) to be too fond of their wives, to dote on them as Senior Deliro on his Fallace,[3] to be too effeminate, or as some do, to be sick for their wives, breed children for them, and like the Tiberini lie in for them; as some birds hatch eggs by turns, they do all women's offices: [4] Cælius Rhodiginus, *Ant. lect. lib.* 6, *cap.* 24, makes mention of a fellow out of Seneca, that was so besotted on his wife, he could not endure a moment out of her company, he wore her scarf when he went abroad next his heart, and would never drink but in that cup she began first.[5] We have many such fondlings that are their wives' packhorses and slaves (*nam grave malum uxor superans virum suum*, as the comical poet hath it, there's no greater misery to a man than to let his wife domineer), to carry her muff, dog, and fan, let her wear the breeches, lay out, spend, and do what she will, go and come whither, when she will, they give consent:

> Here, take my muff, and, do you hear, good man,
> Now give me Pearl, and carry you my fan, etc.

> *Poscit pallam, redimicula, inaures ;*
> *Curre, quid hic cessas? vulgo vult illa videri,*
> *Tu pete lecticas.* [6]

Many brave and worthy men have trespassed in this kind, *multos foras claros domestica hæc destruxit infamia* [many men of great public esteem have been ruined by this domestic disgrace], and many noble senators and soldiers (as Pliny notes [7]) have lost their honour, in being *uxorii*, so sottishly overruled by their wives; and therefore Cato in Plutarch made a bitter jest on his fellow-citizens, the Romans: "We govern all the world abroad, and our wives at home rule us." These offend in one extreme; but too hard and too severe are far more offensive on the other. As just a cause may be long absence of either party, when they must of necessity be much from home, as lawyers, physicians, mariners, by their professions; or otherwise make frivolous, impertinent journeys, tarry long abroad to no purpose, lie out, and are gadding still, upon small occasions, it must needs yield matter of suspicion, when they use their wives unkindly in the meantime, and never tarry at home, it cannot use but engender some such conceit.

> *Uxor si cesses amare te cogitat*
> *Aut tete amari, aut potare, aut animo obsequi,*
> *Et tibi bene esse soli, quum sibi sit male.*[1]

> If thou be absent long, thy wife then thinks,
> Th' art drunk, at ease, or with some pretty minx,
> 'Tis well with thee, or else beloved of some,
> Whilst she, poor soul, doth fare full ill at home.

Hippocrates the physician had a smack of this disease; for when he was to go from home as far as Abdera and some other remote cities of Greece, he writ to his friend Dionysius (if at least those Epistles [2] be his) "to oversee his wife in his absence" (as Apollo set a raven to watch his Coronis), "although she lived in his house with her father and mother, whom he knew would have a care of her; yet that would not satisfy his jealousy, he would have his special friend Dionysius to dwell in his house with her all the time of his peregrination, and to observe her behaviour, how she carried herself in her husband's absence, and that she did not lust after other men.[3] For a woman had need to have an overseer to keep her honest; they are bad by nature, and lightly given all, and if they be not curbed in time, as an unpruned tree, they will be full of wild branches, and degenerate of a sudden." [4] Especially in their husbands' absence: though one Lucretia were trusty, and one Penelope, yet Clytemnestra made Agamemnon cuckold; and no question there be too many of her conditions. If their husbands tarry too long abroad upon unnecessary business, well they may suspect: or if they run one way, their wives at home will fly out another, *quid pro quo*. Or if present, and give them not that content which they ought, *primum ingratæ, mox invisæ noctes quæ per somnum transiguntur*,[5] they cannot endure to lie alone, or to fast long. Peter Godefridus, in his second book of Love, and sixth chapter, hath a story out of St. Anthony's life, of a gentleman, who, by that good man's advice, would not meddle with his wife in the Passion Week, but for his pains she set a pair of horns on his head.[6] Such another he hath out of Abstemius: one persuaded a new-married man "to forbear the three first nights, and he should all his lifetime after be fortunate in cattle," [7] but his impatient wife would not tarry so long: well he might speed in cattle, but not in children.   Such a tale hath Heinsius of an impotent and slack scholar, a mere student, and a friend of his, that seeing by chance a fine damsel sing and dance, would needs marry her; the match was soon made, for he was young and rich, *genis gratus, corpore glabellus, arte multiscius, et fortuna opulentus* [smooth-cheeked, soft-skinned, well edu-cated, and rich], like that Apollo in Apuleius.   The first night, having liberally taken his liquor (as in that country they do) my fine scholar was so fuzzled, that he no sooner was laid in bed but he fell fast asleep, never waked till morning, and then much abashed, *purpureis formosa rosis cum Aurora ruberet* [when the fair morn with purple hue 'gan shine], he made an excuse, I know not what, out of Hippocrates Cous, etc., and for that time it went current:[1] but whenas afterward he did not play the man as he should do, she fell in league with a good fellow, and whilst he sat up late at his study about those criticisms, mending some hard places in Festus or Pollux, came cold to bed, and would tell her still what he had done, she did not much regard what he said, etc.   "She would have another matter mended much rather, which he did not conceive was corrupt":[2] thus he continued at his study late, she at her sport, *alibi enim festivas noctes agitabat* [she was having a gay night somewhere else], hating all scholars for his sake, till at length he began to suspect, and turned a little yellow, as well he might; for it was his own fault; and if men be jealous in such cases (as oft it falls out[3]) the mends is in their own hands, they must thank themselves.   Who will pity them, saith Neander, or be much offended with such wives, *si deceptæ prius viros decipiant, et cornutos reddant*, if they deceive those that cozened them first? A lawyer's wife in Aristænetus, because her husband was negligent in his business, *quando lecto danda opera*, threatened to cornute him, and did not stick to tell Philinna, one of her gossips, as much, and that aloud for him to hear: "If he follow other men's matters and leave his own, I 'll have an orator shall plead my cause,"[4] I care not if he know it.

A fourth eminent cause of jealousy may be this, when he that is deformed and, as Pindarus of Vulcan, *sine gratiis natus* [ugly from birth], hirsute, ragged, yet virtuously given, will marry some fair nice piece, or light huswife, begins to mis-doubt (as well he may) she doth not affect him.   *Lis est cum forma magna pudicitiæ*,[5] beauty and honesty have ever been at odds.   Abraham was jealous of his wife because she was

fair: so was Vulcan of his Venus, when he made her creaking
shoes, saith Philostratus,[1] *ne mœcharetur, sandalio scilicet
deferente,* that he might hear by them when she stirred, which
Mars *indigne ferre,* was not well pleased with.[2] Good cause
had Vulcan to do as he did, for she was no honester than she
should be.   Your fine faces have commonly this fault; and it is
hard to find, saith Francis Philelphus in an epistle to Saxola
his friend, a rich man honest, a proper woman not proud or
unchaste.   "Can she be fair and honest too?"

> *Sæpe etenim occuluit picta sese hydra sub herba,*
> *Sub specie formæ, incauto se sæpe marito*
> *Nequam animus vendit.*[3]

> [For oft is a serpent concealed beneath the verdant
> grass, and often while the husband suspects
> naught, the beautiful but worthless wife has sold
> herself.]

He that marries a wife that is snout-fair alone, let him look,
saith Barbarus,[4] for no better success than Vulcan had with
Venus, or Claudius with Messalina.   And 'tis impossible almost
in such cases the wife should contain, or the good man not be
jealous: for when he is so defective, weak, ill-proportioned,
unpleasing in those parts which women most affect, and she
most absolutely fair and able on the other side, if she be not
very virtuously given, how can she love him? and although she
be not fair, yet if he admire her and think her so, in his conceit
she is absolute, he holds it unpossible for any man living not to
dote as he doth, to look on her and not lust, not to covet, and if
he be in company with her, not to lay siege to her honesty:
or else out of a deep apprehension of his infirmities, deformities,
and other men's good parts, out of his own little worth and
desert, he distrusts himself (for what is jealousy but distrust?),
he suspects she cannot affect him, or be not so kind and loving as
she should, she certainly loves some other man better than
himself.

Nevisanus, *lib.* 4, *num.* 72, will have barrenness to be a main
cause of jealousy.[5] If her husband cannot play the man, some
other shall, they will leave no remedies unassayed, and thereupon the good man grows jealous; I could give an instance,
but be it as it is.

I find this reason given by some men, because they have
been formerly naught themselves, they think they may
be so served by others; they turned up trump before the cards

were shuffled, they shall have therefore *legem talionis*, like
for like.

> *Ipse miser docui, quo posset ludere pacto*
> *Custodes, eheu nunc premor arte mea.*[1]

> Wretch as I was, I taught her bad to be,
> And now mine own sly tricks are put upon me.

Mala mens, malus animus, as the saying is, ill dispositions cause
ill suspicions.

> There is none jealous, I durst pawn my life,
> But he that hath defiled another's wife,
> And for that he himself hath gone astray,
> He straightway thinks his wife will tread that way.[2]

To these two above-named causes, or incendiaries of this rage,
I may very well annex those circumstances of time, place,
persons, by which it ebbs and flows, the fuel of this fury, as
Vives truly observes:[3] and such-like accidents or occasions,
proceeding from the parties themselves or others, which much
aggravate and intend this suspicious humour. For many men
are so lasciviously given, either out of a depraved nature, or
too much liberty, which they do assume unto themselves by
reason of their greatness, in that they are noblemen (for *licentia
peccandi et multitudo peccantium* [liberty to sin and multitude
of sinners] are great motives), though their own wives be
never so fair, noble, virtuous, honest, wise, able, and well
given, they must have change.

> *Qui cum legitimi junguntur fœdere lecti*
> *Virtute egregiis facieque domoque puellis,*
> *Scorta tamen fœdasque lupas in fornice quærunt,*
> *Et per adulterium nova carpere gaudia tentant.*[4]

> Who being match'd to wives most virtuous,
> Noble, and fair, fly out lascivious.

Quod licet ingratum est, that which is ordinary is unpleasant.
Nero (saith Tacitus) abhorred Octavia his own wife, a noble
virtuous lady, and loved Acte, a base quean in respect. Cerin-
thus rejected Sulpicia, a nobleman's daughter, and courted
a poor servant maid,[5] *tanta est aliena in messe voluptas* [so
pleasant it is to enjoy another's harvest], for that "stolen waters
be more pleasant":[6] or, as Vitellius the emperor was wont to
say, *Jucundiores amores qui cum periculo habentur*, like stolen
venison, still the sweetest is that love which is most difficultly
attained: they like better to hunt by stealth in another man's

walk, than to have the fairest course that may be at game
of their own.

Aspice ut in cœlo modo sol, modo luna ministret,
Sic etiam nobis una puella parum est. [1]

As sun and moon in heaven change their course,
So they change loves, though often to the worse.

Or that some fair object so forcibly moves them, they cannot
contain themselves; be it heard or seen, they will be at it.
Nessus, the centaur, was by agreement to carry Hercules and
his wife over the river Evenus; no sooner had he set Deianira
on the other side but he would have offered violence unto her,
leaving Hercules to swim over as he could: and though her
husband was a spectator, yet would he not desist till Hercules
with a poisoned arrow shot him to death.[2] Neptune saw by
chance that Thessalian Tyro, Enipeus' wife; he forthwith in
the fury of his lust counterfeited her husband's habit, and
made him cuckold.[3] Tarquin heard Collatine commend his
wife, and was so far enraged that in the midst of the night to
her he went. Theseus stole Ariadne,[4] *vi rapuit* [forcibly carried
off] that Trœzenian Anaxo, Antiope, and now being old, Helena,
a girl not yet ready for a husband. Great men are most part
thus affected all, as a horse they neigh, saith Jeremiah, after
their neighbours' wives,[5] *ut visa pullus adhinnit equa* [as the
horse neighs at sight of the mare]: and if they be in company
with other women, though in their own wives' presence, they
must be courting and dallying with them. Juno in Lucian
complains of Jupiter that he was still kissing Ganymede before
her face, which did not a little offend her: and besides, he was
a counterfeit Amphitryo, a bull, a swan, a golden shower,
and played many such bad pranks, too long, too shameful to
relate.

Or that they care little for their own ladies, and fear no
laws, they dare freely keep whores at their wives' noses. 'Tis
too frequent with noblemen to be dishonest; *Pietas, probitas,*
fides, privata bona sunt, as he said [6] long since, piety, chastity,
and such-like virtues are for private men: not to be much
looked after in great courts: and which Suetonius [said] of the
good princes of his time, they might be all engraven in one
ring, we may truly hold of chaste potentates of our age. For
great personages will familiarly run out in this kind, and yield
occasion of offence. Montaigne, in his Essays,[7] gives instance
in Cæsar, Mahomet the Turk, that sacked Constantinople, and

Ladislaus, King of Naples, that besieged Florence: great men,
and great soldiers, are commonly great, etc.; *probatum est* [it is
a known fact], they are good doers. Mars and Venus are
equally balanced in their actions:

> *Militis in galea nidum fecere columbæ,*
> *Apparet Marti quam sit amica Venus.*[1]

> A dove within a head-piece made her nest,
> 'Twixt Mars and Venus see an interest.

Especially if they be bald, for bald men have ever been suspicious (read more in Aristotle, *sect.* 4, *prob.* 19), as Galba, Otho,
Domitian, and remarkable Cæsar amongst the rest: *Urbani
servate uxores, mœchum calvum adducimus* [2] [citizens, look to
your wives, we bring along a bald-headed gallant]; besides,
this bald Cæsar, saith Curio in Suetonius, was *omnium mulierum
vir* [ran after every woman he saw]; he made love to Eunoe,
Queen of Mauritania; to Cleopatra; to Posthumia, wife to Sergius
Sulpicius; to Lollia, wife to Gabinius; to Tertulla, of Crassus;
to Mucia, Pompey's wife, and I know not how many besides:
and well he might, for, if all be true that I have read, he had
a licence to lie with whom he list. *Inter alios honores Cæsari
decretos* (as Suetonius, *cap.* 52 *de Julio,* and Dion, *lib.* 44, relate)
jus illi datum, cum quibuscunque feminis se jungendi. Every
private history will yield such variety of instances: otherwise
good, wise, discreet men, virtuous and valiant, but too faulty
in this. Priamus had fifty sons, but seventeen alone lawfully
begotten. Philippus Bonus left fourteen bastards.[3] Laurence
Medices,[4] a good prince and a wise, but, saith Machiavel, prodigiously lascivious.[5] None so valiant as Castruccius Castrucanus, but, as the said author hath it, none so incontinent as
he was.[6] And 'tis not only predominant in grandees, this fault;
but, if you will take a great man's testimony, 'tis familiar with
every base soldier in France (and elsewhere, I think). "This
vice" (saith mine author [7]) "is so common with us in France,
that he is of no account, a mere coward, not worthy the name
of a soldier, that is not a notorious whoremaster." In Italy
he is not a gentleman, that besides his wife hath not a courtesan
and mistress. 'Tis no marvel, then, if poor women in such cases
be jealous, when they shall see themselves manifestly neglected,
contemned, loathed, unkindly used; their disloyal husbands to
entertain others in their rooms, and many times to court ladies
to their faces; other men's wives to wear their jewels: how
shall a poor woman in such a case moderate her passion? *Quis*

tibi nunc, Dido, cernenti talia sensus![1] [What feelings were thine, Dido, at such a sight!]

How, on the other side, shall a poor man contain himself from this feral malady, when he shall see so manifest signs of his wife's inconstancy? whenas, like Milo's wife, she dotes upon every young man she sees, or, as Martial's Sota,[2] *deserto sequitur Clitum marito* [deserts her husband and follows Clitus]. Though her husband be proper and tall, fair and lovely to behold, able to give contentment to any one woman, yet she will taste of the forbidden fruit: Juvenal's Iberina to a hair, she is as well pleased with one eye as one man. If a young gallant come by chance into her presence, a Fastidious Brisk,[3] that can wear his clothes well in fashion, with a lock, jingling spur, a feather, that can cringe, and withal compliment, court a gentlewoman, she raves upon him: "O what a lovely proper man he was," another Hector, an Alexander, a goodly man, a demigod, how sweetly he carried himself, with how comely a grace, *sic oculos, sic ille manus, sic ora ferebat* [such eyes, such hands, such looks], how neatly he did wear his clothes! *Quam sese ore ferens, quam forti pectore et armis*[4] [how nobly he looked, how bravely he bore himself!], how bravely did he discourse, ride, sing, and dance, etc.; and then she begins to loathe her husband, *repugnans osculatur* [she kisses him with loathing], to hate him and his filthy beard, his goatish complexion, as Doris said of Polyphemus, *totus qui saniem, totus ut hircus olet,*[5] he is a rammy fulsome fellow, a goblin-faced fellow, he smells, he stinks, *et cæpas simul alliumque ructat* [he reeks of onion and garlic]; *si quando ad thalamum,* etc. [should he approach the nuptial couch], how like a dizzard, a fool, an ass, he looks, how like a clown he behaves himself! she will not come near him by her own good will, but wholly rejects him, as Venus did her fuliginous Vulcan at last: *Nec deus hunc mensa, dea nec dignata cubili est* [no god honoured him with a seat at his table, nor goddess with her couch]. So did Lucretia, a lady of Senæ,[6] after she had but seen Euryalus, *in Euryalum tota ferebatur, domum reversa,* etc., she would not hold her eyes off him in his presence, *tantum egregio decus enitet ore*[7] [such beauty from his noble presence shone], and in his absence could think of none but him, *odit virum,* she loathed her husband forthwith, might not abide him:

> *Et conjugalis negligens tori, viro*
> *Præsente, acerbo nauseat fastidio;*[8]

> All against the laws of matrimony,
> She did abhor her husband's phis'nomy;

and sought all opportunity to see her sweetheart again. Now
when the good man shall observe his wife so lightly given,
"to be so free and familiar with every gallant, her immodesty
and wantonness" (as Camerarius notes [1]), it must needs yield
matter of suspicion to him, when she still pranks up herself
beyond her means and fortunes, makes impertinent journeys,
unnecessary visitations, stays out so long, with such and such
companions, so frequently goes to plays, masks, feasts, and all
public meetings, shall use such immodest gestures,[2] free speeches,
and withal show some distaste of her own husband; how can he
choose, though he were another Socrates, but be suspicious, and
instantly jealous? *Socraticas tandem faciet transcendere metas* [3]
['twill make him transgress the Socratic bounds]; more especially
when he shall take notice of their more secret and sly tricks,
which to cornute their husbands they commonly use (*dum ludis,
ludos hæc te facit* [while you play, she makes game of you]),
they pretend love, honour, chastity, and seem to respect them
before all men living; saints in show, so cunningly can they
dissemble, they will not so much as look upon another man in
his presence, so chaste, so religious, and so devout, they cannot
endure the name or sight of a quean, an harlot, out upon her![4]
and in their outward carriage are most loving and officious,
will kiss their husband, and hang about his neck (dear husband,
sweet husband), and with a composed countenance salute him,
especially when he comes home; or if he go from home, weep,
sigh, lament, and take upon them to be sick and swoon (like
Jocundo's wife in Ariosto,[5] when her husband was to depart),
and yet arrant, etc., they care not for him:

> Ay me, the thought (quoth she) makes me so 'fraid,
> That scarce the breath abideth in my breast;
> Peace, my sweet love and wife, Jocundo said,
> And weeps as fast, and comforts her his best, etc.
> All this might not assuage the woman's pain,
> Needs must I die before you come again,
> Nor how to keep my life I can devise,
> The doleful days and nights I shall sustain,
> From meat my mouth, from sleep will keep mine eyes, etc.
> That very night that went before the morrow,
> That he had pointed surely to depart,
> Jocondo's wife was sick, and swoon'd for sorrow
> Amid his arms, so heavy was her heart.

And yet for all these counterfeit tears and protestations, Jocundo
coming back in all haste for a jewel he had forgot,

His chaste and [faithful] yoke-fellow he found
Yok'd with a knave, all hor..sty neglected,
The adulterer sleeping very sound,
Yet by his face was easily detected;
A beggar's brat bred by him from his cradle,
And now was riding on his master's saddle.

Thus can they cunningly counterfeit, as Platina describes their customs,[1] "kiss their husbands, whom they had rather see hanging on a gallows, and swear they love him dearer than their own lives, whose soul they would not ransom for their little dog's":

Similis si permutatio detur,
Morte viri cupiunt animam servare catellæ.

Many of them seem to be precise and holy forsooth, and will go to such a church, to hear such a good man by all means, an excellent man, when 'tis for no other intent (as he follows it) than "to see and to be seen, to observe what fashions are in use, to meet some pander, bawd, monk, friar, or to entice some good fellow." [2] For they persuade themselves, as Nevisanus shows,[3] "that it is neither sin nor shame to lie with a lord or a parish priest, if he be a proper man"; "and though she kneel often, and pray devoutly, 'tis" (saith Platina) "not for her husband's welfare, or children's good, or any friend, but for her sweetheart's return, her pander's health." [4] If her husband would have her go, she feigns herself sick, *Et simulat subito condoluisse caput:* [5] her head aches, and she cannot stir; but if her paramour ask as much, she is for him in all seasons, at all hours of the night. In the kingdom of Malabar, and about Goa in the East Indies,[6] the women are so subtle that, with a certain drink they give them to drive away cares as they say, "they will make them sleep for twenty-four hours, or so intoxicate them that they can remember naught of that they saw done or heard, and, by washing of their feet, restore them again, and so make their husbands cuckolds to their faces." [7] Some are ill disposed [8] at all times to all persons they like, others more wary to some few, at such and such seasons, as Augusta Livia *non nisi plena navi vectorem tollebat* [carried no passenger save in a full boat]. But as he said:

No pen could write, no tongue attain to tell,
By force of eloquence, or help of art,
Of women's treacheries the hundredth part.[9]

Both, to say truth, are often faulty; men and women give just occasion in this humour of discontent, aggravate and yield matter of suspicion: but most part of the chief causes proceed from other adventitious accidents and circumstances, though the parties be free, and both well given themselves. The undiscreet carriage of some lascivious gallant (*et e contra* of some light woman) by his often frequenting of an house, bold unseemly gestures, may make a breach, and by his over-familiarity, if he be inclined to yellowness, colour him quite out. If he be poor, basely born, saith Benedetto Varchi, and otherwise unhandsome, he suspects him the less; but if a proper man, such as was Alcibiades in Greece, and Castruccius Castrucanus in Italy, well descended, commendable for his good parts, he taketh on the more, and watcheth his doings. Theodosius the emperor gave his wife Eudocia a golden apple when he was a suitor to her, which she long after bestowed upon a young gallant in the court, of her especial acquaintance. The emperor, espying this apple in his hand, suspected forthwith, more than was, his wife's dishonesty, banished him the court, and from that day following forbare to accompany her any more.[1] A rich merchant had a fair wife; according to his custom he went to travel; in his absence a good fellow tempted his wife; she denied him; yet he, dying a little after, gave her a legacy for the love he bore her. At his return, her jealous husband, because she had got more by land than he had done at sea, turned her away upon suspicion.[2]

Now when those other circumstances of time and place, opportunity and importunity, shall concur, what will they not effect?

Fair opportunity can win the coyest she that is,
So wisely he takes time, as he 'll be sure he will not miss:
Then he that loves her gamesome vein, and tempers toys with art,
Brings love that swimmeth in her eyes to dive into her heart.

As at plays, masks, great feasts and banquets, one singles out his wife to dance, another courts her in his presence, a third tempts her, a fourth insinuates with a pleasing compliment, a sweet smile, ingratiates himself with an amphibological speech, as that merry companion in the satirist[3] did to his Glycerium, *adsidens et interiorem palmam amabiliter concutiens* [sitting by her and lovingly stroking her palm]:

Quod meus hortus habet sumas impune licebit,
Si dederis nobis quod tuus hortus habet;

[You are at liberty to take what is in my garden if you will give me what is in your garden;]

with many such, etc., and then, as he saith,

She may no while in chastity abide,
That is assaid on every side.

For after a great feast, *Vino sæpe suum nescit amica virum* [1]
[in her cups a maid oft knows not her own lover].   Noah (saith
Hierome [2]) "showed his nakedness in his drunkenness, which
for six hundred years he had covered in soberness."   Lot lay
with his daughters in his drink, as Cinyras with Myrrha, *quid
enim Venus ebria curat?* [3] [for what scruples has love when
flown with wine?]   The most continent may be overcome, or
if otherwise they keep bad company, they that are modest of
themselves, and dare not offend, "confirmed by others, grow
impudent, and confident, and get an ill habit." [4]

> *Alia quæstus gratia matrimonium corrumpit,*
> *Alia peccans multas vult morbi habere socias.* [5]

> [One for pelf breaks her marriage vow, another desires
> to have many companions in sin.]

Or if they dwell in suspected places, as in an infamous inn,
near some stews, near monks, friars, Nevisanus adds, where be
many tempters and solicitors, idle persons that frequent their
companies, it may give just cause of suspicion.   Martial [6] of
old inveighed against them that counterfeited a disease to go
to the bath; for so, many times,

> *relicto*
> *Conjuge Penelope venit, abit Helene.*

> [She left her husband a Penelope, she returned a Helen.]

Æneas Sylvius puts in a caveat against princes' courts, because
there be *tot formosi juvenes qui promittunt,* so many brave suitors
to tempt, etc.   "If you leave her in such a place, you shall likely
find her in company you like not; either they come to her, or
she is gone to them." [7]   Kornmannus [8] makes a doubting jest
in his lascivious country: *Virginis illibata censeaturne castitas ad
quam frequentur accedant scholares?* [can a girl be presumed to
have preserved her chastity who is visited by many students?]
And Baldus the lawyer scoffs on; *Quum scholaris, inquit, loquitur
cum puella, non præsumitur ei dicere, Pater noster,* when a scholar
talks with a maid or another man's wife in private, it is presumed
he saith not a paternoster.   Or if I shall see a monk or a friar
climb up a ladder at midnight into a virgin's or widow's chamber-
window, I shall hardly think he then goes to administer the
sacraments, or to take her confession.   These are the ordinary
causes of jealousy, which are intended or remitted as the
circumstances vary.

MEMB. II.

Symptoms of Jealousy: Fear, Sorrow, Suspicion, strange Actions,
Gestures, Outrages, Locking Up, Oaths, Trials, Laws, etc.

OF all passions, as I have already proved, love is most violent,
and of those bitter potions which this love-melancholy affords,
this bastard jealousy is the greatest, as appears by those prodigious symptoms which it hath, and that it produceth. For
besides fear and sorrow, which is common to all melancholy,
anxiety of mind, suspicion, aggravation, restless thoughts,
paleness, meagreness, neglect of business, and the like, these
men are farther yet misaffected, and in a higher strain. 'Tis
a more vehement passion, a more furious perturbation, a bitter
pain, a fire, a pernicious curiosity, a gall corrupting the honey
of our life, madness, vertigo, plague, hell, they are more than
ordinarily disquieted, they lose *bonum pacis* [the boon of peace],
as Chrysostom observes; [1] and though they be rich, keep
sumptuous tables, be nobly allied, yet *miserrimi omnium sunt*,
they are most miserable, they are more than ordinarily discontent, more sad, *nihil tristius*, more than ordinarily suspicious.
Jealousy, saith Vives,[2] "begets unquietness in the mind, night
and day: he hunts after every word he hears, every whisper,
and amplifies it to himself" (as all melancholy men do in other
matters) "with a most unjust calumny of others; he mis-
interprets everything is said or done, most apt to mistake or
misconster," he pries into every corner, follows close, observes
to a hair. 'Tis proper to jealousy so to do,

> Pale hag, infernal fury, pleasure's smart,
> Envy's observer, prying in every part.

Besides those strange gestures of staring, frowning, grinning,
rolling of eyes, menacing, ghastly looks, broken pace, interrupt,
precipitate half-turns. He will sometimes sigh, weep, sob for
anger,

> *Nempe suos imbres etiam ista tonitrua fundunt,*
>
> [These thunders bring their own downpours after them,]

swear and belie, slander any man, curse, threaten, brawl, scold,
fight; and sometimes again flatter and speak fair, ask forgiveness, kiss and coll, condemn his rashness and folly, vow, protest,
and swear he will never do so again; and then eftsoons, impatient
as he is, rave, roar, and lay about him like a madman, thump

her sides, drag her about perchance, drive her out of doors,
send her home, he will be divorced forthwith, she is a whore,
etc.; by and by with all submiss compliment entreat her fair,
and bring her in again, he loves her dearly, she is his sweet,
most kind and loving wife, he will not change, nor leave her for
a kingdom; so he continues off and on, as the toy takes him,
the object moves him, but most part brawling, fretting, unquiet
he is, accusing and suspecting not strangers only, but brothers
and sisters, father and mother, nearest and dearest friends.
He thinks with those Italians,

> *Chi non tocca parentado,*
> *Tocca mai e rado,*

and through fear conceives unto himself things almost incredible
and impossible to be effected. As a heron when she fishes, still
prying on all sides, or as a cat doth a mouse, his eye is never
off hers; he gloats on him, on her, accurately observing on whom
she looks, who looks at her, what she saith, doth, at dinner, at
supper, sitting, walking, at home, abroad, he is the same, still
inquiring, maundering, gazing, listening, affrighted with every
small object; why did she smile, why did she pity him, commend
him? why did she drink twice to such a man? why did she offer
to kiss, to dance? etc.; a whore, a whore, an arrant whore. All
this he confesseth in the poet:

> *Omnia me terrent, timidus sum, ignosce timori,*
> *Et miser in tunica suspicor esse virum.*
> *Me lædit si multa tibi dabit oscula mater,*
> *Me soror, et cum qua dormit amica simul.*[1]

> Each thing affrights me, I do fear,
>   Ah pardon me my fear,
> I doubt a man is hid within
>   The clothes that thou dost wear.

Is 't not a man in woman's apparel? is not somebody in that
great chest, or behind the door, or hangings, or in some of
those barrels? may not a man steal in at the window with a
ladder of ropes, or come down the chimney, have a false key,
or get in when he is asleep? If a mouse do but stir, or the
wind blow, a casement clatter, that 's the villain, there he is:
by his good will no man shall see her, salute her, speak with her,
she shall not go forth of his sight, so much as to do her needs.
Non ita bovem Argus, etc.,[2] Argus did not so keep his cow, that
watchful dragon the golden fleece, or Cerberus the coming in
of hell, as he keeps his wife. If a dear friend or near kinsman

come as a guest to his house, to visit him, he will never let him be out of his own sight and company, lest peradventure, etc. If the necessity of his business be such that he must go from home, he doth either lock her up, or commit her with a deal of injunctions and protestations to some trusty friends, him and her he sets and bribes to oversee: one servant is set in his absence to watch another, and all to observe his wife, and yet all this will not serve; though his business be very urgent, he will when he is half-way come back again in all post-haste, rise from supper, or at midnight, and be gone, and sometimes leave his business undone, and as a stranger court his own wife in some disguised habit. Though there be no danger at all, no cause of suspicion, she live in such a place where Messalina herself could not be dishonest if she would, yet he suspects her as much as if she were in a bawdy-house, some prince's court, or in a common inn, where all comers might have free access. He calls her on a sudden all to naught, she is a strumpet, a light huswife, a bitch, an arrant whore. No persuasion, no protestation can divert this passion, nothing can ease him, secure or give him satisfaction. It is most strange to report what outrageous acts by men and women have been committed in this kind, by women especially, that will run after their husbands into all places and companies, as Jovianus Pontanus' wife did by him,[1] follow him whithersoever he went, it matters not, or upon what business, raving like Juno in the tragedy, miscalling, cursing, swearing, and mistrusting every one she sees. Gomesius in his third book of the life and deeds of Francis Ximenins, sometime Archbishop of Toledo, hath a strange story of that incredible jealousy of Joan Queen of Spain, wife to King Philip, mother of Ferdinand and Charles the Fifth, emperors: when her husband Philip, either for that he was tired with his wife's jealousy, or had some great business, went into the Low Countries, she was so impatient and melancholy upon his departure, that she would scarce eat her meat, or converse with any man; and though she were with child, the season of the year very bad, the wind against her, in all haste she would to sea after him. Neither Isabella her queen mother, the archbishop, or any other friend could persuade her to the contrary, but she would after him. When she was now come into the Low Countries, and kindly entertained by her husband, she could not contain herself, "but in a rage ran upon a yellow-haired wench," with whom she suspected her husband to be naught, "cut off her hair, did beat her black and blue, and so dragged

her about." [1]   It is an ordinary thing for women in such cases
to scratch the faces, slit the noses of such as they suspect; as
Henry the Second's importune Juno did by Rosamond at Wood-
stock: for she complains in a modern poet,[2] she scarce spake,

> But flies with eager fury to my face,
> Offering me most unwomanly disgrace.
> Look how a tigress, etc.
> So fell she on me in outrageous wise,
> As could disdain and jealousy devise.

Or if it be so they dare not or cannot execute any such tyrannical
injustice, they will miscall, rail and revile, bear them deadly
hate and malice, as Tacitus observes, "The hatred of a jealous
woman is inseparable against such as she suspects." [3]

> *Nulla vis flammæ tumidique venti*
> *Tanta, nec teli metuenda torti,*
> *Quanta cum conjux viduata tædis*
> *Ardet et odit.*[4]

> Winds, weapons, flames make not such hurly-burly,
> As raving women turn all topsy-turvy.

So did Agrippina by Lollia, and Calpurnia in the days of Claudius.
But women are sufficiently curbed in such cases; the rage of
men is more eminent, and frequently put in practice.   See but
with what rigour those jealous husbands tyrannize over their poor
wives in Greece, Spain, Italy, Turkey, Africa, Asia, and generally
over all those hot countries.   *Mulieres vestræ terra vestra, arate
sicut vultis,*[5] Mahomet in his Alcoran gives this power to men:
your wives are as your land, till them, use them, entreat them
fair or foul, as you will yourselves.   *Mecastor lege dura vivunt
mulieres* [6] [of a truth, women's lives are governed by a hard
law], they lock them still in their houses, which are so many
prisons to them, will suffer nobody to come at them, or their
wives to be seen abroad, *nec campos liceat lustrare patentes*
[they may not stroll across the open fields].   They must not
so much as look out.   And if they be great persons, they have
eunuchs to keep them, as the Grand Seignior among the Turks,
the Sophies of Persia, those Tartarian Mogors, and Kings of
China.   *Infantes masculos castrant innumeros ut regi serviant,*
saith Riccius,[7] "they geld innumerable infants" to this purpose;
the King of China "maintains 10,000 eunuchs in his family to
keep his wives." [8]   The Xeriffs of Barbary keep their courtesans
in such a strict manner, that if any man come but in sight of
them he dies for it; and if they chance to see a man, and do

not instantly cry out, though from their windows, they must be put to death. The Turks have I know not how many black, deformed eunuchs (for the white serve for other ministries) to this purpose sent commonly from Egypt, deprived in their childhood of all their privities, and brought up in the seraglio at Constantinople to keep their wives; which are so penned up they may not confer with any living man, or converse with younger women, have a cucumber or carrot sent into them for their diet, but sliced, for fear, etc., and so live and are left alone to their unchaste thoughts all the days of their lives. The vulgar sort of women, if at any time they come abroad, which is very seldom, to visit one another or to go to their baths, are so covered that no man can see them, as the matrons were in old Rome, *lectica aut sella tecta vectæ* [riding in a litter or sedan-chair], so Dion[1] and Seneca record, *velatæ totæ incedunt* [they go completely veiled], which Alexander ab Alexandro relates of the Parthians, *lib.* 5, *cap.* 24,[2] which, with Andreas Tiraquellus his commentator, I rather think should be understood of Persians. I have not yet said all; they do not only lock them up, *sed et pudendis seras adhibent*: hear what Bembus relates, *lib.* 6 of his Venetian History, of those inhabitants that dwell about Quiloa in Africa. *Lusitani, inquit, quorundum civitates adierunt, qui natis statim feminis naturam consuunt, quoad urinæ exitus ne impediatur, easque quum adoleverint sic consutas in matrimonium collocant, ut sponsi prima cura sit conglutinatas puellæ oras ferro interscindere.* In some parts of Greece at this day, like those old Jews, they will not believe their wives are honest, *nisi pannum menstruatum prima nocte videant*: our countryman Sandys, in his Peregrination,[3] saith it is severely observed in Zacynthus, or Zante; and Leo Afer in his time at Fez, in Africa: *Non credunt virginem esse nisi videant sanguineam mappam; si non, ad parentes pudore rejicitur.* Those sheets are publicly shown by their parents, and kept as a sign of incorrupt virginity. The Jews of old examined their maids *ex tenui membrana,* called hymen, which Laurentius in his Anatomy, Columbus, *lib.* 12, *cap.* 16, Capivaccius, *lib.* 4, *cap.* 11, *de uteri affectibus,* Vincent. Alsarius Genuensis, *Quæsit. med. cent.* 4, Hieronymus Mercurialis, *Consult.,* Ambros. Pareus, Julius Cæsar Claudinus, *Respons.* 4, as that also *de ruptura venarum ut sanguis fluat,*[4] copiously confute; 'tis no sufficient trial, they contend. And yet others again defend it, Gaspar Bartholinus, *Institut. Anat. lib.* 1, *cap.* 31, Pinæus of Paris, Albertus Magnus, *de secret. mulier. cap.* 9 *et* 10, etc., and think they speak too much in favour of women. *Ludovicus Bonaciolus,*[1] *lib. 2, cap.* 2, *Muliebr., naturalem illam uteri labiorum constrictionem, in qua virginitatem consistere volunt, astringentibus medicinis fieri posse vindicat, et si defloratæ sint, astutæ mulieres (inquit) nos fallunt in his.*[2] *Idem Alsarius Crucius Genuensis iisdem fere verbis. Idem Avicenna, lib.* 3, *fen.* 20, *tract.* 1, *cap.* 47, *Rhasis, Continent. lib.* 24,[3] *Rodericus a Castro, de nat. mul. lib.* 1, *cap.* 3. An old bawdy nurse in Aristænetus[4] (like that Spanish Cælestina, *quæ quinque mille virgines fecit mulieres, totidemque mulieres arte sua virgines*[5]), when a fair maid of her acquaintance wept and made her moan to her, how she had been deflowered, and, now ready to be married, was afraid it would be perceived, comfortably replied, *Noli vereri, filia,* etc.: "Fear not, daughter, I'll teach thee a trick to help it." *Sed hæc extra callem* [but these matters are out of my way]. To what end are all those astrological questions, *an sit virgo, an sit casta, an sit mulier?* and such strange absurd trials in Albertus Magnus, Bap. Porta, *Mag. lib. 2, cap. 21,* in Wecker, *lib. 5 de secret.,* by stones, perfumes, to make them piss, and confess I know not what in their sleep; some jealous brain was the first founder of them. And to what passion may we ascribe those severe laws against jealousy (Num. v, 14), adulterers (Deut. xxii, 22), as amongst the Hebrews, amongst the Egyptians (read Bohemus, *lib.* 1, *cap.* 5, *de mor. gen.*;[6] of the Carthaginians, *cap.* 6; of Turks, *lib.* 2, *cap.* 11), amongst the Athenians of old, Italians at this day, wherein they are to be severely punished, cut in pieces, burned, *vivi-comburio,* buried alive, with several expurgations, etc., are they not as so many symptoms of incredible jealousy? We may say the same of those vestal virgins that fetched water in a sieve, as Tatia did in Rome, *anno ab urbe condita* 800, before senators; and Æmilia, *virgo innocens,* that ran over hot irons,[7] as Emma, Edward the Confessor's mother, did, the king himself being a spectator, with the like. We read in Nicephorus, that Cunegunda, the wife of Henricus Bavarus, emperor, suspected of adultery, *insimulata adulterii per ignitos vomeres illæsa transiit,* trod upon red-hot coulters, and had no harm: such another story we find in Regino, *lib.* 2; in Aventinus and Sigonius, of Charles the Third and his wife Richarda, *an.* 887, that was so purged with hot irons. Pausanias saith that he was once an eye-witness of such a miracle at Diana's temple, a maid without any harm at all walked upon burning coals. Pius Secundus,[8] in his description of Europe, *cap.* 46, relates as much, that it was commonly practised at Diana's temple, for women to go barefoot over hot coals, to try their honesties: Plinius, Solinus, and many writers, make mention of Feronia's temple,[1] and Dionysius Halicarnasseus, *lib.* 3, of Memnon's statue, which were used to this purpose, Tatius, *lib.* 6, of Pan his cave (much like old St. Wilfrid's needle in Yorkshire [2]) wherein they did use to try maids, whether they were honest; [3] when Leucippe went in, *suavissimus exaudiri sonus cœpit* [a wonderfully sweet sound began to make itself heard]. Austin, *de Civ. Dei, lib.* 10, *cap.* 16, relates many such examples, all which Lavater, *de spectr. part.* 1, *cap.* 19, contends to be done by the illusion of devils; though Thomas, *quæst.* 6, *de potentia*, etc., ascribes it to good angels. Some, saith Austin,[4] compel their wives to swear they be honest, as if perjury were a lesser sin than adultery; some consult oracles, as Pheron, that blind king of Egypt.[5] Others reward, as those old Romans used to do; if a woman were contented with one man, *corona pudicitiæ donabatur*, she had a crown of chastity bestowed on her. When all this will not serve, saith Alexander Gaguinus, *cap.* 5 *descript. Muscoviæ*, the Muscovites, if they suspect their wives, will beat them till they confess, and if that will not avail, like those wild Irish, be divorced at their pleasures, or else knock them on the heads, as the old Gauls have done in former ages.[6] Of this tyranny of jealousy read more in Parthenius, *Erot. cap.* 10; Camerarius, *cap.* 53 *Hor. subcis. et cent.* 2, *cap.* 34; Cælia's Epistles; Tho. Chaloner, *de repub. Ang. lib.* 9; Ariosto, *lib.* 31, staff 1; Felix Platerus, *Observat. lib.* 1, etc.

MEMB. III.

Prognostics of Jealousy, Despair, Madness, to make away themselves and others

THOSE which are jealous, most part, if they be not otherwise relieved, "proceed from suspicion to hatred, from hatred to frenzy, madness, injury, murder, and despair." [7]

> A plague by whose most damnable effect,
> Divers in deep despair to die have sought.
> By which a man to madness near is brought,
> As well with causeless as with just suspect.[8]

In their madness many times, saith Vives,[9] they make away themselves and others. Which induceth Cyprian to call it *fecundam et multiplicem perniciem, fontem cladium et seminarium delictorum,* a fruitful mischief, the seminary of offences, and fountain of murders. Tragical examples are too common in this kind, both new and old, in all ages, as of Cephalus and Procris,[1] Pheron of Egypt,[2] Tereus, Atreus, and Thyestes. Alexander Pheræus was murdered of his wife, *ob pellicatus suspicionem,* Tully saith.[3] Antoninus Verus was so made away by Lucilla; Demetrius the son of Antigonus, and Nicanor, by their wives; Hercules poisoned by Deianira, Cæcinna murdered by Vespasian,[4] Justina, a Roman lady, by her husband. Amestris, Xerxes' wife, because she found her husband's cloak in Masista his house, "cut off Masista his wife's paps, and gave them to the dogs, flayed her besides, and cut off her ears, lips, tongue, and slit the nose of Artaynta her daughter."[5] Our late writers are full of such outrages.

Paulus Æmilius, in his History of France,[6] hath a tragical story of Chilpericus the First his death, made away by Fredegunde his queen. In a jealous humour he came from hunting, and stole behind his wife, as she was dressing and combing her head in the sun, gave her a familiar touch with his wand, which she mistaking for her lover, said, "Ah, Landre, a good knight should strike before, and not behind": but when she saw herself betrayed by his presence, she instantly took order to make him away. Hierome Osorius, in the eleventh book of the deeds of Emanuel, King of Portugal, to this effect hath a tragical narration of one Ferdinandus Calderia, that wounded Gotherinus, a noble countryman of his, at Goa in the East Indies, "and cut off one of his legs, for that he looked, as he thought, too familiarly upon his wife, which was afterwards a cause of many quarrels and much bloodshed."[7] Guianerius, *cap. 36 de ægritud. matr.,* speaks of a silly jealous fellow, that seeing his child new-born included in a kell, thought sure a Franciscan that used to come to his house was the father of it, it was so like the friar's cowl, and thereupon threatened the friar to kill him:[8] Fulgosus, of a woman in Narbonne, that cut off her husband's privities in the night, because she thought he played false with her. The story of Jonuses Bassa, and fair Manto his wife, is well known to such as have read the Turkish History; and that of Joan of Spain, of which I treated in my former section. Her jealousy, saith Gomesius, was the cause of both their deaths: King Philip died for grief a little after, as Martian his physician gave it out, "and she for her part after a melancholy discontented life, misspent in lurking-holes and corners, made an end of her miseries."[9]

Felix Plater, in the first book of his Observations, hath many
such instances, of a physician of his acquaintance, "that was
first mad through jealousy, and afterwards desperate": [1] of a
merchant "that killed his wife in the same humour, and after
precipitated himself": [2] of a doctor of law that cut off his
man's nose: of a painter's wife in Basil, *anno* 1600, that was
mother of nine children and had been twenty-seven years
married, yet afterwards jealous, and so impatient that she
became desperate, and would neither eat nor drink in her own
house, for fear her husband should poison her. 'Tis a common
sign this; for when once the humours are stirred, and the
imagination misaffected, it will vary itself in divers forms;
and many such absurd symptoms will accompany, even madness itself. Sckenkius, *Observat. lib. 4, cap. de uter.* hath an
example of a jealous woman that by this means had many
fits of the mother: and in his first book of some that through
jealousy ran mad: of a baker that gelded himself to try his
wife's honesty, etc. Such examples are too common.

MEMB. IV.

SUBSECT. I.—*Cure of Jealousy: by avoiding Occasions, not to
be Idle; by Good Counsel; to contemn it, not to watch or
lock them up; to dissemble it, etc.*

As of all other melancholy, some doubt whether this malady
may be cured or no, they think 'tis like the gout,[3] or Switzers,
whom we commonly call Walloons, those hired soldiers, if once
they take possession of a castle they can never be got out.

> *Qui timet, ut sua sit, ne quis sibi subtrahat illam,*
> *Ille Machaonia vix ope salvus erit.*

> [He who is in constant fear that his wife will be filched
> from him can scarce be cured by any doctor.]

> This is the cruel wound, against whose smart,
> No liquor's force prevails, or any plaster,
> No skill of stars, no depth of magic art,
> Devised by that great clerk Zoroaster;
> A wound that so infects the soul and heart,
> As all our sense and reason it doth master;
> A wound whose pang and torment is so durable,
> As it may rightly called be incurable.[4]

Yet what I have formerly said of other melancholy, I will say again, it may be cured, or mitigated at least, by some contrary passion, good counsel and persuasion, if it be withstood in the beginning, maturely resisted, and as those ancients hold, "the nails of it be pared before they grow too long." [1] No better means to resist or repel it than by avoiding idleness, to be still seriously busied about some matters of importance, to drive out those vain fears, foolish fantasies, and irksome suspicions out of his head, and then to be persuaded by his judicious friends to give ear to their good counsel and advice, and wisely to consider how much he discredits himself, his friends, dishonours his children, disgraceth his family, publisheth his shame, and, as a trumpeter of his own misery, divulgeth, macerates, grieves himself and others; what an argument of weakness it is, how absurd a thing in its own nature, how ridiculous, how brutish a passion, how sottish, how odious; for as Hierome well hath it,[2] *Odium sui facit, et ipse novissime sibi odio est*, others hate him, and at last he hates himself for it; how hare-brain a disease, mad and furious. If he will but hear them speak, no doubt he may be cured. Joan, Queen of Spain, of whom I have formerly spoken, under pretence of changing air was sent to Complutum, or Alcala de las Henares, where Ximenius the Archbishop of Toledo then lived, that by his good counsel (as for the present she was) she might be eased.[3] "For a disease of the soul, if concealed, tortures and overturns it, and by no physic can sooner be removed than by a discreet man's comfortable speeches." [4] I will not here insert any consolatory sentences to this purpose, or forestall any man's invention, but leave it every one to dilate and amplify as he shall think fit in his own judgment: let him advise with Siracides, *cap.* ix, 1: "Be not jealous over the wife of thy bosom"; read that comfortable and pithy speech to this purpose of Ximenius, in the author himself, as it is recorded by Gomesius; consult with Chaloner, *lib.* 9 *de repub. Anglor.*, or Cælia in her Epistles, etc. Only this I will add, that if it be considered aright, which causeth this jealous passion, be it just or unjust, whether with or without cause, true or false, it ought not so heinously to be taken; 'tis no such real or capital matter, that it should make so deep a wound. 'Tis a blow that hurts not, an insensible smart, grounded many times upon false suspicion alone, and so fostered by a sinister conceit. If she be not dishonest, he troubles and macerates himself without a cause; or put case, which is the worst, he be a cuckold, it cannot be helped, the

more he stirs in it, the more he aggravates his own misery.
How much better were it in such a case to dissemble or contemn
it! why should that be feared which cannot be redressed?
Multæ tandem deposuerunt (saith Vives [1]) *quum flecti maritos
non posse vident,* many women, when they see there is no
remedy, have been pacified; and shall men be more jealous than
women? 'Tis some comfort in such a case to have companions,
Solamen miseris socios habuisse doloris. Who can say he is
free? Who can assure himself he is not one *de præterito* [in
the past], or secure himself *de futuro* [for the future]? If it
were his case alone, it were hard; but being as it is almost a
common calamity, 'tis not so grievously to be taken. If a man
have a lock which every man's key will open as well as his own,
why should he think to keep it private to himself? In some
countries they make nothing of it, *ne nobiles quidem,* saith Leo
Afer,[2] in many parts of Africa (if she be past fourteen) there's
not a nobleman that marries a maid, or that hath a chaste
wife; 'tis so common; as the moon gives horns once a month
to the world, do they to their husbands at least. And 'tis most
part true which that Caledonian lady, Argentocoxus a British
prince his wife, told Julia Augusta, which she took her up for
dishonesty: "We Britons are naught at least with some few
choice men of the better sort, but you Romans lie with every
base knave, you are a company of common whores." [3] Severus
the emperor in his time made laws for the restraint of this vice; [4]
and as Dion Nicæus relates in his life, *tria millia mœchorum,*
three thousand cuckold-makers, or *naturæ monetam adulterantes,*
as Philo calls them, false coiners, and clippers of nature's money,
were summoned into the court at once. And yet, *Non omnem
molitor quæ fluit unda videt,* the miller sees not all the water
that goes by his mill; no doubt but, as in our days, these were
of the commonalty, all the great ones were not so much as
called in question for it. Martial's epigram [5] I suppose might
have been generally applied in those licentious times: *Omnia
solus habes,* etc., thy goods, lands, money, wits are thine own,
Uxorem sed habes, Candide, cum populo, but, neighbour Candidus, your wife is common. Husband and cuckold in that age,
it seems, were reciprocal terms; the emperors themselves did
wear Actæon's badge; how many Cæsars might I reckon up
together, and what a catalogue of cornuted kings and princes
in every story! Agamemnon, Menelaus, Philippus of Greece,
Ptolemæus of Ægypt, Lucullus, Cæsar, Pompeius, Cato,
Augustus, Antonius, Antoninus, etc., that wore fair plumes

of bull's feathers in their crests. The bravest soldiers and most
heroical spirits could not avoid it. They have been active and
passive in this business, they have either given or taken horns.
King Arthur,[1] whom we call one of the Nine Worthies, for all
his great valour, was unworthily served by Mardred, one of his
Round-Table knights: and Guithera, or Helena Alba, his fair
wife, as Leland interprets it, was an arrant honest woman.
Parcerem libenter (saith mine author [2]) *heroinarum læsæ majestati,
si non historiæ veritas aurem vellicaret*, I could willingly wink
at a fair lady's faults, but that I am bound by the laws of
history to tell the truth: against his will, God knows, did he
write it, and so do I repeat it. I speak not of our times all this
while, we have good, honest, virtuous men and women, whom
fame, zeal, fear of God, religion and superstition contains: and
yet for all that, we have many knights of this order, so dubbed
by their wives, many good women abused by dissolute husbands.
In some places, and such persons, you may as soon enjoin
them to carry water in a sieve as to keep themselves honest.
What shall a man do now in such a case? What remedy is to
be had? how shall he be eased? By suing a divorce? this is
hard to be effected: *si non caste, tamen caute* [if they act not
chastely, they act warily], they carry the matter so cunningly,
that though it be as common as simony, as clear and as manifest
as the nose in a man's face, yet it cannot be evidently proved,
or they likely taken in the fact: they will have a knave Gallus
to watch, or with that Roman Sulpicia,[3] all made fast and sure,

*Ne se Cadurcis destitutam fasciis,
Nudam Caleno concumbentem videat.*

[Lest he should see her undressed and lying with Calenus.]

She will hardly be surprised by her husband, be he never so
wary. Much better then to put it up; the more he strives in
it, the more he shall divulge his own shame; make a virtue of
necessity, and conceal it. Yea, but the world takes notice of it,
'tis in every man's mouth: let them talk their pleasure, of whom
speak they not in this sense? From the highest to the lowest
they are thus censured all; there is no remedy then but patience.
It may be 'tis his own fault, and he hath no reason to complain,
'tis *quid pro quo*, she is bad, he is worse. "Bethink thyself,
hast thou not done as much for some of thy neighbours? why
dost thou require that of thy wife, which thou wilt not perform
thyself?" [4] Thou rangest like a town bull, "why art thou so
incensed if she tread awry?" [5]

Be it that some woman break chaste wedlock's laws,
And leaves her husband and becomes unchaste:
Yet commonly it is not without cause,
She sees her man in sin her goods to waste,
She feels that he his love from her withdraws,
And hath on some perhaps less worthy placed,
Who strike with sword, the scabbard them may strike,
And sure love craveth love, like asketh like.[1]

Ea semper studebit, saith Nevisanus,[2] *pares reddere vices*, she
will quit it if she can.   And therefore, as well adviseth Siracides,
cap. ix, 1, "teach her not an evil lesson against thyself," which,
as Jansenius, Lyranus, on this text, and Carthusianus interpret,
is no otherwise to be understood than that she do thee not a
mischief.   I do not excuse her in accusing thee; but if both
be naught, mend thyself first; for as the old saying is, A good
husband makes a good wife.

Yea, but, thou repliest, 'tis not the like reason betwixt man
and woman, through her fault my children are bastards, I may
not endure it; *Sit amarulenta, sit imperiosa, prodiga*, etc.,[3]
let her scold, brawl, and spend, I care not, *modo sit casta*, so she
be honest, I could easily bear it; but this I cannot, I may not,
I will not; my faith, my fame, mine eye must not be touched,
as the diverb is, *Non patitur tactum fama, fides, oculus*, I say
the same of my wife, touch all, use all, take all but this.   I
acknowledge that of Seneca to be true, *Nullius boni jucunda
possessio sine socio*, there is no sweet content in the possession
of any good thing without a companion, this only excepted,
I say, *this*.   And why this?   Even this which thou so much
abhorrest, it may be for thy progeny's good, better be any man's
son than thine,[4] to be begot of base Irus, poor Seius, or mean
Mævius, the town swineherd's, a shepherd's son: and well is
he, that like Hercules he hath any two fathers; for thou thyself
hast peradventure more diseases than an horse, more infirmities
of body and mind, a cankered soul, crabbed conditions; make
the worst of it, as it is *vulnus insanabile, sic vulnus insensibile*,
as it is incurable, so it is insensible.   But art thou sure it is so?
res agit ille tuas?[5] [does he do thy business for thee?], doth he so
indeed?   It may be thou art over-suspicious, and without a
cause as some are: if it be *octimestris partus*, born at eight months,
or like him, and him, they fondly suspect he got it; if she speak
or laugh familiarly with such or such men, then presently she
is naught with them; such is thy weakness: whereas charity,
or a well-disposed mind, would interpret all unto the best.   St.
Francis, by chance seeing a friar familiarly kissing another man's

wife, was so far from misconceiving it, that he presently kneeled
down and thanked God there was so much charity left: but they,
on the other side, will ascribe nothing to natural causes, indulge
nothing to familiarity, mutual society, friendship; but out of a
sinister suspicion, presently lock them close, watch them,
thinking by those means to prevent all such inconveniences,
that's the way to help it; whereas by such tricks they do
aggravate the mischief. 'Tis but in vain to watch that which
will away.

> *Nec custodiri si velit ulla potest;*
> *Nec mentem servare potes, licet omnia serves;*
> *Omnibus exclusis, intus adulter erit.*[1]

> None can be kept resisting for her part;
> Though body be kept close, within her heart
> Advoutry lurks, t' exclude it there 's no art.

Argus with an hundred eyes cannot keep her, *et hunc unus sæpe
fefellit amor* [even he was frequently deceived, and by love
alone], as in Ariosto: [2]

> If all our hearts were eyes, yet sure, they said,
> We husbands of our wives should be betrayed.

Hierome holds, *Uxor impudica servari non potest, pudica non
debet, infida custos castitatis est necessitas,* to what end is all
your custody? A dishonest woman cannot be kept, an honest
woman ought not to be kept, necessity is a keeper not to be
trusted. *Difficile custoditur, quod plures amant:* that which
many covet, can hardly be preserved, as Sarisburiensis thinks.[3]
I am of Æneas Sylvius' mind, "Those jealous Italians do very
ill to lock up their wives; for women are of such a disposition,
they will most covet that which is denied most, and offend least
when they have free liberty to trespass."[4] It is in vain to
lock her up if she be dishonest; *et tyrannicum imperium,* as our
great master Aristotle calls it, too tyrannical a task, most
unfit; for when she perceives her husband observes her and
suspects,[5] *liberius peccat* [she sins more freely], saith Nevisanus.
Toxica zelotypo dedit uxor mœcha marito [6] [the adulterous wife
gave poison to her jealous husband], she is exasperated, seeks
by all means to vindicate herself, and will therefore offend,
because she is unjustly suspected. The best course then is
to let them have their own wills, give them free liberty, without
any keeping.

> In vain our friends from this do us dehort,
> For beauty will be where is most resort.

If she be honest as Lucretia to Collatinus, Laodamia to
Protesilaus, Penelope to her Ulysses, she will so continue her
honour, good name, credit: *Penelope conjux semper Ulyssis ero*
[I shall always be Penelope the wife of Ulysses]; and as Phocias'
wife, in Plutarch, called her husband "her wealth, treasure,
world, joy, delight, orb, and sphere," [1] she will hers. The vow
she made unto her goodman, love, virtue, religion, zeal, are
better keepers than all those locks, eunuchs, prisons; she will
not be moved:

> *At mihi vel tellus optem prius ima dehiscat,*
> *Aut pater omnipotens adigat me fulmine ad umbras,*
> *Pallentes umbras Erebi, noctemque profundam,*
> *Ante, pudor, quam te violem, aut tua jura resolvam.* [2]

> First I desire the earth to swallow me,
> Before I violate mine honesty,
> Or thunder from above drive me to hell,
> With those pale ghosts and ugly night to dwell.

She is resolved with Dido to be chaste; though her husband be
false, she will be true; and as Octavia writ to her Antony:

> These walls that here do keep me out of sight,
> Shall keep me all unspotted unto thee,
> And testify that I will do thee right,
> I 'll never stain thine house, though thou shame me. [3]

Turn her loose to all those Tarquins and satyrs, she will not be
tempted. In the time of Valence the emperor, saith St. Austin, [4]
one Archidamus, a consul of Antioch, offered an hundred pound
of gold to a fair young wife, and besides to set her husband free,
who was then *sub gravissima custodia*, a dark prisoner, *pro
unius noctis concubitu* [for one night's intercourse]; but the
chaste matron would not accept of it. When one commended
Theano's fine arm to his fellows, she took him up short: "Sir,
'tis not common"; [5] she is wholly reserved to her husband.
Bilia had an old man to her spouse, and his breath stunk, so
that nobody could abide it abroad; "coming home one day he
reprehended his wife, because she did not tell him of it: she
vowed unto him, she had told him, but she thought every
man's breath had been as strong as his." [6] Tigranes and
Armenia his lady were invited to supper by King Cyrus: when
they came home, Tigranes asked his wife how she liked Cyrus,
and what she did especially commend in him? "she swore she
did not observe him; when he replied again, what then she did
observe, whom she looked on? she made answer, her husband

that said he would die for her sake."¹ Such are the properties
and conditions of good women; and if she be well given, she
will so carry herself; if otherwise she be naught, use all the
means thou canst, she will be naught. *Non deest animus sed
corruptor* [not the will but the seducer is lacking], she hath so
many lies, excuses, as an hare hath muses, tricks, panders, bawds,
shifts to deceive, 'tis to no purpose to keep her up, or to reclaim
her by hard usage. Fair means peradventure may do somewhat.
*Obsequio vinces aptius ipse tuo*² [you will gain better success by
giving in]. Men and women are both in a predicament in this
behalf, so sooner won, and better pacified. *Duci volunt, non
cogi* [they want to be led, not forced]; though she be as arrant
a scold as Xantippe, as cruel as Medea, as clamorous as Hecuba,
as lustful as Messalina, by such means (if at all) she may be
reformed. Many patient Grizels,³ by their obsequiousness in
this kind, have reclaimed their husbands from their wandering
lusts. In Nova Francia⁴ and Turkey (as Leah, Rachel, and
Sarah did to Abraham and Jacob) they bring their fairest damsels
to their husbands' beds; Livia seconded the lustful appetites of
Augustus; Stratonice, wife to King Deiotarus, did not only
bring Electra, a fair maid, to her goodman's bed, but brought
up the children begot on her, as carefully as if they had been
her own. Tertius Æmilius' wife, Cornelia's mother, perceiving
her husband's intemperance, *rem dissimulavit*, made much of
the maid, and would take no notice of it. A new-married man,
when a pickthank friend of his, to curry favour, had showed
him his wife familiar in private with a young gallant, courting
and dallying, etc., "Tush," said he, "let him do his worst, I dare
trust my wife, though I dare not trust him." The best remedy
then is by fair means; if that will not take place, to dissemble
it as I say, or turn it off with a jest: hear Guevara's advice in
this case, *Vel joco excipies, vel silentio eludes* [either make a jest of
it, or ignore it]; for if you take exceptions at everything your
wife doth, Solomon's wisdom, Hercules' valour, Homer's learning,
Socrates' patience, Argus' vigilancy, will not serve turn. Therefore *minus malum*, a less mischief, Nevisanus holds,⁵ *dissimulare* [to dissemble], to be *cunarum emptor*,⁶ a buyer of cradles,
as the proverb is, than to be too solicitous. "A good fellow,
when his wife was brought to bed before her time, bought half
a dozen cradles beforehand for so many children, as if his wife
should continue to bear children every two months."⁷ Pertinax
the emperor, when one told him a fiddler was too familiar
with his empress, made no reckoning of it.⁸ And when that

Macedonian Philip was upbraided with his wife's dishonesty,
cum tot victor regnorum ac populorum esset, etc., a conqueror
of kingdoms could not tame his wife (for she thrust him out of
doors), he made a jest of it. *Sapientes portant cornua in pectore,
stulti in fronte*, saith Nevisanus, wise men bear their horns in
their hearts, fools on their foreheads. Eumenes, King of Pergamus, was at deadly feud with Perseus of Macedonia, insomuch
that Perseus, hearing of a journey he was to take to Delphi, set
a company of soldiers to intercept him in his passage; they did
it accordingly, and as they supposed, left him stoned to death.
The news of this fact was brought instantly to Pergamus;
Attalus, Eumenes' brother, proclaimed himself king forthwith,
took possession of the crown, and married Stratonice the queen.
But by and by, when contrary news was brought, that King
Eumenes was alive and now coming to the city, he laid by his
crown, left his wife, as a private man went to meet him and
congratulate his return. Eumenes, though he knew all particulars passed, yet dissembling the matter, kindly embraced
his brother, and took his wife into his favour again, as if no
such matter had been heard of or done.[1] Jocundo, in Ariosto,
found his wife in bed with a knave, both asleep, went his ways,
and would not so much as wake them, much less reprove them
for it. An honest fellow, finding in like sort his wife had
played false at tables, and borne a man too many, drew his
dagger, and swore if he had not been his very friend, he would
have killed him. Another hearing one had done that for him
which no man desires to be done by a deputy, followed in a rage
with his sword drawn, and having overtaken him, laid adultery
to his charge; the offender, hotly pursued, confessed it was
true; with which confession he was satisfied, and so left him,
swearing that if he had denied it he would not have put it up.[2]
How much better is it to do thus than to macerate himself,
impatiently to rave and rage, to enter an action (as Arnoldus
Tilius did in the court of Toulouse against Martin Guerre his
fellow-soldier, for that he counterfeited his habit and was too
familiar with his wife), so to divulge his own shame, and to
remain for ever a cuckold on record! How much better be
Cornelius Tacitus than Publius Cornutus, to contemn in such
cases, or take no notice of it! *Melius sic errare, quam zelotypiæ
curis*, saith Erasmus, *se conficere* [it is better to make such a
mistake than to become a prey to jealousy], better be a wittol
and put it up, than to trouble himself to no purpose. And
though he will not *omnibus dormire* [sleep for everyone],

be an ass, as he is an ox, yet to wink at it as many do is not
amiss at some times, in some cases, to some parties, if it be for
his commodity, or some great man's sake, his landlord, patron,
benefactor (as Galba the Roman, saith Plutarch,[1] did by
Mæcenas, and Phayllus of Argos did by King Philip, when he
promised him an office on that condition he might lie with
his wife), and so let it pass:

> Pol me haud pœnitet,
> Scilicet boni dimidium dividere cum Jove,[2]

"It never troubles me" (said Amphitryo) "to be cornuted by
Jupiter"; let it not molest thee then; be friends with her;

> Tu cum Alcmena uxore antiquam in gratiam
> Redi; [3]
> [Receive Alcmena to your grace again;]

let it, I say, make no breach of love between you. Howsoever,
the best way is to contemn it, which Henry II, King of France,
advised a courtier of his, jealous of his wife and complaining
of her unchasteness, to reject it, and comfort himself; [4] for he
that suspects his wife's incontinency, and fears the Pope's curse,
shall never live a merry hour or sleep a quiet night: no remedy
but patience. When all is done, according to that counsel of
Nevisanus,[5] *si vitium uxoris corrigi non potest, ferendum est:*
if it may not be helped, it must be endured. *Date veniam et
sustinete taciti* [pardon and say nothing], 'tis Sophocles' advice,
keep it to thyself, and (which Chrysostom calls *palæstram
philosophiæ et domesticum gymnasium,* a school of philosophy),
put it up. There is no other cure but time to wear it out,
injuriarum remedium est oblivio [forgetfulness is the cure of
wrongs], as if they had drunk a draught of Lethe in Trophonius'
den. To conclude, age will bereave her of it, *dies dolorem
minuit,* time and patience must end it.

> The mind's affections patience will appease,
> It passions kills, and healeth each disease.[6]

SUBSECT. II.—*By prevention before or after Marriage, Plato's
    Community, marry a Courtesan, Philters, Stews, to marry
    one equal in years, fortunes, of a good family, education,
    good place, to use them well, etc.*

Of such medicines as conduce to the cure of this malady
I have sufficiently treated; there be some good remedies remaining, by way of prevention, precautions, or admonitions,

which, if rightly practised, may do much good. Plato, in his Commonwealth, to prevent this mischief belike, would have all things common, wives and children, all as one: and which Cæsar in his Commentaries observed of those old Britons that first inhabited this land, they had ten or twelve wives allotted to such a family, or promiscuously to be used by so many men; not one to one, as with us, or four, five, or six to one, as in Turkey. The Nicholaites, a sect that sprung, saith Austin,[1] from Nicholas the Deacon, would have women indifferent; and the cause of this filthy sect was Nicholas the Deacon's jealousy, for which when he was condemned, to purge himself of his offence he broached his heresy that it was lawful to lie with one another's wives, and for any man to lie with his: like to those Anabaptists in Munster,[2] that would consort with other men's wives as the spirit moved them: or as Mahomet,[3] the seducing prophet, would needs use women as he list himself, to beget prophets; two hundred and five, their Alcoran saith, were in love with him, and he as able as forty men.[4] Amongst the old Carthaginians, as Bohemus relates out of Sabellicus,[5] the king of the country lay with the bride the first night, and once in a year they went promiscuously all together. Munster, *Cosmog. lib. 3, cap.* 497, ascribes the beginning of this brutish custom (unjustly) to one Picardus, a Frenchman, that invented a new sect of Adamites, to go naked as Adam did, and to use promiscuous venery at set times. When the priest repeated that of Genesis, "Increase and multiply," out went the candles in the place where they met, "and without all respect of age, persons, conditions, catch that catch may, every man took her that came next,"[6] etc.; some fasten this on those ancient Bohemians and Russians: others on the inhabitants of Mambrium, in the Lucerne valley in Piedmont;[7] and, as I read, it was practised in Scotland amongst Christians themselves, until King Malcolm's time, the king or the lord of the town had their maidenheads. In some parts of India in our age,[8] and those Icelanders,[9] as amongst the Babylonians of old,[10] they will prostitute their wives and daughters (which Chalcocondylas, a Greek modern writer, for want of better intelligence, puts upon us Britons) to such travellers or seafaring men as come amongst them by chance, to show how far they were from this feral vice of jealousy, and how little they esteemed it. The kings of Calicut, as Lod. Vertomannus relates,[11] will not touch their wives, till one of their Biarmi or high priests have lain first with them, to sanctify their wombs. But those Essæi [12] and Montanists, two strange sects of old, were in another extreme, they would not marry at all, or have any society with women, "because of their intemperance they held them all to be naught." [1] Nevisanus the lawyer, *lib. 4, num. 33, Sylv. nupt.*, would have him that is inclined to this malady, to prevent the worst, marry a quean; *Capiens meretricem, hoc habet saltem boni quod non decipitur, quia scit eam sic esse, quod non contingit aliis* [the advantage is that at least he is not deceived, because he knows what she is; which cannot be said of others]. A fornicator in Seneca constuprated two wenches in a night; for satisfaction, the one desired to hang him, the other to marry him. Hieronymus, King of Syracuse in Sicily, espoused himself to Pitho, keeper of the stews; and Ptolemy took Thais, a common whore, to be his wife, had two sons, Leontiscus and Lagus, by her, and one daughter Irene: [2] 'tis therefore no such unlikely thing. A citizen of Eugubine gelded himself to try his wife's honesty, and to be freed from jealousy; [3] so did a baker in Basil, to the same intent. [4] But of all other precedents in this kind, that of Combabus [5] is most memorable; who to prevent his master's suspicion, for he was a beautiful young man, and sent by Seleucus his lord and king, with Stratonice the queen to conduct her into Syria, fearing the worst, gelded himself before he went, and left his genitals behind him in a box sealed up. His mistress by the way fell in love with him, but he, not yielding to her, was accused to Seleucus of incontinency (as that Bellerophon was in like case falsely traduced by Sthenobœa, to King Prœtus her husband, *cum non posset ad coitum inducere*), and that by her, and was therefore at his coming home cast into prison: the day of hearing appointed, he was sufficiently cleared and acquitted, by showing his privities, which to the admiration of the beholders he had formerly cut off. The Lydians used to geld women whom they suspected, saith Leonicus, *Var. hist. lib. 3, cap.* 49, as well as men. To this purpose Saint Francis, because he used to confess women in private, to prevent suspicion, and prove himself a maid, stripped himself before the Bishop of Assisi and others: [6] and Friar Leonard for the same cause went through Viterbium in Italy without any garments.

Our pseudo-Catholics, to help these inconveniences which proceed from jealousy, to keep themselves and their wives honest, make severe laws against adultery, present death; and withal [for] fornication, a venial sin, as a sink to convey that furious and swift stream of concupiscence, they appoint and

permit stews, those punks and pleasant sinners, the more to
secure their wives in all populous cities, for they hold them as
necessary as churches; and howsoever unlawful, yet to avoid a
greater mischief to be tolerated in policy, as usury, for the
hardness of men's hearts; and for this end they have whole
colleges of courtesans in their towns and cities. Of Cato's
mind belike,[1] that would have his servants (*cum ancillis congredi
coitus causa, definito ære, ut graviora facinora evitarent, cæteris
interim interdicens*) familiar with some such feminine creatures,
to avoid worse mischiefs in his house, and made allowance for it.
They hold it unpossible for idle persons, young, rich, and lusty,
so many servants, monks, friars, to live honest, too tyrannical
a burden to compel them to be chaste, and most unfit to suffer
poor men, younger brothers, and soldiers at all to marry, as
those diseased persons, votaries, priests, servants. Therefore,
as well to keep and ease the one as the other, they tolerate and
wink at these kind of brothel-houses and stews. Many probable
arguments they have to prove the lawfulness, the necessity, and
a toleration of them, as of usury; and without question in policy
they are not to be contradicted: but altogether in religion.
Others prescribe philters, spells, charms to keep men and women
honest. *Mulier ut alienum virum non admittat præter suum:
Accipe fel hirci, et adipem, et exsicca, calescat in oleo, etc., et non
alium præter te amabit.*[2] *In Alexi, Porta, etc., plura invenies,
et multo his absurdiora, uti et in Rhasi, ne mulier virum admittat,
et maritum solum diligat, etc.* But these are most part pagan,
impious, irreligious, absurd, and ridiculous devices.
   The best means to avoid these and like inconveniences are to
take away the causes and occasions. To this purpose Varro
writ *Satiram Menippeam*,[3] but it is lost. Patricius [4] prescribes
four rules to be observed in choosing of a wife (which whoso
will may read); Fonseca the Spaniard, in his 45th *cap. Amphitheat. Amoris*, sets down six special cautions for men, four for
women; Sam. Neander, out of Schonbernerus, five for men,
five for women; Anthony Guevara many good lessons;
Cleobulus two alone,[5] others otherwise; as first to make a good
choice in marriage, to invite Christ to their wedding, and which
St. Ambrose adviseth,[6] *Deum conjugii præsidem habere* [to let
God preside over the wedding], and to pray to Him for her
(*A Domino enim datur uxor prudens* [a prudent wife is the gift
of God], Prov. xix), not to be too rash and precipitate in his
election, to run upon the first he meets, or dote on every stout
fair piece he sees, but to choose her as much by his ears as

eyes, to be well advised whom he takes, of what age, etc., and
cautelous in his proceedings. An old man should not marry
a young woman, nor a young woman an old man:

> *Quam male inæquales veniunt ad aratra juvenci!* [1]
>
> [How ill come ill-matched oxen to the plough!]

such matches must needs minister a perpetual cause of suspicion,
and be distasteful to each other.

> *Noctua ut in tumulis, super atque cadavera bubo,*
> *Talis apud Sophoclem nostra puella sedet.* [2]
>
> Night-crows on tombs, owl sits on carcass dead,
> So lies a wench with Sophocles in bed.

For Sophocles, as Athenæus [3] describes him, was a very old
man, as cold as January, a bed-fellow of bones, and doted yet
upon Archippe, a young courtesan, than which nothing can be
more odious. *Senex maritus uxori juveni ingratus est,* [4] an old
man is a most unwelcome guest to a young wench, unable, unfit:

> *Amplexus suos fugiunt puellæ,*
> *Omnis horret Amor Venusque Hymenque.* [5]
>
> [Maidens shun his embraces; Cupid, Venus, and Hymen
> all shudder at him.]

And as in like case a good fellow that had but a peck of corn
weekly to grind, yet would needs build a new mill for it, found
his error eftsoons, for either he must let his mill lie waste, pull
it quite down, or let others grind at it: so these men, etc.

Seneca therefore disallows all such unseasonable matches,
habent enim maledicti locum crebræ nuptiæ [frequent weddings
bring ill-repute]. And as Tully farther inveighs,[6] "'tis unfit
for any, but ugly and filthy in old age." *Turpe senilis amor*
[an old man's love is vile], one of the three things God hateth.[7]
Plutarch, in his book *contra Coloten*, rails downright at such
kind of marriages, which are attempted by old men, *qui jam
corpore impotenti, et a voluptatibus deserti, peccant animo* [who,
being impotent in body and past pleasure, yet sin in their minds],
and makes a question whether in some cases it be tolerable at
least for such a man to marry, *qui Venerem affectat sine viribus,*
that is now past those venereous exercises, "as a gelded man
lies with a virgin and sighs" (Ecclus. xxx, 20), and now complains with him in Petronius, *Funerata est hæc pars jam, quæ
fuit olim Achillea* [this part is dead and buried which was once
Achillean], he is quite done:

*Vixit puellæ nuper idoneus,
Et militavit non sine gloria.*[1]

[He has had his day with the girls, and served with
some credit in the field of love.]

But the question is whether he may delight himself as those
priapean popes, which, in their decrepit age, lay commonly
between two wenches every night, *contactu formosarum et con-
trectatione, num adhuc gaudeat*; and as many doting sires do to
their own shame, their children's undoing, and their families'
confusion: he abhors it, *tanquam ab agresti et furioso domino
fugiendum*, it must be avoided as a bedlam-master, and not
obeyed.

*Alecto
Ipsa faces præfert nubentibus, et malus Hymen
Triste ululat,*

[Alecto herself holds the torch at the nuptials, and
ill-boding Hymen makes sad wail,]

the devil himself makes such matches. Levinus Lemnius [2]
reckons up three things which generally disturb the peace of
marriage: the first is when they marry *intempestive* or unseasonably, "as many mortal men marry precipitately and inconsiderately when they are effete and old; the second, when they
marry unequally for fortunes and birth; the third, when a sick
impotent person weds one that is sound"; *novæ nuptæ spes
frustratur* [the hope of the bride is cheated]: many dislikes
instantly follow. Many doting dizzards, it may not be denied,
as Plutarch confesseth, "recreate themselves with such obsolete,
unseasonable, and filthy remedies" (so he calls them), "with
a remembrance of their former pleasures; against nature they
stir up their dead flesh"; [3] but an old lecher is abominable;
mulier tertio nubens, Nevisanus holds, [4] *præsumitur lubrica et
inconstans*, a woman that marries a third time may be presumed
to be no honester than she should. Of them both, thus Ambrose
concludes in his Comment upon Luke: "They that are coupled
together, not to get children, but to satisfy their lust, are not
husbands, but fornicators"; [5] with whom St. Austin consents:
matrimony without hope of children, *non matrimonium, sed
concubium dici debet*, is not a wedding but a jumbling or coupling
together. In a word, (except they wed for mutual society, help
and comfort one of another, in which respects, though Tiberius
deny it,[6] without question old folks may well marry, for sometimes a man hath most need of a wife, according to Puccius,

when he hath no need of a wife; otherwise it is most odious,
when an old Acherontic dizzard, that hath one foot in his
grave, a *silicernium* [funeral feast], shall flicker after a young
wench that is blithe and bonny,

> *salaciorque*
> *Verno passere, et albulis columbis.*[1]

[And more lustful than the sparrow in spring or the
    snow-white doves.]

What can be more detestable?

> *Tu cano capite amas, senex nequissime?*
> *Jam plenus ætatis, animaque fœtida,*
> *Senex hircosus, tu osculare mulierem?*
> *Utine adiens vomitum potius excutias.*[2]

> Thou old goat, hoary lecher, naughty man,
> With stinking breath, art thou in love?
> Must thou be slavering? she spews to see
> Thy filthy face, it doth so move.

Yet, as some will, it is much more tolerable for an old man to
marry a young woman (Our Lady's match they call it), for
cras erit mulier [she will soon be middle-aged], as he said in
Tully. Cato the Roman, Critobulus in Xenophon,[3] Traquellus
of late,[4] Julius Scaliger, etc., and many famous precedents we
have in that kind; but not *e contra* [of the opposite kind]: 'tis
not held fit for an ancient woman to match with a young man.
For as Varro will, *Anus dum ludit morti delicias facit* [when an
old woman disports herself, she makes Death merry], 'tis
Charon's match between Cascus and Casca,[5] and the devil himself is surely well pleased with it. And therefore, as the poet
inveighs,[6] thou old Vetustilla, bed-ridden quean, that art now
skin and bones,

> *Cui tres capilli, quatuorque sunt dentes,*
> *Pectus cicadæ, crusculumque formicæ,*
> *Rugosiorem quæ geris stola frontem,*
> *Et aranerum cassibus pares mammas.*

> That hast three hairs, four teeth, a breast
> Like grasshopper, an emmet's crest,
> A skin more rugged than thy coat,
> And dugs like spider's web to boot.

Must thou marry a youth again? And yet *ducentas ire nuptum
post mortes amant* [they want to marry again after burying a
hundred husbands]: howsoever it is, as Apuleius [7] gives out of
his Meroe, *congressus annosus, pestilens, abhorrendus*, a pestilent

match, abominable, and not to be endured. In such case how
can they otherwise choose but be jealous? how should they
agree one with another? This inequality is not in years only,
but in birth, fortunes, conditions, and all good qualities:

      Si qua voles apte nubere, nube pari.[1]

      [If you want a suitable match, marry one of your own
          station.]

'Tis my counsel, saith Anthony Guevara, to choose such a one.
Civis civem ducat, nobilis nobilem, let a citizen match with a
citizen, a gentleman with a gentlewoman; he that observes not
this precept (saith he) *non generum sed malum genium, non
nurum sed furiam, non vitæ comitem, sed litis fomitem domi
habebit*, instead of a fair wife shall have a fury, for a fit son-in-
law a mere fiend, etc. Examples are too frequent.

Another main caution fit to be observed is this, that though
they be equal in years, birth, fortunes, and other conditions,
yet they do not omit virtue and good education, which Musonius
and Antipater so much inculcate in Stobæus.

      Dos est magna parentum
      Virtus, et metuens alterius viri
      Certo fœdere castitas.

      [The best dowry is a good parentage, and firm chastity
          that fears a stranger's touch.]

If, as Plutarch adviseth, one must eat *modium salis*, a bushel
of salt with him, before he choose his friend, what care should
be had in choosing a wife, his second self, how solicitous should
he be to know her qualities and behaviour! and when he is
assured of them, not to prefer birth, fortune, beauty, before
bringing up, and good conditions. Cocuage, god of cuckolds,
as one merrily said,[2] accompanies the goddess Jealousy, both
follow the fairest, by Jupiter's appointment, and they sacrifice
to them together: beauty and honesty seldom agree; straight
personages have often crooked manners; fair faces, foul vices;
good complexions, ill conditions. *Suspicionis plena res est, et
insidiarum*, beauty (saith Chrysostom [3]) is full of treachery and
suspicion: he that hath a fair wife cannot have a worse mischief,
and yet most covet it, as if nothing else in marriage but that
and wealth were to be respected. Francis Sforza, Duke of
Milan, was so curious in this behalf, that he would not marry
the Duke of Mantua's daughter, except he might see her naked
first: [4] which Lycurgus appointed in his laws, and Morus in
his Utopian commonwealth approves. In Italy, as a traveller

observes,[1] if a man have three or four daughters, or more, and
they prove fair, they are married eftsoons: if deformed, they
change their lovely names of Lucia, Cynthia, Camæna, call them
Dorothy, Ursula, Bridget, and so put them into monasteries,
as if none were fit for marriage, but such as are eminently fair:
but these are erroneous tenents: a modest virgin, well conditioned, to such a fair stout piece is much to be preferred. If
thou wilt avoid them, take away all causes of suspicion and
jealousy, marry a coarse piece, fetch her from Cassandra's temple,[2]
which was wont in Italy to be a sanctuary of all deformed
maids, and so thou shalt be sure that no man will make thee
cuckold, but for spite. A citizen of Byzance in Thrace had a
filthy, dowdy, deformed slut to his wife, and finding her in bed
with another man, cried out as one amazed: *O miser! quæ te
necessitas huc adegit?* "O thou wretch, what necessity brought
thee hither?" as well he might; for who can affect such a one?
But this is warily to be understood, most offend in another
extreme, they prefer wealth before beauty, and so she be rich,
they care not how she look; but these are all out as faulty as
the rest. *Attendenda uxoris forma,* as Sarisburiensis adviseth,[3]
ne si alteram aspexeris, mox eam sordere putes [pay heed to your
wife's appearance, lest on seeing some other woman you should
find her distasteful], as the knight in Chaucer that was married
to an old woman,

> And all day after hid him as an owl,
> So woe was him his wife looked so foul.

Have a care of thy wife's complexion, lest whilst thou seest
another, thou loathest her, she prove jealous, thou naught:

> *Si tibi deformis conjux, si serva venusta,*
> *Ne utaris serva.*

[If you have an ugly wife and a handsome maid, abstain
from the maid.]

I can perhaps give instance. *Molestum est possidere, quod nemo
habere dignetur,* [it is] a misery to possess that which no man
likes: on the other side, *difficile custoditur quod plures amant* [it is
difficult to keep that which many covet]. And as the bragging
soldier vaunted in the comedy, *nimia est miseria pulchrum esse
hominem nimis* [it is a great misery to be so very handsome].
Scipio did never so hardly besiege Carthage as these young
gallants will beset thine house, one with wit or person, another
with wealth, etc. If she be fair, saith Guazzo, she will be
suspected howsoever. Both extremes are naught, *pulchra cito*

adamatur, fœda facile concupiscit, the one is soon beloved,
the other loves; one is hardly kept, because proud and arrogant,
the other not worth keeping; what is to be done in this case?
Ennius, in *Menelippe*, adviseth thee as a friend to take *statam
formam, si vis habere incolumem pudicitiam*, one of a middle
size, neither too fair, nor too foul:

> *Nec formosa magis quam mihi casta placet;* [1]
>
> [Beauty pleases me not more than chastity;]

with old Cato, though fit, let her beauty be *neque lectissima,
neque illiberalis* [neither too exquisite, nor without charm],
between both. This I approve; but of the other two I resolve
with Sarisburiensis, *cæteris paribus*, both rich alike, endowed
alike, *majori miseria deformis habetur quam formosa servatur*,
I had rather marry a fair one, and put it to the hazard, than
be troubled with a blowze; but do thou as thou wilt, I speak
only of myself.

Howsoever, *quod iterum moneo*, I would advise thee this much,
be she fair or foul, to choose a wife out of a good kindred,
parentage, well brought up, in an honest place.

> *Primum animo tibi proponas quo sanguine creta,
> Qua forma, qua ætate, quibusque ante omnia virgo
> Moribus, in junctos veniat nova nupta penates.* [2]
>
> [Consider first whence she springs, what is her
> appearance, her age, above all her character.]

He that marries a wife out of a suspected inn or alehouse, buys
a horse in Smithfield, and hires a servant in Paul's, as the
diverb is, shall likely have a jade to his horse, a knave for his
man, an arrant honest woman to his wife. *Filia præsumitur
esse matri similis* [the daughter is presumed to be like her
mother], saith Nevisanus,[3] "such a mother, such a daughter"; [4]
mali corvi malum ovum [like crow, like egg], cat to her kind.

> *Scilicet exspectas ut tradat mater honestos
> Atque alios mores quam quos habet?* [5]
>
> [Do you really think that the mother can transmit a
> good character which she has not herself?]

If the mother be dishonest, in all likelihood the daughter will
matrizare, take after her in all good qualities,

> *Creden' Pasiphæ non tauripotente futuram
> Taeuripetam?*

If the dam trot, the foal will not amble. My last caution is,
that a woman do not bestow herself upon a fool, or an apparent

melancholy person; jealousy is a symptom of that disease, and
fools have no moderation. Justina, a Roman lady, was much
persecuted, and after made away by her jealous husband, she
caused and enjoined this epitaph, as a caveat to others, to be
engraven on her tomb:

> *Discite ab exemplo Justinæ, discite patres,*
> *Ne nubat fatuo filia vestra viro,* etc.[1]

> Learn parents all, and by Justina's case,
> Your children to no dizzards for to place.

After marriage, I can give no better admonitions than to use
their wives well, and which a friend of mine told me that was a
married man, I will tell you as good cheap, saith Nicostratus in
Stobæus:[2] to avoid future strife, and for quietness' sake, "when
you are in bed, take heed of your wife's flattering speeches
overnight, and curtain sermons in the morning."   Let them do
their endeavour likewise to maintain them to their means,
which Patricius ingeminates,[3] and let them have liberty with
discretion, as time and place requires: many women turn queans
by compulsion, as Nevisanus observes,[4] because their husbands
are so hard, and keep them so short in diet and apparel, *paupertas
cogit eas meretricari*, poverty and hunger, want of means, makes
them dishonest, or bad usage; their churlish behaviour forceth
them to fly out, or bad examples, they do it to cry quittance.
In the other extreme some are too liberal, as the proverb is,
Turdus malum sibi cacat, they make a rod for their own tails, as
Candaules did to Gyges in Herodotus,[5] commend his wife's
beauty himself, and besides would needs have him see her
naked.   Whilst they give their wives too much liberty to gad
abroad, and bountiful allowance, they are accessory to their
own miseries; *animæ uxorum pessime olent*, as Plautus jibes,
they have deformed souls, and by their painting and colours
procure *odium mariti*, their husband's hate, especially *cum
miseri viscantur labra mariti*[6] [when they make their poor
husband's lips sticky].   Besides, their wives (as Basil notes[7])
*impudenter se exponunt masculorum aspectibus, jactantes tunicas,
et coram tripudiantes*, impudently thrust themselves into other
men's companies, and by their indecent wanton carriage provoke and tempt the spectators.   Virtuous women should keep
house; and 'twas well performed and ordered by the Greeks,

> *Mulier ne qua in publicum*
> *Spectandam se sine arbitro præbeat viro;*

> [That a woman should not show herself in public
> unaccompanied by her husband;]

which made Phidias belike at Elis paint Venus treading on a tortoise, a symbol of women's silence and housekeeping. For a woman abroad and alone is like a deer broke out of a park, *quam mille venatores insequuntur*, whom every hunter follows; and besides in such places she cannot so well vindicate herself, but as that virgin Dinah (Gen. xxxiv, 2), "going for to see the daughters of the land," lost her virginity, she may be defiled and overtaken of a sudden.

Imbelles damæ quid nisi præda sumus?

[We helpless deer are only to be hunted.]

And therefore I know not what philosopher he was, that would have women come but thrice abroad all their time, "to be baptized, married, and buried";[1] but he was too strait-laced. Let them have their liberty in good sort, and go in good sort, *modo non annos viginti ætatis suæ domi relinquant*, as a good fellow said, so that they look not twenty years younger abroad than they do at home, they be not spruce, neat, angels abroad, beasts, dowdies, sluts at home; but seek by all means to please and give content to their husbands: to be quiet above all things, obedient, silent and patient; if they be incensed, angry, chide a little, their wives must not cample again,[2] but take it in good part. An honest woman, I cannot now tell where she dwelt, but by report an honest woman she was, hearing one of her gossips by chance complain of her husband's impatience, told her an excellent remedy for it, and gave her withal a glass of water, which when he brawled she should hold still in her mouth, and that *toties quoties*, as often as he chid; she did so two or three times with good success, and at length seeing her neighbour, gave her great thanks for it, and would needs know the ingredients, she told her in brief what it was, "fair water," and no more: for it was not the water, but her silence which performed the cure.[3] Let every froward woman imitate this example, and be quiet within doors, and (as M. Aurelius prescribes[4]) a necessary caution it is to be observed of all good matrons that love their credits, to come little abroad, but follow their work at home, look to their household affairs and private business, *œconomiæ incumbentes*, be sober, thrifty, wary, circumspect, modest, and compose themselves to live to their husbands' means, as a good housewife should do,

Quæ studiis gavisa coli, partita labores
Fallet opus cantu, formæ assimulata coronæ

Cura puellaris, circum fusosque rotasque
Cum volvet, etc.[1]

[Who delights in the labour of the distaff, beguiling
her work with song, her maids working in a
ring round her, as she turns the wheel and the
spindle.]

Howsoever 'tis good to keep them private, not in prison:

Quisquis custodit uxorem vectibus et seris,
Etsi sibi sapiens, stultus est, et nihil sapit.[2]

[Whoso guards a wife with bolts and bars may think
himself clever, but is really a fool.]

Read more of this subject, *Horol. princ. lib.* 2, *per totum*;
Arnisæus, *Polit.*; Cyprian; Tertullian; Bossus, *de mulier apparat.*;
Godefridus, *de amor. lib.* 2, *cap.* 4; Levinus Lemnius, *cap.* 54, *de
institut. Christ.*; Barbarus, *de re uxor. lib.* 2, *cap.* 2; Franciscus
Patricius, *de institut. reipub. lib.* 4, *tit.* 4 *et* 5, *de officio mariti et
uxoris*; Christ. Fonseca, *Amphitheat. Amor. cap.* 45; Sam.
Neander, etc.

These cautions concern him; and if by those or his own
discretion otherwise he cannot moderate himself, his friends
must not be wanting by their wisdom, if it be possible, to give
the party grieved satisfaction, to prevent and remove the
occasions, objects, if it may be to secure him. If it be one
alone, or many, to consider whom he suspects or at what times,
in what place he is most incensed, in what companies. Nevisanus [3] makes a question whether a young physician ought to
be admitted in cases of sickness, into a new-married man's
house, to administer a julep, a syrup, or some such physic. The
Persians of old would not suffer a young physician to come
amongst women. Apollonides Cous made Artaxerxes cuckold,
and was after buried alive for it.[4] A gaoler in Aristænetus had
a fine young gentleman to his prisoner; in commiseration of his
youth and person he let him loose, to enjoy the liberty of the
prison, but he unkindly made him a cornuto.[5] Menelaus gave
good welcome to Paris a stranger, his whole house and family
were at his command, but he ungently stole away his best-
beloved wife. The like measure was offered to Agis, King of
Lacedæmon, by Alcibiades [6] an exile, for his good entertainment; he was too familiar with Timæa his wife, begetting a
child of her, called Leotychides, and bragging moreover, when
he came home to Athens, that he had a son should be king of
the Lacedemonians. If such objects were removed, no doubt
but the parties might easily be satisfied, or that they could use

them gently and entreat them well, not to revile them, scoff at, hate them, as in such cases commonly they do; 'tis an human infirmity, a miserable vexation, and they should not add grief to grief, nor aggravate their misery, but seek to please, and by all means give them content, by good counsel, removing such offensive objects, or by mediation of some discreet friends. In old Rome there was a temple erected by the matrons to that *Viriplaca Dea*[1] [husband-placating goddess], another to *Venus Verticordia, quæ maritos uxoribus reddebat benevolos* [Venus the Turner of Hearts, who makes husbands well disposed to their wives], whither (if any difference happened between man and wife) they did instantly resort: there they did offer sacrifice, a white hart, Plutarch records, *sine felle*, without the gall (some say the like of Juno's temple), and make their prayers for conjugal peace: before some indifferent arbitrators and friends, the matter was heard between man and wife, and commonly composed.[2] In our times we want no sacred churches or good men to end such controversies, if use were made of them. Some say that precious stone called beryllus,[3] others a diamond, hath excellent virtue, *contra hostium injurias, et conjugatos invicem conciliare*, to reconcile men and wives, to maintain unity and love; you may try this when you will, and as you see cause. If none of all these means and cautions will take place, I know not what remedy to prescribe, or whither such persons may go for ease, except they can get into the same Turkey paradise,[4] "where they shall have as many fair wives as they will themselves, with clear eyes, and such as look on none but their own husbands," no fear, no danger of being cuckolds; or else I would have them observe that strict rule of Alphonsus, to marry a deaf and dumb man to a blind woman.[5] If this will not help, let them, to prevent the worst, consult with an astrologer,[6] and see whether the significators in her horoscope agree with his, that they be not *in signis et partibus odiose intuentibus aut imperantibus, sed mutuo et amice antisciis et obedientibus* [in signs and quarters of hostile aspect and command, but in such as are friendly and mutually obliging], otherwise (as they hold) there will be intolerable enmities between them: or else get him *sigillum Veneris*, a characteristical seal stamped in the day and hour of Venus, when she is fortunate, with such and such set words and charms, which Villanovanus and Leo Suavius prescribe, *ex sigillis magicis Salomonis, Hermetis, Raguelis*, etc., with many such, which Alexis, Albertus, and some of our natural magicians put upon us: *Ut mulier cum aliquo adulterare non possit, incide de capillis ejus, etc.* [to prevent a woman committing adultery, cut from her hair, etc.], and he shall surely be gracious in all women's eyes, and never suspect or disagree with his own wife so long as he wears it. If this course be not approved, and other remedies may not be had, they must in the last place sue for a divorce; but that is somewhat difficult to effect, and not all out so fit. For as Felisacus in his tract *de justa uxore* urgeth, if that law of Constantine the Great, or that of Theodosius and Valentinian, concerning divorce, were in use in our times, *innumeras propemodum viduas haberemus, et cælibes viros*, we should have almost no married couples left. Try therefore those former remedies; or, as Tertullian[1] reports of Democritus, that put out his eyes because he could not look upon a woman without lust, and was much troubled to see that which he might not enjoy, let him make himself blind, and so he shall avoid that care and molestation of watching his wife. One other sovereign remedy I could repeat, an especial antidote against jealousy, an excellent cure, but I am not now disposed to tell it, not that like a covetous empiric I conceal it for any gain, but some other reasons, I am not willing to publish it; if you be very desirous to know it, when I meet you next I will peradventure tell you what it is in your ear. This is the best counsel I can give; which he that hath need of, as occasion serves, may apply unto himself. In the meantime, *Di talem terris avertite pestem* [ye gods, avert such a plague from the earth], as the proverb is; from heresy, jealousy and frenzy, good Lord, deliver us.

SECT IV. MEMB. I.

SUBSECT. I.—*Religious Melancholy. Its Object God; what His Beauty is; how it allureth. The Parts and Parties affected*

THAT there is such a distinct species of love-melancholy, no man hath ever yet doubted; but whether this subdivision of Religious Melancholy[2] be warrantable, it may be controverted.

> *Pergite Pierides, medio nec calle vagantem*
> *Linquite me, qua nulla pedum vestigia ducunt,*
> *Nulla rotæ currus testantur signa priores.*[3]

> [Onward, ye Muses, nor forsake me in the midst of
> my journey where no footsteps guide me, no
> forerunner hath left trace of carriage-wheel.]

I have no pattern to follow as in some of the rest, no man to imitate. No physician hath as yet distinctly written of it as

of the other; all acknowledge it a most notable symptom, some
a cause, but few a species or kind. Aretæus,[1] Alexander, Rhasis,
Avicenna, and most of our late writers, as Gordonius, Fuchsius,
Plater, Bruel, Montaltus, etc., repeat it as a symptom. "Some
seem to be inspired of the Holy Ghost, some take upon them to
be prophets,[2] some are addicted to new opinions, some foretell
strange things *de statu mundi et Antichristi*," saith Gordonius.
Some will prophesy of the end of the world to a day almost,
and the fall of the Antichrist, as they have been addicted or
brought up; for so melancholy works with them, as Laurentius
holds.[3] If they have been precisely given, all their meditations
tend that way, and in conclusion produce strange effects; the
humour imprints symptoms according to their several inclinations and conditions, which makes Guianerius [4] and Felix Plater [5]
put too much devotion, blind zeal, fear of eternal punishment
and that last judgment for a cause of those enthusiastics and
desperate persons; but some do not obscurely make a distinct
species of it, dividing love-melancholy into that whose object
is women, and into the other whose object is God. Plato, *in
Convivio*, makes mention of two distinct furies; and amongst
our neoterics, Hercules de Saxonia, *lib.* 1 *Pract. med. cap.* 16,
cap. de melanch., doth expressly treat of it in a distinct species.
"Love-melancholy" (saith he) "is twofold: the first is that (to
which peradventure some will not vouchsafe this name or species
of melancholy) affection of those which put God for their object,
and are altogether about prayer, fasting, etc.; the other about
women." [6] Peter Forestus in his Observations delivereth as
much in the same words: and Felix Platerus, *de mentis alienat.
cap.* 3, *Frequentissima est ejus species, in qua curanda sæpissime
multum fui impeditus;* 'tis a frequent disease; and they have
a ground of what they say, forth of Aretæus and Plato. Aretæus,
an old author, in his third book, *cap.* 6, doth so divide love-
melancholy, and derives this second from the first, which comes
by inspiration or otherwise.[7] Plato in his *Phædrus* hath these
words: "Apollo's priests in Delphi, and at Dodona, in their
fury do many pretty feats, and benefit the Greeks, but never
in their right wits." [8] He makes them all mad, as well he
might; and he that shall but consider that superstition of old,
those prodigious effects of it (as in its place I will show the several
furies of our *fatidici dii* [prophetic gods], pythonissas, sibyls,
enthusiasts, pseudoprophets, heretics, and schismatics in these
our latter ages), shall instantly confess, that all the world again
cannot afford so much matter of madness, so many stupend

symptoms, as superstition, heresy, schism hath brought out:
that this species alone may be paralleled to all the former,
hath a greater latitude and more miraculous effects; that it
more besots and infatuates men than any other above named
whatsoever, doth more harm, works more disquietness to mankind, and hath more crucified the souls of mortal men (such hath
been the devil's craft) than wars, plagues, sicknesses, dearth,
famine, and all the rest.

Give me but a little leave, and I will set before your eyes in
brief a stupend, vast, infinite ocean of incredible madness and
folly: a sea full of shelves and rocks, sands, gulfs, euripes and
contrary tides, full of fearful monsters, uncouth shapes, roaring
waves, tempests, and siren calms, halcyonian seas, unspeakable
misery, such comedies and tragedies, such absurd and ridiculous,
feral and lamentable fits, that I know not whether they are
more to be pitied or derided, or may be believed, but that we
daily see the same still practised in our days, fresh examples,
nova novitia, fresh objects of misery and madness in this kind
that are still represented unto us, abroad, at home, in the
midst of us, in our bosoms.

But before I can come to treat of these several errors and
obliquities, their cause, symptoms, affections, etc., I must say
something necessarily of the object of this love, God Himself,
what this love is, how it allureth, whence it proceeds, and
(which is the cause of all our miseries) how we mistake, wander
and swerve from it.

Amongst all those divine attributes that God doth vindicate
to Himself, eternity, omnipotency, immutability, wisdom,
majesty, justice, mercy, etc., His beauty is not the least.[1]
"One thing," saith David, "have I desired of the Lord, and that
I will still desire, to behold the beauty of the Lord" (Ps. xxvii, 4).
"And out of Sion, which is the perfection of beauty, hath God
shined" (Ps. l, 2). All other creatures are fair, I confess, and
many other objects do much enamour us, a fair house, a fair
horse, a comely person. "I am amazed," said Austin, "when I
look up to heaven and behold the beauty of the stars, the beauty
of angels, principalities, powers; who can express it? who can
sufficiently commend or set out this beauty which appears in us?
so fair a body, so fair a face, eyes, nose, cheeks, chin, brows, all
fair and lovely to behold; besides the beauty of the soul which
cannot be discerned. If we so labour and be so much affected
with the comeliness of creatures, how should we be ravished
with that admirable lustre of God Himself?"[2] If ordinary

beauty have such a prerogative and power, and what is amiable and fair, to draw the eyes and ears, hearts and affections of all spectators unto it, to move, win, entice, allure, how shall this divine form ravish our souls, which is the fountain and quint-essence of all beauty? *Cælum pulchrum, sed pulchrior cæli fabricator ;* if heaven be so fair, the sun so fair, how much fairer shall He be, that made them fair? "For by the greatness and beauty of the creatures, proportionally the maker of them is seen" (Wisd. xiii, 5). If there be such pleasure in beholding a beautiful person alone, and, as a plausible sermon, he so much affect us, what shall this beauty of God Himself, that is infinitely fairer than all creatures, men, angels, etc.? *Omnis pulchritudo florum, hominum, angelorum, et rerum omnium pulcherrimarum ad Dei pulchritudinem collata, nox est et tenebræ,*[1] all other beauties are night itself, mere darkness, to this our inexplicable, incom-prehensible, unspeakable, eternal, infinite, admirable, and divine beauty. This lustre, *pulchritudo omnium pulcherrima* [a beauty surpassing all other beauties], this beauty and "splendour of the divine Majesty"[2] is it that draws all creatures to it, to seek it, love, admire, and adore it; and those heathens, pagans, philosophers, out of those relics they have yet left of God's image, are so far forth incensed, as not only to acknowledge a God, but, though after their own inventions, to stand in admira-tion of His bounty, goodness, to adore and seek Him; the magnificence and structure of the world itself, and beauty of all His creatures, His goodness, providence, protection, enforceth them to love Him, seek Him, fear Him, though a wrong way to adore Him: but for us that are Christians, regenerate, that are His adopted sons, illuminated by His word, having the eyes of our hearts and understandings opened, how fairly doth He offer and expose Himself! *Ambit nos Deus* (Austin saith) *donis et forma sua,* He woos us by His beauty, gifts, promises, to come unto Him; "the whole Scripture is a message, an exhorta-tion, a love-letter to this purpose,"[3] to incite us and invite us, "God's epistle," as Gregory calls it, "to His creatures."[4] He sets out His Son and His Church in that epithalamium or mystical Song of Solomon, to enamour us the more, comparing His head to fine gold, "His locks curled and black as a raven" (Cant. v, 11); "His eyes like doves on rivers of waters, washed with milk; His lips as lilies, drooping down pure juice; His hands as rings of gold set with chrysolite": and His Church to "a vineyard, a garden enclosed, a fountain of living waters, an orchard of pomegranates, with sweet scents of saffron, spike,

calamus and cinnamon, and all the trees of incense, as the
chief spices, the fairest amongst women, no spot in her, His
sister, His spouse, undefiled, the only daughter of her mother,[1]
dear unto her, fair as the moon, pure as the sun, looking out as
the morning"; that by these figures, that glass, these spiritual
eyes of contemplation, we might perceive some resemblance of
His beauty, the love between His Church and Him. And so
in the forty-fifth Psalm this beauty of His Church is compared
to a "queen in a vesture of gold of Ophir, embroidered raiment
of needlework, that the king might take pleasure in her beauty."
To incense us further yet, John, in his Apocalypse,[2] makes a
description of that heavenly Jerusalem, the beauty of it, and in
it the Maker of it; likening it to "a city of pure gold, like unto
clear glass, shining and garnished with all manner of precious
stones, having no need of sun or moon: for the Lamb is the
light of it, the glory of God doth illuminate it"; to give us to
understand the infinite glory, beauty and happiness of it. Not
that it is no fairer than these creatures to which it is compared,
but that this vision of his, this lustre of His divine Majesty,
cannot otherwise be expressed to our apprehensions, "no tongue
can tell, no heart can conceive it," as Paul saith. Moses himself
(Exod. xxxiii, 18), when he desired to see God in His glory, was
answered that he might not endure it, no man could see His
face and live. *Sensibile forte destruit sensum*, a strong object
overcometh the sight, according to that axiom in philosophy:
fulgorem solis ferre non potes, multo magis Creatoris: if thou
canst not endure the sunbeams, how canst thou endure that
fulgor and brightness of Him that made the sun? The sun
itself, and all that we can imagine, are but shadows of it, 'tis
visio præcellens [a marvellous sight], as Austin calls it,[3] the
quintessence of beauty this, "which far exceeds the beauty of
heavens, sun and moon, stars, angels, gold and silver, woods,
fair fields, and whatsoever is pleasant to behold." All those
other beauties fail, vary, are subject to corruption, to loathing;
"but this is an immortal vision, a divine beauty, an immortal
love, an indefatigable love and beauty," [4] with sight of which
we shall never be tired nor wearied, but still the more we see
the more we shall covet Him." For as one saith,[5] "Where
this vision is, there is absolute beauty; and where is that beauty,
from the same fountain comes all pleasure and happiness;
neither can beauty, pleasure, happiness, be separated from
His vision or sight, or His vision from beauty, pleasure, happiness." In this life we have but a glimpse of this beauty and

happiness: we shall hereafter, as John saith, see Him as He is: thine eyes, as Isaiah promiseth (xxxiii, 17), "shall behold the King in His glory," then shall we be perfectly enamoured, have a full fruition of it, desire, behold and love Him alone as the most amiable and fairest object, or *summum bonum*, or chiefest good.[1]

This likewise should we now have done, had not our will been corrupted; and as we are enjoined to love God with all our heart, and all our soul: for to that end were we born, to love this object, as Melancthon discourseth,[2] and to enjoy it. "And Him our will would have loved and sought alone as our *summum bonum*, or principal good, and all other good things for God's sake: and nature, as she proceeded from it, would have sought this fountain; but in this infirmity of human nature this order is disturbed, our love is corrupt"; and a man is like that monster in Plato,[3] composed of a Scylla, a lion and a man; we are carried away headlong with the torrent of our affections: the world, and that infinite variety of pleasing objects in it, do so allure and enamour us, that we cannot so much as look towards God, seek Him, or think on Him as we should: we cannot, saith Austin, *rempub. cœlestem cogitare* [direct our thoughts to the heavenly state], we cannot contain ourselves from them, their sweetness is so pleasing to us.   Marriage, saith Gualter,[4] detains many, "a thing in itself laudable, good and necessary, but many, deceived and carried away with the blind love of it, have quite laid aside the love of God, and desire of His glory.   Meat and drink hath overcome as many, whilst they rather strive to please, satisfy their guts and belly, than to serve God and nature."   Some are so busied about merchandise to get money, they lose their own souls, whiles covetously carried, and with an unsatiable desire of gain, they forget God; as much we may say of honour, leagues, friendships, health, wealth, and all other profits or pleasures in this life whatsoever.   "In this world there be so many beautiful objects, splendours and brightness of gold, majesty of glory, assistance of friends, fair promises, smooth words, victories, triumphs, and such an infinite company of pleasing beauties to allure us, and draw us from God, that we cannot look after Him."[5]   And this is it which Christ himself, those prophets and apostles, so much thundered against, dehort us from: "Love not the world, nor the things that are in the world" (1 John ii, 15).   "If any man love the world, the love of the Father is not in him" (v. 16).   "For all that is in the world, as lust of the flesh, the lust of the eyes, and pride

of life, is not of the Father, but of the world: and the world
passeth away and the lust thereof; but he that fulfilleth the
will of God abideth for ever" (v. 17) "No man," saith our
Saviour, "can serve two masters, but he must love the one and
hate the other," etc.; *Bonos vel malos mores, boni vel mali
faciunt amores* [a right or wrong love makes a good or bad
character], Austin well infers: and this is that which all the
Fathers inculcate. He cannot (Austin admonisheth[1]) be God's
friend, that is delighted with the pleasures of the world; "make
clean thine heart, purify thine heart; if thou wilt see this beauty,
prepare thyself for it." "It is the eye of contemplation by
which we must behold it, the wing of meditation which lifts us
up and rears our souls with the motion of our hearts and sweetness of contemplation": so saith Gregory, cited by Bonaventure.[2]
And as Philo Judæus seconds him,[3] "He that loves God will
soar aloft and take him wings; and leaving the earth fly up to
heaven, wander with sun and moon, stars, and that heavenly
troop, God Himself being his guide." If we desire to see Him,
we must lay aside all vain objects, which detain us and dazzle
our eyes, and as Ficinus adviseth us,[4] "get us solar eyes, spectacles as they that look on the sun: to see this divine beauty,
lay aside all material objects, all sense, and then thou shalt see
Him as He is." "Thou covetous wretch," as Austin expostulates, "why dost thou stand gaping on this dross, muck-hills,
filthy excrements? behold a far fairer object, God Himself woos
thee; behold Him, enjoy Him." [5] He is sick for love (Cant. v),
He invites thee to His sight, to come into His fair garden, to
eat and drink with Him, to be merry with Him, to enjoy His
presence for ever. Wisdom cries out in the streets besides the
gates, in the top of high places, before the city, at the entry
of the door, and bids them give ear to her instruction, which
is better than gold or precious stones;[6] no pleasures can be
compared to it: leave all then and follow her, *vos exhortor, o amici,
et obsecro* [I exhort and beseech you, friends]. In Ficinus'
words,[7] I exhort and beseech you, "that you would embrace
and follow this divine love with all your hearts and abilities,
by all offices and endeavours make this so loving God propitious
unto you." For whom alone, saith Plotinus,[8] "we must forsake
the kingdoms and empires of the whole earth, sea, land, and air,
if we desire to be engrafted into Him, leave all and follow Him."

Now, forasmuch as this love of God is a habit infused of God,
as Thomas holds, 1, 2, *quæst.* 23, "by which a man is inclined to
love God above all, and his neighbour as himself," [9] we must

pray to God that He will open our eyes, make clear our hearts, that we may be capable of His glorious rays, and perform those duties that He requires of us (Deut. vi and Josh. xxiii), "to love God above all, and our neighbour as ourself," to keep His commandments. "In this we know," saith John (*cap.* v, *2*), "we love the children of God, when we love God and keep His commandments. This is the love of God, that we keep His commandments"; "he that loveth not, knoweth not God, for God is love" (*cap.* iv, 8,) "and he that dwelleth in love, dwelleth in God, and God in him"; for love presupposeth knowledge, faith, hope, and unites us to God Himself, as Leon Hebræus delivereth unto us,[1] and is accompanied with the fear of God, humility, meekness, patience, all those virtues, and charity itself. For if we love God, we shall love our neighbour, and perform the duties which are required at our hands, to which we are exhorted (1 Cor. xiii, 4, 5; Ephes. iv; Coloss. iii; Rom. xii). We shall not be envious or puffed up, or boast, disdain, think evil, or be provoked to anger, but suffer all things; "endeavour to keep the unity of the Spirit in the bond of peace"; forbear one another, forgive one another, clothe the naked, visit the sick, and perform all those works of mercy which Clemens Alexandrinus [2] calls *amoris et amicitiæ impletionem et extensionem*, the extent and complement of love; and that not for fear or worldly respects, but *ordine ad Deum*, for the love of God Himself. This we shall do if we be truly enamoured; but we come short in both, we neither love God nor our neighbour as we should. Our love in spiritual things is too "defective, in worldly things too excessive, there is a jar in both."[3] We love the world too much; God too little; our neighbour not at all, or for our own ends. *Vulgus amicitias utilitate probat* [men usually value friendships for what they can bring]. The chief thing we respect is our commodity: and what we do is for fear of worldly punishment, for vainglory, praise of men, fashion, and such by-respects, not for God's sake. We neither know God aright, nor seek, love, or worship Him as we should. And for these defects, we involve ourselves into a multitude of errors, we swerve from this true love and worship of God: which is a cause unto us of unspeakable miseries; running into both extremes, we become fools, madmen, without sense, as now in the next place I will show you.

The parties affected are innumerable almost, and scattered over the face of the earth, far and near, and so have been in all precedent ages, from the beginning of the world to these times,

of all sorts and conditions. For method's sake I will reduce
them to a twofold division, according to those two extremes of
excess and defect, impiety and superstition, idolatry and
atheism. Not that there is any excess of divine worship or
love of God; that cannot be, we cannot love God too much, or
do our duty as we ought, as papists hold, or have any perfection
in this life, much less supererogate; when we have all done, we
are unprofitable servants. But because we do *aliud agere* [attend
to the wrong thing], zealous without knowledge, and too
solicitous about that which is not necessary, busying ourselves
about impertinent, needless, idle, and vain ceremonies, *populo
ut placerent* [to please the public], as the Jews did about sacrifices, oblations, offerings, incense, new moons, feasts, etc., but as
Isaiah taxeth them (i, 12): "Who required this at your hands?"
We have too great opinion of our own worth, that we can
satisfy the law: and do more than is required at our hands,
by performing those evangelical counsels, and such works of
supererogation, merit for others, which Bellarmine, Gregory
de Valentia, all their Jesuits and champions defend, that if
God should deal in rigour with them, some of their Franciscans
and Dominicans are so pure that nothing could be objected
to them. Some of us again are too dear, as we think, more
divine and sanctified than others, of a better mettle, greater
gifts, and, with that proud Pharisee, contemn others in respect
of ourselves; we are better Christians, better learned, choice
spirits, inspired, know more, have special revelation, perceive
God's secrets, and thereupon presume, say and do many times
which is not befitting to be said or done. Of this number are
all superstitious idolaters, ethnics, Mahometans, Jews, heretics,
enthusiasts, divinators, prophets, sectaries, and schismatics.
Zanchius [1] reduceth such infidels to four chief sects; but I will
insist and follow mine own intended method: all which, with
many other curious persons, monks, hermits, etc., may be
ranged in this extreme, and fight under this superstitious
banner, with those rude idiots and infinite swarms of people
that are seduced by them. In the other extreme or in defect,
march those impious epicures, libertines, atheists, hypocrites,
infidels, worldly, secure, impenitent, unthankful, and carnal-
minded men, that attribute all to natural causes, that will
acknowledge no supreme power; that have cauterized consciences, or live in a reprobate sense; or such desperate persons
as are too distrustful of His mercies. Of these there be many
subdivisions, divers degrees of madness and folly, some more

than other, as shall be showed in the symptoms: and yet all
miserably out, perplexed, doting, and beside themselves for
religion's sake. For as Zanchius well distinguished,[1] and all the
world knows, religion is twofold, true or false; false is that vain
superstition of idolaters, such as were of old, Greeks, Romans,
present Mahometans, etc. *Timorem deorum inanem* [futile fear
of the gods], Tully could term it;[2] or as Zanchius defines it, *ubi
falsi dii, aut falso cultu colitur Deus,* when false gods, or that
God is falsely worshipped. And 'tis a miserable plague, a
torture of the soul, a mere madness, *religiosa insania* [religious
insanity], Meteran calls it,[3] or *insanus error,* as Seneca,[4] a frantic
error; or as Austin, *insanus animi morbus,* a furious disease of
the soul; *insania omnium insanissima,* a quintessence of madness;
for he that is superstitious can never be quiet.[5] 'Tis proper to
man alone, *uni superbia, avaritia, superstitio* [in him alone are
found pride, avarice, and superstition], saith Pliny, *lib. 7, cap. 1,
atque etiam post sævit de futuro,* which wrings his soul for the
present and to come: the greatest misery belongs to mankind,
a perpetual servitude, a slavery, *ex timore timor* [6] [one fear leading
to another], an heavy yoke, the seal of damnation, an intolerable
burden. They that are superstitious are still fearing, suspecting,
vexing themselves with auguries, prodigies, false tales, dreams,
idle, vain works, unprofitable labours, as Boterus observes,[7]
cura mentis ancipite versantur [they are tormented with anxiety],
enemies to God and to themselves. In a word, as Seneca concludes, *Religio Deum colit, superstitio destruit,* superstition
destroys, but true religion honours God. True religion, *ubi
verus Deus vere colitur,* where the true God is truly worshipped,
is the way to heaven, the mother of virtues, love, fear, devotion,
obedience, knowledge, etc. It rears the dejected soul of man,
and amidst so many cares, miseries, persecutions, which this
world affords, it is a sole ease, an unspeakable comfort, a sweet
reposal, *jugum suave, et leve,* a light yoke, an anchor, and an
haven. It adds courage, boldness, and begets generous spirits:
although tyrants rage, persecute, and that bloody lictor or
sergeant be ready to martyr them, *aut lita, aut morere* [either
sacrifice or die] (as in those persecutions of the primitive Church
it was put in practice, as you may read in Eusebius and others),
though enemies be now ready to invade, and all in an uproar,
Si fractus illabatur orbis, impavidum ferient ruinæ,[8] though
heaven should fall on his head, he would not be dismayed.
But as a good Christian prince once made answer to a menacing
Turk, *facile scelerata hominum arma contemnit, qui Dei præsidio*

tutus est [he who is secure in the protection of God can easily despise the impious weapons of men]: or as Phalaris· writ to Alexander in a wrong cause, he nor any other enemy could terrify him, for that he trusted in God.[1] *Si Deus nobiscum, quis contra nos?* [If God is with us, who is against us?] In all calamities, persecutions, whatsoever, as David did (2 Sam. ii, 22), he will sing with him, "The Lord is my rock, my fortress, my strength, my refuge, the tower and horn of my salvation," etc. In all troubles and adversities (Ps. xlvi, 1), "God is my hope and help, still ready to be found, I will not therefore fear," etc.; 'tis a fear expelling fear; he hath peace of conscience, and is full of hope, which is (saith Austin [2]) *vita vitæ mortalis*, the life of this our mortal life, hope of immortality, the sole comfort of our misery: otherwise, as Paul saith, we of all others were most wretched, but this makes us happy, counterpoising our hearts in all miseries; superstition torments, and is from the devil, the author of lies; but this is from God Himself, as Lucian, that Antiochian priest, made his divine confession in Eusebius,[3] *Auctor nobis de Deo Deus est,* God is the author of our religion Himself, His word is our rule, a lanthorn to us, dictated by the Holy Ghost, He plays upon our hearts as so many harp-strings, and we are His temples, He dwelleth in us, and we in Him.

The part affected of superstition is the brain, heart, will, understanding, soul itself, and all the faculties of it, *totum compositum* [the whole composition], all is mad and dotes. Now for the extent, as I say, the world itself is the subject of it (to omit that grand sin of atheism), all times have been misaffected; past, present, "There is not one that doth good, no not one, from the prophet to the priest," etc. A lamentable thing it is to consider, how many myriads of men this idolatry and superstition (for that comprehends all) hath infatuated in all ages, besotted by this blind zeal, which is religion's ape, religion's bastard, religion's shadow, false glass. For where God hath a temple, the devil will have a chapel: where God hath sacrifices, the devil will have his oblations: where God hath ceremonies, the devil will have his traditions: where there is any religion, the devil will plant superstition; and 'tis a pitiful sight to behold and read what tortures, miseries it hath procured, what slaughter of souls it hath made, how it raged amongst those old Persians, Syrians, Egyptians, Greeks, Romans, Tuscans, Gauls, Germans, Britons, etc. *Britannia jam hodie celebrat tam attonite,* saith Pliny,[4] *tantis ceremoniis* (speaking of superstition) *ut dedisse Persis videri possit:* the Britons are so stupendly superstitious

III—* L 888

in their ceremonies, that they go beyond those Persians. He that shall but read in Pausanias alone, those gods, temples, altars, idols, statues, so curiously made with such infinite cost and charge amongst those old Greeks, such multitudes of them and frequent varieties, as Gerbelius truly observes,[1] may stand amazed, and never enough wonder at it; and thank God withal, that by the light of the Gospel we are so happily freed from that slavish idolatry in these our days. But heretofore, almost in all countries, in all places, superstition hath blinded the hearts of men; in all ages what a small portion hath the true Church ever been! *Divisum imperium cum Jove Dæmon habet* [the devil shares authority with Jove]. The patriarchs and their families, the Israelites, a handful in respect, Christ and his apostles, and not all of them, neither. Into what straits hath it been compinged, a little flock! how hath superstition on the other side dilated herself, error, ignorance, barbarism, folly, madness, deceived, triumphed, and insulted over the most wise, discreet, and understanding men! Philosophers, dynasts, monarchs, all were involved and overshadowed in this mist, in more than Cimmerian darkness. *Adeo ignara superstitio mentes hominum depravat, et nonnunquam sapientum animos transversos agit* [2] [superstition has such a hold on the human mind that it sometimes leads astray even the wise]. At this present, *quota pars!* how small a part is truly religious! How little in respect! Divide the world into six parts, and one, or not so much, is Christians; idolaters and Mahometans possess almost Asia, Africa, America, Magellanica. The kings of China, Great Cham, Siam, and Bornay, Pegu, Deccan, Narsinga, Japan, etc., are gentiles, idolaters, and many other petty princes in Asia, Monomotopa, Congo, and I know not how many other petty princes in Africa, all Terra Australis Incognita, most of America pagans, differing all in their several superstitions; and yet all idolaters. The Mahometans extend themselves over the Great Turk's dominions in Europe, Africa, Asia, to the Xeriffs in Barbary, and his territories in Fez, Sus, Morocco, etc. The Tartar, the Great Mogor, the Sophy of Persia, with most of their dominions and subjects, are at this day Mahometans. See how the devil rageth! Those at odds, or differing among themselves, some for Ali, some for Enbocar, for Acmar, and Ozimen,[3] those four doctors, Mahomet's successors, and are subdivided into seventy-two inferior sects, as Leo Afer reports.[4] The Jews, as a company of vagabonds, are scattered over all parts; whose story, present estate, progress from time to time, is fully set down by Mr.

Thomas Jackson, Doctor of Divinity, in his Comment on the Creed.[1] A fifth part of the world, and hardly that, now professeth Christ, but so inlarded and interlaced with several superstitions, that there is scarce a sound part to be found, or any agreement amongst them. Presbyter John in Africa, lord of those Abyssines or Ethiopians, is by his profession a Christian, but so different from us, with such new absurdities and ceremonies, such liberty, such a mixture of idolatry and paganism, that they keep little more than a bare title of Christianity.[2] They suffer polygamy, circumcision, stupend fastings, divorce as they will themselves, etc., and as the papists call on the Virgin Mary, so do they on Thomas Didymus before Christ.[3] The Greek or Eastern Church is rent from this of the West, and as they have four chief patriarchs, so have they four subdivisions, besides those Nestorians, Jacobins, Syrians, Armenians, Georgians, etc., scattered over Asia Minor, Syria, Egypt, etc., Greece, Valachia, Circassia, Bulgary, Bosnia, Albania, Illyricum, Sclavonia, Croatia, Thrace, Servia, Rascia,[4] and a sprinkling amongst the Tartars. The Russians, Muscovites, and most of that Great Duke's subjects, are part of the Greek Church, and still Christians: but as one saith, *temporis successu multas illi addiderunt superstitiones*, in process of time they have added so many superstitions, they be rather semi-Christians than otherwise.[5] That which remains is the Western Church with us in Europe, but so eclipsed with several schisms, heresies and superstitions, that one knows not where to find it. The papists have Italy, Spain, Savoy, part of Germany, France, Poland, and a sprinkling in the rest of Europe. In America, they hold all that which Spaniards inhabit, Hispania Nova, Castella Aurea, Peru, etc. In the East Indies, the Philippinæ, some small holds about Goa, Malacca, Zelan,[6] Ormus, etc., which the Portuguese got not long since, and those land-leaping Jesuits have essayed in China, Japan, as appears by their yearly letters; in Africa they have Melinda, Quiloa, Mombaze, etc., and some few towns; they drive out one superstition with another. Poland is a receptacle of all religions, where Samosetans, Socinians, Photinians (now protected in Transylvania and Poland), Arians, Anabaptists are to be found, as well as in some German cities. Scandia is Christian, but as Damianus à Goes,[7] the Portugal knight, complains, so mixed with magic, pagan rites and ceremonies, they may be as well counted idolaters: what Tacitus formerly said of a like nation is verified in them, "A people subject to superstition, contrary to religion."[8] And some of

them, as about Lapland, and the Pilapians, the devil's possession
to this day, *Misera hæc gens* (saith mine author [1]) *Satanæ
hactenus possessio . . . et quod maxime mirandum et dolendum,*
and which is to be admired and pitied, if any of them be baptized,
which the kings of Sweden much labour, they die within seven
or nine days after, and for that cause they will hardly be brought
to Christianity, but worship still the devil, who daily appears
to them; in their idolatrous courses, *gaudentibus diis patriis,
quos religiose colunt* [rejoicing in their ancestral gods whom they
scrupulously worship], etc. Yet are they very superstitious,
like our wild Irish; though they of the better note, the
kings of Denmark and Sweden govern themselves, that them, be
Lutherans. The remnant are Calvinists, Lutherans, in Germany equally mixed; and yet the emperor himself, dukes of
Lorraine, Bavaria, and the princes electors, are most part
professed papists. And though some part of France and
Ireland, Great Britain, half the cantons in Switzerland, and the
Low Countries be Calvinists, more defecate than the rest, yet
at odds amongst themselves, not free from superstition. And
which Brocard the monk, in his description of the Holy Land,[2]
after he had censured the Greek Church and showed their
errors, concluded at last, *Faxit Deus ne Latinis multa irrepserint
stultitiæ,* I say, God grant there be no fopperies in our Church.
As a dam of water stopped in one place breaks out into another,
so doth superstition. I say nothing of Anabaptists, Socinians,
Brownists, Barrowists, Familists, etc. There is superstition in
our prayers, often in our hearing of sermons, bitter contentions,
invectives, persecutions, strange conceits, besides diversity of
opinions, schisms, factions, etc. But as the Lord (Job xlii, 7)
said to Eliphaz the Temanite and his two friends, "His wrath
was kindled against them, for they had not spoken of him
things that were right," we may justly of these schismatics
and heretics, how wise soever in their own conceits, *non recte
loquuntur de Deo,* they speak not, they think not, they write
not well of God, and as they ought. And therefore, *Quid,
quæso, mi Dorpi,* as Erasmus concludes to Dorpius, *hisce theologis
faciamus, aut quid preceris, nisi forte fidelem medicum, qui cerebro
medeatur?* What shall we wish them, but *sanam mentem* [a
sound mind] and a good physician? But more of their differences,
paradoxes, opinions, mad pranks, in the Symptoms: I now
hasten to the Causes.

SUBSECT. II.—*Causes of Religious Melancholy. From the Devil by miracles, apparitions, oracles. His instruments or factors, Politicians, Priests, Impostors, Heretics, blind guides. In them simplicity, fear, blind zeal, ignorance, solitariness, curiosity, pride, vainglory, presumption, etc. His engines, fasting, solitariness, hope, fear, etc.*

We are taught in Holy Scripture, that the devil "rangeth abroad like a roaring lion, still seeking whom he may devour": and as in several shapes, so by several engines and devices he goeth about to seduce us; sometimes he transforms himself into an angel of light, and is so cunning that he is able, if it were possible, to deceive the very elect. He will be worshipped as God Himself, and is so adored by the heathen, and esteemed.[1] And in imitation of that divine power, as Eusebius observes,[2] to abuse or emulate God's glory, as Dandinus adds,[3] he will have all homage, sacrifices, oblations, and whatsoever else belongs to the worship of God, to be done likewise unto him, *similis erit altissimo* [he will be like the Most High], and by this means infatuates the world, deludes, entraps, and destroys many a thousand souls. Sometimes by dreams, visions (as God to Moses by familiar conference), the devil in several shapes talks with them: in the Indies it is common,[4] and in China nothing so familiar as apparitions, inspirations, oracles; by terrifying them with false prodigies, counterfeit miracles, sending storms, tempests, diseases, plagues (as of old in Athens there was Apollo Alexicacus, Apollo Λοίμιος, *pestifer et malorum depulsor* [plague-bringer and plague-remover]), raising wars, seditions by spectrums, troubling their consciences, driving them to despair, terrors of mind, intolerable pains; by promises, rewards, benefits, and fair means, he raiseth such an opinion of his deity and greatness, that they dare not do otherwise than adore him, do as he will have them, they dare not offend him. And to compel them more to stand in awe of him, "he sends and cures diseases, disquiets their spirits" (as Cyprian saith), "torments and terrifies their souls, to make them adore him; and all his study, all his endeavour is to divert them from true religion to superstition; and because he is damned himself, and in an error, he would have all the world participate of his errors, and be damned with him."[5] The *primum mobile*, therefore, and first mover of all superstition, is the devil, that great enemy of mankind, the principal agent, who in a thousand several shapes, after divers fashions, with several engines,

illusions, and by several names hath deceived the inhabitants
of the earth, in several places and countries, still rejoicing at
their falls. "All the world over before Christ's time he freely
domineered, and held the souls of men in most slavish subjection," saith Eusebius,[1] "in divers forms, ceremonies, and
sacrifices, till Christ's coming," as if those devils of the air
had shared the earth amongst them, which the Platonists held
for gods (*Ludus deorum sumus* [2] [we are the sport of the gods]),
and were our governors and keepers. In several places, they
had several rites, orders, names, of which read Wierus, *de præstigiis dæmonum, lib.* 1, *cap.* 5, Strozzius Cicogna, and others: [3]
Adonided amongst the Syrians; Adramelech amongst the Caper-
naites; Asiniæ amongst the Emathites; Astarte with the Sidonians; Astaroth with the Palestines; Dagon with the Philistines;
Tartary with the Hanæi; Milcom amongst the Ammonites; Bel,
the Babylonians; Beelzebub and Baal with the Samaritans and
Moabites; Apis, Isis, and Osiris amongst the Egyptians; Apollo
Pythius at Delphi, Colophon, Ancyra, Cumæ, Erythræ; Jupiter
in Crete, Venus at Cyprus, Juno at Carthage, Æsculapius at
Epidaurus, Diana at Ephesus, Pallas at Athens, etc. And even
in these our days, both in the East and West Indies, in Tartary,
China, Japan, etc., what strange idols, in what prodigious forms,
with what absurd ceremonies are they adored! What strange
sacraments, like ours of Baptism and the Lord's Supper, what
goodly temples, priests, sacrifices they had in America, when the
Spaniards first landed there, let Acosta the Jesuit relate, *lib.* 5,
cap. 1, 2, 3, 4, etc., and how the devil imitated the Ark and the
children of Israel's coming out of Egypt; with many such. For
as Lipsius well discourseth out of the doctrine of the Stoics,
maxime cupiunt adorationem hominum, now and of old, they
still and most especially desire to be adored by men. See but
what Vertomannus, *lib.* 5, *cap.* 2, Marcus Polus, Lerius, Benzo,
P. Martyr ·in his Ocean Decades, Acosta, and Mat. Riccius,
Expedit. Christ. in Sinas, lib. 1, relate. Eusebius [4] wonders
how that wise city of Athens and flourishing kingdoms of
Greece should be so besotted; and we in our times; how those
witty Chinese, so perspicacious in all other things, should be
so gulled, so tortured with superstition, so blind, as to worship
stocks and stones. But it is no marvel, when we see all out as
great effects amongst Christians themselves; how are those
Anabaptists, Arians, and Papists above the rest, miserably
infatuated! Mars, Jupiter, Apollo, and Æsculapius have resigned their interest, names, and offices to St. George

(*Maxime bellorum rector, quem nostra juventus
Pro Mavorte colit*),[1]

[O great lord of war, whom our youth worship in place
of Mars,]

St. Christopher, and a company of fictitious saints, Venus to
the Lady of Loretto. And as those old Romans had several
distinct gods for divers offices, persons, places, so have they
saints, as Lavater well observes out of Lactantius,[2] *mutato
nomine tantum* [only the name is changed], 'tis the same spirit
or devil that deludes them still. The manner how, as I say, is
by rewards, promises, terrors, affrights, punishments: in a word,
fair and foul means, hope and fear. How often hath Jupiter,
Apollo, Bacchus, and the rest, sent plagues in Greece and Italy,
because their sacrifices were neglected![3]

> *Di multa neglecti dederunt
> Hesperiæ mala luctuosæ,*[4]

[For her neglect of the gods Italy hath been made
grievously to mourn,]

to terrify them, to rouse them up, and the like: see but Livy,
Dionysius Halicarnasseus, Thucydides, Pausanias, Philostratus,
Polybius,[5] before the battle of Cannæ, *prodigiis, signis, ostentis,
templa cuncta, privatæ etiam ædes scatebant* [all the temples, and
even private houses, were full of signs and portents]. Œneus
reigned in Ætolia, and because he did not sacrifice to Diana
with his other gods (see more in Libanius his *Diana*), she sent a
wild boar, *insolitæ magnitudinis, qui terras et homines misere
depascebatur*, to spoil both men and country, which was afterwards killed by Meleager. So Plutarch in the life of Lucullus
relates, how Mithridates, King of Pontus, at the siege of Cyzicum,
with all his navy, was overthrown by Proserpina, for neglecting
of her holy day. She appeared in a vision to Aristagoras in the
night, *Cras, inquit, tibicinem Libycum cum tibicine Pontico
committam* ["To-morrow," said she, "I will cause a contest
between a Libyan and a Pontic piper"], and the day following
this enigma was understood; for with a great south wind which
came from Libya, she quite overwhelmed Mithridates' army.
What prodigies and miracles, dreams, visions, predictions,
apparitions, oracles, have been of old at Delphi, Dodona, Trophonius' Den, at Thebes, and Lebadea,[6] of Jupiter Ammon in
Egypt, Amphiaraus in Attica, etc.! what strange cures performed by Apollo and Æsculapius! Juno's image and that of

Fortune spake,[1] Castor and Pollux fought in person for the
Romans against Hannibal's army,[2] as Pallas, Mars, Juno, Venus,
for Greeks and Trojans, etc. Amongst our pseudo-Catholics
nothing so familiar as such miracles; how many cures done by
our Lady of Loretto, at Sichem! of old at our St. Thomas'
shrine, etc. St. Sabine was seen to fight for Arnulphus, Duke
of Spoleto.[3] St. George fought in person for John the Bastard
of Portugal, against the Castilians;[4] St. James for the Spaniards
in America. In the battle of Bannockburn, where Edward the
Second, our English king, was foiled by the Scots, St. Philanus'
arm was seen to fight (if Hector Boethius doth not impose[5]),
that was before shut up in a silver capcase; another time, in
the same author, St. Magnus fought for them. Now for visions,
revelations, miracles, not only out of the Legend, out of purgatory, but every day comes news from the Indies, and at home;
read the Jesuits' letters, Ribadeneira, Thurselinus, Acosta,
Lippomanus; Xaverius', Ignatius' Lives, etc., and tell me
what difference?

His ordinary instruments or factors which he useth, as God
Himself did good kings, lawful magistrates, patriarchs, prophets,
to the establishing of His Church, are politicians,[6] statesmen,
priests, heretics, blind guides, impostors, pseudo-prophets, to
propagate his superstition. And first to begin with politicians,
it hath ever been a principal axiom with them to maintain
religion or superstition, which they determine of, alter and vary
upon all occasions, as to them seems best; they make religion
mere policy, a cloak, a human invention; *nihil æque valet ad
regendos vulgi animos ac superstitio* [nothing is so effective for
keeping the masses under control as superstition], as Tacitus[7]
and Tully[8] hold. Austin, *lib. 4 de Civitat. Dei, cap.* 9, censures
Scævola saying and acknowledging *expedire civitates religione
falli*, that it was a fit thing cities should be deceived by religion,
according to the diverb, *Si mundus vult decipi, decipiatur*, if
the world will be gulled, let it be gulled, 'tis good howsoever to
keep it in subjection. 'Tis that Aristotle[9] and Plato[10] inculcate
in their Politics, "Religion neglected brings plagues to the city,
opens a gap to all naughtiness." 'Tis that which all our late
politicians ingeminate: Cromerus, *lib. 2 Pol. hist.*; Boterus,
lib. 3 de incrementis urbium; Clapmarius, *lib. 2, cap.* 9, *de arcanis
rerump.*; Arnisæus, *cap.* 4, *lib. 2, Polit.* Captain Machiavel
will have a prince by all means to counterfeit religion, to be
superstitious in show at least, to seem to be devout, frequent
holy exercises, honour divines, love the Church, affect priests, as

Numa, Lycurgus, and such law-makers were and did, *non ut
his fidem habeant, sed ut subditos religionis metu facilius in officio
contineant* [not that he should believe in it, but in order that
his subjects through religious scruples may be more easily kept
in obedience], to keep people in obedience. *Nam naturaliter*
(as Cardan writes) *lex Christiana lex est pietatis, justitiæ, fidei,
simplicitatis*, etc.[1] [for by its nature Christianity is a religion of
piety, justice, faith, simplicity, etc.].   But this error of his,
Innocentius Gentilettus, a French lawyer, *theorem*. 9, *comment*. 1,
de relig., and Thomas Bozius in his book *de ruinis gentium et
regnorum*, have copiously confuted.   Many politicians, I dare
not deny, maintain religion as a true means, and sincerely speak
of it without hypocrisy, are truly zealous and religious themselves.   Justice and religion are the two chief props and supporters of a well-governed commonwealth; but most of them
are but Machiavellians, counterfeits only for political ends;
for *solus rex* [despotism] (which Campanella, *cap*. 18 *Atheismi
Triumphati*, observes), as amongst our modern Turks, *reipub.
finis* [is the end of the State]; as knowing *magnum ejus in
animos imperium* [2] [its great sway over men's minds]; and that,
as Sabellicus delivers, "A man without religion is like a horse
without a bridle." [3]   No way better to curb than superstition,
to terrify men's consciences, and to keep them in awe: they
make new laws, statutes, invent new religions, ceremonies, as
so many stalking-horses, to their ends.   *Hæc enim (religio) si
falsa sit, dummodo vera credatur, animorum ferociam domat,
libidines coercet, subditos principi obsequentes efficit* [4] [a religion,
even if false, as long as it is believed, moderates passion, checks
sensual indulgence, and makes subjects obedient to their prince].
"Therefore" (saith Polybius [5] of Lycurgus), "did he maintain
ceremonies, not that he was superstitious himself, but that he
perceived mortal men more apt to embrace paradoxes than
aught else, and durst attempt no evil things for fear of the
gods."   This was Zamolxis' stratagem amongst the Thracians,
Numa's plot, when he said he had conference with the nymph
Egeria, and that of Sertorius with an hart: to get more credit
to their decrees, by deriving them from the gods; or else they
did all by divine instinct, which Nicholas Damascen well observes
of Lycurgus, Solon, and Minos, they had their laws dictated,
monte sacro, by Jupiter himself.   So Mahomet referred his new
laws to the angel Gabriel, by whose direction he gave out they
were made.[6]   Caligula in Dion feigned himself to be familiar
with Castor and Pollux, and many such, which kept those

Romans under (who, as Machiavel proves, *lib.* 1 *Disput. cap.* 11 *et* 12, were *religione maxime moti*, most superstitious): and did curb the people more by this means than by force of arms or severity of human laws. *Sola plebecula eam agnoscebat* (saith Vaninus, *dial.* 1, *lib.* 4, *de admirandis naturæ arcanis*, speaking of religion), *quæ facile decipitur* [only the common people, which is easily deceived, believed in it], *magnates vero et philosophi nequaquam*, your grandees and philosophers had no such conceit, *sed ad imperii confirmationem et amplificationem, quam sine prætextu religionis tueri non poterant* [save for the strengthenirg and extension of government, which was impossible save under the cloak of religion]; and many thousands in all ages have ever held as much, philosophers especially; *animadvertebant hi semper hæc esse fabellas* [they knew all along that these things were fables], *attamen ob metum publicæ potestatis silere cogebantur*, [but] they were still silent for fear of laws, etc. To this end that Syrian Pherecydes, Pythagoras his master, broached in the East amongst the heathens first the immortality of the soul, as Trismegistus did in Egypt, with a many of feigned gods. Those French and Briton Druids in the West first taught, saith Cæsar,[1] *non interire animas* [that souls did not die], but after death to go [2] from one to another, that so they might encourage them to virtue. 'Twas for a politic end, and to this purpose the old poets feigned those Elysian Fields, their Æacus, Minos, and Rhadamanthus, their infernal judges, and those Stygian lakes, fiery Phlegethons, Pluto's kingdom, and variety of torments after death.[3] Those that had done well went to the Elysian Fields, but evil-doers to Cocytus, and to that burning lake of hell, with fire and brimstone for ever to be tormented.[4] 'Tis this which Plato labours for in his *Phædo*, *et* 3 *de Rep.*,[5] the Turks in their Alcoran, when they set down rewards and several punishments for every particular virtue and vice, when they persuade men that they that die in battle shall go directly to heaven,[6] but wicked livers to eternal torment, and all of all sorts (much like our papistical purgatory) for a set time shall be tortured in their graves, as appears by that tract which John Baptista Alfaqui, that Mauritanian priest, now turned Christian, hath written in his confutation of the Alcoran. After a man's death two black angels, Nunquir and Nequir (so they call them), come to him to his grave and punish him for his precedent sins; if he lived well, they torture him the less; if ill, *per indesinentes cruciatus ad diem judicii*, they incessantly punish him to the day of judgment. *Nemo viventium qui ad*

horum mentionem non totus horret et contremiscit, the thought of
this crucifies them all their lives long, and makes them spend
their days in fasting and prayer, *ne mala hæc contingant* [lest
these ills befall them], etc. A Tartar prince, saith Marcus
Polus, *lib. 1, cap.* 28, called *Senex de Montibus* [the Old Man of
the Mountains], the better to establish his government amongst
his subjects, and to keep them in awe, found a convenient place
in a pleasant valley, environed with hills, in which "he made a
delicious park full of odoriferous flowers and fruits, and a
palace of all worldly contents" [1] that could possibly be devised,
music, pictures, variety of meats, etc., and chose out a certain
young man, whom with a soporiferous potion he so benumbed
that he perceived nothing; "and so, fast asleep as he was,
caused him to be conveyed into this fair garden"; [2] where after
he had lived awhile in all such pleasures a sensual man could
desire, "he cast him into a sleep again, and brought him forth,
that when he awaked he might tell others he had been in
Paradise." [3] The like he did for hell, and by this means brought
his people to subjection. Because heaven and hell are mentioned in the Scriptures, and to be believed necessary by Christians; so cunningly can the devil and his ministers, in imitation
of true religion, counterfeit and forge the like, to circumvent
and delude his superstitious followers. Many such tricks and
impostures are acted by politicians, in China especially, but
with what effect I will discourse in the Symptoms.

Next to politicians, if I may distinguish them, are some of
our priests (who make religion policy), if not far beyond them,
for they domineer over princes and statesmen themselves.
Carnificinam exercent, one saith, they tyrannize over men's
consciences more than any other tormentors whatsoever, partly
for their commodity and gain; *Religionum enim omnium abusus*
(as Postellus holds [4]), *quæstus scilicet sacrificum in causa est*
[the cause of the abuse of all religions is the greed of the priests],
for sovereignty, credit, to maintain their state and reputation,
out of ambition and avarice, which are their chief supporters.
What have they not made the common people believe? Impossibilities in nature, incredible things. What devices, traditions, ceremonies, have they not invented in all ages to keep
men in obedience, to enrich themselves? *Quibus quæstui sunt
capti superstitione animi* [who make their profit out of superstitious persons], as Livy saith.[5] Those Egyptian priests of
old got all the sovereignty into their hands, and knowing, as
Curtius insinuates,[6] *nulla res efficacius multitudinem regit quam*

superstitio; melius vatibus quam ducibus parent, vana religione capti, etiam impotentes feminæ: the common people will sooner obey priests than captains, and nothing so forcible as superstition, or better than blind zeal to rule a multitude; have so terrified and gulled them, that it is incredible to relate. All nations almost have been besotted in this kind; amongst our Britons and old Gauls the Druids; Magi in Persia; philosophers in Greece; Chaldeans amongst the Oriental; Brachmanni in India; Gymnosophists in Ethiopia; the Turdetanes in Spain; augurs in Rome, have insulted; Apollo's priests in Greece, Phœbades and Pythonissæ, by their oracles and phantasms; Amphiaraus and his companions; now Mahometan and pagan priests, what can they not effect? How do they not infatuate the world? *Adeo ubique* (as Scaliger writes of the Mahometan priests [1]), *tum gentium tum locorum, gens ista sacrorum ministra, vulgi secat spes, ad ea quæ ipsi fingunt somnia,* so cunningly can they gull the commons in all places and countries. But above all others, that high priest of Rome, the dam of that monstrous and superstitious brood, the bull-bellowing Pope which now rageth in the West, that three-headed Cerberus, hath played his part. "Whose religion at this day is mere policy, a state wholly composed of superstition and wit, and needs nothing but wit and superstition to maintain it, that useth colleges and religious houses to as good purpose as forts and castles, and doth more at this day"[2]—by a company of scribbling parasites, fiery-spirited friars, zealous anchorites, hypocritical confessors, and those prætorian soldiers, his janissary Jesuits, that dissociable society, as Langius terms it,[3] *postremus diaboli conatus et sæculi excrementum* [the last effort of the devil and the off-scouring of the age], that now stand in the fore-front of the battle, will have a monopoly of, and engross all other learning, but domineer in divinity, *Excipiunt soli totius vulnera belli*[4] [alone they bear the brunt of the whole war], and fight alone almost (for the rest are but his dromedaries and asses)—than ever he could have done by garrisons and armies. What power of prince, or penal law, be it never so strict, could enforce men to do that which for conscience' sake they will voluntarily undergo? As to fast from all flesh, abstain from marriage, rise to their prayers at midnight, whip themselves, with stupend fasting and penance, abandon the world, wilful poverty, perform canonical and blind obedience, to prostrate their goods, fortunes, bodies, lives, and offer up themselves at their Superior's feet, at his command? What so powerful an engine as superstition? which

they right well perceiving, are of no religion at all themselves:
Primum enim (as Calvin rightly suspects, the tenor and practice
of their life proves) *arcanæ illius theologiæ, quod apud eos regnat,
caput est, nullum esse deum,* they hold there is no God, as Leo X
did, Hildebrand the magician,[1] Alexander VI, Julius II, mere
atheists, and which the common proverb amongst them approves:
"The worst Christians of Italy are the Romans, of the Romans
the priests are wildest, the lewdest priests are preferred to be
cardinals, and the baddest man amongst the cardinals is chosen
to be Pope,"[2] that is an epicure, as most part the Popes
are, infidels and Lucianists, for so they think and believe;
and what is said of Christ to be fables and impostures, of
heaven and hell, day of judgment, paradise, immortality of the
soul, are all

> *Rumores vacui, verbaque inania,*
> *Et par sollicito fabula somnio,*[3]

dreams, toys, and old wives' tales.   Yet as so many whetstones
to make other tools cut, but cut not themselves,[4] though they
be of no religion at all, they will make others most devout
and superstitious, by promises and threats compel, enforce
from, and lead them by the nose like so many bears in a line;
whenas their end is not to propagate the Church, advance God's
kingdom, seek His glory or common good, but to enrich themselves, to enlarge their territories, to domineer and compel them
to stand in awe, to live in subjection to the See of Rome.   For
what otherwise care they?   *Si mundus vult decipi, decipiatur*
[if the world wishes to be gulled, let it be gulled], 'tis fit it should
be so.   And [that] for which Austin [5] cites Varro to maintain
his Roman religion, we may better apply to them: *Multa vera,
quæ vulgus scire non est utile; pleraque falsa, quæ tamen aliter
existimare populum expedit;* some things are true, some false,
which for their own ends they will not have the gullish commonalty take notice of.   As well may witness their intolerable
covetousness, strange forgeries, fopperies, fooleries, unrighteous
subtleties, impostures, illusions, new doctrines, paradoxes,
traditions, false miracles, which they have still forged to enthral,
circumvent, and subjugate them, to maintain their own estates.[6]
One while by bulls, pardons, indulgences, and their doctrine of
good works, that they be meritorious, hope of heaven, by that
means they have so fleeced the commonalty, and spurred on
this free superstitious horse, that he runs himself blind, and is an
ass to carry burdens.   They have so amplified Peter's patrimony

that from a poor bishop he is become *Rex regum, Dominus dominantium*, a demigod, as his canonists make him (Felinus and the rest), above God Himself; and for his wealth and temporalties, is not inferior to many kings;[1] his cardinals, princes' companions;[2] and in every kingdom almost, abbots, priors, monks, friars, etc., and his clergy, have engrossed a third part, half, in some places all, into their hands.[3] Three princes electors in Germany, bishops; besides Magdeburg, Spires, Salzburg, Bremen, Bamberg, etc. In France, as Bodine, *lib. de repub.*, gives us to understand, their revenues are twelve millions and three hundred thousand livres; and of twelve parts of the revenues in France the Church possesseth seven. The Jesuits, a new sect begun in this age, have, as Middendorpius[4] and Pelargus[5] reckon up, three or four hundred colleges in Europe, and more revenues than many princes. In France, as Arnoldus proves, in thirty years they have got *bis centum librarum millia annua*, £200,000 [annually]. I say nothing of the rest of their orders. We have had in England, as Armachanus demonstrates, above thirty thousand friars at once, and as Speed collects out of Leland and others,[6] almost six hundred religious houses, and near £200,000 in revenues of the old rent belonging to them, besides images of gold, silver, plate, furniture, goods and ornaments, as Weever calculates,[7] and esteems them, at the dissolution of abbeys, worth a million of gold. How many towns in every kingdom hath superstition enriched! What a deal of money by musty relics, images, idolatry, have their mass-priests engrossed, and what sums have they scraped by their other tricks, Loretto in Italy, Walsingham in England, in those days, *ubi omnia auro nitent* [where everything shines with gold], saith Erasmus, St. Thomas' shrine, etc., may witness. Delphi, so renowned of old in Greece for Apollo's oracle;[8] Delos, *commune conciliabulum et emporium sola religione munitum* [which became a great centre of trade and concourse solely through its religious associations]; Dodona, whose fame and wealth were sustained by religion,[9] were not so rich, so famous. If they can get but a relic of some saint, the Virgin Mary's picture, idols or the like, that city is for ever made, it needs no other maintenance. Now if any of these their impostures or juggling tricks be controverted, or called in question; if a magnanimous or zealous Luther, an heroical Luther, as Dithmarus calls him,[10] dare touch the monks' bellies, all is in a combustion, all is in an uproar: Demetrius and his associates are ready to pull him in pieces, to keep up their trades. "Great is Diana of the

Ephesians": [1] with a mighty shout of two hours long they will roar and not be pacified.

Now for their authority, what by auricular confession, satisfaction, penance, Peter's keys, thunderings, excommunications, etc., roaring bulls, this high priest of Rome, shaking his Gorgon's head, hath so terrified the soul of many a silly man, insulted over majesty itself, and swaggered generally over all Europe for many ages, and still doth to some, holding them as yet in slavish subjection, as never tyrannizing Spaniards did by their poor negroes, or Turks by their galley-slaves. "The Bishop of Rome" (saith Stapleton, a parasite of his, *de mag. Eccles. lib.* 2, *cap.* 1) "hath done that without arms, which those Roman emperors could never achieve with forty legions of soldiers," [2] deposed kings, and crowned them again with his foot, made friends, and corrected at his pleasure, etc. "'Tis a wonder," saith Machiavel, *Florentinæ hist. lib.* 1, "what slavery King Henry the Second endured for the death of Th. Becket, what things he was enjoined by the Pope, and how he submitted himself to do that which in our times a private man would not endure," [3] and all through superstition. Henry the Fourth, deposed of his empire, stood barefooted with his wife at the gates of Canossa.[4] Frederick the Emperor was trodden on by Alexander the Third; [5] another held Adrian's stirrup; King John kissed the knees of Pandulph the Pope's legate, etc. What made so many thousand Christians travel from France, Britain, etc., into the Holy Land, spend such huge sums of money, go a pilgrimage so familiarly to Jerusalem, to creep and crouch, but slavish superstition? What makes them so freely venture their lives, to leave their native countries, to go seek martyrdom in the Indies, but superstition? to be assassinates, to meet death, murder kings, but a false persuasion of merit, of canonical or blind obedience which they instil into them, and animate them by strange illusions, hope of being martyrs and saints? Such pretty feats can the devil work by priests, and so well for their own advantage can they play their parts. And if it were not yet enough by priests and politicians to delude mankind and crucify the souls of men, he hath more actors in his tragedy, more irons in the fire, another scene of heretics, factious, ambitious wits, insolent spirits, schismatics, impostors, false prophets, blind guides, that out of pride, singularity, vainglory, blind zeal, cause much more madness yet, set all in an uproar by their new doctrines, paradoxes, figments, crotchets, make new divisions, subdivisions, new sects, oppose one superstition

to another, one kingdom to another, commit prince and subjects, brother against brother, father against son, to the ruin
and destruction of a commonwealth, to the disturbance of peace,
and to make a general confusion of all estates. How did those
Arians rage of old! how many did they circumvent! Those
Pelagians, Manichees, etc.! their names alone would make a
just volume. How many silly souls have impostors still deluded,
drawn away, and quite alienated from Christ! Lucian's Alexander; Simon Magus, whose statue was to be seen and adored
in Rome, saith Justin Martyr, *Simoni deo sancto*, etc., after his
decease; Apollonius Tyanæus,[1] Cynops, Eumo, who, by counterfeiting some new ceremonies and juggling tricks of that *Dea
Syria* [Syrian Goddess], by spitting fire, and the like, got an
army together of forty thousand men, and did much harm:
with Eudo de Stellis, of whom Nubrigensis speaks, *lib.* 1, *cap.* 19,
that in King Stephen's days imitated most of Christ's miracles,
fed I know not how many people in the wilderness, and built
castles in the air, etc., to the seducing of multitudes of poor
souls. In Franconia, 1476, a base illiterate fellow took upon
him to be a prophet and preach, John Beheim by name, a neat-
herd at Nicholhausen; he seduced thirty thousand persons, and
was taken by the commonalty to be a most holy man, come
from heaven. "Tradesmen left their shops, women their
distaffs, servants ran from their masters, children from their
parents, scholars left their tutors, all to hear him, some for
novelty, some for zeal. He was burnt at last by the Bishop
of Wurtzburg, and so he and his heresy vanished together."[2]
How many such impostors, false prophets, have lived in every
king's reign! what chronicles will not afford such examples!
that as so many *ignes fatui*, have led men out of the way, terrified
some, deluded others, that are apt to be carried about by the
blast of every wind, a rude inconstant multitude, a silly company
of poor souls, that follow all, and are cluttered together like so
many pebbles in a tide. What prodigious follies, madness,
vexations, persecutions, absurdities, impossibilities, these impostors, heretics, etc., have thrust upon the world, what strange
effects, shall be showed in the Symptoms.

Now the means by which, or advantages the devil and his
infernal ministers take, so to delude and disquiet the world
with such idle ceremonies, false doctrines, superstitious fopperies,
are from themselves, innate fear, ignorance, simplicity, hope and
fear, those two battering cannons and principal engines, with
their objects, reward and punishment, purgatory, *limbus patrum*,[3]

etc., which now more than ever tyrannize; "for what province is free from atheism, superstition, idolatry, schism, heresy, impiety, their factors and followers?" [1]   Thence they proceed, and from that same decayed image of God, which is yet remaining in us.

> *Os homini sublime dedit, cœlumque tueri*
> *Jussit.*
>
> [He turned man's gaze upwards and bade him scan
>   the heavens.]

Our own conscience doth dictate so much unto us, we know there is a God, and nature doth inform us. *Nulla gens tam barbara* (saith Tully[2]) *cui non insideat hæc persuasio Deum esse; sed nec Scytha, nec Græcus, nec Persa, nec Hyperboreus dissentiet* (as Maximus Tyrius the Platonist, *Ser.* 1, farther adds), *nec continentis nec insularum habitator*, let him dwell where he will, in what coast soever, there is no nation so barbarous that is not persuaded there is a God.   It is a wonder to read of that infinite superstition amongst the Indians in this kind, of their tenents in America: *Pro suo quisque libitu varias res venerabantur superstitiose, plantas, animalia, montes, etc., omne quod amabant aut horrebant* [they have a superstitious reverence for various things, each according to his taste—plants, animals, mountains, etc., anything that they have loved or feared] (some places excepted, as he grants, that had no God at all).   So "the heavens declare the glory of God, and the firmament declares his handiwork" (Ps. xix).   Every creature will evince it:

> *Præsentemque refert quælibet herba deum.*
>
> [Every blade of grass testifies to the presence of God.]

Nolentes sciunt, fatentur inviti, as the said Tyrius proceeds; will or nill, they must acknowledge it.   The philosophers, Socrates, Plato, Plotinus, Pythagoras, Trismegistus, Seneca, Epictetus, those Magi, Druids, etc., went as far as they could by the light of nature; *multa præclara de natura Dei scripta reliquerunt*,[3] "writ many things well of the nature of God, but they had but a confused light, a glimpse."

> *Quale per incertam lunam sub luce maligna*
> *Est iter in silvis,*[4]

as he that walks by moonshine in a wood, they groped in the dark; they had a gross knowledge, as he in Euripides, *O Deus, quicquid es, sive cœlum, sive terra, sive aliud quid* [O God, whatsoever thou beest, whether sky, earth, or anything else], and that of Aristotle, *Ens entium, miserere mei* [Being of beings, pity me].

And so of the immortality of the soul, and future happiness.
Immortalitatem animæ (saith Hierome) *Pythagoras somniavit,
Democritus non credidit, in consolationem damnationis suæ
Socrates in carcere disputavit; Indus, Persa, Gothus, etc., philosophantur* [Pythagoras dreamed of the immortality of the soul;
Democritus disbelieved it; Socrates under sentence of death
found consolation in discussing it; the Indian, Persian, Goth,
etc., philosophize about it].   So some said this, some that, as
they conceived themselves, which the devil perceiving, led them
farther out (as Lemnius observes [1]) and made them worship
him as their god with stocks and stones, and torture themselves
to their own destruction, as he thought fit himself, inspired his
priests and ministers with lies and fictions to prosecute the
same, which they for their own ends were as willing to undergo,
taking advantage of their simplicity, fear, and ignorance.   For
the common people are as a flock of sheep, a rude, illiterate rout,
void many times of common sense, a mere beast, *bellua multorum
capitum* [a beast of many heads], will go whithersoever they
are led: as you lead a ram over a gap by the horns, all the rest
will follow, *non qua eundum, sed qua itur* [2] [not where they should
go but where they are led], they will do as they see others do,
and as their prince will have them; let him be of what religion
he will, they are for him.   Now for those idolaters, Maxentius
and Licinius, then for Constantine a Christian.   *Qui Christum
negant male pereant, acclamatum est decies* [the cry, "Perish
those who deny Christ," was repeated ten times [3]], for two hours'
space; *qui Christum non colunt, Augusti inimici sunt, acclamatum
est ter decies* [4] [the cry, "Those who do not worship Christ are
enemies of Augustus," was repeated thirty times]; and by and
by idolaters again under that apostate Julianus; all Arians
under Constantius, good Catholics again under Jovinianus.
"And little difference there is between the discretion of men
and children in this case, especially of old folks and women,"
as Cardan discourseth,[5] "whenas they are tossed with fear and
superstition, and with other men's folly and dishonesty."   So
that I may say their ignorance is a cause of their superstition,
a symptom, and madness itself: *Supplicii causa est, suppliciumque sui* [it is a cause of punishment and its own punishment].
Their own fear, folly, stupidity, to-be-deplored lethargy, is that
which gives occasion to the other, and pulls these miseries on
their own heads.   For in all these religions and superstitions
amongst our idolaters, you shall still find that the parties first
affected are silly, rude, ignorant people, old folks, that are

naturally prone to superstition, weak women, or some poor, rude, illiterate persons, that are apt to be wrought upon and gulled in this kind, prone without either examination or due consideration (for they take up religion a-trust, as at mercers' they do their wares) to believe anything. And the best means they have to broach first, or to maintain it when they have done, is to keep them still in ignorance: for "ignorance is the mother of devotion," as all the world knows, and these times can amply witness. This hath been the devil's practice, and his infernal ministers', in all ages; not as our Saviour, by a few silly fishermen, to confound the wisdom of the world, to save publicans and sinners, but to make advantage of their ignorance, to convert them and their associates; and that they may better effect what they intend, they begin, as I say, with poor, stupid, illiterate persons.[1] So Mahomet did when he published his Alcoran, which is a piece of work (saith Bredenbachius [2]) "full of nonsense, barbarism, confusion, without rhyme, reason, or any good composition, first published to a company of rude rustics, hog-rubbers, that had no discretion, judgment, art, or understanding, and is so still maintained." For it is a part of their policy to let no man comment, dare to dispute or call in question to this day any part of it, be it never so absurd, incredible, ridiculous, fabulous as it is, it must be believed *implicite*, upon pain of death no man must dare to contradict it: "God and the emperor," etc. What else do our papists but, by keeping the people in ignorance, vent and broach all their new ceremonies and traditions, when they conceal the Scripture, read it in Latin, and to some few alone, feeding the slavish people in the meantime with tales out of legends, and such-like fabulous narrations? Whom do they begin with but collapsed ladies, some few tradesmen, superstitious old folks, illiterate persons, weak women, discontent, rude, silly companions, or sooner circumvent? So do all our schismatics and heretics. Marcus and Valentinian, heretics in Irenæus,[3] seduced first I know not how many women, and made them believe they were prophets. Friar Cornelius of Dort seduced a company of silly women.[4] What are all our Anabaptists, Brownists, Barrowists, Familists, but a company of rude, illiterate, capricious, base fellows? What are most of our papists, but stupid, ignorant and blind bayards? how should they otherwise be, when as they are brought up and kept still in darkness? "If their pastors" (saith Lavater) "have done their duties, and instructed their flocks as they ought in the principles of

Christian religion, or had not forbidden them the reading of Scriptures, they had not been as they are." [1] But being so misled all their lives in superstition, and carried hoodwinked like hawks, how can they prove otherwise than blind idiots and superstitious asses? what else shall we expect at their hands? Neither is it sufficient to keep them blind, and in Cimmerian darkness, but withal, as a schoolmaster doth by his boys to make them follow their books, sometimes by good hope, promises and encouragements, but most of all by fear, strict discipline, severity, threats and punishment, do they collogue and soothe up their silly auditors, and so bring them into a fools' paradise. *Rex eris, aiunt, si recte facies,* do well, thou shalt be crowned [say they]; but for the most part by threats, terrors, and affrights, they tyrannize and terrify their distressed souls: knowing that fear alone is the sole and only means to keep men in obedience, according to that *hemistichium* of Petronius, *Primus in orbe deos fecit timor* [fear first created gods in the world], the fear of some divine and supreme powers keeps men in obedience, makes the people do their duties: they play upon their consciences; which was practised of old in Egypt by their priests; [2] when there was an eclipse, they made the people believe God was angry, great miseries were to come; they take all opportunities of natural causes, to delude the people's senses, and with fearful tales out of purgatory, feigned apparitions, earthquakes in Japonia or China, tragical examples of devils, possessions, obsessions, false miracles, counterfeit visions, etc. They do so insult over and restrain them, never hobby so dared a lark, that they will not offend the least tradition, tread, or scarce look awry. [3] *Deus bone* (Lavater exclaims [4]), *quot hoc commentum de purgatorio misere afflixit!* good God, how many men have been miserably afflicted by this fiction of purgatory!

To these advantages of hope and fear, ignorance and simplicity, he hath several engines, traps, devices, to batter and enthral, omitting no opportunities, according to men's several inclinations, abilities, to circumvent and humour them, to maintain his superstitions, sometimes to stupefy, besot them; sometimes again by oppositions, factions, to set all at odds and in an uproar; sometimes he infects one man, and makes him a principal agent; sometimes whole cities, countries. If of meaner sort, by stupidity, canonical obedience, blind zeal, etc. If of better note, by pride, ambition, popularity, vainglory. If of the clergy and more eminent, of better parts than the rest, more learned, eloquent, he puffs them up with a vain conceit of their own worth, *scientia inflati*, they begin to swell, and scorn all the world in respect of themselves, and thereupon turn heretics, schismatics, broach new doctrines, frame new crotchets and the like; or else out of too much learning become mad, or out of curiosity they will search into God's secrets, and eat of the forbidden fruit; or out of presumption of their holiness and good gifts, inspirations, become prophets, enthusiasts, and what not? Or else if they be displeased, discontent, and have not (as they suppose) preferment to their worth, have some disgrace, repulse, neglected, or not esteemed as they fondly value themselves, or out of emulation, they begin presently to rage and rave, *cœlum terræ miscent*, they become so impatient in an instant, that a whole kingdom cannot contain them, they will set all in a combustion, all at variance, to be revenged of their adversaries. Donatus, when he saw Cecilianus preferred before him in the bishopric of Carthage, turned heretic,[1] and so did Arius, because Alexander was advanced: we have examples at home, and too many experiments of such persons. If they be laymen of better note, the same engines of pride, ambition, emulation, and jealousy take place, they will be gods themselves: Alexander in India, after his victories, became so insolent, he would be adored for a god:[2] and those Roman emperors came to that height of madness, they must have temples built to them, sacrifices to their deities, Divus Augustus, D. Claudius, D. Hadrianus: Heliogabalus "put out that vestal fire at Rome, expelled the virgins, and banished all other religions all over the world, and would be the sole God himself."[3] Our Turks, China kings, Great Chams, and Mogors do little less, assuming divine and bombast titles to themselves; the meaner sort are too credulous, and led with blind zeal, blind obedience, to prosecute and maintain whatsoever their sottish leaders shall propose; what they in pride and singularity, revenge, vainglory, ambition, spleen, for gain, shall rashly maintain and broach, their disciples make a matter of conscience, of hell and damnation if they do it not, and will rather forsake wives, children, house and home, lands, goods, fortunes, life itself, than omit or abjure the least tittle of it, and to advance the common cause, undergo any miseries, turn traitors, assassinates, pseudo-martyrs, with full assurance and hope of reward in that other world, that they shall certainly merit by it, win heaven, be canonized for saints.

Now when they are truly possessed with blind zeal and misled with superstition, he hath many other baits to inveigle and

infatuate them farther yet, to make them quite mortified and
mad, and that under colour of perfection, to merit by penance,
going woolward, whipping, alms, fastings, etc. *Anno* 1320,
there was a sect of whippers [1] in Germany, that, to the astonishment of the beholders, lashed and cruelly tortured themselves.
I could give many other instances of each particular.   But these
works so done are meritorious, *ex opere operato, ex condigno,*
for themselves and others, to make them macerate and consume
their bodies, *specie virtutis et umbra* [with an outward show of
virtue], those evangelical counsels are propounded, as our
pseudo-Catholics call them, canonical obedience, wilful poverty,
vows of chastity, monkery,[2] and a solitary life, which extend
almost to all religions and superstitions, to Turks, Chinese,
Gentiles, Abyssinians, Greeks, Latins, and all countries. Amongst
the rest, fasting, contemplation, solitariness, are as it were
certain rams by which the devil doth batter and work upon the
strongest constitutions. *Nonnulli* (saith Peter Forestus) *ob
longas inedias, studia et meditationes cælestes, de rebus sacris
et religione semper agitant,* [some] by fasting overmuch, and
divine meditations, are overcome.   Not that fasting is a thing
of itself to be discommended, for it is an excellent means to
keep the body in subjection, a preparative to devotion, the
physic of the soul, by which chaste thoughts are engendered,
true zeal, a divine spirit, whence wholesome counsels do proceed, concupiscence is restrained, vicious and predominant lusts
and humours are expelled. The Fathers are very much in commendation of it, and, as Calvin notes, "sometimes immoderate.
The mother of health, key of heaven, a spiritual wing to erear
us, the chariot of the Holy Ghost, banner of faith," etc.[3]   And
'tis true they say of it, if it be moderately and seasonably used
by such parties, as Moses, Elias, Daniel, Christ, and as his
apostles [4] made use of it; but when by this means they will
supererogate, and as Erasmus well taxeth,[5] *Cælum non sufficere
putant suis meritis,* [think] heaven is too small a reward for it; they
make choice of times and meats, buy and sell their merits,
attribute more to them than to the Ten Commandments, and
count it a greater sin to eat meat in Lent than to kill a man,
and as one sayeth, *Plus respiciunt assum piscem quam Christum
crucifixum, plus salmonem quam Salomonem, quibus in ore
Christus, Epicurus in corde* [pay more respect to a broiled
fish than to Christ crucified, more regard to salmon than to
Solomon, have Christ on their lips but Epicurus in their hearts];
when some counterfeit, and some attribute more to such works

of theirs than to Christ's death and passion, the devil sets in
a foot, strangely deludes them, and by that means makes them
to overthrow the temperature of their bodies, and hazard their
souls.   Never any strange illusions of devils amongst hermits,
anachorites, never any visions, phantasms, apparitions, enthusiasms, prophets, any revelations, but immoderate fasting,
bad diet, sickness, melancholy, solitariness, or some such things
were the precedent causes, the forerunners or concomitants of
them.   The best opportunity and sole occasion the devil takes
to delude them.   Marsilius Cognatus, *lib.* 1 *Cont. cap.* 7, hath
many stories to this purpose, of such as after long fasting have
been seduced by devils; and "'tis a miraculous thing to relate"
(as Cardan writes [1]) "what strange accidents proceed from
fasting; dreams, superstition, contempt of torments, desire of
death, prophecies, paradoxes, madness; fasting naturally prepares men to these things."   Monks, anachorites, and the like,
after much emptiness, become melancholy, vertiginous, they
think they hear strange noises, confer with hobgoblins, devils,
rivel up their bodies, *et dum hostem insequimur*, saith Gregory,
civem quem diligimus trucidamus [in pursuing the enemy we
kill our fellow-citizen and friends], they become bare skeletons,
skin and bones: *carnibus abstinentes proprias carnes devorant,
ut nil præter cutem et ossa sit reliquum.*   Hilarion, as Hierome
reports in his life [2] (and Athanasius of Antonius), was so bare
with fasting "that the skin did scarce stick to the bones"; for
want of vapours he could not sleep, and for want of sleep became
idle-headed, "heard every night infants cry, oxen low, wolves
howl, lions roar (as he thought), clattering of chains, strange
voices, and the like illusions of devils."   Such symptoms are
common to those that fast long, are solitary, given to contemplation, overmuch solitariness and meditation.   Not that
these things (as I said of fasting) are to be discommended of
themselves, but very behoveful in some cases and good: sobriety
and contemplation join our souls to God, as that heathen
Porphyry can tell us.[3]   "Ecstasis is a taste of future happiness,
by which we are united unto God"; [4] "a divine melancholy, a
spiritual wing," Bonaventure terms it, to lift us up to heaven;
but as it is abused, a mere dotage, madness, a cause and symptom
of religious melancholy.   "If you shall at any time see" (saith
Guianerius) "a religious person over-superstitious, too solitary,
or much given to fasting, that man will certainly be melancholy,
thou mayest boldly say it, he will be so." [5]   P. Forestus hath
almost the same words, and Cardan, *Subtil. lib.* 18, *et cap.* 40,

lib. 8, *de rerum varietate,* "Solitariness, fasting, and that melancholy humour, are the causes of all hermits' illusions." [1] Lavater,
de spect. cap. 19, *part.* 1, and *part.* 1, *cap.* 10, puts solitariness a
main cause of such spectrums and apparitions; none, saith he,
so melancholy as monks and hermits—the devil's bath, melancholy—"none so subject to visions and dotage in this kind, as
such as live solitary lives, they hear and act strange things in
their dotage." [2] Polydore Virgil, *lib.* 2 *de prodigiis,* holds that
"those prophecies and monks' revelations, nuns' dreams, which
they suppose come from God, do proceed wholly *ab instinctu
dæmonum,* by the devil's means"; [3] and so those enthusiasts,
Anabaptists, pseudo-prophets from the same cause. Fracastorius, *lib.* 2 *de intellect.,* will have all your pythonisses, sibyls,
and pseudo-prophets to be mere melancholy: [4] so doth Wierus
prove, *lib.* 1, *cap.* 8, *et lib.* 3, *cap.* 7, and Arculanus, *in* 9 *Rhasis,*
that melancholy is a sole cause, and the devil together, with
fasting and solitariness, of such sibylline prophecies, if there were
ever such, which with Casaubon [5] and others I justly except at;
for it is not likely that the Spirit of God should ever reveal
such manifest revelations and predictions of Christ, to those
pythonissæ, witches, Apollo's priests, the devil's ministers (they
were no better), and conceal them from his own prophets; for
these sibyls set down all particular circumstances of Christ's
coming, and many other future accidents, far more perspicuous
and plain than ever any prophet did. But, howsoever there
be no Phœbades or sibyls, I am assured there be other enthusiasts, prophets, *dii fatidici,* Magi (of which read Jo. Boissardus, who hath laboriously collected them into a great
volume [6] of late, with elegant pictures, and epitomized their
lives), etc., ever have been in all ages, and still proceeding
from those causes, *qui visiones suas enarrant, somniant futura,
prophetisant, et ejusmodi deliriis agitati, Spiritum Sanctum sibi
communicari putant* [7] [who recount their visions, see the future
in dreams, prophesy, and have various fantasies which they
think are communicated to them by the Holy Spirit]. That
which is written of Saint Francis' five wounds, and other such
monastical effects, of him and others, may justly be referred
to this our melancholy; and that which Matthew Paris relates
of the monk of Evesham, who saw heaven and hell in a vision; [8]
of Sir Owen, that went down into Saint Patrick's Purgatory in
King Stephen's days, and saw as much; [9] Walsingham of him
that was showed as much by Saint Julian; Beda, *lib.* 5, *cap.* 13,
14, 15, *et* 20, reports of King Sebba, *lib.* 4, *cap.* 11, *Eccles. hist.,*

that saw strange visions;[1] and Stumphius, *Helvet. Cornic.*, a cobbler of Basil, that beheld rare apparitions at Augsburg in Germany; Alexander ab Alexandro, *Gen. dier. lib.* 6, *cap.* 21, of an enthusiastical prisoner (all out as probable as that of Eris [the son of] Armenius, in Plato's tenth dialogue *de Repub.*, that revived again ten days after he was killed in a battle, and told strange wonders, like those tales Ulysses related to Alcinous in Homer, or Lucian's *Vera Historia* itself), was still after much solitariness, fasting, or long sickness, when their brains were addle, and their bellies as empty of meat as their heads of wit. Florilegus hath many such examples; *fol.* 191, one of Saint Guthlac of Crowland that fought with devils, but still after long fasting, overmuch solitariness; the devil persuaded him therefore to fast, as Moses and Elias did, the better to delude him.[2] In the same author is recorded Carolus Magnus' vision, *an.* 785, or ecstasis, wherein he saw heaven and hell after much fasting and meditation.[3] So did the devil of old with Apollo's priests, Amphiaraus and his fellows, those Egyptians, still enjoin long fasting before he would give any oracles, *triduum a cibo et vino abstinerent* [they were to abstain for three days from food and wine], before they gave any answers,[4] as Volaterran, *lib.* 13, *cap.* 4, records, and Strabo, *Geog. lib.* 14, describes Charon's den, in the way between Tralles and Nysa, whither the priests led sick and fanatic men: but nothing performed without long fasting, no good to be done. That scoffing Lucian conducts his Menippus to hell by the directions of that Chaldean Mithrobarzanes, but after long fasting, and such-like idle preparation.[5] Which the Jesuits right well perceiving of what force this fasting and solitary meditation is to alter men's minds, when they would make a man mad, ravish him, improve him beyond himself, to undertake some great business of moment, to kill a king, or the like, they bring him into a melancholy dark chamber, where he shall see no light for many days together, no company, little meat, ghastly pictures of devils all about him, and leave him to lie as he will himself, on the bare floor in this chamber of meditation, as they call it, on his back, side, belly, till by this strange usage they make him quite mad and beside himself.[6] And then after some ten days, as they find him animated and resolved, they make use of him. The devil hath many such factors, many such engines, which what effect they produce, you shall hear in the following Symptoms.

Subsect. III.—*Symptoms general, love to their own sect, hate of
all other religions, obstinacy, peevishness, ready to undergo
any danger or cross for it; Martyrs, blind zeal, blind obedience,
fastings, vows, belief of incredibilities, impossibilities: Particular of Gentiles, Mahometans, Jews, Christians; and in
them, Heretics old and new, Schismatics, Schoolmen, Prophets,
Enthusiasts, etc.*

Fleat Heraclitus, an rideat Democritus? in attempting to speak
of these symptoms, shall I laugh with Democritus, or weep
with Heraclitus? they are so ridiculous and absurd on the one
side, so lamentable and tragical on the other: a mixed scene
offers itself, so full of errors and a promiscuous variety of
objects, that I know not in what strain to represent it. When
I think of that Turkish paradise, those Jewish fables and pontifical rites, those pagan superstitions, their sacrifices, and ceremonies, as to make images of all matter, and adore them when
they have done, to see them kiss the pyx, creep to the cross, etc.,
I cannot choose but laugh with Democritus: but when I see them
whip and torture themselves, grind their souls for toys and
trifles, desperate, and now ready to die, I cannot choose but
weep with Heraclitus. When I see a priest say mass, with all
those apish gestures, murmurings, etc., read the customs of the
Jews' synagogue, or Mahometan meskites, I must needs laugh
at their folly: [1] *Risum teneatis amici?* [Could you restrain your
laughter, friends?]; but when I see them make matters of
conscience of such toys and trifles, to adore the devil, to endanger
their souls, to offer their children to their idols, etc., I must
needs condole their misery. When I see two superstitious
orders contend *pro aris et focis* [as for their very lives], with such
have and hold, *de lana caprina* [about a goat's fleece], some
write such great volumes to no purpose, take so much pains to
so small effect, their satires, invectives, apologies, dull and gross
fictions; when I see grave learned men rail and scold like butter-
women, methinks 'tis pretty sport, and fit for Calphurnius and
Democritus to laugh at.[2] But when I see so much blood spilt,
so many murders and massacres, so many cruel battles fought,
etc., 'tis a fitter subject for Heraclitus to lament. As Merlin [3]
when he sat by the lake-side with Vortigern, and had seen the
white and red dragon fight, before he began to interpret or to
speak, *in fletum prorupit*, fell a-weeping, and then proceeded
to declare to the king what it meant; I should first pity and
bewail this misery of humankind with some passionate preface,

wishing mine eyes a fountain of tears, as Jeremy did, and then
to my task. For it is that great torture, that infernal plague
of mortal men, *omnium pestium pestilentissima superstitio* [super-
stition, the direst of plagues], and able of itself alone to stand
in opposition to all other plagues, miseries, and calamities
whatsoever; far more cruel, more pestiferous, more grievous,
more general, more violent, of a greater extent. Other fears
and sorrows, grievances of body and mind, are troublesome for
the time; but this is for ever, eternal damnation, hell itself, a
plague, a fire: an inundation hurts one province alone, and the
loss may be recovered; but this superstition involves all the
world almost, and can never be remedied. Sickness and sorrows
come and go, but a superstitious soul hath no rest; *superstitione
imbutus animus nunquam quietus esse potest*,[1] no peace, no
quietness. True religion and superstition are quite opposite,
longe diversa carnificina et pietas, as Lactantius describes, the
one erears, the other dejects; *illorum pietas, mera impietas*
[the piety of those people is sheer impiety]; the one is an easy
yoke, the other an intolerable burden, an absolute tyranny;
the one a sure anchor, an haven; the other a tempestuous ocean;
the one makes, the other mars; the one is wisdom, the other is
folly, madness, indiscretion; the one unfeigned, the other a
counterfeit; the one a diligent observer, the other an ape; one
leads to heaven, the other to hell. But these differences will
more evidently appear by their particular symptoms. What
religion is, and of what parts it doth consist, every catechism
will tell you, what symptoms it hath, and what effects it produceth: but for their superstitions, no tongue can tell them,
no pen express, they are so many, so diverse, so uncertain, so
unconstant, and so different from themselves. *Tot mundi superstitiones quot cœlo stellæ*, one saith, there be as many superstitions
in the world as there be stars in heaven, or devils themselves
that are the first founders of them: with such ridiculous, absurd
symptoms and signs, so many several rites, ceremonies, torments
and vexations accompanying, as may well express and beseem
the devil to be the author and maintainer of them. I will
only point at some of them, *ex ungue leonem*, guess at the rest,
and those of the chief kinds of superstition, which beside us
Christians now domineer and crucify the world, Gentiles,
Mahometans, Jews, etc.

Of these symptoms some be general, some particular to each
private sect; general to all are an extraordinary love and
affection they bear and show to such as are of their own sect,

and more than Vatinian hate to such as are opposite in religion, as they call it, or disagree from them in their superstitious rites, blind zeal (which is as much a symptom as a cause), vain fears, blind obedience, needless works, incredibilities, impossibilities, monstrous rites and ceremonies, wilfulness, blindness, obstinacy, etc. For the first, which is love and hate, as Montanus saith,[1] *nulla firmior amicitia quam quæ contrahitur hinc; nulla discordia major, quam quæ a religione fit:* no greater concord, no greater discord than that which proceeds from religion. It is incredible to relate, did not our daily experience evince it, what factions, *quam teterrimæ factiones* (as Rich. Dinoth writes[2]), have been of late for matters of religion in France, and what hurly-burlies all over Europe for these many years. *Nihil est quod tam impotenter rapiat homines, quam suscepta de salute opinio; siquidem pro ea omnes gentes corpora et animas devovere solent, et arctissimo necessitudinis vinculo se invicem colligare* [nothing so completely dominates men's minds as their religious beliefs: for this whole nations will sacrifice themselves body and soul, and enter into the closest bonds of friendship with one another]. We are all brethren in Christ, servants of one Lord, members of one body, and therefore are or should be at least dearly beloved, inseparably allied in the greatest bond of love and familiarity, united partakers not only of the same cross, but coadjutors, comforters, helpers, at all times, upon all occasions: as they did in the primitive Church (Acts iv), they sold their patrimonies, and laid them at the apostles' feet; and many such memorable examples of mutual love we have had under the ten general persecutions, many since. Examples on the other side of discord none like, as our Saviour saith, he came therefore into the world to set father against son, etc. In imitation of whom the devil belike (*nam superstitio irrepsit veræ religionis imitatrix*,[3] superstition is still religion's ape, as in all other things, so in this) doth so combine and glue together his superstitious followers in love and affection, that they will live and die together: and what an innate hatred hath he still inspired to any other superstition opposite! How those old Romans were affected, those ten persecutions may be a witness, and that cruel executioner in Eusebius, *Aut lita aut morere,* sacrifice or die. No greater hate, more continuate, bitter faction, wars, persecution in all ages, than for matters of religion; no such feral opposition, father against son, mother against daughter, husband against wife, city against city, kingdom against kingdom: as of old at Tentyra and Ombos:

Immortale odium, et nunquam sanabile vulnus,
Inde furor vulgo, quod numina vicinorum
Odit uterque locus, quum solos credit habendos
Esse deos quos ipse colit.[1]

Immortal hate it breeds, a wound past cure,
And fury to the commons still to endure:
Because one city t' other's gods as vain
Deride, and his alone as good maintain.

The Turks at this day count no better of us than of dogs, so they
commonly call us giaours, infidels, miscreants, make that their
main quarrel and cause of Christian persecution. If he will
turn Turk, he shall be entertained as a brother, and had in
good esteem, a Mussulman or a believer, which is a greater tie
to them than any affinity or consanguinity. The Jews stick
together like so many burrs; but as for the rest, whom they call
Gentiles, they do hate and abhor, they cannot endure their
Messias should be a common saviour to us all, and rather, as
Luther writes,[2] "than they that now scoff at them, curse them,
persecute and revile them, shall be coheirs and brethren with
them, or have any part or fellowship with their Messias, they
would crucify their Messias ten times over, and God Himself,
His angels, and all His creatures, if it were possible, though they
endure a thousand hells for it." Such is their malice towards
us. Now for papists, what in a common cause for the advancement of their religion they will endure, our traitors and pseudo-
Catholics will declare unto us; and how bitter on the other side
to their adversaries, how violently bent, let those Marian times
record, as those miserable slaughters at Merindol and Cabriers,[3]
the Spanish Inquisition, the Duke of Alva's tyranny in the Low
Countries, the French massacres and civil wars.

Tantum religio potuit suadere malorum.[4]

[So great the evils to which religion could prompt.]

Not there only, but all over Europe, we read of bloody battles,
racks and wheels, seditions, factions, oppositions,

obvia signis
Signa, pares aquilas, et pila minantia pilis,[5]

[Standard against standard, lance facing lance,]

invectives and contentions. They had rather shake hands
with a Jew, Turk, or, as the Spaniards do, suffer Moors to live
amongst them, and Jews, than Protestants; "My name"
(saith Luther[6]) "is more odious to them than any thief or

murderer." So it is with all heretics and schismatics whatsoever: and none so passionate, violent in their tenents, opinions,
obstinate, wilful, refractory, peevish, factious, singular and stiff
in defence of them; they do not only persecute and hate, but
pity all other religions, account them damned, blind, as if
they alone were the true Church, they are the true heirs, have
the fee-simple of heaven by a peculiar donation, 'tis entailed
on them and their posterities, their doctrine sound, *per funem
aureum de cœlo delapsa doctrina* [let down from heaven by a
golden rope], they alone are to be saved. The Jews at this day
are so incomprehensibly proud and churlish, said Luther,[1] that
soli salvari, soli domini terrarum salutari volunt [they think that
they alone are worthy to be saved, to be saluted as lords of the
earth]. And as Buxtorfius adds,[2] "so ignorant and self-willed
withal, that amongst their most understanding rabbins you shall
find naught but gross dotage, horrible hardness of heart, and
stupend obstinacy in all their actions, opinions, conversations:
and yet so zealous withal, that no man living can be more,
and vindicate themselves for the elect people of God." 'Tis
so with all other superstitious sects, Mahometans, Gentiles in
China and Tartary, our ignorant Papists, Anabaptists, Separa-
tists, and peculiar churches of Amsterdam; they alone, and
none but they, can be saved. "Zealous" (as Paul saith, Rom.
x, 2) "without knowledge," [3] they will endure any misery, any
trouble, suffer and do that which the sunbeams will not endure
to see, *religionis acti furiis* [under the influence of religious
frenzy], all extremities, losses and dangers, take any pains, fast,
pray, vow chastity, wilful poverty, forsake all and follow their
idols, die a thousand deaths, as some Jews did to Pilate's
soldiers in like case, *exsertos præbentes jugulos, et manifeste præ
se ferentes* (as Josephus hath it), *cariorem esse rita sibi legis
patriæ observationem* [stretching out their necks to the slayers,
and giving plain proof that the observance of their ancestral
law was dearer to them than life], rather than abjure or deny
the least particle of that religion which their fathers profess
and they themselves have been brought up in, be it never so
absurd, ridiculous, they will embrace it, and without farther
inquiry or examination of the truth, though it be prodigiously
false, they will believe it; they will take much more pains to
go to hell than we shall do to heaven. Single out the most
ignorant of them, convince his understanding, show him his
errors, grossness, and the absurdities of his sect, *non persuadebis
etiansi persuaseris*, he will not be persuaded. As those pagans

told the Jesuits in Japan, they would do as their forefathers
have done;[1] and with Rathold the Frisian prince, go to hell for
company, if most of their friends went thither: they will not
be moved, no persuasion, no torture can stir them. So that
papists cannot brag of their vows, poverty, obedience, orders,
merits, martyrdoms, fastings, alms, good works, pilgrimages:
much and more than all this, I shall show you, is and hath
been done by these superstitious Gentiles, pagans, idolaters and
Jews: their blind zeal and idolatrous superstition in all kinds
is much at one; little or no difference, and it is hard to say
which is the greatest, which is the grossest. For if a man shall
duly consider those superstitious rites amongst the ethnics in
Japan, the Bannians in Guzerat, the Chinese idolaters, Americans
of old,[2] in Mexico especially, Mahometan priests, he shall find
the same government almost, the same orders and ceremonies,
or so like that they may seem all apparently to be derived from
some heathen spirit, and the Roman hierarchy no better than
the rest. In a word, this is common to all superstition, there
is nothing so mad and absurd, so ridiculous, impossible, incredible,
which they will not believe, observe, and diligently perform, as
much as in them lies; nothing so monstrous to conceive, or
intolerable to put in practice, so cruel to suffer, which they will
not willingly undertake. So powerful a thing is superstition.
" O Egypt" (as Trismegistus exclaims), "thy religion is fables,
and such as posterity will not believe."[3]   I know that in true
religion itself, many mysteries are so apprehended alone by
faith, as that of the Trinity, which Turks especially deride,
Christ's incarnation, resurrection of the body at the last day,
quod ideo credendum (saith Tertullian) *quod incredibile* [which is
to be believed just because it is incredible], etc., many miracles
not to be controverted or disputed of. *Mirari non rimari
sapientia vera est* [true wisdom is to admire and not to inquire],
saith Gerhardus;[4] *et in divinis* (as a good Father informs us)
quædam credenda, quædam admiranda, etc. some things are to
be believed, embraced, followed with all submission and
obedience, some again admired. Though Julian the Apostate
scoff at Christians in this point, *quod captivemus intellectum in
obsequium fidei,* saying, that the Christian creed is like the
Pythagorean *Ipse dixit,* we make our will and understanding
too slavishly subject to our faith, without farther examination
of the truth; yet, as Saint Gregory truly answers, our creed is
altioris præstantiæ [of a higher excellence], and much more
divine; and as Thomas will, *pie consideranti semper suppetunt*

rationes, ostendentes credibilitatem in mysteriis supernaturalibus,
we do absolutely believe it, and upon good reasons, for, as
Gregory well informeth us, *Fides non habet meritum, ubi humana
ratio quærit experimentum:* that faith hath no merit, is not
worth the name of faith, that will not apprehend without a
certain demonstration: we must and will believe God's word;
and if we be mistaken or err in our general belief, as Richardus
de Sancto Victore vows he will say to Christ Himself at the day
of judgment; "Lord, if we be deceived, Thou alone hast deceived
us": [1] thus we plead.   But for the rest I will not justify that
pontificial consubstantiation, that which Mahometans [2] and
Jews justly except at, as Campanella confesseth, *Atheismi
triumphat. cap.* 12, *fol.* 125, *difficillimum dogma esse, nec aliud
subjectum magis hæreticorum blasphemiis, et stultis irrisionibus
politicorum reperiri* [it is a most difficult dogma, and particularly
exposed to the blasphemies of the heretics and the scoffing of
men of the world].   They hold it impossible, *Deum in pane
manducari* [that God should be eaten in bread]; and besides
they scoff at it; *Vide gentem comedentem Deum suum, inquit
quidam Maurus* [See the people that eat their own God, saith
a certain Moor].   *Hunc Deum* [3] *muscæ et vermes irrident, quum
ipsum polluunt et devorant; subditus est igni, aquæ, et latrones
furantur; pyxidem auream humi prosternunt, et se tamen non
defendit hic Deus. Qui fieri potest, ut sit integer in singulis
hostiæ particulis, idem corpus numero, tam multis locis, cœlo,
terra, etc.?* [This God is the sport of worms and flies, when they
pollute and consume Him; He is subject to the ravages of fire
and water, and the depredations of thieves.   They cast the
golden pyx on the ground, and yet this God does not defend
Himself.   How is it possible that He should remain whole when
the Host is divided into so many particles, that the same body
should be in so many places, in the sky, the earth, etc.?]   But
he that shall read the Turks' Alcoran, the Jews' Talmud, and
papists' Golden Legend, [4] in the meantime will swear that such
gross fictions, fables, vain traditions, prodigious paradoxes
and ceremonies, could never proceed from any other spirit than
that of the devil himself, which is the author of confusion and
lies; and wonder withal how such wise men as have been of the
Jews, such learned understanding men as Averroes, Avicenna,
or those heathen philosophers, could ever be persuaded to
believe or to subscribe to the least part of them, *aut fraudem
non detegere* [or at least did not expose the deceit]; but that, as
Vaninus answers, [5] *ob publicæ potestatis formidinem allatrare*

philosophi non audebant, they durst not speak for fear of the law.
But I will descend to particulars: read their several symptoms
and then guess.

Of such symptoms as properly belong to superstition, or that
irreligious religion, I may say as of the rest, some are ridiculous,
some again feral to relate. Of those ridiculous, there can be
no better testimony than the multitude of their gods, those
absurd names, actions, offices they put upon them, their feasts,
holy days, sacrifices, adorations, and the like. The Egyptians
that pretended so great antiquity, three hundred kings before
Amasis and, as Mela writes, thirteen thousand years from the
beginning of their chronicles, that bragged so much of their
knowledge of old, for they invented arithmetic, astronomy,
geometry; of their wealth and power, that vaunted of twenty
thousand cities; and yet at the same time their idolatry and
superstition was most gross: they worshipped, as Diodorus
Siculus records, sun and moon under the name of Isis and
Osiris, and after, such men as were beneficial to them, or any
creature that did them good. In the city of Bubastis they
adored a cat, saith Herodotus, ibises and storks, an ox (saith
Pliny), leeks and onions,[1] Macrobius:

> *Porrum et cæpe deos imponere nubibus ausi,*
> *Hos tu, Nile, deos colis.*[2]

> [They did not shrink from making the leek and the
> onion lords of heaven. These are thy gods, O
> Egypt!]

Scoffing Lucian in his *Vera Historia,* which, as he confesseth
himself, was not persuasively written as a truth, but in comical
fashion to glance at the monstrous fictions and gross absurdities
of writers and nations, to deride without doubt this prodigious
Egyptian idolatry, feigns this story of himself: that when he
had seen the Elysian Fields, and was now coming away, Rhadamanthus gave him a mallow root, and bade him pray to that
when he was in any peril or extremity; which he did accordingly; for when he came to Hydramardia in the Island of
Treacherous Women, he made his prayers to his root, and was
instantly delivered. The Syrians, Chaldeans, had as many
proper gods of their own invention; see the said Lucian, *de
Dea Syria;* Mornay, *cap. 22 de veritat. relig.;* Guliel. Stuckius,
Sacrorum Sacrificiorumque Gentil. descript.;[3] Peter Faber,
Semester. lib. 3, *cap.* 1, 2, 3; Selden, *de diis Syris,* Purchas'
Pilgrimage, Rosinus of the Romans,[4] and Lilius Giraldus of the

Greeks. The Romans borrowed from all, besides their own gods, which were *majorum* and *minorum gentium*, as Varro holds, certain and uncertain; some celestial, select, and great ones, others Indigetes and *semi-dei*, Lares, Lemures, Dioscuri, Soteres, and Parastatæ, *dii tutelares* [tutelar deities] amongst the Greeks: gods of all sorts, for all functions; some for the land, some for sea; some for heaven, some for hell; some for passions, diseases, some for birth, some for weddings, husbandry, woods, waters, gardens, orchards, etc.; all actions and offices: Pax, Quies, Salus, Libertas, Felicitas, Strenua, Stimula, Horta, Pan, Sylvanus, Priapus, Flora, Cloacina, Stercutius, Febris, Pallor, Invidia, Protervia, Risus, Angerona, Volupia, Vacuna, Viriplaca, Veneranda, Pales, Neptunia Doris; kings, emperors, valiant men that had done any good offices for them, they did likewise canonize and adore for gods, and it was usually done, *usitatum apud antiquos*, as Jac. Boissardus well observes,[1] *deificare homines qui beneficiis mortales juvarent* [to deify men who had conferred benefits on mankind], and the devil was still ready to second their intents, *statim se ingessit illorum sepulchris, statuis, templis, aris*, etc., he crept into their temples, statues, tombs, altars, and was ready to give oracles, cure diseases, do miracles, etc., as by Jupiter, Æsculapius, Tiresias, Apollo, Mopsus, Amphiaraus, etc., *dii et semi-dii* [gods and demi-gods]. For so they were *semi-dii*, demi-gods, some *medii inter deos et homines* [intermediate between men and gods], as Max. Tyrius, the Platonist, *Ser.* 26 *et* 27, maintains and justifies in many words.[2] "When a good man dies, his body is buried, but his soul *ex homine dæmon evadit*, becomes forthwith a demi-god, nothing disparaged with malignity of air or variety of forms, rejoiceth, exults and sees that perfect beauty with his eyes. Now being deified, in commiseration he helps his poor friends here on earth, his kindred and allies, informs, succours, etc., punisheth those that are bad and do amiss, as a good genius to protect and govern mortal men, appointed by the gods; so they will have it, ordaining some for provinces, some for private men, some for one office, some for another. Hector and Achilles assist soldiers to this day; Æsculapius all sick men, the Dioscuri seafaring men, etc., and sometimes upon occasion they show themselves." The Dioscuri, Hercules, and Æsculapius he saw himself (or the devil in his likeness), *non somnians sed vigilans ipse vidi* [I saw not in a dream but waking]. So far Tyrius. And not good men only do they thus adore, but tyrants, monsters, devils, (as Stuckius inveighs [3]) Neros, Domitians, Heliogables, beastly

women, and arrant whores amongst the rest. For all intents,
places, creatures, they assign gods:

> *Et domibus, tectis, thermis, et equis soleatis*
> *Assignare solent genios,*

> [They are wont to assign protecting spirits to houses,
>   buildings, baths, and horses,]

saith Prudentius. Cuna for cradles, Diverra for sweeping
houses, Nodina knots, Prema, Premunda, Hymen, Hymenæus,
for weddings; Comus the god of good fellows, gods of silence,
of comfort, Hebe goddess of youth, Mena *menstruarum*, etc.,
male and female gods, of all ages, sexes and dimensions, with
beards, without beards, married, unmarried, begot, not born
at all, but as Minerva start out of Jupiter's head. Hesiod
reckons up at least thirty thousand gods, Varro three hundred
Jupiters. As Jeremy told them, their gods were [according]
to the multitude of cities.[1]

> *Quicquid humus, pelagus, cælum miserabile gignit,*
> *Id dixere deos, colles, freta, flumina, flammas.*

> Whatever heavens, sea, and land begat.
> Hills, seas, and rivers, God was this and that.

And which was most absurd, they made gods upon such ridiculous occasions; "As children make babies" (so saith Mornæus [2]),
"their poets make gods," *et quos adorant in templis, ludunt in
theatris* [the gods whom they worship in their temples they
laugh at in their theatres], as Lactantius scoffs. Saturn, a man,
gelded himself, did eat his own children, a cruel tyrant driven
out of his kingdom by his son Jupiter, as good a god as himself,
a wicked lascivious paltry king of Crete, of whose rapes, lusts,
murders, villainies, a whole volume is too little to relate. Venus,
a notorious strumpet, as common as a barber's chair, Mars',
Adonis', Anchises' whore, is a great she-goddess as well as the
rest, as much renowned by their poets; with many such; and
these gods, so fabulously and foolishly made, *cærimoniis,
hymnis, et canticis celebrant* [they honour with ceremonies,
hymns, and chants]; their errors, *luctus et gaudia, amores, iras,
nuptias et liberorum procreationes* (as Eusebius well taxeth [3]),
weddings, mirth and mournings, loves, angers, and quarrelling
they did celebrate in hymns, and sing of in their ordinary songs,
as it were publishing their villainies. But see more of their
originals. When Romulus was made away by the sedition of
the senators, to pacify the people, Julius Proculus gave out that

Romulus was taken up by Jupiter into heaven, and therefore
to be ever after adored for a god amongst the Romans.[1] Syro-
phanes of Egypt had one only son, whom he dearly loved; he
erected his statue in his house, which his servants did adorn
with crowns and garlands, to pacify their master's wrath when
he was angry, so by little and little he was adored for a god.
This did Semiramis for her husband Belus, and Hadrian the
emperor by his minion Antinous.   Flora was a rich harlot in
Rome, and for that she made the commonwealth her heir, her
birthday was solemnized long after; and to make it a more
plausible holiday, they made her goddess of flowers, and sacrificed to her amongst the rest.   The matrons of Rome, as
Dionysius Halicarnasseus relates, because at their entreaty
Coriolanus desisted from his wars, consecrated a church *Fortunæ muliebri* [to the Good Fortune of women]; and Venus
Barbata had a temple erected, for that somewhat was amiss
about hair,[2] and so the rest.[3]   The citizens of Alabanda, a small
town in Asia Minor, to curry favour with the Romans (who
then warred in Greece with Perseus of Macedon, and were
formidable to these parts), consecrated a temple to the City of
Rome, and made her a goddess, with annual games and sacrifices; so a town of houses was deified, with shameful flattery
of the one side to give, and intolerable arrogance on the other
to accept, upon so vile and absurd an occasion.   Tully writes
to Atticus, that his daughter Tulliola might be made a goddess,
and adored as Juno and Minerva, and as well she deserved it.
Their holy days and adorations were all out as ridiculous; those
Lupercals of Pan, Florals of Flora, Bona Dea, Anna Perenna,
Saturnals, etc., as how they were celebrated, with what lascivious
and wanton gestures, bald ceremonies, by what bawdy priests,[4]
how they hang their noses over the smoke of sacrifices, saith
Lucian,[5] and lick blood like flies that was spilled about the
altars.   Their carved idols, gilt images of wood, iron, ivory,
silver, brass, stone (*Olim truncus eram* [once I was a stock], etc.),
were most absurd, as being their own workmanship: for as
Seneca notes, *adorant ligneos deos, et fabros interim qui fecerunt,
contemnunt*, they adore [the] work, contemn the workman; and
as Tertullian follows it, *Si homines non essent diis propitii, non
essent dii*, had it not been for men, they had never been gods,
but blocks still, and stupid statues, in which mice, swallows,
birds made their nests, spiders their webs, and in their very
mouths laid their excrements.   Those images, I say, were all
out as gross as the shapes in which they did represent them:

Jupiter with a ram's head, Mercury a dog's, Pan like a goat,
Hecate with three heads, one with a beard, another without;
see more in Carterius and Verdurius [1] of their monstrous forms
and ugly pictures: and, which was absurder yet, they told
them these images came from heaven, as that of Minerva in
her temple at Athens, *quod e cœlo cecidisse credebant accolæ*
[which the inhabitants believed to have fallen from heaven],
saith Pausanias. They formed some like storks, apes, bulls,
and yet seriously believed; and that which was impious and
abominable, they made their gods notorious whoremasters,
incestuous sodomites (as commonly they were all, as well as
Jupiter, Mars, Apollo, Mercury, Neptune, etc.), thieves, slaves,
drudges (for Apollo and Neptune made tiles in Phrygia), kept
sheep, Hercules emptied stables, Vulcan a blacksmith, unfit
to dwell upon the earth for their villainies, much less in heaven,
as Mornay well saith,[2] and yet they gave them out to be such;
so weak and brutish, some to whine, lament, and roar, as Isis
for her son and Cynocephalus, as also all her weeping priests;
Mars in Homer to be wounded, vexed; Venus run away crying,
and the like; than which what can be more ridiculous? *Nonne
ridiculum lugere quod colas, vel colere quod lugeas?* (which
Minuclus objects [3]) *Si dii, cur plangitis? si mortui, cur adoratis?*
[Is it not absurd to mourn over that which you worship or
worship that which you mourn over? If they are gods, why do
you lament them? If men, why do you worship them?]; that
it is no marvel if Lucian,[4] that adamantine persecutor of superstition, and Pliny could so scoff at them and their horrible
idolatry as they did; if Diagoras took Hercules' image, and
put it under his pot to seethe his pottage, which was, as he
said, his thirteenth labour. But see more of their fopperies in
Cypr., 4 *tract. de Idol. varietat.*; Chrysostom, *advers. Gentil.*;
Arnobius, *adv. Gentes.*; Austin, *de Civ. Dei*; Theodoret, *de curat.
Græc. affect.*; Clemens Alexandrinus, Minucius Felix, Eusebius,
Lactantius, Stuckius, etc. Lamentable, tragical, and fearful
those symptoms are, that they should be so far forth affrighted
with their fictitious gods, as to spend the goods, lives, fortunes,
precious time, best days in their honour, to sacrifice unto
them, to their inestimable loss, such hecatombs,[5] so many
thousand sheep, oxen with gilded horns, goats, as Crœsus, King
of Lydia,[6] Marcus Julianus,[7] surnamed *ob crebras hostias Vic-
timarius, et Tauricremus* [Victimarius and Tauricremas (bull-
burner), on account of the number of his offerings], and the
rest of the Roman emperors usually did with such labour and

cost; and not emperors only and great ones, *pro communi bono*
[for the general good], were at this charge, but private men
for their ordinary occasions. Pythagoras offered an hundred
oxen for the invention of a geometrical problem, and it was an
ordinary thing to sacrifice in Lucian's time, "a heifer for their
good health, four oxen for wealth, an hundred for a kingdom,
nine bulls for their safe return from Troy to Pylos," etc.[1] Every
god almost had a peculiar sacrifice: the Sun horses, Vulcan
fire, Diana a white hart, Venus a turtle, Ceres a hog, Proserpine
a black lamb, Neptune a bull (read more in Stuckius at large [2]),
besides sheep, cocks, corals, frankincense, to their undoings, as
if their gods were affected with blood or smoke. "And surely"
(saith he) "if one should but repeat the fopperies of mortal
men, in their sacrifices, feasts, worshipping their gods, their
rites and ceremonies, what they think of them, of their diet,
houses, orders, etc., what prayers and vows they make; if one
should but observe their absurdity and madness, he would burst
out a-laughing, and pity their folly." [3]   For what can be more
absurd than their ordinary prayers, petitions, requests,[4] sacrifices, oracles, devotions? of which we have a taste in Maximus
Tyrius, *Serm.* 1, Plato's *Alcibiades Secundus*, Persius, *Sat.* 2,
Juvenal, *Sat.* 10, there likewise exploded. *Mactant opimas et
pingues hostias deo quasi esurienti, profundunt vina tanquam
sitienti, lumina accendunt velut in tenebris agenti* (Lactantius,
lib. 2, *cap.* 6): as if their gods were hungry, athirst, in the dark,
they light candles, offer meat and drink.   And what so base
as to reveal their counsels and give oracles *e viscerum ster-
quiliniis*, out `of the bowels and excremental parts of beasts?
Sordidos deos [filthy gods] Varro truly calls them therefore, and
well he might.   I say nothing of their magnificent and sumptuous
temples, those majestical structures: to the roof of Apollo
Didymæus' temple *ad Branchidas*, as Strabo writes,[5] a thousand
oaks did not suffice. Who can relate the glorious splendour,
and stupend magnificence, the sumptuous building of Diana
at Ephesus, Jupiter Ammon's temple in Africa, the Pantheon
at Rome, the Capitol, the Serapeum at Alexandria, Apollo's
temple at Daphne in the suburbs of Antioch? the great temple
at Mexico, so richly adorned, and so capacious (for 10,000
men might stand in it at once), that fair Pantheon of Cusco,
described by Acosta in his Indian History, which eclipse both
Jews and Christians?   There were in old Jerusalem, as some
write, 408 synagogues; but new Cairo reckons up (if Radzivilius
may be believed [6]) 6,800 meskites; Fez 400, whereof 50 are most

magnificent, like St. Paul's in London. Helena built 300 fair
churches in the Holy Land, but one bassa hath built 400
meskites. The Mahometans have 1000 monks in a monastery;
the like saith Acosta of Americans; Riccius of the Chinese, for
men and women, fairly built; and more richly endowed, some
of them, than Arras in Artois, Fulda in Germany, or St. Edmunds-
bury in England with us: who can describe those curious and
costly statues, idols, images, so frequently mentioned in Pausanias? I conceal their donaries, pendants, other offerings,
presents, to these their fictitious gods daily consecrated. Alexander, the son of Amyntas, King of Macedonia, sent two statues
of pure gold to Apollo at Delphi;[1] Croesus, King of Lydia,
dedicated an hundred golden tiles in the same place with a
golden altar:[2] no man came empty-handed to their shrines.
But these are base offerings in respect; they offered men themselves alive. The Leucadians, as Strabo writes, sacrificed every
year a man, *averruncandæ deorum iræ causa*, to pacify their
gods, *de montis præcipitio dejecerunt* [they cast him down a
precipice], etc., and they did voluntarily undergo it. The Decii
did so sacrifice *diis manibus* [to the gods of the Lower World];
Curtius did leap into the gulf. Were they not all strangely
deluded to go so far to their oracles, to be so gulled by them,
both in war and peace, as Polybius relates (which their augurs,
priests, vestal virgins can witness), to be so superstitious, that
they would rather lose goods and lives than omit any ceremonies
or offend their heathen gods? Nicias, that generous and
valiant captain of the Greeks, overthrew the Athenian navy,
by reason of his too much superstition, because the augurs told
him it was ominous to set sail from the haven of Syracuse
whilst the moon was eclipsed; he tarried so long till his enemies
besieged him, he and all his army were overthrown.[3] The
Parthians of old were so sottish in this kind, they would rather
lose a victory, nay, lose their own lives, than fight in the night,
'twas against their religion.[4] The Jews would make no resistance
on the Sabbath, when Pompeius besieged Jerusalem; and some
Jewish Christians in Africa, set upon by the Goths, suffered
themselves upon the same occasion to be utterly vanquished.
The superstition of the Dibrenses, a bordering town in Epirus,
besieged by the Turks, is miraculous almost to report. Because
a dead dog was flung into the only fountain which the city had,
would die of thirst all, rather than drink of that unclean water,[5]
and yield up the city upon any conditions. Though the prætor
and chief citizens began to drink first, using all good persuasions,

their superstition was such, no saying would serve, they must
all forthwith die or yield up the city. *Vix ausim ipse credere*
(saith Barletius [1]) *tantam superstitionem, vel affirmare levissimam
hanc causam tantæ rei vel magis ridiculam, quum non dubitem
risum potius quam admirationem posteris excitaturam* [I could
scarce believe such superstition possible, and hesitate to assign
so trivial a cause, or one even more ridiculous, to so great an
event, for fear of exciting laughter rather than wonder]. The
story was too ridiculous, he was ashamed to report it, because
he thought nobody would believe it. It is stupend to relate
what strange effects this idolatry and superstition hath brought
forth of the latter years in the Indies and those bordering parts:
in what feral shapes the devil is adored,[2] *ne quid mali intentent*
[lest they should plot any harm], as they say;[3] for in the mountains betwixt Scanderoon and Aleppo at this day there are dwelling a certain kind of people called Coords, coming of the race of
the ancient Parthians, who worship the devil, and allege this
reason in so doing: God is a good man and will do no harm, but
the devil is bad and must be pleased, lest he hurt them. It is
wonderful to tell how the devil deludes them, how he terrifies
them, how they offer men and women sacrifices unto him, an
hundred at once, as they did infants in Crete to Saturn of old,
the finest children, like Agamemnon's Iphigenia, etc. At
Mexico,[4] when the Spaniards first overcame them, they daily
sacrificed *viva hominum corda e viventium corporibus extracta*,
the hearts of men yet living, 20,000 in a year (Acosta, *lib.* 5,
cap. 20) to their idols made of flour and men's blood, and every
year 6,000 infants of both sexes: and as prodigious to relate
how they bury their wives with husbands deceased,[5] 'tis fearful
to report and harder to believe,

> *Nam certamen habent leti quæ viva sequatur*
> *Conjugium, pudor est non licuisse mori*,[6]

> [They vie with one another who shall follow him to
> the grave, and feel disgraced if not allowed to die,]

and burn them alive, best goods, servants, horses, when a grandee
dies, twelve thousand at once amongst the Tartars when a Great
Cham departs,[7] or an emperor in America: how they plague themselves, which abstain from all that hath life, like those old
Pythagoreans, with immoderate fastings, as the Bannians about
Surat, they of China, that for superstition's sake never eat
flesh nor fish all their lives, never marry, but live in deserts
and by-places, and some pray to their idols twenty-four hours

together without any intermission, biting off their tongues when they have done, for devotion's sake.[1] Some again are brought to that madness by their superstitious priests (that tell them such vain stories of immortality, and the joys of heaven in that other life), that many thousands voluntarily break their own necks, as Cleombrotus Ambraciotes' auditors of old, precipitate themselves, that they may participate of that unspeakable happiness in the other world.[2] One poisons, another strangles himself, and the King of China had done as much, deluded with this vain hope, had he not been detained by his servant. But who can sufficiently tell of their several superstitions, vexations, follies, torments? I may conclude with Possevinus,[3] *Religio facit asperos mites, homines e feris; superstitio ex hominibus feras*, religion makes wild beasts civil, superstition makes wise men beasts and fools; and the discreetest that are, if they give way to it, are no better than dizzards; nay more if that of Plotinus be true, *is unus religionis scopus, ut ei quem colimus similes fiamus*, that's the drift of religion, to make us like him whom we worship, what shall be the end of idolaters, but to degenerate into stocks and stones? of such as worship these heathen gods, for *dii gentium dæmonia* [the gods of the heathen are devils], but to become devils themselves?[4] 'Tis therefore *exitiosus error, et maxime periculosus*, a most perilous and dangerous error of all others, as Plutarch holds,[5] *turbulenta passio hominem consternans*, a pestilent, a troublesome passion, that utterly undoeth men. Unhappy superstition, Pliny calls it, *morte non finitur*,[6] death takes away life, but not superstition. Impious and ignorant are far more happy than they which are superstitious, no torture like to it, none so continuate, so general, so destructive, so violent.

In this superstitious row, Jews for antiquity may go next to Gentiles: what of old they have done, what idolatries they have committed in their groves and high places, what their Pharisees, Sadducees, Scribes, Essæi, and such sectaries have maintained, I will not so much as mention: for the present, I presume no nation under heaven can be more sottish, ignorant, blind, superstitious, wilful, obstinate, and peevish, tiring themselves with vain ceremonies to no purpose; he that shall but read their rabbins' ridiculous comments, their strange interpretation of scriptures, their absurd ceremonies, fables, childish tales, which they steadfastly believe, will think they be scarce rational creatures; their foolish customs,[7] when they rise in the morning, and how they prepare themselves to prayer, to meat, with what superstitious washings, how to their Sabbath, to their other feasts, weddings, burials, etc. Last of all, the expectation of their Messias, and those figments, miracles, vain pomp that shall attend him, as how he shall terrify the Gentiles, and overcome them by new diseases; how Michael the archangel shall sound his trumpet, how he shall gather all the scattered Jews into the Holy Land, and there make them a great banquet, "wherein shall be all the birds, beasts, fishes, that ever God made, a cup of wine that grew in Paradise, and that hath been kept in Adam's cellar ever since." [1] At the first course shall be served in that great ox in Job xli, 1, "that every day feeds on a thousand hills" (Ps. l, 10), that great Leviathan, and a great bird, that laid an egg so big, "that by chance tumbling out of the nest, it knocked down three hundred tall cedars, and breaking as it fell, drowned an hundred and sixty villages"; [2] this bird stood up to the knees in the sea, and the sea was so deep that a hatchet would not fall to the bottom in seven years: of their Messias' wives and children; [3] Adam and Eve, etc.; and that one stupend fiction amongst the rest: when a Roman prince asked of Rabbi Jehosua ben Hanania, why the Jews' God was compared to a lion, he made answer, he compared himself to no ordinary lion, but to one in the wood Ela, which when he desired to see, the rabbin prayed to God he might, and forthwith the lion set forward. "But when he was four hundred miles from Rome, he so roared that all the great-bellied women in Rome made aborts, the city walls fell down, and when he came an hundred miles nearer, and roared the second time, their teeth fell out of their heads, the emperor himself fell down dead, and so the lion went back." [4] With an infinite number of such lies and forgeries, which they verily believe, feed themselves with vain hope, and in the meantime will by no persuasions be diverted, but still crucify their souls with a company of idle ceremonies, live like slaves and vagabonds, will not be relieved or reconciled.

Mahometans are a compound of Gentiles, Jews, and Christians, and so absurd in their ceremonies, as if they had taken that which is most sottish out of every one of them, full of idle fables in their superstitious law; their Alcoran itself a gallimaufry of lies, tales, ceremonies, traditions, precepts, stolen from other sects, and confusedly heaped up to delude a company of rude and barbarous clowns. As how birds, beasts, stones, saluted Mahomet when he came from Mecca, the moon came down from heaven to visit him, how God sent for him, spake to him, etc., [5]

with a company of stupend figments of the angels, sun, moon,
and stars, etc., of the day of judgment, and three sounds to
prepare to it, which must last fifty thousand years, of Paradise,
which wholly consists in *coeundi et comedendi voluptate* [carnal
and material pleasures], and *pecorinis hominibus scriptum,
bestialis beatitudo* [an animal felicity, fit for men like cattle], is so
ridiculous, that Virgil, Dante, Lucian, nor any poet can be more
fabulous.   Their rites and ceremonies are most vain and superstitious; wine and swine's flesh are utterly forbidden by their
law, they must pray five times a day, and still towards the
south,[1] wash before and after all their bodies over, with many
such.   For fasting, vows, religious orders, peregrinations, they
go far beyond any papists, they fast a month together many
times, and must not eat a bit till sun be set.[2]   Their kalenders,
dervises, and torlachers, etc., are more abstemious,[3] some of
them, than Carthusians, Franciscans, anachorites, forsake all,
live solitary, fare hard, go naked, etc.   Their pilgrimages are
as far as to the river Ganges [4] (which the Gentiles of those tracts
likewise do), to wash themselves, for that river, as they hold,
hath a sovereign virtue to purge them of all sins, and no man
can be saved that hath not been washed in it.[5]   For which
reason they come far and near from the Indies; *maximus gentium
omnium confluxus est* [there is a great concourse from all nations],
and infinite numbers yearly resort to it.   Others go as far as
Mecca to Mahomet's tomb, which journey is both miraculous
and meritorious.   The ceremonies of flinging stones to stone
the devil, of eating a camel at Cairo by the way; their fastings,
their running till they sweat, their long prayers, Mahomet's
temple, tomb, and building of it, would ask a whole volume to
dilate: and for their pains taken in this holy pilgrimage, all
their sins are forgiven, and they reputed for so many saints.
And divers of them with hot bricks, when they return, will put
out their eyes, "that they never after see any profane thing,[6]
bite out their tongues," etc.   They look for their prophet
Mahomet as Jews do for their Messiah.   Read more of their
customs, rites, ceremonies, in Lonicerus, *Turcic. hist. tom.* 1,
from the tenth to the twenty-fourth chapter; Bredenbachius,
cap. 4, 5, 6; Leo Afer, *lib.* 1; Busbequius; Sabellicus; Purchas,
lib. 3, *cap.* 3, *et* 4, 5; Theodorus Bibliander, etc.   Many foolish
ceremonies you shall find in them; and which is most to be
lamented, the people are generally so curious in observing of
them, that if the least circumstance be omitted, they think
they shall be damned, 'tis an irremissible offence, and can hardly

be forgiven. "I kept in my house amongst my followers"
(saith Busbequius, sometime the Turk's orator in Constantinople)
"a Turkey boy, that by chance did eat shell-fish, a meat forbidden by their law, but the next day when he knew what he
had done, he was not only sick to cast and vomit, but very
much troubled in mind, would weep and grieve many days
after, torment himself for his foul offence." [1]   Another Turk,
being to drink a cup of wine in his cellar, first made a huge noise
and filthy faces, "to warn his soul, as he said, that it should not
be guilty of that foul fact which he was to commit." [2]   With
such toys as these are men kept in awe, and so cowed that they
dare not resist, or offend the least circumstance of their law,
for conscience' sake, misled by superstition, which no human
edict otherwise, no force of arms, could have enforced.

In the last place are pseudo-Christians, in describing of whose
superstitious symptoms as a mixture of the rest, I may say
that which St. Benedict once saw in a vision, one devil in the
market-place, but ten in a monastery, because there was more
work; in populous cities they would swear and forswear, lie,
falsify, deceive fast enough of themselves, one devil could circumvent a thousand; but in their religious houses a thousand devils
could scarce tempt one silly monk.   All the principal devils,
I think, busy themselves in subverting Christians; Jews, Gentiles, and Mahometans are *extra callem,* out of the fold, and need
no such attendance, they make no resistance, *eos enim pulsare
negligit, quos quieto jure possidere se sentit* [3] [he is at no pains to
drive those whom he thinks he can take over without effort],
they are his own already: but Christians have that shield of
faith, sword of the Spirit to resist, and must have a great deal
of battery before they can be overcome.   That the devil is
most busy amongst us that are of the true Church, appears by
those several oppositions, heresies, schisms, which in all ages
he hath raised to subvert it, and in that of Rome especially,
wherein Antichrist himself now sits and plays his prize.   This
mystery of iniquity began to work even in the Apostles' time,
many Antichrists and heretics were abroad, many sprung up
since, many now present, and will be to the world's end, to
dementate men's minds, to seduce and captivate their souls.
Their symptoms I know not how better to express than in that
twofold division, of such as lead, and are led.   Such as lead
are heretics, schismatics, false prophets, impostors, and their
ministers: they have some common symptoms, some peculiar.
Common, as madness, folly, pride, insolency, arrogancy,

singularity, peevishness, obstinacy, impudence, scorn and contempt of all other sects, *Nullius addicti jurare in verba magistri*
[binding themselves to follow the teaching of no master]; they
will approve of naught but what they first invent themselves,
no interpretation good but what their infallible spirit dictates:
none shall be *in secundis*, no, not *in tertiis*, they are only wise,
only learned in the truth, all damned but they and their followers;
Cædem scripturarum faciunt ad materiam suam, saith Tertullian,
they make a slaughter of Scriptures, and turn it as a nose of
wax to their own ends.   So irrefragable in the meantime, that
what they have once said, they must and will maintain, in whole
tomes, duplications, triplications, never yield to death, so self-
conceited, say what you can.   As Bernard [1] (erroneously some
say) speaks of P. Aliardus, *Omnes patres sic, atque ego sic*. Though
all the Fathers, councils, the whole world contradict it, they
care not, they are all one: and as Gregory well notes "of such as
are vertiginous, they think all turns round and moves, all err;
whenas the error is wholly in their own brains." [2]   Magallianus
the Jesuit, in his Comment on 1 Tim. vi, 20, and Alphonsus
de Castro, *lib.* 1 *adversus hæreses*, gives two more eminent
notes or probable conjectures to know such men by (they might
have taken themselves by the noses when they said it): "First,
they affect novelties and toys, and prefer falsehood before truth; [3]
secondly, they care not what they say, that which rashness and
folly hath brought out, pride afterward, peevishness and
contumacy shall maintain to the last gasp." [4]   Peculiar
symptoms are prodigious paradoxes, new doctrines, vain
phantasms, which are many and diverse as they themselves.
Nicholaites of old would have wives in common; [5] Montanists
will not marry at all, nor Tatians, forbidding all flesh, Severians
wine; Adamians go naked, because Adam did so in Paradise; [6]
and some barefoot all their lives, because God (Exod. iii and
Joshua v) bid Moses [and Joshua] so to do, and Isaiah (xx) was
bid to put off his shoes; [7] Manichees hold that Pythagorean
transmigration of souls from men to beasts; the Circumcellions
in Africa, "with a mad cruelty made away themselves, some by
fire, water, breaking their necks, and seduced others to do the
like, threatening some if they did not," [8] with a thousand such;
as you may read in Austin [9] (for there were fourscore and eleven
heresies in his times, besides schisms and smaller factions),
Epiphanius, Alphonsus de Castro, Danæus, Gab. Prateolus, etc.
Of prophets, enthusians and impostors, our ecclesiastical
stories afford many examples; of Eliases and Christs, as our

Eudo de Stellis,[1] a Briton in King Stephen's time, that went invisible, translated himself from one to another in a moment, fed thousands with good cheer in the wilderness, and many such; nothing so common as miracles, visions, revelations, prophecies. Now what these brainsick heretics once broach, and impostors set on foot, be it never so absurd, false, and prodigious, the common people will follow and believe. It will run along like murrain in cattle, scab in sheep. *Nulla scabies,* as he said,[2] *superstitione scabiosior* [no scab festers worse than superstition]: as he that is bitten with a mad dog bites others, and all in the end become mad; either out of affection of novelty, simplicity, blind zeal, hope and fear, the giddy-headed multitude will embrace it, and without farther examination approve it.

Sed vetera querimur, these are old, *hæc prius fuere* [things of the past]. In our days we have a new scene of superstitious impostors and heretics, a new company of actors, of Antichrists, that great Antichrist himself: a rope of popes, that by their greatness and authority bear down all before them: who from that time they proclaimed themselves universal bishops, to establish their own kingdom, sovereignty, greatness, and to enrich themselves, brought in such a company of human traditions, purgatory, *limbus patrum, infantum,* and all that subterranean geography, mass, adoration of saints, alms, fastings, bulls, indulgencies, orders, friars, images, shrines, musty relics, excommunications, confessions, satisfactions, blind obediences, vows, pilgrimages, peregrinations, with many such curious toys, intricate subtleties, gross errors, obscure questions, to vindicate the better and set a gloss upon them, that the light of the Gospel was quite eclipsed, darkness over all, the Scriptures concealed, legends brought in, religion banished, hypocritical superstition exalted, and the Church itself obscured and persecuted:[3] Christ and His members crucified more, saith Benzo, by a few necromantical, atheistical popes, than ever it was by Julian the Apostate, Porphyrius the Platonist, Celsus the physician, Libanius the Sophister;[4] by those heathen emperors, Huns, Goths, and Vandals. What each of them did, by what means, at what times, *quibus auxiliis* [by what assistance], superstition climbed to this height, traditions increased, and Antichrist himself came to his estate, let Magdeburgenses, Kemnisius, Osiander, Bale, Mornay, Foxe, Usher, and many others relate. In the meantime, he that shall but see their profane rites and foolish customs, how superstitiously kept,

how strictly observed, their multitude of saints, images, that
rabble of Romish deities, for trades, professions, diseases, persons, offices, countries, places: St. George for England; St. Denis
for France; Patrick, Ireland; Andrew, Scotland; Jago, Spain,
etc.; Gregory for students; Luke for painters; Cosmas and
Damian for philosophers; Crispin, shoemakers; Katherine,
spinners, etc.; Anthony for pigs; Gallus, geese; Wenceslaus,
sheep; Pelagius, oxen; Sebastian, the plague; Valentine, falling
sickness: Apollonia, toothache; Petronella for agues; and the
Virgin Mary for sea and land, for all parties, offices: he that
shall observe these things, their shrines, images, oblations,
pendants, adorations, pilgrimages they make to them, what
creeping to crosses, our Lady of Loretto's rich gowns,[1] her
donaries, the cost bestowed on images, and number of suitors;
St. Nicholas' burg in France; our St. Thomas' shrine of old at
Canterbury; those relics at Rome, Jerusalem, Genoa, Lyons,
Pratum,[2] St. Denis; and how many thousands come yearly to
offer to them, with what cost, trouble, anxiety, superstition
(for forty several masses are daily said in some of their churches,[3]
and they rise at all hours of the night to mass, come barefoot,
etc.), how they spend themselves, times, goods, lives, fortunes,
in such ridiculous observations; their tales and figments, false
miracles, buying and selling of pardons, indulgences for 40,000
years to come, their processions on set days, their strict fastings,
monks, anachorites, friar mendicants, Franciscans, Carthusians,
etc.; their vigils and fasts, their ceremonies at Christmas, Shrove-
tide, Candlemas, Palm-Sunday, St. Blaise, St. Martin, St.
Nicholas' day; their adorations, exorcisms, etc., will think all
those Grecian, pagan, Mahometan superstitions, gods, idols,
and ceremonies, the name, time and place, habit only altered,
to have degenerated into Christians. Whilst they prefer
traditions before Scriptures; those evangelical councils, poverty,
obedience, vows, alms, fasting, supererogations, before God's
commandments; their own ordinances instead of His precepts,
and keep them in ignorance, blindness, they have brought the
common people into such a case by their cunning conveyances,
strict discipline, and servile education, that upon pain of damnation they dare not break the least ceremony, tradition, edict;
hold it a greater sin to eat a bit of meat in Lent than kill a man:
their consciences are so terrified that they are ready to despair
if a small ceremony be omitted; and will accuse their own father,
mother, brother, sister, nearest and dearest friends of heresy
if they do not as they do, will be their chief executioners, and

help first to bring a faggot to burn them. What mulct, what penance soever is enjoined, they dare not but do it, tumble with St. Francis in the mire amongst hogs, if they be appointed, go woolward, whip themselves, build hospitals, abbeys, etc., go to the East or West Indies, kill a king, or run upon a sword-point: they perform all, without any muttering or hesitation, believe all.

> *Ut pueri infantes credunt signa omnia ahena*
> *Vivere, et esse homines, et sic isti omnia ficta*
> *Vera putant, credunt signis cor inesse ahenis.*[1]

> As children think their babies live to be,
> Do they these brazen images they see.

And whilst the ruder sort are so carried headlong with blind zeal, are so gulled and tortured by their superstitions, their own too credulous simplicity and ignorance, their epicurean popes and hypocritical cardinals laugh in their sleeves, and are merry in their chambers with their punks, they do *indulgere genio* [enjoy themselves], and make much of themselves. The middle sort, some for private gain, hope of ecclesiastical prefer-ment (*Quis expedivit psittaco suum* Χαῖρε *?* [Who made the parrot so ready with its "Good day?"]), popularity, base flattery, must and will believe all their paradoxes and absurd tenents, without exception, and as obstinately maintain and put in practice all their traditions and idolatrous ceremonies (for their religion is half a trade) to the death; they will defend all, the Golden Legend itself, with all the lies and tales in it: as that of St. George, St. Christopher, St. Winifred, St. Denis, etc. It is a wonder to see how Nic. Harpsfield, that pharisaical impostor, amongst the rest, *Ecclesiast. Hist. cap. 22, sæc. prim. sex*, puzzles himself to vindicate that ridiculous fable of St. Ursula and the eleven thousand virgins, as when they lived,[2] how they came to Cologne, by whom martyred, etc.; though he can say nothing for it, yet he must and will approve it: *Nobilitavit (inquit) hoc sæculum Ursula cum comitibus, cujus historia utinam tam mihi esset expedita et certa, quam in animo meo certum ac expeditum est, eam esse cum sodalibus beatam in cœlis virginem* [This age, saith he, hath been ennobled by Ursula and her companions, and I wish I could be as sure of the authenticity of the story as I am that she and her companions are enjoying heavenly bliss]. They must and will (I say) either out of blind zeal believe, vary their compass with the rest as the latitude of religion varies, apply themselves to the times and seasons, and for fear and flattery are content to subscribe and do all that in them lies to maintain and defend their present government and slavish religious schoolmen, canonists, Jesuits, friars, priests, orators, sophisters, luxuriant wits who either for that they had nothing else to do, knew not otherwise how to busy themselves in those idle times, for the Church then had few or no open adversaries, or better to defend their lies, fictions, miracles, transubstantiations, traditions, popes' pardons, purgatories, masses, impossibilities, etc., with glorious shows, fair pretences, big words, and plausible wits, have coined a thousand idle questions, nice distinctions, subtleties, obs and sols,[1] such tropological, allegorical expositions, to salve all appearances, objections, such quirks and quiddities, "quodlibetaries," as Bale saith of Ferribrigge and Strode, instances, ampliations, decrees, glosses, canons, that instead of sound commentaries, good preachers, are come in a company of mad sophisters, *primo secundo secundarii*, sectaries, canonists, Sorbonists, Minorites, with a rabble of idle controversies and questions: *An Papa sit Deus, an quasi Deus? An participet utramque Christi naturam?* [Whether the Pope is God or a kind of God? Whether he partakes of each nature of Christ?] Whether it be as possible for God to be an humble-bee or a gourd, as a man?[2] Whether He can produce respect without a foundation or term? make a whore a virgin? fetch Trajan's soul from hell, and how? with a rabble of questions about hell-fire: whether it be a greater sin to kill a man, or to clout shoes upon a Sunday? whether God can make another God like unto Himself? Such, saith Kemnisius, are most of your schoolmen (mere alchemists), 200 commentators on Peter Lombard (Pitseus, *Catal. scriptorum Anglic.*, reckons up 180 English commentators alone, on the matter of the Sentences), Scotists, Thomists, Reals, Nominals, etc., and so perhaps that of St. Austin[3] may be verified, *Indocti rapiunt cœlum, docti interim descendunt ad infernum* [the ignorant attain heaven, the learned meanwhile descend to hell]. Thus they continued in such error, blindness, decrees, sophisms, superstitions; idle ceremonies and traditions were the sum of their new-coined holiness and religion, and by these knaveries and stratagems they were able to involve multitudes, to deceive the most sanctified souls, and, if it were possible, the very elect. In the meantime the true Church, as wine and water mixed, lay hid and obscure to speak of, till Luther's time, who began upon a sudden to defecate, and as another sun to drive away those foggy mists of superstition, to restore it to that purity of the primitive Church. And after him many good and godly men, divine spirits, have done their endeavours, and still do.

> And what their ignorance esteemed so holy,
> Our wiser ages do account as folly.[1]

But see the devil, that will never suffer the Church to be quiet or at rest: no garden so well tilled but some noxious weeds grow up in it, no wheat but it hath some tares: we have a mad giddy company of precisians, schismatics, and some heretics, even in our own bosoms in another extreme (*Dum vitant stulti vitia in contraria currunt* [fools in avoiding one fault rush into the opposite]); that out of too much zeal in opposition to Antichrist, human traditions, those Romish rites and superstitions, will quite demolish all, they will admit of no ceremonies at all, no fasting days, no cross in baptism, kneeling at communion, no church music, etc., no bishops' courts, no church government, rail at all our church discipline, will not hold their tongues, and all for the peace of thee, O Sion! No, not so much as degrees some of them will tolerate, or universities; all human learning ('tis *cloaca diaboli* [the devil's sewer]), hoods, habits, cap and surplice, such as are things indifferent in themselves, and wholly for ornament, decency, or distinction' sake, they abhor, hate, and snuff at, as a stone-horse when he meets a bear: they make matters of conscience of them, and will rather forsake their livings than subscribe to them. They will admit of no holidays, or honest recreations, as of hawking, hunting, etc., no churches, no bells some of them, because papists use them; no discipline, no ceremonies but what they invent themselves; no interpretations of Scriptures, no comments of Fathers, no councils, but such as their own phantastical spirits dictate, or *recta ratio* [right reason], as Socinians; by which spirit misled, many times they broach as prodigious paradoxes as papists themselves. Some of them turn prophets, have secret revelations, will be of privy council with God Himself, and know all His secrets, *per capillos Spiritum Sanctum tenent, et omnia sciunt cum sint asini omnium obstinatissimi* [2] [they hold the Holy Spirit by the hair, and pretend to know everything though they are but a pack of obstinate asses]. A company of giddy heads will take upon them to define how many shall be saved and who damned in a parish, where they shall sit in heaven, interpret apocalypses (*commentatores præcipites et vertiginosos* [headstrong and scatterbrain commentators], one calls them, as well he might) and those hidden mysteries to private persons, times, places, as

their own spirit informs them, private revelations shall suggest,
and precisely set down when the world shall come to an end,
what year, what month, what day.   Some of them again have
such strong faith, so presumptuous, they will go into infected
houses, expel devils, and fast forty days, as Christ Himself did;
some call God and His attributes into question, as Vorstius and
Socinus; some princes, civil magistrates, and their authorities,
as Anabaptists, will do all their own private spirit dictates,
and nothing else.   Brownists, Barrowists, Familists, and those
Amsterdamian sects and sectaries, are led all by so many
private spirits.   It is a wonder to reveal what passages Sleidan
relates in his Commentaries, of Cretink, Knipperdoling, and
their associates, those madmen of Munster in Germany; what
strange enthusiasms, sottish revelations they had, how absurdly
they carried themselves, deluded others; and as profane
Machiavel in his Political Disputations holds of Christian
religion, in general it doth enervate, debilitate, take away
men's spirits and courage from them, *simpliciores reddit homines*
[makes men more simple], breeds nothing so courageous soldiers
as that Roman: we may say of these peculiar sects, their religion
takes away not spirits only, but wit and judgment, and deprives
them of their understanding; for some of them are so far gone
with their private enthusiasms and revelations, that they are
quite mad, out of their wits.   What greater madness can there
be than for a man to take upon him to be a god, as some do?
to be the Holy Ghost, Elias, and what not?   In Poland, 1518,
in the reign of King Sigismund, one said he was Christ, and got
him twelve apostles, came to judge the world, and strangely
deluded the commons.[1]   One David George, an illiterate painter,
not many years since, did as much in Holland, took upon him
to be the Messias, and had many followers.[2]   Benedictus
Victorinus Faventinus, *consil.* 15, writes as much of one Honorius,
that thought he was not only inspired as a prophet, but that
he was a god himself, and had familiar conference with God
and His angels.[3]   Lavater, *de spect. cap.* 2, *part.* 8, hath a story
of one John Sartorius, that thought he was the prophet Elias,
and, *cap.* 7, of divers others that had conference with angels,
were saints, prophets.   Wierus, *lib.* 3 *de lamiis, cap.* 7, makes
mention of a prophet of Groningen that said he was God the
Father; of an Italian and Spanish prophet that held as much.
We need not rove so far abroad, we have familiar examples at
home: Hacket that said he was Christ; Coppinger and Arthing-
ton his disciples; Burchet and Hovatus, burned at Norwich.[4]

We are never likely seven years together without some such
new prophets that have several inspirations, some to convert
the Jews, some fast forty days, go with Daniel to the lions'
den; some foretell strange things, some for one thing, some for
another.   Great precisians of mean conditions and very illiterate,
most part by a preposterous zeal, fasting, meditation, melancholy, are brought into those gross errors and inconveniences.
Of those men I may conclude generally, that howsoever they
may seem to be discreet, and men of understanding in other
matters, discourse well, *læsam habent imaginationem* [they have
a diseased imagination], they are like comets, round in all places
but only where they blaze, *cætera sani* [sane in other respects],
they have impregnable wits many of them, and discreet otherwise, but in this their madness and folly breaks out beyond
measure, *in infinitum erumpit stultitia*.   They are certainly far
gone with melancholy, if not quite mad, and have more need
of physic than many a man that keeps his bed, more need of
hellebore than those that are in Bedlam.

Subsect. IV.—*Prognostics of Religious Melancholy*

You may guess at the prognostics by the symptoms.   What
can these signs foretell otherwise than folly, dotage, madness,
gross ignorance, despair, obstinacy, a reprobate sense, a bad
end?[1]   What else can superstition, heresy produce, but wars,
tumults, uproars, torture of souls, and despair, a desolate land,
as Jeremy teacheth, *cap.* vii, 34, when they commit idolatry,
and walk after their own ways? how should it be otherwise
with them? what can they expect but "blasting, famine, dearth,"
and all the plagues of Egypt, as Amos denounceth, *cap.* iv,
vers. 9, 10; to be led into captivity?   If our hopes be frustrate,
"we sow much and bring in little, eat and have not enough,
drink and are not filled, clothe and be not warm," etc. (Haggai
i, 6); "we look for much and it comes to little, whence is it?
His house was waste, they came to their own houses" (*vers.* 9);
"therefore the heaven stayed his dew, the earth his fruit."
Because we are superstitious, irreligious, we do not serve God
as we ought, all these plagues and miseries come upon us; what
can we look for else but mutual wars, slaughters, fearful ends
in this life, and in the life to come eternal damnation?   What
is it that hath caused so many feral battles to be fought, so
much Christian blood shed, but superstition?   That Spanish

Inquisition, racks, wheels, tortures, torments, whence do they
proceed? from superstition. Bodine the Frenchman in his
Method. hist.[1] accounts Englishmen barbarians, for their civil
wars: but let him read those Pharsalian fields fought of late in
France for religion,[2] their massacres, wherein by their own
relations in twenty-four years I know not how many millions
have been consumed, whole families and cities, and he shall find
ours to be but velitations to theirs. But it hath ever been the
custom of heretics and idolaters, when they are plagued for
their sins, and God's just judgments come upon them, not to
acknowledge any fault in themselves, but still impute it unto
others. In Cyprian's time it was much controverted between
him and Demetrius an idolater, who should be the cause of
those present calamities. Demetrius laid all the fault on
Christians (and so they did ever in the primitive Church, as
appears by the first book of Arnobius [3]), "that there were not
such ordinary showers in winter, the ripening heat in summer,
so seaonable springs, fruitful autumns, no marble mines in the
mountains, less gold and silver than of old; that husbandmen,
seamen, soldiers, all were scanted, justice, friendship, skill in
arts, all was decayed," [4] and that through Christians' default,
and all their other miseries from them, *quod dii nostri a vobis
non colantur*, because they did not worship their gods. But
Cyprian retorts all upon him again, as appears by his tract
against him. 'Tis true the world is miserably tormented and
shaken with wars, dearth, famine, fire, inundations, plagues,
and many feral diseases rage amongst us, *sed non ut tu quereris,
ista accidunt quod dii vestri a nobis non colantur, sed quod a
vobis non colatur Deus, a quibus nec quæritur, nec timetur*, [but]
not as thou complainest, that we do not worship your gods,
but because you are idolaters, and do not serve the true God,
neither seek Him, nor fear Him as you ought. Our papists
object as much to us, and account us heretics, we them; the
Turks esteem of both as infidels, and we them as a company of
pagans; Jews against all; when indeed there is a general fault
in us all, and something in the very best, which may justly
deserve God's wrath, and pull these miseries upon our heads.
I will say nothing here of those vain cares, torments, needless
works, penance, pilgrimages, pseudomartyrdom, etc. We heap
upon ourselves unnecessary troubles, observations; we punish
our bodies, as in Turkey (saith Busbequius, *Leg. Turcic. ep.* 3)[5]
"one did, that was much affected with music, and to hear
boys sing, but very superstitious; an old sibyl coming to his

house, or an holy woman" (as that place yields many), "took him down for it, and told him that in that other world he should suffer for it; thereupon he flung his rich and costly instruments which he had bedecked with jewels, all at once into the fire. He was served in silver plate, and had goodly household stuff: a little after, another religious man reprehended him in like sort, and from thenceforth he was served in earthen vessels. Last of all a decree came forth, because Turks might not drink wine themselves, that neither Jew nor Christian then living in Constantinople might drink any wine at all." In like sort amongst papists, fasting at first was generally proposed as a good thing; after, from such meats at set times, and then last of all so rigorously proposed, to bind the consciences upon pain of damnation. "First Friday," saith Erasmus, "then Saturday, *et nunc periclitatur dies Mercurii*," and Wednesday now is in danger of a fast. "And for such-like toys some so miserably afflict themselves, to despair and death itself, rather than offend, and think themselves good Christians in it, whenas indeed they are superstitious Jews." [1] So saith Leonardus Fuchsius, a great physician in his time. "We are tortured in Germany with these popish edicts, our bodies so taken down, our goods so diminished, that if God had not sent Luther, a worthy man, in time, to redress these mischiefs, we should have eaten hay with our horses before this." [2] As in fasting,[3] so in all other superstitious edicts, we crucify one another without a cause, barring ourselves of many good and lawful things, honest disports, pleasures and recreations; for wherefore did God create them but for our use? Feasts, mirth, music, hawking, hunting, singing, dancing, etc., *non tam necessitatibus nostris Deus inservit, sed in delicias amamur* [were given by God not to serve our necessities, but, out of His great love, for our delectation], as Seneca notes, God would have it so. And as Plato, 2 *de legibus*, gives out, *Deos laboriosam hominum vitam miseratos*, the gods in commiseration of human estate sent Apollo, Bacchus, and the Muses, *qui cum voluptate tripudia et saltationes nobis ducant*, to be merry with mortals, to sing and dance with us; so that he that will not rejoice and enjoy himself, making good use of such things as are lawfully permitted, *non est temperatus* [is not temperate], as he will, *sed superstitiosus* [but superstitious]. "There is nothing better for a man than that he should eat and drink, and that he should make his soul enjoy good in his labour" (Eccles. ii, 24). And as one said of hawking and hunting,[4] *Tot solatia in hac ægri orbis*

calamitate mortalibus tædiis Deus objecit, I say of all honest
recreations, God hath therefore indulged them to refresh, ease,
solace and comfort us. But we are some of us too stern, too
rigid, too precise, too grossly superstitious, and whilst we make a
conscience of every toy, with touch not, taste not, etc., as those
Pythagoreans of old, and some Indians now, that will eat no
flesh, or suffer any living creature to be killed, the Bannians
about Guzerat; we tyrannize over our brother's soul, lose the
right use of many good gifts, honest sports, games and pleasant
recreations,[1] punish ourselves without a cause,[2] lose our liberties,
and sometimes our lives. *Anno* 1270, at Magdeburg in Germany,
a Jew fell into a privy upon a Saturday, and without help could
not possibly get out; he called to his fellows for succour, but they
denied it, because it was their Sabbath, *non licebat opus manuum
exercere* [no manual labour was permitted]; the bishop hearing
of it, the next day forbade him to be pulled out, because it was
our Sunday: in the meantime the wretch died before Monday.[3]
We have myriads of examples in this kind amongst those rigid
sabbatarians, and therefore not without good cause, *intolerabilem
perturbationem* Seneca calls it,[4] as well he might, an intolerable
perturbation, that causeth such dire events, folly, madness,
sickness, despair, death of body and soul, and hell itself.

SUBSECT. V.—*Cure of Religious Melancholy*

To purge the world of idolatry and superstition will require
some monster-taming Hercules, a divine Æsculapius, or Christ
Himself to come in His own person, to reign a thousand years
on earth before the end, as the millenaries will have Him. They
are generally so refractory, self-conceited, obstinate, so firmly
addicted to that religion in which they have been bred and
brought up, that no persuasion, no terror, no persecution can
divert them. The consideration of which hath induced many
commonwealths to suffer them to enjoy their consciences as
they will themselves. A toleration of Jews is in most provinces
of Europe; in Asia they have their synagogues; Spaniards permit
Moors to live amongst them; the Mogullians Gentiles; the Turks
all religions. In Europe, Poland and Amsterdam are the common
sanctuaries. Some are of opinion that no man ought to be
compelled for conscience' sake, but let him be of what religion
he will, he may be saved, as Cornelius was formerly accepted,
Jew, Turk, Anabaptists, etc., if he be an honest man, live soberly
and civilly in his profession (Volkelius, Crellius, and the rest of

the Socinians, that now nestle themselves about Cracow and Rakow in Poland, have renewed this opinion), serve his own God with that fear and reverence as he ought. *Sua cuique civitati (Læli) religio sit, nostra nobis;* Tully thought fit every city should be free in this behalf, adore their own *custodes et topicos deos,* tutelar and local gods, as Symmachus calls them. Isocrates adviseth Demonicus, "when he came to a strange city, to worship by all means the gods of the place," [1] *et unumquemque topicum deum sic coli oportere, quomodo ipse præceperit* [every local deity should be worshipped in the manner he has himself prescribed]: which Cæcilius in Minucius [2] labours, and would have every nation *sacrorum ritus gentiles habere et deos colere municipes,* keep their own ceremonies, worship their peculiar gods, which Pomponius Mela reports of the Africans, *Deos suos patrio more venerantur,* they worship their own gods according to their own ordination. For why should any one nation, as he there pleads, challenge that universality of God, *Deum suum quem nec ostendunt, nec vident, discurrentem scilicet et ubique præsentem, in omnium mores, actus, et occultas cogitationes inquirentem* [their own God whom they neither show nor see, who is supposed to run all ways and be everywhere, and to survey the character, actions, and hidden thoughts of all], etc., as Christians do? let every province enjoy their liberty in this behalf, worship one God, or all as they will, and are informed. The Romans built altars *diis Asiæ, Europæ, Libyæ, diis ignotis et peregrinis* [to the gods of Asia, Europe, Libya, to unknown and foreign gods]: others otherwise, etc. Plinius Secundus, as appears by his epistle to Trajan, would not have the Christians so persecuted, and in some time of the reign of Maximinus, as we find it registered in Eusebius, *lib.* 9, *cap.* 9, there was a decree made to this purpose, *Nullus cogatur invitus ad hunc vel illum deorum cultum* [let no one be compelled against his will to worship any particular deity], and by Constantine in the nineteenth year of his reign, as Baronius informeth us, [3] *Nemo alteri exhibeat molestiam, quod cujusque animus vult, hoc quisque transigat* [let no one interfere with any one else, let each act as he will]; new gods, new lawgivers, new priests, will have new ceremonies, customs and religions, to which every wise man as a good formalist should accommodate himself.

> *Saturnus periit, perierunt et sua jura,*
> *Sub Jove nunc mundus, jussa sequare Jovis.* [4]

> [Saturn is gone, and ended is his sway;
> Jove now is lord, the word of Jove obey.]

The said Constantine the emperor, as Eusebius writes, flung down and demolished all the heathen gods, silver, gold statues, altars, images and temples, and turned them all to Christian churches, *infestus gentilium monumentis ludibrio exposuit* [he hated the monuments of the Gentiles, and subjected them to insult]; the Turk now converts them again to Mahometan meskites. The like edict came forth in the reign of Arcadius and Honorius. Symmachus the orator,[1] in his days, to procure a general toleration, used this argument: "Because God is immense and infinite, and His nature cannot perfectly be known, it is convenient He should be as diversely worshipped as every man shall perceive or understand."[2] It was impossible, he thought, for one religion to be universal: you see that one small province can hardly be ruled by one law, civil or spiritual; and "how shall so many distinct and vast empires of the world be united into one? It never was, never will be." Besides, if there be infinite planetary and firmamental worlds, as some will,[3] there be infinite genii or commanding spirits belonging to each of them; and so, *per consequens* (for they will be all adored), infinite religions. And therefore let every territory keep their proper rites and ceremonies, as their *dii tutelares* will, so Tyrius calls them, "and according to the quarter they hold," their own institutions, revelations, orders, oracles, which they dictate from time to time, or teach their priests or ministers. This tenent was stiffly maintained in Turkey not long since, as you may read in the third epistle of Busbequius, "that all those should participate of eternal happiness, that lived an holy and innocent life, what religion soever they professed."[4] Rustan Bassa was a great patron of it; though Mahomet himself was sent *virtute gladii* [by dint of the sword] to enforce all, as he writes in his Alcoran, to follow him. Some again will approve of this for Jews, Gentiles, infidels, that are out of the fold, they can be content to give them all respect and favour, but by no means to such as are within the precincts of our own Church, and called Christians, to no heretics, schismatics, or the like; let the Spanish Inquisition, that fourth Fury, speak of some of them, the civil wars and massacres in France, our Marian times. Magallianus the Jesuit[5] will not admit of conference with an heretic, but severity and rigour to be used, *non illis verba reddere, sed furcas figere oportet* [we should not argue with them, but erect gallows for them]; and Theodosius is commended in Nicephorus, *lib.* 12, *cap.* 15, "that he put all heretics to silence."[6] Bernard, *Epist.* 190, will have club-law, fire and

sword for heretics, "compel them, stop their mouths, not with
disputations, or refute them with reasons, but with fists";[1] and
this is their ordinary practice. Another company are as mild
on the other side; to avoid all heart-burning and contentious
wars and uproars, they would have a general toleration in every
kingdom, no mulct at all, no man for religion or conscience
be put to death, which Thuanus the French historian much
favours,[2] our late Socinians defend, Vaticanus against Calvin,
in a large treatise in behalf of Servetus, vindicates; Castalio,
etc., Martin Bellius, and his companions maintained this opinion
not long since in France, whose error is confuted by Beza in
a just volume. The medium is best, and that which Paul
prescribes (Gal. vi, 1): "If any man shall fall by occasion, to
restore such a one with the spirit of meekness, by all fair means,
gentle admonitions"; but if that will not take place, *Post unam
et alteram admonitionem hæreticum devita* [after the second
admonition, avoid a heretic], he must be excommunicate, as
Paul did by Hymenæus, delivered over to Satan. *Immedicabile
vulnus ense recidendum est* [an incurable limb must be ampu-
tated]. As Hippocrates said in physic, I may well say in
divinity, *Quæ ferro non curantur, ignis curat* [what is not cured
by the sword is cured by fire]. For the vulgar, restrain them
by laws, mulcts, burn their books, forbid their conventicles;
for when the cause is taken away, the effect will soon cease.
Now for prophets, dreamers, and such rude silly fellows, that
through fasting, too much meditation, preciseness, or by melancholy are distempered, the best means to reduce them *ad sanam
mentem* [to their senses] is to alter their course of life, and with
conference, threats, promises, persuasions, to intermix physic.
Hercules de Saxonia had such a prophet committed to his
charge in Venice, that thought he was Elias, and would fast
as he did; he dressed a fellow in angel's attire, that said he came
from heaven to bring him divine food, and by that means
stayed his fast, administered his physic; so by the mediation of
this forged angel he was cured. Rhasis, an Arabian, *Cont.
lib.* 1, *cap.* 9, speaks of a fellow that in like case complained to
him, and desired his help: "I asked him" (saith he) "what the
matter was; he replied, I am continually meditating of heaven
and hell, and methinks I see and talk with fiery spirits,
smell brimstone, etc., and am so carried away with these conceits that I can neither eat, nor sleep, nor go about my business.
I cured him" (saith Rhasis) "partly by persuasion, partly by
physic, and so have I done by many others."[3]   We have

frequently such prophets and dreamers amongst us, whom we persecute with fire and fagot; I think the most compendious cure, for some of them at least, had been in Bedlam. *Sed de his satis* [but enough of this].

MEMB. II.

SUBSECT. I.—*Religious Melancholy in Defect; Parties affected, Epicures, Atheists, Hypocrites, Worldly Secure, Carnalists, all Impious Persons, Impenitent Sinners, etc.*

IN that other extreme, or defect of this love of God, knowledge, faith, fear, hope, etc., are such as err both in doctrine and manners, Sadducees, Herodians, libertines, politicians; all manner of atheists, epicures, infidels, that are secure, in a reprobate sense, fear not God at all, and such are too distrustful and timorous, as desperate persons be. That grand sin of atheism or impiety, Melancthon [1] calls it, *monstrosam melancholiam*, monstrous melancholy; or *venenatam melancholiam*, poisoned melancholy. A company of Cyclopes or giants, that war with the gods, as the poets feigned, antipodes to Christians, that scoff at all religion, at God Himself, deny Him and all His attributes, His wisdom, power, providence, His mercy and judgment.

> *Esse aliquos manes, et subterranea regna,*
> *Et contum, et Stygio ranas in gurgite nigras,*
> *Atque una transire vadum tot millia cymba,*
> *Nec pueri credunt, nisi qui nondum ære lavantur.* [2]

> [That there are shades and an underworld, and such
> things as Charon's pole and black frogs in the
> Stygian pool, and thousands crossing the strait
> in a single skiff—these tales are not believed even
> by boys, save those who are not yet in their teens.]

That there is either heaven or hell, resurrection of the dead, pain, happiness, or world to come, *credat Judæus Apella* [tell it to the marines]; for their parts they esteem them as so many poet's tales, bugbears; Lucian's Alexander, Moses, Mahomet, and Christ are all as one in their creed. When those bloody wars in France for matters of religion (saith Richard Dinoth [3]) were so violently pursued between Huguenots and papists, there was a company of good fellows laughed them all to scorn for being such superstitious fools to lose their wives and fortunes, accounting faith, religion, immortality of the soul, mere fopperies and illusions. Such loose atheistical spirits are too predominant in all kingdoms.[1] Let them contend, pray, tremble, trouble themselves that will, for their parts, they fear neither God nor devil; but with that Cyclops in Euripides,

Haud ulla numina expavescunt cœlitum,
Sed victimas uni deorum maximo,
Ventri offerunt, deos ignorant cæteros.

They fear no god but one,
They sacrifice to none
But belly, and him adore,
For gods they know no more.

"Their god is their belly," as Paul saith, *Sancta mater saturitas; quibus in solo vivendi causa palato est* [their Holy Mother is satiety; they live only for eating]. The idol which they worship and adore is their mistress; with him in Plautus, *Mallem hæc mulier me amet quam dii*, they had rather have her favour than the gods'. Satan is their guide, the flesh is their instructor, hypocrisy their counsellor, vanity their fellow-soldier, their will their law, ambition their captain, custom their rule; temerity, boldness, impudence their art, toys their trading, damnation their end. All their endeavours are to satisfy their lust and appetite, how to please their genius, and to be merry for the present:

Ede, lude, bibe, post mortem nulla voluptas.

[Eat, drink, and be merry—after death there is no
    pleasure.]

"The same condition is of men and of beasts; as the one dieth, so dieth the other" (Eccles. iii, 19). The world goes round:

Truditur dies die,
Novæque pergunt interire lunæ.[2]

[Day treads on the heels of day, and fresh moons rise
    and wane.]

They did eat and drink of old, marry, bury, bought, sold, planted, built, and will do still.[3] "Our life is short and tedious, and in the death of a man there is no recovery, neither was any man known that hath returned from the grave; for we are born at all adventure, and we shall be hereafter as though we had never been; for the breath is as smoke in our nostrils, etc., and the spirit vanisheth as the soft air.[4] Come let us enjoy the pleasures that are present,[5] let us cheerfully use the creatures as in youth, let us fill ourselves with costly wine and ointments, let not the flower of our life pass by us, let us crown ourselves with rosebuds before they are withered," etc. *Vivamus, mea Lesbia, atque amemus* [1] [my Lesbia, let us live and love], etc. "Come let us take our fill of love, and pleasure in dalliance, for this is our portion, this is our lot." [2]

Tempora labuntur, tacitisque senescimus annis.
[Time glides on, and we age insensibly with the years.]

For the rest of heaven and hell, let children and superstitious fools believe it: for their parts, they are so far from trembling at the dreadful day of judgment that they wish with Nero, *Me vivo fiat*, let it come in their times: so secure, so desperate, so immoderate in lust and pleasure, so prone to revenge, that, as Paterculus said of some caitiffs in his time in Rome, *quod nequiter ausi, fortiter executi:* it shall not be so wickedly attempted, but as desperately performed, whate'er they take in hand. Were it not for God's restraining grace, fear and shame, temporal punishment, and their own infamy, they would Lycaon-like [3] exenterate, as so many cannibals eat up, or [as] Cadmus' soldiers consume one another. These are most impious, and commonly professed atheists, that never use the name of God but to swear by it; that express naught else but Epicurism in their carriage, or hypocrisy; with Pentheus they neglect and contemn these rites and religious ceremonies of the gods; they will be gods themselves, or at least *socii deorum* [colleagues of the gods]. *Divisum imperium cum Jove Cæsar habet* [Cæsar divides the empire with Jove]. Apries, an Egyptian tyrant, grew, saith Herodotus,[4] to that height of pride, insolency and impiety, to that contempt of gods and men, that he held his kingdom so sure, *ut a nemine deorum aut hominum sibi eripi posset*, neither god nor men could take it from him. A certain blasphemous king of Spain [5] (as Lausius reports [6]) made an edict, that no subject of his, for ten years' space, should believe in, call on, or worship any god. And as Jovius relates of Mahomet the Second, that sacked Constantinople, "he so behaved himself, that he believed neither Christ nor Mahomet; and thence it came to pass that he kept his word and promise no farther than for his advantage, neither did he care to commit any offence to satisfy his lust." [7] I could say the like of many princes, many private men (our stories are full of them) in times past, this present age, that love, fear, obey, and perform all civil duties as they shall find them expedient or behoveful to their own ends. *Securi adversus deos, securi adversus homines, votis non est opus*, which Tacitus reports of some Germans,[1] they need not pray, fear, hope, for they are secure, to their thinking, both from God and men. Bulco Opiliensis, sometime Duke of Silesia, was such a one to an hair; he lived (saith Æneas Sylvius [2]) at Uratislavia,[3] "and was so mad to satisfy his lust, that he believed neither heaven nor hell, or that the soul was immortal, but married wives, and turned them up as he thought fit, did murder and mischief, and what he list himself." [4] This duke hath too many followers in our days: say what you can, dehort, exhort, persuade to the contrary, they are no more moved, *quam si dura silex aut stet Marpesia cautes*, than so many stocks and stones; tell them of heaven and hell, 'tis to no purpose, *laterem lavas* [you are washing a brick (i.e. wasting your labour)], they answer as Ataliba, that Indian prince, did Friar Vincent, "when he brought him a book, and told him all the mysteries of salvation, heaven and hell, were contained in it: he looked upon it, and said he saw no such matter, asking withal how he knew it"; [5] they will but scoff at it, or wholly reject it. Petronius in Tacitus, when he was now by Nero's command bleeding to death, *audiebat amicos nihil referentes de immortalitate animæ, aut sapientum placitis, sed levia carmina et faciles versus*, instead of good counsel and divine meditations, he made his friends sing him bawdy verses and scurrile songs. Let them take heaven, paradise, and that future happiness that will, *bonum est esse hic*, it is good being here: there is no talking to such, no hope of their conversion, they are in a reprobate sense, mere carnalists, fleshly-minded men, which howsoever they may be applauded in this life by some few parasites, and held for wordly wise men, "They seem to me" (saith Melancthon) "to be as mad as Hercules was when he raved and killed his wife and children." [6] A milder sort of these atheistical spirits there are that profess religion, but *timide et hæsitanter* [timidly and with hesitation], tempted thereunto out of that horrible consideration of diversity of religions, which are and have been in the world (which argument Campanella, *Atheismi Triumphati cap.* 9, both urgeth and answers), besides the covetousness, imposture, and knavery of priests, *quæ faciunt* (as Postellus observes [7]) *ut rebus sacris minus faciant fidem* [which cause religion to be less believed in], and those religions some of them so phantastical, exorbitant, so violently maintained with equal constancy and assurance; whence they infer, that if there be so many religious sects, and

denied by the rest, why may they not be all false? or why
should this or that be preferred before the rest? The sceptics
urge this, and amongst others it is the conclusion of Sextus
Empiricus, *lib. 8 advers. Mathematicos*: after many philosophical
arguments and reasons pro and con that there are gods, and again
that there are no gods, he so concludes, *cum tot inter se pugnent,*
etc., *una tantum potest esse vera* [there are so many diverse
opinions, and yet one only can be true], as Tully likewise disputes: Christians say they alone worship the true God, pity
all other sects, lament their case; and yet those old Greeks and
Romans that worshipped the devil, as the Chinese now do,
aut deos topicos, [or] their own gods, as Julian the Apostate,
Cæcilius in Minucius,[1] Celsus, and Porphyrius the philosopher
object, and as Machiavel contends, were much more noble,
generous, victorious, had a more flourishing commonwealth,
better cities, better soldiers, better scholars, better wits; their
gods often overcame our gods, did as many miracles, etc. Saint
Cyril, Arnobius, Minucius, with many other ancients, of late
Lessius, Mornæus, Grotius *de verit. relig. Christianæ*, Savonarola
de verit. fidei Christianæ, well defend; but Zanchius, Campanella,[2]
Marinus Marcennus, Bozius, and Gentilettus answer all these
atheistical arguments at large. But this again troubles many
as of old, wicked men generally thrive, professed atheists thrive:

> *Nullos esse deos, inane cœlum,*
> *Affirmat Selius : probatque, quod se*
> *Factum, dum negat hæc, videt beatum.*[3]

> There are no gods, heavens are toys,
> Selius in public justifies;
> Because that whilst he thus denies
> Their deities, he better thrives.

This is a prime argument: and most part your most sincere,
upright, honest, and good men are depressed.[4] "The race is
not to the swift, nor the battle to the strong" (Eccles. ix, 11),
"nor yet bread to the wise, favour nor riches to men of understanding, but time and chance comes to all." There was a
great plague in Athens (as Thucydides, *lib. 2*, relates), in which
at last every man, with great licentiousness, did what he list,
not caring at all for God's or men's laws. "Neither the fear
of God nor laws of men" (saith he) "awed any man, because the
plague swept all away alike, good and bad; they thence concluded it was alike to worship or not worship the gods, since
they perished all alike." Some cavil and make doubts of
Scripture itself: it cannot stand with God's mercy, that so many

should be damned, so many bad, so few good, such have and
hold about religions, all stiff on their side, factious alike, thrive
alike, and yet bitterly persecuting and damning each other.
"It cannot stand with God's goodness, protection, and providence" (as St. Chrysostom [1] in the dialect of such discontented persons) "to see and suffer one man to be lame, another
mad, a third poor and miserable all the days of his life, a fourth
grievously tormented with sickness and aches," to his last hour.
"Are these signs and works of God's providence, to let one man
be deaf, another dumb? A poor honest fellow lives in disgrace,
woe and want, wretched he is; whenas a wicked caitiff abounds
in superfluity of wealth, keeps whores, parasites, and what he
will himself." *Audis, Jupiter, hæc?* [Hearest thou this, O
Jupiter?] *Talia multa connectentes, longum reprehensionis
sermonem erga Dei providentiam contexunt* [they bring many such
instances together, and weave out of them a long screed against
the providence of God]. Thus they mutter and object (see the
rest of their arguments in Marcennus *in Genesin*, and in Campanella, amply confuted), with many such vain cavils, well
known, not worthy the recapitulation or answering: whatsoever
they pretend, they are *interim* of little or no religion.

Cousin-germans to these men are many of our great philosophers and deists, who, though they be more temperate in this
life, give many good moral precepts, honest, upright, and sober
in their conversation, yet in effect they are the same (accounting no man a good scholar that is not an atheist), *nimis altum
sapiunt*, too much learning makes them mad. Whiles they
attribute all to natural causes, contingence of all things, as
Melancthon calls them,[2] *pertinax hominum genus*, a peevish
generation of men, that misled by philosophy and the devil's
suggestion, their own innate blindness, deny God as much as
the rest, hold all religion a fiction, opposite to reason and philosophy, though for fear of magistrates, saith Vaninus,[3] they durst
not publicly profess it. Ask one of them of what religion he is,
he scoffingly replies, a philosopher, a Galenist, an Averroist,[4]
and with Rabelais a physician, a Peripatetic, an Epicure. In
spiritual things God must demonstrate all to sense, leave a pawn
with them, or else seek some other creditor. They will acknowledge nature and fortune, yet not God; though in effect they
grant both: for, as Scaliger defines, Nature signifies God's
ordinary power; or, as Calvin writes, Nature is God's order,
and so things extraordinary may be called unnatural: Fortune
His unrevealed will; and so we call things changeable that are

beside reason and expectation. To this purpose Minucius, *in Octaviano*,[1] and Seneca well discourseth with them, *lib.* 4 *de beneficiis, cap.* 5, 6, 7.[2] "They do not understand what they say; what is Nature but God? call him what thou wilt, Nature, Jupiter, he hath as many names as offices: it comes all to one pass, God is the fountain of all, the first Giver and Preserver, from whom all things depend," *a quo, et per quem omnia*,[3]

Nam quodcunque vides Deus est, quocunque moveris,

God is all in all, God is everywhere, in every place. And yet this Seneca, that could confute and blame them, is all out as much to be blamed and confuted himself, as mad himself; for he holds *fatum Stoicum*, that inevitable necessity in the other extreme, as those Chaldean astrologers of old did, against whom the prophet Jeremy so often thunders, and those heathen mathematicians, Nigidius Figulus, magicians, and Priscillianists, whom St. Austin so eagerly confutes, those Arabian question-aries, *Novem Judices* [the Nine Judges], Albumazar, Dorotheus, etc., and our countryman Estuidus,[4] that take upon them to define out of those great conjunctions of stars, with Ptolemæus, the periods of kingdoms, or religions, of all future accidents, wars, plagues, schisms, heresies, and what not? all from stars, and such things, saith Maginus, *quæ sibi et intelligentiis suis reservavit Deus*, which God hath reserved to Himself and His angels, they will take upon them to foretell, as if stars were immediate, inevitable causes of all future accidents. Cæsar Vaninus, in his book *de admirandis naturæ arcanis, dial.* 52, *de oraculis*, is more free, copious, and open in the explication of this astrological tenent of Ptolemy than any of our modern writers, Cardan excepted, a true disciple of his master Pomponatius; according to the doctrine of Peripatetics, he refers all apparitions, prodigies, miracles, oracles, accidents, alterations of religions, kingdoms, etc. (for which he is soundly lashed by Marinus Marcennus, as well he deserves), to natural causes (for spirits he will not acknowledge), to that light, motion, influences of heavens and stars, and to the intelligences that move the orbs: *Intelligentia quæ movet orbem mediante cœlo*, etc. Intelligences do all: and after a long discourse of miracles done of old, *Si hæc dæmones possint, cur non et intelligentiæ cœlorum motrices?* [If demons can do this, why not the intelligences that move the heavens?] And as these great conjunctions, aspects of planets, begin or end, vary, are vertical and predominant, so have religions, rites, ceremonies, and kingdoms their beginning, progress, periods. *In urbibus, regibus, religionibus, ac in particularibus hominibus, hæc vera ac manifesta sunt, ut Aristoteles innuere videtur, et quotidiana docet experientia, ut historias perlegens videbit; quid olim in Gentili lege Jove sanctius et illustrius? quid nunc vile magis et execrandum? Ita cælestia corpora pro mortalium beneficio religiones ædificant, et cum cessat influxus, cessat lex* [The fact is patent in respect of cities, kings, and religions, and also of ordinary individuals, as Aristotle seems to hint and daily experience teaches, as any one will see who reads history. What is more sacred and noble in the religion of the Gentiles than Jove? What is now more despised and execrated? Thus the heavenly bodies build up religions for the good of mankind, and when their influence ceases, the religion also passes away], etc. And because, according to their tenents, the world is eternal, intelligences eternal, influences of stars eternal, kingdoms, religions, alterations shall be likewise eternal, and run round after many ages; *Atque iterum ad Trojam magnus mittetur Achilles; renascentur religiones et cærimoniæ, res humanæ in idem recident, nihil nunc quod non olim fuit, et post sæculorum revolutiones alias est, erit, etc., idem specie,* saith Vaninus, *non individuo quod Plato significavit* ["Once more to Troy shall great Achilles be sent"; old religions and ceremonies shall be resuscitated; history shall repeat itself, there is nothing now which was not already once on a time, and with the revolution of time shall be again . . . the same in kind but not in the individual, as Plato said]. These (saith mine author [1]), these are the decree of Peripatetics, which though I recite, *in obsequium Christianæ fidei detestor,* as I am a Christian I detest and hate. Thus Peripatetics and astrologians held in former times, and to this effect of old in Rome, saith Dionysius Halicarnasseus, *lib.* 7, when those meteors and prodigies appeared in the air after the banishment of Coriolanus, "men were diversely affected: some said they were God's just judgments for the execution of that good man, some referred all to natural causes, some to stars, some thought they came by chance, some by necessity" [2] decreed *ab initio,* and could not be altered. The two last opinions of necessity and chance were, it seems, of greater note than the rest.

> *Sunt qui in Fortunæ jam casibus omnia ponunt,*
> *Et mundum credunt nullo rectore moveri,*
> *Natura volvente vices,* etc. [3]

[Some ascribe everything to chance, and believe that the world has no ruler, but that it goes on by nature.]

For the first, of chance, as Sallust likewise informeth us,[1] those old Romans generally received. "They supposed fortune alone gave kingdoms and empires, wealth, honours, offices; and that for two causes: first, because every wicked, base, unworthy wretch was preferred, rich, potent, etc.; secondly, because of their uncertainty, though never so good, scarce any one enjoyed them long; but after, they began upon better advice to think otherwise, that every man made his own fortune." The last of necessity was Seneca's tenent, that God was *alligatus causis secundis*, so tied to second causes, to that inexorable necessity, that He could alter nothing of that which was once decreed; *sic erat in fatis*, it cannot be altered, *semel jussit, semper paret Deus, nulla vis rumpit, nullæ preces, nec ipsum fulmen*, God hath once said it, and it must for ever stand good, no prayers, no threats, nor power, nor thunder itself can alter it. Zeno, Chrysippus, and those other Stoics, as you may read in Tully, 2 *de divinatione*, Gellius, *lib. 6, cap.* 2, etc., maintained as much. In all ages, there have been such that either deny God in all or in part; some deride Him, they could have made a better world and rule it more orderly themselves, blaspheme Him, derogate at their pleasure from Him. 'Twas so in Plato's time, "Some say there be no gods, others that they care not for men, a middle sort grant both." [2] *Si non sit Deus, unde bona? si sit Deus, unde mala?* [If there is no God, whence comes good? if there is, whence evil?] So Cotta argues in Tully; why made He not all good, or at least tenders not the welfare of such as are good? As the woman told Alexander, if He be not at leisure to hear causes, and redress them, why doth He reign? Sextus Empiricus hath many such arguments. [3] Thus perverse men cavil. So it will ever be, some of all sorts, good, bad, indifferent, true, false, zealous, ambidexters, neutralists, lukewarm, libertines, atheists, etc. They will see these religious sectaries agree amongst themselves, be reconciled all, before they will participate with, or believe any: they think in the meantime (which Celsus objects, and whom Origen confutes [4]): "We Christians adore a person put to death [5] with no more reason than the barbarous Getes worshipped Zamolxis, the Cilicians Mopsus, the Thebans Amphiaraus, and the Lebadeans Trophonius; one religion is as true as another, new-fangled devices, all for human respects"; great-witted Aristotle's works are as much authentical to them as Scriptures, subtle Seneca's Epistles as canonical as St. Paul's, Pindarus' Odes as good as the Prophet David's Psalms, Epictetus' Enchiridion equivalent to wise Solomon's

Proverbs. They do openly and boldly speak this and more, some of them, in all places and companies. "Claudius the emperor was angry with Heaven, because it thundered, and challenged Jupiter into the field; with what madness! " saith Seneca; "he thought Jupiter could not hurt him, but he could hurt Jupiter." [1] Diagoras, Demonax, Epicurus, Pliny, Lucian, Lucretius,

Contemptorque deum Mezentius,

[And Mezentius, despiser of the gods,]

professed atheists all in their times: though not simple atheists neither, as Cicogna proves, *lib.* 1, *cap.* 1; they scoffed only at those pagan gods, their plurality, base and fictitious offices. Gilbertus Cognatus labours much, and so doth Erasmus, to vindicate Lucian from scandal, and there be those that apologize for Epicurus, but all in vain; Lucian scoffs at all, Epicurus he denies all, and Lucretius his scholar defends him in it:

Humana ante oculos fœde cum vita jaceret,
In terris oppressa gravi cum religione,
Quæ caput a cœli regionibus ostendebat,
Horribili super aspectu mortalibus instans, etc., [2]

When human kind was drench'd in superstition,
With ghastly looks aloft, which frighted mortal men, etc.,

he alone, as another Hercules, did vindicate the world from that monster. Uncle Pliny, *lib.* 2, *cap.* 7, *Nat. Hist.,* and *lib.* 7, *cap.* 55, in express words denies the immortality of the soul. [3] Seneca doth little less, *lib.* 7, *epist.* 55 *ad Lucilium, et lib. de consol. ad Marciam,* or rather more. [4] Some Greek commentators would put as much upon Job, that he should deny resurrection, etc., whom Pineda copiously confutes, in *cap.* vii, Job, *vers.* 9. Aristotle is hardly censured of some, both divines and philosophers—St. Justin, in *Parænetica ad Gentes,* Greg. Nazianzen, in *Disput. adversus Eun.,* Theodoret, *lib.* 5 *de curat. Græc. affec.,* Origen, *lib. de principiis.* Pomponatius justifies in his tract (so styled at least) *de immortalitate animæ,* Scaliger (who would forswear himself at any time, saith Patricius, in defence of his great master Aristotle), and Dandinus, *lib.* 3 *de anima,* acknowledge as much. Averroes oppugns all spirits and supreme powers; of late Brunus (*infelix Brunus* [unhappy Brunus], Kepler calls him [5]), Machiavel, Cæsar Vaninus, lately burned [6] at Toulouse in France, and Pet. Aretine, have publicly maintained such atheistical paradoxes, with that Italian Boccace with his fable of three rings,[1] etc., *ex quo infert haud posse internosci, quæ sit verior religio, Judaica, Mahometana, an Christiana, quoniam eadem signa,*[2] etc. [from which he infers that it cannot be distinguished which is the true religion, Judaism, Mahommedanism, or Christianity, since the same signs, etc.]. Marinus Marcennus [3] suspects Cardan for his Subtleties, Campanella, and Charron's Book of Wisdom, with some other tracts, to savour of atheism: [4] but amongst the rest that pestilent book *de tribus mundi impostoribus, quem sine horrore (inquit) non legas, et Mundi Cymbalum dialogis quatuor contentum, anno* 1538, *auctore Perierio, Parisiis excusum* [about the three impostors of the world, not to be read without shuddering, and the Cymbal of the World, in four dialogues, by Perierius (i.e. Despériers), printed in Paris in 1538], etc.[5]   And as there have been in all ages such blasphemous spirits, so there have not been wanting their patrons, protectors, disciples and adherents. Never so many atheists in Italy and Germany, saith Colerus,[6] as in this age: the like complaint Marcennus makes in France, 50,000 in that one city of Paris.   Frederick the emperor, as Matthew Paris records,[7] *licet non sit recitabile* [though it is not fit to be repeated] (I use his own words) is reported to have said, *Tres præstigiatores, Moses, Christus, et Mahomet, uti mundo dominarentur, totum populum sibi contemporaneum seduxisse* [three swindlers, Moses, Christ, and Mahomet, seduced all their contemporaries, in order that they might rule over the world].   (Henry, the Landgrave of Hesse, heard him speak it.) *Si principes imperii institutioni meæ adhærerent, ego multo meliorem modum credendi et vivendi ordinarem* [if the princes of the empire were willing to follow my advice, I could lay down a much better system of belief and conduct].

To these professed atheists we may well add that impious and carnal crew of worldly-minded men, impenitent sinners, that go to hell in a lethargy, or in a dream; who though they be professed Christians, yet they will *nulla pallescere culpa*, make a conscience of nothing they do, they have cauterized consciences, and are indeed in a reprobate sense, "past all feeling, have given themselves over to wantonness, to work all manner of uncleanness even with greediness" (Ephes. iv, 19).   They do know there is a God, a day of judgment to come, and yet for all that, as Hugo saith, *ita comedunt ac dormiunt, ac si diem judicii evasissent; ita ludunt ac rident, ac si in cælis cum Deo regnarent:* they are as merry for all the sorrow, as if they had escaped all dangers, and were in heaven already;

Metus omnes, et inexorabile fatum
Subjecit pedibus, strepitumque Acherontis avari.[1]

[He has placed himself above fear, he rides roughshod
over inexorable fate and the roar of greedy Acheron.]

Those rude idiots and ignorant persons, that neglect and contemn the means of their salvation, may march on with these;
but above all others, those Herodian temporizing statesmen,
political Machiavellians and hypocrites, that make a show of
religion, but in their hearts laugh at it. *Simulata sanctitas
duplex iniquitas;* they are in a double fault, "that fashion
themselves to this world," which Paul forbids,[2] and like Mercury
the planet, are good with good, bad with bad. When they are
at Rome, they do there as they see done, puritans with puritans,
papists with papists; *omnium horarum homines* [time-servers],
formalists, ambidexters, lukewarm Laodiceans. All their study
is to please,[3] and their god is their commodity, their labour to
satisfy their lusts, and their endeavours to their own ends.
Whatsoever they pretend, or in public seem to do, "With the
fool in their hearts, they say there is no God." [4]　*Heus tu! de
Jove quid sentis?* [Hallo, there! what do you think about Jupiter?]
Their words are as soft as oil, but bitterness is in their hearts;
like Alexander the Sixth,[5] so cunning dissemblers, that what
they think they never speak. Many of them are so close, you
can hardly discern it, or take any just exceptions at them;
they are not factious, oppressors as most are, no bribers, no
simoniacal contractors, no such ambitious, lascivious persons
as some others are, no drunkards, *sobrii solem vident orientem,
sobrii vident occidentem,* they rise sober, and go sober to bed,
plain-dealing, upright, honest men, they do wrong to no man,
and are so reputed in the world's esteem at least, very zealous
in religion, very charitable, meek, humble, peace-makers, keep
all duties, very devout, honest, well spoken of, beloved of all
men; but he that knows better how to judge, he that examines
the heart, saith they are hypocrites, *Cor dolo plenum; sonant
vitium percussa maligne* [their hearts are full of guile; when
struck they sound hollow], they are not sound within. As it
is with writers[6] oftentimes, *plus sanctimoniæ in libello, quam
libelli auctore,* more holiness is in the book than in the author
of it; so 'tis with them: many come to church with great Bibles,
whom Cardan said he could not choose but laugh at, and will
now and then *dare operam Augustino,* read Austin, frequent
sermons, and yet professed usurers, mere gripes, *tota vitæ ratio
epicurea est;* all their life is epicurism and atheism, come to

church all day, and lie with a courtesan at night. *Qui Curios simulant et Bacchanalia vivunt*, they have Esau's hands, and Jacob's voice; yea, and many of those holy friars, sanctified men, *cappam*, saith Hierome, *et cilicium induunt, sed intus latronem tegunt.* They are wolves in sheep's clothing, *Introrsum turpes, speciosi pelle decora*, fair without, and most foul within. *Latet plerumque sub tristi amictu lascivia, et deformis horror vili veste tegitur :*[1] oft-times under a mourning weed lies lust itself, and horrible vices under a poor coat. But who can examine all those kinds of hypocrites, or dive into their hearts? If we may guess at the tree by the fruit, never so many as in these days; show me a plain-dealing true honest man; *Et pudor, et probitas, et timor omnis abest* [there is no self-respect, honesty, or fear of any kind]. He that shall but look into their lives, and see such enormous vices, men so immoderate in lust, unspeakable in malice, furious in their rage, flattering and dissembling (all for their own ends), will surely think they are not truly religious, but of an obdurate heart, most part in a reprobate sense, as in this age. But let them carry it as they will for the present, dissemble as they can, a time will come when they shall be called to an account, their melancholy is at hand, they pull a plague and curse upon their own heads, *thesaurisant iram Dei* [they are storing up the anger of God]. Besides all such as are *in deos contumeliosi*, blaspheme, contemn, neglect God, or scoff at Him, as the poets feign of Salmoneus, that would in derision imitate Jupiter's thunder, he was precipitated for his pains, Jupiter *intonuit contra* [thundered against him], etc., so shall they certainly rue it in the end, (*in se spuit, qui in cælum spuit*[2] [he spits on himself who spits at the sky]), their doom 's at hand, and hell is ready to receive them.

Some are of opinion that it is in vain to dispute with such atheistical spirits in the meantime, 'tis not the best way to reclaim them. Atheism, idolatry, heresy, hypocrisy, though they have one common root, that is indulgence to corrupt affection, yet their growth is different, they have divers symptoms, occasions, and must have several cures and remedies. 'Tis true some deny there is any God; some confess, yet believe it not; a third sort confess and believe, but will not live after His laws, worship and obey Him; others allow God and gods subordinate, but not one God, no such general God, *non talem deum*, but several topic gods for several places, and those not to persecute one another for any difference, as Socinus will, but rather love and cherish.

To describe them in particular, to produce their arguments
and reasons, would require a just volume; I refer them therefore
that expect a more ample satisfaction to those subtle and
elaborate treatises, devout and famous tracts of our learned
divines (schoolmen amongst the rest, and casuists) that have
abundance of reasons to prove there is a God, the immortality
of the soul, etc., out of the strength of wit and philosophy
bring irrefragable arguments to such as are ingenuous and well
disposed; at the least, answer all cavils and objections to confute their folly and madness, and to reduce them, *si fieri posset*
[if possible], *ad sanam mentem*, to a better mind, though to small
purpose many times. Amongst others consult with Julius
Cæsar La Galla, professor of philosophy in Rome, who hath
written a large volume of late to confute atheists; of the immortality of the soul, Hierome; Montanus *de immortalitate animæ*;
Lelius Vincentius of the same subject; Thomas Giaminus, and
Franciscus Collius *de Paganorum animabus post mortem*, a famous
doctor of the Ambrosian College in Milan. Bishop Fotherby in
his Atheomastix, Doctor Dove, Doctor Jackson, Abernethy,
Corderoy, have written well of this subject in our mother
tongue: in Latin, Colerus, Zanchius, Palearius, Illyricus,
Philippus,[1] Faber Faventinus, etc. But *instar omnium*, the
most copious confuter of atheists, is Marinus Marcennus in his
Commentaries on Genesis, with Campanella's *Atheismus Trium-
phatus*.[2] He sets down at large the causes of this brutish
passion (seventeen in number I take it), answers all their
arguments and sophisms, which he reduceth to twenty-six heads,
proving withal his own assertion: "There is a God, such a God,
the true and sole God," by thirty-five reasons. His colophon
is how to resist and repress atheism, and to that purpose he
adds four especial means or ways, which whoso will may
profitably peruse.

SUBSECT. II.—*Despair. Despairs, Equivocations, Definitions,
Parties and Parts affected*

There be many kinds of desperation, whereof some be holy,
some unholy, as one distinguisheth;[3] that unholy he defines out
of Tully to be *ægritudinem animi sine ulla rerum expectatione
meliore*, a sickness of the soul without any hope or expectation
of amendment, which commonly succeeds fear; for whilst evil
is expected, we fear; but when it is certain, we despair. Accord-

ing to Thomas, 2, 2*æ*, *distinct.* 40, *art.* 4, it is *recessus a re desiderata, propter impossibilitatem existimatam,* a restraint from the thing desired, for some impossibility supposed. Because they cannot obtain what they would, they become desperate, and many times either yield to the passion by death itself, or else attempt impossibilities, not to be performed by men. In some cases, this desperate humour is not much to be discommended, as in wars it is a cause many times of extraordinary valour; as Josephus, *lib.* 1 *de bello Jud. cap.* 14, L. Danæus, *in Aphoris. polit. pag.* 226, and many politicians hold. It makes them improve their worth beyond itself, and of a forlorn impotent company become conquerors in a moment. *Una salus victis nullam sperare salutem* [the only hope for the conquered is despair]. In such courses when they see no remedy but that they must either kill or be killed, they take courage, and oftentimes *præter spem,* beyond all hope, vindicate themselves. Fifteen thousand Locrenses fought against an hundred thousand Crotonienses, and seeing now no way but one, they must all die, thought they would not depart unrevenged,[1] and thereupon desperately giving an assault, conquered their enemies. *Nec alia causa victoriæ* (saith Justin, mine author) *quam quod desperaverant* [their victory was due entirely to their despair]. William the Conqueror, when he first landed in England, sent back his ships, that his soldiers might have no hope of retiring back. Bodine[2] excuseth his countrymen's overthrow at that famous battle at Agincourt, in Henry the Fifth his time (*cui simile,* saith Froissart, *tota historia producere non possit,* which no history can parallel almost, wherein one handful of Englishmen overthrew a royal army of Frenchmen), with this refuge of despair, *pauci desperati,* a few desperate fellows being compassed in by their enemies, past all hope of life, fought like so many devils; and gives a caution, that no soldiers hereafter set upon desperate persons, which after Frontinus and Vigetius, Guicciardine likewise admonisheth, *Hypomnes. part.* 2, *pag.* 25, not to stop an enemy that is going his way.[3] Many such kinds there are of desperation, when men are past hope of obtaining any suit, or in despair of better fortune; *Desperatio facit monachum* [despair makes the monk], as the saying is, and desperation causeth death itself; how many thousands in such distress have made away themselves, and many others! For he that cares not for his own, is master of another man's life. A Tuscan soothsayer, as Paterculus tells the story,[4] perceiving himself and Fulvius Flaccus, his dear friend, now both carried to prison by Opimius, and in despair of pardon, seeing the young man weep, *Quin tu potius hoc inquit facis,* [said,] "Do as I do"; and with that knocked out his brains against the door-cheek as he was entering into prison, *protinusque illiso capite in carceris januam effuso cerebro expiravit,* and so desperately died. But these are equivocal, unproper. "When I speak of despair," saith Zanchius,[1] "I speak not of every kind, but of that alone which concerns God. It is opposite to hope, and a most pernicious sin, wherewith the devil seeks to entrap men." Musculus makes four kinds of desperation, of God, ourselves, our neighbour, or anything to be done; but this division of his may be reduced easily to the former: all kinds are opposite to hope, that sweet moderator of passions, as Simonides calls it; I do not mean that vain hope which phantastical fellows feign to themselves, which according to Aristotle is *insomnium vigilantium,* a waking dream; but this divine hope which proceeds from confidence, and is an anchor to a floating soul; *spes alit agricolas* [hope sustains the farmers], even in our temporal affairs hope revives us, but in spiritual it further animateth; and were it not for hope, "we of all others were the most miserable," as Paul saith, in this life; were it not for hope, the heart would break; "for though they be punished in the sight of men" (Wisdom iii, 4), "yet is their hope full of immortality"; yet doth it not so rear, as despair doth deject; this violent and sour passion of despair is of all perturbations most grievous, as Patricius holds.[2] Some divide it into final and temporal; final is incurable, which befalleth reprobates;[2] temporal is a rejection of hope and comfort for a time, which may befall the best of God's children, and it commonly proceeds "from weakness of faith,"[3] as in David, when he was oppressed he cried out, "O Lord, thou hast forsaken me," but this for a time. This ebbs and flows with hope and fear; it is a grievous sin howsoever: although some kind of despair be not amiss, when, saith Zanchius, we despair of our own means, and rely wholly upon God: but that species is not here meant. This pernicious kind of desperation is the subject of our discourse, *homicida animæ,* the murderer of the soul, as Austin terms it, a fearful passion, wherein the party oppressed thinks he can get no ease but by death, and is fully resolved to offer violence unto himself; so sensible of his burthen, and impatient of his cross, that he hopes by death alone to be freed of his calamity (though it prove otherwise), and chooseth with Job (vi, 8, 9; vii, 15) "rather to be strangled and die than to be in his bonds."

The part affected is the whole soul, and all the faculties of it;[1] there is a privation of joy, hope, trust, confidence, of present and future good, and in their place succeed fear, sorrow, etc., as in the Symptoms shall be showed. The heart is grieved, the conscience wounded, the mind eclipsed with black fumes arising from those perpetual terrors.

SUBSECT. III.—*Causes of Despair, the Devil, Melancholy, Meditation, Distrust, Weakness of Faith, Rigid Ministers, Misunderstanding Scriptures, Guilty Consciences, etc.*

The principal agent and procurer of this mischief is the devil; those whom God forsakes, the devil by His permission lays hold on. Sometimes he persecutes them with that worm of conscience, as he did Judas, Saul,[2] and others. The poets call it Nemesis, but it is indeed God's just judgment, *sero sed serio,* He strikes home at last, and setteth upon them "as a thief in the night" (1 Thess. v, 2). This temporary passion made David cry out,[3] "Lord, rebuke me not in thine anger, neither chasten me in thine heavy displeasure; for thine arrows have light upon me, etc., there is nothing sound in my flesh, because of thine anger." Again, "I roar for the very grief of my heart" and (Psalm xxii), "My God, my God, why hast thou forsaken me, and art so far from my health, and the words of my crying? I am like to water poured out, my bones are out of joint, mine heart is like wax, that is molten in the midst of my bowels." So Psalm lxxxvii, vers. 15 and 16, and Psalm cii: "I am in misery at the point of death, from my youth I suffer thy terrors, doubting for my life; thine indignations have gone over me, and thy fear hath cut me off." Job doth often complain in this kind; and those God doth not assist, the devil is ready to try and torment, "still seeking whom he may devour." If he find them merry, saith Gregory, "he tempts them forthwith to some dissolute act; if pensive and sad, to a desperate end." *Aut suadendo blanditur, aut minando terret,* sometimes by fair means, sometimes again by foul, as he perceives men severally inclined. His ordinary engine by which he produceth this effect, is the melancholy humour itself, which is *balneum diaboli,* the devil's bath; and as in Saul, those evil spirits get in, as it were, and take possession of us.[4] Black choler is a shoeing-horn, a bait to allure them, insomuch that many writers make melancholy an ordinary cause and a symptom of despair, for that such men are most apt, by reason of their ill-disposed temper, to distrust, fear, grief, mistake, and amplify whatsoever they preposterously conceive or falsely apprehend. *Conscientia scrupulosa nascitur ex vitio naturali complexione melancholica* [an over-scrupulous conscience springs from a natural defect, from a melancholic disposition] (saith Navarrus, *cap.* 27, *num.* 282, *tom.* 2, *Cas. conscien.*). The body works upon the mind, by obfuscating the spirits and corrupted instruments, which Perkins [1] illustrates by simile of an artificer that hath a bad tool; his skill is good, ability correspondent, by reason of ill tools his work must needs be lame and unperfect. But melancholy and despair, though often, do not always concur; there is much difference: melancholy fears without a cause, this upon great occasion; melancholy is caused by fear and grief, but this torment procures them and all extremity of bitterness; much melancholy is without affliction of conscience, as Bright [2] and Perkins illustrate by four reasons; and yet melancholy alone again may be sometimes a sufficient cause of this terror of conscience. Felix Plater so found it in his Observations,[3] *E melancholicis alii damnatos se putant, Deo curæ non sunt, nec prædestinati*, etc., "they think they are not predestinate, God hath forsaken them"; and yet otherwise very zealous and religious; and 'tis common to be seen, "melancholy for fear of God's judgment and hell-fire, drives men to desperation; fear and sorrow, if they be immoderate, end often with it." Intolerable pain and anguish, long sickness, captivity, misery, loss of goods, loss of friends, and those lesser griefs, do sometimes effect it, or such dismal accidents. *Si non statim relevantur*, saith Marcennus,[4] *dubitant an sit Deus*, if they be not eased forthwith, they doubt whether there be any God, they rave, curse, "and are desperately mad because good men are oppressed, wicked men flourish, they have not as they think to their desert," and through impatience of calamities are so misaffected. Democritus put out his eyes, *ne malorum civium prosperos videret successus*, because he could not abide to see wicked men prosper, and was therefore ready to make away himself, as A. Gellius writes of him.[5] Felix Plater hath a memorable example in this kind, of a painter's wife in Basil, that was melancholy for her son's death, and for melancholy became desperate; she thought God would not pardon her sins, "and for four months still raved that she was in hell-fire, already damned." [6] When the humour is stirred up, every small object aggravates and incenseth it, as the parties are addicted. The

same author hath an example of a merchant-man, that for the
loss of a little wheat, which he had overlong kept, was troubled
in conscience,[1] for that he had not sold it sooner or given it to
the poor, yet a good scholar and a great divine; no persuasion
would serve to the contrary, but that for this fact he was
damned: in other matters very judicious and discreet. Solitariness, much fasting, divine meditations, and contemplations
of God's judgments, most part accompany this melancholy,
and are main causes, as Navarrus holds;[2] to converse with
such kind of persons so troubled is sufficient occasion of trouble
to some men. *Nonnulli ob longas inedias, studia et meditationes
cœlestes, de rebus sacris et religione semper agitant,* etc.: Many
(saith P. Forestus) through long fasting, serious meditations of
heavenly things, fall into such fits; and as Lemnius adds, *lib.* 4,
cap. 21, "if they be solitary given, superstitious, precise, or
very devout; seldom shall you find a merchant, a soldier, an
innkeeper, a bawd, an host, a usurer so troubled in mind, they
have cheverel consciences that will stretch, they are seldom
moved in this kind or molested: young men and middle age
are more wild and less apprehensive; but old folks, most part,
such as are timorous and religiously given."[3] Pet. Forestus,
Observat. lib. 10, *cap.* 12, *de morbis cerebri,* hath a fearful example
of a minister, that through precise fasting in Lent, and overmuch meditation, contracted this mischief, and in the end
became desperate, thought he saw devils in his chamber, and
that he could not be saved; he smelled nothing, as he said,
but fire and brimstone, was already in hell, and would ask
them still if they did not smell as much.[4] "I told him he was
melancholy, but he laughed me to scorn, and replied that he
saw devils, talked with them in good earnest, would spit in my
face and ask me if I did not smell brimstone"; but at last he
was by him cured. Such another story I find in Plater, *Observat.
lib.* 1. A poor fellow had done some foul offence, and for
fourteen days would eat no meat, in the end became desperate,
the divines about him could not ease him, but so he died.[5]
Continual meditation of God's judgments troubles many; *Multi
ob timorem futuri judicii,* saith Guatinerius, *cap.* 5, *tract.* 15,
et suspicionem desperabundi sunt [many fall into despair through
fear of the last judgment]. David himself complains that God's
judgments terrified his soul, Psalm cxix, part. 15, vers. 8: "My
flesh trembleth for fear of thee, and I am afraid of thy judgments." *Quoties diem illum cogito* (saith Hierome[6]) *toto corpore
contremisco,* I tremble as often as I think of it. The terrible

meditation of hell-fire and eternal punishment much torments a sinful silly soul. What's a thousand years to eternity? *Ubi mœror, ubi fletus, ubi dolor sempiternus; mors sine morte, finis sine fine* [the home of sorrow, weeping, eternal pain; death undying, end unending]; a finger burnt by chance we may not endure, the pain is so so grievous, we may not abide an hour, a night is intolerable; and what shall this unspeakable fire then be that burns for ever, innumerable infinite millions of years, *in omne œvum, in æternum!* O eternity!

> *Æternitas est illa vox,*
> *Vox illa fulminatrix,*
> *Tonitruis minacior,*
>   *Fragoribusque cœli,*
> *Æternitas est illa vox, . . .*
>   *Meta carens et ortu,* etc.
> *Tormenta nulla territant,*
>   *Quæ finiuntur annis;*
> *Æternitas, æternitas*
>   *Versat coquitque pectus.*
> *Auget hæc pœnas indies,*
>   *Centuplicatque flammas,* etc.[1]

> [Eternity is the dreadful word of doom, more terrifying than thunder and the crashes of the sky. Eternity is the dread word, without end or beginning. Those torments affright us not which are bounded by a span of years, but Eternity, Eternity agitates and torments the breast; daily it makes the sufferings more dire, and increases the flames a hundredfold.]

This meditation terrifies these poor distressed souls, especially if their bodies be predisposed by melancholy, they religiously given, and have tender consciences, every small object affrights them, the very inconsiderate reading of Scripture itself, and misinterpretation of some places of it, as: "Many are called, few are chosen." "Not every one that saith Lord. . . ." "Fear not, little flock." "He that stands, let him take heed lest he fall." "Work out your salvation with fear and trembling." "That night two shall be in a bed, one received, the other left." "Strait is the way that leads to heaven, and few there are that enter therein." The Parable of the Seed and of the Sower, "Some fell on barren ground, some was choked." "Whom he hath predestinated, he hath chosen." "He will have mercy on whom he will have mercy." *Non est volentis nec currentis, sed miserentis Dei* ["It is not of him that willeth, nor of him that runneth, but of God that showeth mercy"]. These and the like places terrify the souls of many; election, predestination,

reprobation, preposterously conceived, offend divers, with a deal
of foolish presumption, curiosity, needless speculation, contemplation, solicitude, wherein they trouble and puzzle themselves
about those questions of grace, free will, perseverance, God's
secrets; they will know more than is revealed of God in His
Word, human capacity or ignorance can apprehend, and too
importunate inquiry after that which is revealed; mysteries,
ceremonies, observation of Sabbaths, laws, duties, etc., with
many such which the casuists discuss, and schoolmen broach,
which divers mistake, misconster, misapply to themselves to
their own undoing, and so fall into this gulf. "They doubt of
their election, how they shall know it, by what signs; and so
far forth," saith Luther, "with such nice points, torture and
crucify themselves, that they are almost mad, and all they get
by it is this, they lay open a gap to the devil by desperation to
carry them to hell." But the greatest harm of all proceeds
from those thundering ministers, a most frequent cause they
are of this malady; "and do more harm in the Church" (saith
Erasmus [1]) "than they that flatter; great danger on both sides,
the one lulls them asleep in carnal security, the other drives
them to despair." Whereas St. Bernard well adviseth,[2] "We
should not meddle with the one without the other, nor speak
of judgment without mercy; the one alone brings desperation,
the other security." But these men are wholly for judgment; of a rigid disposition themselves, there is no mercy with
them, no salvation, no balsam for their diseased souls, they can
speak of nothing but reprobation, hell-fire, and damnation; as
they did (Luke xi, 46) lade men with burdens grievous to be
borne, which they themselves touch not with a finger. 'Tis
familiar with our papists to terrify men's souls with purgatory,
tales, visions, apparitions, to daunt even the most generous
spirits, "to require charity," as Brentius observes,[3] "of others,
bounty, meekness, love, patience, when they themselves breathe
naught but lust, envy, covetousness." They teach others to
fast, give alms, do penance, and crucify their mind with superstitious observations, bread and water, haircloths, whips, and
the like, when they themselves have all the dainties the world
can afford, lie on a down-bed with a courtesan in their arms.
Heu quantum patimur pro Christo! as he [4] said; what a cruel
tyranny is this, so to insult over and terrify men's souls! Our
indiscreet pastors, many of them, come not far behind, whilst
in their ordinary sermons they speak so much of election, predestination, reprobation *ab æterno* [from the beginning of the

world], subtraction of grace, preterition, voluntary permission, etc., by what signs and tokens they shall discern and try themselves, whether they be God's true children elect, *an sint reprobi*, *prædestinati*, etc., with such scrupulous points, they still aggravate sin, thunder out God's judgments without respect, intempestively rail at and pronounce them damned in all auditories, for giving so much to sports and honest recreations, making every small fault and thing indifferent an irremissible offence, they so rent, tear and wound men's consciences, that they are almost mad, and at their wits' end.

"These bitter potions" (saith Erasmus [1]) "are still in their mouths, nothing but gall and horror, and a mad noise, they make all their auditors desperate": many are wounded by this means, and they commonly that are most devout and precise, have been formerly presumptuous, and certain of their salvation; they that have tender consciences, that follow sermons, frequent lectures, that have indeed least cause, they are most apt to mistake, and fall into these miseries. I have heard some complain of Parsons' Resolution, and other books of like nature (good otherwise), they are too tragical, too much dejecting men, aggravating offences: great care and choice, much discretion is required in this kind.

The last and greatest cause of this malady is our own conscience, sense of our sins, and God's anger justly deserved, a guilty conscience for some foul offence formerly committed.

> *O miser Oreste, quid morbi te perdit?*
> Or. *Conscientia, sum enim mihi conscius de malis*
> *perpetratis.* [2]

> [Hapless Orestes, say, what ill consumes thee?
> *Or.* Conscience, which pricks me for my evil deeds.]

"A good conscience is a continual feast," but a galled conscience is as great a torment as can possibly happen, a still baking oven (so Pierius in his *Hieroglyph.* compares it), another hell. Our conscience, which is a great ledger-book, wherein are written all our offences, a register to lay them up (which those Egyptians in their hieroglyphics expressed by a mill, as well for the continuance as for the torture of it [3]), grinds our souls with the remembrance of some precedent sins, makes us reflect upon, accuse and condemn our own selves. "Sin lies at door," etc. [4] I know there be many other causes assigned by Zanchius, Musculus, [5] and the rest; as incredulity, infidelity, presumption, ignorance, blindness, ingratitude, discontent, those five grand miseries in Aristotle, ignominy, need, sickness, enmity, death, etc.; but this of conscience is the greatest, *instar ulceris corpus jugiter percellens*[1] [torturing the body like an ulcer]: this scrupulous conscience (as Peter Forestus calls it) which tortures so many, that either out of a deep apprehension of their unworthiness, and consideration of their own dissolute life, "accuse themselves and aggravate every small offence, when there is no such cause, misdoubting in the meantime God's mercies, they fall into these inconveniences."[2] The poets call them Furies, Diræ,[3] but it is the conscience alone which is a thousand witnesses to accuse us,

> *Nocte dieque suum gestant in pectore testem.*[4]
>
> [Night and day they carry the accusing witness in their own breast.]

A continual testor to give in evidence, to empanel a jury to examine us, to cry guilty, a persecutor with hue and cry to follow, an apparitor to summon us, a bailiff to carry us, a serjeant to arrest, an attorney to plead against us, a gaoler to torment, a judge to condemn, still accusing, denouncing, torturing and molesting. And as the statue of Juno in that holy city near Euphrates in Assyria[5] will look still towards you, sit where you will in her temple, she stares full upon you, if you go by, she follows with her eye, in all sites, places, conventicles, actions, our conscience will be still ready to accuse us. After many pleasant days and fortunate adventures, merry tides, this conscience at last doth arrest us. Well he may escape temporal punishment, bribe a corrupt judge,[6] and avoid the censure of law, and flourish for a time; for "who ever saw" (saith Chrysostom) "a covetous man troubled in mind when he is telling of his money, an adulterer mourn with his mistress in his arms? we are then drunk with pleasure, and perceive nothing":[7] yet as the prodigal son had dainty fare, sweet music at first, merry company, jovial entertainment, but a cruel reckoning in the end, as bitter as wormwood, a fearful visitation commonly follows. And the devil that then told thee that it was a light sin, or no sin at all, now aggravates on the other side, and telleth thee that it is a most irremissible offence, as he did by Cain and Judas, to bring them to despair; every small circumstance before neglected and contemned will now amplify itself, rise up in judgment, and accuse the dust of their shoes, dumb creatures, as to Lucian's tyrant *lectus et candela*, the bed and candle, did bear witness, to torment their souls for their sins past. Tragical examples in this kind are too familiar and common: Hadrian, Galba, Nero, Otho, Vitellius, Caracalla, were in such horror of conscience for their offences committed, murders, rapes, extortions, injuries, that they were weary of their lives, and could get nobody to kill them. Kennetus, King of Scotland,[1] when he had murdered his nephew Malcolm, King Duff's son, Prince of Cumberland, and with counterfeit tears and protestations dissembled the matter a long time, "at last his conscience accused him, his unquiet soul could not rest day or night, he was terrified with fearful dreams, visions, and so miserably tormented all his life." [2] It is strange to read what Comineus [3] hath written of Louis XI, that French king; of Charles VIII; of Alphonsus, King of Naples; in the fury of his passion how he came into Sicily, and what pranks he played. Guicciardine, a man most unapt to believe lies, relates how that Ferdinand his father's ghost, who before had died for grief, came and told him that he could not resist the French king, he thought every man cried France, France; the reason of it (saith Comineus) was because he was a vile tyrant, a murderer, an oppressor of his subjects, he bought up all commodities, and sold them at his own price, sold abbeys to Jews and falconers; both Ferdinand his father and he himself never made conscience of any committed sin; and to conclude, saith he, it was impossible to do worse than they did. Why was Pausanias, the Spartan tyrant, Nero, Otho, Galba, so persecuted with spirits in every house they came, but for their murders which they had committed? [4] Why doth the devil haunt many men's houses after their deaths, appear to them living, and take possession of their habitations, as it were, of their palaces, but because of their several villainies? Why had Richard the Third such fearful dreams, saith Polydore, but for his frequent murders? Why was Herod so tortured in his mind? because he had made away Mariamne his wife. Why was Theodoricus, the King of the Goths, so suspicious, and so affrighted with a fish-head alone, but that he had murdered Symmachus, and Boethius his son-in-law, those worthy Romans? (Cælius, *lib.* 27, *cap.* 22). See more in Plutarch, in his tract *de his qui sero a Numine puniuntur*, and in his book *de tranquillitate animi*, etc. Yea, and sometimes God Himself hath a hand in it, to show His power, humiliate, exercise, and to try their faith (divine temptation, Perkins calls it, *Cas. Cons. lib.* 1, *cap.* 8, *sect.* 1), to punish them for their sins; God the avenger, as David terms Him,[5] *ultor a tergo Deus*; His wrath is apprehended of a guilty soul, as by Saul and Judas, which the poets expressed by Adrastea, or Nemesis:

> *Assequitur Nemesisque virum vestigia servat,*
> *Ne male quid facias.*

[Nemesis follows in the track of man, therefore sin not.]

And she is, as Ammianus, *lib.* 14, describes her,[1] "the queen of causes, and moderator of things," now she pulls down the proud, now she rears and encourageth those that are good; he gives instance in his Eusebius; Nicephorus, *lib.* 10, *cap.* 35, *Eccles. Hist.*, in Maximinus and Julian. Fearful examples of God's just judgment, wrath and vengeance, are to be found in all histories, of some that have been eaten to death with rats and mice, as Popelius the second King of Poland, *anno* 830, his wife and children;[2] the like story is of Hatto, Archbishop of Mentz, *anno* 969, so devoured by these vermin, which howsoever Serrarius the Jesuit, *Mogunt. rerum lib.* 4, *cap.* 5, impugn by twenty-two arguments, Trithemius, Munster, Magdeburgenses,[3] and many others relate for a truth. Such another example I find in Giraldus Cambrensis, *Itin. Camb. lib.* 2, *cap.* 2, and where not?

And yet for all these terrors of conscience, affrighting punishments which are so frequent, or whatsoever else may cause or aggravate this fearful malady in other religions, I see no reason at all why a papist at any time should despair, or be troubled for his sins; for let him be never so dissolute a caitiff, so notorious a villain, so monstrous a sinner, out of that treasure of indulgences and merits of which the Pope is dispensator he may have free pardon and plenary remission of all his sins. There be so many general pardons for ages to come, forty thousand years to come, so many jubilees, so frequent gaol-deliveries out of purgatory for all souls now living, or after dissolution of the body so many particular masses daily said in several churches, so many altars consecrated to this purpose, that if a man have either money or friends, or will take any pains to come to such an altar, hear a mass, say so many paternosters, undergo such and such penance, he cannot do amiss, it is impossible his mind should be troubled, or he have any scruple to molest him. Besides that *Taxa Cameræ Apostolicæ* [tax of the Apostolic Chamber], which was first published to get money in the days of Leo Decimus, that sharking pope, and since divulged to the same ends, sets down such easy rates and dispensations for all offences, for perjury, murder, incest, adultery, etc., for so many grosses or dollars (able to invite any man to sin, and provoke him to offend, methinks, that otherwise would not), such comfortable remission, so gentle and parable a pardon, so ready at hand, with so small cost and suit obtained, that I cannot see how he that hath any friends amongst them (as I say), or money in his purse, or will at least to ease himself, can anyway miscarry or be misaffected, how he should be desperate, in danger of damnation, or troubled in mind. Their ghostly fathers can so readily apply remedies, so cunningly string and unstring, wind and unwind their devotions, play upon their consciences with plausible speeches and terrible threats, for their best advantage settle and remove, erect with such facility and deject, let in and out, that I cannot perceive how any man amongst them should much or often labour of this disease, or finally miscarry. The causes above named must more frequently therefore take hold in others.

SUBSECT. IV.—*Symptoms of Despair, Fear, Sorrow, Suspicion, Anxiety, Horror of Conscience, Fearful Dreams and Visions*

As shoemakers do when they bring home shoes, still cry leather is dearer and dearer, may I justly say of those melancholy symptoms: these of despair are most violent, tragical, and grievous, far beyond the rest, not to be expressed but negatively, as it is privation of all happiness, not to be endured; "for a wounded spirit who can bear it?" (Prov. xviii, 14). What, therefore, Timanthes did in his picture of Iphigenia,[1] now ready to be sacrificed, when he had painted Calchas mourning, Ulysses sad, but most sorrowful Menelaus, and showed all his art in expressing variety of affections, he covered the maid's father Agamemnon's head with a veil, and left it to every spectator to conceive what he would himself; for that true passion and sorrow in *summo gradu*,[2] such as his was, could not by any art be deciphered: what he did in his picture, I will do in describing the symptoms of despair; imagine what thou canst, fear, sorrow, furies, grief, pain, terror, anger, dismal, ghastly, tedious, irksome, etc., it is not sufficient, it comes far short, no tongue can tell, no heart conceive it. 'Tis an epitome of hell, an extract, a quintessence, a compound, a mixture of all feral maladies, tyrannical tortures, plagues, and perplexities. There is no sickness almost but physic provideth a remedy for it; to every sore chirurgery will provide a salve; friendship helps poverty; hope of liberty easeth imprisonment; suit and favour revoke banishment; authority and time wear away reproach: but what physic, what chirurgery, what wealth, favour, authority can relieve, bear out, assuage, or expel a troubled conscience? A quiet mind cureth all them, but all they cannot comfort a distressed soul: who can put to silence the voice of desperation? All that is single in other melancholy, *horribile, dirum, pestilens, atrox, ferum* [horrible, terrible, loathsome, cruel, barbarous], concur in this, it is more than melancholy in the highest degree; a burning fever of the soul; so mad, saith Jacchinus,[1] by this misery; fear, sorrow, and despair he puts for ordinary symptoms of melancholy. They are in great pain and horror of mind, distraction of soul, restless, full of continual fears, cares, torments, anxieties, they can neither eat, drink, nor sleep for them, take no rest:

> *Perpetua impietas, nec mensæ tempore cessat,*
> *Exagitat vesana quies, somnique furentes.*[2]

> Neither at bed, nor yet at board,
> Will any rest despair afford.

Fear takes away their content, and dries the blood, wasteth the marrow, alters their countenance, "even in their greatest delights, singing, dancing, dalliance," they are still (saith Lemnius[3]) tortured in their souls. It consumes them to naught: "I am like a pelican in the wilderness" (saith David of himself, temporally afflicted), "an owl, because of thine indignation" (Ps. cii, 6, 10); and (Ps. lv, 4), "My heart trembleth within me, and the terrors of death have come upon me; fear and trembling are come upon me," etc.; "at death's door" (Ps. cvii, 18) "their soul abhors all manner of meats." Their sleep is (if it be any) unquiet, subject to fearful dreams and terrors.[4] Peter in his bonds slept secure, for he knew God protected him; and Tully makes it an argument of Roscius Amerinus' innocency, that he killed not his father, because he so securely slept. Those martyrs in the primitive Church were most cheerful and merry in the midst of their persecutions;[5] but it is far otherwise with these men, tossed in a sea, and that continually without rest or intermission; they can think of naught that is pleasant, "their conscience will not let them be quiet,"[6] in perpetual fear, anxiety, if they be not yet apprehended, they are in doubt still they shall be ready to betray themselves, as Cain did, he thinks every man will kill him; "and roar for the grief of heart" (Ps. xxxviii, 8), as David did; as Job did (iii, 20, 21, 22, etc.):

"Wherefore is light given to him that is in misery, and life to them that have heavy hearts? which long for death, and if it come not, search it more than treasures, and rejoice when they can find the grave." They are generally weary of their lives, a trembling heart they have, a sorrowful mind, and little or no rest: *Terror ubique tremor, timor undique et undique terror*, fears, terrors, and affrights in all places, at all times and seasons. *Cibum et potum pertinaciter aversantur multi, nodum in scirpo quæritantes, et culpam imaginantes ubi nulla est*, as Wierus writes, *de lamiis, lib.* 3, *cap.* 7, they refuse many of them meat and drink, cannot rest, aggravating still and supposing grievous offences where there are none. God's heavy wrath is kindled in their souls, and notwithstanding their continual prayers and supplications to Christ Jesus, they have no release or ease at all, but a most intolerable torment, and insufferable anguish of conscience, and that makes them, through impatience, to murmur against God many times, to rave, to blaspheme, turn atheists, and seek to offer violence to themselves. Deut. xxviii, 65, 66, 67: "In the morning they wish for evening, and for morning in the evening, for the sight of their eyes which they see, and fear of hearts." Marinus Marcennus, in his Comment on Genesis,[1] makes mention of a desperate friend of his, whom, amongst others, he came to visit and exhort to patience, that broke out into most blasphemous atheistical speeches, too fearful to relate, when they wished him to trust in God. *Quis est ille Deus (inquit) ut serviam illi, quid proderit si oraverim; si præsens est, cur non succurrit? cur non me carcere, inedia, squalore confectum liberat? quid ego feci? etc. Absit a me hujus-modi Deus.* [Who is that God that I should serve Him, what will it help me if I pray to Him? If He exists, why does He not help me? Why does He not rescue me from prison, starvation, and misery? What have I done? Far be from me such a God.] Another of his acquaintance broke out into like atheistical blasphemies upon his wife's death, raved, cursed, said and did he cared not what. And so for the most part it is with them all; many of them in their extremity think they hear and see visions, outcries, confer with devils, that they are tormented, possessed, and in hell-fire, already damned, quite forsaken of God, they have no sense or feeling of mercy or grace, hope of salvation, their sentence of condemnation is already past and not to be revoked, the devil will certainly have them. Never was any living creature in such torment before, in such a miserable estate, in such distress of mind, no hope, no faith, past cure, reprobate, continually tempted to make away themselves. Something talks with them, they spit fire and brimstone, they cannot but blaspheme, they cannot repent, believe, or think a good thought, so far carried, *ut cogantur ad impia cogitandum etiam contra voluntatem* [they are constrained to harbour impious thoughts against their will], said Felix Plater,[1] *ad blasphemiam erga Deum, ad multa horrenda perpetranda, ad manus violentas sibi inferendas* [to blaspheming God, doing horrible things, laying violent hands upon themselves], etc., and in their distracted fits and desperate humours to offer violence to others, their familiar and dear friends sometimes, or to mere strangers, upon very small or no occasion; for he that cares not for his own is master of another man's life. They think evil against their wills, that which they abhor themselves, they must needs think, do, and speak. He gives instance in a patient of his, that when he would pray, had such evil thoughts still suggested to him, and wicked meditations.[2] Another instance he hath, of a woman that was often tempted to curse God, to blaspheme and kill herself. Sometimes the devil (as they say) stands without and talks with them, sometimes he is within them, as they think, and there speaks and talks as to such as are possessed: so Apollodorus, in Plutarch, thought his heart spake within him. There is a most memorable example of Francis Spira,[3] an advocate of Padua, *anno* 1545, that being desperate, by no counsel of learned men could be comforted: he felt (as he said) the pains of hell in his soul; in all other things he discoursed aright, but in this most mad. Frisimelica, Bullovat, and some other excellent physicians, could neither make him eat, drink, nor sleep, no persuasion could ease him. Never pleaded any man so well for himself as this man did against himself, and so he desperately died. Springer, a lawyer, hath written his life. Cardinal Crescence died so likewise desperate at Verona; still he thought a black dog followed him to his death-bed, no man could drive the dog away (Sleidan, *Com. cap.* 23, *lib.* 3). "Whilst I was writing this treatise," saith Montaltus, *cap.* 2 *de mel.*, "a nun came to me for help, well for all other matters, but troubled in conscience for five years last past; she is almost mad, and not able to resist, thinks she hath offended God, and is certainly damned."[4] Felix Plater hath store of instances of such as thought themselves damned, forsaken of God, etc.;[5] one amongst the rest, that durst not go to church, or come near the Rhine, for fear to make away himself, because then he was most especially tempted. These and such-like symptoms are intended and remitted, as the malady itself is more or less; some will hear good counsel, some will not; some desire help, some reject all, and will not be eased.

SUBSECT. V.—*Prognostics of Despair, Atheism, Blasphemy, Violent Death, etc.*

Most part, these kind of persons make away themselves;[1] some are mad, blaspheme, curse, deny God, but most offer violence to their own persons, and sometimes to others: "A wounded spirit who can bear?" (Prov. xviii, 14); as Cain, Saul, Achitophel, Judas, blasphemed and died. Bede saith, Pilate died desperate, eight years after Christ. Felix Plater hath collected many examples.[2] "A merchant's wife, that was long troubled with such temptations,"[3] in the night rose from her bed, and out of the window broke her neck into the street; another drowned himself, desperate as he was, in the Rhine; some cut their throats, many hang themselves. But this needs no illustration. It is controverted by some, whether a man so offering violence to himself, dying desperate, may be saved, ay or no? If they die so obstinately and suddenly that they cannot so much as wish for mercy, the worst is to be suspected, because they die impenitent. If their death had been a little more lingering, wherein they might have some leisure in their hearts to cry for mercy, charity may judge the best;[4] divers have been recovered out of the very act of hanging and drowning themselves, and so brought *ad sanam mentem* [to their senses], they have been very penitent, much abhorred their former act, confessed that they have repented in an instant, and cried for mercy in their hearts. If a man put desperate hands upon himself by occasion of madness or melancholy, if he have given testimony before of his regeneration, in regard he doth this not so much out of his will as *ex vi morbi* [on account of his disease], we must make the best construction of it, as Turks do, that think all fools and madmen go directly to heaven.[5]

SUBSECT. VI.—*Cure of Despair by Physic, Good Counsel, Comforts, etc.*

Experience teacheth us, that though many die obstinate and wilful in this malady, yet multitudes again are able to resist and overcome, seek for help and find comfort, are taken *e*

faucibus Erebi, from the chops of hell, and out of the devil's
paws, though they have by obligation given themselves to him.[1]
Some out of their own strength, and God's assistance—"Though
He kill me" (saith Job), "yet will I trust in Him"—out of
good counsel, advice and physic. Bellovacus cured a monk
by altering his habit and course of life;[2] Plater many by physic
alone. But for the most part they must concur; and they take
a wrong course that think to overcome this feral passion by sole
physic; and they are as much out, that think to work this
effect by good advice alone; though both be forcible in themselves, yet *vis unita fortior* [their combined force is greater],
they must go hand in hand to this disease: *Alterius sic altera
poscit opem* [one requires the assistance of the other]. For
physic, the like course is to be taken with this as in other
melancholy: diet, air, exercise; all those passions and perturbations of the mind, etc., are to be rectified by the same means.
They must not be left solitary, or to themselves, never idle,
never out of company. Counsel, good comfort is to be applied,
as they shall see the parties inclined, or to the causes, whether
it be loss, fear, grief, discontent, or some such feral accident,
a guilty conscience, or otherwise by frequent meditation, too
grievous an apprehension, and consideration of his former life;
by hearing, reading of Scriptures, good divines, good advice
and conference, applying God's Word to their distressed souls,
it must be corrected and counterpoised. Many excellent exhortations, parænetical discourses, are extant to this purpose, for
such as are anyway troubled in mind: Perkins, Greenham,
Hayward, Bright, Abernethy, Bolton, Culmannus, Hemmingius,
Cælius Secundus, Nicholas Laurentius, are copious on this subject; Azorius, Navarrus, Sayrus, etc., and such as have written
cases of conscience amongst our pontifical writers. But because
these men's works are not to all parties at hand, so parable
at all times, I will for the benefit and ease of such as are afflicted,
at the request of some friends,[3] recollect out of their voluminous
treatises some few such comfortable speeches, exhortations,
arguments, advice, tending to this subject, and out of God's
Word, knowing, as Culmannus saith upon the like occasion,
"how unavailable and vain men's counsels are to comfort an
afflicted conscience, except God's Word concur and be annexed,
from which comes life, ease, repentance,"[4] etc. Presupposing
first that which Beza, Greenham, Perkins, Bolton, give in charge,
the parties to whom counsel is given be sufficiently prepared,
humbled for their sins, fit for comfort, confessed, tried how they

are more or less afflicted, how they stand affected, or capable of good advice, before any remedies be applied: to such therefore as are so throughly searched and examined, I address this following discourse.

Two main antidotes, Hemmingius observes,[1] opposite to despair: good hope out of God's Word, to be embraced; perverse security and presumption from the devil's treachery, to be rejected; *Illa salus animæ, hæc pestis:* one saves, the other kills, *occidit animam*, saith Austin, and doth as much harm as despair itself, Navarrus the casuist [2] reckons up ten special cures out of Anton., 1 *part. tit.* 3, *cap.* 10: 1. God. 2. Physic. 3. Avoiding such objects as have caused it.[3] 4. Submission of himself to other men's judgments. 5. Answer of all objections, etc. All which Cajetan, Gerson, *lib. de vit. spirit.*, Sayrus, *lib.* 1 *Cas. cons. cap.* 14, repeat and approve out of Emanuel Roderiques, *cap.* 51 *et* 52. Greenham prescribes six special rules, Culmannus seven. First, to acknowledge all help come from God. 2. That the cause of their present misery is sin. 3. To repent and be heartily sorry for their sins. 4. To pray earnestly to God they may be eased. 5. To expect and implore the prayers of the Church, and good men's advice. 6. Physic. 7. To commend themselves to God, and rely upon His mercy: others otherwise, but all to this effect. But forasmuch as most men in this malady are spiritually sick, void of reason almost, overborne by their miseries and too deep an apprehension of their sins, they cannot apply themselves to good counsel, pray, believe, repent, we must, as much as in us lies, occur and help their peculiar infirmities, according to their several causes and symptoms, as we shall find them distressed and complain.

The main matter which terrifies and torments most that are troubled in mind, is the enormity of their offences, the intolerable burthen of their sins, God's heavy wrath and displeasure so deeply apprehended, that they account themselves reprobates, quite forsaken of God, already damned, past all hope of grace, uncapable of mercy, *diaboli mancipia*, slaves of sin, and their offences so great they cannot be forgiven. But these men must know there is no sin so heinous which is not pardonable in itself, no crime so great but by God's mercy it may be forgiven. "Where sin aboundeth, grace aboundeth much more" (Rom. v, 20). And what the Lord said unto Paul in his extremity (2 Cor. xii, 9), "My grace is sufficient for thee, for my power is made perfect through weakness," concerns every man in like case. His promises are made indefinite to all believers, generally spoken to all, touching remission of sins, that are truly penitent, grieved for their offences, and desire to be reconciled; Matt. ix, 12, 13: "I came not to call the righteous, but sinners to repentance," that is, such as are truly touched in conscience for their sins. Again, Matt. xi, 28: "Come unto me all ye that are heavy laden, and I will ease you"; Ezek. xviii, 27: "At what time soever a sinner shall repent him of his sins from the bottom of his heart, I will blot out all his wickedness out of my remembrance, saith the Lord"; Is. xliii, 25: "I, even I, am he that put away thine iniquity for mine own sake, and will not remember thy sins." "As a father" (saith David, Ps. ciii, 13) "hath compassion on his children, so hath the Lord compassion on them that fear Him"; and will receive them again as the prodigal son was entertained (Luke xv), if they shall so come with tears in their eyes, and a penitent heart. *Peccator agnoscat, Deus ignoscit* [if the sinner confesses, God forgives]. "The Lord is full of compassion and mercy, slow to anger, of great kindness" (Ps. ciii, 8). "He will not always chide, neither keep His anger for ever" (v. 9). "As high as the heaven is above the earth, so great is His mercy towards them that fear Him" (v. 11). "As far as the east is from the west, so far hath He removed our sins from us" (v. 12). Though Cain cry out in the anguish of his soul, My punishment is greater than I can bear, 'tis not so; "Thou liest, Cain" (saith Austin), "God's mercy is greater than thy sins." "His mercy is above all His works" (Ps. cxlv, 9), able to satisfy for all men's sins, *antilutron* (1 Tim. ii, 6). His mercy is a panacea, a balsam for an afflicted soul, a sovereign medicine, an alexipharmacum for all sin, a charm for the devil; His mercy was great to Solomon, to Manasseh, to Peter, great to all offenders, and whosoever thou art, it may be so to thee. For why should God bid us pray (as Austin infers) "Deliver us from all evil," *nisi ipse misericors perseveraret*, if He did not intend to help us? He therefore that doubts of the remission of his sins, denies God's mercy, and doth Him injury, saith Austin.[1] Yea, but, thou repliest, I am a notorious sinner, mine offences are not so great as infinite. Hear Fulgentius: "God's invincible goodness cannot be overcome by sin, His infinite mercy cannot be terminated by any: the multitude of His mercy is equivalent to His magnitude."[2] Hear Chrysostom: "Thy malice may be measured, but God's mercy cannot be defined; thy malice is circumscribed, His mercy's infinite."[3] As a drop of water is to the sea, so are thy misdeeds to His mercy: nay, there is no such proportion to be given; for the sea, though great, yet may be measured, but God's mercy cannot be circumscribed. Whatsoever thy sins be then in quantity or quality, multitude or magnitude, fear them not, distrust not. "I speak not this," saith Chrysostom, "to make thee secure and negligent, but to cheer thee up." [1] Yea, but thou urgest again, I have little comfort of this which is said, it concerns me not: *inanis pœnitentia quam sequens culpa coinquinat*, 'tis to no purpose for me to repent, and to do worse than ever I did before, to persevere in sin, and to return to my lusts as a dog to his vomit, or a swine to the mire: to what end is it to ask forgiveness of my sins, and yet daily to sin again and again, to do evil out of an habit? [2] I daily and hourly offend in thought, word, and deed, in a relapse by mine own weakness and wilfulness: my *bonus genius*, my good protecting angel is gone, I am fallen from that I was or would be, worse and worse, "my latter end is worse than my beginning." *Si quotidie peccas, quotidie*, saith Chrysostom, *pœnitentiam age*, if thou daily offend, daily repent; "if twice, thrice, an hundred, an hundred thousand times, twice, thrice, an hundred thousand times repent." [3] As they do by an old house that is out of repair, still mend some part or other; so do by thy soul, still reform some vice, repair it by repentance, call to Him for grace, and thou shalt have it; "for we are freely justified by His grace" (Rom. iii, 24). If thine enemy repent, as our Saviour enjoined Peter, forgive him seventy-seven times; and why shouldst thou think God will not forgive thee? Why should the enormity of thy sins trouble thee? God can do it, He will do it. "My conscience" (saith Anselm) "dictates to me that I deserve damnation, my repentance will not suffice for satisfaction: but Thy mercy, O Lord, quite overcomes all my transgressions." [4] The gods once (as the poets feign) with a gold chain would pull Jupiter out of heaven, but all they together could not stir him, and yet he could draw and turn them as he would himself; maugre all the force and fury of these infernal fiends, and crying sins, "His grace is sufficient." Confer the debt and the payment; Christ and Adam; sin and the cure of it; the disease and the medicine; confer the sick man to his physician, and thou shalt soon perceive that His power is infinitely beyond it. God is better able, as Bernard informeth us, "to help, than sin to do us hurt; Christ is better able to save, than the devil to destroy." [5] If He be a skilful physician, as Fulgentius adds, "He can cure all diseases; if merciful, He will." [6] *Non est perfecta bonitas, a qua non omnis malitia vincitur*, His goodness is not absolute

and perfect, if it be not able to overcome all malice. Submit thyself
unto Him, as St. Austin adviseth, "He knoweth best what he
doth; and be not so much pleased when He sustains thee, as
patient when He corrects thee; He is omnipotent, and can cure
all diseases when He sees his own time." [1] He looks down from
heaven upon earth, that He may hear the "mourning of
prisoners, and deliver the children of death" (Ps. cii, 19, 20).
"And though our sins be as red as scarlet, He can make them
as white as snow" (Is. i, 18).   Doubt not of this, or ask how it
shall be done: He is all-sufficient that promiseth; *Qui fecit
mundum de immundo*, saith Chrysostom, He that made a fair
world of naught, can do this and much more for His part: do
thou only believe, trust in Him, rely on Him, be penitent and
heartily sorry for thy sins.   Repentance is a sovereign remedy
for all sins, a spiritual wing to erear us, a charm for our miseries,
a protecting amulet to expel sin's venom, an attractive loadstone to draw God's mercy and graces unto us.   *Peccatum vulnus,
pænitentia medicinam:* [2] sin made the breach, repentance must
help it; howsoever thine offence came, by error, sloth, obstinacy,
ignorance, *exitur per pænitentiam*, this is the sole means to be
relieved.   Hence comes our hope of safety, by this alone sinners
are saved, God is provoked to mercy.   "This unlooseth all
that is bound, enlighteneth darkness, mends that is broken, puts
life to that which was desperately dying": [3] makes no respect of
offences, or of persons.   "This doth not repel a fornicator,
reject a drunkard, resist a proud fellow, turn away an idolater,
but entertains all, communicates itself to all." [4]   Who persecuted the Church more than Paul, offended more than Peter?
and yet by repentance (saith Chrysologus) they got both
magisterium et ministerium sanctitatis, the magistery [and
ministry] of holiness.   The prodigal son went far, but by
repentance he came home at last.   "This alone will turn a
wolf into a sheep, make a publican a preacher, turn a thorn
into an olive, make a debauched fellow religious," [5] a blasphemer
sing hallelujah, make Alexander the coppersmith truly devout,
make a devil a saint, "and him that polluted his mouth with
calumnies, lying, swearing, and filthy tunes and tones, to
purge his throat with divine psalms." [6]   Repentance will effect
prodigious cures, make a stupend metamorphosis.   "An hawk
came into the ark and went out again an hawk; a lion came in,
went out a lion; a bear, a bear; a wolf, a wolf; but if an hawk
come into this sacred temple of repentance, he will go forth a
dove" (saith Chrysostom), "a wolf go out a sheep, a lion a

lamb." [1] "This gives sight to the blind, legs to the lame, cures all diseases, confers grace, expels vice, inserts virtue, comforts and fortifies the soul." [2] Shall I say, let thy sin be what it will, do but repent, it is sufficient? *Quem pœnitet peccasse pene est innocens* [3] [he who repents of his sin is wellnigh innocent]. 'Tis true indeed, and all-sufficient this, they do confess, if they could, repent; but they are obdurate, they have cauterized consciences, they are in a reprobate sense, they cannot think a good thought, they cannot hope for grace, pray, believe, repent, or be sorry for their sins, they find no grief for sin in themselves, but rather a delight, no groaning of spirit, but are carried headlong to their own destruction, "heaping wrath to themselves against the day of wrath" (Rom. ii, 5). 'Tis a grievous case this, I do yield, and yet not to be despaired; God of His bounty and mercy calls all to repentance (Rom. ii, 4); thou mayst be called at length, restored, taken to His grace, as the thief upon the cross at the last hour, as Mary Magdalen and many other sinners have been, that were buried in sin. "God" (saith Fulgentius) "is delighted in the conversion of a sinner, He sets no time"; [4] *prolixitas temporis Deo non prœjudicat, aut gravitas peccati*, deferring of time or grievousness of sin do not prejudicate His grace, things past and to come are all one to Him, as present: 'tis never too late to repent. "This heaven of repentance is still open for all distressed souls"; [5] and howsoever as yet no signs appear, thou mayst repent in good time. Hear a comfortable speech of St. Austin: "Whatsoever thou shalt do, how great a sinner soever, thou art yet living; if God would not help thee, He would surely take thee away; but in sparing thy life, He gives thee leisure, and invites thee to repentance." [6] Howsoever as yet, I say, thou perceivest no fruit, no feeling, findest no likelihood of it in thyself, patiently abide the Lord's good leisure, despair not, or think thou art a reprobate; He came to call sinners to repentance, (Luke v, 32), of which number thou art one; He came to call thee, and in His time will surely call thee. And although as yet thou hast no inclination to pray, to repent, thy faith be cold and dead, and thou wholly averse from all divine functions, yet it may revive, as trees are dead in winter, but flourish in the spring; these virtues may lie hid in thee for the present, yet hereafter show themselves, and peradventure already bud, howsoever thou dost not perceive it. 'Tis Satan's policy to plead against, suppress and aggravate, to conceal those sparks of faith in thee. Thou dost not believe, thou sayest, yet thou

wouldst believe if thou couldst, 'tis thy desire to believe;
then pray, "Lord, help mine unbelief";[1] and hereafter thou
shalt certainly believe: *Dabitur sitienti*,[2] it shall be given to him
that thirsteth.   Thou canst not yet repent, hereafter thou shalt;
a black cloud of sin as yet obnubilates thy soul, terrifies thy
conscience, but this cloud may conceive a rainbow at the last,
and be quite dissipated by repentance.   Be of good cheer; a
child is rational in power, not in act; and so art thou penitent
in affection, though not yet in action.   'Tis thy desire to
please God, to be heartily sorry; comfort thyself, no time is
overpast, 'tis never too late.   A desire to repent is repentance
itself, though not in nature, yet in God's acceptance; a willing
mind is sufficient.   "Blessed are they that hunger and thirst
after righteousness" (Matt. v, 6).   He that is destitute of
God's grace, and wisheth for it, shall have it.   "The Lord"
(saith David, Ps. x, 17) "will hear the desire of the poor," that
is, of such as are in distress of body and mind.   'Tis true thou
canst not as yet grieve for thy sin, thou hast no feeling of faith,
I yield; yet canst thou grieve thou dost not grieve?   It troubles
thee, I am sure, thine heart should be so impenitent and hard,
thou wouldst have it otherwise; 'tis thy desire to grieve, to
repent and believe.   Thou lovest God's children and saints
in the meantime, hatest them not, persecutest them not, but
rather wishest thyself a true professor, to be as they are, as thou
thyself hast been heretofore; which is an evident token thou art
in no such desperate case.   'Tis a good sign of thy conversion,
thy sins are pardonable, thou art, or shalt surely be reconciled,
"The Lord is near them that are of a contrite heart" (Luke iv,
18).   A true desire of mercy in the want of mercy, is mercy
itself; a desire of grace in the want of grace, is grace itself; a
constant and earnest desire to believe, repent, and to be reconciled to God, if it be in a touched heart, is an acceptation of
God, a reconciliation, faith and repentance itself.[3]   For it is
not thy faith and repentance, as Chrysostom truly teacheth,
that is available, but God's mercy that is annexed to it,[4] He
accepts the will for the deed.   So that I conclude, to feel in
ourselves the want of grace, and to be grieved for it, is grace
itself.   I am troubled with fear my sins are not forgiven,
Careless objects: but Bradford answers they are; "for God
hath given thee a penitent and believing heart, that is, an heart
which desireth to repent and believe; for such a one is taken of
Him (He accepting the will for the deed) for a truly penitent
and believing heart."

All this is true, thou repliest, but yet it concerns not thee,
'tis verified in ordinary offenders, in common sins, but thine
are of an higher strain, even against the Holy Ghost Himself,
irremissible sins, sins of the first magnitude, written with a pen
of iron, engraven with the point of a diamond. Thou art
worse than a pagan, infidel, Jew, or Turk, for thou art an
apostate and more, thou hast voluntarily blasphemed, renounced God and all religion, thou art worse than Judas himself, or they that crucified Christ: for they did offend out of
ignorance, but thou hast thought in thine heart there is no
God. Thou hast given thy soul to the devil, as witches and
conjurors do, *explicite* and *implicite*, by compact, band, and
obligation (a desperate, a fearful case), to satisfy thy lust or
to be revenged of thine enemies; thou didst never pray, come
to church, hear, read, or do any divine duties with any devotion,
but for formality and fashion sake, with a kind of reluctancy,
'twas troublesome and painful to thee to perform any such
thing, *præter voluntatem*, against thy will. Thou never mad'st
any conscience of lying, swearing, bearing false witness, murder,
adultery, bribery, oppression, theft, drunkenness, idolatry,
but hast ever done all duties for fear of punishment, as they
were most advantageous, and to thine own ends, and committed all such notorious sins with an extraordinary delight,
hating that thou shouldst love, and loving that thou shouldst
hate. Instead of faith, fear and love of God, repentance, etc.,
blasphemous thoughts have been ever harboured in his mind,
even against God Himself, the blessed Trinity; the Scripture
false,[1] rude, harsh, immethodical; heaven, hell, resurrection,
mere toys and fables, incredible, impossible, absurd, vain, ill
contrived;[2] religion, policy and human invention, to keep men
in obedience, or for profit, invented by priests and lawgivers
to that purpose. If there be any such supreme power, He takes
no notice of our doings, hears not our prayers, regardeth them
not, will not, cannot help, or else He is partial, an excepter of
persons, author of sin, a cruel, a destructive God, to create our
souls and destinate them to eternal damnation, to make us
worse than our dogs and horses; why doth He not govern
things better, protect good men, root out wicked livers? why
do they prosper and flourish? as she raved in the tragedy,[3]
Pellices cœlum tenent [concubines are throned in heaven], there
they shine, *Suasque Perseus aureas stellas habet* [and Perseus
hath his own golden stars]; where is His providence? how
appears it?

Marmoreo Licinus tumulo jacet, at Cato parvo,
    Pomponius nullo.   Quis putet esse Deos?
    [Licinus is buried in a marble tomb, Cato in a common
        grave, and Pomponius lies unburied.   Can you
        believe there is a God?]

Why doth He suffer Turks to overcome Christians, the enemy
to triumph over His Church, paganism to domineer in all places
as it doth, heresies to multiply, such enormities to be committed, and so many such bloody wars, murders, massacres,
plagues, feral diseases? why doth He not make us all good,
able, sound? why makes He venomous creatures, rocks, sands,
deserts, this earth itself the muck-hill of the world, a prison, an
house of correction? [1] *Mentimur regnare Jovem* [we feign
that Jove rules], etc., with many such horrible and execrable
conceits, not fit to be uttered; *terribilia de fide, horribilia de
Divinitate* [terrible things about the faith, horrible things about
the Divinity].   They cannot some of them but think evil,
they are compelled, *volentes nolentes,* to blaspheme, especially
when they come to church and pray, read, etc., such foul and
prodigious suggestions come into their hearts.

    These are abominable, unspeakable offences, and most oppo-
site to God, *tentationes fœdæ et impiæ* [foul and impious tempta-
tions], yet in this case, he or they that shall be tempted and
so affected, must know that no man living is free from such
thoughts in part, or at some times, the most divine spirits have
been so tempted in some sort, evil custom, omission of holy
exercises, ill company, idleness, solitariness, melancholy or
depraved nature, and the devil is still ready to corrupt, trouble,
and divert our souls, to suggest such blasphemous thoughts
into our phantasies, ungodly, profane, monstrous and wicked
conceits.   If they come from Satan, they are more speedy,
fearful and violent, the parties cannot avoid them: they are
more frequent, I say, and monstrous when they come; for the
devil he is a spirit, and hath means and opportunity to mingle
himself with our spirits, and sometimes more slyly, sometimes
more abruptly and openly, to suggest such devilish thoughts
into our hearts; he insults and domineers in melancholy distempered phantasies and persons especially; melancholy is
balneum diaboli, as Serapio holds, the devil's bath, and invites
him to come to it.   As a sick man frets, raves in his fits, speaks
and doth he knows not what, the devil violently compels such
crazed souls to think such damned thoughts against their wills,
they cannot but do it; sometimes more continuate, or by fits,
he takes his advantage, as the subject is less able to resist, he

III—*O   888 aggravates, extenuates, affirms, denies, damns, confounds the spirits, troubles heart, brain, humours, organs, senses, and wholly domineers in their imaginations. If they proceed from themselves, such thoughts, they are remiss and moderate, not so violent and monstrous, not so frequent. The devil commonly suggests things opposite to nature, opposite to God and His Word, impious, absurd, such as a man would never of himself, or could not conceive, they strike terror and horror into the parties' own hearts. For if he or they be asked whether they do approve of such-like thoughts or no, they answer (and their own souls truly dictate as much) they abhor them as hell and the devil himself, they would fain think otherwise if they could; he hath thought otherwise, and with all his soul desires so to think again; he doth resist, and hath some good motions intermixed now and then: so that such blasphemous, impious, unclean thoughts are not his own, but the devil's; they proceed not from him, but from a crazed phantasy, distempered humours, black fumes which offend his brain: [1] they are thy crosses, the devil's sins, and he shall answer for them, he doth enforce thee to do that which thou dost abhor, and didst never give consent to: and although he hath sometimes so slyly set upon thee, and so far prevailed as to make thee in some sort to assent to such wicked thoughts, to delight in [them], yet they have not proceeded from a confirmed will in thee, but are of that nature which thou dost afterwards reject and abhor. Therefore be not overmuch troubled and dismayed with such kind of suggestions, at least if they please thee not, because they are not thy personal sins, for which thou shalt incur the wrath of God, or His displeasure: contemn, neglect them, let them go as they come, strive not too violently, or trouble thyself too much, but as our Saviour said to Satan in like case, say thou, "Avoid, Satan," I detest thee and them. *Satanæ est mala ingerere* (saith Austin), *nostrum non consentire:* as Satan labours to suggest, so must we strive not to give consent, and it will be sufficient: the more anxious and solicitous thou art, the more perplexed, the more thou shalt otherwise be troubled and entangled. Besides, they must know this, all so molested and distempered, that although these be most execrable and grievous sins, they are pardonable yet, through God's mercy and goodness they may be forgiven, if they be penitent and sorry for them. Paul himself confesseth (Rom. xvii, 19): "He did not the good he would do, but the evil which he would not do; 'tis not I, but sin that dwelleth in me." 'Tis not thou, but

Satan's suggestions, his craft and subtlety, his malice. Comfort thyself then, if thou be penitent and grieved, or desirous to be so, these heinous sins shall not be laid to thy charge; God's mercy is above all sins, which if thou do not finally contemn, without doubt thou shalt be saved. "No man sins against the Holy Ghost, but he that wilfully and finally renounceth Christ, and contemneth Him and His word to the last, without which there is no salvation, from which grievous sin, God of His infinite mercy deliver us." [1] Take hold of this to be thy comfort, and meditate withal on God's word, labour to pray, to repent, to be renewed in mind, "keep thine heart with all diligence" (Prov. iv, 13), resist the devil, and he will fly from thee, pour out thy soul unto the Lord with sorrowful Hannah, "pray continually," as Paul enjoins, and, as David did (Ps. i), "meditate on His law day and night."

Yea, but this meditation is that mars all, and mistaken makes many men far worse, misconceiving all they read or hear, to their own overthrow; the more they search and read Scriptures, or divine treatises, the more they puzzle themselves, as a bird in a net, the more they are entangled and precipitated into this preposterous gulf. "Many are called, but few are chosen" (Matt. xx, 16, and xxii, 14), with such-like places of Scripture misinterpreted, strike them with horror; they doubt presently whether they be of this number or no: God's eternal decree of predestination, absolute reprobation, and such fatal tables, they form to their own ruin, and impinge upon this rock of despair. How shall they be assured of their salvation? by what signs? "If the righteous scarcely be saved, where shall the ungodly and sinners appear?" (1 Pet. iv, 18). Who knows, saith Solomon, whether he be elect? This grinds their souls; how shall they discern they are not reprobates? But I say again, how shall they discern they are? From the devil can be no certainty, for he is a liar from the beginning; if he suggests any such thing, as too frequently he doth, reject him as a deceiver, an enemy of humankind, dispute not with him, give no credit to him, obstinately refuse him, as St. Anthony did in the wilderness, whom the devil set upon in several shapes; or as the collier did, so do thou by him. For when the devil tempted him with the weakness of his faith, and told him he could not be saved, as being ignorant in the principles of religion, and urged him moreover to know what he believed, what he thought of such and such points and mysteries: the collier told him he believed as the Church did; "But what" (said the devil again) "doth the Church believe?" "As I do" (said the collier); "And what's that thou believest?" "As the Church doth," etc.; when the devil could get no other answer, he left him. If Satan summon thee to answer, send him to Christ: He is thy liberty, thy protector against cruel death, raging sin, that roaring lion; He is thy righteousness, thy Saviour, and thy life. Though he say thou art not of the number of the elect, a reprobate, forsaken of God, hold thine own still, *hic murus aheneus esto*, let this be as a bulwark, a brazen wall to defend thee, stay thyself in that certainty of faith; let that be thy comfort, Christ will protect thee, vindicate thee, thou art one of His flock, He will triumph over the law, vanquish death, overcome the devil, and destroy hell. If he say thou art none of the elect, no believer, reject him, defy him, thou hast thought otherwise, and mayst so be resolved again; comfort thyself; this persuasion cannot come from the devil, and much less can it be grounded from thyself; men are liars, and why shouldest thou distrust? A denying Peter, a persecuting Paul, an adulterous cruel David, have been received; an apostate Solomon may be converted; no sin at all but impenitency can give testimony of final reprobation. Why shouldest thou then distrust, misdoubt thyself, upon what ground, what suspicion? This opinion alone of particularity? Against that, and for the certainty of election and salvation on the other side, see God's good will toward men, hear how generally His grace is proposed to him, and him, and them, each man in particular, and to all; 1 Tim. ii, 4: "God will that all men be saved, and come to the knowledge of the truth." 'Tis an universal promise, "God sent not His Son into the world to condemn the world, but that through Him the world might be saved" (John iii, 17). He that acknowledgeth himself a man in the world, must likewise acknowledge he is of that number that is to be saved; Ezek. xxxiii, 11: "I will not the death of a sinner, but that he repent and live." But thou art a sinner; therefore He will not thy death. "This is the will of Him that sent me, that every man that believeth in the Son should have everlasting life" (John vi, 40). "He would have no man perish, but all come to repentance" (2 Pet. iii, 9). Besides, remission of sins is to be preached, not to a few, but universally to all men, "Go therefore and tell all nations, baptizing them," etc. (Matt. xxviii, 19). "Go into all the world, and preach the Gospel to every creature" (Mark xvi, 15). Now there cannot be contradictory wills in God; He will have all saved, and not all, how can this stand together? be secure then, believe, trust in Him, hope well, and be saved. Yea, that's the main matter, how shall I believe, or discern my security from carnal presumption? my faith is weak and faint, I want those signs and fruits of sanctification, sorrow for sin, thirsting for grace, groanings of the spirit, love of Christians as Christians, avoiding occasion of sin, endeavour of new obedience, charity, love of God, perseverance.[1] Though these signs be languishing in thee, and not seated in thine heart, thou must not therefore be dejected or terrified; the effects of the faith and spirit are not yet so fully felt in thee; conclude not therefore thou art a reprobate, or doubt of thine election, because the elect themselves are without them before their conversion. Thou mayst in the Lord's good time be converted; some are called at the eleventh hour. Use, I say, the means of thy conversion, expect the Lord's leisure; if not yet called, pray thou mayst be, or at least wish and desire thou mayst be.

Notwithstanding all this which might be said to this effect to ease their afflicted minds, what comfort our best divines can afford in this case, Zanchius, Beza, etc., this furious curiosity, needless speculation, fruitless meditation about election, reprobation, free will, grace, such places of Scripture preposterously conceived, torment still, and crucify the souls of too many, and set all the world together by the ears. To avoid which inconveniences, and to settle their distressed minds, to mitigate those divine aphorisms (though in another extreme some), our late Arminians have revived that plausible doctrine of universal grace, which many Fathers, our late Lutherans and modern papists do still maintain, that we have free will of ourselves, and that grace is common to all that will believe.[2] Some again, though less orthodoxal, will have a far greater part saved than shall be damned (as Cælius Secundus stiffly maintains in his book *de amplitudine regni cœlestis*, or some impostor under his name), *beatorum numerus multo major quam damnatorum.* He calls that other tenent of special election and reprobation "a prejudicate, envious, and malicious opinion, apt to draw all men to desperation."[3][4] "Many are called, few chosen," etc. He opposeth some opposite parts of Scripture to it, "Christ came into the world to save sinners," etc. And four especial arguments he produceth, one from God's power. If more be damned than saved, he erroneously concludes, the devil hath the greater sovereignty; for what is power but to protect? and majesty consists in multitude.[5] "If the devil have the greater part, where is His mercy, where is His power?

how is He *Deus Optimus Maximus, misericors*? etc.; where is
His greatness, where His goodness?" He proceeds, "We
account him a murderer that is accessary only, or doth not help
when he can; which may not be supposed of God without great
offence, because He may do what He will, and is otherwise
accessary, and the author of sin. The nature of good is to be
communicated, God is good, and will not then be contracted in
His goodness: for how is He the Father of mercy and comfort,
if His good concern but a few? O envious and unthankful
men to think otherwise!" [1] "Why should we pray to God that
are Gentiles, and thank Him for His mercies and benefits, that
hath damned us all innocuous for Adam's offence, one man's
offence, one small offence, eating of an apple? why should we
acknowledge Him for our governor that hath wholly neglected
the salvation of our souls, contemned us, and sent no prophets
or instructors to teach us, as He hath done to the Hebrews?" [2]
So Julian the Apostate objects. Why should these Christians
(Cælius urgeth) reject us and appropriate God unto themselves,
Deum illum suum unicum, etc.? But to return to our forged
Cælius. At last he comes to that, he will have those saved
that never heard of, or believed in Christ, *ex puris naturalibus*
[because they were still in their natural state], with the Pelagians, and proves it out of Origen and others. "They" (saith
Origen) "that never heard God's word, are to be excused for
their ignorance; we may not think God will be so hard, angry,
cruel or unjust as to condemn any man *indicta causa* [unheard].
They alone (he holds) are in the state of damnation that refuse
Christ's mercy and grace, when it is offered.[3] Many worthy
Greeks and Romans, good moral honest men, that kept the law
of nature, did to others as they would be done to themselves, are
as certainly saved, he concludes, as they were that lived uprightly
before the law of Moses. They were acceptable in God's sight,
as Job was, the Magi, the Queen of Sheba, Darius of Persia,
Socrates, Aristides, Cato, Curius, Tully, Seneca, and many
other philosophers, upright livers, no matter of what religion,
as Cornelius, out of any nation, so that he live honestly, call on
God, trust in Him, fear Him, he shall be saved. This opinion
was formerly maintained by the Valentinian and Basilidian
heretics, revived of late in Turkey,[4] of what sect Rustan Bassa
was patron, defended by Galeatius, Martius, and some ancient
Fathers,[5] and of later times favoured by Erasmus,[6] by Zuinglius
in exposit. fidei ad Regem Galliæ, whose tenent Bullinger vindicates, and Gualter approves in a just apology with many argu-

ments. There be many Jesuits that follow these Calvinists in
this behalf, Franciscus Buchsius Moguntinus, Andradius *Consil.
Trident.*, many schoolmen that out of 1 Rom. ii, 14, 15, are verily
persuaded that those good works of the Gentiles did so far please
God, that they might *vitam æternam promereri* [earn eternal
life], and be saved in the end. Sesellius, and Benedictus
Justinianus in his Comment on the first of the Romans, Matthias
Ditmarsh the politician, with many others, hold a mediocrity,
they may be *salute non indigni* [not unworthy of salvation], but
they will not absolutely decree it. Hoffmannus, a Lutheran
professor of Helmstadt, and many of his followers, with most of
our Church, and papists, are stiff against it. Franciscus Collius
hath fully censured all opinions in his five books *de Paganorum
animabus post mortem*, and amply dilated this question, which
whoso will may peruse. But to return to my author; his conclusion is, that not only wicked livers, blasphemers, reprobates,
and such as reject God's grace, "but that the devils themselves
shall be saved at last," [1] as Origen himself long since delivered
in his works, and our late Socinians defend,[2] Ostorodius, *cap.* 41
Institut., Smaltius, etc. Those terms of "all" and "for ever"
in Scripture are not eternal, but only denote a longer time,
which by many examples they prove. The world shall end like
a comedy, and we shall meet at last in heaven, and live in bliss
altogether, or else in conclusion, *in nihil evanescere* [vanish into
nothing]. For how can he be merciful that shall condemn
any creature to eternal unspeakable punishment, for one small
temporary fault, all posterity, so many myriads for one and
another man's offence, *quid meruistis oves ?* [what have you sheep
done?] But these absurd paradoxes are exploded by our
Church, we teach otherwise. That this vocation, predestination, election, reprobation, *non ex corrupta massa, prævisa fide*
[not from the corruption of the material, from faith foreseen],
as our Arminians, or *ex prævisis operibus* [from works foreseen],
as our papists, *non ex præteritione* [not from our omission],
but God's absolute decree *ante mundum creatum* (as many of our
Church hold), was from the beginning, before the foundation of
the world was laid, or *homo conditus* [man was fashioned] (or
from Adam's fall, as others will, *homo lapsus objectum est repro-
bationis* [man through sin is an object of reprobation]) with
perseverantia sanctorum [the perseverance of the saints], we
must be certain of our salvation, we may fall, but not finally,
which our Arminians will not admit. According to His immutable, eternal, just decree and counsel of saving men and angels,

God calls all, and would have all to be saved according to the
efficacy of vocation: all are invited, but only the elect apprehended: the rest that are unbelieving, impenitent, whom God
in His just judgment leaves to be punished for their sins, are in
a reprobate sense; yet we must not determine who are such,
condemn ourselves or others, because we have an universal invitation; all are commanded to believe, and we know not how soon or
how late before our end we may be received. I might have said
more of this subject; but forasmuch as it is a forbidden question,
and in the Preface or Declaration to the Articles of the Church,
printed 1633, to avoid factions and altercations, we that are
university divines especially, are prohibited "all curious search,
to print or preach, or draw the article aside by our own sense
and comments, upon pain of ecclesiastical censure," I will
surcease, and conclude with Erasmus [1] of such controversies:
*Pugnet qui volet, ego censeo leges majorum reverenter suscipiendas,
et religiose observandas, velut a Deo profectas ; nec esse tutum, nec
esse pium, de potestate publica sinistram concipere aut serere
suspicionem. Et siquid est tyrannidis, quod tamen non cogat ad
impietatem, satius est ferre, quam seditiose reluctari* [Let him
dispute who will, I hold that the laws of our ancestors are to
be treated with reverence and scrupulously observed, as
originating from God; and that it is neither safe nor pious to
harbour and spread suspicions of the public authority. It is
better to endure tyranny, so long as it does not drive us to
impiety, than seditiously to resist].

But to my former task. The last main torture and trouble
of a distressed mind is not so much this doubt of election, and
that the promises of grace are smothered and extinct in them,
nay quite blotted out, as they suppose, but withal God's heavy
wrath, a most intolerable pain and grief of heart seizeth on them:[2]
to their thinking they are already damned, they suffer the pains
of hell, and more than possibly can be expressed, they smell
brimstone, talk familiarly with devils, hear and see chimeras,
prodigious, uncouth shapes, bears, owls, antics, black dogs,
fiends, hideous outcries, fearful noises, shrieks, lamentable complaints; they are possessed, and through impatience they roar
and howl, curse, blaspheme, deny God, call His power in
question, abjure religion, and are still ready to offer violence
unto themselves, by hanging, drowning, etc.; never any miserable wretch from the beginning of the world was in such a woeful
case. To such persons I oppose God's mercy and His justice;
judicia Dei occulta, non injusta: His secret counsel and just

judgment, by which He spares some, and sore afflicts others again in this life; His judgment is to be adored, trembled at, not to be searched or inquired after by mortal men: He hath reasons reserved to Himself, which our frailty cannot apprehend. He may punish all if He will, and that justly for sin; in that He doth it in some, is to make a way for His mercy that they repent and be saved, to heal them, to try them, exercise their patience, and make them call upon Him, to confess their sins and pray unto Him, as David did (Ps. cxix, 137), "Righteous art Thou, O Lord, and just are Thy judgments," as the poor publican (Luke xviii, 13), "Lord have mercy upon me a miserable sinner"; to put confidence and have an assured hope in Him, as Job had (xiii, 15), "Though He kill me I will trust in Him." *Ure, seca, occide, O Domine,* (saith Austin) *modo serves animam,* kill, cut in pieces, burn my body (O Lord), to save my soul. A small sickness; one lash of affliction, a little misery, many times will more humiliate a man, sooner convert, bring him home to know himself, than all those parænetical discourses, the whole theory of philosophy, law, physic, and divinity, or a world of instances and examples. So that this, which they take to be such an insupportable plague, is an evident sign of God's mercy and justice, of His love and goodness: *periisent nisi periissent,* had they not thus been undone, they had finally been undone. Many a carnal man is lulled asleep in perverse security, foolish presumption, is stupefied in his sins, and hath no feeling at all of them; "I have sinned" (he saith), "and what evil shall come unto me?" (Ecclus. v, 4), and "Tush, how shall God know it?" and so in a reprobate sense goes down to hell. But here, *Cynthius aurem vellit,* God pulls them by the ear, by affliction He will bring them to heaven and happiness; "Blessed are they that mourn, for they shall be comforted" (Matt. v, 4); a blessed and an happy state, if considered aright, it is, to be so troubled. "It is good for me that I have been afflicted" (Ps. cxix); "before I was afflicted I went astray, but now I keep Thy word." "Tribulation works patience, patience hope" (Rom. v, 3, 4), and by such-like crosses and calamities we are driven from the stake of security. So that affliction is a school or academy, wherein the best scholars are prepared to the commencements of the Deity. And though it be most troublesome and grievous for the time, yet know this, it comes by God's permission and providence; He is a spectator of thy groans and tears, still present with thee; the very hairs of thy head are numbered, not one of them can fall to the ground

without the express will of God: He will not suffer thee to be
tempted above measure, He corrects us all, *numero, pondere,
et mensura* [1] [by number, weight, and measure], the Lord will
not quench the smoking flax, or break the bruised reed, *Tentat*
(saith Austin) *non ut obruat, sed ut coronet*, He suffers thee to
be tempted for thy good. And as a mother doth handle her
child sick and weak, not reject it, but with all tenderness observe
and keep it, so doth God by us, not forsake us in our miseries,
or relinquish us for our imperfections, but with all piety and
compassion support and receive us; whom He loves, He loves to
the end. Rom. viii: "Whom He hath elected, those He hath
called, justified, sanctified, and glorified." Think not then
thou hast lost the Spirit, that thou art forsaken of God, be not
overcome with heaviness of heart, but as David said, "I will
not fear, though I walk in the shadows of death." We must all
go, *non a deliciis ad delicias* [not from delights to delights],
but from the cross to the crown, by hell to heaven, as the old
Romans put Virtue's temple in the way to that of Honour:
we must endure sorrow and misery in this life. 'Tis no new
thing this, God's best servants and dearest children have been
so visited and tried. Christ in the garden cried out, "My God,
my God, why hast Thou forsaken me?" His son by nature,
as thou art by adoption and grace. Job, in his anguish, said,
"The arrows of the Almighty God were in him" (Job vi, 4),
"His terrors fought against him, the venom drank up his spirit."
Cap. xiii, 26, he saith, "God was his enemy, writ bitter things
against him, (xvi, 9) hated him," His heavy wrath had so
seized on his soul. David complains, "his eyes were eaten up,
sunk into his head" (Ps. vi, 7), "his moisture became as the
drought in summer, his flesh was consumed, his bones vexed";
yet neither Job nor David did finally despair. Job would not
leave his hold, but still trust in Him, acknowledging Him to
be his good God. "The Lord gives, the Lord takes, blessed
be the name of the Lord" (Job. i, 21). "Behold I am vile,
I abhor myself, repent in dust and ashes" (Job xlii, 6). David
humbled himself (Ps. xxxi), and upon his confession received
mercy. Faith, hope, repentance, are the sovereign cures and
remedies, the sole comforts in this case; confess, humble thyself,
repent, it is sufficient. *Quod purpura non potest, saccus potest*
[what the purple cannot effect, the sackcloth can], saith
Chrysostom; the King of Nineveh's sackcloth and ashes did
that which his purple robes and crown could not effect;
quod diadema non potuit, cinis perfecit. Turn to Him, He

will turn to thee; the Lord is near those that are of a
contrite heart, and will save such as be afflicted in spirit
(Ps. xxxiv, 18). "He came to the lost sheep of Israel"
(Matt. xv, 24). *Si cadentem intuetur, clementiæ manum protendit* [if He sees one falling, He holds out the hand of kind-
ness], He is at all times ready to assist. *Nunquam spernit
Deus pænitentiam, si sincere et simpliciter offeratur,* He never
rejects a penitent sinner; though he have come to the full
height of iniquity, wallowed and delighted in sin, yet if he
will forsake his former way, *libenter amplexatur,* He will receive
him. *Parcam huic homini,* saith Austin [1] (*ex persona Dei*),
quia sibi ipsi non pepercit; ignoscam quia peccatum agnovit: I
will spare him because he hath not spared himself; I will pardon
him because he doth acknowledge his offence: let it be never
so enormous a sin, "His grace is sufficient" (2 Cor. xii, 9).
Despair not then, faint not at all, be not dejected, but rely on
God, call on Him in thy trouble, and He will hear thee, He will
assist, help, and deliver thee: "Draw near to Him, He will
draw near to thee" (James iv, 8). Lazarus was poor and full
of boils, and yet still he relied upon God; Abraham did hope
beyond hope.

Thou exceptest, These were chief men, divine spirits, *Deo
cari,* beloved of God, especially respected; but I am a contemptible and forlorn wretch, forsaken of God, and left to the
merciless fury of evil spirits. I cannot hope, pray, repent, etc.
How often shall I say it? thou mayst perform all these duties,
Christian offices, and be restored in good time. A sick man
loseth his appetite, strength and ability, his disease prevaileth
so far that all his faculties are spent, hand and foot perform not
their duties, his eyes are dim, hearing dull, tongue distastes
things of pleasant relish, yet nature lies hid, recovereth again,
and expelleth all those feculent matters by vomit, sweat, or
some such-like evacuations. Thou art spiritually sick, thine
heart is heavy, thy mind distressed, thou mayst happily
recover again, expel those dismal passions of fear and grief;
God did not suffer thee to be tempted above measure; whom He
loves (I say) He loves to the end; hope the best. David in his
misery prayed to the Lord, remembering how He had formerly
dealt with him; and with that meditation of God's mercy confirmed his faith, and pacified his own tumultuous heart in his
greatest agony. "O my soul, why art thou so disquieted within
me?" etc. Thy soul is eclipsed for a time, I yield, as the sun
is shadowed by a cloud; no doubt but those gracious beams of

God's mercy will shine upon thee again, as they have formerly
done: those embers of faith, hope and repentance, now buried
in ashes, will flame out afresh, and be fully revived.   Want of
faith, no feeling of grace for the present, are not fit directions;
we must live by faith, not by feeling; 'tis the beginning of grace
to wish for grace: we must expect and tarry.   David, a man
after God's own heart, was so troubled himself: "Awake, why
sleepest thou?   O Lord, arise, cast me not off; wherefore hidest
Thou Thy face, and forgettest mine affliction and oppression?
My soul is bowed down to the dust.   Arise, redeem us," etc.
(Ps. xliv, 23).   He prayed long before he was heard, *expectans
expectavit*; endured much before he was relieved.   Ps. lxix, 3,
he complains, "I am weary of crying, and my throat is dry,
mine eyes fail, whilst I wait on the Lord"; and yet he perseveres.
Be not dismayed, thou shalt be respected at last.   God often
works by contrarieties, He first kills and then makes alive,
He woundeth first and then healeth, He makes man sow in
tears, that he may reap in joy; 'tis God's method: he that is
so visited must with patience endure and rest satisfied for the
present.   The paschal lamb was eaten with sour herbs; we shall
feel no sweetness of His blood, till we first feel the smart of our
sins.   Thy pains are great, intolerable for the time; thou art
destitute of grace and comfort, stay the Lord's leisure, He will
not (I say) suffer thee to be tempted above that thou art able
to bear (1 Cor. x, 13), but will give an issue to temptation.   He
works all for the best to them that love God (Rom. viii, 28).
Doubt not of thine election, it is an immutable decree; a mark
never to be defaced: you have been otherwise, you may and
shall be.   And for your present affliction, hope the best, it will
shortly end.   "He is present with His servants in their affliction" (Ps. xci, 15).   "Great are the troubles of the righteous,
but the Lord delivereth them out of all" (Ps. xxxiv, 19).   "Our
light affliction, which is but for a moment, worketh in us an
eternal weight of glory" (2 Cor. iv, 17), "not answerable to that
glory which is to come"; "Though now in heaviness," saith
1 Pet. i, 6, "you shall rejoice."
    Now last of all to those external impediments, terrible objects,
which they hear and see many times, devils, bugbears, and
mormoluches, noisome smells, etc.   These may come, as I have
formerly declared in my precedent discourse of the Symptoms
of Melancholy, from inward causes; as a concave glass reflects
solid bodies, a troubled brain for want of sleep, nutriment, and
by reason of that agitation of spirits to which Hercules de

Saxonia attributes all symptoms almost, may reflect and show prodigious shapes, as our vain fear and crazed phantasy shall suggest and feign, as many silly weak women and children in the dark, sick folks, and frantic for want of repast and sleep, suppose they see that they see not: many times such terriculaments may proceed from natural causes, and all other senses may be deluded. Besides, as I have said, this humour is *balneum diaboli*, the devil's bath, by reason of the distemper of humours, and infirm organs in us: he may so possess us inwardly to molest us, as he did Saul and others, by God's permission: he is prince of the air, and can transform himself into several shapes, delude all our senses for a time, but his power is determined, he may terrify us, but not hurt; God hath given "His angels charge over us, He is a wall round about His people" (Ps. xci, 11, 12). There be those that prescribe physic in such cases, 'tis God's instrument and not unfit. The devil works by mediation of humours, and mixed diseases must have mixed remedies. Levinus Lemnius, *cap*. 57 *et* 58, *Exhort. ad vit. opt. instit.*, is very copious on this subject, besides that chief remedy of confidence in God, prayer, hearty repentance, etc., of which, for your comfort and instruction, read Lavater *de spectris*, *part*. 3, *cap*. 5 *et* 6, Wierus *de præstigiis dæmonum, lib*. 5, Philip Melancthon, and others, and that Christian armour which Paul prescribes; he sets down certain amulets, herbs, and precious stones, which have marvellous virtues all, *profligandis dæmonibus*, to drive away devils and their illusions: sapphires, chrysolites, carbuncles, etc., *quæ mira virtute pollent ad lemures, striges, incubos, genios aereos arcendos, si veterum monumentis habenda fides* [which are wonderfully effective for keeping off ghosts, spirits, etc., if we may believe the ancient records]. Of herbs, he reckons us pennyroyal, rue, mint, angelica, peony; Rich. Argentine, *de præstigiis dæmonum, cap*. 20, adds *hypericon* or St. John's wort, *perforata herba* [the perforate herb], which by a divine virtue drives away devils, and is therefore *fuga dæmonum*: all which rightly used, by their suffitus *dæmonum vexationibus obsistunt, afflictas mentes a dæmonibus relevant, et venenatis fumis*, expel devils themselves, and all devilish illusions. Anthony Musa, the Emperor Augustus his physician, *cap*. 6, *de betonia*, approves of betony to this purpose; the ancients used therefore to plant it in churchyards, because it was held to be an holy herb, and good against fearful visions, did secure such places as it grew in, and sanctified those persons that carried it about them.[1] *Idem fere Matthiolus in Dioscoridem.*

Others commend accurate music; so Saul was helped by David's
harp. Fires to be made in such rooms where spirits haunt,
good store of lights to be set up, odours, perfumes, and suffumigations, as the angel taught Tobias, of brimstone and bitumen,
thus, myrrha, [frankincense, myrrh], bryony-root, with many
such simples which Wecker hath collected, *lib.* 15 *de secretis,
cap.* 15. *R sulphuris drachmam unam, recoquatur in vitis albæ
aqua, ut dilutius sit sulphur; detur ægro: nam dæmones sunt
morbi* [take one dram of sulphur, dilute it by heating in water
of white bryony, and administer it to the patient; for devils
are only diseases] (saith Rich. Argentine, *lib. de præstigiis
dæmonum, cap. ult.*). Vigetus hath a far larger receipt to this
purpose, which the said Wecker cites out of Wierus: *R sulphuris,
vini, bituminis, opoponacis, galbani, castorei,* etc. Why sweet
perfumes, fires and so many lights should be used in such places,
Ernestus Burgravius, *Lucerna vitæ et mortis,* and Fortunius
Licetus assigns this cause, *quod his boni genii provocentur, mali
arceantur*: because good spirits are well pleased with, but evil
abhor them. And therefore those old Gentiles, present Mahometans, and papists have continual lamps burning in their
churches all day and all night, lights at funerals and in their
graves; *lucernæ ardentes ex auro liquefacto* [lamps fed with
liquefied gold] for many ages to endure (saith Lazius), *ne
dæmones corpus lædant* [to prevent evil spirits from molesting
the body]; lights ever burning as those vestal virgins, pythonissæ maintained heretofore, with many such, of which read
Tostatus, *in* 2 *Reg. cap.* 6, *quæst.* 43; Thyreus, *cap.* 57, 58, 62,
etc., *de locis infestis*; Pictorius, *Isagog. de dæmonibus,* etc.; see
more in them. Cardan would have the party affected wink
altogether in such a case, if he see aught that offends him, or
cut the air with a sword in such places they walk and abide,
gladiis enim et lanceis terrentur [for they are afraid of swords and
spears]; shoot a pistol at them, for being aerial bodies (as
Cælius Rhodiginus, *lib.* 1, *cap.* 29, Tertullian, Origen, Psellas,
and many hold), if stroken, they feel pain. Papists commonly
enjoin and apply crosses, holy-water, sanctified beads, amulets,
music, ringing of bells, for to that end are they consecrated
and by them baptized, characters, counterfeit relics, so many
masses, peregrinations, oblations, adjurations, and what not?
Alexander Albertinus à Rocha, Petrus Thyræus, and Hieronymus Mengus, with many other pontificial writers, prescribe and
set down several forms of exorcisms, as well to houses possessed
with devils as to demoniacal persons; but I am of Lemnius'

mind,[1] 'tis but *damnosa adjuratio, aut potius ludificatio*, a mere
mockage, a counterfeit charm, to no purpose, they are fopperies
and fictions, as that absurd story [2] is amongst the rest, of a
penitent woman seduced by a magician in France, at St. Bawne,
exorcised by Domphius, Michaelis, and a company of circum-
venting friars. If any man (saith Lemnius) will attempt such
a thing, without all those juggling circumstances, astrological
elections of time, place, prodigious habits, fustian, big, sesqui-
pedal words, spells, crosses, characters, which exorcists ordinarily
use, let him follow the example of Peter and John, that without
any ambitious swelling terms cured a lame man (Acts iii): "In
the name of Christ Jesus rise and walk." His name alone is
the best and only charm against all such diabolical illusions;
so doth Origen advise, and so Chrysostom: *Hæc erit tibi baculus,
hæc turris inexpugnabilis, hæc armatura* [this shall be your staff,
your impregnable fortress, your armour]. *Nos quid ad hæc
dicemus, plures fortasse expectabunt*, saith St. Austin. Many
men will desire my counsel and opinion what is to be done in
this behalf; I can say no more, *quam ut vera fide, quæ per dilectionem operatur* [than that, in the true faith which works through
love], *ad Deum unum fugiamus*, let them fly to God alone for
help. Athanasius, in his book *de variis quæst.*, prescribes as a
present charm against devils, the beginning of the sixty-eighth
Psalm, *Exsurgat Deus, dissipentur inimici* [Let God arise, let
His enemies be scattered], etc. But the best remedy is to fly
to God, to call on Him, hope, pray, trust, rely on Him, to
commit ourselves wholly to Him. What the practice of the
primitive Church was in this behalf, *et quis dæmonia ejiciendi
modus* [and what its method was of casting out devils] read
Wierus at large, *lib.* 5 *de curat. Lam. malef. cap.* 38 *et deinceps.*
    Last of all: If the party affected shall certainly know this
malady to have proceeded from too much fasting, meditation,
precise life, contemplation of God's judgments (for the devil
deceives many by such means), in that other extreme he circumvents melancholy itself, reading some books, treatises, hearing
rigid preachers, etc. If he shall perceive that it hath begun
first from some great loss, grievous accident, disaster, seeing
others in like case, or any such terrible object, let him speedily
remove the cause, which to the cure of this disease Navarrus
so much commends, *avertat cogitationem a re scrupulosa* [3] [let
him avert his thoughts from the painful subject], by all opposite
means, art, and industry, let him *laxare animum*, by all honest
recreations refresh and recreate his distressed soul; let him direct

his thoughts, by himself and other of his friends. Let him read no more such tracts or subjects, hear no more such fearful tones, avoid such companies, and by all means open himself, submit himself to the advice of good physicians and divines, which is *contraventio scrupulorum* [a relief in uneasiness], as he [1] calls it, hear them speak to whom the Lord hath given the tongue of the learned, to be able to minister a word to him that is weary,[2] whose words are as flagons of wine. Let him not be obstinate, headstrong, peevish, wilful, self-conceited (as in this malady they are), but give ear to good advice, be ruled and persuaded; and no doubt but such good counsel may prove as prosperous to his soul as the angel was to Peter, that opened the iron gates, loosed his bands, brought him out of prison, and delivered him from bodily thraldom; they may ease his afflicted mind, relieve his wounded soul, and take him out of the jaws of hell itself. I can say no more, or give better advice to such as are anyway distressed in this kind, than what I have given and said. Only take this for a corollary and conclusion, as thou tenderest thine own welfare in this and all other melancholy, thy good health of body and mind, observe this short precept, give not way to solitariness and idleness. "Be not solitary, be not idle."

SPERATE MISERI,
CAVETE FELICES.

[Hope, ye unhappy ones; ye happy ones, fear.]

Vis a dubio liberari? vis quod incertum est evadere? Age pœnitentiam dum sanus es; sic agens, dico tibi quod securus es, quod pœnitentiam egisti eo tempore quo peccare potuisti. [Do you wish to be freed from doubt? do you desire to escape uncertainty? Be penitent while of sound mind: by so doing I assert that you are safe, because you have devoted that time to penitence in which you might have been guilty of sin.]—Austin.

NOTES

PAGE 3

[1] Encom. Moriæ. Leviores esse nugas quam ut theologum deceant.
[2] Lib. 8 Eloquent. cap. 14, de affectibus. Mortalium vitio fit qui præclara quæque in pravos usus vertunt.
[3] Quoties de amatoriis mentio facta est, tam vehementer excandui; tam severa tristitia violari aures meas obscœno sermone nolui, ut me tanquam unam ex philosophis intuerentur.
[4] Martial.   [5] Lib. 4 of Civil Conversation.

PAGE 4

[1] Si male locata est opera scribendo, ne ipsi locent in legendo.
[2] Med. epist. lib. 1, ep. 14. Cadmus Milesius, teste Suida, de hoc erotico amore 14 libros scripsit, nec me pigebit in gratiam adolescentum hanc scribere epistolam.
[3] Comment. in 2 Æneid.
[4] Meros amores meram impudicitiam sonare videtur nisi, etc.

PAGE 5

[1] Ser. 8.   [2] Quod risum et eorum amores commemoret.
[3] Quum multa ei objecissent quod Critiam tyrannidem docuisset, quod Platonem juraret loquacem sophistam, etc., accusationem amoris nullam fecerunt. Ideoque honestus amor, etc.

PAGE 6

[1] Carpunt alii Platonicam majestatem quod amori nimium indulserit, Dicæarchus et alii; sed male. Omnis amor honestus et bonus, et amore digni qui bene dicunt de amore.
[2] Med. obser. lib. 2, cap. 7. De admirando amoris affectu dicturus; ingens patet campus et philosophicus, quo sæpe homines ducuntur ad insaniam, libeat modo vagari, etc. Quæ non ornent modo, sed fragrantia et succulentia jucunda plenius alant, etc.
[3] Lib. 1, præfat. de amoribus agens relaxandi animi causa laboriosissimis studiis fatigati; quando et theologi se his juvari et juvare illæsis moribus volunt.
[4] Hist. lib. 12, cap. 34.
[5] Quid quadragenario convenit cum amore? Ego vero agnosco amatorium scriptum mihi non convenire: qui jam meridiem prætergressus in vesperem feror.—Æneas Sylvius, præfat.
[6] [Mateo Aleman's picaresque story, Guzman de Alfarache.]
[7] Ut severiora studia iis amœnitatibus lector condire possit.—Accius.
[8] Discum quam philosophum audire malunt.
[9] In Som. Scip. E sacrario suo tum ad cunas nutricum sapientes eliminarunt, solas aurium delicias profitentes.
[10] Babylonius et Ephesius, qui de amore scripserunt, uterque amores Myrrhæ, Cyrenes, et Adonidis.—Suidas.
[11] Pet. Aretine, dial. Ital.

433

PAGE 7

[1] Hor.   [2] Legendi cupidiores, quam ego scribendi, saith Lucian.
[3] Plus capio voluptatis inde, quam spectandis in theatro ludis.
[4] Prooemio in Isaiam.   Multo major pars Milesias fabulas revolventium quam Platonis libros.
     In vita philosophus, in epigrammatis amator, in epistolis petulans, in præceptis severus. [Madaurensis = Apuleius, who was a native of Madaura.]

PAGE 8

[1] Mart.   [2] Ovid.
[3] Martianus Capella, lib. 1 de nupt. philol.   Virginali suffusa rubore oculos peplo obnubens, etc.
[4] Isago. ad sac. Scrip. cap. 13.
[5] Barthius, notis in Cælestinam, ludum Hisp.
[6] Ficinus, Comment. cap. 17.   Amore incensi inveniendi amoris, amorem quæsivimus et invenimus.

PAGE 9

[1] Auctor Cælestinæ, Barth. interprete.
[2] Hor. lib. 1, Ode 34.
[3] Hæc prædixi ne quis temere nos putaret scripsisse de amorum leno-ciniis, de praxi, fornicationibus, adulteriis, etc.
[4] Taxando et ab his deterrendo humanam lasciviam et insaniam, sed et remedia docendo: non igitur candidus lector nobis succenseat, etc. Commonitio erit juvenibus hæc, hisce ut abstineant magis, et omissa las-civia quæ homines reddit insanos, virtutis incumbant studiis (Æneas Sylv.), et curam amoris si quis nescit hinc poterit scire.
[5] Catullus.   [6] Viros nudos castæ feminæ nihil a statuis distare.
[7] Hony soit qui mal y pense.

PAGE 10

[1] Præf. Suid.
[2] Exerc. 301.   Campus amoris maximus et spinis obsitus, nec levissimo pede transvolandus.

PAGE 11

[1] Grad. 1, cap. 29, ex Platone.   Primæ et communissimæ perturbationes ex quibus ceteræ oriuntur et earum sunt pedisequæ.
[2] Amor est voluntarius affectus et desiderium re bona fruendi.
[3] Desiderium optantis, amor eorum quibus fruimur; amoris principium, desiderii finis, amatum adest.
[4] Principio lib de amore..   Operæ pretium est de amore considerare, utrum deus, an dæmon, an passio quædam animæ, an partim deus, partim dæmon, passio partim, etc.   Amor est actus animi bonum desiderans.
[5] Magnus dæmon, Convivio.
[6] Boni pulchrique fruendi desiderium.
[7] Godefridus, lib. 1, cap. 2.   Amor est delectatio cordis alicujus ad aliquid, propter aliquod desiderium in appetendo, et gaudium perfruendo per desiderium currens, requiescens per gaudium.
[8] Non est amor desiderium aut appetitus ut ab omnibus hactenus traditum; nam cum potimur amata re, non manet appetitus; est igitur affectus quo cum re amata aut unimur, aut unionem perpetuamus.
[9] Omnia appetunt bonum.

PAGE 12

[1] Terram non vis malam, malam segetem, sed bonam arborem, equum bonum, etc.
[2] Nemo amore capitur nisi qui fuerit ante forma specieque delectatus.

[3] Amabile objectum amoris et scopus, cujus adeptio est finis, cujus gratia amamus. Animus enim aspirat ut eo fruatur, et formam boni habet et praecipue videtur et placet.—Piccolomineus, grad. 7, cap. 2, et grad. 8, cap. 35.

[4] Forma est vitalis fulgor ex ipso bono manans per ideas, semina, rationes, umbras effusus, animos excitans ut per bonum in unum redigantur.

[5] Pulchritudo est perfectio compositi ex congruente ordine, mensura et ratione partium consurgens, et venustas inde prodiens gratia dicitur et res omnes pulchrae gratiosae.

[6] Gratia et pulchritudo ita suaviter animos demulcent, ita vehementer alliciunt, et admirabiliter connectuntur, ut in unum confundant et distingui non possunt, et sunt tanquam radii et splendores divini solis in rebus variis vario modo fulgentes.

[7] Species pulchritudinis hauriuntur oculis, auribus, aut concipiuntur interna mente.

[8] Nihil hinc magis animos conciliat quam musica, pulchrae aedes, etc.

PAGE 13

[1] In reliquis sensibus voluptas, in his pulchritudo et gratia.

[2] Lib. 4 de divinis.

[3] Convivio Platonis. Duae Veneres duo amores; quarum una antiquior et sine matre, coelo nata, quam coelestem Venerem nuncupamus; altera vero junior a Jove et Dione prognata, quam vulgarem Venerem vocamus.

[4] Alter ad superna erigit, alter deprimit ad inferna.

[5] Alter excitat hominem ad divinam pulchritudinem lustrandam, cujus causa philosophiae studia et justitiae, etc.

PAGE 14

[1] Omnis creatura cum bona sit, et bene amari potest et male.

[2] Duas civitates duo faciunt amores; Jerusalem facit amor Dei, Babylonem amor saeculi; unusquisque se quid amet interroget, et inveniet unde sit civis.

[3] Alter mari ortus, ferox, varius, fluctuans, inanis, juvenum, mare referens, etc. Alter aurea catena coelo demissa bonum furorem mentibus mittens, etc.

PAGE 15

[1] Tria sunt, quae amari a nobis bene vel male possunt; Deus, proximus, mundus; Deus supra nos; juxta nos proximus; infra nos mundus. Tria Deus, duo proximus, unum mundus habet, etc.

[2] Ne confundam vesanos et foedos amores beatis, sceleratum cum puro, divino, et vero, etc.

[3] Fonseca, cap. 1 Amor., ex Augustini forsan lib. 11 de Civit. Dei. Amore inconcussus stat mundus, etc.   [4] Alciat.

[5] Porta. Vitis laurum non amat, nec ejus odorem; si prope crescat, enecat. Lappa lenti adversatur.

PAGE 16

[1] Sympathia olei et myrti ramorum et radicum se complectentium.—Mizaldus, Secret. cent. 1, 47.

[2] Theocritus, Idyll. 9.   [3] Mantuan.

[4] Caritas munifica, qua mercamur de Deo regnum Dei.

[5] Polanus, Partit. Zanchius, de natura Dei, cap. 3, copiose de hoc amore Dei agit.

PAGE 17

[1] Nich. Bellus, discurs. 28, de amatoribus. Virtutem provocat, conservat pacem in terra, tranquillitatem in aere, ventis lætitiam, etc.
[2] Camerarius, Emb. 100, cen. 2.
[3] Dial. 3.   [4] Juven.   [5] Gen. i.
[6] Caussinus.   [7] Theodoret e Plotino.

PAGE 18

[1] Affectus nunc appetitivæ potentiæ, nunc rationalis; alter cerebro residet, alter hepate, corde, etc.
[2] Cor varie inclinatur, nunc gaudens, nunc mœrens; statim ex timore nascitur zelotypia, furor, spes, desperatio.
[3] Ad utile sanitas refertur; utilium est ambitio, cupido, desiderium potius quam amor, excessus, avaritia.
[4] Piccolom. grad. 7, cap. 1.
[5] Lib. de amicit. Utile mundanum, carnale jucundum, spirituale honestum.
[6] Ex singulis tribus fit caritas et amicitia, quæ respicit Deum et proximum.

PAGE 19

[1] Benefactores præcipue amamus.—Vives, 3 de anima.
[2] Josh. vii, 21.   [3] Petronius Arbiter.
[4] Juvenalis.   [5] Joh. Secund. lib. silvarum.

PAGE 20

[1] Lucianus, Timon.
[2] [The comparison of a group of friends to the triple-bodied Geryon is Lucian's (Toxaris, 63).]
[3] Pers. [1, 25; an allusion to the splitting of stones by the roots of the wild fig-tree.]

PAGE 21

[1] Part. 1, sect. 2, memb. 2, subs. 11.   [2] 1 Tim. i, 8.
[3] Lips. epist. Camdeno.   [4] Leland of St. Edmondsbury.
[5] Cœlum serenum, cœlum visum fœdum.—Polyd. lib. 1 de Anglia.
[6] Credo equidem vivos ducent e marmore vultus.
[7] Max. Tyrius, ser. 9.

PAGE 22

[1] Part. 1, sect. 2, memb. 3.   [2] Mart.
[3] Omnif. mag. lib. 12, cap. 3.
[4] De sale geniali, lib. 3, cap. 15.
[5] Theod. Prodromus, Amor. lib. 3.
[6] Similitudo morum parit amicitiam.
[7] Vives, 3 de anima.
[8] Qui simul fecere naufragium, aut una pertulere vincula, vel consilii conjurationisve societate junguntur, invicem amant: Brutum et Cassium invicem infensos Cæsarianus dominatus conciliavit. Æmilius Lepidus et Julius Flaccus, quum essent inimicissimi, censores renunciati simultates illico deposuere.—Scultet. cap. 4, de causa amor.
[9] Papinius.

PAGE 23

[1] Isocrates Demonico præcipit ut quum alicujus amicitiam vellet, illum laudet, quod laus initium amoris sit, vituperatio simultatum.
[2] Suspect. lect. lib. 1, cap. 2.   [3] Isa. xlix.
[4] Rara est concordia fratrum.

Page 24

[1] Grad. 1, cap. 22.
[2] Vives, 3 de anima. Ut paleam succinum, sic formam amor trahit.
[3] [Gnatho is the parasite in Terence's Eunuchus.]
[4] Sect. seq.   [5] Nihil divinius homine probo.

Page 25

[1] James iii, 17.
[2] Gratior est pulchro veniens e corpore virtus.
[3] Orat. 18. Deformes plerumque philosophi ad id quod in aspectum cadit, ea parte elegantes quæ oculos fugit.
[4] [A reference to Alcibiades' comparison of Socrates to the grotesque figures of satyrs which, when opened, were found to contain images of the gods. See Plato's Banquet.]   [5] 43 de consol.

Page 26

[1] Causa ei paupertatis, philosophia, sicut plerisque probitas fuit.
[2] Ablue corpus et cape regis animum, et in eam fortunam qua dignu res continentiam istam profer.   [3] Vita ejus.
[4] Qui præ divitiis humana spernunt, nec virtuti locum putant nisi opes affluant. Q. Cincinnatus consensu patrum in dictatorem Romanum electus.   [5] Curtius.
[6] Edgar Etheling, England's darling.
[7] Morum suavitas, obvia comitas, prompta officia mortalium animos demerentur.
[8] Epist. lib. 8. Semper amavi, ut tu scis, M. Brutum propter ejus summum ingenium, suavissimos mores, singularem probitatem et constantiam; nihil est, mihi crede, virtute formosius, nihil amabilius.
[9] Ardentes amores excitaret, si simulacrum ejus ad oculos penetraret.—Plato, Phædone.
[10] Epist. lib. 4. Validissime diligo virum rectum, disertum, quod apud me potentissimum est.
[11] Est quædam pulchritudo justitiæ quam videmus oculis cordis, amamus, et exardescimus, ut in martyribus, quum eorum membra bestiæ lacerarent, etsi alias deformes, etc.
[12] Lipsius, Manuduc. ad Phys. Stoic. lib. 3, diff. 17. Solus sapiens pulcher.
[13] Fortitudo et prudentia pulchritudinis laudem præcipue merentur.

Page 27

[1] Franc. Belforest. in Hist. an. 1430.
[2] Erat autem fœde deformis, et ea forma, qua citius pueri terreri possent, quam invitari ad osculum puellæ.
[3] Deformis iste etsi videatur senex, divinum animum habet.
[4] Fulgebat vultu suo: fulgor et divina majestas homines ad se trahens.
[5] Præfat. Bib. vulgar.
[6] Pars inscrip. Tit. Livii statuæ Patavii.

Page 28

[1] A true-love's knot.   [2] Stobæus e Græco.
[3] Solinus. Pulchri nulla est facies.
[4] O dulcissimi laquei, qui tam feliciter devinciunt, ut etiam a vinctis diligantur, qui a gratiis vincti sunt, cupiunt arctius deligari et in unum redigi.   [5] [Silius Italicus.]
[6] "He loved him as he loved his own soul" (1 Sam. xv, 1), "beyond the love of women" [2 Sam. i, 26].
[7] Virg. 9 Æn. Qui super exanimem sese conjecit amicum Confossus.

[8] Amicus animæ dimídium.—Austin, Confess. 4, cap. 6. Quod de Virgilio Horatius: Et serves animæ dimidium meæ.
[9] Plinius.

PAGE 29

[1] Illum argento et auro, illum ebore, marmore affingit, et nuper ingenti adhibito auditorio ingentem de vita ejus librum recitavit.—Epist. lib. 4, epist. 68.
[2] Lib. 3, ep. 21, Prisco suo.
[3] Dedit mihi quantum potuit maximum, daturus amplius si potuisset. Tametsi quid homini dari potest majus quam gloria, laus, et æternitas? At non erunt fortasse quæ scripsit. Ille tamen scripsit tanquam essent futura.
[4] For, genus irritabile vatum.
[5] Lib. 13 de legibus. Magnam enim vim habent, etc.
[6] Pari tamen studio et pietate conscribendæ vitæ ejus munus suscepi, et postquam sumptuosa condere pro fortuna non licuit, exiguo sed eo forte liberalis ingenii monumento justa sanctissimo cineri solventur.

PAGE 30

[1] 1 Sam. xxv, 3.   [2] Esther iii, 2.   [3] [See vol. i, p. 282, note 1.]
[4] Amm. Marcellinus, lib. 22.
[5] Ut mundus duobus polis sustentatur: ita lex Dei, amore Dei et proximi; duobus his fundamentis vincitur; machina mundi corruit, si una de polis turbatur; lex perit divina si una ex his.

PAGE 31

[1] 8 et 9 libro.   [2] Ter. Adelph. 4, 5.
[3] De amicit. Caritas parentum dilui nisi detestabili scelere non potest.
[4] Lapidum fornicibus simillima, casura, nisi se invicem sustentaret.—Seneca.
[5] Dii immortales, dici non potest quantum caritatis nomen illud habet.
[6] Ovid. Fast.   [7] Anno 1347. Jacob Mayer, Annal. Fland. lib. 12.
[8] Tully.   [9] Lucianus Toxari. Amicitia ut sol in mundo, etc.
[10] Vit. Pompon. Attici.

PAGE 32

[1] Spenser, Faerie Queene, lib. 4, cant. 9, staff 1, 2.
[2] Siracides.   [3] Plutarch, pretiosum numisma.
[4] Xenophon. Verus amicus præstantissima possessio.   [5] Epist. 52.

PAGE 33

[1] Greg. Per amorem Dei, proximi gignitur; et per hunc amorem proximi, Dei nutritur.
[2] Piccolomineus, grad. 7, cap. 27. Hoc felici amoris nodo ligantur familiæ, civitates, etc.
[3] Veras absolutas hæc parit virtutes, radix omnium virtutum, mens et spiritus.
[4] Divino calore animos incendit, incensos purgat, purgatos elevat ad Deum, Deum placat, hominem Deo conciliat.—Bernard.
[5] Ille inficit, hic perficit, ille deprimit, hic elevat; hic tranquillitatem, ille curas parit; hic vitam recte informat, ille deformat, etc.

PAGE 34

[1] Boethius, lib. 2, met. 8.
[2] Deliquium patitur caritas, odium ejus loco succedit.—Basil, 1 ser. de instit. mon.
[3] Nodum in scirpo quærentes [seeking a knot in a bulrush].

PAGE 35

[1] Hyrcanæque admorunt ubera tigres.   [2] Heraclitus.
[3] Si in Gehennam abit, pauperem qui non alat: quid de eo fiet qui pauperem denudat?—Austin.

PAGE 37

[1] Jovius, vita ejus.
[2] Immortalitatem beneficio literarum, immortali gloriosa quadam cupiditate concupivit. Quod cives quibus benefecisset perituri, mœnia ruitura, etsi regio sumptu ædificata, non libri.
[3] Plutarch, Pericle.   [4] Tullius, lib. 1 de legibus.
[5] Gen. xxxv, 8.   [6] Hor.   [7] Durum genus sumus.

PAGE 38

[1] Tull. pro Rosc. Mentiri vis causa mea? ego vero cupide et libenter mentiar tua causa; et si quando me vis perjurare, ut paululum tu compendii facias, paratum fore scito.
[2] Gallienus. in Treb. Pollio. Lacera, occide, mea mente irascere. Rabie jecur incendente feruntur præcipites. Vopiscus of Aurelian. Tantum fudit sanguinis quantum quis vini potavit.
[3] Evangelii tubam belli tubam faciunt; in pulpitis pacem, in colloquiis bellum suadent.   [4] Ps. xiv, 1.

PAGE 39

[1] De bello Judaico, lib. 6, cap. 16. Puto si Romani contra nos venire tardassent, aut hiatu terræ devorandam fuisse civitatem, aut diluvio perituram, aut fulmina ao Sodoma cum incendio passuram, ob desperatum populi, etc.
[2] Benefacit animæ suæ vir misericors.
[3] Concordia magnæ [parvæ] res crescunt, discordia maximæ dilabuntur.

PAGE 40

[1] Lipsius.   [2] Memb. 1, subs. 2.   [3] Amor er amicitia.
[4] Phædrus, orat. in laudem amoris Platonis Convivio.
[5] Vide Boccac. de Geneal. deorum.
[6] See the moral in Plutarch of that fiction.   [7] Affluentiæ Deus.

PAGE 41

[1] Cap. 7 Comment. in Plat. Convivium.
[2] See more in Valesius, lib. 3 Cont. med. et cont. 13.
[3] Vives, 3 de anima. Oramus te ut tuis artibus et caminis nos refingas, et ex duobus unum facias; quod et fecit, et exinde amatores unum sunt et unum esse petunt.
[4] See more in Natalis Comes, Imag. deorum; Philostratus, de imaginibus; Lilius Giraldus, Syntag. de diis; Phornutus, etc.
[5] Juvenis pingitur quod amore plerumque juvenes capiuntur; sic et mollis, formosus, nudus, quod simplex et apertus hic affectus; ridet quod oblectamentum præ se ferat, cum pharetra, etc.
[6] A petty Pope, claves habet superorum et inferorum, as Orpheus, etc.
[7] Lib. 13, cap. 5, Deipnosoph.
[8] Regnat et in superos jus habet ille deos.—Ovid.
[9] Plautus.   [10] Selden, proleg. 3 cap. de diis Syris.

PAGE 42

[1] Dial. 3.
[2] A concilio deorum rejectus et ad majorem ejus ignominiam, etc.
[3] Fulmine concitatior.   [4] Sophocles.   [5] Tom. 4.

⁶ Dial. deorum, tom. 3.

⁷ Quippe matrem ipsius quibus modis me afficit, nunc in Idam adigens Anchisæ causa, etc.

⁸ Jampridem et plagas ipsi in nates incussi sandalio.

PAGE 43

¹ Altopilus, fol. 79.

² Nullis amor est medicabilis herbis.

³ Plutarch, in Amatorio. Dictator quo creato cessant reliqui magistratus.

⁴ Claudian, descript. vener. anulæ.

⁵ Neque prius in iis desiderium cessat dum dejectus consoletur; videre enim est ipsam arborem incurvatam, ultro ramis ab utrisque vicissim ad osculum exporrectis. Manifesta dant mutui desiderii signa.

⁶ Multas palmas contingens quæ simul crescunt, rursusque ad amantem regrediens, eamque manu attingens, quasi osculum mutuo ministrare videtur, et expediti concubitus gratiam facit.

⁷ Quam vero ipsa desideret affectu ramorum significat, et ad illam respicit; amantur, etc.

PAGE 44

¹ Virg. Georg. 3.   ² Propertius.

³ Dial. deorum. Confide, mater, leonibus ipsis familiaris jam factus sum, et sæpe conscendi eorum terga et apprehendi jubas; equorum more insidens eos agito, et illi mihi caudis adblandiuntur.

⁴ Leones præ amore furunt. Plin. lib. 8, cap. 16; Arist. lib. 6 Hist. animal.

⁵ Cap. 17 of his book of hunting.   ⁶ Lucretius.

⁷ De sale, lib. 1, cap. 21. Pisces ob amorem marcescunt, pallescunt, etc.

PAGE 45

¹ Hauriendæ aquæ causa venientes ex insidiis a Tritone comprehensæ, etc.

² Plin. lib. 10, cap. 5. Quumque aborta tempestate periisset Hernias in sicco piscis expiravit.

³ Postquam puer morbo abiit, et ipse delphinus periit.

⁴ Pleni sunt libri quibus feræ in homines inflammatæ fuerunt, in quibus ego quidem semper assensum sustinui, veritus ne fabulosa crederem; donec vidi lyncem quem habui ab Assyria, sic affectum erga unum de meis hominibus, etc.

⁵ Desiderium suum testatus post inediam aliquot dierum interiit.

⁶ Orpheus, Hymno Ven.

PAGE 46

¹ Qui hæc in atræ bilis aut imaginationis vim referre conati sunt, nihil faciunt.

² Cantantem audies et vinum bibes, quale antea nunquam bibisti; te rivalis turbabit nullus; pulchra autem pulchro contente vivam, et moriar.

PAGE 47

¹ Multi factum hoc cognovere, quod in media Græcia gestum sit.

² Rem curans domesticam, ut ante, peperit aliquot liberos, semper tamen tristis et pallida.

³ Hæc audivi a multis fide dignis qui asseverabant Ducem Bavariæ eadem retulisse Duci Saxoniæ pro veris.

Page 48

[1] Fabula Damarati et Aristonis in Herodoto, lib. 6, Erato.
[2] Interpret. Mersio.
[3] Deus angelos misit ad tutelam cultumque generis humani; sed illos cum hominibus commorantes, dominator ille terræ salacissimus paulatim ad vitia pellexit, et mulierum congressibus inquinavit.
[4] Quidam ex illo capti sunt amore virginum, et libidine victi defecerunt, ex quibus gigantes qui vocantur nati sunt.
[5] Pererius in Gen. lib. 8, cap. 6, ver. 1; Zanc., etc.
[6] Purchas, Hakl. Posth. par. 1, lib. 4, cap. 1, s. 7.
[7] In Clio.   [8] Deus ipse hoc cubili requiescens.
[9] Physiologiæ Stoicorum lib. 1, cap. 20.   Si spiritus unde semen iis, etc., at exempla turbant nos; mulierum quotidianæ confessiones de mistione omnes asserunt, et sunt in hac urbe Lovanio exempla.
[10] Unum dixero, non opinari me ullo retro ævo tantam copiam satyrorum et salacium istorum geniorum sc ostendisse, quantum nunc quotidianæ narrationes, et judiciales sententiæ proferunt.

Page 49

[1] Virg.
[2] "For it is a shame to speak of those things which are done of them in secret," Eph. v, 12.
[3] Plutarch, Amator. lib.   [4] Lib. 13.

Page 50

[1] Rom. i, 27.   [2] Lilius Giraldus, vita ejus.
[3] Pueros amare solis philosophis relinquendum vult Lucianus, dial. Amorum.   [4] Busbequius.
[5] Lucianus, Charidemo.   [6] Achilles Tatius, lib. 2.

Page 51

[1] Non est hæc mentula demens?—Mart.
[2] Jovius, Musc.
[3] Præfat. lectori lib. de vitis pontif.
[4] Mercurialis, cap. de Priapismo.   Cælius, lib. 11 Antiq. lect. cap. 14. Galenus, 6 de locis aff.
[5] De morb. mulier. lib. 1, cap. 15.
[6] Herodotus, lib. 2, Euterpe. Uxores insignium virorum non statim vita functas tradunt condendas, ac ne eas quidem feminas quæ formosæ sunt, sed quatriduo ante defunctas, ne cum iis salinarii concumbant, etc.
[7] Metam. 10.   [8] Seneca, de ira, lib. 11, cap. 18.
[9] Nullus est meatus ad quem non pateat aditus impudicitiæ.—Clem. Alex. Pædag. lib. 3, cap. 3.
[10] Seneca, 1, Nat. quæst.   [11] Tom. P. Gryllo.

Page 52

[1] De morbis mulierum, lib. 1, cap. 15.
[2] Amphitheat. amor. cap. 4, interprete Curtio.
[3] Æneas Sylvius. Juvenal.
[4] Tertul. Prover. lib. 4 adversus Marc. cap. 40.   [5] Chaucer.
[6] Tom. 1, Dial. Deorum, Lucianus. Amore non ardent Musæ.
[7] In Amator. dialog.

Page 53

[1] Hor.   [2] Lucretius.   [3] Fonseca.   [4] Hor.
[5] Propert.   [6] Simonides, Græc.   [7] Ausonius.

PAGE 54

[1] Geryon amicitiæ symbolum. [2] Propert. lib. 2.
[3] Plutarch, cap. 30, Rom. Hist.
[4] Junonem habeam iratam, si unquam meminerim me virginem fuisse.
Infans enim paribus inquinata sum, et subinde majoribus me applicui,
donec ad ætatem perveni: ut Milo vitulum, etc.
[5] Pornoboscodidasc. dial. lat. interp. Gasp. Barthio ex Ital.
[6] Angelico Scriptur. Concentu.

PAGE 55

[1] Epictetus, cap. 42.   Mulieres statim ab anno 14 movere incipiunt, etc.
attrectari se sinunt et exponunt.—Levinus Lemnius.
[2] Lib. 3, fol. 126.   [3] Catullus.   [4] [Propertius].
[5] De mulierum inexhausta libidine luxuque insatiabili omnes æque
regiones conqueri posse existimo.—Steph.   [6] Euripides.

PAGE 56

[1] Plautus.
[2] Oculi caligant, aures graviter audiunt, capilli fluunt, cutis arescit,
flatus olet, tussis, etc.—Cyprian.
[3] Lib. 8 Epist. Rufinus.
[4] Hiatque turpis inter aridas nates podex.
[5] Cadaverosa adeo ut ab inferis reversa videri possit, vult adhuc catulire.
[6] Nam et matrimoniis est despectum senium.—Æneas Silvius.
[7] Quid toto terrarum orbe communius? quæ civitas, quod oppidum,
quæ familia vacat amatorum exemplis?—Æneas Sylvius. Quis trigesimum annum natus nullum amoris causa peregit insigne facinus? ego de
me facio conjecturam, quem amor in mille pericula misit.
[8] Forestus, Plato.
[9] Pract. major, tract. 6, cap. 1, rub. 11, de ægrit. cap. Quod his multum
contingat.

PAGE 57

[1] Hæc ægritudo est sollicitudo melancholica in qua homo applicat sibi
continuam cogitationem super pulchritudine ipsius quam amat, gestuum,
morum.
[2] Animi forte accidens quo quis rem habere nimia aviditate concupiscit,
ut ludos venatores, aurum et opes avari.
[3] Assidua cogitatio super rem desideratam, cum confidentia obtinendi,
ut spe apprehensum delectabile, etc.
[4] Morbus corporis potius quam animi.
[5] Amor est passio melancholica.
[6] Ob calefactionem spirituum pars anterior capitis laborat ob consumptionem humiditatis.
[7] Affectus animi concupiscibilis e desiderio rei amatæ per oculos in mente
concepto, spiritus in corde et jecore incendens.
[8] Odyss. et Metamor. 4 Ovid.
[9] Quod talem carnificinam in adolescentum visceribus amor faciat
inexplebilis.
[10] Testiculi quoad causam conjunctam, hepar antecedentem, possunt
esse subjectum.

PAGE 58

[1] Proprie passio cerebri est ob corruptam imaginationem.
[2] Cap. de affectibus.
[3] Est corruptio imaginativæ et æstimativæ facultatis, ob formam
fortiter affixam, corruptumque judicium, ut semper de eo cogitet, ideoque

recte melancholicus appellatur. Concupiscentia vehemens ex corrupto judicio æstimativæ virtutis.

[4] Comment. in Convivium Platonis. Irretiuntur cito quibus nascentibus Venus fuerit in Leone, vel Luna Venerem vehementer aspexerit, et qui eadem complexione sunt præditi.

[5] Plerumque amatores sunt, et si feminæ meretrices.—Lib. de audiend.

[6] Comment. in Genes. cap. 3.

[7] Et si in hoc parum a præclara infamia stultitiaque abero, vincit tamen amor veritatis.

PAGE 59

[1] Edit. Basil. 1553, cum commentar. in Ptolemæi Quadripartitum.

[2] Fol. 445, Basil. edit.   [3] Dial. amorum.

PAGE 60

[1] Citius maris fluctus et nives cœlo delabentes numeraris quam amores meos; alii amores aliis succedunt, ac priusquam desinant priores, incipiunt sequentes. Adeo humidis oculis meus inhabitat asylus omnem formam ad se rapiens, ut nulla satietate expleatur. Quænam hæc ira Veneris, etc.

[2] Num. 32.   [3] Qui calidum testiculorum crasin habent, etc.

[4] Printed at Paris 1628, seven years after my first edition.

[5] Ovid de art.

PAGE 61

[1] Gerbelius, Descript. Græciæ. Rerum omnium affluentia et loci mira opportunitas, nullo non die hospites in portas advertebant. Templo Veneris mille meretrices se prostituebant.

[2] Tota Cypri insula deliciis incumbit, et ob id tantum luxuriæ dedita ut sit olim Veneri sacrata.—Ortelius. Lampsacus, olim Priapo sacer ob vinum generosum, et loci delicias.—Idem.

[3] Agri Neapolitani delectatio, elegantia, amœnitas, vix intra modum humanum consistere videtur; unde, etc.—Leander Albertus, in Campania.

[4] Lib. de laud. urb. Neap.

[5] Disputat. de morbis animi, Reinoldo interprete.

[6] Lampridius. Quod decem noctibus centum virgines fecisset mulieres.

[7] Vita ejus.

PAGE 62

[1] If they contain themselves, many times it is not virtutis amore; non deest voluntas sed facultas.

[2] In Muscov.   [3] Catullus ad Lesbiam.   [4] Hor.

[5] Polit. 8, num. 28. Ut naptha ad ignem, sic amor ad illos qui torpescunt otio.

[6] Pausanias, Attic. lib. 1. Cephalus egregiæ formæ juvenis ab Aurora raptus quod ejus amore capta esset.

[7] In Amatorio.

PAGE 63

[1] E Stobæo, ser. 62.

[2] Amor otiosæ cura est sollicitudinis.

[3] Principes plerumque ob licentiam et adfluentiam divitiarum istam passionem solent incurrere.

[4] Ardenter appetit qui otiosam vitam agit, et communiter incurrit hæc passio solitarios deliciose viventes, incontinentes, religiosos, etc.

[5] Plutarch, vit. ejus.   [6] Vina parant animos veneri.

[7] Sed nihil erucæ faciunt bulbique salaces; Improba nec prosit jam satureia tibi. [Martial.]

Page 64

[1] Petronius. Curavi me mox cibis validioribus, etc.

[2] Uti ille apud Sckenkium, qui post potionem, uxorem et quatuor ancillas proximo cubiculo cubantes compressit.

[3] Pers. Sat. 1.

[4] Siracides. Nox et amor vinumque nihil moderabile suadent.

[5] Ep. ad Olympiam.   [6] Hymno.

[7] Hor. lib. 3, Od. 25.   [8] De sale lib. cap. 21.

[9] Kornmannus, lib. de virginitate.

[10] Garcias ab Horto, Aromatum lib. 1, cap. 28.

[11] Surax radix ad coitum summe facit; si quis comedat, aut infusionem bibat, membrum subito erigitur.—Leo Afer, lib. 9, cap. ult.

[12] Quæ non solum edentibus sed et genitale tangentibus tantum valet, ut coire summe desiderent; quoties fere velint, possint; alios duodecies profecisse, alios ad 60 vices pervenisse refert.

Page 65

[1] Lucian, tom. 4, Dial. amorum.

[2] Ea enim hominum intemperantium libido est ut etiam fama ad amandum impellantur, et audientes æque afficiuntur ac videntes.

[3] Formosam Sostrato filiam audiens, uxorem cupit, et sola illius auditione ardet.

[4] Quoties de Panthea Xenophontis locum perlego, ita animo affectus ac si coram intuerer.

[5] Pulchritudinem sibi ipsis confingunt.—Imagines.

[6] De aulico, lib. 2, fol. 116. 'Tis a pleasant story, and related at large by him.

[7] Gratia venit ab auditu æque ac visu, et species amoris in phantasiam recipiunt sola relatione.—Piccolomineus, grad. 8, cap. 38.

[8] Lips. cent. 2, epist. 22. Beauty's Encomions.

[9] Propert.

[10] Amoris primum gradum visus habet, ut aspiciat rem amatam.

[11] Achilles Tatius, lib. 1. Forma telo quovis acutior ad inferendum vulnus, perque oculos amatorio vulneri aditum patefaciens in animum penetrat.

Page 66

[1] In tota rerum natura nihil forma divinius, nihil augustius, nihil pretiosius, cujus vires hinc facile intelliguntur, etc.

[2] Christ. Fonseca.   [3] S. L.

[4] Bruys, prob. 11 de forma, e Luciano.

[5] Lib. de calumnia. Formosi calumnia vacant; dolemus alios meliore loco positos, fortunam nobis novercam, illis, etc.

[6] Invidemus sapientibus, justis, nisi beneficiis assidue amorem extorquent; solos formosos amamus et primo velut aspectu benevolentia conjungimur, et eos tanquam deos colimus, libentius iis servimus quam aliis imperamus, majoremque, etc.

Page 67

[1] Formæ majestatem barbari verentur, nec alii majores quam quos eximia forma natura donata est.   Heliod. lib 5, Curtius 6, Arist. Polit.

[2] Serm. 63.   [3] Plutarch, vit. ejus.   [4] Brisonius, Strabo.

[5] Lib. 6, cap. 5. Magnorumque operum non alios capaces putant quam quos eximia specie natura donavit.

[6] Lib. de vitis pontificum Rom.   [7] Lib. 2, cap. 6.

Page 68

[1] Dial. amorum, cap. 2, de magia; lib. 2 Connub. cap. 27.
[2] Virgo formosa etsi oppido pauper, abunde est dotata.
[3] Isocrates. Plures ob formam immortalitatem adepti sunt quam ob reliquas omnes virtutes.
[4] Lucian, tom. 4, Charidemus. Qui pulchri, merito apud deos et apud homines honore affecti. Muta commendatio, quavis epistola ad commendandum efficacior.
[5] Lib. 9 Var. Hist. Tanta formæ elegantia ut ab ea nuda, etc.

Page 69

[1] Esdras iv, 29.
[2] Origen, hom. 23 in Numb. In ipsos tyrannos tyrannidem exercet.
[3] Illud certe magnum ob quod gloriari possunt formosi, quod robustis necessarium sit laborare, fortem periculis se objicere, sapientem, etc.
[4] Majorem vim habet ad commendandum forma, quam accurate scripta epistola.—Arist.
[5] Heliodor. lib. 1. [6] Knolles, Hist. Turcica.
[7] Daniel, in Complaint of Rosamond.

Page 70

[1] Stroza filius, Epig. [2] Sect. 2, memb. 1, subs. 1.
[3] Stromatum lib. Post captam Trojam cum impetu ferretur ad occidendam Helenam, stupore adeo pulchritudinis correptus ut ferrum excideret, etc.
[4] Tantæ formæ fuit ut cum vincta loris feris exposita foret, equorum calcibus obterenda, ipsis jumentis admirationi fuit; lædere noluerunt.
[5] Lib. 8 Miles.

Page 71

[1] Æthiop. lib. 3. [2] Athenæus, lib. 8. [3] Apuleius, Aur. asino.
[4] Shakespeare. [5] Marlowe. [6] Ov. Met. 1.

Page 72

[1] Ovid. Met. lib. 5. [2] Leland. [3] Angerianus.
[4] Si longe aspiciens hæc urit lumine divos atque homines prope, cur urere lina nequit?—Angerianus.

Page 73

[1] Idem Angerianus.
[2] Obstupuit mirabundus membrorum elegantiam, etc.—Ep. 7.
[3] Stobæus, e Græco.
[4] Parum abfuit quo minus saxum ex homine factus sum, ipsis statuis immobiliorem me fecit.
[5] Veteres Gorgonis fabulam confinxerunt, eximium formæ decus stupidos reddens.
[6] Hor. Ode 5. [7] Marlowe's Hero.
[8] Aspectum virginis sponte fugit insanus fere, et impossibile existimans ut simul eam aspicere quis possit, et intra temperantiæ metas se continere.
[9] Apuleius, lib. 4. Multi mortales longis itineribus, etc.

Page 74

[1] Nic. Gerbel. lib. 5, Achaia.
[2] J. Secundus, Basiorum lib.
[3] Musæus. Illa autem bene morata, per ædem quocunque vagabatur, sequentem mentem habebat, et oculos, et corda virorum.
[4] Homer. [5] Marlowe.

[6] Pornoboscodidascalo, dial. Ital. Latin. donat. a Gasp. Barthio Germano.
[7] Propertius.
[8] Vestium splendore et elegantia ambitione incessus, donis, cantilenis, etc., gratiam adipisci.
[9] Præ cæteris corporis proceritate et egregia indole mirandus apparebat, cæteri autem capti ejus amore videbantur, etc.

PAGE 75

[1] Aristænetus, Ep. 10.
[2] Tom. 4, Dial. meretr.   Respicientes et ad formam ejus obstupescentes.
[3] In Charidemo.   Sapientiæ merito pulchritudo præfertur et opibus.
[4] Indignum nihil est Troas fortes et Achivos tempore tam longo perpessos esse labores.
[5] Digna quidem facies pro qua vel obiret Achilles, Vel Priamo bell causa probanda fuit.—Proper. lib. 2.
[6] Cæcus qui Helenæ formam carpserat.
[7] Those mutinous Turks that murmured at Mahomet, when they saw Irene, excused his absence.—Knolles.
[8] In laudem Helenæ erat.
[9] Apul. Miles. lib. 4.   [10] Secundus, Bas. 13.   [11] Curtius, lib. 10.

PAGE 76

[1] Confessions.   [2] Seneca.   Amor in oculis oritur.
[3] Ovid, Fast.   [4] Plutarch.
[5] Lib. de pulchrit. Jesu et Mariæ.
[6] Lucian, Charidemus.   Supra omnes mortales felicissimum si hac frui possit.

PAGE 77

[1] Lucian, Amores.   Insanum quiddam ac furibundum exclamans, O fortunatissime deorum Mars qui propter hanc vinctus fuisti.
[2] Ov. Met. lib. 4.
[3] Omnes dii complexi sunt, et in uxorem sibi petierunt.—Nat. Comes, de Venere.
[4] Ut cum lux noctis affulget, omnium oculos incurrit: sic Autolycus, etc.
[5] Delevit omnes ex animo mulieres.
[6] Nam vincit et vel ignem, ferrumque si qua pulchra est.—Anacreon, 2.
[7] Spenser in his Faerie Queene.
[8] Achilles Tatius, lib. 1.
[9] Statim ac eam contemplatus sum, occidi; oculos a virgine avertere conatus sum, sed illi repugnabant.

PAGE 78

[1] Pudet dicere, non celabo tamen.   Memphim veniens me vicit, et continentiam expugnavit, quam ad senectutem usque servaram, oculis corporis, etc.
[2] Nunc primum circa hanc anxius animi hæreo.—Aristænetus, Ep. 17.
[3] Virg. Æn. 4.   [4] Amaranto dial.
[5] Comasque ad speculum disposuit.
[6] Imag. Polystrato.   Si illam saltem intuearis, statuis immobiliorem te faciet: si conspexeris eam, non relinquetur facultas oculos ab ea amovendi; abducet te alligatum quocunque voluerit, ut ferrum ad se trahere ferunt adamantem.

PAGE 79

[1] Plaut. Merc.   [2] In the Knight's Tale.
[3] Ex debita totius proportione aptaque partium compositione.—Piccolomineus.
[4] Hor. Od. 19, lib. 1.

PAGE 80

[1] Ter. Eunuch. Act. 2, sc. 3. [2] Petronius, Catal.
[3] Sophocles, Antigone.
[4] Jo. Secundus, Bas. 19. [5] Lœchæus.
[6] Arandus. Vallis amœnissima e duobus montibus composita niveis.

PAGE 81

[1] Ovid. [2] Fol. 77. Dapsiles hilares amatores, etc.
[3] When Cupid slept. Cæsariem auream habentem, ubi Psyche vidit, mollemque ex ambrosia cervicem inspexit, crines crispos, purpureas genas candidasque, etc.—Apuleius.
[4] In laudem calvitii. Splendida coma quisque adulter est; allicit aurea coma.
[5] Venus ipsa non placeret comis nudata, capite spoliata, si qualis ipsa Venus cum fuit virgo omni gratiarum choro stipata, et toto cupidinum populo concinnata, balteo suo cincta, cinnama fragrans, et balsama, si calva processerit, placere non potest Vulcano suo.
[6] Arandus. Capilli retia Cupidinis, sylva cædua, in qua nidificat Cupido, sub cujus umbra amores mille modis se exercent.
[7] Theod. Prodromus, Amor. lib. 1.

PAGE 82

[1] Epist. 27. Ubi pulchram tibiam, bene compactum tenuemque pedem vidi.
[2] Plaut. Cas. [3] Claudus optime rem agit.
[4] Fol. 5. Si servum viderint, aut statorem altius cinctum, aut pulvere perfusum, aut histrionem in scenam traductum, etc.
[5] Me pulchra fateor carere forma, verum luculenta —— nostra est.— Petronius, Catal. de Priapo. [6] Galen.
[7] Calcagninus Apologis. Quæ pars maxime desiderabilis? Alius frontem, alius genas, etc.
[8] Interfemineum. [9] Heinsius.

PAGE 83

[1] Amoris hami, duces, judices et indices qui momento insanos sanant, sanos insanire cogunt, oculatissimi corporis excubitores, quid non agunt? Quid non cogunt?
[2] Sunt enim oouli, præcipuæ pulchritudinis sedes.—Lib. 6.
[3] Ocelli, carm. 17, cujus et Lipsius, Epist. Quæst. lib. 3, cap. 11, meminit ob elegantiam.
[4] Cynthia prima suis miserum me cepit ocellis, Contactum nullis ante cupidinibus.—Propert. lib. 1.
[5] In Catalect. [6] De Sulpicia, lib. 4.
[7] Pulchritudo ipsa per occultos radios in pectus amantis dimanans amatæ rei formam insculpsit.—Tatius, lib. 5.

PAGE 84

[1] Jacob Cornelius, Ammon Tragœd. Act. 1, sc. 1.
[2] Rosæ formosarum oculis nascuntur, et hilaritas vultus elegantiæ corona.—Philostratus, Deliciis.
[3] Epist., et in Deliciis. Abi et oppugnationem relinque, quam flamma non extinguit; nam ab amore ipsa flamma sentit incendium: quæ corporum penetratio, quæ tyrannis hæc? etc.
[4] Lœchæus, Panthea. [5] Propertius.

Page 85

[1] Ovid. Amorum lib. 2, eleg. 4.
[2] Scut. Hercul.   [3] Calcagninus, dial.
[4] Iliad 1.   [5] Hist. lib. 1.
[6] Sandys' Relation, fol. 67.   [7] Mantuan.
[8] Amor per oculos, nares, poros influens, etc.
[9] Mortales tum summopere fascinantur quando frequentissimo intuitu aciem dirigentes, etc.

Page 86

[1] Ideo si quis nitore polleat oculorum, etc.
[2] Spiritus puriores fascinantur, oculus a se radios emittit, etc.
[3] Lib. de pulch. Jes. et Mar.
[4] Lib. 2, cap. 23. Colore triticum referente, crine flava, acribus oculis.
[5] Lippi solo intuitu alios lippos faciunt, et patet una cum radio vaporem corrupti sanguinis emanare, cujus contagione oculus spectantis inficitur.
[6] Vita Apollon.   [7] Comment. in Aristot. Probl.
[8] Sic radius a corde percutientis missus, regimen proprium repetit, cor vulnerat, per oculos et sanguinem inficit et spiritus, subtili quadam vi. —Castil. lib. 3 de aulico.
[9] Lib. 10. Causa omnis et origo omnis præsentis doloris tute es; isti enim tui oculi, per meos oculos ad intima delapsi præcordia, acerrimum meis medullis commovent incendium; ergo miserere tui causa pereuntis.

Page 87

[1] Lycias in Phædri vultum inhiat, Phædrus in oculos Lyciæ scintillas suorum defigit oculorum; cumque scintillis, etc. Sequitur Phædrus Lyciam, quia cor suum petit spiritum; Phædrum Lycias, quia spiritus propriam sedem postulat. Verum Lycias, etc.
[2] Dæmonia, inquit, quæ in hoc eremo nuper occurrebant.
[3] Castilio, de aulico, lib. 3, fol. 228. Oculi ut milites in insidiis semper recubant, et subito ad visum sagittas emittunt, etc.
[4] Nec mirum si reliquos morbos qui ex contagione nascuntur consideremus, pestem, pruritum, scabiem, etc.
[5] Lucretius.

Page 88

[1] In beauty, that of favour is preferred before that of colours, and decent motion is more than that of favour.—Bacon's Essays.
[2] Martialis.
[3] Multi tacite opinantur commercium illud adeo frequens cum barbaris. nudis, ac presertim cum feminis, ad libidinem provocare, àt minus multo noxia illorum nuditas quam nostrarum feminarum cultus.
[4] Ausim asseverare splendidum illum cultum, fucos, etc.

Page 89

[1] Harmo. Evangel. lib. 6, cap. 6.
[2] Serm. de concep. Virg. Physiognomia Virginis omnes movet ad castitatem.
[3] 3 sent. d. 3, q. 3. Mirum, virgo formosissima, sed a nemine concupita.
[4] Met. 10.
[5] Rosamond's Complaint, by Sam. Daniel.

Page 90

[1] Æneas Sylvius.
[2] Heliodor. lib. 2. Rhodopis Thracia tam inevitabili fascino instructa, tam exacte oculis intuens attraxit, ut si in illam quis incidisset, fieri non posset quin caperetur.

³ Lib. 3 de providentia: Animi fenestræ oculi, et omnis improba cupiditas per ocellos tanquam canales introit.
⁴ Buchanan.   ⁵ Ovid, de arte amandi.
⁶ Pers. Sat. 3.   ⁷ Vel centum Charites ridere putaret.—Musæus, of Hero.
⁸ Hor. Od. 22, lib. 1.

PAGE 91

¹ Eustathius, lib. 5.   ² Mantuan.
³ Tom. 4, Meretr. dial. Exornando seipsam eleganter, facilem et hilarem se gerendo erga cunctos, ridendo suave ac blandum quid, etc.
⁴ Angerianus.
⁵ Vel si forte vestimentum de industria elevetur, ut pedum ac tibiarum pars aliqua conspiciatur, dum templum aut locum aliquem adierit.

PAGE 92

¹ Sermone, quod non feminæ viris cohabitent.   Non locuta es lingua, sed locuta es gressu: non locuta es voce, sed oculis locuta es clarius quam voce.
² Jovianus Pontanus, Baiar. lib. 1, ad Hermionem.
³ De luxu vestium discurs. 6.   Nihil aliud deest nisi ut præco vos præcedat, etc.
⁴ If you can tell how, you may sing this to the tune a sow-gelder blows.
⁵ Auson. Epig. 39.
⁶ Plin. lib. 33, cap. 10.   Campaspen nudam picturus Apelles, amore ejus illaqueatus est.
⁷ [Charles the Bold, Duke of Burgundy.]

PAGE 93

¹ In Tyrrhenis conviviis nudæ mulieres ministrabant.
² Epist. 7, lib. 2.
³ Amatoria miscentes vidit, et in ipsis complexibus audit, etc.; emersit inde cupido in pectus virginis.
⁴ Spartian.   ⁵ Sidney's Arcadia.
⁶ De immod. mulier. cultu.   ⁷ Discurs. 6, de luxu vestium.

PAGE 94

¹ Petronius, fol. 95.   Quo spectant flexæ comæ? quo facies medicamine attrita et oculorum mollis petulantia? quo incessus tam compositus, etc.
² Ter.
³ P. Aretine.   Hortulanus non ita exercetur visendis hortis, eques equis, armis, nauta navibus, etc.
⁴ Epist. 4.   Sonus armillarum bene sonantium, odor unguentorum, etc.
⁵ Tom. 4, Dial. Amor.   Vascula plena multæ infelicitatis omnem maritorum opulentiam in hæc impendunt, dracones pro monilibus habent, qui utinam vere dracones essent.—Lucian.
⁶ Seneca.

PAGE 95

¹ Castilio, de aulic. lib. 1.   Mulieribus omnibus hoc imprimis in votis est, ut formosæ sint, aut si reipsa non sint, videantur tamen esse; et si qua parte natura defuit, artis suppetias adjungunt: unde illæ faciei unctiones, dolor et cruciatus in arctandis corporibus, etc.
² Ovid. Epist. Med. Jasoni.
³ Modo caudatas tunicas, etc.—Bossus.
⁴ Scribanius, Philos. Christ. cap. 6.
⁵ Ter. Eunuc. Act. 2, scen. 3.
⁶ Stroza fil.   ⁷ Ovid.

PAGE 96

[1] S. Daniel.

[2] Lib. de victimis. Fracto incessu, obtuitu lascivo, calamistrata, cincinnata, fucata, recens lota, purpurissata, pretiosoque amicta palliolo, spirans unguenta, ut juvenum animos circumveniat.

[3] Orat. in ebrios. Impudenter se masculorum aspectibus exponunt, insolenter comas jactantes, trahunt tunicas pedibus collidentes, oculoque petulanti, risu effuso, ad tripudium insanientes, omnem adolescentum intemperantiam in se provocantes, idque in templis memoriæ martyrum consecratis; pomœrium civitatis officinam fecerunt impudentiæ.

[4] Hymno Veneri dicato.

PAGE 97

[1] Argonaut. lib. 3.   [2] Vit. Anton.

[3] Regia domo ornatuque certantes, sese ac formam suam Antonio offerentes, etc. Cum ornatu et incredibili pompa per Cydnum fluvium navigarent aurata puppi, ipsa ad similitudinem Veneris ornata, puellæ Gratiis similes, pueri Cupidinibus, Antonius ad visum stupefactus.

[4] Amictum chlamyde et coronis, quum primum aspexit Cnemonem, ex potestate mentis excidit.

[5] Lib. de lib. prop.   [6] Ruth iii, 3.   [7] Cap. x, 3.
[8] Juv. Sat. 4.   [9] Hor. lib. 2. Od. 11.

PAGE 98

[1] Cap. 27.   [2] Epist. 90.

[3] Quicquid est boni moris levitate extinguitur, et politura corporis muliebres munditias antecessimus, colores meretricios viri sumimus, tenero et molli gradu suspendimus gradum, non ambulamus.—Nat. quæst. lib. 7, cap. 31.

[4] Liv. lib. 4, dec. 4.

[5] Quid exultas in pulchritudine panni? Quid gloriaris in gemmis ut facilius invites ad libidinosum incendium?—Mat. Bossus, de immoder. mulier. cultu.

[6] Epist. 113. Fulgent monilibus, moribus sordent, purpurata vestis, conscientia pannosa, cap. 3, 17.

[7] De virginali habitu. Dum ornari cultius, dum evagari virgines volunt, desinunt esse virgines. Clemens Alexandrinus, lib. de pulchr. animæ, ibid.

PAGE 99

[1] Lib. 2 de cultu mulierum. Oculos depictos verecundia, inferentes in aures sermonem Dei, annectentes crinibus jugum Christi, caput maritis subjicientes, sic facile et satis eritis ornatæ: vestite vos serico probitatis, byssino sanctitatis, purpura pudicitiæ; taliter pigmentatæ Deum habebitis amatorem.

[2] Suas habeant Romanæ lascivias; purpurissa ac cerussa ora perungant, fomenta libidinum, et corruptæ mentis indicia; vestrum ornamentum Deus sit, pudicitia, virtutis studium.—Bossus.

[3] Plautus.

[4] Sollicitiores de capitis sui decore quam de salute, inter pectinem et speculum diem perdunt, concinniores esse malunt quam honestiores, et rempublicam minus turbari curant quam comam.—Seneca.

[5] Lucian.

[6] Non sic Furius de Gallis, non Papirius de Samnitibus, Scipio de Numantia triumphavit, ac illa se vincendo in hac parte.

PAGE 100

[1] Anacreon, 4. Solum intuentur aurum.

[2] Asses tecum si vis vivere mecum.

[3] Theognis.   [4] Chaloner, lib. 9 de Repub. Ang.

Page 101

[1] Uxorem ducat Danaen, etc.   [2] Ovid.

[3] Epist. 14.   Formam spectant alii per gratias, ego pecuniam, etc.; ne mihi negotium facesse.

[4] Qui caret argento, frustra utitur argumento.

[5] Juvenalis.

[6] Tom. 4, Meret. dial.   Multos amatores rejecit, quia pater ejus nuper mortuus, ac dominus ipse factus bonorum omnium.

[7] Lib. 3, cap. 14.   Quis nobilium eo tempore, sibi aut filio aut nepoti uxorem accipere cupiens, oblatam sibi aliquam propinquarum ejus non acciperet obviis manibus?   Quarum turbam acciverat e Normannia in Angliam ejus rei gratia.

[8] Alexander Gaguinus, Sarmat. Europ. descript.

[9] Tom. 3 Annal.

Page 102

[1] Libido statim deferbuit, fastidium cœpit, et quod in ea tantopere adamavit aspernatur, et ab ægritudine liberatus in angorem incidit.

[2] De puellæ voluntate periculum facere solis oculis non est satis, sed efficacius aliquid agere oportet, ibique etiam machinam alteram adhibere: itaque manus tange, digitos constringe, atque inter stringendum suspira; si hæc agentem æquo te animo feret, neque facta hujusmodi aspernabitur, tum vero dominam appella, ejusque collum suaviare.

Page 103

[1] Hungry dogs will eat dirty puddings.

[2] Shakespeare.

[3] Tatius, lib. 1.

[4] In mammarum attractu, non aspernanda inest jucunditas, et attrectatus, etc.

[5] Ovid, Met. 1.   [6] Mantuan.

Page 104

[1] Manus ad cubitum nuda, coram astans, fortius intuita, tenuem de pectore spiritum ducens, digitum meum pressit, et bibens pedem pressit; mutuæ compressiones corporum, labiorum commixtiones, pedum connexiones, etc.   Et bibit eodem loco, etc.

[2] Epist. 4.   Respexi, respexit et illa subridens, etc.

[3] Virgil, Æn. 4.   [4] Propertius.

[5] Ovid. Amor. lib. 2, eleg. 2.

Page 105

[1] Romæ vivens flore fortunæ, et opulentiæ meæ, ætas, forma, gratia conversationis, maxime me fecerunt expetibilem, etc.

[2] De aulic. lib. 1, fol. 63.

[3] Ut adulterini mercatorum panni.   [4] Busbeq. Epist.

[5] Paranympha in cubiculum adducta capillos ad cutim referebat; sponsus inde ad eam ingressus cingulum solvebat, nec prius sponsam aspexit interdiu quam ex illa factus esset pater.

Page 106

[1] Serm. cont. concub.

[2] Lib. 2, Epist. ad filium et virginem et matrem viduam, epist. 10. Dabit tibi barbatulus quispiam manum, sustentabit lassam, et pressis digitis aut tentabitur aut tentabit, etc.

[3] Loquetur alius nutibus, et quicquid metuit dicere, significabit affectibus. Inter has tantas voluptatum illecebras etiam ferreas mentes libido domat. Difficile inter epulas servatur pudicitia.

⁴ Clamore vestium ad se juvenes vocat; capilli fasciolis comprimuntur crispati, cingulo pectus arctatur, capilli vel in frontem, vel in aures defluunt: palliolum interdum cadit, ut nudet humeros, et quasi videri noluerit, festinans celat, quod volens detexerit.

⁵ Serm. cont. concub. In sancto et reverendo sacramentorum tempore multas occasiones, ut illis placeant qui eas vident, præbent.

⁶ Pont. Baia. lib. 1.

PAGE 107

¹ Descr. Brit.

² Res est blanda canor, discunt cantare puellæ pro facie, etc.—Ovid, 3 de art. amandi.

³ Epist. lib. 1. Cum loquitur Lais, quanta, O dii boni, vocis ejus dulcedo!

⁴ Aristænetus, lib. 2, epist. 5. Quam suave canit! verbum audax dixi, omnium quos vidi formosissimus; utinam amare me dignetur!

⁵ Imagines. Si cantantem audieris, ita demulcebere, ut parentum et patriæ statim obliviscaris.

⁶ Idyll. 18. Neque sane ulla sic citharam pulsare novit.

⁷ Amatorio Dialogo.

⁸ Puellam cithara canentem vidimus.

PAGE 108

¹ Apollonius, Argonaut, lib. 3. ² Catullus.

³ Pornoboscodidascalo, dial. Ital. Latin. interp. Gaspar. Barthio, Germ. Fingebam honestatem plusquam virginis vestalis, intuebar oculis uxoris, addebam gestus, etc.

PAGE 109

¹ Tom. 4, Dial. meretr.

² Amatorius sermo vehemens vehementis cupiditatis incitatio est.— Tatius, lib. 1.

³ De luxuria et deliciis compositi.

⁴ Æneas Sylvius. Nulla machina validior quam lectio lascivæ historiæ: sæpe etiam hujusmodi fabulis ad furorem incenduntur.

⁵ Martial, lib. 3. ⁶ Lib. 1, cap. 7.

PAGE 110

¹ Eustathius, lib. 1. Picturæ parant animum ad Venerem, etc. Horatius ad res venereas intemperantior traditur; nam cubiculo suo sic specula dicitur habuisse disposita, ut quocunque respexisset imaginem coitus referrent.—Suetonius, vit. ejus.

² Osculum ut phalangium inficit. ³ Hor. ⁴ Heinsius.

⁵ Applico me illi proximius et spisse deosculata sagum peto.

⁶ Petronius, Catalect.

⁷ Catullus ad Lesbiam: Da mihi basia mille, deinde centum, etc.

⁸ Petronius. ⁹ Apuleius, lib. 10, et Catalect.

¹⁰ Petronius. ¹¹ Apuleius.

¹² Petronius, Proselios ad Circen.

PAGE 111

¹ Petronius.

² Animus conjungitur, et spiritus etiam noster per osculum effiuit; alternatim se in utriusque corpus infundentes commiscent; animæ potius quam corporis connectio.

³ Catullus. ⁴ Lucian, tom. 4.

5 Non dat basia, dat Neæra nectar, dat rores animæ suaveolentes, dat nardum, thymumque, cinnamumque et mel, etc.—Secundus, Bas. 4.
6 Eustathius, lib. 3.　　　　　7 Catullus.　　　　　8 Buchanan.
9 Ovid. Am. Eleg. 18.　　　　10 Ovid.
11 Cum capita liment solitis morsiunculis, et cum mammillarum pressiunculis.—Lip. od. ant. lec. lib. 3.
12 Tom. 4, Dial. meretr.

Page 112

1 Apuleius, Miles. 6. Et unum blandientis linguæ admulsum longe mellitum; et post, lib. 11: Arctius eam complexus cœpi suaviari jamque pariter patentis oris inhalitu cinnameo et occursantis linguæ illisu nectareo, etc.
2 Lib. 1 advers. Jovin. cap. 30.
3 Oscula qui sumpsit, si non et cetera sumpsit, etc.

Page 113

1 Corpus placuit mariti sui tolli ex arca, atque illi quæ vocabat cruci adfigi.
2 Novi ingenium mulierum, nolunt ubi velis, ubi nolis cupiunt ultro.—Ter. Eunuc. Act. 4, sc. 7.　　　　　3 Marlowe.

Page 114

1 Pornoboscodidascalo, dial. Ital. Latin. donat. a Gasp. Barthio Germano. Quanquam natura et arte eram formosissima, isto tamen astu tanto speciosior videbar, quod enim oculis cupitum ægre præbetur, multo magis affectus humanos incendit.
2 Quo majoribus me donis propitiabat, eo pejoribus illum modis tractabam, ne basium impetravit, etc.
3 Comes de monte Turco Hispanus has de venatione sua partes misit, jussitque peramanter orare, ut hoc qualecunque donum suo nomine accipias.
4 His artibus hominem ita excantabam, ut pro me ille ad omnia paratus, etc.　　　　　5 Tom. 4, Dial. meretr.
6 Relicto illo, ægre ipsi interim faciens, et omnino difficilis.

Page 115

1 Si quis enim nec zelotypus irascitur, nec pugnat aliquando amator, nec perjurat, non est habendus amator, etc. Totus hic ignis zelotypia constat, etc.; maximi amores inde nascuntur. Sed si persuasum illi fuerit te solum habere, elanguescit illico amor suus.
2 Venientem videbis ipsum denuo inflammatum et prorsus insanientem.
3 Et sic cum fere de illo desperassem, post menses quatuor ad me rediit.

Page 116

1 Petronius, Catal.
2 Imagines deorum. fol. 327. Varios amores facit, quos aliqui interpretantur multiplices affectus et illecebras, alios puellos, puellas, alatos, alios poma aurea, alios sagittas, alios laqueos, etc.
3 Epist. lib. 3, vita Pauli Eremitæ.
4 Meretrix speciosa cœpit delicatius stringere colla complexibus, et corpore in libidinem concitato, etc.
5 Camden, in Gloucestershire. Huic præfuit nobilis et formosa abbatissa, Godwinus comes indole subtilis, non ipsam, sed sua cupiens, reliquit nepotem suum forma elegantissimum, tanquam infirmum donec reverteretur; instruit, etc.

PAGE 117

[1] Ille impiger regem adit, abbatissam et suas prægnantes edocet, exploratoribus missis probat, et iis ejectis, a domino suo manerium accepit.

[2] Post sermones de casu suo suavitate sermonis conciliat animum hominis, manumque inter colloquia et risus ad barbam protendit et palpare cœpit cervicem suam et osculari; quid multa? Captivum ducit militem Christi. Complexura evanescit, dæmones in aere monachum riserunt.

[3] Choræa circulus, cujus centrum diabolus.

[4] Multæ inde impudicæ domum rediere, plures ambiguæ, melior nulla.

[5] Turpium deliciarum comes est externa saltatio; neque certe facile dictu quæ mala hinc visus hauriat, et quæ pariat, colloquia, monstrosos, inconditos gestus, etc. [6] Juv. Sat. 11.

PAGE 118

[1] Justin, lib. 30. Adduntur instrumenta luxuriæ, tympana et tripudia; nec tam spectator rex, sed nequitiæ magister, etc.

[2] Hor. lib. 3, Od. 6. [3] Havarde, vita ejus.

[4] Of whom he begat William the Conqueror; by the same token she tore her smock down, saying, etc.

[5] Epist. 26. Quis non miratus est saltantem? Quis non vidit et amavit? veterem et novam vidi Romam, sed tibi similem non vidi, Panareta; felix qui Panareta fruitur, etc.

PAGE 119

[1] Principio Ariadne velut sponsa prodit, ac sola recedit; prodiens illico Dionysus ad numeros cantante tibia saltabat; admirati sunt omnes saltantem juvenem, ipsaque Ariadne, ut vix potuerit conquiescere; postea vero cum Dionysus eam aspexit, etc. Ut autem surrexit Dionysus, erexit simul Ariadnem, licebatque spectare gestus osculantium, et inter se complectentium; qui autem spectabant, etc. Ad extremum videntes eos mutuis amplexibus implicatos et jamjam ad thalamum ituros; qui non duxerant uxores jurabant uxores se ducturos; qui autem duxerant conscensis equis et incitatis, ut iisdem fruerentur, domum festinarunt.

[2] Lib. 4, de contemnend. amoribus.

[3] Ad Anysium, epist. 57.

[4] Intempestivum enim est, et a nuptiis abhorrens, inter saltantes podagricum videre senem, et episcopum.

[5] Rem omnium in mortalium vita optimam innocenter accusare.

[6] Quæ honestam voluptatem respicit, aut corporis exercitium, contemni non debet.

[7] Elegantissima res est, quæ et mentem acuet, corpus exerceat, et spectantes oblectet, multos gestus decoros docens, oculos, aures, animum ex æquo demulcens.

PAGE 120

[1] Ovid. [2] System. moralis philosophiæ.

[3] Apuleius, 10. Puelli puellæque virenti florentes ætatula, forma conspicui, veste nitidi, incessu gratiosi, Græcanicam saltantes Pyrrhicam, dispositis ordinationibus, decoros ambitus inerrabant, nunc in orbem flexi, nunc in obliquam seriem connexi, nunc in quadrum cuneati, nunc inde separati, etc.

[4] Lib. 1, cap. 11. [5] Vit. Epaminondæ. [6] Lib. 5.

PAGE 121

[1] Read P. Martyr's Ocean Decades, Benzo, Lerius, Hakluyt, etc.

[2] Angerianus, Erotopægnium.

[3] 5 Leg. Τῆς γὰρ τοιαύτης σπεδῆς ἕνεκα, etc., hujus causa oportuit

disciplinam constitui, ut tam pueri quam puellæ choreas celebrent, spectenturque ac spectent, etc.

[4] Aspectus enim nudorum corporum tam mares quam feminas irritare solet ad enormes lasciviæ appetitus.

[5] Camden, Annal. anno 1578, fol. 276.   Amatoriis facetiis et illecebris exquisitissimus.

[6] Met. 1, Ovid.

[7] Erasmus, Ecl.   Mille mei Siculis errant in montibus agni.

[8] Virg.   [9] Lœchæus.

PAGE 122

[1] Tom. 4, Meretr. dial.   Amare se jurat et lacrimatur dicitque uxorem me ducere velle, quum pater oculos clausisset.

[2] Quum dotem alibi multo majorem aspiciet, etc.

[3] Or upper garment.   Quem Juno miserata veste contexit.

[4] Hor.

[5] Dejeravit illa secundum supra trigesimum ad proximum Decembrem completuram se esse.   [6] Ovid.

PAGE 123

[1] Nam donis vincitur omnis amor.—Tibullus, 1, el. 5.

[2] Fox, Act. 3, sc. 3.   [3] Catullus.

[4] Perjuria ridet amantum Jupiter, et ventos irrita ferre jubet.—Tibul. lib. 3, 6.

[5] In Philebo.   Pejerantibus his dii soli ignoscunt.

[6] Catullus.

PAGE 124

[1] Lib. 1 de contemnendis amoribus.

[2] Dial. Ital.   Argentum ut paleas projiciebat.

[3] Biliosum habui amatorem qui supplex flexis genibus, etc.

[4] Nullus recens allatus terræ fructus, nullum cupediarum genus tam carum erat, nullum vinum Creticum pretiosum, quin ad me ferret illico; credo alterum oculum pignori daturus, etc.

[5] Post musicam opiperas epulas, et tantis juramentis, donis, etc.

[6] Nunquam aliquis umbrarum conjurator tanta attentione, tamque potentibus verbis usus est, quam ille exquisitis mihi dictis, etc.

[7] Chaucer.

[8] Ah crudele genus nec fidum femina nomen!—Tibul. lib. 3, eleg. 4.

[9] Jovianus Pontanus.

PAGE 125

[1] Aristænetus, lib. 2, epist. 13.

[2] Suaviter flebam, ut persuasum habeat lacrimas præ gaudio illius reditus mihi emanare.

[3] Lib. 3.   His accedunt, vultus subtristis, color pallidus, gemebunda vox, ignita suspiria, lacrimæ prope innumerabiles.   Istæ se statim umbræ offerunt tanto squalore et in omni fere diverticulo tanta macie, ut illas jamjam moribundas putes.   [4] Petronius.

[5] Cælestina, Act. 7, Barthio interprete.   Omnibus arridet, et a singulis amari se solam dicit.   [6] Ovid.

PAGE 126

[1] Seneca Hippol.

[2] Tom. 4, Dial. meretr.   Tu vero aliquando mærore afficieris ubi audieris me a meipsa laqueo tui causa suffocatam aut in puteum præcipitatam.

[3] Epist. 20, lib. 2.

[4] Matronæ fient duobus oculis, moniales quatuor, virgines uno, meretrices nullo. [5] Ovid.

[6] Imagines deorum, fol. 332, e Moschi Amore fugitivo, quem Politianus Latinum fecit.

[7] Lib. 3. Mille vix anni sufficerent ad omnes illas machinationes dolosque commemorandos, quos viri et mulieres, ut se invicem circumveniant, excogitare solent.

Page 127

[1] Petronius. [2] Plautus.

[3] Trithemius [Abbot of Spanheim. Wrote Polygraphia (pub. 1518), the first important work on cryptography. Steganographia, on the same subject, was also attributed to him].

[4] [A reference, probably, to Nuntius Inanimatus (The Inanimate Messenger) by Francis Godwin (1562–1633) Bishop of Hereford.]

[5] De Magnet. Philos. lib. 4, cap. 10.

[6] Tibullus, Eleg. 5, lib. 1. Venit in exitium callida lena meum.

[7] Ovid, Met. 10. [8] Pornobosc. Barthii.

[9] De vit. Erem. cap. 3. Ad sororem vix aliquam reclusarum hujus temporis solam invenies, ante cujus fenestram non anus garrula, vel nugigerula mulier sedet, quæ eam fabulis occupet, rumoribus pascat, hujus vel illius monachi, etc.

Page 128

[1] Agreste olus anus vendebat, et Rogo inquam, mater, nunquid scis ubi ego habitem? Delectata illa urbanitate tam stulta, Et quid nesciam? inquit; consurrexitque et cœpit me præcedere; divinam ego putabam, etc.; nudas video meretrices et in lupanar me adductum, sero execratus aniculæ insidias. [2] Plautus, Menæch.

[3] Promissis everberant, molliunt dulciloquiis, et opportunum tempus aucupantes laqueos ingerunt quos vix Lucretia vitaret, escam parant quam vel satur Hippolytus sumeret, etc. Hæ sane sunt virgæ soporiferæ quibus contactæ animæ ad Orcum descendunt; hoc gluten quo compactæ mentium alæ evolare nequeunt, dæmonis ancillæ, quæ sollicitant, etc.

[4] See the Practices of the Jesuits, Anglice, edit. 1630.

Page 129

[1] Æn. Sylv.

[2] *Such* appears to be corrupt, but the Editor has failed to amend it satisfactorily. Shilleto puts *use.*

[3] Chaucer, in the Wife of Bath's Tale.

[4] H. Stephanus, Apol. Herod. lib. 1, cap. 21.

[5] Bale. Puellæ in lectis dormire non poterant.

[6] Idem Josephus, lib. 18, cap. 4.

[7] Liber edit. Augustæ Vindelicorum, an. 1608.

[8] Quarum animas lucrari debent Deo, sacrificant diabolo.

Page 130

[1] M. Drayton, Her. Epist.

[2] Pornoboscodidascalo, dial. Ital. Latin. fact. a Gasp. Barthio. Plus possum quam omnes philosophi, astrologi, necromantici, etc., sola saliva inungens, 1 amplexu et basiis tam furiose furere, tam bestialiter obstupefieri coegi, ut instar idoli me adorarint.

[3] Sagæ omnes sibi arrogant notitiam, et facultatem in amorem alliciendi quos velint; odia inter conjuges serendi, tempestates excitandi, morbos infligendi, etc. [4] Juvenalis Sat.

[5] Idem refert Hen. Kornmannus de mir. mort. lib. 1, cap. 14. Perdite amavit mulierculam quandam, illius amplexibus acquiescens, summa cum indignatione suorum et dolore.

[1] Et inde totus in episcopum furere, illum colere.
[2] Aquisgranum, vulgo Aix. [Aachen, Aix-la-Chapelle.]
[3] Immenso sumptu templum et ædes, etc.
[4] Apolog. Quod Pudentillam viduam ditem et provectioris ætatis feminam cantaminibus in amorem sui pellexisset.
[5] Philopseudes, tom. 3.
[6] Impudicæ mulieres opera veneficarum, diaboli coquarum, amatores suos ad se noctu ducunt et reducunt, ministerio hirci in aere volantis. Multos novi qui hoc fassi sunt, etc.

[1] Mandrake apples, Lemnius, lib. herb. bib. cap. 2.
[2] Of which read Plin. lib. 8, cap. 22, et lib. 13, cap. 25 et Quintilianum, lib. 7.
[3] Lib. 11, cap. 8. Venere implicat eos, qui ex eo bibunt. Idem Ov. Met. 4; Strabo, Geog. lib. 14.
[4] Lod. Guicciardine's Descript. Ger. in Aquisgrano.
[5] Balteus Veneris, in quo suavitas, et dulcia colloquia, benevolentiæ, et blanditiæ, suasiones, fraudes et veneficia includebantur.

[1] Ovid. Facit hunc amor ipse colorem.—Met. 4.
[2] Signa ejus profunditas oculorum, privatio lacrimarum, suspiria, sæpe rident sibi, ac si quod delectabile viderent, aut audirent.
[3] Seneca, Hip. [4] Seneca, Hip.
[5] De morbis cerebri, de erot. amore. Ob spirituum distractionem hepar officio suo non fungitur, nec vertit alimentum in sanguinem, ut debeat. Ergo membra debilia, et penuria alibilis succi marcescunt, squalentque ut herbæ in horto meo hoc mense Maio Zeriscæ, ob imbrium defectum.
[6] Faerie Queene, lib. 3, cant. 11.

[1] Amator. Emblem. 3.
[2] Lib. 4. Animo errat, et quidvis obvium loquitur, vigilias absque causa sustinet, et succum corporis subito amisit.
[3] Apuleius. [4] Chaucer, in the Knight's Tale. [5] Virg. Æn. 4.

[1] Dum vaga passim sidera fulgent, numerat longas tetricus horas, et sollicito nixus cubito suspirando viscera rumpit.
[2] Saliebat crebro tepidum cor ad aspectum Ismenes.
[3] Gordonius, cap. 20. Amittunt sæpe cibum, potum, et maceratur inde totum corpus.
[4] Ter. Eunuch. Dii boni, quid hoc est, adeone homines mutari ex amore, ut non cognoscas eundem esse!
[5] Ovid, Met. 4.
[6] Ad ejus nomen rubebat, et ad aspectum pulsus variebatur.—Plutarch.
[7] Epist. 13.
[8] Barclay, lib. 1. Oculi medico tremore errabant.
[9] Pulsus eorum velox et inordinatus, si mulier quam amat forte transeat.

[1] Signa sunt cessatio ab omni opere insueto, privatio somni, suspiria crebra, rubor cum sit sermo de re amata, et commotio pulsus.
[2] Si noscere vis an homines suspecti tales sint, tangito eorum arterias.

[3] Amor facit inæquales, inordinatos.
[4] In nobilis cujusdam uxore quum subolfacerem adulteri amore fuisse correptam et quam maritus, etc.
[5] Cœpit illico pulsus variari et ferri celerius et sic inveni.
[6] Eunuch. Act. 1, sc. 2.
[7] Epist. 7, lib. 2. Tener sudor et creber anhelitus, palpitatio cordis, etc.
[8] Lib. 1.   [9] Lexoviensis episcopus [Bishop of Lisieux].

PAGE 137

[1] Theodorus Prodromus, Amaranto dial., Gaulmino interpret.
[2] Petron. Catal.
[3] Sed unum ego usque et unum Petam a tuis labellis, postque unum et unum et unum, dari rogabo. Lœchæus, Anacreon.
[4] Jo. Secundus, Bas. 7.
[5] Translated or imitated by Mr. B. Johnson, our arch-poet, in his 119th ep. [The Forest, 6].   [6] Lucret. lib. 4.

PAGE 138

[1] Lucian, tom. 4, Dial. meretr. Sed et aperientes, etc.
[2] Epist. 16.   [3] Deducto ore longo me basio demulcet.
[4] In Deliciis. Mammas tuas tango, etc.   [5] Terent.
[6] Attente adeo in me aspexit, et interdum ingemiscebat, et lacrimabatur. Et si quando bibens, etc.
[7] Quique omnia cernere debes Leucothoen spectas, et virgine figis in una Quos mundo debes oculos.—Ovid, Met. 4.

PAGE 139

[1] Lucian tom. 3. Quoties ad Cariam venis currum sistis, et desuper aspectas.
[2] Ex quo te primum vidi, Pythias, alio oculos vertere non fuit.
[3] Lib. 1.   [4] Dial. amorum.
[5] Ad occasum solis ægre domum rediens, atque totum diem ex adverso deæ sedens recta, in ipsam perpetuo oculorum ictus direxit, etc.
[6] Lib. 3.
[7] Regum palatium non tam diligenti custodia septum fuit, ac ædes meas stipabant, etc.

PAGE 140

[1] Uno et eodem die sexties vel septies ambulant per eandem plateam ut vel unico amicæ suæ fruantur aspectu.—Lib. 3, Theat. Mundi.
[2] Hor.   [3] Ovid.   [4] Ovid.
[5] Hyginus, Fab. 59. Eo die dicitur nonies ad littus currisse.
[6] Chaucer.

PAGE 141

[1] Gen. xxix, 20.   [2] Plautus, Cistel.   [3] Stobæus, e Græco.
[4] Plautus: Credo ego ad hominis carnificinam amorem inventum esse.

PAGE 142

[1] De Civitate Dei, lib. 22, cap. 20. Ex eo oriuntur mordaces curæ, perturbationes, mærores, formidines, insana gaudia, discordiæ, lites, bella, insidiæ, iracundiæ, inimicitiæ, fallaciæ, adulatio, fraus, furtum, nequitia, impudentia.
[2] Marullus, lib. 1.   [3] Ter. Eunuch.
[4] Plautus, Mercat.   [5] Ovid.
[6] Adelphi, Act. 4, sc. 5. M. Bono animo es, duces uxorem hanc. Æ. Hem, pater, num tu ludis me nunc? M. Egone te, quamobrem? Æ. Quod tam misere cupio, etc.

Page 143

[1] Tom. 4, Dial. amorum.
[2] Aristotle, 2 Rhet., puts love therefore in the irascible part.
[3] Ter. Eunuch. Act. 1, sc. 2.
[4] Plautus.   [5] Tom. 3.
[6] Scis quod posthac dicturus fuerim.
[7] Tom. 4, Dial. meretr. Tryphæna, amor me perdit, neque malum hoc amplius sustinere possum.
[8] Aristænetus, lib. 2, epist. 8.

Page 144

[1] Cælestinæ Act 1. Sancti majora lætitia non fruuntur. Si mihi Deus omnium votorum mortalium summam concedat, non magis, etc.
[2] Catullus de Lesbia.   [3] Hor. Ode 9, lib. 3.
[4] Act 3, sc. 5, Eunuch. Ter.   [5] Act. 5, sc. 8.

Page 145

[1] Mantuan.   [2] Ter. Andria, 3, 4.
[3] Lib. 1, de contemn. amoribus. Si quem respexerit amica suavius, et familiarius, si quem alloquuta fuerit, si nutu, nuntio, etc., statim cruciatur.
[4] Callisto in Cælestina.
[5] Pornoboscodidasc. dial. Ital. Patre et matre se singuli orbos censebant, quod meo contubernio carendum esset.
[6] Ter.
[7] Si responsum esset dominam occupatam esse aliisque vacaret, ille statim vix hoc audito velut in armor obriguit, alii se damnare, etc., at cui favebam, in campis Elysiis esse videbatur, etc.
[8] Mantuan.

Page 146

[1] Lœchæus.
[2] Sole se occultante, aut tempestate veniente, statim clauditur ac languescit.
[3] Emblem. amat. 13.   [4] Callisto de Melibœa.
[5] Anima non est ubi animat, sed ubi amat.
[6] Cælestina, Act. 1. Credo in Melibœam, etc.
[7] Ter. Eunuch. Act. 1, sc. 2.

Page 147

[1] Virg. Æn. 4.
[2] Tota hac nocte somnum hisce oculis non vidi.—Ter.
[3] Interdiu oculi, et aures occupatæ distrahunt animum, at noctu solus jactor, ad auroram somnus paulum misertus, nec tamen ex animo puella abiit, sed omnia mihi de Leucippe somnia erant.
[4] Buchanan, Silv.
[5] Æn. Sylv. Te dies noctesque amo, te cogito, te desidero, te voco, te expecto, te spero, tecum oblecto me, totus in te sum.
[6] Hor. lib. 2, Ode 9.

Page 148

[1] Petronius.   [2] Tibullus, lib. 3, Eleg. 3.   [3] Ovid, Fast. 2, ver. 777.
[4] Virg. Æn. 4.   [5] De Pythonissa.
[6] Juno, nec ira deum tantum, nec tela, nec hostes, Quantum tute noces animis illapsa.—Silius Ital. 15 Bel. Punic. de amore.

PAGE 149

[1] Philostratus, vita ejus. Maximum tormentum quod excogitare, vel docere te possum, est ipse amor.

[2] Ausonius, cap. 35.

[3] Et cæco carpitur igni. At mihi sese offert ultra meus ignis Amyntas.

[4] Ter. Eunuc.   [5] Sen. Hippol.

[6] Theocritus, Idyl. 2.   Levibus cor est violabile telis.

[7] Ignis tangentes solum urit, at forma procul astantes inflammat·

[8] Nonius.

[9] Major illa flamma quæ consumit unam animam, quam quæ centum millia corporum.

[10] Mant. Ecl. 2.

PAGE 150

[1] Marullus, Epig. lib. 1.   [2] Imagines deorum.

[3] Ovid.   [4] Æneid 4.   [5] Seneca.

[6] Cor totum combustum, jecur suffumigatum, pulmo arefactus, ut credam miseram illam animam bis elixam aut combustam, ob maximum ardorem quem patiuntur ob ignem amoris.

[7] Embl. Amat. 4 et 5.   [8] Grotius.

PAGE 151

[1] Lib. 4.   Nam istius amoris neque principia neque media aliud habent quid, quam molestias, dolores, cruciatus, defatigationes, adeo ut miserum esse mærore, gemitu, solitudine torqueri, mortem optare, semperque debacchari, sint certa amantium signa et certæ actiones.

[2] Virg. Æn. 4.   [3] Seneca, Hip.

[4] Eclog. 1.   [5] Idyl. 10.

[6] Mant. Eclog. 2.   Ov. Met. 13, de Polyphemo: Uritur oblitus pecorum, antrorumque suorum; jamque tibi formæ, etc.

[7] Ter. Eunuch.

PAGE 152

[1] Qui, quæso?   Amo.   [2] Ter. Eunuch.

[3] Qui olim cogitabat quæ vellet, et pulcherrimis philosophiæ præceptis operam insumpsit, qui universi circuitiones cœlique naturam, etc., hanc unam intendit operam, de sola cogitat, noctes et dies se componit ad hanc, et ad acerbam servitutem redactus animus, etc.

[4] Pars epitaphii ejus.   [5] Epist. prima.

[6] Boethius, lib. 3, met. ult.

[7] Epist. lib. 2.   Valeat pudor, valeat honestas, valeat honor.

[8] Theodor. Prodromus, lib. 3. Amor Mystyli genibus obvolutus, ubertimque lacrimans, etc.   Nihil ex tota præda præter Rhodanthen virginem accipiam.

PAGE 153

[1] Lib. 3.   Certe vix credam, et bona fide fateare, Aretine, te non amasse adeo vehementer; si enim vere amasses, nihil prius aut potius optasses, quam amatæ mulieri placere.   Ea enim amoris lex est idem velle et nolle.

[2] Stroza fil. Epig.

[3] Quippe hæc omnia ex atra bile et amore proveniunt.—Jason Pratensis.

[4] Immensus amor ipse stultitia est.—Cardan, lib. 1 de sapientia.

[5] Mantuan.

[6] [A proverbial expression, implying perplexity and indecision.]

[7] Virg. Æn. 4.

PAGE 154

[1] Seneca, Hippol.   [2] Met. 10.   [3] Buchanan.

[4] An immodest woman is like a bear.

Page 155

[1] Feram induit dum rosas comedat, idem ad se redeat.
[2] Alciatus, de upupa embl. Animal immundum upupa stercora amans; ave hac nihil fœdius, nihil libidinosius.—Sabin. in Ovid. Met.
[3] Love is like a false glass, which represents everything fairer than it is.

Page 156

[1] Hor. Ser. lib. sat. 1, 3.
[2] The daughter and heir of Carolus Pugnax [Charles the Bold].
[3] Seneca in Octavia.   [4] Lœchæus.
[5] Mantuan, Ecl. 1.   [6] Angerianus.
[7] Faerie Queene, cant. 2, lib. 4.

Page 157

[1] Epist. 12. Quis unquam formas vidit orientis, quis occidentis? veniant undique omnes, et dicant veraces, an tam insignem viderint formam.
[2] Nulla vox formam ejus possit comprehendere.
[3] Calcagnini dial. Galat.   [4] Catullus.
[5] Petronii Catalecta.   [6] Chaucer, in the Knight's Tale.

Page 158

[1] Ovid, Met. 13.
[2] Plutarch. Sibi dixit tam pulchram non videri, etc.
[3] Quanto te, Lucifer, aurea Phœbe, tanto virginibus conspectior omnibus Herse.—Ovid.

Page 159

[1] M[ichael] D[rayton], Son. 30.
[2] Martial, lib. 5, Epig. 37.   [3] Ariosto.
[4] Tully, lib 1 de nat. deor. Pulchrior deo, et tamen erat oculis perversissimis.
[5] Marullus ad Neæram, epig. lib. 1.
[6] Barthius.   [7] Ariosto, lib. 29, st. 8.

Page 160

[1] Tibullus.   [2] Marul. lib. 2.
[3] Tibullus, lib. 4, de Sulpicia.   [4] Aristœnetus, Epist. 1.
[5] Epist. 24. Veni cito, carissime Lysia, cito veni; præ te satyri omnes videntur non homines, nullo loco solus es, etc.
[6] Lib. 3 de aulico. Alterius affectui se totum componit, totus placere studet, et ipsius animam amatæ pedissequam facit.

Page 161

[1] Cyropæd. lib. 5. Amor servitus, et qui amant optant eo liberari non secus ac alio quovis morbo, neque liberari tamen possunt, sed validiori necessitate ligati sunt quam si in ferrea vincula confecti forent.
[2] In Paradoxis. An ille mihi liber videtur cui mulier imperat? cui leges imponit, præscribit, jubet, vetat quod videtur? qui nihil imperanti negat, nihil audet, etc.; poscit? dandum; vocat? veniendum; minatur? extimiscendum.
[3] Illane parva est servitus amatorum singulis fere horis pectine capillum, calamistroque barbam componere, faciem aquis redolentibus diluere, etc.
[4] Si quando in pavimentum incautius quid mihi excidisset, elevare inde quam promptissime, nec nisi osculo compacto mihi commendare, etc.

Page 162

[1] Plutarchus, Amat. dial.
[2] Lib. 1 de contem. amor. Quid referam eorum pericula et clades, qui in amicarum ædes per fenestras ingressi stillicidiaque egressi indeque deturbati, sed aut præcipites, membra frangunt, collidunt, aut animam amittunt.

Page 163

[1] Ter. Eunuch. Act. 5, sc. 8.
[2] Paratus sum ad obeundum mortem, si tu jubeas; hanc sitim æstuantis seda, quam tuum sidus perdidit, aquæ et fontes non negant, etc.
[3] Si occidere placet, ferrum meum vides, si verberibus contenta es, curro nudus ad pœnam.
[4] Act. 15, 18. Impera mihi; occidam decem viros, etc.
[5] Gaspar Ens. Puellam misere deperiens, per jocum ab ea in Padum desilire jussus statim e ponte se præcipitavit. Alius Ficino insano amore ardens ab amica jussus se suspendere, illico fecit.

Page 164

[1] Intelligo pecuniam rem esse jucundissimam, meam tamen libentius darem Cliniæ quam ab aliis acciperem; libentius huic servirem, quam aliis imperarem, etc. Noctem et somnum accuso, quod illum non videam, luci autem et soli gratiam habeo quod mihi Cliniam ostendant. Ego etiam cum Clinia in ignem currerem; et scio vos quoque mecum ingressuros si videretis.
[2] Impera quidvis; navigare jube, navem conscendo; plagas accipere, plector; animum profundere, in ignem currere, non recuso, lubens facio.
[3] Hujus ero vivus, mortuus hujus ero.—Propert. lib. 2. Vivam si vivat; si cadat illa, cadam.—Id.
[4] Seneca, in Hipp. Act. 2.
[5] Dial. Amorum. Mihi, o dii cœlestes, ultra sit vita hæc perpetua ex adverso amicæ sedere, et suave loquentem audire, etc.; si moriatur, vivere non sustinebo, et idem erit sepulchrum utrisque.
[6] Buchanan.
[7] Epist. 21. Sit hoc votum a diis amare Delphidem, ab ea amari adloqui pulchram et loquentem audire. [8] Hor.

Page 165

[1] Mart. [2] Lege Calamitates Pet. Abelhardi, Epist. prima.
[3] Ariosto. [4] Chaucer, in the Knight's Tale.
[5] Theodorus Prodromus, Amorum lib. 6, interprete Gaulmino.

Page 166

[1] Ovid, 10 Met.; Hyginus, Fab. 185.
[2] Ariosto, lib. 1, cant. 1, staff 5. [3] Plut. Dial. amor.
[4] Faerie Queene, cant. 1, lib. 4, and cant. 3, lib. 4.
[5] Dum cassis pertusa, ensis instar serræ excisus, scutum, etc.—Barthius, Cælestina.
[6] Lesbia sex cyathis, septem Justina bibatur.
[7] As Xanthus, for the love of Erippe, omnem Europam peragravit.—Parthenius, Erot. cap. 8.
[8] Beroaldus, e Boccaccio.

Page 167

[1] Epist. 17, lib. 2. [2] Lucretius.
[3] Æneas Sylvius. Lucretia quum accepit Euryali literas hilaris statim milliesque papyrum basiavit.

⁴ Mediis inseruit papillis litteram ejus, mille prius pangens suavia.—Arist. 2, epist. 13.
⁵ Plautus, Asinar.   ⁶ Hor.

PAGE 168

¹ Illa domi sedens imaginem ejus fixis oculis assidue conspicata.
² Buchanan, Silvæ.   ³ Fracastorius Naugerio.
⁴ Happy servants that serve her, happy men that are in her company!
⁵ Non ipsos solum sed ipsorum memoriam amant.—Lucian.
⁶ Epist. O ter felix solum! beatus ego, si me calcaveris; vultus tuus amnes sistere potest, etc.

PAGE 169

¹ Idem, Epist. In prato cum sit flores superat; illi pulchri see unius tantum diei; fluvius gratus sed evanescit; at tuus fluvius mari major. Si cœlum aspicio, solem existimo cecidisse, et in terra ambulare, etc.
² Si civitate egrederis, sequentur te dii custodes, spectaculo commoti; si naviges sequentur; quis fluvius salum tuum non rigaret?
³ [Amorum] 2, el. 15.   ⁴ Carm. 22.
⁵ Englished by Mr. B. Holliday, in his Technogamia, Act. 1, sc. 7.

PAGE 170

¹ Ovid. Met. lib. 4.   ² Plautus de milite.
³ Xenophon, Cyropæd, lib. 5.   ⁴ Lucian.
⁵ Petronius.   ⁶ E Græco Ruf.
⁷ Lod. Vertomannus, Navig. lib. 2, cap. 5. O deus, hunc creasti sole candidiorem, e diverso me et conjugem meum et natos meos nigricantes. Utinam hic, etc. Ibit [?] Gazella, Tegeia, Galzerana, et promissis oneravit, et donis, etc.

PAGE 171

¹ M[ichael] D[rayton].   ² Hor. Ode 9. lib. 3.
³ Ov. Met. 10.   ⁴ Buchanan, Hendecasyl.

PAGE 172

¹ Petrarch.
² Cardan, lib. 2 de sap. Ex vilibus generosos efficere solet, ex timidis audaces, ex avaris splendidos, ex agrestibus civiles, ex crudelibus mansuetos, ex impiis religiosos, ex sordidis nitidos atque oultos, ex duris misericordes, ex mutis eloquentes.
³ Anima hominis amore capti tota referta suffitibus et odoribus; pæanes resonat, etc.   ⁴ Ovid.
⁵ In Convivio. Amor Veneris Martem detinet, et fortem facit; adolescentem maxime erubescere cernimus quum amatrix eum turpe quid committentem ostendit.
⁶ Plutarch, Amator. dial.

PAGE 173

¹ Si quo pacto fieri civitas aut exercitus posset partim ex his qui amant, partim ex his, etc.
² Angerianus.   ³ Faerie Queene, lib. 4, cant. 2.
⁴ Zenod. Proverb. cont. 6.   ⁵ Plat. Conviv.
⁶ Lib. 3 de aulico. Non dubito quin is qui talem exercitum haberet, totius orbis statim victor esset, nisi forte cum aliquo exercitu confligendum esset in quo omnes amatores essent.
⁷ Hyginus de cane et lepore cœlesti, et Decimator.
⁸ Vix dici potest quantam inde audaciam assumerent Hispani, inde pauci infinitas Maurorum copias superarunt.

PAGE 174

[1] Lib. 5 de legibus.
[2] Spenser's Faerie Queene, book 3, cant. 8.
[3] Hyginus, lib. 2.   [4] Aratus in Phænom.   [5] Virg.
[6] Hanc ubi conspicatus est Cymon, baculo innixus, immobilis stetit, et mirabundus, etc.

PAGE 175

[1] Plautus, Casina, Act. 2, sc. 4.   [2] Plautus.
[3] Ovid, Met. 2.   [4] Ovid. Met. 4.   [5] Virg. Æn. 1.

PAGE 176

[1] [Severus.]   [2] Ovid. Met. 13.   [3] Virg. Ecl. 2.
[4] Epist. An uxor literato sit ducenda. Noctes insomnes traducendæ, literis renunciandum, sæpe gemendum, nonnunquam et illacrimandum sorti et conditioni tuæ. Videndum quæ vestes, quis cultus te deceat, quis in usu sit, utrum latus barbæ, etc. Cum cura loquendum, incedendum, bibendum et cum cura insaniendum.

PAGE 177

[1] Mart. Epig. 8.   [2] Chil. 4, cent. 5, prov. 16.
[3] Martianus Capella, lib. 1 de nupt. Philol. Jam illum sentio amore teneri, ejusque studio plures habere comparatas in famulitio disciplinas, etc.
[4] Lib. 3 de aulico. Quis choreis insudaret, nisi feminarum causa? Quis musicæ tantam navaret operam nisi quod illius dulcedine permulcere speret? Quis tot carmina componeret, nisi ut inde affectus suos in mulieres explicaret?
[5] Craterem nectaris evertit saltans apud deos, qui in terram cadens, rosam prius albam rubore infecit.
[6] Puellas choreantes circa juvenilem Cupidinis statuam fecit.—Philostrat. Imag. lib. 3, de statuis. Exercitium amori aptissimum.

PAGE 178

[1] Lib. 6 Met.   [2] Tom. 4.
[3] Kornman. de cur. mort. part. 5, cap. 28. Sat. puellæ dormienti insultantium, etc.   [4] View of France.
[5] Vita ejus. Puellæ amore septuagenarius senex usque ad insaniam correptus, multis liberis susceptis: multi non sine pudore conspexerunt senem et philosophum podagricum, non sine risu saltantem ad tibiæ modos.
[6] Anacreon, Carm. 31.

PAGE 179

[1] Joach. Bellius, Epig.
[2] De taciturno loquacem facit, et de verecundo officiosum reddit, de negligente industrium, de socorde impigrum.
[3] Gellius, lib. 1, cap. 8. Pretium noctis centum sestertia.
[4] Josephus, Antiq. Jud. lib. 18, cap. 4.
[5] Ipsi enim volunt suarum amasiarum pulchritudinis præcones ac testes esse, eas laudibus, et cantilenis et versibus exornare, ut auro statuas, ut memorentur, et ab omnibus admirentur.

PAGE 180

[1] Tom. 2, Ant. Dialogo.   [2] Flores Hist. fol. 298.
[3] Per totum annum cantarunt, pluvia super illos non cecidit; non frigus, non calor, non sitis, nec lassitudo illos affecit, etc.
[4] His eorum nomina inscribuntur de quibus quærunt.

PAGE 181

[1] Huic munditias, ornatum, leporem, delicias, ludos, elegantiam, omnem denique vitæ suavitatem debemus.
[2] Hyginus, cap. 272. [3] E Græco. [4] Angerianus.
[5] Fransus, lib. 3 de symbolis. Qui primus symbolum excogitavit voluit nimirum hac ratione implicatum animum evolvere, eumque vel dominæ vel aliis intuentibus ostendere.
[6] Lib. 4, tit. 11, de prin. instit.
[7] Plin. lib. 35, cap. 12. [8] Gerbelius, lib. 6 descript. Gr.

PAGE 182

[1] Lib. 4, num. 102, Sylvæ nuptialis. Poetæ non inveniunt fabulas, aut versus laudatos faciunt, nisi qui ab amore fuerint excitati.
[2] Martial, Ep. 73, lib. 9. [3] Virg. Eclog. 4.

PAGE 183

[1] Teneris arboribus amicarum nomina inscribentes ut simul crescant. —Hædus.
[2] S[amuel] R[owlands], 1600. [3] Lib. 13, cap. Deipnosophist.
[4] See Putean. Epist. 33, de sua Margareta, Beroaldus, etc.
[5] Hen. Steph. Apol. pro Herod.

PAGE 184

[1] Tully, Orat. 3 Verr. [2] Esther v, 6. [3] Matt. xiv, 7.
[4] Gravissimis regni negotiis nihil sine amasiæ suæ consensu fecit, omnesque actiones suas scortillo communicavit, etc.—Nich. Bellus, discurs. 26 de amat.
[5] Amoris famulus omnem scientiam diffitetur, amandi tamen se scientissimum doctorem agnoscit. [6] Serm. 8.
[7] Quis horum scribere molestias potest, nisi qui et is aliquantum insanit?
[8] Lib. 1 de contemnendis amoribus. Opinor hac de re neminem aut disceptare recte posse aut judicare qui non in ea versatur, aut magnum fecerit periculum.

PAGE 185

[1] Semper moritur, nunquam mortuus est qui amat.—Æn. Sylv.
[2] Euryal. ep. ad Lucretiam, apud Æneam Sylvium. Rogas ut amare desistam? roga montes ut in planum deveniant, ut fontes flumina repetant; tam possum te non amare ac suum Phœbus relinquere cursum.
[3] Buchanan, Syl. [4] Propert. lib. 2, Eleg. 1.
[5] Est orcus illa vis, est immedicabilis, est rabies insana. [6] Lib. 2.

PAGE 186

[1] Virg. Ecl. 10. [2] R[obert] T[ofte].
[3] Qui quidem amor utrosque et totam Ægyptum extremis calamitatibus involvit. [4] Plautus.
[5] Ut corpus pondere, sic animus amore præcipitatur. — Austin, lib. 2 de Civ. Dei, cap. 28.
[6] Dial. Hinc oritur pœnitentia, desperatio, et non vident ingenium se cum re simul amisisse.
[7] Idem Savonarola, et plures alii, etc. Rabidam facturus Orexin.—Juven.
[8] Cap. de Heroico Amore. Hæc passio durans sanguinem torridum et atrabiliarum reddit; hic vero ad cerebrum delatus insaniam parat, vigilia et crebro desiderio exsiccans. [9] Virg. Ecl. 2.

[10] Insani fiunt aut sibi ipsis desperantes mortem afferunt. Languentes cito mortem aut maniam patiuntur. [11] Calcagninus.
[12] Lucian, Imag. So for Lucian's mistress, all that saw her and could not enjoy her, ran mad or hanged themselves.

PAGE 187

[1] Musæus. [2] Ovid. Met. 10. [3] Anacreon.
[4] Æneas Sylvius. Ad ejus decessum nunquam visa Lucretia ridere, nullis facetiis, jocis, nullo gaudio potuit ad lætitiam renovari, mox in ægritudinem incidit, et sic brevi contabuit.
[5] Pausanias, Achaicis, lib. 7.
[6] Megarensis amore flagrans.—Lucian, tom. 4. [7] Ovid. Met. 4.

PAGE 188

[1] Furibundus putavit se videre imaginem puellæ, et coram loqui blandiens illi, etc. [2] Juvenis Hebræus.
[3] Juvenis medicinæ operam dans doctoris filiam deperibat, etc.
[4] Gotardus Arthus Gallobelgicus. Nund. vernal. 1615, collum novacula aperuit, et inde expiravit.
[5] Cum renuente parente utroque et ipsa virgine frui non posset, ipsum et ipsam interfecit, hoc a magistratu petens, ut in eodem sepulchro sepeliri possent. [6] Boccaccio.
[7] Sedes eorum qui pro amoris impatientia pereunt.—Virg. 6 Æneid.
[8] Sall., Val. Max. [9] Sabel. lib. 3, En. 6.
[10] Curtius, lib. 5.
[11] Chalcocondylas de reb. Tuscicis, lib. 9. Nerei uxor Athenarum domina, etc.
[12] Nicephorus Greg. Hist. lib. 8. Uxorem occidit, liberos et Michaelem filium videre abhorruit. Thessalonicæ amore captus pronotarii filiæ, etc.

PAGE 189

[1] Parthenius, Erot. lib. cap. 5.
[2] Idem, cap. 21. Gubernatoris filia Achillis amore capta civitatem prodidit.
[3] Idem, cap. 9. [4] Virg. Æn. 6.
[5] Otium naufragium castitatis.—Austin.

PAGE 190

[1] Buchanan, Hendecasyl. [2] Ovid. Remed.
[3] Cap. 16. Circa res arduas exerceri.
[4] Part 2, cap. 23, Reg. San. His, præter horam somni, nulla per otium transeat.
[5] Hor. lib. 1, epist. 2. [6] Seneca.

PAGE 191

[1] Tract. 16, cap. 18. Sæpe nuda carne cilicium portent tempore frigido sine caligis, et nudis pedibus incedant, in pane et aqua jejunent, sæpius se verberibus cædant, etc.
[2] Dæmonibus referta sunt corpora nostra, illorum præcipue qui delicatis vescuntur eduliis, advolitant, et corporibus inhærent; hanc ob rem jejunium impendio probatur ad pudicitiam.
[3] Victus sit attenuatus, balnei frequens usus et sudationes; cold baths, not hot, saith Magninus, part. 3, cap. 23, to dive over head and ears in a cold river, etc.
[4] Ser. de gula. Fames amica virginitati est, inimica lasciviæ: saturitas vero castitatem perdit, et nutrit illecebras.

[5] Vita Hilarionis, lib. 3, epist. Cum tentasset eum dæmon titillatione inter cætera, Ego inquit, aselle, ad corpus suum, faciam, etc.
[6] Strabo, lib. 15 Geog. Sub pellibus cubant, etc.
[7] Cap. 2, part. 2. Si sit juvenis, et non vult obœdire, flagelletur frequenter et fortiter, dum incipiat fœtere.
[8] Laertius, lib. 6, cap. 5. Amori medetur fames; sin aliter, tempus; sin non hoc, laqueus.
[9] Vina parant animos Veneri, etc.   [10] 2 de Legibus.

Page 192

[1] Non minus si vinum bibissent ac si adulterium admisissent.—Gellius, lib. 10, cap. 23.
[2] Reg. San. part. 3, cap. 23. Mirabilem vim habet.
[3] Cum muliere aliqua gratiosa sæpe coire erit utilissimum. Idem Laurentius, cap. 11.   [4] Hor.

Page 193

[1] Cap. 29 de morb. cereb.
[2] Beroaldus, Orat. de amore.
[3] Amatori, cujus est pro impotentia mens amota, opus est ut paulatim animus velut a peregrinatione domum revocetur per musicam, convivia, etc., per aucupium, fabulas, et festivas narrationes, labore usque ad sudorem, etc.
[4] Cælestinæ Act. 2, Barthio interpret.
[5] Cap de Ilishi. Multus hoc affectu sanat cantilena, lætitia, musica; et quidam sunt quos hæc angent.
[6] This author came to my hands since the third edition of this book.

Page 194

[1] Cent. 3, curat. 56. Syrupo helleborato et aliis quæ ad atram bilem pertinent.
[2] Purgetur si ejus dispositio venerit ad adust. humoris, et phlebotomizetur.
[3] Amantium morbus ut pruritus solvitur, venæ sectione et cucurbitulis.
[4] Cura a venæ sectione per aures, unde semper steriles.

Page 195

[1] Seneca.
[2] Cum in mulierem inciderit, quæ cum forma morum suavitatem conjunctam habet, et jam oculos persenserit formæ ad se imaginem cum aviditate quadam rapere cum eadem, etc.
[3] Ovid, Rem.   [4] Æneas Sylvius.   [5] Plautus, Curculio.

Page 196

[1] Tom. 2, lib. 4, cap. 10, Syntag. med. arc. mira. Vitentur oscula, tactus, sermo, et scripta impudica, literæ, etc.
[2] Lib. de singul. cler.
[3] Tam admirabilem splendorem declinet, gratiam, scintillas, amabiles risus, gestus suavissimos, etc.
[4] Lipsius, Hort. leg. lib. 3, antiq. lec.
[5] Lib. 3 de vit. cœlitus compar. cap. 6.
[6] Lucretius.   [7] Lib. 4, eleg. 21.
[8] Job xxxi. Pepigi fœdus cum oculis meis ne cogitarem de virgine.
[9] Dial. 3, de contemptu mundi. Nihil facilius recrudescit quam amor; ut pompa visa renovat ambitionem, auri species avaritiam, spectata corporis forma incendit luxuriam.
[10] Seneca, Cont. lib. 2, cont. 9.

PAGE 197

[1] Ovid.
[2] Met. 7. Ut solet a ventis alimenta assumere, quæque Parva sub inducta latuit scintilla favilla, Crescere et in veteres agitata resurgere flammas.
[3] Eustathii lib. 3. Aspectus amorem incendit, ut marcescentem in palea ignem ventus; ardebam interea majore concepto incendio.
[4] Heliodorus, lib. 4. Inflammat mentem novus aspectus, perinde ac gnis materiæ admotus. Chariclea, etc.
[5] Epist. 16, lib. 2.   [6] Epist. 4, lib. 2.
[7] Curtius, lib. 3. Cum uxorem Darii laudatam audivisset, tantum cupiditati suæ frænum injecit, ut illam vix vellet intueri.
[8] Cyropædia. Cum Pantheæ formam evexisset Araspes, tanto magis, inquit Cyrus, abstinere oportet, quanto pulchrior est.

PAGE 198

[1] Livius. Cum eam regulo cuidam desponsatam audivisset, muneribus cumulatam remisit.
[2] Ep. 39, lib. 7.
[3] Et ea loqui posset quæ soli amatores loqui solent.
[4] Platonis Convivio.
[5] Heliodorus, lib. 4. Expertem esse amoris beatitudo est; at quum captus sis, ad moderationem revocare animum prudentia singularis.
[6] Lucretius, lib. 4.
[7] Hædus, lib. 1, de amor. contem.

PAGE 199

[1] Loci mutatione tanquam non convalescens curandus est.
[2] Amorum lib. 2.
[3] Quisquis amat, loca nota nocent; dies ægritudinem adimit, absentia delet. Ire libet procul hinc patriæque relinquere fines.—Ovid.
[4] Lib. 3, eleg. 20.
[5] Lib. 1 Socrat. Memor. Tibi, O Critobule, consulo ut integrum annum absis, etc.
[6] Proximum est ut esurias; 2, ut moram temporis opponas; 3, ut locum mutes; 4, ut de laqueo cogites.
[7] Philostratus de vita Sophistarum.

PAGE 200

[1] Virg. Æn. 6.   [2] Buchanan.
[3] Annuncientur valde tristia, ut major tristitia possit minorem obfuscare.
[4] Aut quod sit factus senescallus, aut habeat honorem magnum.

PAGE 201

[1] Adolescens Græcus erat in Ægypti cœnobio qui nulla operis magnitudine, nulla persuasione flammam poterat sedare: monasterii pater hac arte servavit. Imperat cuidam e sociis, etc. Flebat ille, omnes adversabantur; solus pater callide opponere, ne abundantia tristitiæ absorberetur; quid multa? hoc invento curatus est, et a cogitationibus pristinis avocatus.
[2] Tom. 4.   [3] Ter.
[4] Hypatia Alexandrina quendam se adamantem prolatis muliebribus pannis, et in eum conjectis ab amoris insania laboravit.—Suidas et Eunapius.

PAGE 202

[1] Savonarola, reg. 5.   [2] Virg. Ecl. 3.
[3] Distributio amoris fiat in plures, ad plures amicas animum applicet.
[4] Ovid.   [5] Hyginus, fab. 43.   [6] Petronius.
[7] Lib. de salt.
[8] E theatro egressus hilaris, ac si pharmacum oblivionis bibisset.
[9] Mus in cista natus, etc.

PAGE 203

[1] In quem e specu subterraneo modicum lucis illabitur.
[2] Deplorabant eorum miseriam qui subterraneis illis locis vitam degunt.
[3] Tatius, lib. 6.   [4] Aristænetus, Epist. 4.
[5] Calcagninus, Dial. Galat. Mox aliam prætulit, aliam prælaturus quam primum occasio arriserit.
[6] Epist. lib. 2, 16. Philosophi sæculi veterem amorem novo, quasi clavum clavo repellere, quod et Assuero regi septem principes Persarum fecere, ut Vasthi reginæ desiderium amore compensarent.
[7] Ovid.

PAGE 204

[1] Lugubri veste indutus, consolationes non admisit, donec Cæsar ex ducali sanguine, virginem matrimonio conjunxi. — Æneas Sylvius, Hist. de Euryalo et Lucretia.
[2] Ter.   [3] Virg. Ecl. 2.   [4] Lib. de beat. vit. cap. 14.

PAGE 205

[1] Longo ucu dioimus, longa desuetudine dediscendum est.—Petrarch, Epist. lib. 5, 8.
[2] Tom. 4, Dial. meretr. Fortasse etiam ipsa ad amorem istum nonnihil contulero.
[3] Quid enim meretrix nisi juventutis expilatrix, virorum rapina seu mors; patrimonii devoratrix, honoris pernicies, pabulum diaboli, janua mortis, inferni supplementum?
[4] Sanguinem hominum sorbent.
[5] Contemplatione Idiotæ, cap. 34. Discrimen vitæ, mors blanda, mel felleum, dulce venenum, pernicies delicata, malum spontaneum, etc.
[6] Pornoboscodidasc. dial. Ital. Gula, ira, invidia, superbia, sacrilegia, latrocinia, cædes, eo die nata sunt, quo primum meretrix professionem fecit. Superbia major quam opulenti rustici, invidia quam luis venereæ, inimicitia nocentior melancholia, avaritia in immensum profunda.
[7] Qualis extra sum vides, qualis intra novit Deus.

PAGE 206

[1] Virg.   [2] Tom. 2, in Votis. Calvus cum sis, nasum habeas simum, etc.

PAGE 207

[1] Petronius.   [2] Ovid.   [3] In Catharticis, lib. 2.
[4] Si ferveat deformis, ecce formosa est; si frigeat formosa, jam sis informis.—Th. Morus, Epigram.

PAGE 208

[1] Amorum dial. tom. 4. Si quis ad auroram contempletur multas mulieres a nocte lecto surgentes, turpiores putabit esse bestiis.
[2] Hugo, de claustro animæ, lib. 1, cap. 1.
[3] Hist. nat. 11, cap. 35. A fly that hath golden wings but a poisoned body.   [4] Buchanan, Hendecasyl.
[5] Apol. pro Raim. Seb.   [6] Ovid, Rem.

PAGE 209

[1] Post unam noctem incertum unde offensam cepit, propter fœtentem ejus spiritum alii dicunt, vel latentem fœditatem repudiavit, rem faciens plane illicitam, et regiæ personæ multum indecoram.

[2] Hall and Grafton belike.

[3] Juvenal.   [4] Martial.   [5] Hor. Ode 13, lib. 4.

[6] Tully in Catilinam.   [7] Lœchæus.

[8] Qualis fuit Venus cum fuit virgo, balsamum spirans, etc.

PAGE 210

[1] Seneca.   [2] Seneca, Hippol.

[3] Camerarius, Emb. 68, cent. 1.   Flos omnium pulcherrimus statim languescit, formæ typus.

[4] Bernar. Bauhusius, Ep. lib. 4.

[5] Pausanias, Lacon. lib. 3.   Uxorem duxit Spartæ mulierum omnium post Helenam formosissimam, at ob mores omnium turpissimam.

[6] Epist. 76.   Gladium bonum dices, non cui deauratus est balteus, nec cui vagina gemmis distinguitur, sed cui ad secandum subtilis acies et mucro munimentum omne rupturus.

[7] Pulchritudo corporis, temporis et morbi ludibrium.—Orat. 2.

[8] Florum mutabilitate fugacior, nec sua natura formosas facit, sed spectantium infirmitas.

[9] Epist. 11.   Quem ego depereo juvenis mihi pulcherrimus videtur; sed forsan amore percita de amore non recte judico.

[10] Luc. Brugensis.

PAGE 211

[1] Idem.   [2] Bebelius adagiis Ger.   [3] Petron. Cat.

[4] [Proverbial for "care has come upon her."]

PAGE 212

[1] M. Drayton.   [2] Senec. Act. 2, Herc. Œtæus.

[3] Vides venustam mulierem, fulgidum habentem oculum, vultu hilari, coruscantem eximium quendam aspectum et decorum præ se ferentem, urentem mentem tuam, et concupiscentiam agentem; cogita terram esse id quod amas, et quod admiraris stercus, et quod te urit, etc., cogita illam jam senescere, jam rugosam cavis genis, ægrotam; tantis sordibus intus plena est, pituita, stercore; reputa quid intra nares, oculos, cerebrum gestat, quas sordes, etc.

PAGE 213

[1] Subtil. 13.   [2] Cardan, Subtil. lib. 13.

PAGE 214

[1] Lib. de contem. amoribus.   Earum mendas volvant animo, sæpe ante oculos constituant, sæpe damnent.

[2] In Deliciis.

[3] Quum amator annulum se amicæ optaret, ut ejus amplexu frui posset, etc., O te miserum, ait annulus, si meas vices obires, videres, audires, etc., nihil non odio dignum observares.

PAGE 215

[1] Lœchæus.   [2] See our English Tatius, lib. 1.

[3] Chaucer, in Romaunt of the Rose.

[4] Qui se facilem in amore probarit, hanc succendito.   At qui succendat, ad hunc diem repertus nemo.—Calcagninus.

[5] Ariosto.   [6] Hor.

[7] [The description of Viraginia, or Virago-land, in Hall's Mundus Alter et Idem.]

PAGE 216

[1] Christoph. Fonseca.   [2] Encom. Demosthen.
[3] Febris hectica uxor, et non nisi morte avellenda.
[4] Synesius. Libros ego liberos genui; Lipsius, Antiq. lect. lib.

PAGE 217

[1] Plautus, Asin. Act. 1.   [2] Senec. in Hercul.
[3] Seneca.   [4] Amator. Emblem.

PAGE 218

[1] [To wear yellow hose = to be jealous.]
[2] De rebus Hibernicis, lib. 3.
[3] Gemmea pocula, argentea vasa, cælata candelabra, aurea, etc. Conchileata aulæa, buccinarum clangorem, tibiarum cantum, et symphoniæ suavitatem, majestatemque principis coronati cum vidissent sella deaurata, etc.
[4] Eubulus, in Chrysilla. Athenæus, Deipnosophist. lib. 13, cap. 3.

PAGE 219

[1] Translated by my brother, Ralph Burton.
[2] Juvenal.   [3] Hæc in speciem dicta cave ut credas.
[4] Bachelors always are the bravest men.—Bacon. Seek eternity in memory, not in posterity, like Epaminondas, that instead of children, left two great victories behind him, which he called his two daughters.
[5] Ecclus. xxv, 1.   [6] Euripides, Androm.
[7] Ælius Verus, imperator. Spar. vita ejus.   [8] Hor.

PAGE 220

[1] Quod licet, ingratum est.
[2] For better for worse, for richer for poorer, in sickness and in health, etc., 'tis durus sermo [a hard saying] to a sensual man.
[3] Ter. Act. 1, sc. 2, Eunuch.
[4] Lucian, tom. 4. Neque cum una aliqua rem habere contentus forem.
[5] Juvenal.   [6] Lib. 28.

PAGE 221

[1] Camerar. 82, cent. 3.   [2] Simonides.
[3] Children make misfortunes more bitter.—Bacon.
[4] Heinsius, Epist. Primerio. Nihil miserius quam procreare liberos ad quos nihil ex hæreditate tua pervenire videas præter famem et sitim.
[5] Chris. Fonseca.   [6] Liberi sibi carcinomata.
[7] Melius fuerat eos sine liberis discessisse.

PAGE 222

[1] Lemnius, cap. 6, lib. 1. Si morosa, si non in omnibus obsequaris, omnia impacata in ædibus, omnia sursum misceri videas, multæ tempestates, etc.
[2] Lib. 2, numer. 101, Sylv. nup.   [3] Juvenal.
[4] Tom. 4, Amores. Omnem mariti opulentiam profundet, totam Arabiam capillis redolens.
[5] Idem, et quis sanæ mentis sustinere queat, etc.
[6] Subegit ancillas quod uxor ejus deformior esset.
[7] Sylv. nup. 1. 2, num. 25. Dives inducit tempestatem, pauper curam; ducens viduam se inducit in laqueum.
[8] Sic quisque dicit, alteram ducit tamen.

Page 223

[1] The male falcon (tassel, tercel, or tiercel) is smaller than the female.]
[2] Si dotata erit, imperiosa, continuoque viro inequitare conabitur.—Petrarch.
[3] If a woman nourish her husband, she is angry and impudent, and full of reproach.—Ecclus. xxv, 22. Scilicet uxori nubere nolo meæ.
[4] Plautus, Mil. Glor. Act. 3, sc. 1.
[5] Stobæus, Ser. 66; Alex. ab. Alexand. lib. 4, cap. 8.
[6] [Thales.]
[7] They shall attend the Lamb in heaven, because they were not defiled with women.—Apoc. xiv, 4.

Page 224

[1] Nuptiæ replent terram, virginitas Paradisum.—Hierome.
[2] Daphne in laurum semper virentem, immortalem docet gloriam paratam virginibus pudicitiam servantibus.
[3] Catul. Car. nuptiali.
[4] [Ben Jonson's translation in The Barriers.]
[5] Diet. salut. cap. 22. Pulcherrimum sertum infiniti pretii, gemma, et pictura speciosa. [6] Mart.

Page 225

[1] Lib. 24. Qua obsequiorum diversitate colantur homines sine liberis.
[2] Hunc alii ad cœnam invitant, princeps huic famulatur, oratores gratis patrocinantur.—Lib. de amore prolis.
[3] Annal. 11. [4] De benefic. 6, 38.
[5] E Græco.

Page 226

[1] Ter. Adelph.
[2] Itineraria in Psalmos, instructione ad lectorem.
[3] Bruson. lib. 7, cap. 22. Si uxor deesset, nihil mihi ad summam felicitatem defuisset.
[4] Extinguitur virilitas ex incantamentorum maleficiis; neque enim fabula est, nonnulli reperti sunt, qui ex veneficiis amore privati sunt, ut ex multis historiis patet.

Page 227

[1] Curat omnes morbos, phthises, hydropes et oculorum morbos, et febre quartana laborantes et amore captos, miris artibus eos demulcet.
[2] [The Leucadian Rock. Cape Ducado, in the island of Leucadia or Santa Maura.]
[3] The moral is, vehement fear expels love. [4] Catullus.
[5] Quum Junonem deperiret Jupiter impotenter, ibi solitus lavare, etc.
[6] Menander. [7] Ovid. Ep. 21.

Page 228

[1] Apud antiquos amor Lethes olim fuit; is ardentes faces in profluentem inclinabat; hujus statua Veneris Erycinæ templo visebatur, quo amantes confluebant, qui amicæ memoriam deponere volebant.
[2] Lib. 10. Vota ei nuncupant amatores, multis de causis, sed imprimis viduæ mulieres, ut sibi alteras a dea nuptias exposcant.
[3] Rhodiginus, Ant. lect. lib. 16, cap. 25, calls it Selenus. Omni amore liberat.
[4] [Publius Syrus] [5] Cupido crucifixus: lepidum poema.
[6] Cap. 19 de morb. cerebri.

PAGE 229

[1] Patiens potiatur re amata, si fieri possit, optima cura.—Cap 16, in 9 Rhasis.

[2] Si nihil aliud, nuptiæ et copulatio cum ea.

[3] Petronius, Catal.

[4] Cap. de Ilishi. Non invenitur cura, nisi regimen connexionis inter eos, secundum modum promissionis, et legis, et sic vidimus ad carnem restitutum, qui jam venerat ad arefactionem; evanuit cura postquam sensit, etc.

[5] Fama est melancholicum quendam ex amore insanabiliter se habentem, ubi puellæ se conjunxisset, restitutum, etc.

[6] Jovian. Pontanus, Basi. lib. 1.

PAGE 230

[1] Speed's Hist. e MS. Ber. Andreæ.

[2] Lucretia in Cælestina, Act. 19, Barthio interpret.

[3] Virg. 4 Æn.

[4] [Roofing-slates were called, according to their sizes, Ladies, Countesses, Duchesses, Queens, etc.]

PAGE 231

[1] E Græco Moschi.   [2] Ovid. Met. 1.

[3] Pausanias, Achaicis, lib. 7. Perdite amabat Callirhoen virginem, et quanto erat Coresi amor vehementior, tanto erat puellæ animus ab ejus amore alienior.

[4] Virg. 6 Æn.   [5] Erasmus, Ecl. Galatea.

[6] Angerianus, Erotopægnion.   [7] Virg.   [8] Lœchæus.

PAGE 232

[1] Ovid, Met. 1.   [2] Erot. lib. 2.   [3] T. H.

PAGE 233

[1] Virg. 4 Æn.   [2] Metamor. 3.   [3] Fracastorius, Dial. de anim.

PAGE 234

[1] Dial. Am.   [2] Ausonius.   [3] Ovid. Met.

PAGE 235

[1] Hom. 5, in 1 Epist. Thess. cap. 4, ver. 1.   [2] Ter.

PAGE 236

[1] Ter. Heaut. scen. ult.

[2] Plebeius et nobilis ambiebant puellam, puellæ certamen in partes venit, etc.

[3] Apuleius, Apol.   [4] Gen. xxvi.

[5] Non peccat venialiter qui mulierem ducit ob pulchritudinem.

[6] Lib. 6 de leg. Ex usu reipub. est ut in nuptiis juvenes neque pauperum affinitatem fugiant, neque divitum sectentur.

[7] Philost. ep. Quoniam pauper sum, idcirco contemptior et abjectior tibi videar? Amor ipse nudus est, gratiæ et astra; Hercules pelle leonina indutus.

PAGE 237

[1] Juvenal.   [2] Lib. 2, ep. 7.

[3] Ejulans inquit, non mentem una addixit mihi fortuna servitute.

[4] De repub. cap. de period. rerumpub.

[5] Com. in Car. Chron.   [6] Plin. in Paneg.   [7] Declam. 306.

474 NOTES

Page 238

[1] Puellis imprimis nulla danda occasio lapsus.—Lemn. lib. 1, 54, de vit. instit.

[2] See more, part. 1, sec. 2, mem. 2, subs. 4.

[3] Filia excedens annum 25 potest inscio patre nubere, licet indignus sit maritus, et eum cogere ad congrue dotandum.

[4] Ne appetentiæ procacioris reputetur auctor.

[5] Expetita enim magis debet videri a viro quam ipsa virum expetisse.

[6] Mulier apud nos 24 annorum vetula est et projectitia.

[7] Comœd. Lysistrat. And. Divo interpr.

[8] Ausonius, Idyll. 14.

Page 239

[1] Idem. [2] Catullus.

[3] Translated by Mr. B. Jonson.

[4] Hom. 5 in 1 Thess. cap. 4, 1.

[5] Plautus. [6] Ovid.

[7] Epist. 12, lib. 2. Eligit conjugem pauperem, indotatam, et subito deamavit, ex commiseratione ejus inopiæ.

Page 240

[1] Virg. Æn.

[2] Fabius Pictor. Amor ipse conjunxit populos, etc.

[3] Lipsius, Polit.; Sebast. Mayer. Select. sect. 1, cap. 13.

Page 241

[1] Mayerus, Select. sect. 1, cap. 14, et Ælian. lib. 13, cap. 33. Cum famulæ lavantis vestes incuriosius custodirent, etc.; mandavit per universam Ægyptum ut femina quæreretur, cujus is calceus esset; eamque sic inventam in matrimonium accepit.

[2] Pausanias, lib. 3, de Laconicis. Dimisit qui nunciarunt, etc., optionem puellis dedit, ut earum quælibet eum sibi virum deligeret, cujus maxime esset forma complacita.

[3] Illius conjugium abominabitur.

[4] Socero quinque circiter annos natu minor.

Page 242

[1] Vit. Galeat. Secundi.

[2] Apuleius, in Catal. Nobis cupido velle dat, posse abnegat.

[3] Anacreon, 56.

Page 243

[1] Continentiæ donum ex fide postulet quia certum sit eum vocari ad cœlibatum cui demis, etc.

[2] Acts xvi, 7. [3] Rom. i, 13. [4] Præfix. gen. Leovitii.

Page 244

[1] Idem Wolfius, dial.

[2] That is, make the best of it, and take his lot as it falls.

[3] Ovid, Met. 1. [4] Mercurialis de Priapismo.

[5] Memorabile quod Ulricus epistola refert Gregorium quum ex piscina quadam allata plus quam sex mille infantum capita vidisset, ingemuisse et decretum de cœlibatu tantam cædis causam confessus, condigno illud pœnitentiæ fructu purgasse.—Kemnisius ex Concil. Trident. part. 3, de cœlibatu sacerdotum.

[1] Si nubat, quam si domi concubinam alat.
[2] Alphonsus Cicaonius, lib. de gest. pontificum.
[3] Cum medici suaderent ut aut nuberet aut coitu uteretur, sic mortem vitari posse, mortem potius intrepidus expectavit, etc.
[4] Epist. 30.   [5] Vide vitam ejus edit. 1623, by Dr. T. James.

[1] Lydgate, in Chaucer's Flower of Curtesie.
[2] 'Tis not multitude but idleness which causeth beggary.
[3] Or to set them awork, and bring them up in some honest trades.
[4] [An allegory in praise of Newfoundland, by Sir William Vaughan, who founded a Welsh colony there.]
[5] Dion Cassius, lib. 56.   [6] Sardus, Buxtorfius.
[7] Claude Albaville, in his History of the Frenchmen to the Isle of Maragnan, an. 1614.
[8] Rara quidem dea tu es, o castitas, in his terris, nec facile perfecta, rarius perpetua; cogi nonnunquam potes, ob naturæ defectum, vel si disciplina pervaserit, censura compresserit.

[1] Peregrin. Hierosol.
[2] Plutarch, vita ejus.   Adolescentiæ medio constitutus.
[3] Ancillas duas egregia forma et ætatis flore.
[4] Alex. ab. Alex. lib. 4, cap. 8.
[5] Tres filii patrem ab excubiis, quinque ab omnibus officiis liberabant.
[6] Nic. Hill, Epic. philos.
[7] Præcepto primo, cogatur nubere aut mulctetur et pecunia templo Junonis dedicetur et publica fiat.
[8] Consol. 3, pros. 7.

[1] Qui se capistro matrimonii alligari non patiuntur.—Lemn. lib. 4, 13, de occult. nat.   Abhorrent multi a matrimonio, ne morosam, querulam, acerbam, amaram uxorem perferre cogantur.
[2] Seneca, Hippol.
[3] Cœlebs enim vixerat nec ad uxorem ducendam unquam induci potuit.
[4] Seneca, Hippol.   [5] Hor.
[6] Æneas Sylvius, de dictis Sigismundi; Heinsius Primerio.

[1] Habeo uxorem ex animi sententia, Camillam Paleotti jurisconsulti filiam.
[2] Legentibus et meditantibus candelas et candelabrum tenuerunt.
[3] Hor.   [4] Ovid.   [5] Aphranius.

[1] Lœchæus.   [2] Bacon's Essays.   [3] Euripides.
[4] Cum juxta mare agrum coleret.

[1] Omnis enim miseriæ immemorem, conjugalis amor eum fecerat.
[2] Non sine ingenti admiratione, tanta hominis caritate motus rex liberos esse jussit, etc.
[3] Qui vult vitare molestias, vitet mundum.

[4] Τί δὲ βίος, τί δὲ τερπνὸν ἄτερ χρυσῆς 'Αφροδίτης; quid vita est quæso quidve est sine Cypride dulce?—Mimnermus.

[5] Erasmus.	[6] E Stobæo.	[7] Menander.
[8] Seneca, Hippol.	[9] Lib. 3, num. 1.	[10] Hist. lib. 4.
[11] Palingenius.	[12] Bruson. lib. 7, cap. 23.	

[13] Noli societatem habere, etc.

PAGE 252

[1] Lib. 1. cap. 6. Si, inquit, Quirites, sine uxore esse possemus, omnes careremus; sed quoniam sic est, saluti potius publicæ quam voluptati consulendum.

[2] Beatum foret si liberos auro et argento mercari, etc.

[3] Seneca, Hippol.

[4] Gen. ii. Adjutorium simile, etc.

PAGE 253

[1] Ovid.

PAGE 254

[1] Euripides.   [2] E Græco, Valerius, lib. 7, cap. 7.

[3] Pervigilium Veneris e vetere poeta.

[4] Domus non potest consistere sine uxore.—Nevisanus, lib. 2, num. 18.

[5] Nemo in severissima Stoicorum familia qui non barbam quoque et supercilium amplexibus uxoris submiserit, aut in ista parte a reliquis dissenserit.—Heinsius Primerio.

[6] Quid libentius homo masculus videre debet quam bellam uxorem?

PAGE 255

[1] Chaucer.   [2] Conclusio Theod. Prodromi 9 lib. Amor.   [3] Ovid.

[4] The conclusion of [the third book of] Chaucer's poem of Troilus and Creseida.

[5] [i.e. got out of danger. Proverbial.]

[6] Epist. 4, lib. 2. Jucundiores multo et suaviores longe post molestas turbas amantium nuptiæ.

[7] Olim meminisse juvabit.

[8] Quid expectatis, intus fiunt nuptiæ, the music, guests, and all the good cheer is within.

[9] Catullus.   [10] Catullus.

[11] J. Secundus, Sylvar. lib. Jam virgo thalamum subibit unde ne virgo redeat, marite, cura.

[12] Ecclus. xxxix. 14.

PAGE 256

[1] Gallieni Epithal.

[2] O noctem quater et quater beatam!

[3] Theocritus, Idyl. 18.

[4] Erasmus, Epithal. P. Ægidii.

[5] [Ibid.] Nec saltent modo sed duo carissima pectora indissolubili mutuæ benevolentiæ nodo copulent, ut nihil unquam eos incedere possit iræ vel tædii. Illa perpetuo nihil audiat nisi, mea lux: ille vicissim nihil nisi, anime mi: atque huic jucunditati ne senectus detrahat, imo potius aliquid adaugeat.

PAGE 257

[1] Kornmannus, de linea amoris.

[2] Third book of Troilus and Creseid.

[3] In his Oration of Jealousy, put out by Fr. Sansovinus.

PAGE 258

[1] Benedetto Varchi.
[2] Exercitat. 317. Cum metuimus ne amatæ rei exturbemur possessione.
[3] Zelus de forma est invidentiæ species ne quis forma quam amamus fruatur.
[4] 3 de anima.
[5] 3 de anima. Tangimur zelotypia de pupillis, liberis carisque curæ nostræ concreditis, non de forma, sed ne male sit iis, aut ne nobis sibique parent ignominiam.
[6] Plutarch.   [7] Seneca, in Herc. Fur.   [8] Exod. xx.

PAGE 259

[1] Lucan.
[2] Danæus, Aphoris. Polit. Semper metuunt ne eorum auctoritas minuatur.
[3] Belli Neapol. lib. 5.
[4] Dici non potest quam tenues et infirmas causas habent mœroris et suspicionis, et hic est morbus occultus, qui in familiis principum regnat.
[5] Omnes æmulos interfecit.—Lampridius.
[6] Constant. Agricult. lib. 10, cap. 5. Cyparissæ, Eteoclis filiæ, saltantes ad æmulationem dearum, in puteum demolitæ sunt, sed terra miserata cupressos inde produxit.
[7] Ovid. Met.   [8] Seneca.

PAGE 260

[1] Quis autem carnifex addictum supplicio crudelius afficiat, quam metus? Metus inquam mortis, infamiæ, cruciatus, sunt illæ ultrices furiæ quæ tyrannos exagitant, etc. Multo acerbius sauciant et pungunt, quam crudeles domini servos vinctos fustibus ac tormentis exulcerare possunt.
[2] Lonicerus, tom. 1 Turc. hist. cap. 24.
[3] Jovius, vita ejus.
[4] Knolles; Busbequius; Sandys, fol. 52.
[5] Nicephorus, lib. 11, cap. 45. Socrates, lib. 7, cap. 35. Neque Valens alicui pepercit qui Theo cognomine vocaretur.
[6] Alexand. Gaguin. Muscov. hist. descrip. cap. 5.
[7] D. Fletcher. Timet omnes ne insidiæ essent.
[8] Herodian, lib. 7. Maximinus invisum se sentiens, quod ex infimo loco in tantam fortunam venisset moribus ac genere barbarus, metuens ne natalium obscuritas objiceretur, omnes Alexandri prædecessoris ministros ex aula ejecit, pluribus interfectis quod mœsti essent ad mortem Alexandri, insidias inde metuens.
[9] Lib. 8. Tanquam feræ solitudine vivebant, terrentes alios, timentes.

PAGE 261

[1] Serres, fol. 56.
[2] Neap. belli, lib. 5. Nulli prorsus homini fidebat, omnes insidiari sibi putabat.
[3] Camden's Remains.   [4] Mat. Paris.
[5] R[obert] T[ofte], notis in Blazon of Jealousy.
[6] Daniel, in his Panegyric to the King.
[7] 3 de anima, cap. de zel. Animalia quædam zelotypia tanguntur, ut olores, columbæ, galli, tauri, etc., ob metum communionis.
[8] Seneca.

478 NOTES

Page 262

[1] Lib. 11 Cyneget.   [2] Chaucer, in his Assembly of Fowls.
[3] Aldrovandus.   [4] Lib. 12.
[5] Sibi timens circa res venereas, solitudines amat quo solus sola femina fruatur.
[6] Crocodili zelotypi et uxorum amantissimi, etc.
[7] Qui dividit agrum communem; inde deducitur ad amantes.

Page 263

[1] Erasmus, chil. 1, cent. 9, adag. 99.
[2] Ter. Eun. Act. 1, sc. 1. Munus nostrum ornato verbis, et illum æmulum, quoad poteris, ab ea pellito.
[3] Pinus puella quondam fuit, etc.
[4] Mars zelotypus Adonidem interfecit.

Page 264

[1] 1 Sam. i, 6.   [2] R. T., Blazon of Jealousy.
[3] Mulierum conditio misera; nullam honestam credunt nisi domo conclusa vivat.
[4] Fynes Moryson.
[5] Nomen zelotypiæ apud istos locum non habet.—Lib. 3, cap. 8.

Page 265

[1] Fynes Moryson, part. 3, cap. 2.   [2] Busbequius, Sandys.
[3] Præ amore et zelotypia sæpius insaniunt.
[4] Australes ne sacra quidem publica fieri patiuntur, nisi uterque sexus pariete medio dividatur: et quum in Angliam, inquit, legationis causa profectus essem, audivi Mendozam legatum Hispaniarum dicentem turpe esse viros et feminas in, etc.

Page 266

[1] Idea. Mulieres præterquam quod sunt infidæ, suspicaces, inconstantes, insidiosæ, simulatrices, superstitiosæ, et si potentes, intolerabiles, amore zelotypæ supra modum.
[2] Ovid, 2 de arte amandi.
[3] Bartello.   [4] R. T.   [5] R. T.
[6] Lib. 2, num. 8. Mulier otiosa facile præsumitur luxuriosa, et sæpe zelotypa.

Page 267

[1] Lib. 2, num. 4.
[2] Quum omnibus infideles feminæ, senibus infidelissimæ.
[3] Mimnermus.
[4] Vix aliqua non impudica, et quam non suspectam merito quis habeat.
[5] Lib. 5 de aur. asino. At ego misera patre meo seniorem maritum nacta sum, eundem cucurbita calviorem et quovis puero pumiliorem, cunctam domum seris et catenis obditam custodientem.
[6] Chaloner.

Page 268

[1] Lib. 4, num. 80.   [2] Ovid, 2 de art. amandi.
[3] Every Man out of his Humour.
[4] Calcagninus, Apol. Tiberini ab uxorum partu earum vices subeunt, ut aves per vices incubant, etc.
[5] Exiturus fascia uxoris pectus alligabat, nec momento præsentia ejus carere poterat, potumque non hauriebat nisi prægustatum labris ejus.
[6] Chaloner.   [7] Panegyr. Trajano.

Page 269

[1] Ter. Adelph. Act. i, sc. i.

[2] Fab. Calvo Ravennate interprete.

[3] Dum rediero domum meam habitabis, et licet cum parentibus habitet hac mea peregrinatione; eam tamen et ejus mores observabis uti absentia viri sui probe degat, nec alios viros cogitet aut quærat.

[4] Femina semper custode eget qui se pudicam contineat; suapte enim natura nequitias insitas habet, quas nisi indies comprimat, ut arbores stolones emittunt, etc.

[5] Heinsius.

[6] Uxor cujusdam nobilis quum debitum maritale sacro passionis hebdomada non obtineret, alterum adiit.

[7] Ne tribus prioribus noctibus rem haberet cum ea, ut esset in pecoribus fortunatus, ab uxore moræ impatiente, etc.

Page 270

[1] Totam noctem bene et pudice nemini molestus dormiendo transegit; mane autem quum nullius conscius facinoris sibi esset, et inertiæ puderet, audisse se dicebat cum dolore calculi solere eam conflictari. Duo præcepta juris una nocte expressit, neminem læserat et honeste vixerat, sed an suum cuique reddidisset, quæri poterat. Mucius opinor et Trebatius hoc negassent.—Lib. i.

[2] Alterius loci emendationem serio optabat, quem corruptum esse ille non invenit.

[3] Such another tale is in Neander de Jocoseriis, his first tale.

[4] Lib. 2, Ep. 3. Si pergit alienis negotiis operam dare sui negligens, erit alius mihi orator qui rem meam agat.

[5] Ovid. Rara est concordia formæ atque pudicitiæ.

Page 271

[1] Epist.   [2] Quod strideret ejus calceamentum.

[3] Hor. Epist. 15.   [4] De re uxoria, lib. i, cap. 5.

[5] Cum steriles sunt, ex mutatione viri se putant concipere.

Page 272

[1] Tibullus, Eleg. 6.   [2] Wither's Sat.

[3] 3 de anima. Crescit ac decrescit zelotypia cum personis, locis, temporibus, negotiis.

[4] Marullus.   [5] Tibullus, Epig.   [6] Prov. ix, 17.

Page 273

[1] Propert. Eleg. 2.

[2] Ovid., lib. 9 Met.; Pausanias; Strabo: Quum crevit imbribus hiemalibus Deianiram suscipit, Herculem nando sequi jubet.

[3] Lucian, tom. 4.   [4] Plutarch.

[5] Cap. v, 8.   [6] Seneca.   [7] Lib. 2, cap. 33.

Page 274

[1] Petronius, Catal.   [2] Suetonius.

[3] Pontus Heuter, vita ejus.

[4] [Lorenzo de' Medici.]

[5] Lib. 8 Flor. hist. Dux omnium optimus et sapientissimus, sed in re venerea prodigiosus.

[6] Vita Castruccii. Idem uxores maritis abalienavit.

[7] Sesellius, lib. 2 de Repub. Gallorum. Ita nunc apud infimos obtinuit hoc vitium, ut nullius fere pretii sit, et ignavus miles qui non in scortatione maxime excellat, et adulterio.

Page 275

[1] Virg. Æn. 4.   [2] Epig. 9, lib. 4.
[3] [A character in Jonson's Every Man out of his Humour.]
[4] Virg. Æn. 4.   [5] Secundus, Silv.
[6] Æneas Sylvius.   [7] Virg. Æn. 4.
[8] E Græco Simonidis.

Page 276

[1] Cont. 2, cap. 38, Oper. subcis. Mulieris liberius et familiarius communicantis cum omnibus licentia et immodestia, sinistri sermonis et suspicionis materiam viro præbet.

[2] Voces liberæ, oculorum colloquia, contractationes parum verecundæ, motus immodici, etc.—Heinsius.

[3] Chaloner.

[4] What is here said is not prejudicial to honest women.

[5] Lib. 28, st. 13.

Page 277

[1] Dial. amor. Pendet fallax et blanda circa oscula mariti, quem in cruce, si fieri posset, deosculari velit: illius vitam cariorem esse sua jurejurando affirmat: quem certe non redimeret anima catelli si posset.

[2] Adeunt templum ut rem divinam audiant, ut ipsæ simulant, sed vel ut monachum fratrem, vel adulterum lingua, oculis, ad libidinem provocent.

[3] Lib. 4, num. 81. Ipsæ sibi persuadent, quod adulterium cum principe vel cum præsule, non est pudor, nec peccatum.

[4] Deum rogat, non pro salute mariti, filii, cognati vota suscipit, sed pro reditu mœchi si abest, pro valetudine lenonis si ægrotet.

[5] Tibullus.

[6] Gotardus Arthus, descrip. Indiæ Orient.; Linschoten.

[7] Garcias ab Horto, Hist. lib. 2, cap. 24, daturam herbam vocat et describit. Tam proclives sunt ad venerem mulieres ut viros inebrient per 24 horas, liquore quodam, ut nihil videant, recordentur, at dormiant, et post lotionem pedum, ad se restituunt, etc.

[8] [i.e. wantonly disposed.]

[9] Ariosto, lib. 28, st. 75.

Page 278

[1] Lipsius, Polit.   [2] Seneca, lib. 2, controv. 8.   [3] Bodicher, Sat.

Page 279

[1] [Propertius.]

[2] Epist. 85, ad Oceanum. Ad unius horæ ebrietatem nudat femora, quæ per sexcentos annos sobrietate contexerat.

[3] Juv. Sat. 6.

[4] Nihil audent primo, post ab aliis confirmatæ, audaces et confidentes sunt, ubi semel verecundiæ limites transierint.

[5] Euripides.   [6] 1, 62.

[7] De miser. curialium. Aut alium cum ea invenies, aut isse [illam ad] alium reperies.   [8] Cap. 18 de Virg.

Page 280

[1] Hom. 38, in cap. 17 Gen. Etsi magnis affluunt divitiis, etc.

[2] 3 de anima. Omnes voces, auras, omnes susurros captat zelotypus, et amplificat apud se cum iniquissima de singulis calumnia. Maxime suspiciosi, et ad pejora credendum proclives.

Page 281

[1] Propertius.   [2] Æneas Sylvius.

PAGE 282

[1] Ant. Dial.

PAGE 283

[1] Rabie concepta, cæsariem abrasit, puellæque mirabiliter insultans faciem vibicibus fœdavit.   [2] Daniel.
[3] Annal. lib. 12. Principis mulieris zelotypæ est in alias mulieres quas suspectas habet, odium inseparabile.
[4] Seneca, in Medea.
[5] Alcoran, cap. Bovis, interprete Ricardo præd. cap. 8 Confutationis.
[6] Plautus.   [7] Expedit. in Sinas, lib. 3, cap. 9.
[8] Decem eunuchorum millia numerantur in regia familia, qui servant uxores ejus.

PAGE 284

[1] Lib. 57, ep. 81.
[2] Semotis a viris servant in interioribus, ab eorum conspectu immunes.
[3] Lib. 1, fol. 7.
[4] Diruptiones hymenis sæpe fiunt a propriis digitis vel ab aliis instrumentis.

PAGE 285

[1] Idem Rhasis Arab., Cont.
[2] Ita clausæ pharmacis ut non possunt coitum exercere.
[3] Qui et pharmacum præscribit docetque.
[4] Epist. 6, Mercero interp.
[5] Barthius. Ludus illi temeratum pudicitiæ florem mentitis machinis pro integro vendere. Ego docebo te, qui mulier ante nuptias sponso te probes virginem.
[6] Qui mulierem violasset, virilia exsecabant, et mille virgas dabant.
[7] Dion. Halic.   [8] [Pope Pius II (Æneas Sylvius).]

PAGE 286

[1] Viridi gaudens Feronia luco.—Virg.
[2] [In the crypt of Ripon Cathedral.]
[3] Ismene was so tried by Diana's well, in which maids did swim, unchaste were drowned.—Eustathius, lib. 8.
[4] Contra mendac. ad confess. 21. cap.
[5] Pheron, Ægypti rex, captus oculis per decennium, oraculum consuluit de uxoris pudicitia.—Herod. Euterp.
[6] Cæsar, lib 6, bello Gall. Vitæ necisque in uxores habuerunt potestatem.
[7] Animi dolores et zelotypia si diutius perseverent, dementes reddunt. Acad. comment. in par. art. Galeni.
[8] Ariosto, lib. 31, staff 6.
[9] 3 de anima, cap. 3, de zelotyp. Transit in rabiem et odium, et sibi et aliis violentas sæpe manus injiciunt.

PAGE 287

[1] Hyginus, cap. 189, Ovid, etc.
[2] Pheron Ægypti rex, de cæcitate oraculum consulens, visum ei rediturum accepit, si oculos abluisset lotio mulieris quæ aliorum virorum esset expers; uxoris urinam expertus nihil profecit, et aliarum frustra, eas omnes (ea excepta per quam curatus fuit) unum in locum coactas concremavit.—Herod. Euterp.
[3] Offic. lib. 2.   [4] Aurelius Victor.
[5] Herod. lib. 9, in Calliope. Masistæ uxorem excarnificat, mammillas præscindit, easque canibus abjicit, filiæ nares præscindit, labra, linguam, etc.
[6] Lib. 1. Dum formæ curandæ intenta capillum in sole pectit, a marito per lusum leviter percussa furtim superveniente virga, risu suborto,

III—*Q888

Mi Landrice, dixit, frontem vir fortis petet, etc. Marito conspecto attonita, cum Landrico mox in ejus mortem conspirat, et statim inter venandum efficit.

[7] Qui Goæ uxorem habens, Gotherinum principem quendam virum quod uxori suæ oculos adjecisset, ingenti vulnere deformavit in facie, et tibiam adscidit, unde mutuæ cædes.

[8] Eo quod infans natus involutus esset panniculo, credebat eum filium fratris Francisci, etc.

[9] Zelotypia reginæ regis mortem acceleravit paulo post, ut Martianus medicus mihi retulit. Illa autem atra bile inde exagitata in latebras se subducens præ ægritudine animi reliquum tempus consumpsit.

Page 288

[1] A zelotypia redactus ad insaniam et desperationem.
[2] Uxorem interemit, inde desperabundus ex alto se præcipitavit.
[3] Tollere nodosam nescit medicina podagram.
[4] Ariosto, lib. 31, staff 5.

Page 289

[1] Veteres mature suadent ungues amoris esse radendos, priusquam producant se nimis.
[2] In Jovianum.   [3] Gomesius, lib. 3 de reb. gestis Ximenii.
[4] Urit enim præcordia ægritudo animi compressa, et in angustiis adducta mentem subvertit, nec alio medicamine facilius erigitur, quam cordati hominis sermone.

Page 290

[1] 3 de anima.   [2] Lib. 3.
[3] Argentocoxi Caledoni reguli uxor, Juliæ Augustæ cum ipsam morderet quod inhoneste versaretur, respondet, Nos cum optimis viris consuetudinem habemus; vos Romanas autem occulte passim homines constuprant.
[4] Leges de mœchis fecit, ex civibus plures in jus vocati.
[5] Lib. 3, Epig. 26.

Page 291

[1] Assert. Arthuri: Parcerem libenter heroinarum læsæ majestati, si non historiæ veritas aurem vellicaret.—Leland.
[2] Lelandus, Assert. Arthuri.   [3] Epigram.
[4] Cogita an sic aliis tu unquam feceris; an hoc tibi nunc fieri dignum sit? severus aliis, indulgens tibi, cur ab uxore exigis quod non ipse præstas?—Plutarch.
[5] Vaga libidine cum ipse quovis rapiaris, cur si vel modicum aberret ipsa insanias?

Page 292

[1] Ariosto, lib. 28, staff 80.
[2] Sylvæ nupt. lib. 4, num. 72.
[3] Lemnius, lib. 4, cap. 13, de occult. nat. mir.
[4] Optimum bene nasci.   [5] Mart.

Page 293

[1] Ovid, Amor. lib. 3, eleg. 4.   [2] Lib. 28, st. 72.
[3] Polycrat. lib. 8, cap. 11, de amor.
[4] Euryal. et Lucret. Qui uxores occludunt, meo judicio minus utiliter faciunt; sunt enim eo ingenio mulieres ut id potissimum cupiant, quod maxime denegatur; si liberas habent habenas, minus delinquunt; frustra seram adhibes, si non sit sponte casta.
[5] Quando cognoscunt maritos hoc advertere.   [6] Ausonius.

Page 294

[1] Opes suas, mundum suum, thesaurum suum, etc.
[2] Virg. Æn.   [3] Daniel.
[4] 1 de serm. d. in monte ros. 16.
[5] O quam formosus lacertus hic! quidam inquit, ad æquales conversus; at illa, Publicus, inquit, non est.
[6] Bilia Duillium virum senem habuit et spiritum fœtidum habentem, quem quum quidam exprobrasset, etc.

Page 295

[1] Numquid tibi, Armenia, Tigranes videbatur esse pulcher? Et illum, inquit, edepol, etc.—Xenoph. Cyropæd. lib. 3.   [2] Ovid.
[3] Read Petrarch's tale of Patient Grizel in Chaucer.
[4] [New France, i.e. Canada.]
[5] Sylv. nup. lib. 4, num. 80.   [6] Erasmus.
[7] Quum accepisset uxorem peperisse secundo a nuptiis mense, cunas quinas vel senas coemit, ut si forte uxor singulis bimensibus pareret.
[8] Julius Capitol. vita ejus. Quum palam citharædus uxorem diligeret, minime curiosus fuit.

Page 296

[1] Disposuit armatos qui ipsum interficerent: hi protenus mandatum exsequentes, etc. Ille et rex declaratur, et Stratonicem quæ fratri nupserat, uxorem ducit; sed postquam audivit fratrem vivere, etc. Attalum comiter accepit, pristinamque uxorem complexus, magno honore apud se habuit.
[2] See John Harington's notes in 28th book of Ariosto.

Page 297

[1] Amator. dial.   [2] Plautus, scen. ult. Amphit.
[3] Idem.   [4] T. Daniel, conjurat. French.
[5] Lib. 4, num. 80.   [6] R. T.

Page 298

[1] Lib. de heres. Quum de zele culparetur, purgandi se causa permisisse fertur ut ea qui vellet uteretur; quod ejus factum in sectam turpissimam versum est, qua placet usus indifferens feminarum.
[2] Sleidan, Com.   [3] Alcoran.
[4] Alcoran edit. et Bibliandro.
[5] De mor. gent. lib. 1, cap. 6. Nupturæ regi devirginandæ exhibentur.
[6] Lumina extinguebantur, nec personæ et ætatis habita reverentia, in quam quisque per tenebras incidit, mulierem cognoscit.
[7] Leander Albertus. Flagitioso ritu cuncti in ædem convenientes post impuram concionem, extinctis luminibus in Venerem ruunt.
[8] Lod. Vertomannus, Navig. lib. 6, cap. 8, et Marcus Polus, lib. 1, cap. 46. Uxores viatoribus prostituunt.
[9] Dithmarus Bleskenius. Ut Agetus Aristoni, pulcherrimam uxorem habens prostituit.
[10] Herodot. in Erato. Mulieres Babyloni cæcum hospite permiscentur ob argentum quod post Veneri sacrum. Bohemus, lib. 2.
[11] Navigat. lib. 5, cap. 4. Prius torum non init, quam a digniore sacerdote nova nupta deflorata sit.   [12] [Essenes.]

Page 299

[1] Bohemus, lib. 2, cap. 3. Ideo nubere nollent ob mulierum intemperantiam, nullam servare viro fidem putabant.
[2] Stephanus, præfat. Herod. Alius e lupanari meretricem, Pitho dictam,

in uxorem duxit; Ptolemæus Thaidem nobile scortum duxit et ex ea duos filios suscepit, etc.
   [3] Poggius Florentinus.   [4] Felix Plater.
   [5] Plutarch, Lucian, Salmuth, tit. 2, de porcellanis, com. in Pancirol. de nov. repert., et Plutarchus.
   [6] Stephanus, e lib. confor. Bonavent. cap. 6, vit. Francisci.

PAGE 300

   [1] Plutarch, vit. ejus.   [2] Wecker, lib. 7 Secret.   [3] Citatur a Gellio.
   [4] Lib. 4, tit. 4, de instit. reipub. de officio mariti.
   [5] Ne cum ea blande nimis agas, ne objurges præsentibus extraneis.
   [6] Epist. 70.

PAGE 301

   [1] Ovid.   [2] Alciat. Emb. 116.
   [3] Deipnosoph. lib. 13, cap. 7.   [4] Euripides.
   [5] Pontanus, Biarum lib. 1.
   [6] Offic. lib.   Luxuria cum omni ætati turpis, tum senectuti fœdissima.
   [7] Ecclus. xxv, 1.   An old man that dotes, etc.

PAGE 302

   [1] Hor. lib. 3, Ode 26.
   [2] Cap. 5 Instit. ad optimam vitam.   Maxima mortalium pars præcipitanter et inconsiderate nubit, idque ea ætate quæ minus apta est, quum senex adolescentulæ, sanus morbidæ, dives pauperi, etc.
   [3] Obsoleto, intempestivo, turpi remedio fatentur se uti; recordatione pristinarum voluptatum se recreant, et adversante natura, pollinctam carnem et enectam excitant.
   [4] Lib. 2, num. 25.
   [5] Qui vero non procreandæ prolis, sed explendæ libidinis causa sibi invicem copulantur, non tam conjuges quam fornicarii habentur.
   [6] Lex Papia.   Sueton. Claud. cap. 23.

PAGE 303

   [1] Pontanus, Biarum lib. 1.   [2] Plautus, Mercator.
   [3] Symposio.   [4] Vide Thuani historiam.
   [5] Calalect vet. poetarum.   [6] Martial. lib. 3, Epig. 62.
   [7] Lib. 1 Miles.

PAGE 304

   [1] Ovid.
   [2] Rabelais, Hist. Pantagruel, lib. 3, cap. 33.
   [3] Hom. 80.   Qui pulchram habet uxorem, nihil pejus habere potest.
   [4] Arnisæus.

PAGE 305

   [1] Itinerar. Ital. Coloniæ edit. 1620, nomine trium Ger. fol. 304.   Displicuit quod dominæ filiabus immutent nomen inditum in baptismo, et pro Catharina, Margareta, etc., ne quid desit ad luxuriam, appellant ipsas nominibus Cynthiæ, Camænæ, etc.
   [2] Leonicus de var. lib. 3, cap. 43.   Asylum virginum deformium Cassandræ templum.   Plutarch.
   [3] Polycrat. lib. 8, cap. 11.

PAGE 306

   [1] Marullus.   [2] Chaloner, lib. 9 de repub. Ang.
   [3] Lib. 2, num. 159.
   [4] Si genetrix caste, caste quoque filia vivit; si meretrix mater, filia talis erit.   [5] Juven. Sat. 6.

[1] Camerarius, cent. 2, cap. 54, Oper. subcis.
[2] Ser. 72.   Quod amicus quidam uxorem habens mihi dixit, dicam vobis; in cubili cavendæ adulationes vesperi, mane clamores.
[3] Lib. 4, tit. 4, de institut. reipub., cap. de officio mariti et uxoris.
[4] Lib. 4 Syl. nup. num. 81.   Non curant de uxoribus, nec volunt iis subvenire de victu, vestitu, etc.
[5] In Clio.   Speciem uxoris supra modum extollens, fecit ut illam nudam coram aspiceret.   [6] Juven. Sat. 6.   [7] Orat. contra ebr.

[1] Ad baptismum, matrimonium et tumulum.
[2] Non vociferatur illa si maritus obganniat.
[3] Fraudem aperiens ostendit ei non aquam sed silentium iracundiæ moderari.
[4] Horol. princip. lib. 2, cap. 8.   Diligenter cavendum feminis illustribus ne frequenter exeant.

[1] Chaloner.   [2] Menander.   [3] Lib. 5, num. 11.
[4] Ctesias in Persicis.   Finxit vulvæ morbum esse, nec curari posse nisi cum viro concumberet, hac arte voti compos, etc.
[5] Exsolvit vinculis solutumque demisit, at ille inhumanus stupravit conjugem.   [6] Plutarch, vita ejus.

[1] Rosinus, lib. 2, 19.   Valerius, lib. 2, cap. 1.
[2] Alexander ab Alexandro, lib. 4, cap. 8, Gen. dier.
[3] Fr. Rueus de gemmis, lib. 2, cap. 8 et 15.
[4] Strozzius Cicogna, lib. 2, cap. 15, spirit. et incan.   Habent ibidem uxores quot volunt cum oculis clarissimis, quos nunquam in aliquem præter maritum fixuri sunt, etc.   Bredenbachius idem et Bohemus, etc.
[5] Uxor cæca ducat maritum surdum, etc.
[6] See Valent. Nabod. differ. com. in Alcabitium, ubi plura.

[1] Cap. 46 Apol.   Quod mulieres sine concupiscentia aspicere non posset, etc.
[2] Called religious because it is still conversant about religion and such divine objects.   [3] Grotius.

[1] Lib. 1, cap. 16.   Nonnulli opinionibus addicti sunt, et futura se prædicere arbitrantur.
[2] Aliis videtur quod sunt prophetæ et inspirati a Spiritu Sancto, et, incipiunt prophetare, et multa futura prædicunt.
[3] Cap. 6 de melanch.
[4] Cap. 5 Tractat.   Multi ob timorem Dei sunt melancholici, et timorem gehennæ.   They are still troubled for their sins.
[5] Plater, cap. 13.
[6] Melancholia Erotica, vel quæ cum amore est, duplex est: prima quæ ab aliis forsan non meretur nomen melancholiæ, est affectio eorum quæ pro objecto proponunt Deum, et ideo nihil aliud curant aut cogitant quam Deum, jejunia, vigilias; altera ob mulieres.
[7] Alia reperitur furoris species a prima vel a secunda, deorum rogantium, vel afflatu numinum furor hic venit.
[8] Qui in Delphis futura prædicunt vates, et in Dodona sacerdotes furentes quidem multa jocunda Græcis deferunt, sani vero exigua aut nulla.

PAGE 313

[1] Deus bonus, justus, pulcher, juxta Platonem.

[2] Miror et stupeo cum cœlum aspicio et pulchritudinem siderum, angelorum, etc.; et quis digne laudet quod in nobis viget, corpus tam pulchrum, frontem pulchram, nares, genas, oculos, intellectum, omnia pulchra; si sic in creaturis laboramus, quid in ipso Deo?

PAGE 314

[1] Drexelius Nicet. lib. 2, cap. 11.

[2] Fulgor divinæ majestatis.—Aug.

[3] In Ps. lxiv. Misit ad nos epistolas et totam scripturam, quibus nobis faceret amandi desiderium.

[4] Epist. 48, lib. 4. Quid est tota scriptura nisi epistola omnipotentis Dei ad creaturam suam?

PAGE 315

[1] Cap. vi, 9.   [2] Cap. xxi, 10.

[3] In Ps. lxxxv. Omnes pulchritudines terrenas auri, argenti, nemorum et camporum, pulchritudinem solis et lunæ, stellarum, omnia pulchra superans.

[4] Immortalis hæc visio, immortalis amor, indefessus amor et visio.

[5] Osorius: Ubicunque visio et pulchritudo divini aspectus, ibi voluptas ex eodem fonte omnisque beatitudo, nec ab ejus aspectu voluptas, nec ab illa voluptate aspectus separari potest.

PAGE 316

[1] Leon Hebræus. Dubitatur an humana felicitas Deo cognoscendo an amando terminetur.

[2] Lib. de anima. Ad hoc objectum amandum et fruendum nati sumus; et hunc expetisset, unicum hunc amasset humana voluntas, ut summum bonum, et cæteras res omnes eo ordine.

[3] 9 de Repub.

[4] Hom. 9 in Epist. Johannis, cap. 2. Multos conjugium decepit, res alioqui salutaris et necessaria, eo quod cæco ejus amore decepti, divini amoris et gloriæ studium in universum abjecerunt; plurimos cibus et potus perdit.

[5] In mundo splendor opum, gloriæ majestas, amicitiarum præsidia, verborum blanditiæ, voluptatum omnis generis illecebræ, victoriæ, triumphi, et infinita alia ab amore Dei nos abstrahunt, etc.

PAGE 317

[1] In Ps. xxxii. Dei amicus esse non potest qui mundi studiis delectatur; ut hanc formam videas munda cor, serena cor, etc.

[2] Contemplationis pluma nos sublevat, atque inde erigimur intentione cordis, dulcedine contemplationis.—Distinct. 6, de 7 Itineribus.

[3] Lib de victimis. Amans Deum, sublimia petit, sumptis alis et in cœlum recte volat, relicta terra, cupidus aberrandi cum sole, luna, stellarumque sacra militia, ipso Deo duce.

[4] In com. Plat. cap. 7. Ut solem videas oculis, fieri debes solaris: ut divinam aspicias pulchritudinem, demitte materiam, demitte sensum, et Deum qualis sit videbis.

[5] Avare, quid inhias his, etc.? pulchrior est qui te ambit ipsum visurus, ipsum habiturus.   [6] Prov. viii.

[7] Cap. 18 Rom. Amorem hunc divinum totis viribus amplexamini; Deum vobis omni officiorum genere propitium facite.

[8] Cap. 7 de pulchritudine. Regna et imperia totius terræ et maris et cœli oportet abjicere si ad ipsum conversus velis inseri.

[9] Habitus a Deo infusus, per quem inclinatur homo ad diligendum Deum super omnia.

NOTES

PAGE 318

[1] Dial. 1.   Omnia convertit amor in ipsius pulchri naturam.
[2] Stromatum lib. 2.   [3] Greenham.

PAGE 319

[1] De primo præcepto.

PAGE 320

[1] De relig. lib. 2, thes. 1.   [2] De nat. deorum.
[3] Hist. Belgic. lib. 8.
[4] Superstitio error insanus est.—Epist. 123.
[5] Nam qui superstitione imbutus est, quietus esse nunquam potest.
[6] Greg.   [7] Polit. lib. 1, cap. 13.   [8] Hor.

PAGE 321

[1] Epist. Phalar.   [2] In Ps. iii.
[3] Lib. 9, cap. 6.   [4] Lib. 30.

PAGE 322

[1] Lib. 6 Descrip. Græc.   Nulla est via qua non innumeris idolis est referta.   Tantum tunc temporis in miserrimos mortales potentiæ et crudelis tyrannidis Satan exercuit.
[2] Alex. ab. Alex. lib. 6, cap. 26.
[3] Purchas' Pilgrim. lib. 1, cap. 3.   [Ali, Abu Bakr, Omar, Othman.]
[4] Lib. 3.

PAGE 323

[1] 2 part. sect. 3, lib. 1, cap. et deinceps.
[2] Titelmannus, Maginus, Bredenbachius; Fr. Alvaresius, Itin. de Abyssinis.   Herbis solum vescuntur votarii, aquis mento tenus dormiunt, etc.
[3] Bredenbachius, Joh. a Meggen.
[4] [The ancient home of the Serbs, situated between Bosnia, Dalmatia, and Albania.
[5] See Passevinus, Herbastein, Maginus, Dr. Fletcher, Jovius, Hakluyt, Purchas, etc., of their errors.   [6] [Ceylon.]
[7] Deplorat. Gentis Lapp.
[8] Gens superstitioni obnoxia, religionibus adversa.

PAGE 324

[1] Doissardus de magia.   Intra septimum aut nonum a baptismo diem moriuntur.   Hinc fit, etc.
[2] Cap. de incolis Terræ Sanctæ.

PAGE 325

[1] Plato in Crit. Dæmones custodes sunt hominum et eorum domini, ut nos animalium; nec hominibus, sed et regionibus imperant, vaticiniis, auguriis, nos regunt.   Idem fere Max. Tyrius, ser. 1, et 26, 27, medios vult dæmones inter deos et homines deorum ministros, præsides hominum, a cœlo ad homines descendentes.
[2] De præparat. Evangel.
[3] Vel in abusum Dei vel in æmulationem.—Dandinus, Com. in lib. 2 Arist. de anima, text. 29.
[4] Dæmones consulunt, et familiares habent dæmones plerique sacerdotes.—Riccius, lib. 1, cap. 10. Expedit. in Sinas.
[5] Vitam turbant, somnos inquietant, irrepentes etiam in corpora mentes terrent, valetudinem frangunt, morbos lacessunt, ut ad cultum sui cogant, nec aliud his studium, quam ut a vera religione ad superstitionem vertant; cum sint ipsi pœnales, quærunt sibi ad pœnas comites, ut habeant erroris participes.

PAGE 326

[1] Lib. 4 Præparat. Evangel. cap. Tantamque victoriam amentia hominum consecuti sunt, ut si colligere in unum velis, universum orbem istis scelestibus spiritibus subjectum fuisse invenies. Usque ad Salvatoris adventum hominum cæde perniciossisimos dæmones placabant, etc.
[2] Plato.
[3] Strozzius Cicogna, Omnif. mag. lib. 3, cap. 7. Ezek. viii, 4; 1 Reg. xi, 4; 2 Reg. iii et xvii, 16; Jer. xlix; Num. xi, 3; Reg. xiii.
[4] Lib. 4, cap. 8, Præpar.

PAGE 327

[1] Bapt. Mant. 4 Fast. de Sancto Georgio.
[2] Part. 1, cap. 1, et lib. 2, cap. 9.
[3] Polyd. Virg. lib. 1 de prodig.
[4] Hor. lib. 3, Od. 6.   [5] Lib. 3 Hist.
[6] [The cave of Trophonius at Lebadea in Bœotia. See Pausanias, 9, 39.]

PAGE 328

[1] Orata lege me dicastis mulieres.—Dion Halicarn.
[2] Tully, de nat. deorum, lib. 2. Æqua Venus Teucris, Pallas iniqua fuit.
[3] Jo. Molanus, lib. 3, cap. 59.
[4] Pet. Oliver. De Johanne primo Portugalliæ rege strenue pugnans, et diversæ partis ictus clypeo excipiens.
[5] Lib. 14. Loculos sponte aperuisse et pro iis pugnasse.
[6] Religion, as they hold, is policy, invented alone to keep men in awe.
[7] 1 Annal.   [8] Omnes religione moventur.—5 in Verrem.
[9] Zaleucus, præfat. legis. Qui urbem aut regionem inhabitant, persuasos esse oportet esse deos.
[10] 10 de legibus. Religio neglecta maximam pestem in civitatem infert, omnium scelerum fenestram aperit.

PAGE 329

[1] Cardanus, Com. in Ptolemæum quadripart.
[2] Lipsius, lib. 1, cap. 3.
[3] Homo sine religione, sicut equus sine fræno.
[4] Vaninus, dial. 52, de oraculis.
[5] Lib. 10. Ideo Lycurgus, etc., non quod ipse superstitiosus, sed quod videret mortales paradoxa facilius amplecti, nec res graves audere sine periculo deorum.
[6] Cleonardus, Epist. 1. Novas leges suas ad Angelum Gabrielem referebat, quo monitore mentiebatur omnia se gerere.

PAGE 330

[1] Lib. 6 belli Gallici. Ut metu mortis neglecto, ad virtutem incitarent.
[2] [i.e. went. Burton is continuing the Latin construction with infinitive.]
[3] De his lege Lucianum de luctu, tom. 1; Homer. Odyss. 11; Virg. Æn. 6.
[4] Barathro sulfure et flamma stagnante æternum demergebantur.
[5] Et 3 de repub. Omnis institutio adolescentum eo referenda ut de deo bene sentiant ob commune bonum.   [6] Boterus.

PAGE 331

[1] Citra aquam, viridarium plantavit maximum et pulcherrimum, floribus odoriferis et suavibus plenum, etc.
[2] Potum quendam dedit quo inescatus, et gravi sopore oppressus, in viridarium interim ducebatur, etc.

³ Atque iterum memoratum potum bibendum exhibuit, et sic extra Paradisum reduxit, ut cum evigilaret, sopore soluto, etc.
⁴ Lib. 1 de orb. concord. cap. 7.
⁵ Lib. 4. ⁶ Lib. 4.

Page 332

¹ Exerc. 228. ² Sir Ed. Sandys.
³ In consult. de princ. inter provinc. Europ. ⁴ Lucan.

Page 333

¹ [Gregory VII.]
² Sir Ed. Sandys in his Relation. ³ Seneca.
⁴ Vice cotis, acutum Reddere quæ ferrum valet, exors ipsa secandi.
⁵ De Civ. Dei, lib. 4, cap. 31.
⁶ Seeking their own, saith Paul, not Christ's.

Page 334

¹ He hath the Duchy of Spoleto in Italy, the Marquisate of Ancona, beside Rome and the territories adjacent, Bologna, Ferrara, etc., Avignon in France, etc.
² Estote fratres mei, et principes hujus mundi.
³ The laity suspect their greatness, witness those Statutes of Mortmain.
⁴ Lib. 8 de Academ.
⁵ Præfat. lib. de paradox. Jesuit. Rom. provincia habet col. 36, Neapol. 23. Veneta 13, Lusit. 15, India orient. 27, Brasil 20, etc.
⁶ In his Chronic. vit. Hen. 8.
⁷ 15th cap. of his Funeral Monuments.
⁸ Pausanias in Laconicis, lib. 3.
⁹ Idem de Achaicis, lib. 7. Cujus summæ opes, et valde inclyta fama.
¹⁰ Exercit. Eth. colleg. 3, disp. 3.

Page 335

¹ Acts xix, 28.
² Pontifex Romanus prorsus inermis regibus terræ jura dat, ad regna evehit, ad pacem cogit, et peccantes castigat, etc., quod imperatores Romani 40 legionibus armati non effecerunt.
³ Mirum quanta passus sit Henricus 2, quomodo se submisit, ea se acturum pollicitus, quorum hodie ne privatus quidem partem faceret.
⁴ Sigonius, 9 Hist. Ital.
⁵ Curio, lib. 4; Foxe, Martyrol.

Page 336

¹ Hierocles contends Apollonius to have been as great a prophet as Christ, whom Eusebius confutes.
² Munster, Cosmog. lib. 3, cap. 37. Artifices ex officinis, arator e stiva, feminæ e colo, etc., quasi numine quodam rapti, nesciis parentibus et dominis recta adeunt, etc. Combustus demum ab Herbipolensi Episcopo; hæresis evanuit.
³ [The "limbo of the fathers," where the souls of good men who died before the coming of Christ were confined.]

Page 337

¹ Nulla non provincia hæresibus, atheismis, etc., plena. Nullus orbis angulus ab hisce belluis immunis.
² Lib. 1 de nat. deorum. ³ Zanchius. ⁴ Virg. 6 Æn.

PAGE 338

[1] Superstitio ex ignorantia divinitatis emersit, ex vitiosa æmulatione et dæmonis illecebris, inconstans, timens, fluctuans, et cui se addicat nesciens, quem imploret, cui se committat, a dæmone facile decepta.—Lemnius, lib. 3, cap. 8.   [2] Seneca.
[3] [i.e. an indefinitely large number of times.]
[4] Vide Baronium, 3 Annalium, ad annum 324, vita Constantini.
[5] De rerum varietate, lib. 3, cap. 38. Parum vero distat sapientia virorum a puerili, multo minus senum et mulierum, cum metu et superstitione et aliena stultitia et improbitate simplices agitantur.

PAGE 339

[1] In all superstition wise men follow fools.—Bacon's Essays.
[2] Peregrin. Hieros. cap. 5. Totum scriptum confusum sine ordine vel colore, absque sensu et ratione ad rusticissimos idem dedit, rudissimos, et prorsus agrestes, qui nullius erant discretionis, ut dijudicare possent.
[3] Lib. 1, cap. 9, Valent. hæres. 9.
[4] Meteranus, lib. 8 Hist. Belg.

PAGE 340

[1] Si doctores suum fecissent officium, et plebem fidei commissam recte instituissent de doctrinæ christianæ capitibus, nec sacris scripturis interdixissent, de multis proculdubio recte sensissent.
[2] Curtius, lib. 4.
[3] See more in Kemnisius' Examen Concil. Trident. de Purgatorio.
[4] Part. 1, cap. 16; part. 3, cap. 18 et 14.

PAGE 341

[1] Austin.   [2] Curtius, lib. 8.
[3] Lampridius vita ejus. Virgines vestales, et sacrum ignem Romæ extinxit, et omnes ubique per orbem terræ religiones, unum hoc studens ut solus deus coleretur.

PAGE 342

[1] Flagellatorum secta. Munster, lib. 3 Cosmog. cap. 19.
[2] Votum cœlibatus, monachatus.
[3] Mater sanitatis, clavis cœlorum, ala animæ quæ leves pennas producat, ut in sublime ferat; currus Spiritus Sancti, vexillum fidei, porta paradisi, vita angelorum, etc.
[4] Castigo corpus meum.—Paul.   [5] Moriæ Encom.

PAGE 343

[1] Lib. 8, cap. 10, de rerum varietate. Admiratione digna sunt quæ per jejunium hoc modo contingunt: somnia, superstitio, contemptus tormentorum, mortis desiderium, obstinata opinio, insania: jejunium naturaliter præparat ad hæc omnia.
[2] Epist. lib. 3. Ita attenuatus fuit jejunio et vigiliis, in tantum exeso corpore ut ossibus vix hærebat, unde nocte infantum vagitus, balatus pecorum, mugitus boum, voces et ludibria dæmonum, etc.
[3] Lib. de abstinentia. Sobrietas et continentia mentem Deo conjungunt.
[4] Extasis nihil est aliud quam gustus futuræ beatitudinis, in qua toti absorbemur in Deum.—Erasmus, Epist. ad Dorpium.
[5] Si religiosum nimis jejunia videris observantem, audaciter melancholicum pronunciabis.—Tract. 5, cap. 5.

PAGE 344

[1] Solitudo ipsa, mens ægra laboribus anxiis et jejuniis, tum temperatura cibis mutata agrestibus, et humor melancholicus eremitis illusionum causæ sunt.

[2] Solitudo est causa apparitionum; nulli visionibus et hinc delirio magis obnoxii sunt quam qui collegiis et eremo vivunt monachi; tales plerumque melancholici ob victum, solitudinem.

[3] Monachi sese putant prophetare ex Deo, et qui solitariam agunt vitam, quum sit instinctu dæmonum; et sic falluntur fatidicæ; a malo genio habent, quæ putant a Deo, et sic enthusiastæ.

[4] Sibyllæ, Pythii, et prophetæ qui divinare solent, omnes fanatici sunt melancholici.

[5] Exercit. cap. 1.

[6] De divinatione et magicis præstigiis.   [7] Idem.

[8] Post 15 dierum preces et jejunia, mirabiles videbat visiones.

[9] Fol. 84, vita Stephani, et fol. 177. Post trium mensium inediam et languorem per 9 dies nihil comedens aut bibens.

PAGE 345

[1] After contemplation in an ecstasis; so Hierome was whipped for reading Tully; see millions of examples in our annals: Bede, Gregory, Jacobus de Voragine, Lippomanus, Hieronymus, John Major de vitis patrum, etc.

[2] Fol. 199. Post abstinentiæ curas miras illusiones dæmonum audivit.

[3] Fol. 155. Post seriam meditationem in vigilia diei dominicæ visionem habuit de purgatorio.

[4] Ubi multos dies manent jejuni consilio sacerdotum auxilia invocantes.

[5] In Necyomant. Et cibus quidem glandes erant, potus aqua, lectus sub divo, etc.

[6] John Everardus, Britanno-Romanus, lib. edit. 1611, describes all the manner of it.

PAGE 346

[1] Varius mappa compescere risum vix poterat.

[2] Pleno ridet Calphurnius ore.—Hor.   [3] Alanus de Insulis.

PAGE 347

[1] Cicero, lib. de finibus.

PAGE 348

[1] In Micah comment.   [2] Gall. hist. lib. 1.   [3] Lactantius.

PAGE 349

[1] Juv. Sat. 15.

[2] Comment. in Micah. Ferre non possunt ut illorum Messias communis servator sit, nostrum gaudium, etc. Messias vel decem decies crucifixuri essent, ipsumque Deum si id fieri posset, una cum angelis et creaturis omnibus, nec absterrentur ab hoc facto etsi mille inferna subeunda forent.

[3] [? Cahors.]   [4] Lucretius.   [5] Lucan.

[6] Ad. Galat. Comment. Nomen odiosius meum quam ullus homicida aut fur.

PAGE 350

[1] Comment. in Micah. Adeo incomprehensibilis et aspera eorum superbia, etc.

[2] Synagog. Judæorum, cap. 1. Inter eorum intelligentissimos Rabbinos nil præter ignorantiam et insipientiam grandem invenies, horrendam indurationem, et obstinationem, etc.

[3] Great is Diana of the Ephesians.—Acts xix.

Page 351

[1] Malunt cum illis insanire, quam cum aliis bene sentire.
[2] Acosta, lib. 5.
[3] O Ægypte, religionis tuæ solæ supersunt fabulæ, eæque incredibiles posteris tuis.
[4] Meditat. 19 de cœna Domin.

Page 352

[1] Lib. 1 de Trin. cap. 2.   Si decepti sumus, etc.
[2] Vide Samsatis Isphocanis objectiones in monachum Milesium.
[3] Lege Hoffman. Mus exenteratus.
[4] As true as Homer's Iliads, Ovid's Metamorphoses, Æsop's Fables.
[5] Dial. 52 de oraculis.

Page 353

[1] O sanctas gentes quibus hæc nascuntur in horto Numina!—Juven. Sat. 15.
[2] Prudentius.   [3] Tiguri, fol. 1494.
[4] Rosin. Antiq. Rom. lib. 2, cap. 1 et deinceps.

Page 354

[1] Lib. de divinatione et magicis præstigiis, in Mopso.
[2] Cosmo Paccio interpret.   Nihil ab aeris caligine aut figurarum varietate impeditus meram pulchritudinem meruit, exultans et misericordia motus, cognatos amicos qui adhuc morantur in terra tuetur, errantibus succurrit, etc.   Deus hoc jussit ut essent genii dii tutelares hominibus, bonos juvantes, malos punientes, etc.
[3] Sacrorum gent. descript.   Non bene meritos solum, sed et tyrannos pro diis colunt, qui genus humanum horrendum in modum portentosa immanitate divexarunt, etc., fœdas meretrices, etc.

Page 355

[1] [Jer. xi, 13.]
[2] Cap. 22 de ver. rel.   Deos finxerunt eorum poetæ, ut infantium puppas.
[3] Proem. lib. contra philos.

Page 356

[1] Livius, lib. 1.   Deus vobis in posterum propitius, Quirites.
[2] Anth. Verdur. Imag. deorum.
[3] Mulieris candido splendentes amicimine varioque lætantes gestimine, verno florentes conamine, solum sternentes, etc.—Apuleius, lib. 11 de asino aureo.
[4] Magna religione quæritur quæ possit adulteria plura numerare.—Minucius.
[5] Lib. de sacrificiis.   Fumo inhiantes, et muscarum in morem sanguinem exugentes circum aras effusum.

Page 357

[1] Imagines Deorum, lib. sic inscript.
[2] De ver. relig. cap. 22.   Indigni qui terram calcent, etc.
[3] Octaviano.
[4] Jupiter Tragœdus, de sacrificiis, et passim alias.
[5] 666 several kinds of sacrifices in Egypt Major reckons up, tom. 2 coll., of which read more in cap. 1 of Laurentius Pignorius his Egypt Characters, a cause of which Sanubius gives, Subcis. lib. 3, cap. 1.

NOTES

493

[6] Herod. Clio.   Immolavit lecta pecora ter mille Delphis, una cum lectis phialis tribus.
[7] Superstitiosus Julianus innumeras sine parsimonia pecudes mactavit. Ammianus, 22. Boves albi M. Cæsari salutem, si tu viceris perimus, lib. 3. Romani observantissimi sunt ceremoniarum, bello præsertim.

PAGE 358

[1] De sacrificiis: buculam pro bona valetudine, boves quatuor pro divitiis, centum pro regno, novemque tauros pro sospite a Troja reditu, etc.
[2] De sacris Gentil. et sacrific. Tig. 1596.
[3] Enimvero si quis recenseret quæ stulti mortales in festis, sacrificiis, diis adorandis, etc., quæ vota faciant, quid de iis statuant, etc., haud scio an risurus, etc.
[4] Max. Tyrius, Ser. 1.   Crœsus regum omnium stultissimus de lebete consulit, alius de numero arenarum, dimensione maris, etc.
[5] Lib. 14.   [The Branchidæ were hereditary priests of Apollo, serving in his temple at Miletus.]
[6] Peregr. Hierosol.

PAGE 359

[1] Solinus.   [2] Herodotus.   [3] Boterus, Polit. lib. 2, cap. 16.
[4] Plutarch. vit. Crassi.   [5] They were of the Greek Church.

PAGE 360

[1] Lib. 5 de gestis Scanderbegis.
[2] In templis immania idolorum monstra conspiciuntur, marmorea, lignea, lutea, etc.—Riccius.
[3] Deum enim placare non est opus, quia non nocet; sed dæmonem sacrificiis placant, etc.   [4] Fer. Cortesius.
[5] M. Polus; Lod. Vertomannus, Navig. lib. 6, cap. 9; P. Martyr, Ocean Dec.
[6] Propertius, lib. 3, eleg. 12.   [7] Matthias a Michou.

PAGE 361

[1] Epist. Jesuit. anno 1549, a Xaverio et sociis. Idemque Riccius, Expedit. ad Sinas, lib. 1 per totum.   Jejunatores apud eos toto die carnibus abstinent et piscibus ob religionem, nocte et die idola colentes; nusquam egredientes.
[2] Ad immortalitatem morte aspirant summi magistratus, etc. Et multi mortales hac insania, et præpostero immortalitatis studio laborant, et misere pereunt: rex ipse clam venenum hausisset, nisi a servo fuisset detentus.
[3] Cantione in lib. 10 Bonini de repub. fol. 111.
[4] Quin ipsius diaboli ut nequitiam referant.
[5] Lib. de superstit.
[6] Hominibus vitæ finis mors, non autem superstitionis, profert hæc suos terminos ultra vitæ finem.
[7] Buxtorfius, Synagog. Jud. cap. 4.   Inter precandum nemo pediculos attingat, vel pulicem, aut per guttur inferius ventum emittat, etc. Id. cap. 5 et seq., cap. 36.

PAGE 362

[1] Illic omnia animalia, pisces, aves, quos Deus unquam creavit mactabuntur, et vinum generosum, etc.
[2] Cujus lapsu cedri altissimi 300 dejecti sunt, quumque e lapsu ovum fuerat confractum, pagi 160 inde submersi, et alluvione inundati.

[3] Every king of the world shall send him one of his daughters to be his wife, because it is written (Ps. xlv, 9), "Kings' daughters shall attend on him," etc.

[4] Quum quadringentis adhuc milliaribus ab imperatore leo hic abesset, tam fortiter rugiebat, ut mulieres Romanæ abortierint omnes, muriquè, etc.

[5] Strozzius Cicogna, Omnif. mag. lib. 1, cap. 1.   Putida multa recenset ex Alcorano, de cœlo, stellis, angelis, Lonicerus, cap. 21, 22, lib. 1.

PAGE 363

[1] Quinquies in die orare Turcæ tenentur ad meridiem.—Bredenbachius, cap. 5.

[2] In quolibet anno mensem integrum jejunant interdiu, nec comedentes nec bibentes, etc.

[3] Nullis unquam multi per totam ætatem carnibus vescuntur.—Leo Afer.

[4] Lonicerus, tom. 1, cap. 17, 18.

[5] Gotardus Arthus, cap. 33, Hist. Orient. Indiæ.   Opinio est expiatorium esse Gangem; et nec mundum ab omni peccato nec salvum fieri posse, qui non hoc flumine se abluat; quam ob causam ex tota India, etc.

[6] Quia nil volunt deinceps videre.

PAGE 364

[1] Nullum se conflictandi finem facit.

[2] Ut in aliquem angulum se reciperet, ne reus fieret ejus delicti quod ipse erat admissurus.   [3] Gregor. Hom.

PAGE 365

[1] Epist. 190.

[2] Orat. 8.   Ut vertigine correptis videntur omnia moveri, omnia iis falsa sunt, quum error in ipsorum cerebro sit.

[3] Res novas affectant et inutiles, falsa veris præferunt.   2. Quod temeritas effutierit, id superbia postmodum tuebitur et contumaciæ, etc.

[4] See more in Vincent. Lyrin.

[5] Aust. de hæres.   Usus mulierum indifferens.

[6] Quod ante peccavit Adam, nudus erat.

[7] Alii nudis pedibus semper ambulant.

[8] Insana feritate sibi non parcunt, nam per mortes varias præcipitiorum, aquarum et ignium, seipsos necant, et in istum furorem alios cogunt, mortem minantes ni faciant.

[9] Elench. hæret. ab orbe condito.

PAGE 366

[1] Nubrigensis lib. cap. 19.   [2] Jovian. Pont. Ant. Dial.

[3] Cum per paganos nomen ejus persequi non poterat, sub specie religionis fraudulenter subvertere disponebat.

[4] That writ de professo against Christians, et Palestinum deum (ut Socrates, lib. 3, cap. 19), Scripturam nugis plenam, etc.   Vide Cyrillum in Julianum, Origenem in Celsum, etc.

PAGE 367

[1] One image had one gown worth 400 crowns and more.

[2] [Prato, near Florence.   Its cathedral possesses the Virgin's girdle.]

[3] As at Our Lady's Church at Bergamo in Italy.

PAGE 368

[1] Lucilius, lib. 1, cap. 22, de falsa religione.   [2] An. 441.

PAGE 369

[1] [Objections and solutions, so marked in the margins of old controversial works.]

[2] Hospinian, Osiander. An hæc propositio Deus sit cucurbita vel scarabæus, sit æque possibilis ac Deus et homo? An possit respectum producere sine fundamento et termino? An levius sit hominem jugulare quam die dominico calceum consuere?

[3] De doct. Christian.

PAGE 370

[1] Daniel.   [2] Agrip. ep. 29.

PAGE 371

[1] Alex. Gaguin. 22. Discipulis ascitis mirum in modum populum decepit.

[2] Guicciard. descrip. Belg. Complures habuit asseclas ab iisdem honoratus.

[3] Hen. Nicholas at Leyden, 1580, such a one.

[4] See Camden's Annals, fol. 242 et 285.

PAGE 372

[1] Arius his bowels burst, Montanus hanged himself, etc. Eudo de Stellis his disciples ardere potius quam ad vitam corrigi maluerunt; tanta vis infixi semel erroris, they died blaspheming.—Nubrigensis, cap. 9, lib. 1. Jer. vii, 23. Amos v, 5.

PAGE 373

[1] Cap. 5.   [2] Poplinerius Lerius, præf. Hist. Rich. Dinoth.

[3] Advers. gentes, lib. 1. Postquam in mundo Christiana gens cœpit, terrarum orbem periisse, et multis malis affectum esse genus humanum videmus.

[4] Quod nec hieme, nec æstate tanta imbrium copia, nec frugibus torrendis solita flagrantia, nec vernali temperie sata tam læta sint, nec arboreis fœtibus autumni fœcundi, minus de montibus marmor eruatur, minus aurum, etc.

[5] Solitus erat oblectare se fidibus, et voce musica canentium; sed hoc omne sublatum Sibyllæ cujusdam interventu, etc. Inde quicquid erat instrumentorum symphoniacorum, auro gemmisque egregio opere distinctorum comminuit, et in ignem injecit, etc.

PAGE 374

[1] Ob id genus observantiuncularum videmus homines misere affligi, et denique mori, et sibi ipsis Christianos videri quum revera sint Judæi.

[2] Ita in corpora nostra fortunasque decretis suis sæviit ut parum obfuerat nisi Deus Lutherum virum perpetua memoria dignissimum excitasset, quin nobis fœno mox communi cum jumentis cibo utendum fuisset.

[3] The Gentiles in India will eat no sensible creatures, or aught that hath blood in it.

[4] Vandormilius de aucupio, cap. 27.

PAGE 375

[1] Some explode all human authors, arts, and sciences, poets, histories, etc., so precise, their zeal overruns their wits; and so stupid, they oppose all human learning, because they are ignorant themselves and illiterate, nothing must be read but Scriptures; but these men deserve to be pitied rather than confuted. Others are so strict, they will admit of no honest

game and pleasure, no dancing, singing, other plays, recreations and games, hawking, hunting, cock-fighting, bear-baiting, etc., because to see one beast kill another is the fruit of our rebellion against God, etc.

[2] Nuda ac tremebunda cruentis Irrepet genibus si candida jusserit Io.—Juvenalis, Sat. 6.

[3] Munster, Cosmog. lib. 3, cap. 444. Incidit in cloacam, unde se non possit eximere, implorat opem sociorum, sed illi negant, etc.

[4] De benefic. 7, 2.

PAGE 376

[1] Numen venerare præsertim quod civitas colit.   [2] Octaviano dial.

[3] Annal. tom. 3, ad annum 324, 1.   [4] Ovid.

PAGE 377

[1] In Epist. Sym.

[2] Quia Deus immensum quiddam est et infinitum, cujus natura perfecte cognosci non potest, æquum ergo est, ut diversa ratione colatur, prout quisque aliquid de Deo percipit aut intelligit.

[3] Campanella, Calcagninus, and others.

[4] Æternæ beatitudinis consortes fore, qui sancte innocenterque hanc vitam traduxerint, quamcunque illi religionem secuti sunt.

[5] Comment. in 1 Tim. vi, ver. 20 et 21. Severitate cum hæreticis agendum, et non aliter.

[6] Quod silentium hæreticis indixerit.

PAGE 378

[1] Igne et fuste potius agendum cum hæreticis quam cum disputationibus; os alia loquens, etc.   [2] Præfat. Hist.

[3] Quidam conquestus est mihi de hoc morbo, et deprecatus est ut ego illum curarem; ego quæsivi ab eo quid sentiret; respondit, Semper imaginor et cogito de Deo et angelis, etc., et ita demersus sum hac imaginatione, ut nec edam nec dormiam, nec negotiis, etc. Ego curavi medicina et persuasione; et sic plures alios.

PAGE 379

[1] De anima, cap. de humoribus.   [2] Juvenal.

[3] Lib. 5 Gal. hist. Quamplurimi reperti sunt qui tot pericula subeuntes irridebant; et quæ de fide, religione, etc., dicebant, ludibrio habebant, nihil eorum admittentes de futura vita.

PAGE 380

[1] Fifty thousand atheists at this day in Paris, Marcennus thinks.

[2] Hor. lib. 2, Od. 18.   [3] Luke xvii.

[4] Wisd. ii, 2.   [5] Vers. 6, 7, 8.

PAGE 381

[1] Catullus, 5.   [2] Prov. vii, 18.

[3] [Lycaon was changed into a wolf.]   [4] Lib. 2.

[5] M. Montan. lib. 1, cap. 4.

[6] Orat. cont. Hispan. Ne proximo decennio deum adorarent, etc.

[7] Talem se exhibuit, ut nec in Christum, nec Mahometem crederet, unde effectum ut promissa nisi quatenus in suum commodum cederent minime servaret, nec ullo scelere peccatum statueret, ut suis desideriis satisfaceret.

PAGE 382

[1] Lib. de mor. Germ.   [2] Europæ Hist. cap. 24.   [3] Or Breslau.

[4] Usque adeo insanus, ut nec inferos, nec superos esse dicat, animasque cum corporibus interire credat, etc.

⁵ Fratres a Bry, Amer. part. 6. Librum a Vincentio monacho datum abjecit, nihil se videre ibi hujusmodi dicens, rogansque unde hæc sciret, quum de cœlo et Tartaro contineri ibi diceret.

⁶ Non minus hi furunt quam Hercules, qui conjugem et liberos interfecit; habet hæc ætas plura hujusmodi portentosa monstra.

⁷ De orbis con. lib. 1, cap. 7.

PAGE 383

¹ Nonne Romani sine deo vestro regnant et fruuntur orbe toto, et vos et deos vestros captivos tenent, etc.—Minucius Octaviano.

² Comment. in Genesin copiosus in hoc subjecto.

³ Martial, lib. 4, epig. 21.

⁴ Ecce pars vestrum et major et melior alget, fame laborat, et deus patitur, dissimulat, non vult, non potest opitulari suis, et vel invalidus vel iniquus est.—Cæcilius in Minuc. Cum rapiunt mala fata bonos, ignoscite fasso, Sollicitor nullos esse putare deos.—Ovid. Vidi ego diis fretos, multos decipi.—Plautus, Casina, Act. 2, sc. 5.

PAGE 384

¹ Ser. 30, in 5 cap. ad Ephes. Hic fractis est pedibus, alter furit, alius ad extremam senectam progressus omnem vitam paupertate peragit, ille morbis gravissimis: sunt hæc Providentiæ opera? hic surdus, ille mutus, etc.

² Omnia contingenter fieri volunt.—Melancthon in præceptum primum.

³ Dial. 1, lib. 4, de admir. nat. arcanis.

⁴ Anima mea sit cum animis philosophorum.

PAGE 385

¹ Deum unum multis designant nominibus, etc.

² Non intelligis te quum hæc dicis, negare te ipsum nomen Dei: quid enim est aliud Natura quam Deus? etc.; tot habet appellationes quot munera.

³ Austin.   ⁴ Principio Ephemer.

PAGE 386

¹ Vaninus, dial. 52, de oraculis.

² Varie homines affecti, alii dei judicium ad tam pii exilium, alii ad naturam referebant, nec ab indignatione dei, sed humanis causis, etc, —12 Natural. quæst. 33, 39.   ⁵ Juv. Sat. 13.

PAGE 387

¹ Epist. ad C. Cæsar. Romani olim putabant fortunam regna et imperia dare; credebant antea mortales fortunam solam opes et honores largiri idque duabus de causis: primum quod indignus quisque dives, honoratus, potens; alterum, vix quisquam perpetuo bonis iis frui visus. Postea prudentiores didicere fortunam suam quemque fingere.

² 10 de legibus. Alii negant esse deos, alii deos non curare res humanas, alii utraque concedunt.   ³ Lib. 8, ad mathem.

⁴ Origen, contra Celsum, lib. 3. Hos immerito nobiscum conferri fuse declarat.

⁵ Crucifixum deum ignominiose Lucianus vita Peregrini Christum vocat.

PAGE 388

¹ De ira, 16, 34. Iratus cœlo quod obstreperet, ad pugnam. vocans Jovem, quanta dementia! putavit sibi nocere non posse, et se nocere tamen Jovi posse.   ² Lib. 1.

³ Idem status post mortem, ac fuit antequam nasceremur. Et Seneca: Idem erit post me quod ante me fuit.

⁴ Lucernæ eadem conditio quum extinguitur, ac fuit antequam accenderetur; ita et hominis.
⁵ Dissert. cum. nuncio sidereo. [Giordano Bruno, "unhappy Brunus," was burnt at the stake, 1600.]
⁶ [Vanini, strangled and burned, 1619.]

Page 389

¹ [Decameron, Day 1, Tale 3.]
² Campanella, cap. 18 Atheism. Triumphat.
³ Comment. in Gen. cap. 7.
⁴ So that a man may meet an atheist as soon in his study as in the street.
⁵ Simonis Religio incerto auctore, Cracoviæ edit. 1588. Conclusio libri est, Ede itaque, bibe, lude, etc., jam Deus figmentum est.
⁶ Lib. de immortalitate animæ.
⁷ Pag. 645, an. 1238, ad finem Henrici tertii. Idem Pistorius, pag. 743 in compilat. sua.

Page 390

¹ Virg. ² Rom. xii, 2.
³ Omnis Aristippum decuit color, et status, et res.
⁴ Ps. xiv, 1. ⁵ Guicciardine. ⁶ Erasmus.

Page 391

¹ Hierome. ² Senec. Consol. ad Polyb. cap. 21.

Page 392

¹ Disput. 4 Philosophiæ adver. Atheos, Venetiis 1627, quarto.
² Edit. Romæ, fol. 1631.
³ Abernethy, cap. 24 of his Physic of the Soul.

Page 393

¹ Omissa spe victoriæ in destinatam mortem conspirant, tantusque ardor singulos cepit, ut victores se putarent si non inulti morerentur.—Justin, lib. 20.
² Method. hist. cap. 5.
³ Hosti abire volenti iter minime interscindas, etc.
⁴ Poster. volum.

Page 394

¹ Super præceptum primum de relig. et partibus ejus. Non loquor de omni desperatione, sed tantum de ea qua desperare solent homines de Deo; opponitur spei, et est peccatum gravissimum, etc.
² Lib. 5, tit. 21, de regis institut. Omnium perturbationum deterrima.
³ Reprobi usque ad finem pertinaciter persistunt.—Zanchius.
⁴ Vitium ab infidelitate proficiscens.

Page 395

¹ Abernethy. ² 1 Sam. xvi, 14.
³ Ps. xxxviii. vers. 1, 2, 3, 8.
⁴ Immiscent se mali genii.—Lem. lib. 1, cap. 16.

Page 396

¹ Cases of Conscience, lib. 1, 16. ² Tract. Melan. cap. 33 et 34.
³ Cap. 3 de mentis alien. Deo minus se curæ esse, nec ad salutem prædestinatos esse. Ad desperationem sæpe ducit hæc melancholia, et est frequentissima ob supplicii metum æternumque judicium; mœror et metus in desperationem plerumque desinunt.

⁴ Comment. in 1 cap. Gen. artic. 3. Quia impii florent, boni 'opprimuntur, etc., alius ex consideratione hujus seria desperabundus.
⁵ Lib. 10, cap. 17.
⁶ Damnatam se putavit, et per quatuor menses Gehennæ pœnam sentire.

PAGE 397

¹ 1566. Ob triticum diutius servatum conscientiæ stimulis agitatur, etc.
² Tom. 2, cap. 27, num. 282. Conversatio cum scrupulosis, vigiliæ, jejunia.
³ Solitarios et superstitiosos plerumque exagitat conscientia, non mercatores, lenones, caupones, fœneratores, etc., largiorem hi nacti sunt conscientiam. Juvenes plerumque conscientiam negligunt, senes autem, etc.
⁴ Annon sentis sulphur? inquit.
⁵ Desperabundus misere periit.
⁶ In 17 Johannis. Non pauci se cruciant, et excarnificant in tantum, ut non parum absint ab insania; neque tamen aliud hac mentis anxietate efficiunt quam ut diabolo potestatem faciant ipsos per desperationem ad inferos producendi.

PAGE 398

¹ Drexelius, Nicet. lib. 2, cap. 11.

PAGE 399

¹ Ecclesiast. lib. 1. Haud scio an majus discrimen ab his qui blandiuntur, an ab his qui territant; ingens utrinque periculum: alii ad securitatem ducunt, alii afflictionum magnitudine mentem absorbent, et in desperationem trahunt.
² Bern. sup. 16 Cant. 1. Alterum sine altero proferre non expedit; recordatio solius judicii in desperationem præcipitat, et misericordiæ fallax ostentatio pessimam generat securitatem.
³ In Luc. hom. 103. Exigunt ab aliis caritatem, beneficentiam, cum ipsi nil spectent præter libidinem, invidiam, avaritiam.
⁴ Leo Decimus.

PAGE 400

¹ De futuro judicio, de damnatione horrendum crepunt, et amaras illas potationes in ore semper habent, ut multos inde in desperationem cogant.
² Euripides.   ³ Pierius.   ⁴ Gen. iv.
⁵ Nine causes Musculus makes.

PAGE 401

¹ Plutarch.
² Alios misere castigat plena scrupulis conscientia, nodum in scirpo quærunt, et ubi nulla causa subest, misericordiæ divinæ diffidentes, se Orco destinant.
³ Cælius, lib. 6.   ⁴ Juvenal.
⁵ Lucian. de dea Syria. Si adstiteris, te aspicit; si transeas, visu te sequitur.
⁶ Prima hæc est ultio, quod se Judice nemo nocens absolvitur, improba quamvis Gratia fallaci prætoris vicerit urna.—Juvenal.
⁷ Quis unquam vidit avarum ringi dum lucrum adest, adulterum dum potitur voto, lugere in perpetrando scelere? voluptate sumus ebrii, proinde non sentimus, etc.

PAGE 402

[1] Buchanan, lib. 6 Hist. Scot. [Kenneth III.]
[2] Animus conscientia sceleris inquietus, nullum admisit gaudium, sed semper vexatus noctu et interdiu per somnum visis horrore plenis pertremefactus, etc.
[3] De bello Neapol.
[4] Thyreus de locis infestis, part. 1, cap. 2. Nero's mother was still in his eyes.   [5] Ps. xliv. 1.

PAGE 403

[1] Regina causarum et arbitra rerum, nunc erectas cervices opprimit, etc.
[2] Alex. Gaguinus, Catal. reg. Pol.
[3] Cosmog. Munster. et Magdeb.

PAGE 404

[1] Plinius, cap. 10, lib. 35. Consumptis affectibus, Agamemnonis caput velavit, ut omnes quem possent maximum mœrorem in virginis patre cogitarent.   [2] [The highest degree.]

PAGE 405

[1] Cap. 15, in 9 Rhasis.   [2] Juv. Sat. 13.
[3] Mentem eripit timor hic, vultum, totumque corporis habitum immutat, etiam in deliciis, in tripudiis, in symposiis, in amplexu conjugis carnificinam exercet.—Lib. 4, cap. 21.
[4] Non sinit conscientia tales homines recta verba proferre, aut rectis quenquam oculis aspicere, ab omni hominum cœtu eosdem exterminat, et dormientes perterrefacit.—Philost. lib. 1 de vita Apollonii.
[5] Eusebius; Nicephorus, Eccles. hist. lib. 4, cap. 17.
[6] Seneca, lib. 18, epist. 106. Conscientia aliud agere non patitur, perturbatam vitam agunt, nunquam vacant, etc.

PAGE 406

[1] Artic. 3, cap. 1, fol. 230. Quod horrendum dictu, desperabundus quidam me præsente cum ad patientiam hortaretur, etc.

PAGE 407

[1] Lib. 1 Observ. cap. 3.
[2] Ad maledicendum Deo.   [3] Goulart.
[4] Dum hæc scribo, implorat opem meam monacha, in reliquis sana, et judicio recta, per 5 annos melancholica; damnatam se dicit, conscientiæ stimulis oppressa, etc.
[5] Alios conquerentes audivi se esse ex damnatorum numero, Deo non esse curæ, aliaque infinita quæ proferre non audebant, vel abhorrebant.

PAGE 408

[1] Musculus, Patricius: ad vim sibi inferendam cogit homines.
[2] 3 de mentis alienat. observ. lib. 1.
[3] Uxor mercatoris diu vexationibus tentata, etc.
[4] Abernethy.   [5] Busbequius.

PAGE 409

[1] John Major, vitis Patrum. Quidam negavit Christum per chirographum post restitutus.
[2] Trincavellius, lib. 3, consil. 46.
[3] My brother, George Burton, Mr. James Whitehall, rector of Checkley

in Staffordshire, my quondam chamber-fellow and late fellow-student in Christ Church, Oxon.

[4] Scio quam vana sit et inefficax humanorum verborum penes afflictos consolatio, nisi verbum Dei audiatur, a quo vita, refrigeratio, solatium, pænitentia.

PAGE 410

[1] Antid. adversus desperationem.
[2] Tom. 2, cap. 27, num. 282.
[3] Aversio cogitationis a re scrupulosa, contraventio scrupulorum.

PAGE 411

[1] Magnam injuriam Deo facit qui diffidit de ejus misericordia.
[2] Bonitas invicti non vincitur; infiniti misericordia non finitur.
[8] Hom. 3, de pænitentia: Tua quidem malitia mensuram habet. Dei autem misericordia mensuram non habet. Tua malitia circumscripta est, etc. Pelagus etsi magnum, mensuram habet; Dei autem, etc.

PAGE 412

[1] Non ut desidiores vos faciam, sed ut alacriores reddam.
[2] Pro peccatis veniam poscere, et mala de novo iterare.
[3] Si bis, si ter, si centies, si centies millies, toties pænitentiam age.
[4] Conscientia mea meruit damnationem, pænitentia non sufficit ad satisfactionem: sed tua misericordia superat omnem offensionem.
[5] Multo efficacior Christi mors in bonum, quam peccata nostra in malum. Christus potentior ad salvandum, quam dæmon ad perdendum.
[6] Peritus medicus potest omnes infirmitates sanare; si misericors, vult.

PAGE 413

[1] Omnipotenti medico nullus languor insanabilis occurrit: tu tantum doceri te sine, manum ejus ne repelle: novit quid agat; non tantum delecteris cum fovet, sed toleres quum secat.
[2] Chrys. hom. 3, de pænit.
[3] Spes salutis per quam peccatores salvantur, Deus ad misericordiam provocatur. Isidor. Omnia ligata tu solvis, contrita sanas, confusa lucidas, desperata animas.
[4] Chrys. hom. 5. Non fornicatorem abnuit, non ebrium avertit, non superbum repellit, non aversatur Idololatram, non adulterum, sed omnes suscipit, omnibus communicat.
[5] Chrys. hom. 5.
[6] Qui turpibus cantilenis aliquando inquinavit os, divinis hymnis animum purgabit.

PAGE 414

[1] Hom. 5. Introivit hic quis accipiter, columba exit; introivit lupus, ovis egreditur, etc.
[2] Omnes languores sanat, cæcis visum, claudis gressum, gratiam confert, etc. [3] Seneca.
[4] Delectatur Deus conversione peccatoris; omne tempus vitæ conversioni deputatur; pro præsentibus habentur tam præterita quam futura.
[5] Austin. Semper pænitentiæ portus apertus est ne desperemus.
[6] Quicquid feceris, quantumcunque peccaveris, adhuc in vita es, unde te omnino si sanare te nollet Deus, auferret; parcendo clamat ut redeas, etc.

PAGE 415

[1] Mark ix, 24. [2] Rev. xxi, 6.
[3] Abernethy, Perkins.
[4] Non est pænitentia, sed Dei misericordia annexa.

PAGE 416

[1] Cæcilius Minucio: Omnia ista figmenta male sanæ religionis, et inepta solatia a poetis inventa, vel ab aliis ob commodum, superstitiosa mysteria, etc.
[2] These temptations and objections are well answered in John Downam's Christian Warfare.   [3] Seneca.

PAGE 417

[1] Vid. Campanella, cap. 6 Atheis. Triumphat. et cap. 2, ad argumentum 12, ubi plura. Si Deus bonus, unde malum? etc.

PAGE 418

[1] Perkins.

PAGE 419

[1] Hemmingius. Nemo peccat in Spiritum Sanctum nisi qui finaliter et voluntarie renunciat Christum, eumque et ejus verbum extreme contemnit, sine qua nulla salus; a quo peccato liberet nos Dominus Jesus Christus. Amen.

PAGE 421

[1] Abernethy.   [2] See whole books of these arguments.
[3] Lib. 3, fol. 122. Præjudicata opinio, invida, maligna, et apta ad impellendos animos in desperationem.
[4] See the antidote in Chamier's tom. 3, lib. 7, Downam's Christian Warfare, etc.
[5] Potentior est Deo diabolus, et mundi princeps, et in multitudine hominum sita est majestas.

PAGE 422

[1] Homicida qui non subvenit quum potest; hoc de Deo sine scelere cogitari non potest, utpote quum quod vult licet. Boni natura communicari. Bonus Deus, quomodo misericordiæ pater, etc.
[2] Vide Cyrillum, lib. 4 adversus Julianum. Qui poterimus illi gratias agere qui nobis non misit Mosen et prophetas, et contempsit bona animarum nostrarum?
[3] Venia danda est iis qui non audiunt ob ignorantiam. Non est tam iniquus Judex Deus, ut quenquam indicta causa damnare velit. Ii solum damnantur, qui oblatam Christi gratiam rejiciunt.
[4] Busbequius; Lonicerus, Tur. Hist. tom. 1, lib. 2.
[5] Clem. Alex.   [6] Paulus Jovius, Elog. vir. illust.

PAGE 423

[1] Non homines sed et ipsi dæmones aliquando servandi.
[2] Vid. Pelsii Harmoniam, art. 22, p. 2.

PAGE 424

[1] Epist. Erasmi de utilitate colloquior. ad lectorem.
[2] Vastata conscientia sequitur sensus iræ divinæ (Hemmingius), fremitus cordis, ingens animæ cruciatus, etc.

PAGE 426

[1] Austin.

PAGE 427

[1] Super Ps. lii. Convertar ad liberandum eum, quia conversus est ad peccatum suum puniendum.

[1] Antiqui soliti sunt hanc herbam ponere in cœmeteriis ideo quod, etc.

[1] Non desunt nostra ætate sacrificuli, qui tale quid attentant, sed a cacodæmone irrisi pudore suffecti sunt et re infecta abierunt.

[2] Done into English by W. B., 1613.

[3] Tom. 2, cap. 27, num. 282.

[1] Navarrus.   [2] Is. l, 4.

GLOSSARY

Volume and page references are appended to words and phrases of special interest, and to instances of words used in a special sense.

A few definitions are quoted from the 1755 edition of Bailey's English Dictionary.

A

abdicate, to expel, dethrone, i, 301.

abort, an abortion.

Abraham-men, beggars who counterfeited lunacy (named after one of the wards in Bedlam), i, 355.

absolute, perfect, faultless.

absolve, to complete, ii, 57.

Acherontic, moribund; "an old Acherontic dizzard," iii, 303.

adamant, a lodestone.

adust, burnt up, having much heat, a supposed condition of the four "humours" of the body; *adustion*, heating to dryness.

advoutry, adultery, iii, 293.

affect, to feel affection for; "affected with," fond of, ii, 73.

affright, affrighted, i, 336.

afternoon-men, tipplers.

alexipharmacum, an antidote for poison, a sovereign remedy.

alicant (old edd. *allegant*), a strong, sweet Spanish wine.

alkermes, a compound cordial, coloured with kermes.

all out, in every respect, altogether, quite.

almuten (astrol.), the planet of chief influence in a horoscope.

ambidexter, a double-dealer, time-server.

ammi, a genus of umbelliferous plants (bishop-weeds), used in medicine.

amphibological, ambiguous.

ampliation, amplification.

angust, rarefied, ii, 49.

annexed, bound together, iii, 12.

antic, a buffoon; a grotesque figure.

apologer, *apologist*, a writer of apologues, a fabulist.

apophlegmatisms, expectorants.

approve, to put to the test; to prove.

aristolochy, birthwort.

ascendant (astrol.), the sign of the zodiac which rises above the horizon at the time of one's birth.

assassinate, an assassin.

Atellanes, popular farces.

Austrian planets, supposed satellites of Saturn, iii, 120.

available, of avail, efficacious, iii, 102.

B

bable, a bauble.

baby, a doll, puppet; "babies of clouts," rag-dolls, i, 46; "look babies in one another's eyes" (iii, 229) refers to the minute reflection of oneself, visible when one looks closely into another's eyes.

ballet, a ballad.

balloon, a kind of football.

bangle, to waste by little and little, to fritter (away), i, 273.

barley-break, an ancient catching game.

bassa, a pasha.

bastard, a sweet, heady Spanish wine, white or brown.

Bavarian chin, or *poke*, goitre.

bayard, blind, one blinded with self-conceit, iii, 339. An allusion to the proverbial saying, "As bold as blind Bayard."

bedlam, a bedlamite, lunatic.

bewray, to betray; to befoul; "all-to bewrayed," befouled all over, iii, 207.

bezoar's (or *bezoar*) *stone*, a calcular concretion found in the stomachs of certain animals.

bird, a nestling, young bird, iii, 23.

black guard, the scullions, etc., connected with a great household, i, 185.

bloody-fallen, chilblained, iii, 155.

bole, a bolus, ii, 234.

bona-roba, a well-dressed woman, iii, 215.

box (in gaming), the bank, ii, 198.

brach, a deerhound, i, 331.

Brachmanni, Brahmins.

brachygraphy, shorthand, ii, 95.

brangling, wrangling, quarrelsome, ii, 195.

brief, an epitome, précis, i, 311.

brise, the land- and sea-breeze in the tropics, ii, 45.

Brontes, a Cyclops who laboured in Vulcan's workshop; hence, a blacksmith, iii, 82.

bull's feathers, insignia of cuckoldom, iii, 291.

Burbonian planets, sunspots, mistaken for planets by early observers, iii, 120.

busk-point, a stay-lace.

by-respects, private ends or views.

C

calamistrate, to curl the hair with tongs; *calamistration*, the act of so curling.

cample, to wrangle, iii, 308.

canvas, dismissal, "sack," ii, 192; "have a canvas," get the sack, be disappointed, i, 282.

capcase, a small portable case, a cash-box.

capital, belonging to or concerning the head; "capital herbs," herbs used in head-medicine, ii, 31.

card, a chart.
careful, full of care.
cari, caraway.
carl, to act like a churl; to talk gruffly, to snarl, i, 210.
caroche, a coach.
cast, discredited, cashiered.
casting-counters, counters used in reckoning, i, 110.
castril, a kestrel.
catholic, universal; "catholic medicine," a catholicon, panacea, ii, 248.
caul, a membrane enclosing viscera, i, 138; a hair-net, iii, 94.
cautelous, wary.
censure (n.), opinion, judgment; "I 'll stand to your censure," I 'll abide by your judgment, i, 72.
censure (v.t.), to judge, criticize.
cerotes, wax plasters.
ceruse, white lead, used as a cosmetic.
ceterach, a species of spleenwort.
chalastic, laxative.
character, a distinguishing mark, characteristic, i, 144; a charm in the form of an inscription, ii, 5, etc.
chequin (old edd. *chickine*), a sequin, a Venetian gold coin, iii, 124.
china, *china-root*, the root of *Smilax China*, a sort of sarsaparilla; *china-broth*, a decoction of the same.
chitty, meagre, iii, 155.
choler, bile, the humour supposed to cause bad temper.
chuff, a surly fellow, a niggard.
cicliminus, cyclamen, sow-bread.
circumforanean, strolling from market to market, itinerant.
civilian, a professor of civil law.
clancular, secret.
cloth (sing. of *clothes*), a garment, iii, 160.
clothing, cloth-making, i, 91.
coal, charcoal, iii, 181.
cockney-like, effeminate, i, 230.
cog, to wheedle; to cheat.
coll, to embrace about the neck, to cuddle.
collapsed, ruined; "collapsed ladies," decayed gentlewomen, iii, 339.
collogue, to wheedle, flatter.
colly, the soot of coal or burned wood.
colone, a husbandman, i, 67.
colt's evil, a distemper affecting young horses; metaphorically, youthful wantonness, iii, 59.
combust (astron.), burnt, i.e. so near the sun as to be obscured by it.
come off, to pay up, i, 322, iii, 115.
comical, pertaining to comedy; "that comical old man," that old man in the comedy, iii, 239.
commencements, degree-conferring ceremonies; "the commencements of the Deity," iii, 425.
commodity, advantage, expediency, profit.
commons, food, regular diet.
compinged, confined, compressed.

complement, an ornamental quality, accomplishment; a fulfilling, iii, 318.

complexion, natural habit, constitution.

complicate, to form by complication, ii, 95.

composed, ordered, sedate (of looks).

conceit, imagination; understanding.

conceited, witty, amusing.

concent, concord, harmony, ii, 118.

concoct, to digest; *concoction*, digestion.

condite, preserved, candied.

conditions, moral state, character.

confer, to compare.

confine (adj.), neighbouring; "confine places," i, 425.

consisting, more or less dense or viscous, ii, 223, 224.

constantly, with a steadfast mind; "constantly died," i, 436.

constellations (astrol.), stellar conjunctions, i. 205.

constringe, to draw together, contract.

contract, concisely, i, 30.

controvert, to deliver contrary opinions; to argue for and against.

convented, convened, come together, ii, 158.

conversions, revolutions (of the heavenly bodies), ii, 129.

cony-catching, cheating, gulling.

cornute, to cuckold; *cornuto*, a cuckold.

coronet, an ornamental head-dress.

corrivate, to draw together in one stream; *corrivation*, the running of streams into one.

corsive, a corrosive, a vexation, i, 107.

cowl-staff, the pole on which a water-vessel was slung.

crack, to boast; *cracker*, a boaster.

crowned (Lat. *coronatus*), sovereign; "a crowned medicine," ii, 239.

crucify, to torment.

cubbed up, cooped up, confined.

curious, requiring care and nicety; particular, difficult to please.

curr, the golden-eye duck, i, 219.

curranto, a courant, a newsletter.

cuscuta, dodder.

cushion-dance, a lively, romping dance, in which a cushion figured, ii, 121.

cut-works, embroidery.

D

Dædalian, maze-constructing, ii, 56.

damnified, injured, i, 230.

dare, to daze, stupefy with terror; "never hobby so dared a lark," iii, 340.

day-net, a net for catching small birds.

daysman, an arbitrator (cf. Job ix, 33), i, 85.

debility (astrol.), a weakness of a planet in influence.

deboshed, debauched.

deducted, drawn off, i, 35.

defecate (v.t.), to purify; (adj.) pure, free from dregs.

defect, deficiency; "for defect," in default, ii, 105.
dehort, to dissuade.
deliquium, a fainting-fit.
descry, to discover, make known; "Jupiter descried himself," i, 179.
detect, to reveal, ii, 191.
detracted, subtracted, iii, 209.
detriment (astrol.), the sign directly opposite that which is a planet's house.
dia- (med.), prefixed to the name of the principal ingredient in a compound medicine, e.g. *diascordium*.
dictery, a witty saying, iii, 249.
dilate, to treat at length.
dilling, darling, iii, 26.
diminutives, medicines that lessen or abate.
disprove, to disallow, disapprove of, ii, 64.
distillation (med.), catarrh.
dittander, pepperwort.
diverb, an antithetical saying or proverb.
divulge, to publish in the vernacular.
dizzard (old edd. *disard*), a blockhead.
dodecatemories, the twelve signs of the zodiac, ii, 44.
dorp, a thorp, village.
draught, a privy.
dropax, a pitch-plaster.
drugger, a druggist, i, 102.
dummerer, a feigner of dumbness, i, 355.
dust-worm, a money-grubber.

E

earth-spine, the ground-pine (*Ajuga champæitys*), ii, 215.
eclegm (med.), an electuary.
economical, pertaining to a household or family, i, 107, 109
eloge, elogium, a panegyric.
eminent, prominent, conspicuous; "eminent notes," distinguishing marks, iii, 365.
enarration, an exposition.
encyclopædian, a circle of knowledge, i, 308.
end, a fragment; "players' ends," tags from plays, iii, 108.
engine, a device, instrument.
entreat, to treat.
enula campana, elecampane (*Inula helenium*).
epicure, an Epicurean, follower of Epicurus.
epithyme, the dodder of thyme.
equant circles (astron.), circles used for determining the motions of the planets.
erear, to carry aloft; "a spiritual wing to erear us," iii, 342, 413.
err, to cause to err, to mislead, i, 197.
escape, an oversight, mistake, i, 33.
ethnics, heathen, pagans.
euripe, euripus, a narrow channel.
evirate, to emasculate.

exaggerate, to heap up, accumulate.
exagitate, to disturb.
exhaust, exhausted.
exolete, obsolete.
exonerate, to discharge, unburden.
exornation, embellishment, adornment.
explode, to drive off the stage, decry, reject, refute.
expostulate, to argue about, call in question, ii, 160; to demand with
    emphasis, iii, 161.
extent, extension, i, 355, iii, 318.
extenuation, belittlement.

F

fabulous, fabulizing; "our fabulous poets," i, 131; cf. ii, 42.
facete, witty.
fact, a thing done, a deed.
fairybabe, a fear-babe, bogy; "fairybabes of tombs," i, 414.
fall, a falling-band, neck-band.
falling sickness, epilepsy.
familiar, of frequent occurrence, habitual; *familiarly*, regularly,
    habitually.
fay, to clean out, i, 350.
feral, deadly, fatal, dangerous, terrible; (astrol.) of the moon "when,
    being separated from one planet, she applies to no other
    while she continues in the same sign" (Bailey), ii, 130.
fieldone, fielden, field-country, ii, 63.
finger-fern, a kind of spleenwort, probably the hard fern.
fitches, vetches, i, 222.
flaggy, drooping, flabby, i, 383.
fleer, to leer, i, 281, 383.
flirt, a hussy, a baggage, i, 109, 417.
fly out, to break out into licence.
foal-foot, colt's-foot.
foot : "every foot," on every occasion, at every step, iii, 124.
foot-clothes, horses' housings, reaching to the ground.
forspoken, bewitched, ill-wished.
fortunately, with success, ii, 239.
fox, to intoxicate, i, 226.
freckons, freckles, iii, 213.
fucate, rouged, counterfeit, iii, 24.
fumadoes, smoked pilchards.
funge (=*fungus*), a dolt, soft-head.
fustilugs, "a sluttish woman who smells rank" (Bailey), iii, 155.
fuzzled (old edd. *fusled*), fuddled.

G

galanga, galingale, an aromatic root resembling ginger.
genethliacal (astrol.), pertaining to the casting of nativities.
genist, genista, broom.
geniture (astrol.), a nativity, horoscope.

ghost, to haunt, i, 45.
good cheap, cheaply.
goosecap, a silly person, i, 349.
Grobian, a sloven (from Dedekind's *Grobianus*, Englished by Dekker in his *Gull's Hornbook*), iii, 156, 174.
grosses, groschens, iii, 403.
gryphes, griffins.
guarded, trimmed with lace, etc.
gubber-tushed, with irregularly projecting teeth.
gymnics, athletic exercises.

H

haberdine, dried and salted cod.
hacker, a slasher, a bully, i, 228.
have and hold, tenacity, iii, 346, 384.
hemrods (*hæmrods*, *emrods*), hæmorrhoids, piles.
hodœporicon, a wayfaring, journey, itinerary.
hold, to maintain the existence of; "he held antipodes," ii, 42.
homocentric, concentric.
hone, to moan; to long (after).
horoscope, the sign of the zodiac that is rising at a person's birth, i, 207.
horrid, bristling; wild, savage.
hot-house, a bathing-house to which one went to be sweated and cupped.
husband, a husbandman, agriculturist, i, 305.
husbandman, a writer on husbandry, i, 221.
huswife, a hussy.
hylech (astrol.), "a planet which in a man's nativity becomes the moderator and significator of life" (Bailey), i, 208.

I

idle-headed, light-headed, iii, 343.
imbonity, inconvenience, i, 434.
immund, uncleanly.
impassionate, without passion, dull, i, 400.
impolite, unpolished.
importune (Lat. *importunus*), cruel, savage, iii, 283.
imposthume, an abscess.
impress, a device; a motto; a seal.
incend, *incense*, to kindle, inflame.
incondite, confused, irregular, clumsy.
incubus, a nightmare.
indefinite, without qualification, iii, 410.
indifferent, held in common, iii, 298; impartial, iii, 310.
indulge to, to give way to, indulge in, i, 249.
Indy bone, ivory, iii, 88.
inescate, to entice, lay baits for, iii, 129.
inform, to shape, fashion, ii, 183.
ingeminate, to reiterate, insist on.

ingenite, inborn.
insensible, imperceptible, i, 292.
insist, to follow (in), i, 180; to dwell (on), ii, 63.
insuavity, unpleasantness, i, 434.
insult, to behave with insolence.
intempestive, untimely, unseasonable.
intend, to intensify; to fix the attention on.
intensive, intense.
intention, intensification (of symptoms), i, 423.
intentive, intent.
interrupt, interrupted.
intricable, entangling, intricate.
irrefragable, stubborn, impervious to argument.

J

jack, the slip of wood that holds the plectrum in the virginal, iii, 179.
jet, to strut, swagger.
Jovial (astrol.), born under Jupiter.
jument, a beast of burden.
just, adequate, suitable, complete.

K

keelpins, ninepins.
keep up, to keep shut up, keep in.
kell, a caul.
kill up, to kill off, i, 56.
knights of the post, hireling witnesses, i, 282.

L

labdanum, ladanum, a resin collected from a species of cistus.
lamia, a sorceress, a vampire.
landleaper, a wanderer, a vagabond.
lapis Armenus, Armenian stone, blue carbonate of copper.
laplolly, loblolly, water-gruel, ii, 154.
lask, a flux, diarrhœa, i, 263.
lave-eared, lop-eared, iii, 155.
lee, a lye, a detergent.
let, a hindrance, obstacle.
libertine, an antinomian.
lie down, to lie in, i, 20.
likely, probably.
limbec, an alembic.
litargy, litharge.
litigious, subject to litigation, iii, 20.
livor, envy, ill-will, malignity.
long square, an oblong, i, 98.
lurch, an ambush; "lying at lurch," lying in wait, lurking, i, 55.
lusorious, appertaining to games; "lusorious lots," games of chance, ii, 82.

M

macerate, to subject to hardships; to harass, mortify.
made, artificial; "made flowers," iii, 81.
magistery, mastership, authority.
magistral, a sovereign remedy.
make away, to murder, make away with.
mala insana, mad-apples, a kind of egg-fruit.
maleficiate, to bewitch.
mancipate, to enslave.
many, a retinue, rout, bevy.
mard, a lump of excrement.
marish, marshy.
maukin, a kitchen-wench, slattern, scarecrow.
Medicean stars, Jupiter's satellites, iii, 120.
mediocrity, middle position; moderation.
mends, amends, remedy.
mere, unadulterated; absolute; unprompted.
meskite (*meschite*), a mosque.
metoposcopy, the art of discovering character from the lines of the
    face, especially the forehead.
minion, minium or red lead, used as a cosmetic.
misconster, to misconstrue.
mithridate, an antidote against poison.
Mogor, Mogul.
moldiwarp, *mouldwarp*, a mole.
moll (old edd. *maule*), a wench, a prostitute, i, 301.
momentany, momentary, ephemeral.
monocerot, a unicorn.
monomachy, a single combat, duel.
moorish, marshy.
mope, a stupid fellow.
mormoluches, bogies, iii, 428 (Gk. μορμολυκεῖα, cf. i, 336).
morphew, a scurfy eruption.
mother: "mother of the maids," a housekeeper, i, 307; "the mother,"
    hysteria, i, 381, etc.
motion, a puppet-show; a moving device; an impulse; a proposition.
mummia, mummy; a distillation from mummies or dead bodies;
    a medicinal liquor or gum.
muscadine, muscadel.
muse, a meuse, a gap through which a hare runs; "as many
    excuses as a hare hath muses" (proverbial), iii, 295.
mushato, a moustache.

N

nænia, *nenia*, a funeral song, a dirge.
næves, *nævi*, birth-marks.
naughtiness, wickedness.
naughty, worthless; "a naughty tree," iii, 12.
nectarine, a sweet drink.
neoteric, modern, favouring modern doctrine.

nodule, a small quantity of medicine in a bag.
noise, a band (of musicians), i, 334.

O

oaf (old edd. *aufe*), a changeling; a deformed person; a dolt.
object, aspect, sight, iii, 109, 110, 118
oblige, to bind, secure the attachment of, i, 203.
obnubilate, to cloud, obscure.
obtrectation, detraction.
occur (v.t.), to counteract, remedy, iii, 410
occurse, a meeting, falling in with, i, 425.
ocyme (*ochyme*), basil.
oilet-holes, eyelet-holes, iii, 261.
opinative, opinionated.
opiparous, sumptuous, ii, 76.
oppugner, an assailant.
orbities, bereavements, ii, 128.
origan (*organ*), marjoram.
otacousticon, an ear-trumpet, ii, 46.
ouch, a brooch, clasped necklace.
outside, one who is all outward show.
overseen, mistaken, iii, 5.

P

painful, painstaking, hard-working.
paint out, to depict.
pantofle, a slipper.
parable, easily procurable.
paraenetical, persuasory.
parietines, ruined walls, ii, 31.
particular, an individual, iii, 125.
partile (astrol.), full, complete.
passenger, a wayfarer, passer by, ii, 75.
peckled, speckled.
peculiar, particular, special.
period, end, sum; "period of all philosophy," i, 133.
personate, masked; impersonated; "personate old man," old man in the play, iii, 225.
perspective: "perspective glass," a telescope; "the perspectives," the various branches of the art of perspective.
perstringe, to glance at, censure, i, 343; to dazzle, iii, 92.
philosopher's game, a kind of chess.
pickitivant, a pointed beard.
pickthank, a flatterer, toady.
pigsney, a term of endearment.
pill, to pillage.
pina, a pine-apple.
pistick nuts, pistachio-nuts.

pittivanted, wearing a pointed beard.

plashed, pleached, woven.

plunged, embarrassed, baffled, i, 176.

points, tagged laces.

poke, a bag; "Bavarian poke," goitre, iii, 155.

politicians, writers on politics.

poll, to plunder.

polyanthean, pertaining to *Polyanthea* and similar collections of commonplaces, used by students of rhetoric, i 316.

polygraphy, cipher-writing, iii, 127.

pontifical, pontifical, papistical.

poor-john, a coarse fish of the cod kind, dried and salted.

popular, studious of popular favour, ii, 204.

portuous, a portess or portass (Fr. *porte-hors*), a breviary, iii, 182.

positively, in orthodox fashion, defending the tenets of the Fathers of the Church, i, 35.

powdered (meat), salted, corned.

precise, puritanical, i, 322, iii, 312.

presently, at once.

press, to inflict the *peine forte et dure*; "I am content to be pressed," i, 22.

pretend, to put forward, allege.

preterition (theol.), the passing over of the non-elect, iii, 400.

prevent, to anticipate.

prick, a skewer, iii, 99.

print, in, in careful, precise fashion, iii, 177.

prize, to play one's, to contend in earnest, i, 264, iii, 364.

probable, plausible.

procession, a litany, i, 271.

produce, to draw out, prolong.

promissors (astrol.), directing influences which foreshadow some event.

propend, to weigh down, incline, iii, 60.

propugner, defender, champion.

prosecute, to follow up, pursue.

prospective, a view, prospect.

prune (falconry), to preen, iii, 94.

pullen, poultry, iii, 132.

purly-hunter, a purlieu-hunter, a freeholder of land within the borders of a forest, licensed to hunt therein, i, 374.

purposes, the game of cross-purposes, ii, 81.

put case, suppose, in case.

put down, to bring into disuse; (p.p.) demoded.

put to, to put out, extend, i, 277.

put up, to put up with.

putid, worthless.

pythonissa, a pythoness, an oracular priestess of Apollo.

Q

quit, to requite, iii, 292.

R

rabato, a rabat, a stiff collar supporting a ruff.
rack, a neck or scrag of mutton, i, 230.
ramshead, the chick-pea.
range, rank, i, 192.
rascetta (*rasceta*), in palmistry, the lines that isolate the hand from the fore-arm.
redshanks, Scotch Highlanders, iii, 191.
refel, to refute.
regiment, regimen, rule of health, ii, 71.
rejourn, to refer, i, 164.
remit, to abate (of a disease).
rent, to rend, iii, 400
respect, in, in comparison.
respective, considerate, ii, 204.
respectless, unregardful, discourteous, i, 307.
rhododaphne, the rose-bay or oleander.
rivel, to shrivel.
roaring-meg, a name for a cannon.
Rosy-cross men, Rosicrucians.
round (in the ear), to whisper, i, 342.
rude, in a rough state; "rude matter," raw material, i, 90.
rumney, a heavy, sweet, white Greek wine.
rustics, writers of books on rural matters.

S

sallet, a salad.
salvatella, the vein that runs into the little finger.
sanded, driven on a sand-bank, i, 339.
sanders, sandal-wood.
Saturnine (astrol.), born under Saturn.
satyrion, an aphrodisiac, iii, 128; the male orchis, ii, 248.
scald, scaly, scurfy, scabbed.
scale, a step of a ladder; "Gemonian scales," *see* i, 282, note 1.
scamble, to struggle; to get along somehow, ii, 192.
scant, to stint.
schede (old edd. *scede*), a sheet of paper, i, 85.
scolopendria, a spleenwort, probably the hart's-tongue fern.
scordium, the water-germander.
scrat, to scratch, i, 286.
secure (v.t.), to reassure; (adj.), careless, reckless.
selenites, the moonstone, i, 373.
sensible, capable of sensation; "sensible creatures," the animal kingdom. *See* i, 155, 157.
serjeant, a bailiff, a constable.
serves, sorb-apples, fruit of the service-tree, i, 221.
setting-stick, an instrument for adjusting the plaits of ruffs.
shadow, a woman's head-dress with projecting brim, shading the face, iii, 94.
shut up, to conclude.

significator (astrol.), "a planet which signifies something remarkable in nativities" (Bailey).
site (n.), position, attitude; "at that site," in that position, iii, 216.
site, sited (p.p.), situated.
skill of, to understand, have skill in, iii, 130.
sleeveless (of errands), trifling, silly, iii, 140.
smell-feast, a parasite, sponger.
snite, a snipe, ii, 73.
Sophy, the Persian monarch, Shah.
spagirically, chemically.
speculation, a viewing, exploration, ii, 67.
spike, spikenard, iii, 314.
spital, a hospital; in particular, a lazar-house.
stale, a decoy-bird, i, 84.
stand to, to abide by, i, 72.
stare, a starling.
steganography, secret writing, iii, 127.
stern, a star, iii, 146.
stick-free, immune from sticking or stabbing, i, 204.
stigmatize, to brand with a hot iron.
still, habitually, continually.
stœchas, stœchado, French lavender.
stramineous, strawy, without pith, i, 340, 367.
stupend, stupendous.
stut, to stutter.
submiss, submissive.
substance, bulk, large quantities; "hellebore in substance," i, 232, ii, 20.
suffite, suffitus, smoke from a fumigation.
superparticular, of a ratio where the greater term exceeds the less by a unit, i, 405.

T

table, a medicinal cake or tablet.
tables, backgammon.
take place, to take effect.
tassel, a male falcon, iii, 223.
temperature, temperament, bodily constitution.
tempestively, seasonably.
tender, to value, have a regard for.
tenent, a tenet.
tenter-bellies, gluttons, iii, 191.
terms (astrol.), "certain degrees of the signs in which planets are observed to have their virtues increased" (Bailey), i, 208.
terriculaments, frights, terrors, iii, 429.
terse, neat.
testor, an attestor, a witness.
tetric, harsh, gloomy.
theologaster, a petty or contemptible theologian.
thistlewarp, a goldfinch.
tire, attire, dress; a woman's head-dress, a tiara.

tit, a chit, iii, 155.
tobacconist, a smoker of tobacco, iii, 264.
topic, local.
torlachers, Mohammedan mendicants, iii, 363.
treacle, a theriac, antidote against poisons; a medicine composed of
　　vipers and other ingredients.
trencher-chaplain, a domestic chaplain, i, 322.
trenchmore, a lively, romping dance, iii, 179.
trivant, a truant, idler, i, 27; *trivantly*, idly, i, 316.
trivial, ordinary.
trunks, a game in which balls were rolled through small arches.
tulipant, a tulip.
turbith, turpeth, the root of *Ipoma turpetha*.
tympany, an abdominal swelling.

U

uncivil, uncivilized, i, 86.
unguentum armarium, the weapon-salve, which cured by "sym-
　　pathy" when applied to the weapon that had made the
　　wound.
union, a large pearl.
upright shoe, a shoe of the same shape for either foot.
urchin, a hedgehog, ii, 201.

V

vastity, desolation, ruin, i, 360.
Vatinian.　*See* i, 268, note 3.
vegetal, vegetable; (pl.) the vegetable kingdom; "vegetal faculty,"
　　see i, 155.
velitation, a skirmish, iii, 373.
venditate, to cry up, boast of, i, 293.
veneres, veneries, beauties, charms.
vent, to vend, sell, i, 24.
village, a villa, country residence, i, 117, ii, 62.
voluntary, a volunteer, i, 60.

W

walk, a hunting district, iii, 273.
want (v.t.), to lack, be free from, do without; (v.i.), to be lacking.
wasters, cudgel-play.
watchet, pale-blue.
wearish, withered, wizened.
weel, a fish-trap.
wesel, the windpipe, weasand.
wether's-head, the ramshead, chick-pea.
whenas, when; whereas; while.
whether, which (of two).

winch, to wince, i, 121.
wistly, wistfully, yearningly.
withy-wind, the wild clematis or traveller's joy, iii, 158.
wolf, a malignant ulcer, iii, 201.
woolward, wearing wool next the skin, for penance.
wreeks (=*reaks*), pranks; "play wreeks," iii, 214.
writhen, twisted, deformed.

Y

yellow, jealous, iii, 270; *yellowness*, jealousy, iii, 278.

INDEX

With a few exceptions, principally the entry under the name of Burton himself, the Index is confined to references to the subject-matter of the *Anatomy of Melancholy*. Major references to place-names and nationalities, however, are also included.

TITLES IN SERIES